FIRST AID THE®

USMLE STEP 1 2021

TAO LE, MD, MHS
Founder, ScholarRx
Associate Clinical Professor, Department of Medicine
University of Louisville School of Medicine

VIKAS BHUSHAN, MD
Founder, *First Aid for the USMLE Step 1*
Boracay, Philippines

MATTHEW SOCHAT, MD
Physician, Hematology/Oncology
Southeastern Medical Oncology Center

HUMOOD BOQAMBAR, MB BCh BAO
Assistant Registrar, Department of Orthopedic Surgery
Farwaniya Hospital

KRISTINA DAMISCH, MD
University of Iowa Carver College of Medicine
Class of 2020

CONNIE QIU
Lewis Katz School of Medicine at Temple University
MD/PhD Candidate

JORDAN ABRAMS, MD
Resident, Department of Anesthesiology,
Perioperative and Pain Medicine
Mount Sinai West and Mount Sinai Morningside Hospitals

CAROLINE COLEMAN, MD
Resident, Department of Medicine
Emory University School of Medicine

KIMBERLY KALLIANOS, MD
Assistant Professor, Department of Radiology and Biomedical Imaging
University of California, San Francisco School of Medicine

Mc Graw Hill

New York / Chicago / San Francisco / Athens / London / Madrid / Mexico City
Milan / New Delhi / Singapore / Sydney / Toronto

First Aid for the® USMLE Step 1 2021: A Student-to-Student Guide

Copyright © 2021 by Tao Le and Vikas Bhushan. All rights reserved. Printed in the United States of America. Except as permitted under the United States Copyright Act of 1976, no part of this publication may be reproduced or distributed in any form or by any means, or stored in a data base or retrieval system, without the prior written permission of the publisher.

Previous editions copyright © 1991 through 2020 by Tao Le and Vikas Bhushan. First edition copyright © 1990, 1989 by Vikas Bhushan, Jeffrey Hansen, and Edward Hon.

Photo and line art credits for this book begin on page 753 and are considered an extension of this copyright page.
Portions of this book identified with the symbol Rx are copyright © USMLE-Rx.com (MedIQ Learning, LLC).
Portions of this book identified with the symbol RU are copyright © Dr. Richard Usatine.
Portions of this book identified with the symbol * are under license from other third parties. Please refer to page 753 for a complete list of those image source attribution notices.

First Aid for the® is a registered trademark of McGraw Hill.

1 2 3 4 5 6 7 8 9 LMN 25 24 23 22 21 20

ISBN 978-1-260-46752-9
MHID 1-260-46752-X

Notice

Medicine is an ever-changing science. As new research and clinical experience broaden our knowledge, changes in treatment and drug therapy are required. The authors and the publisher of this work have checked with sources believed to be reliable in their efforts to provide information that is complete and generally in accord with the standards accepted at the time of publication. However, in view of the possibility of human error or changes in medical sciences, neither the authors nor the publisher nor any other party who has been involved in the preparation or publication of this work warrants that the information contained herein is in every respect accurate or complete, and they disclaim all responsibility for any errors or omissions or for the results obtained from use of the information contained in this work. Readers are encouraged to confirm the information contained herein with other sources. For example and in particular, readers are advised to check the product information sheet included in the package of each drug they plan to administer to be certain that the information contained in this work is accurate and that changes have not been made in the recommended dose or in the contraindications for administration. This recommendation is of particular importance in connection with new or infrequently used drugs.

This book was set in Electra LT Std by GW Inc.
The editors were Bob Boehringer and Christina M. Thomas.
Project management was provided by GW Inc.
The production supervisor was Jeffrey Herzich.
LSC Communications was printer and binder.

This book is printed on acid-free paper.

Copyright © 2021. Exclusive rights by McGraw Hill for manufacture and export. This book cannot be reexported from the country to which it is consigned by McGraw Hill. The International Edition is not available in North America.

McGraw Hill books are available at special quantity discounts to use as premiums and sales promotions, or for use in corporate training programs. To contact a representative please visit the Contact Us pages at www.mhprofessional.com.

Dedication

To all healthcare workers and first responders worldwide leading the fight against COVID-19. We salute your ongoing efforts and honor those who have lost their lives in service to others.

Contents

▸ SECTION III HIGH-YIELD ORGAN SYSTEMS 283

▸ SECTION IV TOP-RATED REVIEW RESOURCES 737

Contributing Authors

LILIT ASLANYAN, DO
Resident, Department of Medicine
New York University Winthrop Hospital

ANUP CHALISE, MBBS
Resident, Department of General Surgery
Nepal Medical College and Teaching Hospital

WEELIC CHONG
Sidney Kimmel Medical College at Thomas Jefferson University
MD/PhD Candidate

PANAGIOTIS KAPARALIOTIS, MD
Resident, Department of Pathology
St. Sophia's Children's Hospital, Greece

MITCHELL A. KATONA, MD, MPH
Resident, Division of Emergency Medicine
Dell Medical School

ANDREA LEAL LOPEZ, MD
ITESM School of Medicine Ignacio A. Santos, Mexico

VASILY OVECHKO, MD
Resident, Department of Pediatric Oncology
Dmitry Rogachev National Medical Research Center of Pediatric Hematology, Oncology and Immunology

VIVEK PODDER, MBBS
Tairunnessa Memorial Medical College and Hospital, Bangladesh

ROHAN BIR SINGH, MD
Fellow, Department of Ophthalmology
Massachusetts Eye and Ear, Harvard Medical School

Image and Illustration Team

YOOREE GRACE CHUNG
Emory University School of Medicine
MD/PhD Candidate

STEPHANIE JONES, PhD
Emory University Laney Graduate School

VICTOR JOSE MARTINEZ LEON, MD
Resident, Department of Medicine
Einstein Medical Center Philadelphia

ANGEL XIAO, MSE
Emory University School of Medicine
Class of 2022

ALIREZA ZANDIFAR, MD
Research Fellow, Department of Radiology
Children's Hospital of Philadelphia

Associate Authors

ERIC L. BARASH
Wake Forest School of Medicine
Class of 2022

LAUREN CLAUS
Johns Hopkins University School of Medicine
Class of 2021

CHRISTIAN FAABORG-ANDERSEN
Emory University School of Medicine
Class of 2022

ELIE FLATOW
Touro College of Osteopathic Medicine - Harlem
Class of 2021

SAMIRA RAHIM IBRAHIM
West Virginia School of Osteopathic Medicine
Class of 2021

TROY KLEBER
Emory University School of Medicine
MD/MSCR Candidate

MARGARET C. SLACK
University of Washington School of Medicine
Class of 2022

REBECCA H. YU
Saba University School of Medicine
Class of 2022

MATTHEW WELLS, DO
Resident, Department of Orthopedic Surgery
William Beaumont Army Medical Center

Image and Illustration Team

SEAN EVANS
Emory University School of Medicine
Class of 2022

Faculty Advisors

DIANA ALBA, MD
Assistant Professor, Division of Endocrinology, Diabetes, and Metabolism
University of California, San Francisco School of Medicine

MARK A.W. ANDREWS, PhD
Professor of Physiology
Lake Erie College of Osteopathic Medicine at Seton Hill

MARIA ANTONELLI, MD
Assistant Professor, Division of Rheumatology
MetroHealth Medical Center, Case Western Reserve University

HERMAN SINGH BAGGA, MD
Urologist, Allegheny Health Network
University of Pittsburgh Medical Center Passavant

SHIN C. BEH, MD
Assistant Professor, Department of Neurology & Neurotherapeutics
UT Southwestern Medical Center at Dallas

CARRIE BOHNERT, MPA
Standardized Patient Educator

SHELDON CAMPBELL, MD, PhD
Professor of Laboratory Medicine
Yale School of Medicine

BROOKS D. CASH, MD
Chief, Gastroenterology, Hepatology, and Nutrition
University of Texas Health Science Center at Houston

DIMITRI CASSIMATIS, MD
Associate Professor, Department of Medicine
Emory University School of Medicine

CATHERINE CHILES, MD
Associate Clinical Professor of Psychiatry
Yale School of Medicine

BRADLEY COLE, MD
Assistant Professor of Neurology
Loma Linda University School of Medicine

SAKINA FARHAT, MD
Consultant Gastroenterologist and Hepatologist
State University of New York Downstate Medical Center

CONRAD FISCHER, MD
Associate Professor, Medicine, Physiology, and Pharmacology
Touro College of Medicine

RAYUDU GOPALAKRISHNA, PhD
Associate Professor, Department of Integrative Anatomical Sciences
Keck School of Medicine of University of Southern California

MEREDITH K. GREER, MD
Fellow, Department of Medicine
Emory University School of Medicine

SUSAN HADLER, MD, MS
Professor Emerita of Pathology and Laboratory Medicine
University of North Carolina School of Medicine

MELANIE SCHORR HAINES, MD
Assistant Professor, Department of Medicine
Harvard Medical School

AMBER J. HECK, PhD
Associate Professor, Department of Medical Education
TCU and UNTHSC School of Medicine

JEFFREY W. HOFMANN, MD, PhD
Fellow, Department of Pathology
University of California, San Francisco School of Medicine

CLARK KEBODEAUX, PharmD
Clinical Associate Professor, Pharmacy Practice and Science
University of Kentucky College of Pharmacy

KRISTINE KRAFTS, MD
Assistant Professor, Department of Basic Sciences
University of Minnesota School of Medicine

MATTHEW KRAYBILL, PhD
Clinical Neuropsychologist
Cottage Health, Santa Barbara, California

GERALD LEE, MD
Associate Professor, Departments of Pediatrics and Medicine
Emory University School of Medicine

KACHIU C. LEE, MD, MPH
Assistant Clinical Professor, Department of Dermatology
The Warren Alpert Medical School of Brown University

WARREN LEVINSON, MD, PhD
Professor, Department of Microbiology and Immunology
University of California, San Francisco School of Medicine

JAMES LYONS, MD
Professor of Pathology and Family Medicine
Alabama College of Osteopathic Medicine

CARL MARFURT, PhD
Professor Emeritus, Department of Anatomy, Cell Biology and Physiology
Indiana University School of Medicine Northwest, Gary

PETER MARKS, MD, PhD
Center for Biologics Evaluation and Research
US Food and Drug Administration

DOUGLAS A. MATA, MD, MPH
Department of Pathology
Memorial Sloan Kettering Cancer Center

KRISTEN L. PAGEL, MD, MPH
Assistant Professor, Department of Psychiatry
University of Utah School of Medicine

VICKI M. PARK, PhD, MS
Assistant Dean
University of Tennessee College of Medicine

DIANE E.S. PAYNE, MD, MPT
Assistant Professor, Department of Orthopedic Surgery
Emory University School of Medicine

SOROUSH RAIS-BAHRAMI, MD
Associate Professor of Urology and Radiology
University of Alabama at Birmingham School of Medicine

RICHARD P. RAMONELL, MD
Fellow, Department of Medicine
Emory University School of Medicine

JOHN C. ROSE, DO
Clinical Instructor, Department of Anesthesiology
Mount Sinai Morningside-West

SASAN SAKIANI, MD
Professor, Department of Medicine
University of Maryland Medical Center

SHIREEN MADANI SIMS, MD
Chief, Division of Gynecology, Gynecologic Surgery, and Obstetrics
University of Florida School of Medicine

HOWARD M. STEINMAN, PhD
Assistant Dean, Biomedical Science Education
Albert Einstein College of Medicine

RICHARD P. USATINE, MD
Professor, Dermatology and Cutaneous Surgery
University of Texas Health Science Center San Antonio

TISHA WANG, MD
Associate Clinical Professor, Department of Medicine
David Geffen School of Medicine at UCLA

SYLVIA WASSERTHEIL-SMOLLER, PhD
Professor Emerita, Department of Epidemiology and Population Health
Albert Einstein College of Medicine

ADAM WEINSTEIN, MD
Associate Professor of Medical Education and Pediatric Nephrology
Geisel School of Medicine at Dartmouth

ABHISHEK YADAV, MBBS, MSc
Associate Professor of Anatomy
Geisinger Commonwealth School of Medicine

KRISTAL YOUNG, MD
Clinical Instructor, Department of Cardiology
Huntington Hospital, Pasadena, California

DONG ZHANG, PhD
Associate Professor of Biochemistry and Cancer Biology
New York Institute of Technology College of Osteopathic Medicine

Foreword

"If you see something that is not right, not fair, not just, you have a moral obligation to do something."

Congressman John Lewis

First Aid for the USMLE Step 1 began over 30 years ago as a resource to prepare aspiring physicians for their first medical board exam. Since then, it has become one of the most well-known textbooks used by medical students worldwide. While we closely follow the USMLE's lead in most respects, the widespread use of our book also provides an opportunity for us to be leaders in medical education.

In prior editions, there has been an unfortunate absence of diversity in both the text and images. This year, we strongly affirm that representing a broad spectrum of patients is essential for preparing for a successful medical career. The practice of medicine is inextricably intertwined with social determinants of health, and sociocultural understanding complements scientific knowledge for the future physician. Failing to provide representation of a diversity of people limits the educational experience and is to the detriment of future patients. We here describe our approach to improving the representation of race, ethnicity, sex, and gender, recognizing that we are neither experts nor authorities on diversity, equity, and inclusion.

We first surveyed our existing visual depictions of patients and pathologies. Of nearly 70 illustrations showing skin tone or sex in the 2020 edition, every single one showed pink/light beige skin, and all but one was male-appearing, excluding reproductive anatomy illustrations. To address this lack of diversity, we revised our illustrations to better reflect Fitzpatrick skin types I-VI and introduced more female-appearing and gender-neutral illustrations.

We also reviewed our use of language in the text. With respect to race and ethnicity, we transitioned from using "African-American" to "Black," as not all Black patients are American or have African ancestry. We now capitalize "Black" in accordance with major journalistic organizations. We also switched from "Caucasian" to "White," which we hope will be more accurate and inclusive.

We found many opportunities to improve the language used to describe disabled and ill patients as well. We now use person-first language such as "patients with diabetes" instead of "diabetic patients." Dated references to "mental retardation" have been replaced with "intellectual disability." We also removed other stigmatizing terms such as "alcoholics," "smokers," "epileptics," and "bulimics" and replaced with appropriate person-first language.

Finally, we reviewed our use of terminology surrounding sex and gender identity. We opted for more neutral language by changing most uses of gendered pronouns to "they/them/theirs," as well as changing "mother" to "pregnant patient." We also removed gendered terms such as "girl," "boy," "woman," and "man" in favor of "female" and "male" when referring to biological sex.

We acknowledge that our approach is imperfect and challenges remain. We also recognize that there may be differing perspectives that need to be addressed and balanced. However, just as the medical community learns invaluable lessons from its patients, we greatly value input from our peers and colleagues. We enthusiastically encourage feedback on our efforts to better represent all people. If you have comments or suggestions, please submit them via our website at **www.firstaidteam.com**. Alternatively, you can email us at **firstaid@scholarrx.com**. Thank you for your help in making *First Aid for the USMLE Step 1* an increasingly inclusive and useful resource.

Louisville	Tao Le
Boracay	Vikas Bhushan
Goldsboro, NC	Matthew Sochat
Kuwait	Humood Boqambar
Iowa City	Kristina Damisch
Philadelphia	Connie Qiu
New York City	Jordan Abrams
Atlanta	Caroline Coleman
San Francisco	Kimberly Kallianos

Preface

With the 31st edition of *First Aid for the USMLE Step 1*, we continue our commitment to providing students with the most useful and up-to-date preparation guide for the USMLE Step 1. This edition represents an outstanding revision in many ways, including:

- 104 entirely new or heavily revised high-yield topics reflecting evolving trends in the USMLE Step 1.
- Updated ethics section and introduction of new communications skills section to reflect the recently changed Step 1 exam.
- Extensive text revisions, new mnemonics, clarifications, and corrections curated by a team of 25 medical student and resident physician authors who excelled on their Step 1 examinations and verified by a team of expert faculty advisors and nationally recognized USMLE instructors.
- Updated with 179 new and revised diagrams and illustrations as part of our ongoing collaboration with USMLE-Rx and ScholarRx (MedIQ Learning, LLC).
- Updated with 62 new and revised photos to help visualize various disorders, descriptive findings, and basic science concepts. Additionally, revised imaging photos have been labeled and optimized to show both normal anatomy and pathologic findings.
- Updated exam preparation advice for USMLE Step 1 pass/fail, Step 1 blueprint changes, and COVID-19 impacts.
- Revised language to support diversity, equity, and inclusion.
- Updated study tips on the opening page of each chapter.
- Improved organization and integration of text, illustrations, clinical images, and tables throughout for focused review of high-yield topics.
- Revised and expanded ratings of current, high-yield review resources, with clear explanations of their relevance to USMLE review.
- Real-time Step 1 updates and corrections can be found exclusively on our blog, www.firstaidteam.com.

We invite students and faculty to share their thoughts and ideas to help us continually improve *First Aid for the USMLE Step 1* through our blog and collaborative editorial platform. (See How to Contribute, p. xvii.)

Louisville	Tao Le
Boracay	Vikas Bhushan
Goldsboro, NC	Matthew Sochat
Kuwait	Humood Boqambar
Iowa City	Kristina Damisch
Philadelphia	Connie Qiu
New York City	Jordan Abrams
Atlanta	Caroline Coleman
San Francisco	Kimberly Kallianos

Special Acknowledgments

This has been a collaborative project from the start. We gratefully acknowledge the thousands of thoughtful comments, corrections, and advice of the many medical students, international medical graduates, and faculty who have supported the authors in our continuing development of *First Aid for the USMLE Step 1*.

We provide special acknowledgment and thanks to the following individuals who made exemplary contributions to this edition through our voting, proofreading, and crowdsourcing platform: Moatasem Al-Janabi, Syeda Akila Ally, Grigory Davidov, Harpreet Dhanjal, Lucia Dominguez, Chinedum Enete, Emma Fenske, Heather Finlay-Morreale, Louna Ftouni, Margaret Ginoza, Fariah Asha Haque, E. Paige Hart, Zeid Hassan, I-Chun Hung, Karawan Hussein, Urma Jalil, Dana Jorgenson, Alvin Jose, Alec Kacew, Clara Kerwin, Shaima Khandaker, Joanna Liao, Annalisa Lopez, Freda Quimba Malanyaon, Jessica Marks, Juliana Maya, Tuba Mirza, Mardochere Morisset, Waneeza Mughees, Billis Paras, Neesirg Patel, Gabrielle Pierce, Faateh Ahmad Rauf, Amitoz Saini, Danusha Sanchez, Andrea Sánchez, Emily Charlotte Sparks, John Spikes II, James Ting, Collin Weintraub, and María Daniela Orellana Zambrano.

For support and encouragement throughout the process, we are grateful to Thao Pham, Jinky Flang, and Jonathan Kirsch, Esq. Thanks to Louise Petersen for organizing and supporting the project. Thanks to our publisher, McGraw Hill, for the valuable assistance of its staff, including Bob Boehringer, Jeffrey Herzich, Christina Thomas, Kristian Sanford, and Don Goyette.

We are also very grateful to Dr. Fred Howell and Dr. Robert Cannon of Textensor Ltd for providing us extensive customization and support for their powerful Annotate.co collaborative editing platform (www.annotate.co), which allows us to efficiently manage thousands of contributions. Thanks to Dr. Richard Usatine and Dr. Kristine Krafts for their outstanding image contributions. Thanks also to Jean-Christophe Fournet (www.humpath.com), Dr. Ed Uthman, and Dr. Frank Gaillard (www.radiopaedia.org) for generously allowing us to access some of their striking photographs.

For exceptional editorial leadership, enormous thanks to Megan Chandler, Mauri Loemker, Julie Mangoff, and Emma D. Underdown. Special thanks to our indexer, Dr. Anne Fifer. We are also grateful to our illustrators, Susan Mazik, Artemisa Gogollari, and Marvin Bundo, for their creative work on the new and updated illustrations. Lastly, tremendous thanks to GW Inc., especially Anne Banning, Victoria Brown, Gary Clark, Cindy Geiss, and Denise Smith.

Louisville	Tao Le
Boracay	Vikas Bhushan
Goldsboro, NC	Matthew Sochat
Kuwait	Humood Boqambar
Iowa City	Kristina Damisch
Philadelphia	Connie Qiu
New York City	Jordan Abrams
Atlanta	Caroline Coleman
San Francisco	Kimberly Kallianos

General Acknowledgments

Each year we are fortunate to receive the input of thousands of medical students and graduates who provide new material, clarifications, and potential corrections through our website and our collaborative editing platform. This has been a tremendous help in clarifying difficult concepts, correcting errata from the previous edition, and minimizing new errata during the revision of the current edition. This reflects our long-standing vision of a true, student-to-student publication. We have done our best to thank each person individually below, but we recognize that errors and omissions are likely. Therefore, we will post an updated list of acknowledgments at our website, www.firstaidteam.com/bonus/. We will gladly make corrections if they are brought to our attention.

For submitting contributions and corrections, many thanks to Raed Ababneh, Nursultan Abdreyev, Youni Abdul, Lana Abusalem, Bradley Acott, Temiloluwa Adejuyigbe, Gauri Adhikari, Ather Adnan, Rasim Agaev, Huzaifa Ahmad, Rija Ahmad, Oluwabukola Ajagbe, Tongwa B. Aka, Nataly Kobra Akbarshahi, Shahad Aladnan, Amr Alalwani, Nida Alam, Qutaiba Al-bustanji, Jose Alfonso, Maged Algazzar, Majed Alghamdi, Ahmed Al-Maidama, Abdulmajeed Almehmadi, Feras Al-Moussally, Maria Alwan, Salman Alyahya, Hamza Amin, Chelsea Amo-Tweneboah, Cara Anderson, Gina Andraos, Akanksha Reddy Annadi, Lordsfavour Anukam, Ali Arafa, Amalia Ardeljan, Amalia Doris Ardeljan, Stephanie Asdell, Christopher Azzam, Wardah Bajwa, Brayton Ballenger, Charlotte Banayan, Dileni C. Bandarage, Alyssa Barré, Isabella Batki, Jeffrey Baum, Tal Bavli, Jerrin Bawa, Alex Belaia, Dimitri Benner, Alexandra Bennett, Ashley Best, Alexandros Bestavasvili, Rohan Bhan, Krish Bharat, Saeed Bhuiyan, Pavit Bhullar, Jennifer Black, Lisle Blackbourn, William Bloom, Alina Bobrova, Luisa Brito, Chrys Buckley, Olena Budarina, Jessica Budiselic, Eamonn Byrnes, Alfonso Caetta, Gabriela Maria Calderon, Santiago Callegari, Sergio Camba, Xi Cao, Cristian Agapito Rosa Carrasquillo, Katie Carsky, Alicia Casella, Yasmin Chaiep, Tina Chen, Santosh Cherian, Devina Chintaman, Akshit Chitkara, Maruf Chowdhury, Matthew J. Christensen, Meaghan Clark, Courtney Cleveland, Aravind R. D., Yann Dacquay, Mohammed Dairywala, Jonathan Daou, Aimen Asim Dar, Naveena Daram, Joe Demian, Andres Diaz, Amin Dice, Taurah Dizadare, Andreea Bianca Dobre, Courtney Duckworth, Ismail Faruk Durmus, Manasa Dutta, Nikolas Echeverry, Matthew Eli, Awab Elnaeem, Mohamed Kamal El-Naeim, Karim Eltaib, Holly Everett, Sarrah Fadul, Amin Farsani, Samia Fatima, Yasmin Fazli, Kristina Flores, Farrar Ford, Katy Franks, Kyle Fratta, Shany Freund, Racha Ftouni, Ron Gadot, Don Galinea-Faigao, Abhishek Gami, Henriette De La Garza, Daniel Gatazka, Nicolas Curi Gawlinski, Leo Georges, Ashley Ghaemi, Paola Ghanem, Ahmad Munir Gharaibeh, Elie Ghasb, Brennan Gibson, Sam Gieg, Aastha Gohil, Sanya Goswami, Sourabh Goyal, Jan Andre Grauman, Shreya Gulati, Avni Gupta, Nanditha Guruvaiah, Rossy Guzman, Noon Hagmusa, Natalie Hassell, Christine Laura Heisen, Ghayda Hemadneh, Aryan Hemani, Trevor Henderson, Briana Hernandez, Sarah Hossain, Sarahbeth Howes, Janie Hu, Vivian Hu, Jonathan Hunter, Lisa Hysa, Ebuka Ibuoka, Mina Iskandar, Beck Jacobsen, Yamna Jadoon, Saira Jahangir, Ala Jamal, Tesmol James, Salem Jaramne, Prayag Jariwala, Chloe Jensen, Hassan El Jesr, Bijay Jeswani, Ankit Juneja, Simrat Kahlon, Nabyl Kalaf, Anastasia Kalantarova, Mohammed Kamareddine, Nivedita Kar, Arneet Kaur, Wajiha Kazmi, Azmeer Khamisani, Ahmed Ali Khan, Jawad Khan, Sunil Babu Khanal, Bhumika Khanna, David S. Kim, Alex Kinzer, Anna Kislik, Ramya Kommidi, Nicholas Koutrakis, Kushal Kriplani, Jonas Kruse, Mariia Kukushkina, Nimisha Kumar, Natalie

LaBossier, Nery y Mara Lamothe, Megan Lane, Joanna Lee, Victor Lee, Chime Lhatso, Xiantian Lin, Alwyn Louis, Joshua St. Louise, Alexander Lu, Lisa-Qiao MacDonald, Divya Madhavarapu, Osama Magableh, Jalal Maghfour, Reema Mahdi, Jainil Maheshwari, Rose Maisner, Freda Malanyaon, Mayra Malik, Mahir Mameledzija, Nikhil Mankuzhy, Abdul Mannan, Yusra Mansour, Rebecca Irene Marshall, Bridget Martinez, Penelope Martinez, Shielah Mauntana, O'Brian Mbakwe, Ashley McNeal, Bryan Medina, Mario Mekhail, Sherin Menachery, David Merkley, Ibrahim El Mikati, Stephan A. Miller, Damir Mingaleev, Sarim Mirza, Niall James Moffett, Deena Mohamed, Mahmoud Mohamed, Kompal Mohan, John Moon, Mohammad Murcy, Sakthi Murugan, Youjin Na, Geraldine Nabeta, Rahul Nachnani, Shamsun Nahar, Zaid R. Kh Najdawi, Alice Nassar, Zachary Nelson, Judith Nnah, Ahmed Noor, Ahmen Noor, Eric Nturibi, Anuli Nwankwo, Ahmad Obeidat, Ross O'Hagan, Cristal Osborne, Olga Ostrovetsky, Ademola Osundeko, Majd Oteibi, Reinis Ozolins, Sophia Padelford, Andrew Palosaari, Zonghao Pan, Niranjan Pandey, Mark Parker, Harshita Pasupuleti, Anmol Patel, Dharmik Patel, Krunal Patel, Manan Patel, Neha Patel, Austin Patrick, Harry Paul, Dmytro Pavlenko, Matthew Pavlica, Dorian Perez, Samantha Perovski, Sahir Pervaiz, Sofia Phirtskhalava, Mark Pilarski, Fanny Pimentel, Denise Powell, Shannon Powell, Meenu Prasad, Jacob Proaño, Kevin Pruitt, Laith Rahabneh, Masum Rahman, Juhi Ramchandani, Lisnaldy Ramirez, Naresa Ramjohn, Vaishnavi Rao, Adel Rasheed, Samyukta Ravi, Sreeram Ravi, Vishnu VB Reddy, Rafey Rehman, Jose Issac Reyes, Kyle Robbins, Samuel Roberts, Quayd Robertson, Pedro Garcia Rodriguez, Helio Manuel Grullón Rodríguez, Gessel Romero, Ariel Rucker, Angelica Maria Sanchez Ruiz, Megan Ryon, Bradley Ryva, Chantal Saberian, George Saboura, Sumeet Saini, Allie Sakowicz, Vishad Samami, Jasneet Sandhu, Omar Sanduka, Prakriti Sapkota, Dhruv Sarwal, Abeer Sarwar, M. Sathyanarayanan, Emma Schulte, Michael Schwarz, Justin Sedgewick, Jessica Sefen, Neha Sehgal, Sirous Seifirad, Nicole Sequeira, Muhanad Shaib, Fahad Shaikh, Ahmed Shakir, Jeffrey Shapiro, Muhammad Usman Sharif, Kanika Sharma, Manisha Sharma, Tina Sharma, Michelle Sheena, Emily Sherry, Minghan Shi, Sami Shoura, Melanie Shpigel, Robert Shvarts, Naomi Siddiquee, Christina Siems, Anantha Singarajah, Manik Inder Singh, Ramzi Y. Skaik, Bryn Smith, Emilie Song, Rishabh Soni, Luke Sorensen, Suganiya Srikanthan, Abhinav Srinath, Hala M. Staitieh, Brett Stark, Hafsa Omer Sulaiman, Saranya Sundaram, Michael Syrett, Nikolaos Syrigos, Basel Tamimi, Hamza Tariq, Aalap K. Trivedi, Amy Tsai, Athanasios Tsimpouras, Shannon Tung, Akemini Udoro, Sheela Vaswani, Jasmine Vatani, Sandra Azareli Garcia Velázquez, Allen Wang, Shelly Wang, Kaystin Weisenberger, Andrew White, Peter Williams, Stephanie Wottrich, Maria Yan, Hafsa Yaseen, Forrest Yeh, Hsinyu Yin, Susan Yohannan, Jamie Yoon, Zurabi Zaalishvili, Syed Zeeshan Haider Zaidi, Caroline Zhao, Michael Zheng, and Patrick Ziarnowski.

How to Contribute

This edition of *First Aid for the USMLE Step 1* incorporates thousands of contributions and improvements suggested by student and faculty advisors. We invite you to participate in this process. Please send us your suggestions for:

- Study and test-taking strategies for the USMLE Step 1
- New facts, mnemonics, diagrams, and clinical images
- High-yield topics that may appear on future Step 1 exams
- Personal ratings and comments on review books, question banks, apps, videos, and courses

For each new entry incorporated into the next edition, you will receive **up to a $20 Amazon.com gift card** as well as personal acknowledgment in the next edition. Significant contributions will be compensated at the discretion of the authors. Also, let us know about material in this edition that you feel is low yield and should be deleted.

All submissions including potential errata should ideally be supported with hyperlinks to a dynamically updated Web resource such as UpToDate, AccessMedicine, and ClinicalKey.

We welcome potential errata on grammar and style if the change improves readability. Please note that *First Aid* style is somewhat unique; for example, we have fully adopted the AMA *Manual of Style* recommendations on eponyms ("We recommend that the possessive form be omitted in eponymous terms") and on abbreviations (no periods with eg, ie, etc). We also avoid periods in tables unless required for full sentences. Kindly refrain from submitting "style errata" unless you find specific inconsistencies with the AMA *Manual of Style* or our diversity initiative as discussed in the Foreword.

The preferred way to submit new entries, clarifications, mnemonics, or potential corrections with a valid, authoritative reference is via our website: **www.firstaidteam.com**.

This website will be continuously updated with validated errata, new high-yield content, and a new online platform to contribute suggestions, mnemonics, diagrams, clinical images, and potential errata.

Alternatively, you can email us at: **firstaid@scholarrx.com.**

Contributions submitted by **May 15, 2021**, receive priority consideration for the 2022 edition of *First Aid for the USMLE Step 1*. We thank you for taking the time to share your experience and apologize in advance that we cannot individually respond to all contributors as we receive thousands of contributions each year.

▶ NOTE TO CONTRIBUTORS

All contributions become property of the authors and are subject to editing and reviewing. Please verify all data and spellings carefully. Contributions should be supported by at least two high-quality references.

Check our website first to avoid duplicate submissions. In the event that similar or duplicate entries are received, only the first complete entry received with valid, authoritative references will be credited. Please follow the style, punctuation, and format of this edition as much as possible.

▶ JOIN THE FIRST AID TEAM

The *First Aid*/ScholarRx team is pleased to offer paid editorial and coaching positions. We are looking for passionate, experienced, and dedicated medical students and recent graduates. Participants will have an opportunity to work on a wide variety of projects, including the popular *First Aid* series and the growing line of USMLE-Rx/ScholarRx products, including Rx Bricks. Please use our webform at https://www.usmle-rx.com/join-the-first-aid-team/ to apply, and include a CV and writing examples.

For 2021, we are actively seeking passionate medical students and graduates with a specific interest in improving our medical illustrations, expanding our database of photographs (including clinical images depicting diverse skin types), and developing the software that supports our crowdsourcing platform. We welcome people with prior experience and talent in these areas. Relevant skills include clinical imaging, digital photography, digital asset management, information design, medical illustration, graphic design, tutoring, and software development.

How to Use This Book

CONGRATULATIONS: You now possess the book that has guided nearly two million students to USMLE success for over 30 years. With appropriate care, the binding should last the useful life of the book. Keep in mind that putting excessive flattening pressure on any binding will accelerate its failure. If you purchased a book that you believe is defective, please **immediately** return it to the place of purchase. If you encounter ongoing issues, you can also contact Customer Service at our publisher, McGraw Hill.

START EARLY: Use this book as early as possible while learning the basic medical sciences. The first semester of your first year is not too early! Devise a study plan by reading Section I: Guide to Efficient Exam Preparation, and make an early decision on resources to use by checking Section IV: Top-Rated Review Resources. Note that *First Aid* is neither a textbook nor a comprehensive review book, and it is not a panacea for inadequate preparation.

CONSIDER *FIRST AID* YOUR ANNOTATION HUB: Annotate material from other resources, such as class notes or comprehensive textbooks, into your book. This will keep all the high-yield information you need in one place. Other tips on keeping yourself organized:

- For best results, use fine-tipped ballpoint pens (eg, BIC Pro+, Uni-Ball Jetstream Sports, Pilot Drawing Pen, Zebra F-301). If you like gel pens, try Pentel Slicci, and for markers that dry almost immediately, consider Staedtler Triplus Fineliner, Pilot Drawing Pen, and Sharpies.
- Consider using pens with different colors of ink to indicate different sources of information (eg, blue for USMLE-Rx Step 1 Qmax, green for UWorld Step 1 Qbank).
- Choose highlighters that are bright and dry quickly to minimize smudging and bleeding through the page (eg, Tombow Kei Coat, Sharpie Gel).
- Many students de-spine their book and get it 3-hole-punched. This will allow you to insert materials from other sources, including curricular materials.

INTEGRATE STUDY WITH CASES, FLASH CARDS, AND QUESTIONS: To broaden your learning strategy, consider integrating your *First Aid* study with case-based reviews (eg, *First Aid Cases for the USMLE Step 1*), flash cards (eg, USMLE-Rx Step 1 Flash Facts), and practice questions (eg, the USMLE-Rx Step 1 Qmax). Read the chapter in the book, then test your comprehension by using cases, flash cards, and questions that cover the same topics. Maintain access to more comprehensive resources (eg, ScholarRx Bricks and USMLE-Rx Step 1 Express videos) for deeper review as needed.

PRIME YOUR MEMORY: Return to your annotated Sections II and III several days before taking the USMLE Step 1. The book can serve as a useful way of retaining key associations and keeping high-yield facts fresh in your memory just prior to the exam. The Rapid Review section includes high-yield topics to help guide your studying.

CONTRIBUTE TO FIRST AID: Reviewing the book immediately after your exam can help us improve the next edition. Decide what was truly high and low yield and send us your comments. Feel free to send us scanned images from your annotated *First Aid* book as additional support. Of course, always remember that **all examinees are under agreement with the NBME to not disclose the specific details of copyrighted test material.**

Selected USMLE Laboratory Values

* = Included in the Biochemical Profile (SMA-12)

Blood, Plasma, Serum	Reference Range	SI Reference Intervals
*Alanine aminotransferase (ALT, GPT at 30°C)	10–40 U/L	10–40 U/L
*Alkaline phosphatase	25–100 U/L	25–100 U/L
Amylase, serum	25–125 U/L	25–125 U/L
*Aspartate aminotransferase (AST, GOT at 30°C)	12–38 U/L	12–38 U/L
Bilirubin, serum (adult) Total // Direct	 0.1–1.0 mg/dL // 0.0–0.3 mg/dL	 2–17 µmol/L // 0–5 µmol/L
*Calcium, serum (Total)	8.4–10.2 mg/dL	2.1–2.6 mmol/L
*Cholesterol, serum (Total)	Rec: < 200 mg/dL	< 5.2 mmol/L
*Creatinine, serum (Total)	0.6–1.2 mg/dL	53–106 µmol/L
Electrolytes, serum Sodium (Na^+) Chloride (Cl^-) * Potassium (K^+) Bicarbonate (HCO_3^-) Magnesium (Mg^{2+})	 136–146 mEq/L 95–105 mEq/L 3.5–5.0 mEq/L 22–28 mEq/L 1.5–2 mEq/L	 136–146 mmol/L 95–105 mmol/L 3.5–5.0 mmol/L 22–28 mmol/L 0.75–1.0 mmol/L
Gases, arterial blood (room air) P_{O_2} P_{CO_2} pH	 75–105 mm Hg 33–45 mm Hg 7.35–7.45	 10.0–14.0 kPa 4.4–5.9 kPa $[H^+]$ 36–44 nmol/L
*Glucose, serum	Fasting: 70–100 mg/dL	3.8–6.1 mmol/L
Growth hormone – arginine stimulation	Fasting: < 5 ng/mL Provocative stimuli: > 7 ng/mL	< 5 µg/L > 7 µg/L
Osmolality, serum	275–295 mOsmol/kg H_2O	275–295 mOsmol/kg H_2O
*Phosphorus (inorganic), serum	3.0–4.5 mg/dL	1.0–1.5 mmol/L
Prolactin, serum (hPRL)	Male: < 17 ng/mL Female: < 25 ng/mL	< 17 µg/L < 25 µg/L
*Proteins, serum Total (recumbent) Albumin Globulins	 6.0–7.8 g/dL 3.5–5.5 g/dL 2.3–3.5 g/dL	 60–78 g/L 35–55 g/L 23–35 g/L
Thyroid-stimulating hormone, serum or plasma	0.4–4.0 µU/mL	0.4–4.0 mIU/L
*Urea nitrogen, serum (BUN)	7–18 mg/dL	25–64 nmol/L
*Uric acid, serum	3.0–8.2 mg/dL	0.18–0.48 mmol/L

(continues)

Cerebrospinal Fluid	Reference Range	SI Reference Intervals
Cell count	0–5/mm^3	0–5 × 10^6/L
Glucose	40–70 mg/dL	2.2–3.9 mmol/L
Proteins, total	< 40 mg/dL	< 0.40 g/L
Hematologic		
Erythrocyte count	Male: 4.3–5.9 million/mm^3 Female: 3.5–5.5 million/mm^3	4.3–5.9 × 10^{12}/L 3.5–5.5 × 10^{12}/L
Erythrocyte sedimentation rate (Westergen)	Male: 0–15 mm/hr Female: 0–20 mm/hr	0–15 mm/hr 0–20 mm/hr
Hematocrit	Male: 41–53% Female: 36–46%	0.41–0.53 0.36–0.46
Hemoglobin, blood	Male: 13.5–17.5 g/dL Female: 12.0–16.0 g/dL	135–175 g/L 120–160 g/L
Hemoglobin, plasma	< 4 mg/dL	< 0.62 μmol/L
Leukocyte count and differential		
Leukocyte count	4,500–11,000/mm^3	4.5–11.0 × 10^9/L
Segmented neutrophils	54–62%	0.54–0.62
Band forms	3–5%	0.03–0.05
Eosinophils	1–3%	0.01–0.03
Basophils	0–0.75%	0–0.0075
Lymphocytes	25–33%	0.25–0.33
Monocytes	3–7%	0.03–0.07
Mean corpuscular hemoglobin	25–35 pg/cell	0.39–0.54 fmol/cell
Mean corpuscular hemoglobin concentration	31%–36% Hb/cell	4.8–5.6 mmol Hb/L
Mean corpuscular volume	80–100 μm^3	80–100 fL
Partial thromboplastin time (activated)	25–40 sec	25–40 sec
Platelet count	150,000–400,000/mm^3	150–400 × 10^9/L
Prothrombin time	11–15 sec	11–15 sec
Reticulocyte count	0.5–1.5% of RBCs	0.005–0.015
Urine		
Creatinine clearance	Male: 97–137 mL/min Female: 88–128 mL/min	97–137 mL/min 88–128 mL/min
Osmolality	50–1200 mOsmol/kg H_2O	50–1200 mOsmol/kg H_2O
Proteins, total	< 150 mg/24 hr	< 0.15 g/24 hr
Other		
Body mass index	Adult: 19–25 kg/m^2	19–25 kg/m^2

First Aid Checklist for the USMLE Step 1

This is an example of how you might use the information in Section I to prepare for the USMLE Step 1. Refer to corresponding topics in Section I for more details.

Years Prior

- ☐ Use top-rated review resources for first-year medical school courses.
- ☐ Ask for advice from those who have recently taken the USMLE Step 1.

Months Prior

- ☐ Review computer test format and registration information.
- ☐ Register six months in advance.
- ☐ Carefully verify name and address printed on scheduling permit. Make sure the name on scheduling permit matches the name printed on your photo ID. Be familiar with COVID-19 cancellation and rescheduling policies.
- ☐ Go online for test date ASAP.
- ☐ Define your exam goals (pass comfortably, beat the mean, ace the test)
- ☐ Set up a realistic timeline for study. Cover less crammable subjects first.
- ☐ Evaluate and choose study materials (review books, question banks).
- ☐ Use a question bank to simulate the USMLE Step 1 to pinpoint strengths and weaknesses in knowledge and test-taking skills.

Weeks Prior

- ☐ Do test simulations in question banks.
- ☐ Assess how close you are to your goal.
- ☐ Pinpoint remaining weaknesses. Stay healthy (exercise, sleep).
- ☐ Verify information on admission ticket (eg, location, date).

One Week Prior

- ☐ Remember comfort measures (loose clothing, earplugs, etc).
- ☐ Work out test site logistics (eg, location, transportation, parking, lunch).
- ☐ Print or download your Scheduling Permit and Scheduling Confirmation to your phone.

One Day Prior

- ☐ Relax.
- ☐ Lightly review short-term material if necessary. Skim high-yield facts.
- ☐ Get a good night's sleep.

Day of Exam

- ☐ Relax.
- ☐ Eat breakfast.
- ☐ Minimize bathroom breaks during exam by avoiding excessive morning caffeine.

After Exam

- ☐ Celebrate, regardless of how well you feel you did.
- ☐ Send feedback to us on our website at **www.firstaidteam.com**.

SECTION I

Guide to Efficient Exam Preparation

"One important key to success is self-confidence. An important key to self-confidence is preparation."

—Arthur Ashe

"Wisdom is not a product of schooling but of the lifelong attempt to acquire it."

—Albert Einstein

"Finally, from so little sleeping and so much reading, his brain dried up and he went completely out of his mind."

—Miguel de Cervantes Saavedra, *Don Quixote*

"Sometimes the questions are complicated and the answers are simple."

—Dr. Seuss

"He who knows all the answers has not been asked all the questions."

—Confucius

"The expert in anything was once a beginner."

—Helen Hayes

"It always seems impossible until it's done."

—Nelson Mandela

▶ INTRODUCTION

Relax.

This section is intended to make your exam preparation easier, not harder. Our goal is to reduce your level of anxiety and help you make the most of your efforts by helping you understand more about the United States Medical Licensing Examination, Step 1 (USMLE Step 1). As a medical student, you are no doubt familiar with taking standardized examinations and quickly absorbing large amounts of material. When you first confront the USMLE Step 1, however, you may find it all too easy to become sidetracked from your goal of studying with maximal effectiveness. Common mistakes that students make when studying for Step 1 include the following:

- Starting to study (including *First Aid*) too late
- Starting to study intensely too early and burning out
- Starting to prepare for boards before creating a knowledge foundation
- Using inefficient or inappropriate study methods
- Buying the wrong resources or buying too many resources
- Buying only one publisher's review series for all subjects
- Not using practice examinations to maximum benefit
- Not understanding how scoring is performed or what the score means
- Not using review books along with your classes
- Not analyzing and improving your test-taking strategies
- Getting bogged down by reviewing difficult topics excessively
- Studying material that is rarely tested on the USMLE Step 1
- Failing to master certain high-yield subjects owing to overconfidence
- Using *First Aid* as your sole study resource
- Trying to prepare for it all alone

In this section, we offer advice to help you avoid these pitfalls and be more productive in your studies.

▶ *The test at a glance:*

- *8-hour exam*
- *Up to a total of 280 multiple choice items*
- *7 test blocks (60 min/block)*
- *Up to 40 test items per block*
- *45 minutes of break time, plus another 15 if you skip the tutorial*

▶ USMLE STEP 1—THE BASICS

The USMLE Step 1 is the first of three examinations that you would normally pass in order to become a licensed physician in the United States. The USMLE is a joint endeavor of the National Board of Medical Examiners (NBME) and the Federation of State Medical Boards (FSMB). The USMLE serves as the single examination system domestically and internationally for those seeking medical licensure in the United States.

The Step 1 exam includes test items that can be grouped by the organizational constructs outlined in Table 1 (in order of tested frequency). In late 2020, the NBME increased the number of items assessing communication skills. While pharmacology is still tested, they are focusing on drug mechanisms rather than on pharmacotherapy. You will generally not be required to identify specific medications indicated for a specific condition. Instead, you will be asked more about mechanisms and side effects.

TABLE 1. Frequency of Various Constructs Tested on the USMLE Step 1.*

Competency	Range, %	System	Range, %
Medical knowledge: applying foundational science concepts	60–70	General principles	12–16
Patient care: diagnosis	20–25	Behavioral health & nervous systems/special senses	9–13
Communication and interpersonal skills	6–9	Respiratory & renal/urinary systems	9–13
Practice-based learning & improvement	4–6	Reproductive & endocrine systems	9–13
Discipline	**Range, %**	Blood & lymphoreticular/immune systems	7–11
Pathology	44–52	Multisystem processes & disorders	6–10
Physiology	25–35	Musculoskeletal, skin & subcutaneous tissue	6–10
Pharmacology	15–22	Cardiovascular system	5–9
Biochemistry & nutrition	14–24	Gastrointestinal system	5–9
Microbiology	10–15	Biostatistics & epidemiology/population health	4–6
Immunology	6–11	Social sciences: communication skills/ethics	6–9
Gross anatomy & embryology	11–15		
Histology & cell biology	8–13		
Behavioral sciences	8–15		
Genetics	5–9		

*Percentages are subject to change at any time. www.usmle.org

How Is the Computer-Based Test (CBT) Structured?

The CBT Step 1 exam consists of one "optional" tutorial/simulation block and seven "real" question blocks of up to 40 questions per block with no more than 280 questions in total, timed at 60 minutes per block. A short 11-question survey follows the last question block. The computer begins the survey with a prompt to proceed to the next block of questions.

Once an examinee finishes a particular question block on the CBT, he or she must click on a screen icon to continue to the next block. Examinees **cannot** go back and change their answers to questions from any previously completed block. However, changing answers is allowed **within** a block of questions as long as the block has not been ended and if time permits.

What Is the CBT Like?

Given the unique environment of the CBT, it's important that you become familiar ahead of time with what your test-day conditions will be like. You can access a 15-minute tutorial and practice blocks at http://orientation.nbme.org/Launch/USMLE/STPF1. This tutorial interface is very similar to the one you will use in the exam; learn it now and you can skip taking it during the exam, giving you up to 15 extra minutes of break time. You can gain experience with the CBT format by taking the 120 practice questions (3 blocks with 40 questions each) available online or by signing up for a practice session at a test center for a fee.

For security reasons, examinees are not allowed to bring any personal electronic equipment into the testing area. This includes both digital and analog watches, cell phones, tablets, and calculators. Examinees are also prohibited from carrying in their books, notes, pens/pencils, and scratch paper. Food and beverages are also prohibited in the testing area. The testing centers are monitored by audio and video surveillance equipment. However, most testing centers allot each examinee a small locker outside the testing area in which he or she can store snacks, beverages, and personal items.

- *Keyboard shortcuts:*
  - *A, B, etc—letter choices*
  - *Esc—exit pop-up Calculator and Notes windows*

Questions are typically presented in multiple choice format, with 4–5 possible answer options. There is a countdown timer on the lower left corner of the screen as well. There is also a button that allows the examinee to mark a question for review. If a given question happens to be longer than the screen (which occurs very rarely), a scroll bar will appear on the right, allowing the examinee to see the rest of the question. Regardless of whether the examinee clicks on an answer choice or leaves it blank, he or she must click the "Next" button to advance to the next question.

- *Heart sounds are tested via media questions. Make sure you know how different heart diseases sound on auscultation.*

- *Be sure to test your headphones during the tutorial.*

The USMLE features a small number of media clips in the form of audio and/or video. There may even be a question with a multimedia heart sound simulation. In these questions, a digital image of a torso appears on the screen, and the examinee directs a digital stethoscope to various auscultation points to listen for heart and breath sounds. The USMLE orientation materials include several practice questions in these formats. During the exam tutorial, examinees are given an opportunity to ensure that both the audio headphones and the volume are functioning properly. If you are already familiar with the tutorial and planning on skipping it, first skip ahead to the section where you can test your headphones. After you are sure the headphones are working properly, proceed to the exam.

- *Familiarize yourself with the commonly tested lab values (eg, Hb, WBC, platelets, Na^+, K^+).*

The examinee can call up a window displaying normal laboratory values. In order to do so, he or she must click the "Lab" icon on the top part of the screen. Afterward, the examinee will have the option to choose between "Blood," "Cerebrospinal," "Hematologic," or "Sweat and Urine." The normal values screen may obscure the question if it is expanded. The examinee may have to scroll down to search for the needed lab values. You might want to memorize some common lab values so you spend less time on questions that require you to analyze these.

- *Illustrations on the test include:*
  - *Gross specimen photos*
  - *Histology slides*
  - *Medical imaging (eg, x-ray, CT, MRI)*
  - *Electron micrographs*
  - *Line drawings*

The CBT interface provides a running list of questions on the left part of the screen at all times. The software also permits examinees to highlight or cross out information by using their mouse. There is a "Notes" icon on the top part of the screen that allows students to write notes to themselves for review at a later time. Finally, the USMLE has recently added new functionality including text magnification and reverse color (white text on black background). Being familiar with these features can save time and may help you better view and organize the information you need to answer a question.

For those who feel they might benefit, the USMLE offers an opportunity to take a simulated test, or "CBT Practice Session" at a Prometric center. Students are eligible to register for this three-and-one-half-hour practice session after they have received their scheduling permit.

The same USMLE Step 1 sample test items (120 questions) available on the USMLE website, www.usmle.org, are used at these sessions. **No new items will be presented.** The practice session is available at a cost of $75 ($155 if taken outside of the US and Canada) and is divided into a short tutorial and three 1-hour blocks of ~40 test items each. Students receive a printed percent-correct score after completing the session. **No explanations of questions are provided.**

▶ *You can take a shortened CBT practice test at a Prometric center.*

You may register for a practice session online at www.usmle.org. A separate scheduling permit is issued for the practice session. Students should allow two weeks for receipt of this permit.

How Do I Register to Take the Exam?

Prometric test centers offer Step 1 on a year-round basis, except for the first two weeks in January and major holidays. The exam is given every day except Sunday at most centers. Some schools administer the exam on their own campuses. Check with the test center you want to use before making your exam plans.

▶ *The Prometric website will display a calendar with open test dates.*

US students can apply to take Step 1 at the NBME website. This application allows you to select one of 12 overlapping three-month blocks in which to be tested (eg, April–May–June, June–July–August). Choose your three-month eligibility period wisely. If you need to reschedule outside your initial three-month period, you can request a one-time extension of eligibility for the next contiguous three-month period, and pay a rescheduling fee. The application also includes a photo ID form that must be certified by an official at your medical school to verify your enrollment. After the NBME processes your application, it will send you a scheduling permit.

The scheduling permit you receive from the NBME will contain your USMLE identification number, the eligibility period in which you may take the exam, and two additional numbers. The first of these is known as your "scheduling number." You must have this number in order to make your exam appointment with Prometric. The second number is known as the "candidate identification number," or CIN. Examinees must enter their CINs at the Prometric workstation in order to access their exams. However, you will not be allowed to bring your permit into the exam and will be asked to copy your CIN onto your scratch paper. Prometric has no access to the codes. **Make sure to bring a paper or electronic copy of your permit with you to the exam!** Also bring an unexpired, government-issued photo ID that includes your signature (such as a driver's license or passport). Make sure the name on your photo ID exactly matches the name that appears on your scheduling permit.

> ▶ *Be familiar with Prometric's policies for cancellation and rescheduling due to COVID-19.*

Once you receive your scheduling permit, you may access the Prometric website or call Prometric's toll-free number to arrange a time to take the exam. You may contact Prometric two weeks before the test date if you want to confirm identification requirements. Be aware that your exam may be canceled because of circumstances related to the COVID-19 pandemic or other unforeseen events. If that were to happen, you should receive an email from Prometric containing notice of the cancellation and instructions on rescheduling. Visit www.prometric.com for updates regarding their COVID-19 cancellation and rescheduling policies.

> ▶ *Test scheduling is done on a "first-come, first-served" basis. It's important to schedule an exam date as soon as you receive your scheduling permit.*

Although requests for taking the exam may be completed more than six months before the test date, examinees will not receive their scheduling permits earlier than six months before the eligibility period. The eligibility period is the three-month period you have chosen to take the exam. Most medical students choose the April–June or June–August period. Because exams are scheduled on a "first-come, first-served" basis, it is recommended that you book an exam date on the Prometric website as soon as you receive your permit. Prometric will provide appointment confirmation on a print-out and by email. Be sure to read the latest *USMLE Bulletin of Information* for further details.

What If I Need to Reschedule the Exam?

You can change your test date and/or center by contacting Prometric at 1-800-MED-EXAM (1-800-633-3926) or www.prometric.com. Make sure to have your CIN when rescheduling. If you are rescheduling by phone, you must speak with a Prometric representative; leaving a voicemail message will not suffice. To avoid a rescheduling fee, you will need to request a change at least 31 calendar days before your appointment. Please note that your rescheduled test date must fall within your assigned three-month eligibility period.

> ▶ *Register six months in advance for seating and scheduling preference.*

When Should I Register for the Exam?

You should plan to register as far in advance as possible ahead of your desired test date (eg, six months), but, depending on your particular test center, new dates and times may open closer to the date. Scheduling early will guarantee that you will get either your test center of choice or one within a 50-mile radius of your first choice. For most US medical students, the desired testing window is in June, since most medical school curricula for the second year end in May or June. Thus, US medical students should plan to register before January in anticipation of a June test date. The timing of the exam is more flexible for IMGs, as it is related only to when they finish exam preparation. Talk with upperclassmen who have already taken the test so you have real-life experience from students who went through a similar curriculum, then formulate your own strategy.

Where Can I Take the Exam?

Your testing location is arranged with Prometric when you book your test date (after you receive your scheduling permit). For a list of Prometric locations nearest you, visit www.prometric.com.

How Long Will I Have to Wait Before I Get My Scores?

The USMLE reports scores in three to four weeks, unless there are delays in score processing. Examinees will be notified via email when their scores are available. By following the online instructions, examinees will be able to view, download, and print their score report online for ~120 days after score notification, after which scores can only be obtained through requesting an official USMLE transcript. Additional information about score timetables and accessibility is available on the official USMLE website.

What About Time?

Time is of special interest on the CBT exam. Here's a breakdown of the exam schedule:

15 minutes	Tutorial (skip if familiar with test format and features)
7 hours	Seven 60-minute question blocks
45 minutes	Break time (includes time for lunch)

▶ *Gain extra break time by skipping the tutorial, or utilize the tutorial time to add personal notes to your scratch paper.*

The computer will keep track of how much time has elapsed on the exam. However, the computer will show you only how much time you have remaining in a given block. Therefore, it is up to you to determine if you are pacing yourself properly (at a rate of approximately one question per 90 seconds).

The computer does not warn you if you are spending more than your allotted time for a break. You should therefore budget your time so that you can take a short break when you need one and have time to eat. You must be especially careful not to spend too much time in between blocks (you should keep track of how much time elapses from the time you finish a block of questions to the time you start the next block). After you finish one question block, you'll need to click to proceed to the next block of questions. If you do not click within 30 seconds, you will automatically be entered into a break period.

Break time for the day is 45 minutes, but you are not required to use all of it, nor are you required to use any of it. You can gain extra break time (but not extra time for the question blocks) by skipping the tutorial or by finishing a block ahead of the allotted time. Any time remaining on the clock when you finish a block gets added to your remaining break time. Once a new question block has been started, you may not take a break until you have reached the end of that block. If you do so, this will be recorded as an "unauthorized break" and will be reported on your final score report.

▶ *Be careful to watch the clock on your break time.*

Finally, be aware that it may take a few minutes of your break time to "check out" of the secure resting room and then "check in" again to resume testing, so plan accordingly. The "check-in" process may include fingerprints, pocket checks, and metal detector scanning. Some students recommend pocketless clothing on exam day to streamline the process.

If I Freak Out and Leave, What Happens to My Score?

Your scheduling permit shows a CIN that you will need to enter to start your exam. Entering the CIN is the same as breaking the seal on a test book, and you are considered to have started the exam when you do so. However, no score will be reported if you do not complete the exam. In fact, if you leave at any time from the start of the test to the last block, no score will be reported. The fact that you started but did not complete the exam, however, will appear on your USMLE score transcript. Even though a score is not posted for incomplete tests, examinees may still get an option to request that their scores be calculated and reported if they desire; unanswered questions will be scored as incorrect.

The exam ends when all question blocks have been completed or when their time has expired. As you leave the testing center, you will receive a printed test-completion notice to document your completion of the exam. To receive an official score, you must finish the entire exam.

What Types of Questions Are Asked?

▸ *Nearly three fourths of Step 1 questions begin with a description of a patient.*

All questions on the exam are **one-best-answer multiple choice items.** Most questions consist of a clinical scenario or a direct question followed by a list of five or more options. You are required to select the single best answer among the options given. There are no "except," "not," or matching questions on the exam. A number of options may be partially correct, in which case you must select the option that best answers the question or completes the statement. Additionally, keep in mind that experimental questions may appear on the exam, which do not affect your score.

How Is the Test Scored?

▸ *Determine if the impending transition to Pass/Fail scoring impacts your optimal testing date.*

The USMLE will be transitioning to a Pass/Fail scoring system no earlier than January 1, 2022. Results from Step 1 exams taken prior to the transition date will be reported using a three-digit test score. Changes will not be made to transcripts containing a three-digit test score after the switch to Pass/Fail grading. Should you consider delaying your exam until Pass/Fail scoring is implemented? At the moment, we don't think so in most situations. First, at press time, the actual implementation date has not been announced. Second, and more importantly, the test date should be driven by your readiness relative to your curriculum and school schedule. On the other hand, there are a number of possible reasons that you might want to consider taking your exam in 2021 and getting a 3-digit score. These may include interest in a competitive specialty, IMG status, and enrollment at a less competitive medical school. In these situations, the USMLE Step 2 CK can provide an additional opportunity to score well and demonstrate a strong fund of knowledge. Consult with your school advisors and follow us on social media for timely updates.

Examinees taking the current test will receive an electronic report that includes the examinee's pass/fail status, a three-digit test score, a bar chart comparing the examinee's performance to that of other examinees', and a graphic depiction of the examinee's performance by physician task, discipline and organ system.

The USMLE score report (see Figure 1) highlights the examinee's strength and weaknesses by providing an overview of their performance by physician task, discipline and organ system compared to their overall performance on the exam. Each of the questions (minus experimental questions) is tagged according to any or all relevant content areas. Yellow-colored boxes (lower, same, higher) on your score report indicate your performance in each specific content area **relative to your overall performance** on the exam.

The NBME provides a three-digit test score based on the total number of items answered correctly on the examination, which corresponds to a particular percentile (see Figure 2). Your three-digit score will be qualified by the mean and standard deviation of US and Canadian medical school first-time examinees.

Since some questions may be experimental and are not counted, it is possible to get different scores for the same number of correct answers. In 2018, the mean score was 231 with a standard deviation of 19.

▶ *The mean Step 1 score for US medical students continues to rise, from 200 in 1991 to 231 in 2018.*

The passing score for Step 1 is 194. The NBME does not report the minimum number of correct responses needed to pass, but estimates that it is roughly 60–70%. The NBME may adjust the minimum passing score in the future, so please check the USMLE website or www.firstaidteam.com for updates.

FIGURE 1. Samples from the USMLE Step 1 Performance Profile.

Your Performance

Test Result: **PASS**

Test Score: **256**

Your Performance Compared to Other Examinees

The chart below represents the distribution of scores for examinees from US and Canadian medical schools taking Step 1 for the first time between January 1, 2018 and December 31, 2018. Reported scores range from 1-300 with a mean of 231 and a standard deviation of 20.

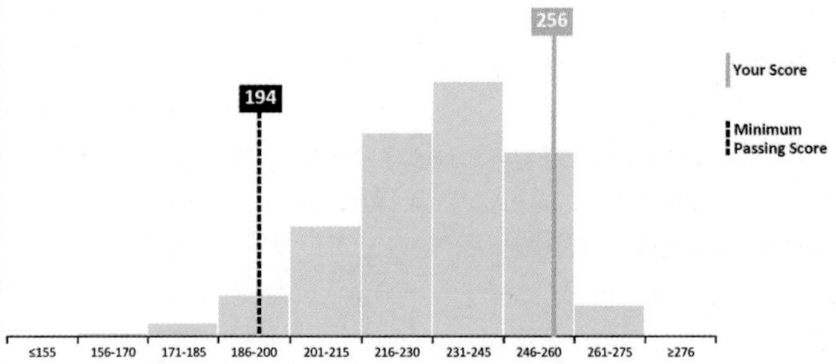

If you tested repeatedly under the same conditions on a different set of items covering the same content, without learning or forgetting, your score would fall within one standard error of the estimate (SEE) of your current score two-thirds of the time. The SEE on this exam is 8 points.

Your score +/- SEE: 248 – 264

Performance by System Relative to Your Overall Step 1 Performance

	(% Items Per Test)	Lower	Same	Higher
General Principles	(13 - 17%)			
Behavioral Health & Nervous Systems/Special Senses	(9 - 13%)			
Reproductive & Endocrine Systems	(9 - 13%)			
Respiratory & Renal/Urinary Systems	(9 - 13%)			
Blood & Lymphoreticular/Immune Systems	(7 - 11%)			
Multisystem Processes & Disorders	(7 - 11%)			
Cardiovascular System	(6 - 10%)			
Musculoskeletal, Skin & Subcutaneous Tissue	(6 - 10%)			
Gastrointestinal System	(5 - 9%)			
Biostatistics & Epidemiology/Population Health	(5 - 7%)			

Performance by Discipline Relative to Your Overall Step 1 Performance

	(% Items Per Test)	Lower	Same	Higher
Pathology	(45 - 52%)			
Physiology	(26 - 34%)			
Pharmacology	(16 - 23%)			
Biochemistry & Nutrition	(12 - 15%)			
Gross Anatomy & Embryology	(11 - 15%)			
Microbiology	(11 - 15%)			
Histology & Cell Biology	(9 - 13%)			
Behavioral Sciences	(8 - 12%)			
Immunology	(7 - 11%)			
Genetics	(5 - 9%)			

FIGURE 2. Score and Percentile for First-time Step 1 Takers.

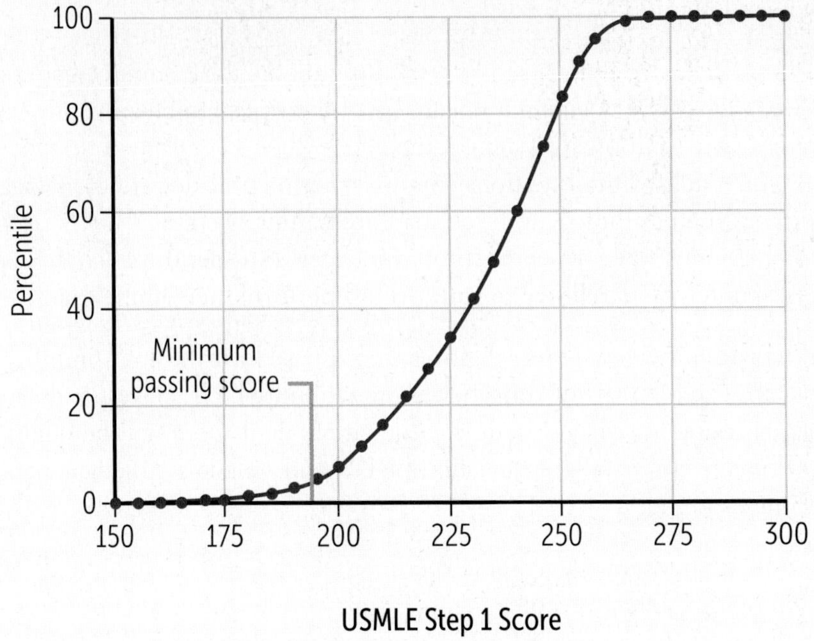

N=72,473 including US and Canadian medical school students testing between January 1, 2016–December 31, 2018. www.usmle.org.

According to the USMLE, medical schools receive a listing of total scores and pass/fail results plus group summaries by discipline and organ system. Students can withhold their scores from their medical school if they wish. Official USMLE transcripts, which can be sent on request to residency programs, include only total scores, not performance profiles.

Consult the USMLE website or your medical school for the most current and accurate information regarding the examination.

TABLE 2. Passing Rates for the 2018–2019 USMLE Step 1.[2]

	2018		2019	
	No. Tested	% Passing	No. Tested	% Passing
Allopathic 1st takers	20,670	96%	21,308	97%
Repeaters	941	67%	838	66%
Allopathic total	21,611	95%	22,146	96%
Osteopathic 1st takers	4,092	96%	4,794	96%
Repeaters	44	73%	43	67%
Osteopathic total	4,136	96%	4,837	96%
Total US/Canadian	**25,747**	**94%**	**26,983**	**96%**
IMG 1st takers	14,332	80%	14,046	82%
Repeaters	2,111	44%	2,019	45%
IMG total	**16,443**	75%	**16,065**	78%
Total Step 1 examinees	**42,190**	87%	**43,048**	89%

What Does My Score Mean?

The most important point with the Step 1 score, while they still report it, is passing versus failing. Passing essentially means, "Hey, you're on your way to becoming a fully licensed doc." As Table 2 shows, the majority of students pass the exam, so remember, we told you to relax.

Beyond that, the main point of having a quantitative score is to give you a sense of how well you've done on the exam and to help schools and residencies rank their students and applicants, respectively.

Official NBME/USMLE Resources

The NBME offers a Comprehensive Basic Science Examination (CBSE) for practice that is a shorter version of the Step 1. The CBSE contains four blocks of 50 questions each and covers material that is typically learned during the basic science years. Scores range from 45 to 95 and correlate with a Step 1 equivalent (see Table 3). The standard error of measurement is approximately 3 points, meaning a score of 80 would estimate the student's proficiency is somewhere between 77 and 83. In other words, the actual Step 1 score could be predicted to be between 218 and 232. Of course, these values do not correlate exactly, and they do not reflect different test preparation methods. Many schools use this test to gauge whether a student is expected to pass Step 1. If this test is offered by your school, it is usually conducted at the end of regular didactic time before any dedicated Step 1 preparation. If you do not encounter the CBSE before your dedicated study time, you need not worry about taking it. Use the information to help set realistic goals and timetables for your success.

The NBME also offers six forms of Comprehensive Basic Science Self-Assessment (CBSSA). Students who prepared for the exam using this web-based tool reported that they found the format and content highly indicative of questions tested on the actual exam. In addition, the CBSSA is a fair predictor of USMLE performance (see Table 4). The test interface, however, does not match the actual USMLE test interface, so practicing with these forms alone is not advised.

The CBSSA exists in two formats: standard-paced and self-paced, both of which consist of four sections of 50 questions each (for a total of 200 multiple choice items). The standard-paced format allows the user up to 75 minutes to complete each section, reflecting time limits similar to the actual exam. By contrast, the self-paced format places a 5-hour time limit on answering all multiple choice questions. Every few years, a new form is released and an older one is retired, reflecting changes in exam content. Therefore, the newer exams tend to be more similar to the actual Step 1, and scores from these exams tend to provide a better estimation of exam day performance.

Keep in mind that this bank of questions is available only on the web. The NBME requires that users start and complete the exam within 90 days of purchase. Once the assessment has begun, users are required to complete the sections within 20 days. Following completion of the questions, the

▸ *Practice questions may be easier than the actual exam.*

TABLE 3. CBSE to USMLE Score Prediction.

CBSE Score	Step 1 Equivalent
≥ 94	≥ 260
92	255
90	250
88	245
86	240
84	235
82	230
80	225
78	220
76	215
74	210
72	205
70	200
68	195
66	190
64	185
62	180
60	175
58	170
56	165
54	160
52	155
50	150
48	145
46	140
≤ 44	≤ 135

TABLE 4. CBSSA to USMLE Score Prediction.

CBSSA Score	Approximate USMLE Step 1 Score
150	155
200	165
250	175
300	186
350	196
400	207
450	217
500	228
550	238
600	248
650	259
700	269
750	280
800	290

CBSSA provides a performance profile indicating the user's relative strengths and weaknesses, much like the report profile for the USMLE Step 1 exam. The profile is scaled with an average score of 500 and a standard deviation of 100. In addition to the performance profile, examinees will be informed of the number of questions answered incorrectly. You will have the ability to review the text of the incorrect question with the correct answer. Explanations for the correct answer, however, will not be provided. The NBME charges $60 for assessments with expanded feedback. The fees are payable by credit card or money order. For more information regarding the CBSE and the CBSSA, visit the NBME's website at www.nbme.org.

The NBME scoring system is weighted for each assessment exam. While some exams seem more difficult than others, the score reported takes into account these inter-test differences when predicting Step 1 performance. Also, while many students report seeing Step 1 questions "word-for-word" out of the assessments, the NBME makes special note that no live USMLE questions are shown on any NBME assessment.

Lastly, the International Foundations of Medicine (IFOM) offers a Basic Science Examination (BSE) practice exam at participating Prometric test centers for $200. Students may also take the self-assessment test online for $35 through the NBME's website. The IFOM BSE is intended to determine an examinee's relative areas of strength and weakness in general areas of basic science—not to predict performance on the USMLE Step 1 exam—and the content covered by the two examinations is somewhat different. However, because there is substantial overlap in content coverage and many IFOM items were previously used on the USMLE Step 1, it is possible to roughly project IFOM performance onto the USMLE Step 1 score scale. More information is available at http://www.nbme.org/ifom/.

▶ DEFINING YOUR GOAL

▶ *Some competitive residency programs place more weight on Step 1 scores when choosing candidates to interview.*

It is useful to define your own personal performance goal when approaching the USMLE Step 1. Your style and intensity of preparation can then be matched to your goal. Furthermore, your goal may depend on your school's requirements, your specialty choice, your grades to date, and your personal assessment of the test's importance. Do your best to define your goals early so that you can prepare accordingly.

▶ *Fourth-year medical students have the best feel for how Step 1 scores factor into the residency application process.*

The value of the USMLE Step 1 score in selecting residency applicants remains controversial, and some have called for less emphasis to be placed on the score when selecting or screening applicants.[3] For the time being, however, it continues to be an important part of the residency application, and it is not uncommon for some specialties to implement filters that screen out applicants who score below a certain cutoff. This is more likely to be seen in competitive specialties (eg, orthopedic surgery, ophthalmology, dermatology, otolaryngology). Independent of your career goals, you can maximize your future options by doing your best to obtain the highest score possible (see Figure 3). At the same time, your Step 1 score is only one of a number of

FIGURE 3. Median USMLE Step 1 Score by Specialty for Matched US Seniors.[a,b]

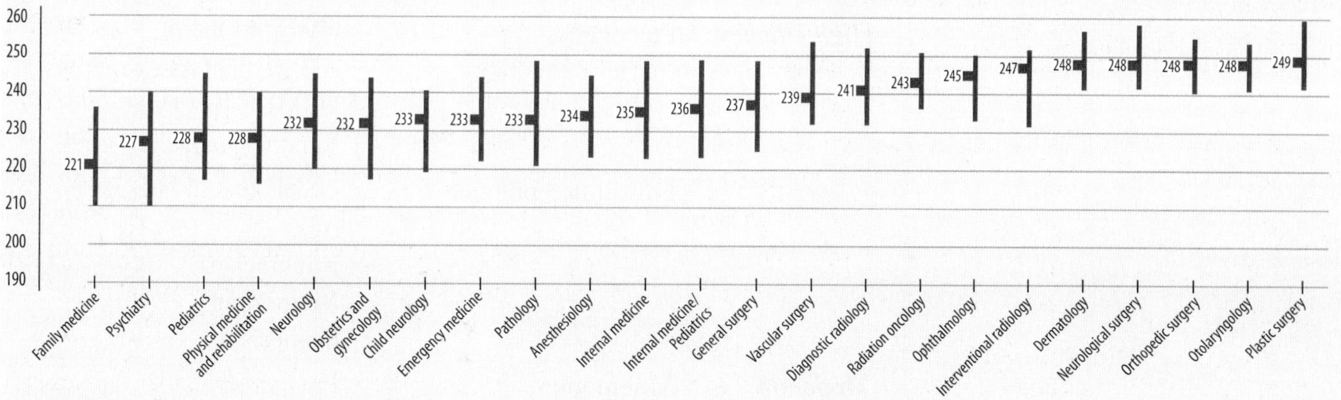

[a]Vertical lines show interquartile range.
[b]Data from National Resident Matching Program. Charting outcomes in the match. https://mk0nrmp3oyqui6wqfm.kinstacdn.com/wp-content/uploads/2020/07/Charting-Outcomes-in-the-Match-2020_MD-Senior_final.pdf. Published July 2020.

factors that are assessed when you apply for residency. In fact, many residency programs value other criteria such as letters of recommendation, third-year clerkship grades, honors, and research experience more than a high score on Step 1. Fourth-year medical students who have recently completed the residency application process can be a valuable resource in this regard.

▶ LEARNING STRATEGIES

Many students feel overwhelmed during the preclinical years and struggle to find an effective learning strategy. Table 5 lists several learning strategies you can try and their estimated effectiveness for Step 1 preparation based on the literature (see References). These are merely suggestions, and it's important to take your learning preferences into account. Your comprehensive learning approach will contain a combination of strategies (eg, elaborative interrogation followed by practice testing, mnemonics review using spaced repetition, etc). Regardless of your choice, the foundation of knowledge you build during your basic science years is the most important resource for success on the USMLE Step 1.

> ▶ *The foundation of knowledge you build during your basic science years is the most important resource for success on the USMLE Step 1.*

HIGH EFFICACY

Practice Testing

Also called "retrieval practice," practice testing has both direct and indirect benefits to the learner.[4] Effortful retrieval of answers does not only identify weak spots—it directly strengthens long-term retention of material.[5] The more effortful the recall, the better the long-term retention. This advantage has been shown to result in higher test scores and GPAs.[6] In fact, research has shown a positive correlation between the number of boards-style practice questions completed and Step 1 scores among medical students.[7]

> ▶ *Research has shown a positive correlation between the number of boards-style practice questions completed and Step 1 scores among medical students.*

TABLE 5. Effective Learning Strategies.

EFFICACY	STRATEGY	EXAMPLE RESOURCES
High efficacy	Practice testing (retrieval practice)	UWorld Qbank NBME Self-Assessments USMLE-Rx QMax Kaplan Qbank
	Distributed practice	USMLE-Rx Flash Facts Anki Firecracker Memorang Osmosis
Moderate efficacy	Mnemonics	*Pre-made:* SketchyMedical Picmonic *Self-made:* Mullen Memory
	Elaborative interrogation/ self-explanation	
	Concept mapping	Coggle FreeMind XMind MindNode
Low efficacy	Rereading	
	Highlighting/underlining	
	Summarization	

Practice testing should be done with "interleaving" (mixing of questions from different topics in a single session). Question banks often allow you to intermingle topics. Interleaved practice helps learners develop their ability to focus on the relevant concept when faced with many possibilities. Practicing topics in massed fashion (eg, all cardiology, then all dermatology) may seem intuitive, but there is strong evidence that interleaving correlates with longer-term retention and increased student achievement, especially on tasks that involve problem solving.[5]

In addition to using question banks, you can test yourself by arranging your notes in a question-answer format (eg, via flash cards). Testing these Q&As in random order allows you to reap the benefit of interleaved practice. Bear in mind that the utility of practice testing comes from the practice of information retrieval, so simply reading through Q&As will attenuate this benefit.

Distributed Practice

Also called "spaced repetition," distributed practice is the opposite of massed practice or "cramming." Learners review material at increasingly spaced out intervals (days to weeks to months). Massed learning may produce more short-term gains and satisfaction, but learners who use distributed practice have better mastery and retention over the long term.[5,9]

Flash cards are a simple way to incorporate both distributed practice and practice testing. Studies have linked spaced repetition learning with flash cards to improved long-term knowledge retention and higher exam scores.[6,8,10] Apps with automated spaced-repetition software (SRS) for flash cards exist for smartphones and tablets, so the cards are accessible anywhere. Proceed with caution: there is an art to making and reviewing cards. The ease of quickly downloading or creating digital cards can lead to flash card overload (it is unsustainable to make 50 flash cards per lecture!). Even at a modest pace, the thousands upon thousands of cards are too overwhelming for Step 1 preparation. Unless you have specific high-yield cards (and have checked the content with high-yield resources), stick to pre-made cards by reputable sources that curate the vast amount of knowledge for you.

▸ Studies have linked spaced repetition learning with flash cards to improved long-term knowledge retention and higher exam scores.

If you prefer pen and paper, consider using a planner or spreadsheet to organize your study material over time. Distributed practice allows for some forgetting of information, and the added effort of recall over time strengthens the learning.

MODERATE EFFICACY

Mnemonics

A "mnemonic" refers to any device that assists memory, such as acronyms, mental imagery (eg, keywords with or without memory palaces), etc. Keyword mnemonics have been shown to produce superior knowledge retention when compared with rote memorization in many scenarios. However, they are generally more effective when applied to memorization-heavy, keyword-friendly topics and may not be broadly suitable.[5] Keyword mnemonics may not produce long-term retention, so consider combining mnemonics with distributed, retrieval-based practice (eg, via flash cards with SRS).

Self-made mnemonics may have an advantage when material is simple and keyword friendly. If you can create your own mnemonic that accurately represents the material, this will be more memorable. When topics are complex and accurate mnemonics are challenging to create, pre-made mnemonics may be more effective, especially if you are inexperienced at creating mnemonics.[11]

Elaborative Interrogation/Self-Explanation

Elaborative interrogation ("why" questions) and self-explanation (general questioning) prompt learners to generate explanations for facts. When reading passages of discrete facts, consider using these techniques, which have been shown to be more effective than rereading (eg, improved recall and better problem-solving/diagnostic performance).[5,12,13]

▸ Elaborative interrogation and self-explanation prompt learners to generate explanations for facts, which improves recall and problem solving.

Concept Mapping

Concept mapping is a method for graphically organizing knowledge, with concepts enclosed in boxes and lines drawn between related concepts. Creating or studying concept maps may be more effective than other activities (eg, writing or reading summaries/outlines). However, studies have reached mixed conclusions about its utility, and the small size of this effect raises doubts about its authenticity and pedagogic significance.[14]

LOW EFFICACY

Rereading

While the most commonly used method among surveyed students, rereading has not been shown to correlate with grade point average.[9] Due to its popularity, rereading is often a comparator in studies on learning. Other strategies that we have discussed (eg, practice testing) have been shown to be significantly more effective than rereading.

Highlighting/Underlining

Because this method is passive, it tends to be of minimal value for learning and recall. In fact, lower-performing students are more likely to use these techniques.[9] Students who highlight and underline do not learn how to actively recall learned information and thus find it difficult to apply knowledge to exam questions.

Summarization

While more useful for improving performance on generative measures (eg, free recall or essays), summarization is less useful for exams that depend on recognition (eg, multiple choice). Findings on the overall efficacy of this method have been mixed.[5]

▶ TIMELINE FOR STUDY

Before Starting

Your preparation for the USMLE Step 1 should begin when you enter medical school. Organize and commit to studying from the beginning so that when the time comes to prepare for the USMLE, you will be ready with a strong foundation.

Make a Schedule

After you have defined your goals, map out a study schedule that is consistent with your objectives, your vacation time, the difficulty of your ongoing

FIGURE 4. Typical Timeline for the USMLE Step 1.

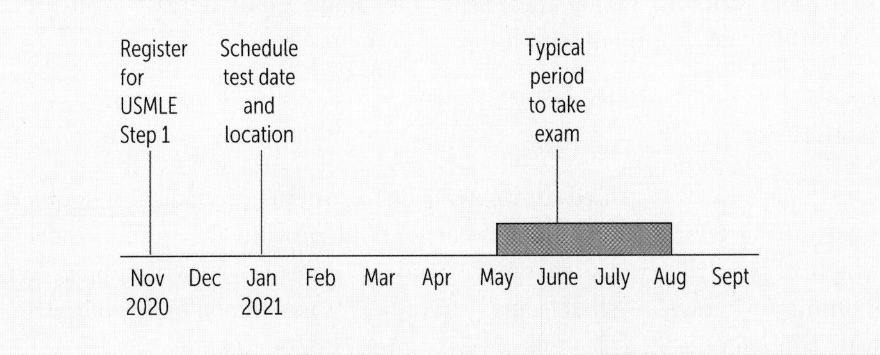

▶ *Customize your schedule. Tackle your weakest section first.*

coursework, and your family and social commitments (see Figure 4). Determine whether you want to spread out your study time or concentrate it into 14-hour study days in the final weeks. Then factor in your own history in preparing for standardized examinations (eg, SAT, MCAT). Talk to students at your school who have recently taken Step 1. Ask them for their study schedules, especially those who have study habits and goals similar to yours. Sample schedules can be found at https://firstaidteam.com/schedules/.

Typically, US medical schools allot between four and eight weeks for dedicated Step 1 preparation. The time you dedicate to exam preparation will depend on your target score as well as your success in preparing yourself during the first two years of medical school. Some students reserve about a week at the end of their study period for final review; others save just a few days. When you have scheduled your exam date, do your best to adhere to it. Studies show that a later testing date does not translate into a higher score, so avoid pushing back your test date without good reason.[15]

Make your schedule realistic, and set achievable goals. Many students make the mistake of studying at a level of detail that requires too much time for a comprehensive review—reading *Gray's Anatomy* in a couple of days is not a realistic goal! Have one catch-up day per week of studying. No matter how well you stick to your schedule, unexpected events happen. But don't let yourself procrastinate because you have catch-up days; stick to your schedule as closely as possible and revise it regularly on the basis of your actual progress. Be careful not to lose focus. Beware of feelings of inadequacy when comparing study schedules and progress with your peers. **Avoid others who stress you out.** Focus on a few top-rated resources that suit your learning style—not on some obscure books your friends may pass down to you. Accept the fact that you cannot learn it all.

▶ *Avoid burnout. Maintain proper diet, exercise, and sleep habits.*

You will need time for uninterrupted and focused study. Plan your personal affairs to minimize crisis situations near the date of the test. Allot an adequate number of breaks in your study schedule to avoid burnout. Maintain a healthy lifestyle with proper diet, exercise, and sleep.

Another important aspect of your preparation is your studying environment. **Study where you have always been comfortable studying.** Be sure to include everything you need close by (review books, notes, coffee, snacks, etc). If you're the kind of person who cannot study alone, form a study group with other students taking the exam. The main point here is to create a comfortable environment with minimal distractions.

Year(s) Prior

▶ *Buy review books early (first year) and use while studying for courses.*

The knowledge you gained during your first two years of medical school and even during your undergraduate years should provide the groundwork on which to base your test preparation. Student scores on NBME subject tests (commonly known as "shelf exams") have been shown to be highly correlated with subsequent Step 1 scores.[16] Moreover, undergraduate science GPAs as well as MCAT scores are strong predictors of performance on the Step 1 exam.[17]

We also recommend that you buy highly rated review books early in your first year of medical school and use them as you study throughout the two years. When Step 1 comes along, these books will be familiar and personalized to the way in which you learn. It is risky and intimidating to use unfamiliar review books in the final two or three weeks preceding the exam. Some students find it helpful to personalize and annotate *First Aid* throughout the curriculum.

Months Prior

Review test dates and the application procedure. Testing for the USMLE Step 1 is done on a year-round basis. If you have disabilities or special circumstances, contact the NBME as early as possible to discuss test accommodations (see the Section I Supplement at www.firstaidteam.com/bonus).

▶ *Simulate the USMLE Step 1 under "real" conditions before beginning your studies.*

Use this time to finalize your ideal schedule. Consider upcoming breaks and whether you want to relax or study. Work backward from your test date to make sure you finish at least one question bank. Also add time to redo missed or flagged questions (which may be half the bank). This is the time to build a structured plan with enough flexibility for the realities of life.

Begin doing blocks of questions from reputable question banks under "real" conditions. Don't use tutor mode until you're sure you can finish blocks in the allotted time. It is important to continue balancing success in your normal studies with the Step 1 test preparation process.

Weeks Prior (Dedicated Preparation)

Your dedicated prep time may be one week or two months. You should have a working plan as you go into this period. Finish your schoolwork strong, take a day off, and then get to work. Start by simulating a full-length USMLE Step 1 if you haven't yet done so. Consider doing one NBME CBSSA and the free questions from the NBME website. Alternatively, you could choose 7 blocks of randomized questions from a commercial question bank. Make sure you get feedback on your strengths and weaknesses and adjust your studying accordingly. Many students study from review sources or comprehensive programs for part of the day, then do question blocks. Also, keep in mind that reviewing a question block can take upward of two hours. Feedback from CBSSA exams and question banks will help you focus on your weaknesses.

- *In the final two weeks, focus on review, practice questions, and endurance. Stay confident!*

One Week Prior

Make sure you have your CIN (found on your scheduling permit) as well as other items necessary for the day of the examination, including a current driver's license or another form of photo ID with your signature (make sure the name on your **ID exactly** matches that on your scheduling permit). Confirm the Prometric testing center location and test time. Work out how you will get to the testing center and what parking and traffic problems you might encounter. Drive separately from other students taking the test on the same day, and exchange cell phone numbers in case of emergencies. If possible, visit the testing site to get a better idea of the testing conditions you will face. Determine what you will do for lunch. Make sure you have everything you need to ensure that you will be comfortable and alert at the test site. It may be beneficial to adjust your schedule to start waking up at the same time that you will on your test day. And of course, make sure to maintain a healthy lifestyle and get enough sleep.

- *One week before the test:*
  - *Sleep according to the same schedule you'll use on test day*
  - *Review the CBT tutorial one last time*
  - *Call Prometric to confirm test date and time*

One Day Prior

Try your best to relax and rest the night before the test. Double-check your admissions and test-taking materials as well as the comfort measures discussed earlier so that you will not have to deal with such details on the morning of the exam. At this point it will be more effective to review short-term memory material that you're already familiar with than to try to learn new material. The Rapid Review section at the end of this book is high yield for last-minute studying. Remember that regardless of how hard you have studied, you cannot know everything. There will be things on the exam that you have never even seen before, so do not panic. Do not underestimate your abilities.

Many students report difficulty sleeping the night prior to the exam. This is often exacerbated by going to bed much earlier than usual. Do whatever it takes to ensure a good night's sleep (eg, massage, exercise, warm milk, no back-lit screens at night). Do not change your daily routine prior to the exam. Exam day is not the day for a caffeine-withdrawal headache.

Morning of the Exam

On the morning of the Step 1 exam, wake up at your regular time and eat a normal breakfast. If you think it will help you, have a close friend or family member check to make sure you get out of bed. Make sure you have your scheduling permit admission ticket, test-taking materials, and comfort measures as discussed earlier. Wear loose, comfortable clothing. Plan for a variable temperature in the testing center. Arrive at the test site 30 minutes

- *No notes, books, calculators, pagers, cell phones, recording devices, or watches of any kind are allowed in the testing area, but they are allowed in lockers.*

▶ *Arrive at the testing center 30 minutes before your scheduled exam time. If you arrive more than half an hour late, you will not be allowed to take the test.*

before the time designated on the admission ticket; however, do not come too early, as doing so may intensify your anxiety. When you arrive at the test site, the proctor should give you a USMLE information sheet that will explain critical factors such as the proper use of break time. Seating may be assigned, but ask to be reseated if necessary; you need to be seated in an area that will allow you to remain comfortable and to concentrate. Get to know your testing station, especially if you have never been in a Prometric testing center before. Listen to your proctors regarding any changes in instructions or testing procedures that may apply to your test site.

Finally, remember that it is natural (and even beneficial) to be a little nervous. Focus on being mentally clear and alert. Avoid panic. When you are asked to begin the exam, take a deep breath, focus on the screen, and then begin. Keep an eye on the timer. Take advantage of breaks between blocks to stretch, maybe do some jumping jacks, and relax for a moment with deep breathing or stretching.

After the Test

After you have completed the exam, be sure to have fun and relax regardless of how you may feel. Taking the test is an achievement in itself. Remember, you are much more likely to have passed than not. Enjoy the free time you have before your clerkships. Expect to experience some "reentry" phenomena as you try to regain a real life. Once you have recovered sufficiently from the test (or from partying), we invite you to send us your feedback, corrections, and suggestions for entries, facts, mnemonics, strategies, resource ratings, and the like (see p. xvii, How to Contribute). Sharing your experience will benefit fellow medical students.

▶ STUDY MATERIALS

Quality Considerations

Although an ever-increasing number of review books and software are now available on the market, the quality of such material is highly variable. Some common problems are as follows:

- Certain review books are too detailed to allow for review in a reasonable amount of time or cover subtopics that are not emphasized on the exam.
- Many sample question books were originally written years ago and have not been adequately updated to reflect recent trends.
- Some question banks test to a level of detail that you will not find on the exam.

▶ *If a given review book is not working for you, stop using it no matter how highly rated it may be or how much it costs.*

Review Books

In selecting review books, be sure to weigh different opinions against each other, read the reviews and ratings in Section IV of this guide, examine the books closely in the bookstore, and choose carefully. You are investing not only money but also your limited study time. Do not worry about finding the "perfect" book, as many subjects simply do not have one, and different students prefer different formats. Supplement your chosen books with personal notes from other sources, including what you learn from question banks.

There are two types of review books: those that are stand-alone titles and those that are part of a series. Books in a series generally have the same style, and you must decide if that style works for you. However, a given style is not optimal for every subject.

▶ *Charts and diagrams may be the best approach for physiology and biochemistry, whereas tables and outlines may be preferable for microbiology.*

You should also find out which books are up to date. Some recent editions reflect major improvements, whereas others contain only cursory changes. Take into consideration how a book reflects the format of the USMLE Step 1.

Apps

With the explosion of smartphones and tablets, apps are an increasingly popular way to review for the Step 1 exam. The majority of apps are compatible with both iOS and Android. Many popular Step 1 review resources (eg, UWorld, USMLE-Rx) have apps that are compatible with their software. Many popular web references (eg, UpToDate) also now offer app versions. All of these apps offer flexibility, allowing you to study while away from a computer (eg, while traveling).

Practice Tests

Taking practice tests provides valuable information about potential strengths and weaknesses in your fund of knowledge and test-taking skills. Some students use practice examinations simply as a means of breaking up the monotony of studying and adding variety to their study schedule, whereas other students rely almost solely on practice. You should also subscribe to one or more high-quality question banks.

▶ *Most practice exams are shorter and less clinical than the real thing.*

Additionally, some students preparing for the Step 1 exam have started to incorporate case-based books intended primarily for clinical students on the wards or studying for the Step 2 CK exam. *First Aid Cases for the USMLE Step 1* aims to directly address this need.

After taking a practice test, spend time on each question and each answer choice whether you were right or wrong. There are important teaching points in each explanation. Knowing why a wrong answer choice is incorrect is just as important as knowing why the right answer is correct. Do not panic if your practice scores are low as many questions try to trick or distract you to highlight a certain point. Use the questions you missed or were unsure about to develop focused plans during your scheduled catch-up time.

▶ *Use practice tests to identify concepts and areas of weakness, not just facts that you missed.*

Textbooks and Course Syllabi

Limit your use of textbooks and course syllabi for Step 1 review. Many textbooks are too detailed for high-yield review and include material that is generally not tested on the USMLE Step 1 (eg, drug dosages, complex chemical structures). Syllabi, although familiar, are inconsistent across medical schools and frequently reflect the emphasis of individual faculty, which often does not correspond to that of the USMLE Step 1. Syllabi also tend to be less organized than top-rated books and generally contain fewer diagrams and study questions.

▸ TEST-TAKING STRATEGIES

▸ *Practice! Develop your test-taking skills and strategies well before the test date.*

Your test performance will be influenced by both your knowledge and your test-taking skills. You can strengthen your performance by considering each of these factors. Test-taking skills and strategies should be developed and perfected well in advance of the test date so that you can concentrate on the test itself. We suggest that you try the following strategies to see if they might work for you.

Pacing

You have seven hours to complete up to 280 questions. Note that each one-hour block contains up to 40 questions. This works out to approximately 90 seconds per question. We recommend following the "1 minute rule" to pace yourself. Spend no more than 1 minute on each question. If you are still unsure about the answer after this time, mark the question, make an educated guess, and move on. Following this rule, you should have approximately 20 minutes left after all questions are answered, which you can use to revisit all of your marked questions. Remember that some questions may be experimental and do not count for points (and reassure yourself that these experimental questions are the ones that are stumping you). In the past, pacing errors have been detrimental to the performance of even highly prepared examinees. The bottom line is to keep one eye on the clock at all times!

▸ *Time management is an important skill for exam success.*

Dealing with Each Question

There are several established techniques for efficiently approaching multiple choice questions; find what works for you. One technique begins with identifying each question as easy, workable, or impossible. Your goal should be to answer all easy questions, resolve all workable questions in a reasonable amount of time, and make quick and intelligent guesses on all impossible questions. Most students read the stem, think of the answer, and turn immediately to the choices. A second technique is to first skim the answer choices to get a context, then read the last sentence of the question (the lead-in), and then read through the passage quickly, extracting only information relevant to answering the question. This can be particularly helpful for questions with long clinical vignettes. Try a variety of techniques on practice exams and see what works best for you. If you get overwhelmed, remember that a 30-second time out to refocus may get you back on track.

Guessing

There is **no penalty** for wrong answers. Thus, **no test block should be left with unanswered questions.** If you don't know the answer, first eliminate incorrect choices, then guess among the remaining options. **Note that dozens of questions are unscored experimental questions** meant to obtain statistics for future exams. Therefore, some questions will seem impossible simply because they are part of the development process for future exams.

Changing Your Answer

The conventional wisdom is not to change answers that you have already marked unless there is a convincing and logical reason to do so—in other words, go with your "first hunch." Many question banks tell you how many questions you changed from right to wrong, wrong to wrong, and wrong to right. Use this feedback to judge how good a second-guesser you are. If you have extra time, reread the question stem and make sure you didn't misinterpret the question.

> ▶ *Go with your first hunch, unless you are certain that you are a good second-guesser.*

▶ CLINICAL VIGNETTE STRATEGIES

In recent years, the USMLE Step 1 has become increasingly clinically oriented. This change mirrors the trend in medical education toward introducing students to clinical problem solving during the basic science years. The increasing clinical emphasis on Step 1 may be challenging to those students who attend schools with a more traditional curriculum.

> ▶ *Be prepared to read fast and think on your feet!*

What Is a Clinical Vignette?

A clinical vignette is a short (usually paragraph-long) description of a patient, including demographics, presenting symptoms, signs, and other information concerning the patient. Sometimes this paragraph is followed by a brief listing of important physical findings and/or laboratory results. The task of assimilating all this information and answering the associated question in the span of one minute can be intimidating. So be prepared to read quickly and think on your feet. Remember that the question is often indirectly asking something you already know.

> ▶ *Practice questions that include case histories or descriptive vignettes are critical for Step 1 preparation.*

Strategy

Remember that Step 1 vignettes usually describe diseases or disorders in their most classic presentation. So look for cardinal signs (eg, malar rash for SLE or nuchal rigidity for meningitis) in the narrative history. Be aware that the question will contain classic signs and symptoms instead of buzzwords. Sometimes the data from labs and the physical exam will help you confirm or reject possible diagnoses, thereby helping you rule answer choices in or out. In some cases, they will be a dead giveaway for the diagnosis.

▶ *Step 1 vignettes usually describe diseases or disorders in their most classic presentation.*

Making a diagnosis from the history and data is often not the final answer. Not infrequently, the diagnosis is divulged at the end of the vignette, after you have just struggled through the narrative to come up with a diagnosis of your own. The question might then ask about a related aspect of the diagnosed disease. Consider skimming the answer choices and lead-in before diving into a long stem. However, be careful with skimming the answer choices; going too fast may warp your perception of what the vignette is asking.

▶ IF YOU THINK YOU FAILED

After the test, many examinees feel that they have failed, and most are at the very least unsure of their pass/fail status. There are several sensible steps you can take to plan for the future in the event that you do not achieve a passing score. First, save and organize all your study materials, including review books, practice tests, and notes. Familiarize yourself with the reapplication procedures for Step 1, including application deadlines and upcoming test dates.

Make sure you know both your school's and the NBME's policies regarding retakes. The NBME allows a maximum of six attempts to pass each Step examination.[18] You may take Step 1 no more than three times within a 12-month period. Your fourth and subsequent attempts must be at least 12 months after your first attempt at that exam and at least six months after your most recent attempt at that exam. No earlier than July 1, 2021, the total number of attempts an examinee may take per Step examination will be reduced to four attempts.

▶ *If you pass Step 1 (score of 194 or above), you are not allowed to retake the exam.*

The performance profiles on the back of the USMLE Step 1 score report provide valuable feedback concerning your relative strengths and weaknesses. Study these profiles closely. Set up a study timeline to strengthen gaps in your knowledge as well as to maintain and improve what you already know. Do not neglect high-yield subjects. It is normal to feel somewhat anxious about retaking the test, but if anxiety becomes a problem, seek appropriate counseling.

TESTING AGENCIES

- **National Board of Medical Examiners (NBME) / USMLE Secretariat**
  Department of Licensing Examination Services
  3750 Market Street
  Philadelphia, PA 19104-3102
  (215) 590-9500 (operator) or
  (215) 590-9700 (automated information line)
  Email: webmail@nbme.org
  www.nbme.org

- **Educational Commission for Foreign Medical Graduates (ECFMG)**
  3624 Market Street
  Philadelphia, PA 19104-2685
  (215) 386-5900
  Email: info@ecfmg.org
  www.ecfmg.org

REFERENCES

1. United States Medical Licensing Examination. Available from: https://www.usmle.org/pdfs/step-1/content_step1.pdf. Accessed October 9, 2020.
2. United States Medical Licensing Examination. 2019 Performance Data. Available from: https://www.usmle.org/performance-data/default.aspx#2019_step-1. Accessed October 9, 2020.
3. Prober CG, Kolars JC, First LR, et al. A plea to reassess the role of United States Medical Licensing Examination Step 1 scores in residency selection. *Acad Med.* 2016;91(1):12–15.
4. Roediger HL, Butler AC. The critical role of retrieval practice in long-term retention. *Trends Cogn Sci.* 2011;15(1):20–27.
5. Dunlosky J, Rawson KA, Marsh EJ, et al. Improving students' learning with effective learning techniques: promising directions from cognitive and educational psychology. *Psychol Sci Publ Int.* 2013;14(1):4–58.
6. Larsen DP, Butler AC, Lawson AL, et al. The importance of seeing the patient: test-enhanced learning with standardized patients and written tests improves clinical application of knowledge. *Adv Health Sci Educ.* 2013;18(3):409–425.
7. Panus PC, Stewart DW, Hagemeier NE, et al. A subgroup analysis of the impact of self-testing frequency on examination scores in a pathophysiology course. *Am J Pharm Educ.* 2014;78(9):165.
8. Deng F, Gluckstein JA, Larsen DP. Student-directed retrieval practice is a predictor of medical licensing examination performance. *Perspect Med Educ.* 2015;4(6):308–313.
9. McAndrew M, Morrow CS, Atiyeh L, et al. Dental student study strategies: are self-testing and scheduling related to academic performance? *J Dent Educ.* 2016;80(5):542–552.

10. Augustin M. How to learn effectively in medical school: test yourself, learn actively, and repeat in intervals. *Yale J Biol Med.* 2014;87(2):207–212.
11. Bellezza FS. Mnemonic devices: classification, characteristics, and criteria. *Rev Educ Res.* 1981;51(2):247–275.
12. Dyer J-O, Hudon A, Montpetit-Tourangeau K, et al. Example-based learning: comparing the effects of additionally providing three different integrative learning activities on physiotherapy intervention knowledge. *BMC Med Educ.* 2015;15:37.
13. Chamberland M, Mamede S, St-Onge C, et al. Self-explanation in learning clinical reasoning: the added value of examples and prompts. *Med Educ.* 2015;49(2):193–202.
14. Nesbit JC, Adesope OO. Learning with concept and knowledge maps: a meta-analysis. *Rev Educ Res.* 2006;76(3):413–448.
15. Pohl CA, Robeson MR, Hojat M, et al. Sooner or later? USMLE Step 1 performance and test administration date at the end of the second year. *Acad Med.* 2002;77(10):S17–S19.
16. Holtman MC, Swanson DB, Ripkey DR, et al. Using basic science subject tests to identify students at risk for failing Step 1. *Acad Med.* 2001;76(10):S48–S51.
17. Basco WT, Way DP, Gilbert GE, et al. Undergraduate institutional MCAT scores as predictors of USMLE Step 1 performance. *Acad Med.* 2002;77(10):S13–S16.
18. United States Medical Licensing Examination. 2021 USMLE Bulletin of Information. Available from: https://www.usmle.org/pdfs/bulletin/2021bulletin.pdf. Accessed October 9, 2020.

SECTION I SUPPLEMENT

Special Situations

Please visit **www.firstaidteam.com/bonus/** to view this section.

- First Aid for the International Medical Graduate
- First Aid for the Osteopathic Medical Student
- First Aid for the Podiatric Medical Student
- First Aid for the Student Requiring Test Accommodations

▶ NOTES

SECTION II

High-Yield General Principles

"I've learned that I still have a lot to learn."

—Maya Angelou

"Never regard study as a duty, but as the enviable opportunity to learn."

—Albert Einstein

"Live as if you were to die tomorrow. Learn as if you were to live forever."

—Gandhi

"Success is the maximum utilization of the ability that you have."

—Zig Ziglar

▶ HOW TO USE THE DATABASE

The 2021 edition of *First Aid for the USMLE Step 1* contains a revised and expanded database of basic science material that students, student authors, and faculty authors have identified as high yield for board review. The information is presented in a partially organ-based format. Hence, Section II is devoted to the foundational principles of biochemistry, microbiology, immunology, basic pathology, basic pharmacology, and public health sciences. Section III focuses on organ systems, with subsections covering the embryology, anatomy and histology, physiology, clinical pathology, and clinical pharmacology relevant to each. Each subsection is then divided into smaller topic areas containing related facts. Individual facts are generally presented in a three-column format, with the **Title** of the fact in the first column, the **Description** of the fact in the second column, and the **Mnemonic** or **Special Note** in the third column. Some facts do not have a mnemonic and are presented in a two-column format. Others are presented in list or tabular form in order to emphasize key associations.

The database structure used in Sections II and III is useful for reviewing material already learned. These sections are **not** ideal for learning complex or highly conceptual material for the first time.

The database of high-yield facts is not comprehensive. Use it to complement your core study material and not as your primary study source. The facts and notes have been condensed and edited to emphasize the high-yield material, and as a result, each entry is "incomplete" and arguably "over-simplified." Often, the more you research a topic, the more complex it becomes, with certain topics resisting simplification. Determine your most efficient methods for learning the material, and do not be afraid to abandon a strategy if it is not working for you.

Our database of high-yield facts is updated annually to keep current with new trends in boards emphasis, including clinical relevance. However, we must note that inevitably many other high-yield topics are not yet included in our database.

We actively encourage medical students and faculty to submit high-yield topics, well-written entries, diagrams, clinical images, and useful mnemonics so that we may enhance the database for future students. We also solicit recommendations of alternate tools for study that may be useful in preparing for the examination, such as charts, flash cards, apps, and online resources (see How to Contribute, p. xvii).

Image Acknowledgments

All images and diagrams marked with ℞ are © USMLE-Rx.com (MedIQ Learning, LLC) and reproduced here by special permission. All images marked with RU are © Dr. Richard P. Usatine, author of *The Color Atlas of Family Medicine*, *The Color Atlas of Internal Medicine*, and *The Color Atlas of Pediatrics*, and are reproduced here by special permission (www.usatinemedia.com). Images and diagrams marked with * are adapted or reproduced with permission of other sources as listed on page 753. Images and diagrams with no acknowledgment are part of this book.

Disclaimer

The entries in this section reflect student opinions on what is high yield. Because of the diverse sources of material, no attempt has been made to trace or reference the origins of entries individually. We have regarded mnemonics as essentially in the public domain. Errata will gladly be corrected if brought to the attention of the authors, either through our online errata submission form at www.firstaidteam.com or directly by email to firstaid@scholarrx.com.

NOTES

HIGH-YIELD PRINCIPLES IN

Biochemistry

"The nitrogen in our DNA, the calcium in our teeth, the iron in our blood, the carbon in our apple pies were made in the interiors of collapsing stars. We are made of starstuff."

—Carl Sagan

"Biochemistry is the study of carbon compounds that crawl."

—Mike Adams

"We think we have found the basic mechanism by which life comes from life."

—Francis H. C. Crick

DNA was the first three-dimensional Xerox machine.

—Kenneth Ewart Boulding

This high-yield material includes molecular biology, genetics, cell biology, and principles of metabolism (especially vitamins, cofactors, minerals, and single-enzyme-deficiency diseases). When studying metabolic pathways, emphasize important regulatory steps and enzyme deficiencies that result in disease, as well as reactions targeted by pharmacologic interventions. For example, understanding the defect in Lesch-Nyhan syndrome and its clinical consequences is higher yield than memorizing every intermediate in the purine salvage pathway.

Do not spend time learning details of organic chemistry, mechanisms, or physical chemistry. Detailed chemical structures are infrequently tested; however, many structures have been included here to help students learn reactions and the important enzymes involved. Familiarity with the biochemical techniques that have medical relevance—such as ELISA, immunoelectrophoresis, Southern blotting, and PCR—is useful. Review the related biochemistry when studying pharmacology or genetic diseases as a way to reinforce and integrate the material.

▶ BIOCHEMISTRY—MOLECULAR

Chromatin structure

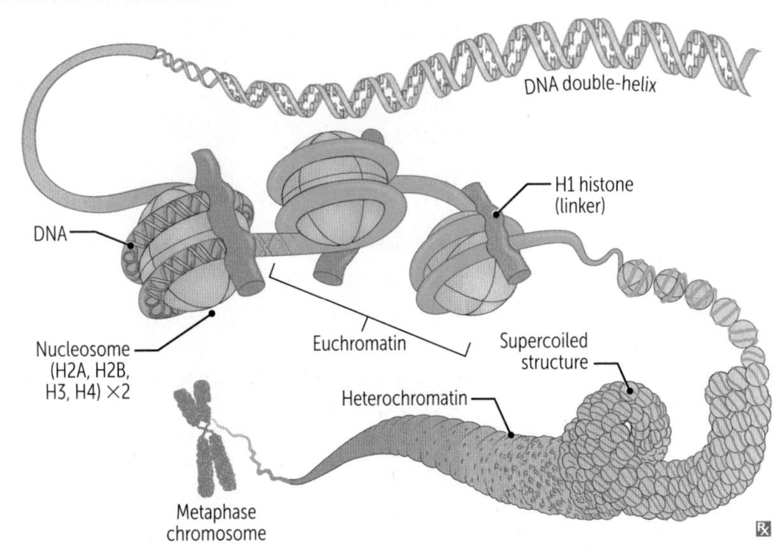
DNA double-helix
H1 histone
(linker)
DNA
Nucleosome
(H2A, H2B,
H3, H4) ×2
Euchromatin
Supercoiled
structure
Heterochromatin
Metaphase
chromosome

DNA exists in the condensed, chromatin form to fit into the nucleus. DNA loops twice around a histone octamer to form a nucleosome ("beads on a string"). H1 binds to the nucleosome and to "linker DNA," thereby stabilizing the chromatin fiber.

Phosphate groups give DNA a ⊖ charge. Lysine and arginine give histones a ⊕ charge.

In mitosis, DNA condenses to form chromosomes. DNA and histone synthesis occurs during S phase.

Mitochondria have their own DNA, which is circular and does not utilize histones.

Heterochromatin 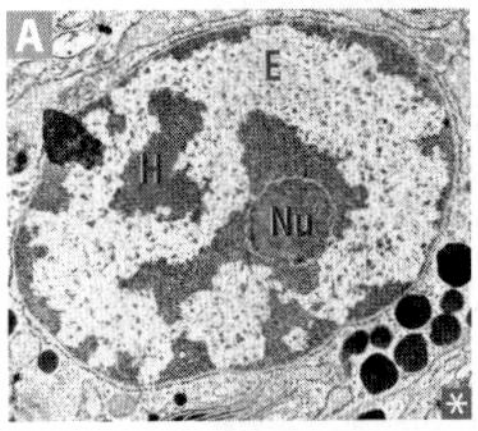 A E H Nu	Condensed, appears darker on EM (labeled H in A; Nu, nucleolus). Sterically inaccessible, thus transcriptionally inactive. ↑ methylation, ↓ acetylation.	**H**eterochromatin = **h**ighly condensed. Barr bodies (inactive X chromosomes) may be visible on the periphery of nucleus.
Euchromatin	Less condensed, appears lighter on EM (labeled E in A). Transcriptionally active, sterically accessible.	*Eu* = true, "truly transcribed." **E**uchromatin is **e**xpressed.
DNA methylation	Changes the expression of a DNA segment without changing the sequence. Involved with aging, carcinogenesis, genomic imprinting, transposable element repression, and X chromosome inactivation (lyonization).	DNA is methylated in imprinting. Methylation within gene promoter (CpG islands) typically represses (silences) gene transcription. CpG **m**ethylation **m**akes DNA **m**ute.
Histone methylation	Usually causes reversible transcriptional suppression, but can also cause activation depending on location of methyl groups.	Histone **m**ethylation **m**ostly **m**akes DNA **m**ute.
Histone acetylation	Removal of histone's ⊕ charge → relaxed DNA coiling → ↑ transcription.	Thyroid hormone receptors alter thyroid hormone synthesis by acetylation. Dysregulated acetylation is implicated in Huntington disease. Histone **a**cetylation makes DNA **a**ctive.
Histone deacetylation	Removal of acetyl groups → tightened DNA coiling → ↓ transcription.	

Nucleotides

Nucleoside = base + (deoxy)ribose (sugar).
Nucleotide = base + (deoxy)ribose + phosphate; linked by 3′-5′ phosphodiester bond.

5′ end of incoming nucleotide bears the triphosphate (energy source for the bond). α-Phosphate is target of 3′ hydroxyl attack.

Purines (**A**,**G**)—2 rings.
Pyrimidines (**C**,**U**,**T**)—1 ring.

Pure As Gold.
CUT the **py**ramid.
Thymine has a **methy**l.

Deamination reactions:
- Cytosine → uracil
- Adenine → hypoxanthine
- Guanine → xanthine
- 5-methylcytosine → thymine

C-G bond (3 H bonds) stronger than A-T bond (2 H bonds). ↑ C-G content → ↑ melting temperature of DNA. "**C-G** bonds are like **C**razy **G**lue."

Uracil found in RNA; thymine in DNA. Methylation of uracil makes thymine.

Amino acids necessary for **purine** synthesis (cats **purr** until they **GAG**):
- **G**lycine
- **A**spartate
- **G**lutamine

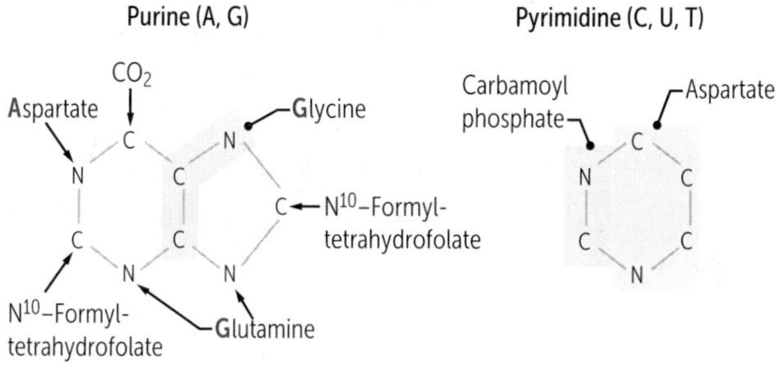
Purine (A, G)
CO_2
Aspartate
Glycine
N^{10}–Formyl-tetrahydrofolate
N^{10}–Formyl-tetrahydrofolate
Glutamine
Pyrimidine (C, U, T)
Carbamoyl phosphate
Aspartate

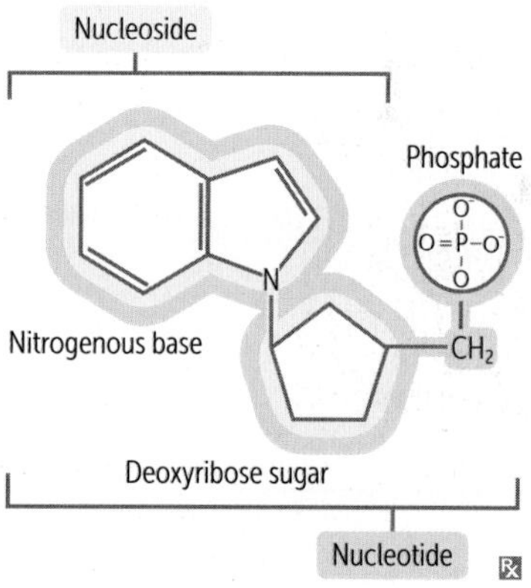
Nucleoside
Phosphate
Nitrogenous base
CH_2
Deoxyribose sugar
Nucleotide

De novo pyrimidine and purine synthesis

Various immunosuppressive, antineoplastic, and antibiotic drugs function by interfering with nucleotide synthesis:

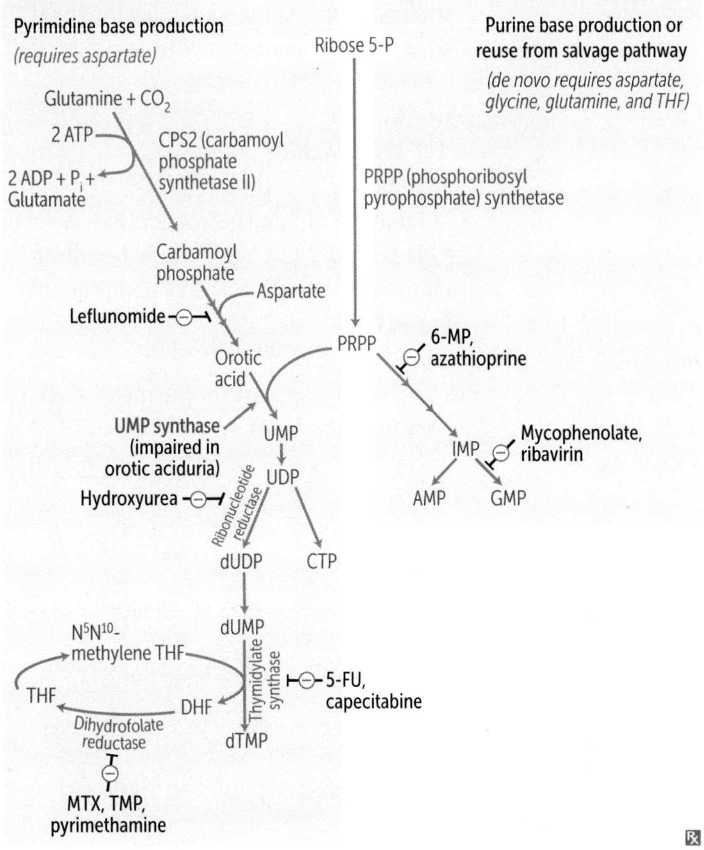

Pyrimidine synthesis:
- Leflunomide: inhibits dihydroorotate dehydrogenase
- 5-fluorouracil (5-FU) and its prodrug capecitabine: form 5-F-dUMP, which inhibits thymidylate synthase (↓ dTMP)

Purine synthesis:
- 6-mercaptopurine (6-MP) and its prodrug azathioprine: inhibit de novo purine synthesis
- Mycophenolate and ribavirin: inhibit inosine monophosphate dehydrogenase

Purine and pyrimidine synthesis:
- Hydroxyurea: inhibits ribonucleotide reductase
- Methotrexate (MTX), trimethoprim (TMP), and pyrimethamine: inhibit dihydrofolate reductase (↓ deoxythymidine monophosphate [dTMP]) in humans, bacteria, and protozoa, respectively

CPS1 = m1tochondria (urea cycle)
CPS2 = cytwosol

℞

Purine salvage deficiencies

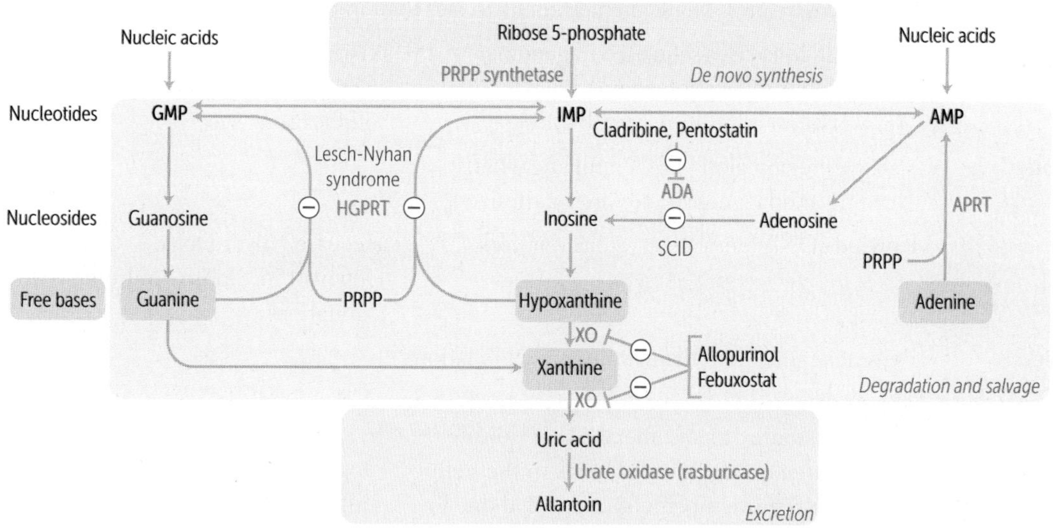

ADA, adenosine deaminase; APRT, adenine phosphoribosyltransferase; HGPRT, hypoxanthine guanine phosphoribosyltransferase, XO, xanthine oxidase; SCID, severe combined immune deficiency (autosomal recessive inheritance)

Adenosine deaminase deficiency	ADA is required for degradation of adenosine and deoxyadenosine. ↓ ADA → ↑ dATP → ↓ ribonucleotide reductase activity → ↓ DNA precursors in cells → ↓ lymphocytes.	One of the major causes of autosomal recessive SCID.
Lesch-Nyhan syndrome	Defective purine salvage due to absent **HGPRT**, which converts hypoxanthine to IMP and guanine to GMP. ↑ purine synthesis (↑ PRPP aminotransferase activity) → excess uric acid production. X-linked recessive. Findings: intellectual disability, self-mutilation, aggression, hyperuricemia (red/orange "sand" [sodium urate crystals] in diaper), gout, dystonia, macrocytosis.	**HGPRT**: **H**yperuricemia **G**out **P**issed off (aggression, self-mutilation) **R**ed/orange crystals in urine **T**ense muscles (dystonia) Treatment: allopurinol or febuxostat (2nd line).

Genetic code features

Unambiguous	Each codon specifies only 1 amino acid.	
Degenerate/ redundant	Most amino acids are coded by multiple codons. **Wobble**—codons that differ in 3rd ("wobble") position may code for the same tRNA/amino acid. Specific base pairing is usually required only in the first 2 nucleotide positions of mRNA codon.	Exceptions: methionine (AUG) and tryptophan (UGG) encoded by only 1 codon.
Commaless, nonoverlapping	Read from a fixed starting point as a continuous sequence of bases.	Exceptions: some viruses.
Universal	Genetic code is conserved throughout evolution.	Exception in humans: mitochondria.

DNA replication	Occurs in 5′ → 3′ direction ("5ynth3sis") in continuous and discontinuous (Okazaki fragment) fashion. Semiconservative. More complex in eukaryotes than in prokaryotes, but shares analogous enzymes.	
Origin of replication A	Particular consensus sequence in genome where DNA replication begins. May be single (prokaryotes) or multiple (eukaryotes).	AT-rich sequences (such as TATA box regions) are found in promoters and origins of replication.
Replication fork B	Y-shaped region along DNA template where leading and lagging strands are synthesized.	
Helicase C	Unwinds DNA template at replication fork.	**H**elicase **h**alves DNA. Deficient in **Bloom** syndrome (***BLM*** gene mutation).
Single-stranded binding proteins D	Prevent strands from reannealing or degradation by nucleases.	
DNA topoisomerases E	Creates a **single-** (topoisomerase **I**) or **double-** (topoisomerase **II**) stranded break in the helix to add or remove supercoils (as needed due to underwinding or overwinding of DNA).	In eukaryotes: irinotecan/topotecan inhibit topoisomerase (TOP) I, etoposide/teniposide inhibit TOP II. In prokaryotes: fluoroquinolones inhibit TOP II (DNA gyrase) and TOP IV.
Primase F	Makes an RNA primer on which DNA polymerase III can initiate replication.	
DNA polymerase III G	Prokaryotes only. Elongates leading strand by adding deoxynucleotides to the 3′ end. Elongates lagging strand until it reaches primer of preceding fragment.	DNA polymerase III has 5′ → 3′ synthesis and proofreads with 3′ → 5′ exonuclease. Drugs blocking DNA replication often have a modified 3′ OH, thereby preventing addition of the next nucleotide ("chain termination").
DNA polymerase I H	Prokaryotes only. Degrades RNA primer; replaces it with DNA.	Same functions as DNA polymerase III, also excises RNA primer with 5′ → 3′ exonuclease.
DNA ligase I	Catalyzes the formation of a phosphodiester bond within a strand of double-stranded DNA.	Joins Okazaki fragments. **L**igase **l**inks DNA.
Telomerase	Eukaryotes only. A reverse transcriptase (RNA-dependent DNA polymerase) that adds DNA (**TTAGGG**) to 3′ ends of chromosomes to avoid loss of genetic material with every duplication.	Often upregulated in cancer, downregulated in aging and progeria. Telomerase **TAG**s for **G**reatness and **G**lory.

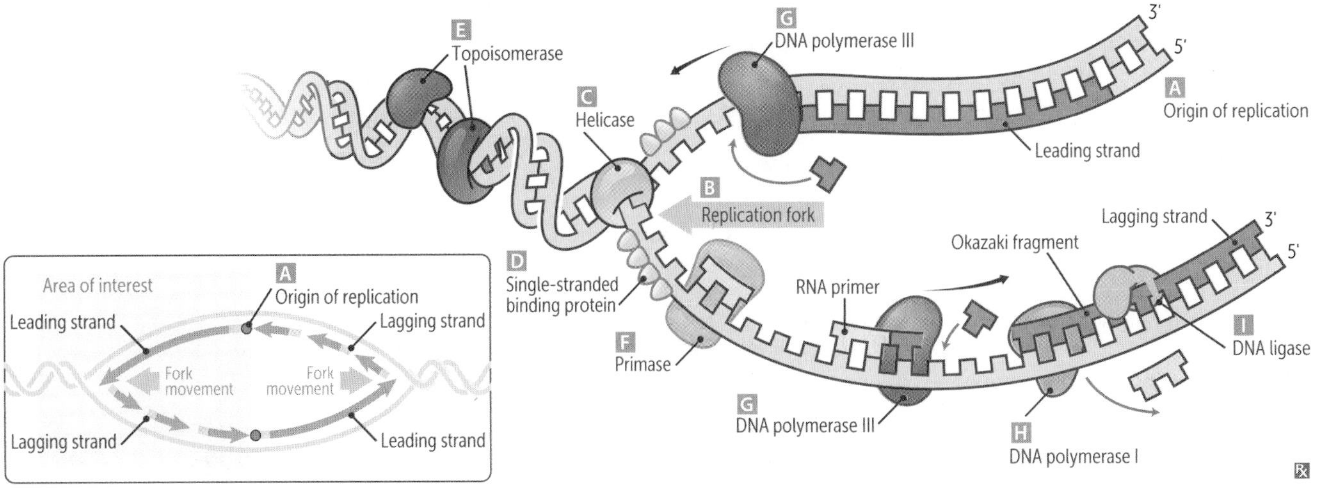

DNA repair

Double strand		
Nonhomologous end joining	Brings together 2 ends of DNA fragments to repair double-stranded breaks. Defective in ataxia-telangiectasia. Homology not required. Some DNA may be lost.	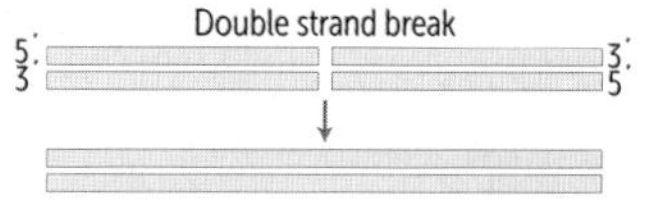 Nonhomologous end joining
Homologous recombination	Requires 2 homologous DNA duplexes. A strand from damaged dsDNA is repaired using a complementary strand from intact homologous dsDNA as a template. Defective in breast/ovarian cancers with *BRCA1* mutation and in Fanconi anemia. Restores duplexes accurately without loss of nucleotides.	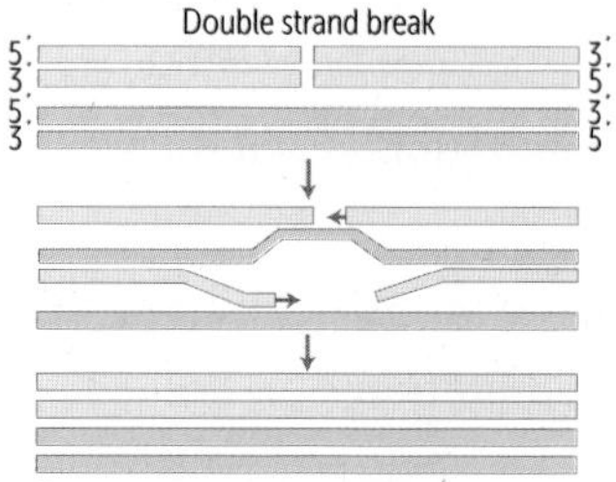 Homologous recombination
Single strand		
Nucleotide excision repair	Specific endonucleases release the oligonucleotides containing damaged bases; DNA polymerase and ligase fill and reseal the gap, respectively. Repairs bulky helix-distorting lesions.	Occurs in G_1 phase of cell cycle. Defective in xeroderma pigmentosum (inability to repair DNA pyrimidine dimers caused by UV exposure). Presents with dry skin, photosensitivity, skin cancer.
Base excision repair	Base-specific Glycosylase removes altered base and creates AP site (apurinic/apyrimidinic). One or more nucleotides are removed by AP-Endonuclease, which cleaves 5′ end. AP-Lyase cleaves 3′ end. DNA Polymerase-β fills the gap and DNA ligase seals it.	Occurs throughout cell cycle. Important in repair of spontaneous/toxic deamination. "GEL Please."
Mismatch repair	Mismatched nucleotides in newly synthesized (unmethylated) strand are removed and gap is filled and resealed.	Occurs predominantly in S phase of cell cycle. Defective in Lynch syndrome (hereditary nonpolyposis colorectal cancer [HNPCC]).

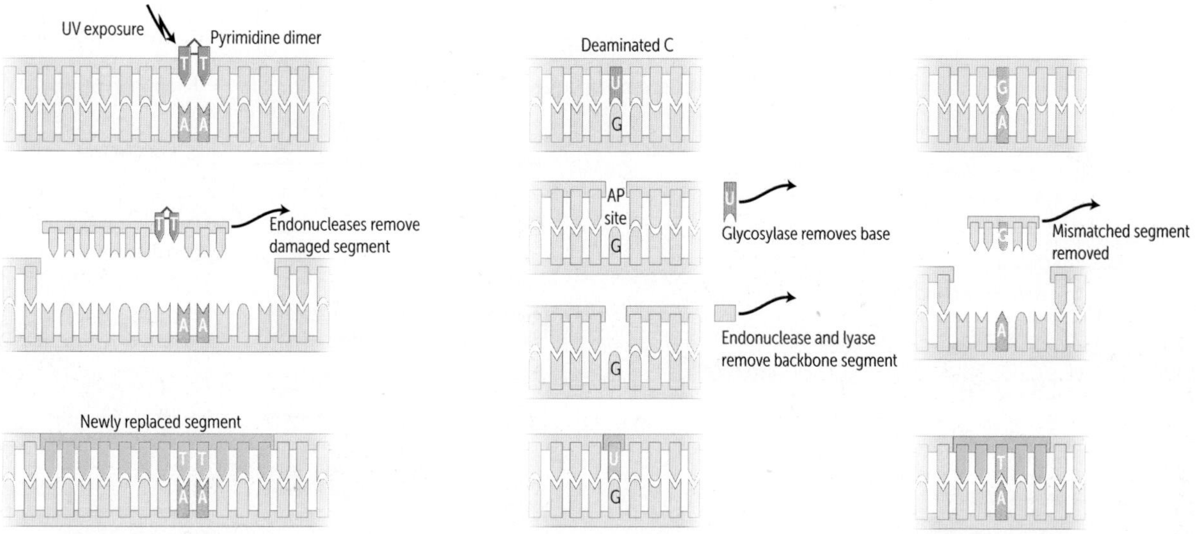

Nucleotide excision repair | Base excision repair | Mismatch repair

Mutations in DNA

Degree of change: silent << missense < nonsense < frameshift. Single nucleotide substitutions are repaired by DNA polymerase and DNA ligase. Types of single nucleotide (point) mutations:
- Transition—purine to purine (eg, A to G) or pyrimidine to pyrimidine (eg, C to T).
- Transversion—purine to pyrimidine (eg, A to T) or pyrimidine to purine (eg, C to G).

Single nucleotide substitutions	
Silent mutation	Codes for same (synonymous) amino acid; often involves 3rd position of codon (tRNA wobble).
Missense mutation	Results in changed amino acid (called conservative if new amino acid has similar chemical structure). Examples: sickle cell disease (substitution of glutamic acid with valine).
Nonsense mutation	Results in early **stop** codon (UGA, UAA, UAG). Usually generates nonfunctional protein. **Stop** the **nonsense**!
Other mutations	
Frameshift mutation	Deletion or insertion of any number of nucleotides not divisible by 3 → misreading of all nucleotides downstream. Protein may be shorter or longer, and its function may be disrupted or altered. Examples: Duchenne muscular dystrophy, Tay-Sachs disease.
Splice site mutation	Retained intron in mRNA → protein with impaired or altered function. Examples: rare causes of cancers, dementia, epilepsy, some types of β-thalassemia, Gaucher disease, Marfan syndrome.

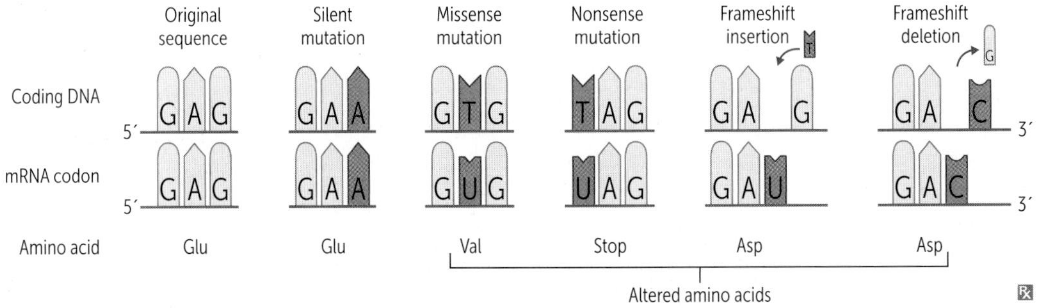

Lac operon

Classic example of a genetic response to an environmental change. Glucose is the preferred metabolic substrate in *E coli*, but when glucose is absent and lactose is available, the *lac* operon is activated to switch to lactose metabolism. Mechanism of shift:
- Low glucose → ↑ adenylate cyclase activity → ↑ generation of cAMP from ATP → activation of catabolite activator protein (CAP) → ↑ transcription.
- High lactose → unbinds repressor protein from repressor/operator site → ↑ transcription.

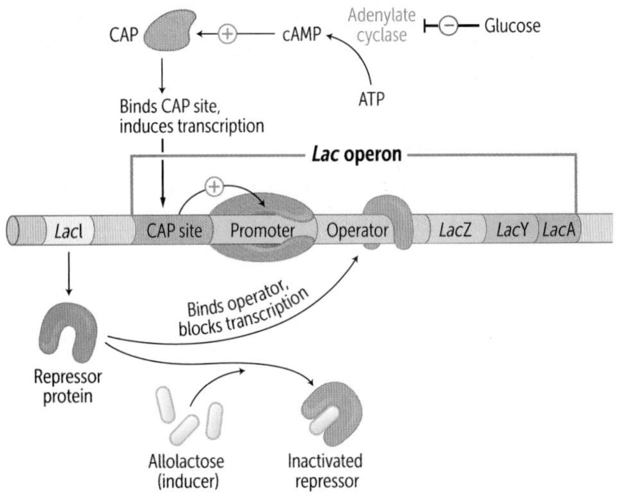

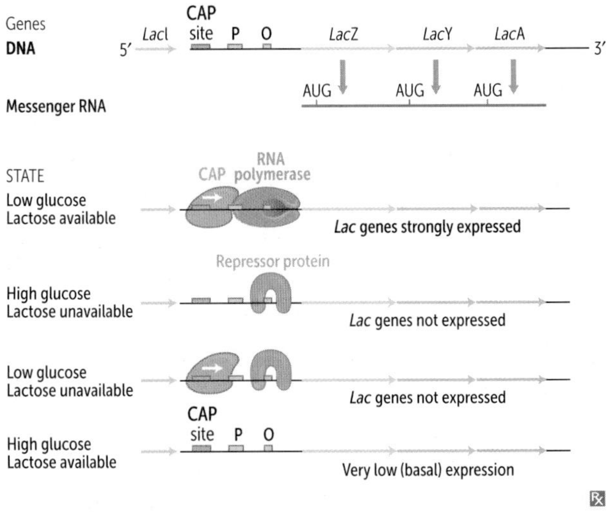

Functional organization of a eukaryotic gene

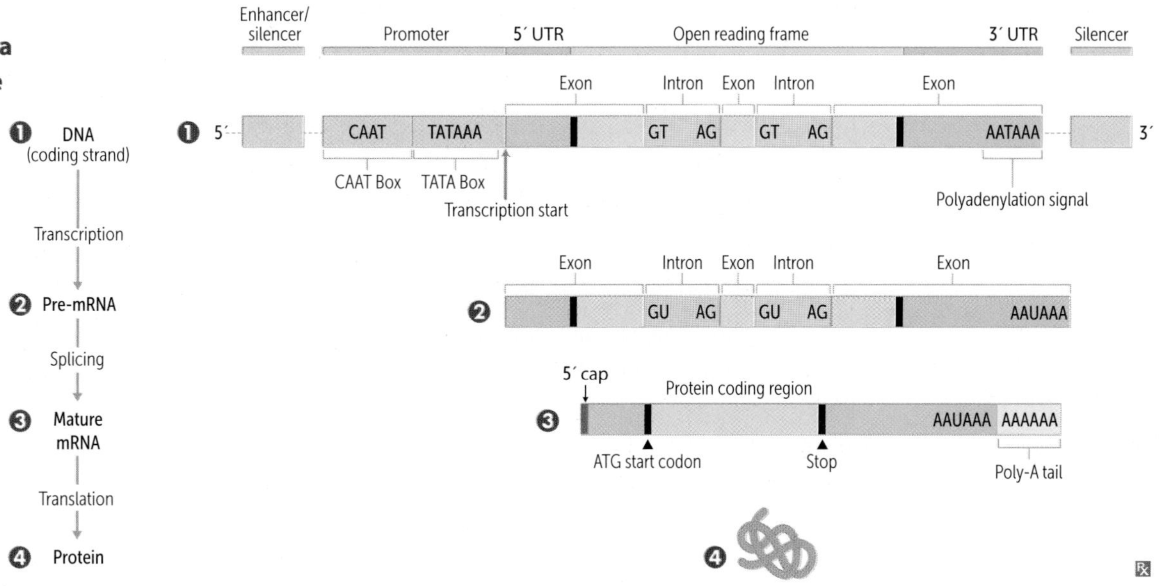

Regulation of gene expression

Promoter	Site where RNA polymerase II and multiple other transcription factors bind to DNA upstream from gene locus (AT-rich upstream sequence with TATA and CAAT boxes, which differ between eukaryotes and prokaryotes).	Promoter mutation commonly results in dramatic ↓ in level of gene transcription.
Enhancer	DNA locus where regulatory proteins ("**activators**") bind, **increasing** expression of a gene on the same chromosome.	Enhancers and silencers may be located close to, far from, or even within (in an intron) the gene whose expression they regulate.
Silencer	DNA locus where regulatory proteins ("**repressors**") bind, **decreasing** expression of a gene on the same chromosome.	

RNA processing (eukaryotes)

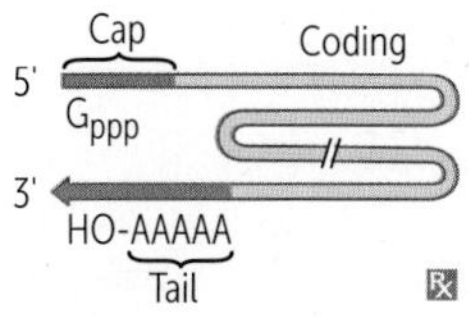

Initial transcript is called heterogeneous nuclear RNA (hnRNA). hnRNA is then modified and becomes mRNA.

The following processes occur in the nucleus:

- Capping of 5′ end (addition of 7-methylguanosine cap)
- Polyadenylation of 3′ end (~ 200 A's → poly-A tail)
- Splicing out of introns

Capped, tailed, and spliced transcript is called mRNA.

mRNA is transported out of nucleus to be translated in cytosol.

mRNA quality control occurs at cytoplasmic processing bodies (P-bodies), which contain exonucleases, decapping enzymes, and microRNAs; mRNAs may be degraded or stored in P-bodies for future translation.

Poly-A polymerase does not require a template.

AAUAAA = polyadenylation signal.

RNA polymerases

Eukaryotes	RNA polymerase I makes **r**RNA, the most common (**r**ampant) type; present only in nucleolus. RNA polymerase II makes **m**RNA (**m**assive), **m**icroRNA (**mi**RNA), and small **n**uclear RNA (**sn**RNA). RNA polymerase III makes 5S rRNA, **t**RNA (**t**iny). No proofreading function, but can initiate chains. RNA polymerase II opens DNA at promoter site.	I, II, and III are numbered in the same order that their products are used in protein synthesis: rRNA, mRNA, then tRNA. α-amanitin, found in *Amanita phalloides* (death cap mushrooms), inhibits RNA polymerase II. Causes dysentery and severe hepatotoxicity if ingested. Actinomycin D, also called dactinomycin, inhibits RNA polymerase in both prokaryotes and eukaryotes.
Prokaryotes	1 RNA polymerase (multisubunit complex) makes all 3 kinds of RNA.	Rifamycins (rifampin, rifabutin) inhibit DNA-dependent RNA polymerase in prokaryotes.

Splicing of pre-mRNA Part of process by which precursor mRNA (pre-mRNA) is transformed into mature mRNA. Alterations in snRNP assembly can cause clinical disease; eg, in spinal muscular atrophy, snRNP assembly is affected due to ↓ SMN protein → congenital degeneration of anterior horns of spinal cord → symmetric weakness (hypotonia, or "floppy baby syndrome").

Anti-U1 snRNP antibodies are associated with SLE, mixed connective tissue disease, other rheumatic diseases.

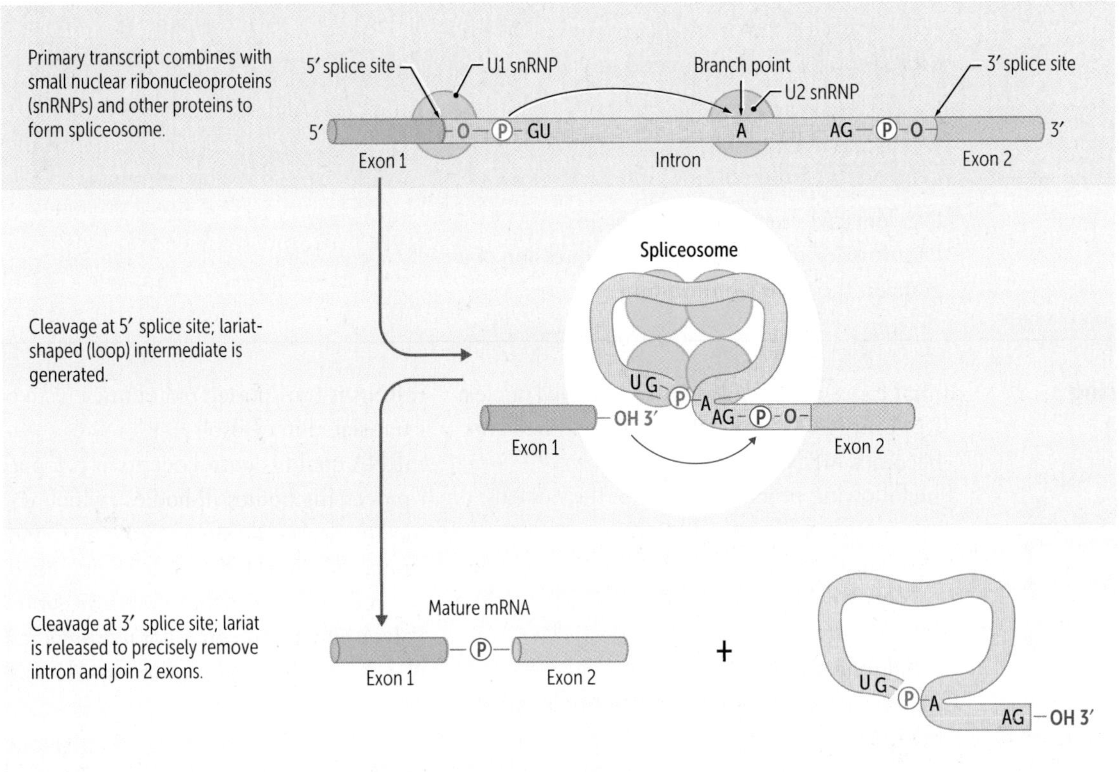
Primary transcript combines with small nuclear ribonucleoproteins (snRNPs) and other proteins to form spliceosome.
5′ splice site
U1 snRNP
Branch point
U2 snRNP
3′ splice site
5′
O—P—GU
A
AG—P—O
3′
Exon 1
Intron
Exon 2
Spliceosome
Cleavage at 5′ splice site; lariat-shaped (loop) intermediate is generated.
UG
P
A
OH 3′
AG—P—O
Exon 1
Exon 2
Cleavage at 3′ splice site; lariat is released to precisely remove intron and join 2 exons.
Mature mRNA
P
Exon 1
Exon 2
+
UG
P
A
AG—OH 3′
℞

Introns vs exons

Exons contain the actual genetic information coding for protein.
Introns do not code for protein, but are important in regulation of gene expression.
Different exons are frequently combined by alternative splicing to produce a larger number of unique proteins.
Alternative splicing can produce a variety of protein products from a single hnRNA (heterogenous nuclear RNA) sequence (eg, transmembrane vs secreted Ig, tropomyosin variants in muscle, dopamine receptors in the brain, host defense evasion by tumor cells).

Introns are **in**tervening sequences and stay **in** the nucleus, whereas **ex**ons **ex**it and are **ex**pressed.

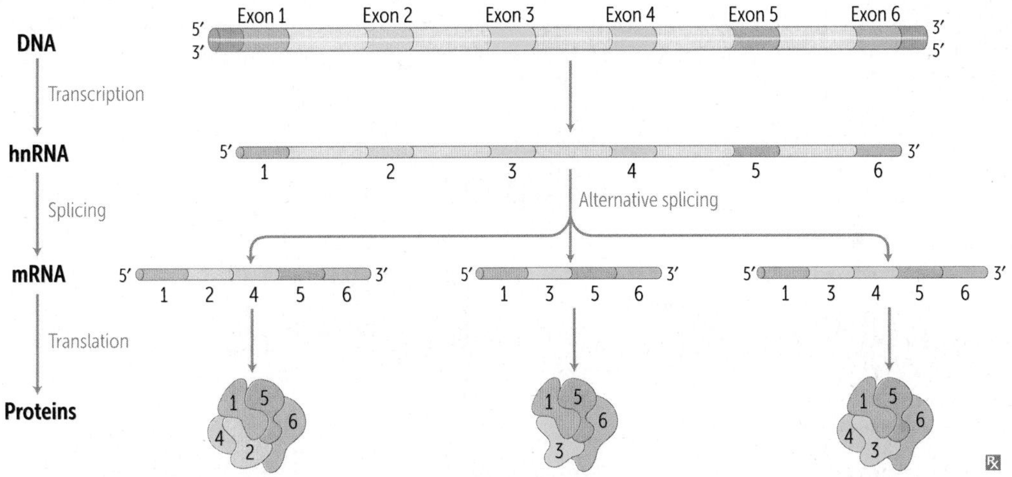

tRNA

Structure	75–90 nucleotides, 2° structure, cloverleaf form, anticodon end is opposite 3′ aminoacyl end. All tRNAs, both eukaryotic and prokaryotic, have CCA at 3′ end along with a high percentage of chemically modified bases. The amino acid is covalently bound to the 3′ end of the tRNA. **CCA Can Carry Amino** acids. T-arm: contains the TΨC (ribothymidine, pseudouridine, cytidine) sequence necessary for tRNA-ribosome binding. **T**-arm **T**ethers tRNA molecule to ribosome. D-arm: contains **D**ihydrouridine residues necessary for tRNA recognition by the correct aminoacyl-tRNA synthetase. **D**-arm allows **D**etection of the tRNA by aminoacyl-tRNA synthetase. Attachment site: 3′-**ACC**-5′ is the amino acid **ACC**eptor site.
Charging	Aminoacyl-tRNA synthetase (uses ATP; 1 unique enzyme per respective amino acid) and binding of charged tRNA to the codon are responsible for the accuracy of amino acid selection. Aminoacyl-tRNA synthetase matches an amino acid to the tRNA by scrutinizing the amino acid before and after it binds to tRNA. If an incorrect amino acid is attached, the bond is hydrolyzed. A mischarged tRNA reads the usual codon but inserts the wrong amino acid.

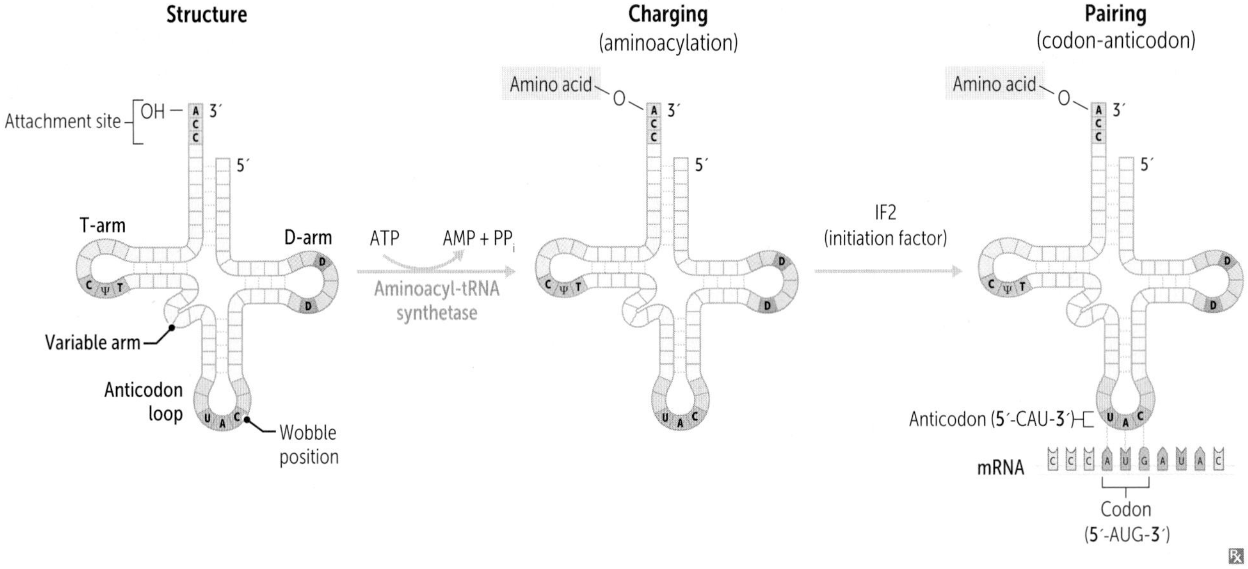

Start and stop codons

mRNA start codons	AUG.	**AUG** in**AUG**urates protein synthesis.
Eukaryotes	Codes for methionine, which may be removed before translation is completed.	
Prokaryotes	Codes for N-formylmethionine (fMet).	fMet stimulates neutrophil chemotaxis.
mRNA stop codons	UGA, UAA, UAG.	**UGA** = **U G**o **A**way. **UAA** = **U A**re **A**way. **UAG** = **U A**re **G**one.

Protein synthesis

Initiation	1. Eukaryotic initiation factors (eIFs) identify the 5′ cap. 2. eIFs help assemble the 40S ribosomal subunit with the initiator tRNA. 3. eIFs released when the mRNA and the ribosomal 60S subunit assemble with the complex. Requires GTP.	Eukaryotes: 40S + 60S → 80S (even). Prokaryotes: 30S + 50S → 70S (prime). Synthesis occurs from N-terminus to C-terminus. ATP—tRNA Activation (charging). GTP—tRNA Gripping and Going places (translocation).
Elongation	❶ Aminoacyl-tRNA binds to A site (except for initiator methionine, which binds the P site), requires an elongation factor and GTP. ❷ rRNA ("ribozyme") catalyzes peptide bond formation, transfers growing polypeptide to amino acid in A site. ❸ Ribosome advances 3 nucleotides toward 3′ end of mRNA, moving peptidyl tRNA to P site (translocation).	Think of "going APE": A site = incoming Aminoacyl-tRNA. P site = accommodates growing Peptide. E site = holds Empty tRNA as it Exits. Elongation factors are targets of bacterial toxins (eg, *Diphtheria*, *Pseudomonas*). Shine-Dalgarno sequence—ribosomal binding site in prokaryotic mRNA. Enables protein synthesis initiation by aligning the ribosome with the start codon so that code is read correctly.
Termination	Eukaryotic release factors (eRFs) recognize the stop codon and halt translation → completed polypeptide is released from ribosome. Requires GTP.	

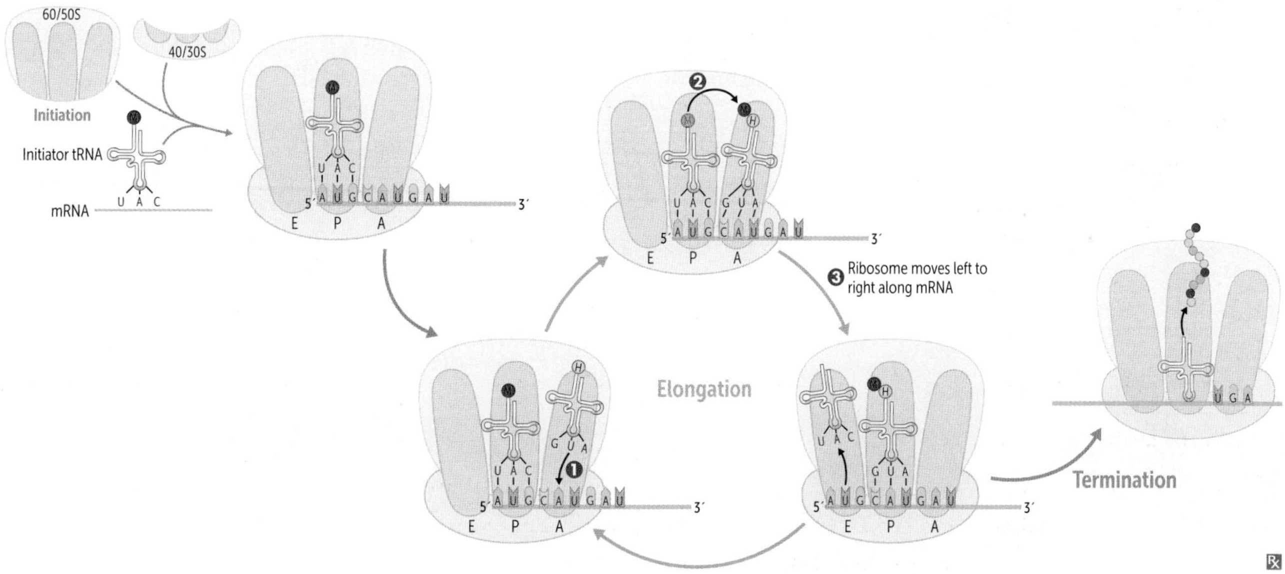

Posttranslational modifications

Trimming	Removal of N- or C-terminal propeptides from zymogen to generate mature protein (eg, trypsinogen to trypsin).
Covalent alterations	Phosphorylation, glycosylation, hydroxylation, methylation, acetylation, and ubiquitination.

Chaperone protein	Intracellular protein involved in facilitating and maintaining protein folding. In yeast, heat shock proteins (eg, HSP60) are constitutively expressed, but expression may increase with high temperatures, acidic pH, and hypoxia to prevent protein denaturing/misfolding.

▶ BIOCHEMISTRY—CELLULAR

Cell cycle phases	Checkpoints control transitions between phases of cell cycle. This process is regulated by cyclins, cyclin-dependent kinases (CDKs), and tumor suppressors. M phase (shortest phase of cell cycle) includes mitosis (prophase, prometaphase, metaphase, anaphase, telophase) and cytokinesis (cytoplasm splits in two). G_1 and G_0 are of variable duration.
REGULATION OF CELL CYCLE	
Cyclin-dependent kinases	Constitutively expressed but inactive when not bound to cyclin.
Cyclin-CDK complexes	Cyclins are phase-specific regulatory proteins that activate CDKs when stimulated by growth factors. The cyclin-CDK complex can then phosphorylate other proteins (eg, Rb) to coordinate cell cycle progression. This complex must be activated/inactivated at appropriate times for cell cycle to progress.
Tumor suppressors	p53 → p21 induction → CDK inhibition → Rb hypophosphorylation (activation) → G_1-S progression inhibition. Mutations in tumor suppressor genes can result in unrestrained cell division (eg, Li-Fraumeni syndrome). Growth factors (eg, insulin, PDGF, EPO, EGF) bind tyrosine kinase receptors to transition the cell from G_1 to S phase.

CELL TYPES		
Permanent	Remain in G_0, regenerate from stem cells.	Neurons, skeletal and cardiac muscle, RBCs.
Stable (quiescent)	Enter G_1 from G_0 when stimulated.	Hepatocytes, lymphocytes, PCT, periosteal cells.
Labile	Never go to G_0, divide rapidly with a short G_1. Most affected by chemotherapy.	Bone marrow, gut epithelium, skin, hair follicles, germ cells.

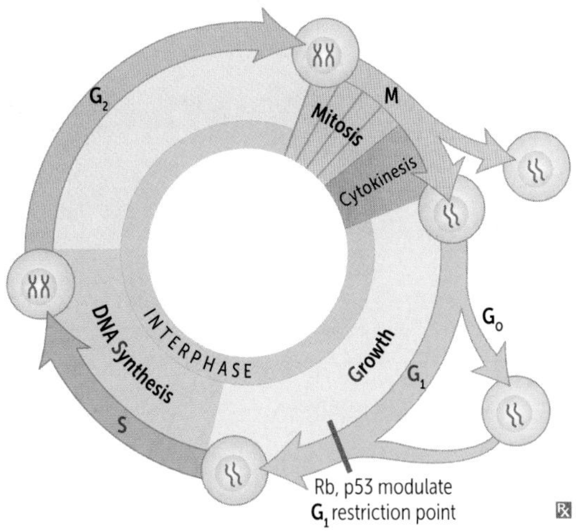

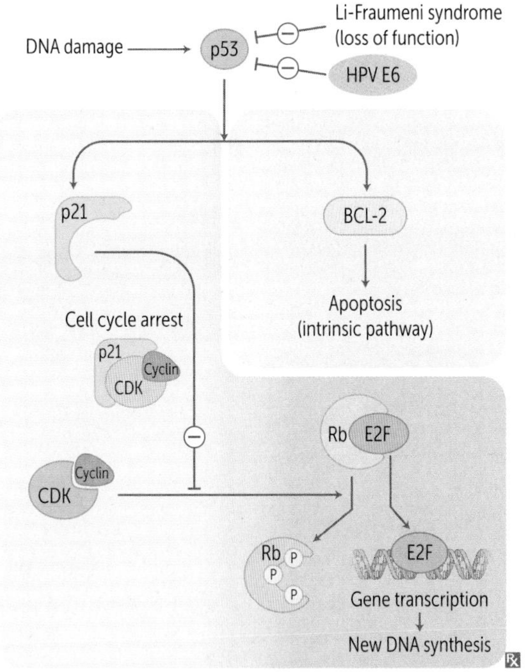

Rough endoplasmic reticulum

Site of synthesis of secretory (exported) proteins and of N-linked oligosaccharide addition to lysosomal and other proteins.
Nissl bodies (RER in neurons)—synthesize peptide neurotransmitters for secretion.
Free ribosomes—unattached to any membrane; site of synthesis of cytosolic, peroxisomal, and mitochondrial proteins.

N-linked glycosylation occurs in the eNdoplasmic reticulum.
Mucus-secreting goblet cells of small intestine and antibody-secreting plasma cells are rich in RER.
Proteins within organelles (eg, ER, Golgi bodies, lysosomes) are formed in RER.

Smooth endoplasmic reticulum

Site of steroid synthesis and detoxification of drugs and poisons. Lacks surface ribosomes. Location of glucose-6-phosphatase (last step in both glycogenolysis and gluconeogenesis).

Liver hepatocytes and steroid hormone–producing cells of the adrenal cortex and gonads are rich in SER.

Cell trafficking

GOlgi is distribution center for proteins and lipids from ER to vesicles and plasma membrane. Posttranslational events in O-oligosaccharides include modifying N-oligosaccharides on asparagine, adding O-oligosaccharides on serine and threonine, and adding mannose-6-phosphate to proteins for lysosomal and other proteins.
Endosomes are sorting centers for material from outside the cell or from the Golgi, sending it to lysosomes for destruction or back to the membrane/Golgi for further use.

I-cell disease (inclusion cell disease/mucolipidosis type II)—inherited lysosomal storage disorder (autosomal recessive); defect in N-acetylglucosaminyl-1-phosphotransferase → failure of the Golgi to phosphorylate mannose residues (↓ mannose-6-phosphate) on glycoproteins → enzymes secreted extracellularly rather than delivered to lysosomes → lysosomes deficient in digestive enzymes → build-up of cellular debris in lysosomes (inclusion bodies). Results in coarse facial features, gingival hyperplasia, corneal clouding, restricted joint movements, claw hand deformities, kyphoscoliosis, and ↑ plasma levels of lysosomal enzymes. Often fatal in childhood.

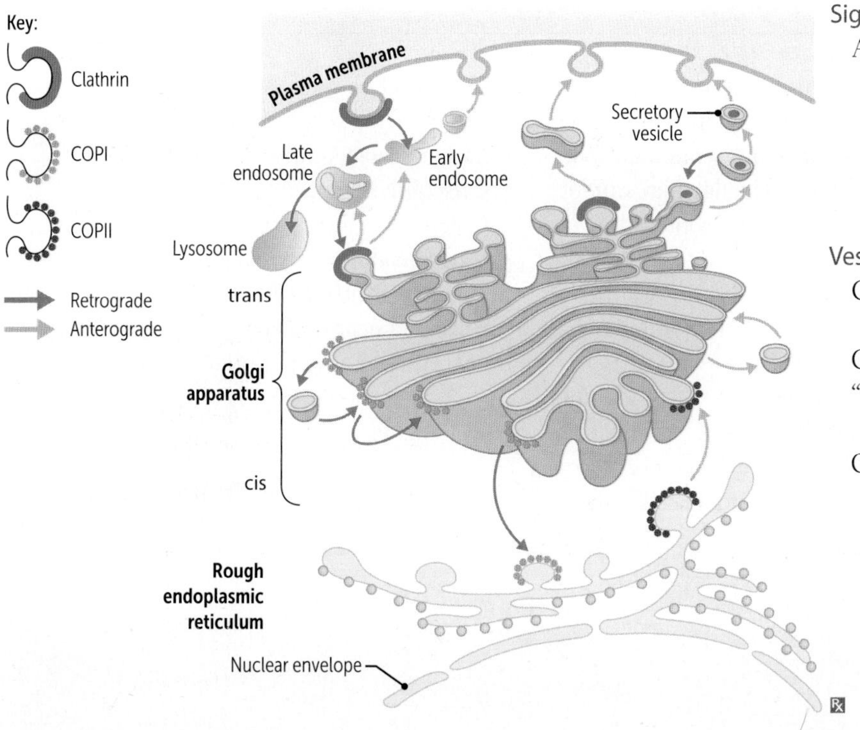
Key:
Clathrin
COPI
COPII
Retrograde
Anterograde
Plasma membrane
Secretory vesicle
Late endosome
Early endosome
Lysosome
trans
Golgi apparatus
cis
Rough endoplasmic reticulum
Nuclear envelope

Signal recognition particle (SRP)

Abundant, cytosolic ribonucleoprotein that traffics polypeptide-ribosome complex from the cytosol to the RER. Absent or dysfunctional SRP → accumulation of protein in cytosol.

Vesicular trafficking proteins

COPI: Golgi → Golgi (retrograde); *cis*-Golgi → ER.
COPII: ER → *cis*-Golgi (anterograde).
"Two (COPII) steps forward (anterograde); one (COPI) step back (retrograde)."
Clathrin: *trans*-Golgi → lysosomes; plasma membrane → endosomes (receptor-mediated endocytosis [eg, LDL receptor activity]).

Peroxisome

Membrane-enclosed organelle involved in:
- β-oxidation of very-long-chain fatty acids (VLCFA) (strictly peroxisomal process)
- α-oxidation of branched-chain fatty acids (strictly peroxisomal process)
- Catabolism of amino acids and ethanol
- Synthesis of cholesterol, bile acids, and plasmalogens (important membrane phospholipid, especially in white matter of brain)

Zellweger syndrome—autosomal recessive disorder of peroxisome biogenesis due to mutated *PEX* genes. Hypotonia, seizures, hepatomegaly, early death.

Refsum disease—autosomal recessive disorder of α-oxidation → buildup of phytanic acid due to inability to degrade it. Scaly skin, ataxia, cataracts/night blindness, shortening of 4th toe, epiphyseal dysplasia. Treatment: diet, plasmapheresis.

Adrenoleukodystrophy—X-linked recessive disorder of β-oxidation due to mutation in *ABCD1* gene → VLCFA buildup in **adrenal** glands, white (**leuko**) matter of brain, testes. Progressive disease that can lead to adrenal gland crisis, progressive loss of neurologic function, death.

Proteasome

Barrel-shaped protein complex that degrades damaged or ubiquitin-tagged proteins. Defects in the ubiquitin-proteasome system have been implicated in some cases of Parkinson disease.

Cytoskeletal elements

A network of protein fibers within the cytoplasm that supports cell structure, cell and organelle movement, and cell division.

TYPE OF FILAMENT	PREDOMINANT FUNCTION	EXAMPLES
Microfilaments	Muscle contraction, cytokinesis	Actin, microvilli.
Intermediate filaments	Maintain cell structure	Vimentin, desmin, cytokeratin, lamins, glial fibrillary acidic protein (GFAP), neurofilaments.
Microtubules	Movement, cell division	Cilia, flagella, mitotic spindle, axonal trafficking, centrioles.

Microtubule

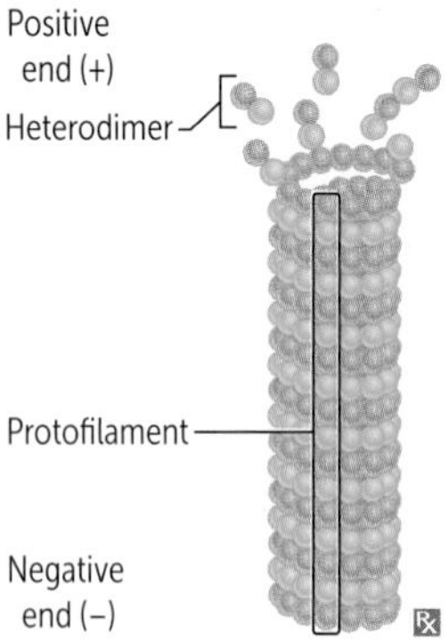
Positive end (+)
Heterodimer
Protofilament
Negative end (–)

Cylindrical outer structure composed of a helical array of polymerized heterodimers of α- and β-tubulin. Each dimer has 2 GTP bound. Incorporated into flagella, cilia, mitotic spindles. Also involved in slow axoplasmic transport in neurons.

Molecular motor proteins—transport cellular cargo toward opposite ends of microtubule.
- Retrograde to microtubule (+ → –)—dynein.
- Anterograde to microtubule (– → +)—kinesin.

Clostridium tetani toxin, herpes simplex virus, poliovirus, and rabies virus use dynein for retrograde transport to the neuronal cell body.

Drugs that act on microtubules (**m**icrotubules **g**et **c**onstructed **v**ery **t**erribly):
- Mebendazole (antihelminthic)
- Griseofulvin (antifungal)
- Colchicine (antigout)
- Vinca alkaloids (anticancer)
- Taxanes (anticancer)

Negative end **n**ear **n**ucleus.
Positive end **p**oints to **p**eriphery.

Ready? **A**ttack!

Cilia structure

9 doublet + 2 singlet arrangement of microtubules A.

Basal body (base of cilium below cell membrane) consists of 9 microtubule triplets B with no central microtubules.

Axonemal dynein—ATPase that links peripheral 9 doublets and causes bending of cilium by differential sliding of doublets.

Gap junctions enable coordinated ciliary movement.

Kartagener syndrome—autosomal recessive dynein arm defect → immotile cilia → dysfunctional ciliated epithelia. Findings: developmental abnormalities due to impaired migration and orientation (eg, situs inversus C, hearing loss due to dysfunctional eustachian tube cilia); recurrent infections (eg, sinusitis, ear infections, bronchiectasis due to impaired ciliary clearance of debris/pathogens); infertility (↑ risk of ectopic pregnancy due to dysfunctional fallopian tube cilia, immotile spermatozoa). Lab findings: ↓ nasal nitric oxide (used as screening test).

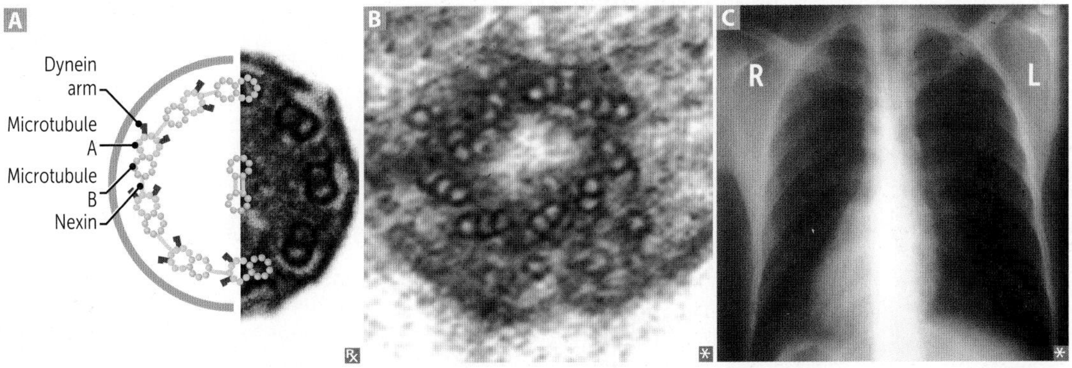
A
Dynein arm
Microtubule A
Microtubule B
Nexin
B
C
R
L

Sodium-potassium pump

Na^+-K^+ ATPase is located in the plasma membrane with ATP site on cytosolic side. For each ATP consumed, **2 K^+** go **in** to the cell (pump dephosphorylated) and **3 Na^+** go **out** of the cell (pump phosphorylated).

2 strikes? **K**, you're still **in**. **3** strikes? **Nah**, you're **out**!

Cardiac glycosides (digoxin and digitoxin) directly inhibit Na^+-K^+ ATPase → indirect inhibition of Na^+/Ca^{2+} exchange → ↑ $[Ca^{2+}]_i$ → ↑ cardiac contractility.

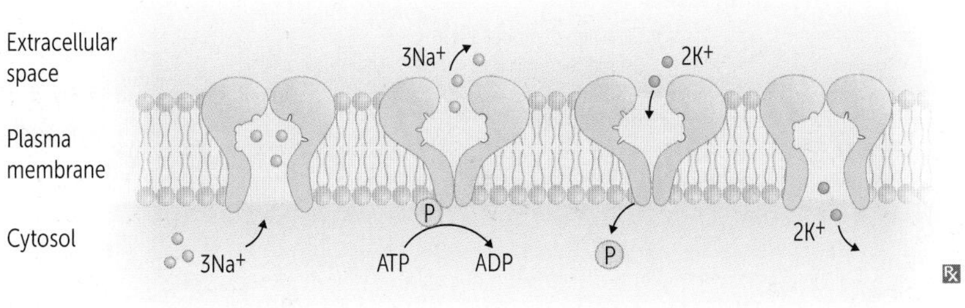
Extracellular space
Plasma membrane
Cytosol
3Na+
2K+
P
3Na+
ATP
ADP
P
2K+

Collagen	Most abundant protein in the human body. Extensively modified by posttranslational modification. Organizes and strengthens extracellular matrix.	Type I - Skeleton Type II - Cartilage Type III - Arteries Type IV - Basement membrane SCAB
Type I	Most common (90%)—Bone (made by osteoblasts), Skin, Tendon, dentin, fascia, cornea, **late** wound repair.	Type **I**: b**one**, tend**one**. ↓ production in osteogenesis imperfecta type I.
Type II	Cartilage (including hyaline), vitreous body, nucleus pulposus.	Type **II**: car**two**lage.
Type III	Reticulin—skin, **blood vessels**, uterus, fetal tissue, **early** wound repair.	Type **III**: deficient in **vascular** type of Ehlers-Danlos syndrome (**threE D**).
Type IV	Basement membrane (basal lamina), lens.	Type **IV**: under the **floor** (basement membrane). Defective in Alport syndrome; targeted by autoantibodies in Goodpasture syndrome.

Collagen synthesis and structure

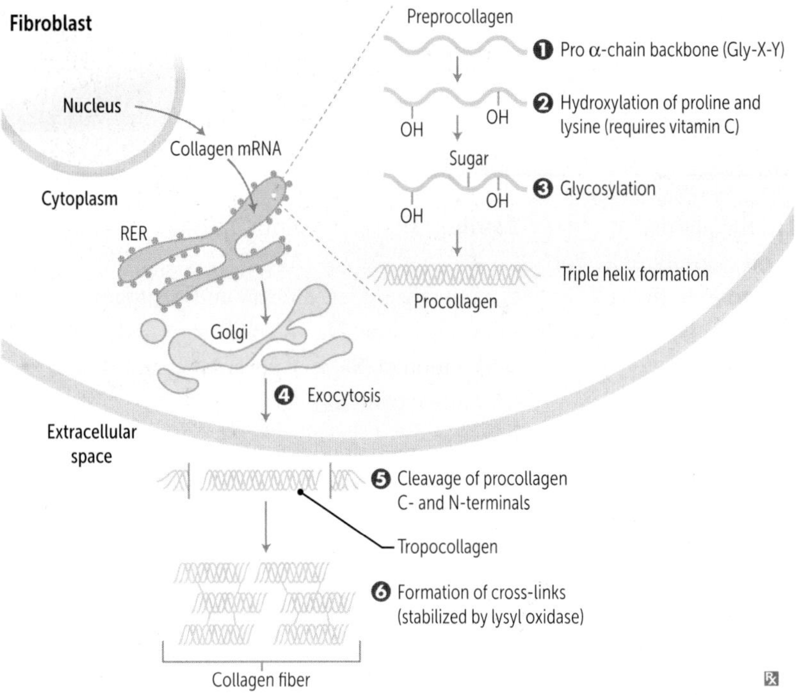

❶ Synthesis—translation of collagen α chains (preprocollagen)—usually Gly-X-Y (X and Y are proline or lysine). Collagen is ⅓ glycine; glycine content of collagen is less variable than that of lysine and proline. Hydroxyproline is used for lab quantification of collagen.

❷ Hydroxylation—hydroxylation ("hydroxCylation") of specific proline and lysine residues. Requires vitamin C; deficiency → scurvy.

❸ Glycosylation—glycosylation of pro-α-chain hydroxylysine residues and formation of procollagen via hydrogen and disulfide bonds (triple helix of 3 collagen α chains). Problems forming triple helix → osteogenesis imperfecta.

❹ Exocytosis—exocytosis of procollagen into extracellular space.

❺ Proteolytic processing—cleavage of disulfide-rich terminal regions of procollagen → insoluble tropocollagen.

❻ Cross-linking—reinforcement of many staggered tropocollagen molecules by covalent lysine-hydroxylysine cross-linkage (by copper-containing lysyl oxidase) to make collagen fibrils. Cross-linking of collagen increases with age. Problems with cross-linking → Menkes disease.

Osteogenesis imperfecta

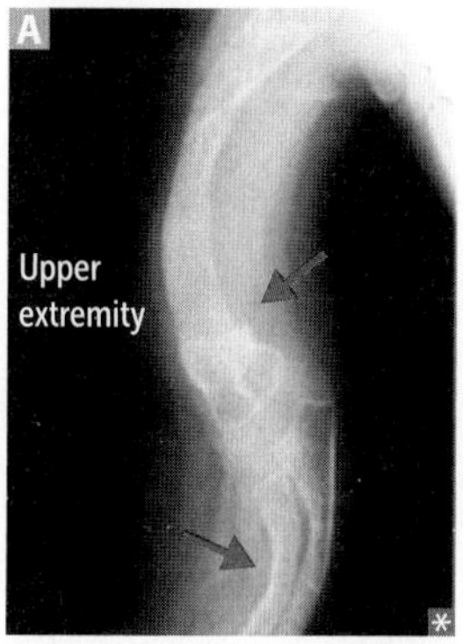
A
Upper extremity

Genetic bone disorder (brittle bone disease) caused by a variety of gene defects (most commonly *COL1A1* and *COL1A2*).

Most common form is autosomal dominant with ↓ production of otherwise normal type I collagen (altered triple helix formation). Manifestations include:

- Multiple fractures and bone deformities (arrows in A) after minimal trauma (eg, during birth)
- Blue sclerae B due to the translucent connective tissue over choroidal veins
- Some forms have tooth abnormalities, including opalescent teeth that wear easily due to lack of dentin (dentinogenesis imperfecta)
- Conductive hearing loss (abnormal ossicles)

May be confused with child abuse.

Treat with bisphosphonates to ↓ fracture risk.

Patients can't **BITE**:

Bones = multiple fractures
I (eye) = blue sclerae
Teeth = dental imperfections
Ear = hearing loss

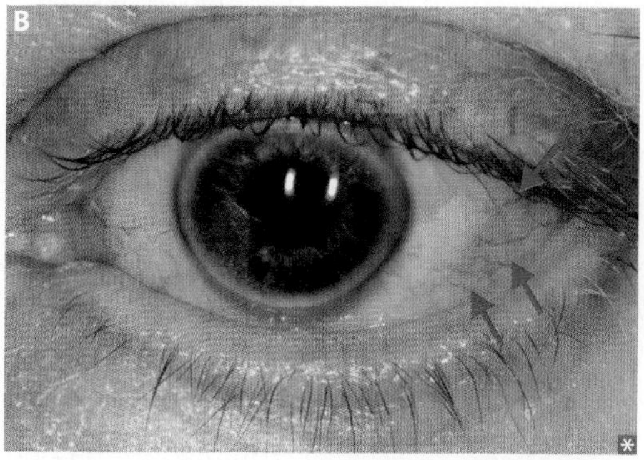
B

Ehlers-Danlos syndrome

Faulty collagen synthesis causing hyperextensible skin A, hypermobile joints B, and tendency to bleed (easy bruising).

Multiple types. Inheritance and severity vary. Can be autosomal dominant or recessive. May be associated with joint dislocation, berry and aortic aneurysms, organ rupture.

Hypermobility type (joint instability): most common type.

Classical type (joint and skin symptoms): caused by a mutation in type V collagen (eg, *COL5A1*, *COL5A2*).

Vascular type (fragile tissues including vessels [eg, aorta], muscles, and organs that are prone to rupture [eg, gravid uterus]): mutations in type III procollagen (eg, *COL3A1*).

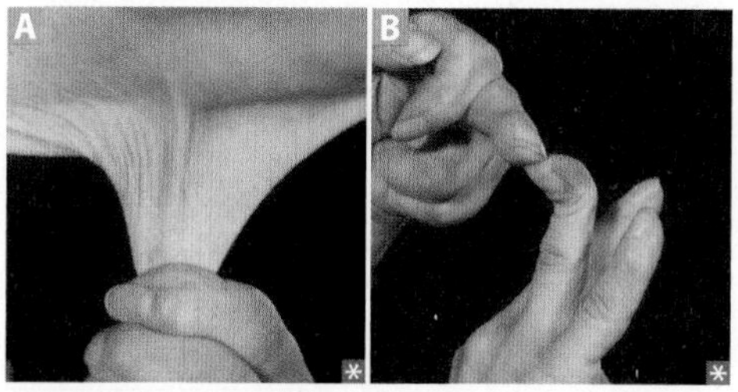
A
B

Menkes disease

X-linked recessive connective tissue disease caused by impaired copper absorption and transport due to defective Menkes protein *ATP7A* (**A**bsent copper), vs *ATP7B* in Wilson disease (copper **B**uildup). Leads to ↓ activity of lysyl oxidase (copper is a necessary cofactor) → defective collagen. Results in brittle, "kinky" hair, growth and developmental delay, hypotonia, ↑ risk of cerebral aneurysms.

Elastin

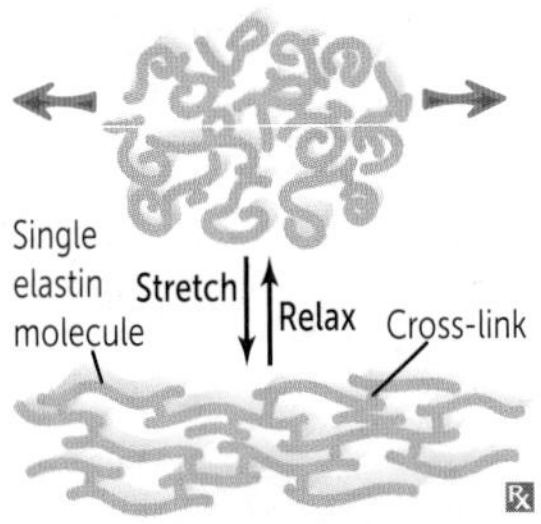
Single elastin molecule
Stretch
Relax
Cross-link

Stretchy protein within skin, lungs, large arteries, elastic ligaments, vocal cords, epiglottis, ligamenta flava (connect vertebrae → relaxed and stretched conformations).
Rich in nonhydroxylated proline, glycine, and lysine residues, vs the hydroxylated residues of collagen.
Tropoelastin with fibrillin scaffolding.
Cross-linking takes place extracellularly and gives elastin its elastic properties.
Broken down by elastase, which is normally inhibited by α_1-antitrypsin.
α_1-Antitrypsin deficiency results in unopposed elastase activity, which can cause COPD.
Changes with aging: ↓ dermal collagen and elastin, ↓ synthesis of collagen fibrils; cross-linking remains normal.

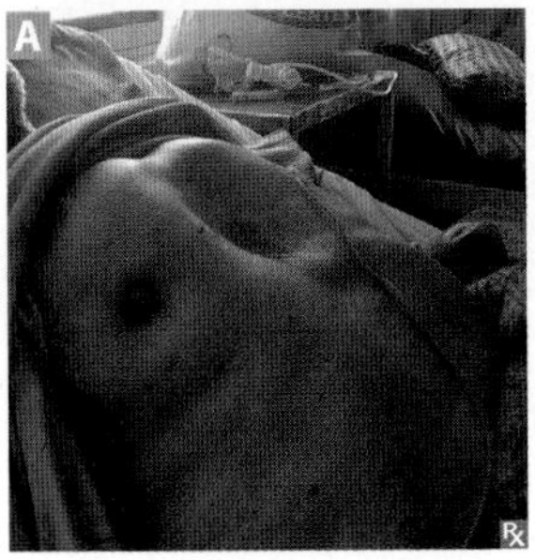

Marfan syndrome—autosomal dominant (with variable expression) connective tissue disorder affecting skeleton, heart, and eyes. *FBN1* gene mutation on chromosome 15 (fifteen) results in defective fibrillin-1, a glycoprotein that forms a sheath around elastin and sequesters TGF-β. Findings: tall with long extremities; chest wall deformity (pectus carinatum [pigeon chest] or pectus excavatum A); hypermobile joints; long, tapering fingers and toes (arachnodactyly); cystic medial necrosis of aorta; aortic root aneurysm rupture or dissection (most common cause of death); mitral valve prolapse; ↑ risk of spontaneous pneumothorax.

Homocystinuria—presentation similar to Marfan syndrome with pectus deformity, tall stature, ↑ arm:height ratio, ↓ upper:lower body segment ratio, arachnodactyly, joint hyperlaxity, skin hyperelasticity, scoliosis.

	Marfan syndrome	Homocystinuria
INHERITANCE	Autosomal dominant	Autosomal recessive
INTELLECT	Normal	Decreased
VASCULAR COMPLICATIONS	Aortic root dilatation	Thrombosis
LENS DISLOCATION	Upward (**Mar**fan **fans** out)	Downward

▶ BIOCHEMISTRY—LABORATORY TECHNIQUES

Polymerase chain reaction

Molecular biology lab procedure used to amplify a desired fragment of DNA. Useful as a diagnostic tool (eg, neonatal HIV, herpes encephalitis).

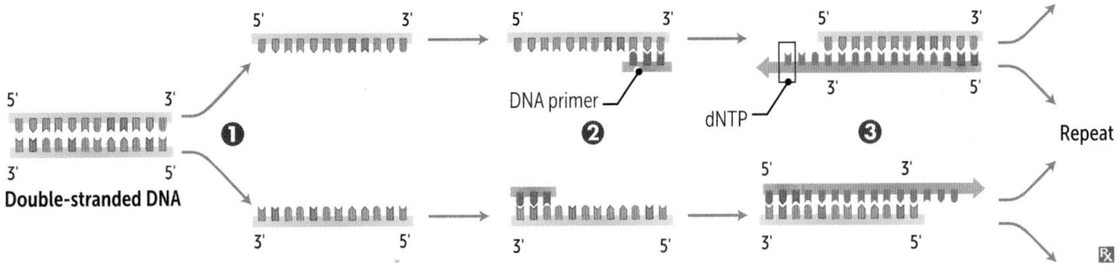
5'
3'
Double-stranded DNA
DNA primer
dNTP
❶
❷
❸
Repeat

❶ **Denaturation**—DNA is heated to ~95°C to separate the strands.
❷ **Annealing**—Sample is cooled to ~55°C. DNA primers, a heat-stable DNA polymerase *(Taq)*, and deoxynucleotide triphosphates (dNTPs) are added. DNA primers anneal to the specific sequence to be amplified on each strand.
❸ **Elongation**—Temperature is increased to ~72°C. DNA polymerase attaches dNTPs to the strand to replicate the sequence after each primer.

Heating and cooling cycles continue until the amount of DNA is sufficient.

CRISPR/Cas9

A genome editing tool derived from bacteria. Consists of a guide RNA (gRNA) ❶, which is complementary to a target DNA sequence, and an endonuclease (Cas9), which makes a single- or double-strand break at the target site ❷. Break imperfectly repaired by nonhomologous end joining (NHEJ) → accidental frameshift mutations ("knock-out") 3A, or a donor DNA sequence can be added to fill in the gap using homology-directed repair (HDR) 3B.

Not used clinically. Potential applications include removing virulence factors from pathogens, replacing disease-causing alleles of genes with healthy variants, and specifically targeting tumor cells.

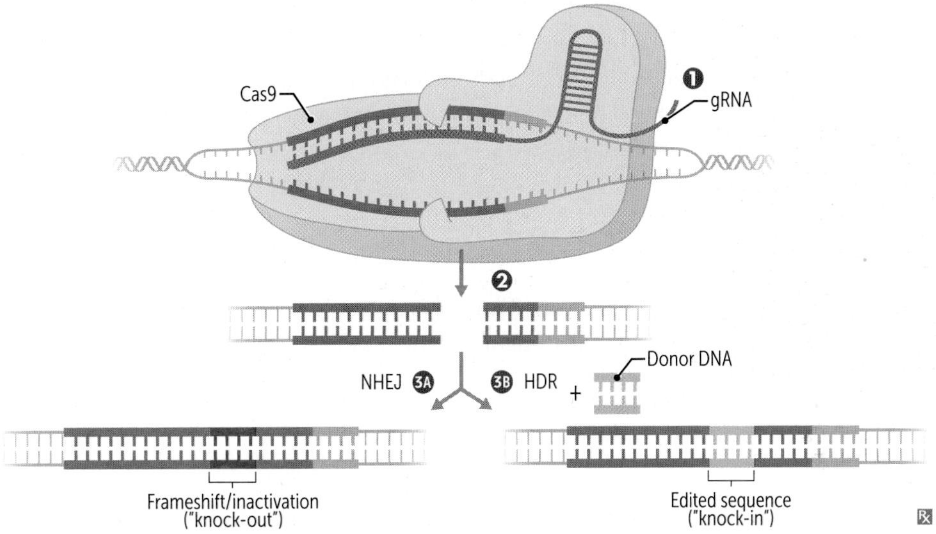

Blotting procedures

Southern blot

1. **DNA** sample is enzymatically cleaved into smaller pieces, which are separated on a gel by electrophoresis, and then transferred to a filter.
2. Filter is exposed to radiolabeled DNA probe that recognizes and anneals to its complementary strand.
3. Resulting double-stranded, labeled piece of DNA is visualized when filter is exposed to film.

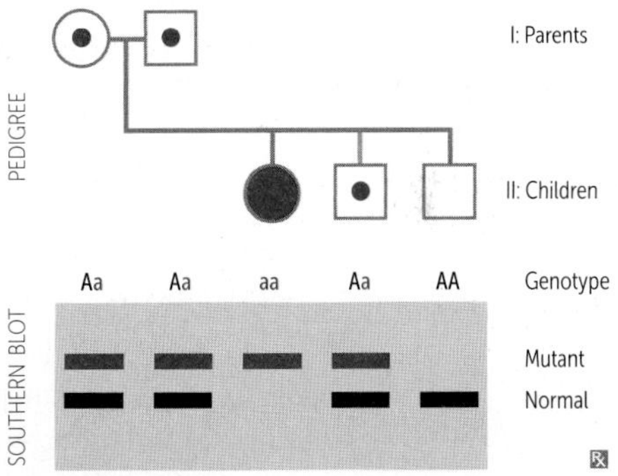

Northern blot

Similar to Southern blot, except that an **RNA** sample is electrophoresed. Useful for studying mRNA levels, which are reflective of gene expression.

SNoW DRoP:
Southern = DNA
Northern = RNA
Western = Protein

Northern blots detect splicing errors.

Western blot

Sample protein is separated via gel electrophoresis and transferred to a membrane. Labeled antibody is used to bind to relevant **protein.**

Southwestern blot

Identifies **DNA-binding proteins** (eg, c-Jun, c-Fos [leucine zipper motif]) using labeled double-stranded DNA probes.

Flow cytometry

Laboratory technique to assess size, granularity, and protein expression (immunophenotype) of individual cells in a sample.

Commonly used in workup of hematologic abnormalities (eg, leukemia, paroxysmal nocturnal hemoglobinuria, fetal RBCs in pregnant person's blood) and immunodeficiencies (eg, $CD4^+$ cell count in HIV).

Cells are tagged with antibodies specific to surface or intracellular proteins. Antibodies are then tagged with a unique fluorescent dye. Sample is analyzed one cell at a time by focusing a laser on the cell and measuring light scatter and intensity of fluorescence.

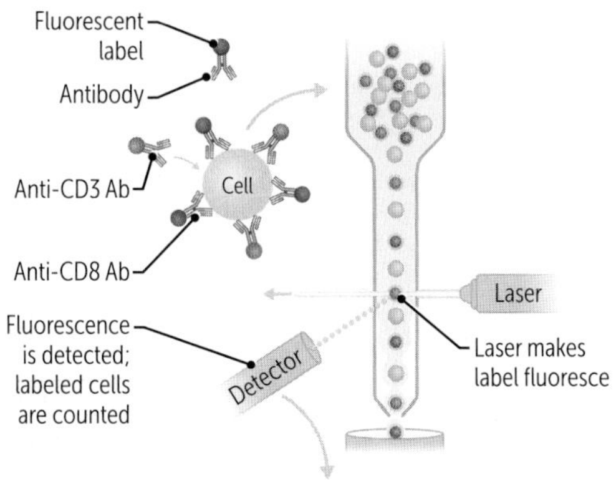

Data are plotted either as histogram (one measure) or scatter plot (any two measures, as shown). In illustration:
- Cells in left lower quadrant $\ominus$ for both CD8 and CD3.
- Cells in right lower quadrant $\oplus$ for CD8 and $\ominus$ for CD3. In this example, right lower quadrant is empty because all CD8-expressing cells also express CD3.
- Cells in left upper quadrant $\oplus$ for CD3 and $\ominus$ for CD8.
- Cells in right upper quadrant $\oplus$ for both CD8 and CD3.

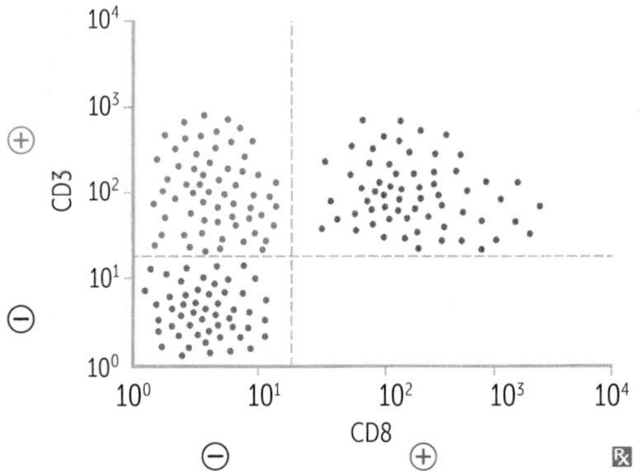

Microarrays

Array consisting of thousands of DNA oligonucleotides arranged in a grid on a glass or silicon chip. The DNA or RNA samples being compared are attached to different fluorophores and hybridized to the array. The ratio of fluorescence signal at a particular oligonucleotide reflects the relative amount of the hybridizing nucleic acid in the two samples.

Used to compare the relative expression of genes in two samples. Can detect single nucleotide polymorphisms (SNPs) and copy number variants (CNVs) for genotyping, clinical genetic testing, forensic analysis, and cancer mutation and genetic linkage analysis.

Enzyme-linked immunosorbent assay

Immunologic test used to detect the presence of either a specific antigen or antibody in a patient's blood sample. Detection involves the use of an antibody linked to an enzyme. Added substrate reacts with enzyme, producing a detectable signal. Can have high sensitivity and specificity, but is less specific than Western blot. Often used to screen for HIV infection.

Karyotyping

Colchicine is added to cultured cells to halt chromosomes in metaphase. Chromosomes are stained, ordered, and numbered according to morphology, size, arm-length ratio, and banding pattern (arrows in A point to extensive abnormalities in a cancer cell).

Can be performed on a sample of blood, bone marrow, amniotic fluid, or placental tissue.

Used to diagnose chromosomal imbalances (eg, autosomal trisomies, sex chromosome disorders).

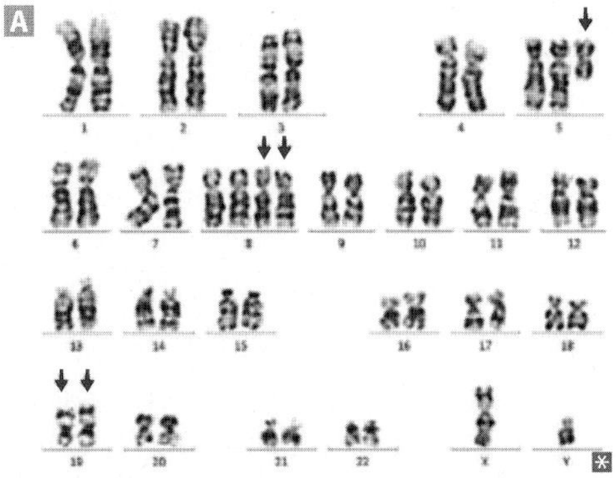

Fluorescence in situ hybridization

Fluorescent DNA or RNA probe binds to specific gene site of interest on chromosomes (arrows in A point to abnormalities in a cancer cell; each fluorescent color represents a chromosome-specific probe).

Used for specific localization of genes and direct visualization of chromosomal anomalies at the molecular level.

- Microdeletion—no fluorescence on a chromosome compared to fluorescence at the same locus on the second copy of that chromosome.
- Translocation—fluorescence signal that corresponds to one chromosome is found in a different chromosome (two white arrows in A show fragments of chromosome 17 that have translocated to chromosome 19).
- Duplication—a second copy of a chromosome, resulting in a trisomy or tetrasomy (two blue arrows in A duplicated chromosomes 8, resulting in a tetrasomy).

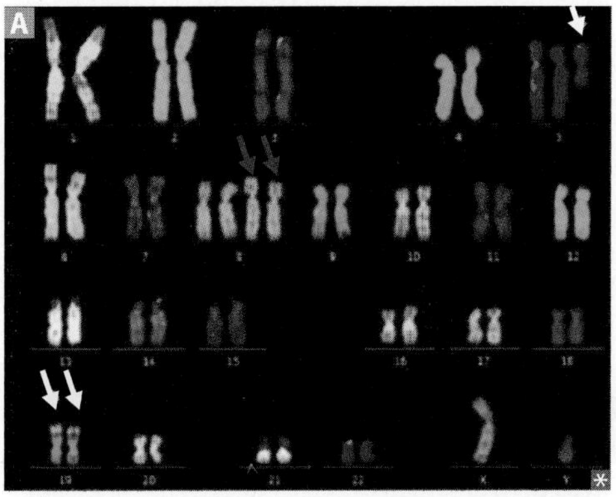

Molecular cloning

Production of a recombinant DNA molecule in a bacterial host.

Steps:

1. Isolate eukaryotic mRNA (post-RNA processing) of interest.
2. Add reverse transcriptase (an RNA-dependent DNA polymerase) to produce complementary DNA (cDNA, lacks introns).
3. Insert cDNA fragments into bacterial plasmids containing antibiotic resistance genes.
4. Transform (insert) recombinant plasmid into bacteria.
5. Surviving bacteria on antibiotic medium produce cloned DNA (copies of cDNA).

Gene expression modifications	Transgenic strategies in mice involve: ▪ Random insertion of gene into mouse genome ▪ Targeted insertion or deletion of gene through homologous recombination with mouse gene	Knock-**out** = removing a gene, taking it **out**. Knock-**in** = **in**serting a gene. Random insertion—constitutive expression. Targeted insertion—conditional expression.
RNA interference	Process whereby small non-coding RNA molecules target mRNAs to inhibit gene expression.	
MicroRNA	Naturally produced by cell as hairpin structures. Loose nucleotide pairing allows broad targeting of related mRNAs. When miRNA binds to mRNA, it blocks translation of mRNA and sometimes facilitates its degradation.	Abnormal expression of miRNAs contributes to certain malignancies (eg, by silencing an mRNA from a tumor suppressor gene).
Small interfering RNA	Usually derived from exogenous dsRNA source (eg, virus). Once inside a cell, siRNA requires complete nucleotide pairing, leading to highly specific mRNA targeting. Results in mRNA cleavage prior to translation.	Can be produced by in vitro transcription for gene "knockdown" experiments.

▶ BIOCHEMISTRY—GENETICS

Genetic terms

TERM	DEFINITION	EXAMPLE
Codominance	Both alleles contribute to the phenotype of the heterozygote.	Blood groups A, B, AB; α_1-antitrypsin deficiency; HLA groups.
Variable expressivity	Patients with the same genotype have varying phenotypes.	2 patients with neurofibromatosis type 1 (NF1) may have varying disease severity.
Incomplete penetrance	Not all individuals with a mutant genotype show the mutant phenotype. % penetrance × probability of inheriting genotype = risk of expressing phenotype.	*BRCA1* gene mutations do not always result in breast or ovarian cancer.
Pleiotropy	One gene contributes to multiple phenotypic effects.	Untreated phenylketonuria (PKU) manifests with light skin, intellectual disability, and musty body odor.
Anticipation	Increased severity or earlier onset of disease in succeeding generations.	Trinucleotide repeat diseases (eg, Huntington disease).
Loss of heterozygosity	If a patient inherits or develops a mutation in a tumor suppressor gene, the wild type allele must be deleted/mutated before cancer develops. This is not true of oncogenes.	Retinoblastoma and the "two-hit hypothesis," Lynch syndrome (HNPCC), Li-Fraumeni syndrome.

Genetic terms *(continued)*

TERM	DEFINITION	EXAMPLE
Dominant negative mutation	Exerts a dominant effect. A heterozygote produces a nonfunctional altered protein that also prevents the normal gene product from functioning.	A single mutated *p53* tumor suppressor gene results in a protein that is able to bind DNA and block the nonmutated p53 from binding to the promoter.
Linkage disequilibrium	Tendency for certain alleles at 2 linked loci to occur together more or less often than expected by chance. Measured in a population, not in a family, and often varies in different populations.	
Mosaicism 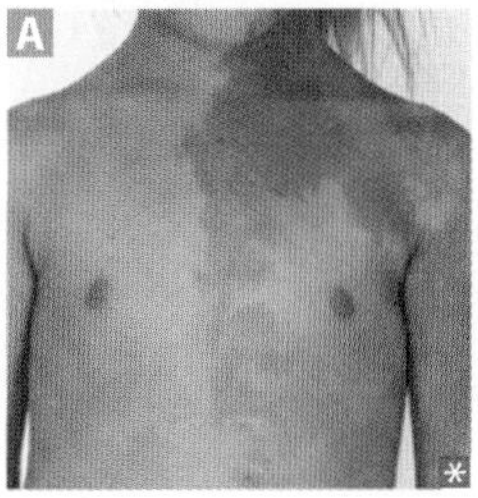	Presence of genetically distinct cell lines in the same individual. Somatic mosaicism—mutation arises from mitotic errors after fertilization and propagates through multiple tissues or organs. Gonadal mosaicism—mutation only in egg or sperm cells. If parents and relatives do not have the disease, suspect gonadal (or germline) mosaicism.	**McCune-Albright syndrome**—due to G_s-protein activating mutation. Presents with unilateral café-au-lait spots A with ragged edges, polyostotic fibrous dysplasia (bone is replaced by collagen and fibroblasts), and at least one endocrinopathy (eg, precocious puberty). Lethal if mutation occurs before fertilization (affecting all cells), but survivable in patients with mosaicism.
Locus heterogeneity	Mutations at different loci can produce a similar phenotype.	Albinism, retinitis pigmentosa, familial hypercholesteremia.
Allelic heterogeneity	Different mutations in the same locus produce the same phenotype.	β-thalassemia.
Heteroplasmy	Presence of both normal and mutated mtDNA, resulting in variable expression in mitochondrially inherited disease.	mtDNA passed from mother to all children.
Uniparental disomy	Offspring receives 2 copies of a chromosome from 1 parent and no copies from the other parent. HeterodIsomy (heterozygous) indicates a meiosis I error. IsodIsomy (homozygous) indicates a meiosis II error or postzygotic chromosomal duplication of one of a pair of chromosomes, and loss of the other of the original pair.	Uniparental is euploid (correct number of chromosomes). Most occurrences of uniparental disomy (UPD) → normal phenotype. Consider isodisomy in an individual manifesting a recessive disorder when only one parent is a carrier. Examples: Prader-Willi and Angelman syndromes.

Hardy-Weinberg population genetics

	A (p)	a (q)
A (p)	AA (p^2)	Aa (pq)
a (q)	Aa (pq)	aa (q^2)

If p and q represent the frequencies of alleles A and a, respectively, in a population, then $p + q = 1$:

- p^2 = frequency of homozygosity for allele A
- q^2 = frequency of homozygosity for allele a
- $2pq$ = frequency of heterozygosity (carrier frequency, if an autosomal recessive disease)

Therefore, the sum of the frequencies of these genotypes is $p^2 + 2pq + q^2 = 1$.

The frequency of an X-linked recessive disease in males = q and in females = q^2.

Hardy-Weinberg law assumptions include:

- No mutation occurring at the locus
- Natural selection is not occurring
- Completely random mating
- No net migration
- Large population

If a population is in Hardy-Weinberg equilibrium, then the values of p and q remain constant from generation to generation.

Disorders of imprinting Imprinting—one gene copy is silenced by methylation, and only the other copy is expressed → parent-of-origin effects.

	Prader-Willi syndrome	**Angelman syndrome**
WHICH GENE IS SILENT?	Maternally derived genes are silenced Disease occurs when the paternal allele is deleted or mutated	Paternally derived *UBE3A* is silenced Disease occurs when the maternal allele is deleted or mutated
SIGNS AND SYMPTOMS	Hyperphagia, obesity, intellectual disability, hypogonadism, hypotonia	Seizures, Ataxia, severe Intellectual disability, inappropriate Laughter Set SAIL for Angel Island
CHROMOSOMES INVOLVED	Chromosome 15 of paternal origin	*UBE3A* on maternal copy of chromosome 15
NOTES	25% of cases are due to maternal uniparental disomy	5% of cases are due to paternal uniparental disomy
	POP: Prader-Willi, Obesity/overeating, Paternal allele deleted	MAMAS: Maternal allele deleted, Angelman syndrome, Mood, Ataxia, Seizures

Prader Will
nl: mom quiet, dad works
2nd: deleted
opp in Angel

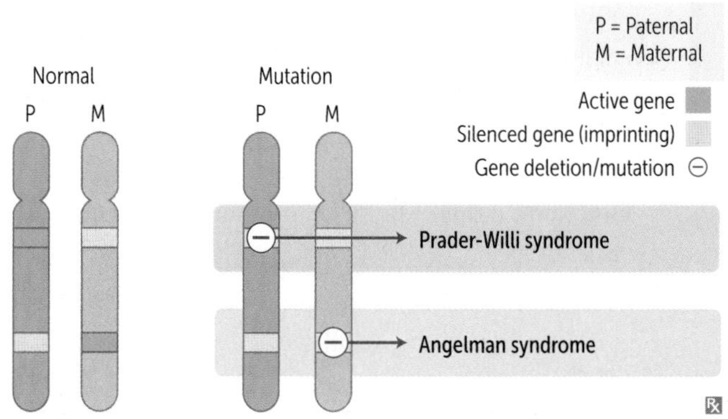
P = Paternal
M = Maternal
Normal
Mutation
P
M
P
M
Active gene
Silenced gene (imprinting)
Gene deletion/mutation
Prader-Willi syndrome
Angelman syndrome

Modes of inheritance

Autosomal dominant

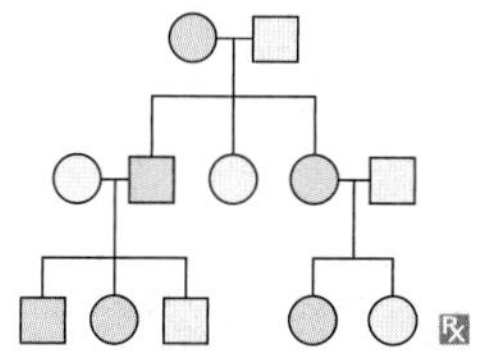

Often due to defects in structural genes. Many generations, both males and females are affected.

	A	a
a	Aa	aa
a	Aa	aa

Often pleiotropic (multiple apparently unrelated effects) and variably expressive (different between individuals). Family history crucial to diagnosis. With one affected (heterozygous) parent, on average, ½ of children affected.

Autosomal recessive

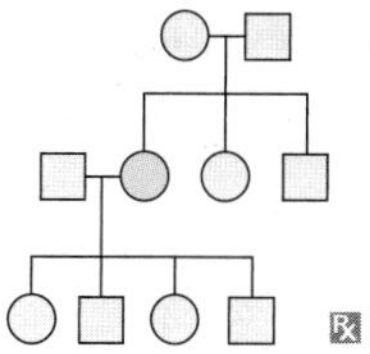

With 2 carrier (heterozygous) parents, on average: ¼ of children will be affected (homozygous), ½ of children will be carriers, and ¼ of children will be neither affected nor carriers.

	A	a
A	AA	Aa
a	Aa	aa

Often due to enzyme deficiencies. Usually seen in only 1 generation. Commonly more severe than dominant disorders; patients often present in childhood.

↑ risk in consanguineous families.

Unaffected individual with affected sibling has 2/3 probability of being a carrier.

X-linked recessive

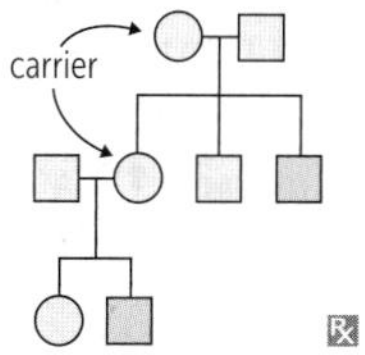

Sons of heterozygous mothers have a 50% chance of being affected. No male-to-male transmission. Skips generations.

	X	X
X	XX	XX
Y	XY	XY

	X	X
X	XX	XX
Y	XY	XY

Commonly more severe in males. Females usually must be homozygous to be affected.

X-linked dominant

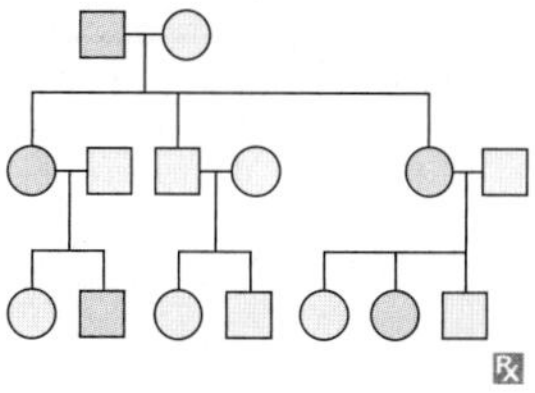

Transmitted through both parents. Mothers transmit to 50% of daughters and sons; fathers transmit to all daughters but no sons.

	X	X
X	XX	XX
Y	XY	XY

	X	X
X	XX	XX
Y	XY	XY

Examples: fragile X syndrome, Alport syndrome, **hypophosphatemic rickets** (also called X-linked hypophosphatemia)—phosphate wasting at proximal tubule → rickets-like presentation.

Mitochondrial inheritance

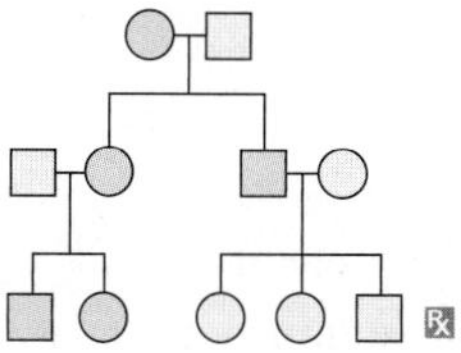

Transmitted only through the mother. All offspring of affected females may show signs of disease.

Variable expression in a population or even within a family due to heteroplasmy.

Mitochondrial myopathies—rare disorders; often present with myopathy, lactic acidosis, and CNS disease, eg, MELAS syndrome (mitochondrial encephalomyopathy, lactic acidosis, and stroke-like episodes). 2° to failure in oxidative phosphorylation. Muscle biopsy often shows "ragged red fibers" (due to accumulation of diseased mitochondria in the subsarcolemma of the muscle fiber).

Leber hereditary optic neuropathy (LHON)—cell death in optic nerve neurons → subacute bilateral vision loss in teens/young adults, 90% males. Usually permanent. Also leads to neurologic dysfunction, cardiac conduction defects.

□ = unaffected male; ■ = affected male; ○ = unaffected female; ● = affected female.

Autosomal dominant diseases

Achondroplasia, autosomal dominant polycystic kidney disease, familial adenomatous polyposis, familial hypercholesterolemia, hereditary hemorrhagic telangiectasia (Osler-Weber-Rendu syndrome), hereditary spherocytosis, Huntington disease, Li-Fraumeni syndrome, Marfan syndrome, multiple endocrine neoplasias, myotonic muscular dystrophy, neurofibromatosis type 1 (von Recklinghausen disease), neurofibromatosis type 2, tuberous sclerosis, von Hippel-Lindau disease.

Autosomal recessive diseases

Oculocutaneous albinism, phenylketonuria, cystic fibrosis, sickle cell disease, Wilson disease, sphingolipidoses (except Fabry disease), hemochromatosis, glycogen storage diseases, thalassemia, mucopolysaccharidoses (except Hunter syndrome), Friedreich ataxia, Kartagener syndrome, ARPKD. Oh please! Can students who score high grades tell me features of the kidney disorder Autosomal Recessive Polycystic Kidney Disease?

Cystic fibrosis

GENETICS

Autosomal recessive; defect in *CFTR* gene on chromosome 7; commonly a deletion of Phe508. Most common lethal genetic disease in patients with European ancestry.

PATHOPHYSIOLOGY

CFTR encodes an ATP-gated Cl^- channel that secretes Cl^- in lungs and GI tract, and reabsorbs Cl^- in sweat glands. Phe508 deletion → misfolded protein → improper protein trafficking and protein retention in RER → protein absent from cell membrane → ↓ Cl^- (and H_2O) secretion; ↑ intracellular Cl^- results in compensatory ↑ Na^+ reabsorption via epithelial Na^+ channels (ENaC) → ↑ H_2O reabsorption → abnormally thick mucus secreted into lungs and GI tract. ↑ Na^+ reabsorption also causes more negative transepithelial potential difference.

DIAGNOSIS

↑ Cl^- concentration in pilocarpine-induced sweat test is diagnostic. Can present with contraction alkalosis and hypokalemia (ECF effects analogous to a patient taking a loop diuretic) because of ECF H_2O/Na^+ losses via sweating and concomitant renal K^+/H^+ wasting. ↑ immunoreactive trypsinogen (newborn screening) due to clogging of pancreatic duct.

COMPLICATIONS

Recurrent pulmonary infections (eg, *S aureus* [infancy and early childhood], *P aeruginosa* [adulthood], allergic bronchopulmonary aspergillosis [ABPA]), chronic bronchitis and bronchiectasis → reticulonodular pattern on CXR, opacification of sinuses. Nasal polyps, nail clubbing.

Pancreatic insufficiency, malabsorption with steatorrhea, and fat-soluble vitamin deficiencies (A, D, E, K) progressing to endocrine dysfunction (CF-related diabetes), biliary cirrhosis, liver disease. Meconium ileus in newborns.

Infertility in males (absence of vas deferens, spermatogenesis may be unaffected) and subfertility in females (amenorrhea, abnormally thick cervical mucus).

TREATMENT

Multifactorial: chest physiotherapy, albuterol, aerosolized dornase alfa (DNase), and inhaled hypertonic saline facilitate mucus clearance. Azithromycin used as anti-inflammatory agent. Ibuprofen slows disease progression. Pancreatic enzyme replacement therapy (pancrelipase) for pancreatic insufficiency.

Combination of lumacaftor or tezacaftor (each corrects misfolded proteins and improves their transport to cell surface) with ivacaftor. (opens Cl^- channels → improved chloride transport).

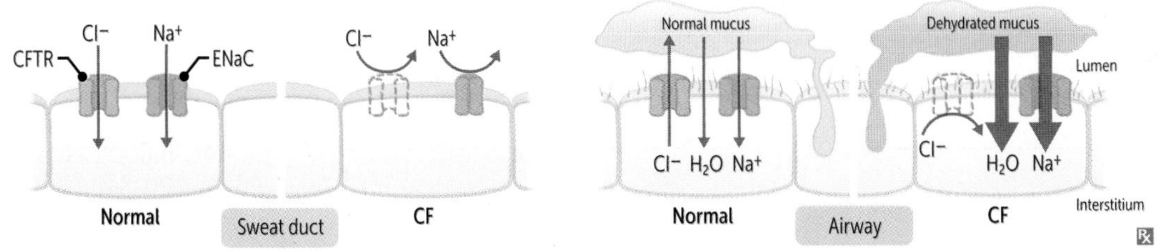

X-linked recessive diseases	Bruton agammaglobulinemia, Duchenne and Becker muscular dystrophies, Fabry disease, G6PD deficiency, hemophilia A and B, Hunter syndrome, Lesch-Nyhan syndrome, ocular albinism, ornithine transcarbamylase deficiency, Wiskott-Aldrich syndrome. Females with Turner syndrome (45,XO) are more likely to have an X-linked recessive disorder. X-inactivation (lyonization)—during development, one of the X chromosomes in each XX cell is randomly deactivated and condensed into a Barr body (methylated heterochromatin). If skewed inactivation occurs, XX individuals may express X-linked recessive diseases (eg, G6PD); penetrance and severity of X-linked dominant diseases in XX individuals may also be impacted.

Muscular dystrophies

Duchenne

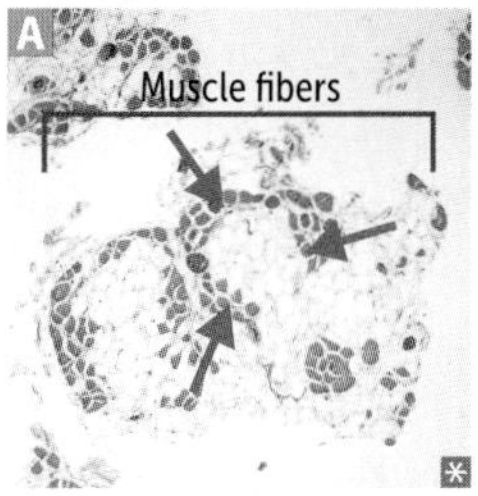

X-linked recessive disorder typically due to **frameshift** deletions or nonsense mutations → truncated or absent dystrophin protein → progressive myofiber damage. Weakness begins in pelvic girdle muscles and progresses superiorly. Pseudohypertrophy of calf muscles due to fibrofatty replacement of muscle A. Waddling gait.

Onset before 5 years of age. Dilated cardiomyopathy is common cause of death.

Gowers sign—patient uses upper extremities to help stand up. Classically seen in Duchenne muscular dystrophy, but also seen in other muscular dystrophies and inflammatory myopathies (eg, polymyositis).

Duchenne = deleted dystrophin.

Dystrophin gene (*DMD*) is the largest protein-coding human gene → ↑ chance of spontaneous mutation. Dystrophin helps anchor muscle fibers, primarily in skeletal and cardiac muscle. It connects the intracellular cytoskeleton (actin) to the transmembrane proteins α- and β-dystroglycan, which are connected to the extracellular matrix (ECM). Loss of dystrophin → myonecrosis.

↑ CK and aldolase; genetic testing confirms diagnosis.

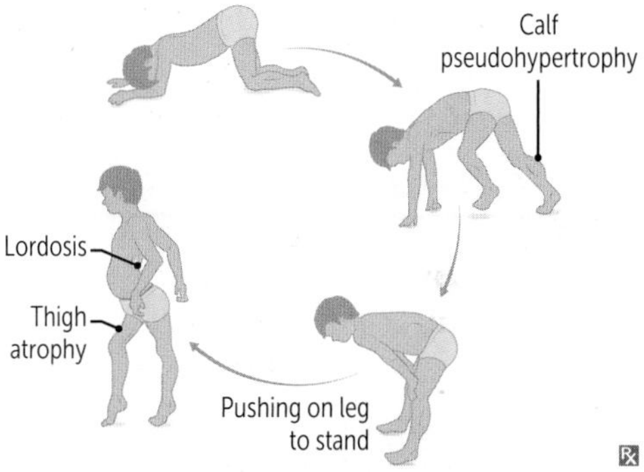

Becker

X-linked recessive disorder typically due to **non-frameshift** deletions in dystrophin gene (partially functional instead of truncated). Less severe than Duchenne (Becker is better). Onset in adolescence or early adulthood.

Deletions can cause both Duchenne and Becker muscular dystrophies. ⅔ of cases have large deletions spanning one or more exons.

Myotonic dystrophy

Autosomal dominant. Onset 20–30 years. CTG trinucleotide repeat expansion in the *DMPK* gene → abnormal expression of myotonin protein kinase → myotonia (eg, difficulty releasing hand from handshake), muscle wasting, cataracts, testicular atrophy, frontal balding, arrhythmia.

Cataracts, Toupee (early balding in males), Gonadal atrophy.

Rett syndrome

Sporadic disorder seen almost exclusively in females (affected males die in utero or shortly after birth). Most cases are caused by de novo mutation of *MECP2* on X chromosome. Symptoms of **Rett** syndrome usually appear between ages 1–4 and are characterized by regression ("**rett**urn") in motor, verbal, and cognitive abilities; ataxia; seizures; growth deceleration; and stereotyped hand-wringing.

Fragile X syndrome

X-linked dominant inheritance. Trinucleotide repeats in FMR1 → hypermethylation of cytosine residues → ↓ expression.

Most common inherited cause of intellectual disability (Down syndrome is most common genetic cause, but most cases occur sporadically).

Trinucleotide repeat expansion [$(CGG)_n$] occurs during oogenesis.

Premutation (50-200 repeats) → tremor, ataxia, 1° ovarian insufficiency.

Full mutation (>200 repeats) → postpubertal macroorchidism (enlarged testes), long face with large jaw, large everted ears, autism, mitral valve prolapse, hypermobile joints.

Self-mutilation is common and can be confused with Lesch-Nyhan syndrome.

Trinucleotide repeat expansion diseases

May show genetic anticipation (disease severity ↑ and age of onset ↓ in successive generations).

DISEASE	TRINUCLEOTIDE REPEAT	MODE OF INHERITANCE	MNEMONIC
Huntington disease	$(CAG)_n$	AD	Caudate has ↓ ACh and GABA
Myotonic dystrophy	$(CTG)_n$	AD	Cataracts, Toupee (early balding in males), Gonadal atrophy in males, reduced fertility in females
Fragile X syndrome	$(CGG)_n$	XD	Chin (protruding), Giant Gonads
Friedreich ataxia	$(GAA)_n$	AR	Ataxic GAAit

Autosomal trisomies

Autosomal monosomies are incompatible with life due to a high chance of expression of recessive traits for that chromosome.

Down syndrome (trisomy 21)

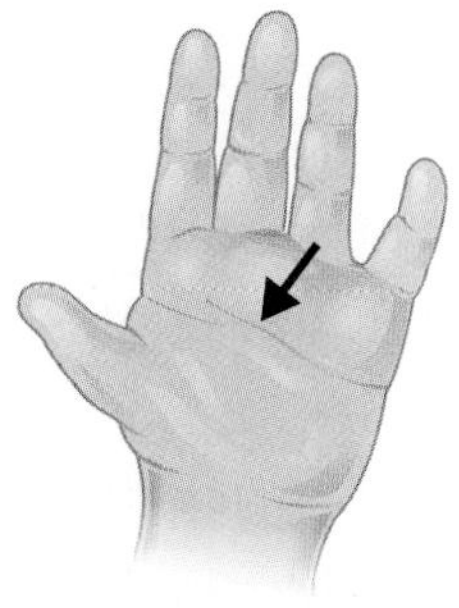

Single palmar crease

Findings: intellectual disability, flat facies, prominent epicanthal folds, single palmar crease, incurved 5th finger, gap between 1st 2 toes, duodenal atresia, Hirschsprung disease, congenital heart disease (eg, ASD), Brushfield spots (whitish spots at the periphery of the iris). Associated with early-onset Alzheimer disease (chromosome 21 codes for amyloid precursor protein), ↑ risk of AML/ALL.

95% of cases due to meiotic nondisjunction, most commonly during meiosis I (↑ with advanced maternal age: from 1:1500 in females < 20 to 1:25 in females > 45).

4% of cases due to unbalanced Robertsonian translocation, most typically between chromosomes 14 and 21. Only 1% of cases are due to postfertilization mitotic error.

Incidence 1:700.

Drinking age (**21**).

Most common viable chromosomal disorder and most common cause of genetic intellectual disability.

First-trimester ultrasound commonly shows ↑ nuchal translucency and hypoplastic nasal bone. Markers for Down syndrome are **hi** up: ↑ **h**CG, ↑ **i**nhibin.

The **5 A's** of Down syndrome:

- Advanced maternal age
- Atresia (duodenal)
- Atrioventricular septal defect
- Alzheimer disease (early onset)
- AML/ALL

Edwards syndrome (trisomy 18)

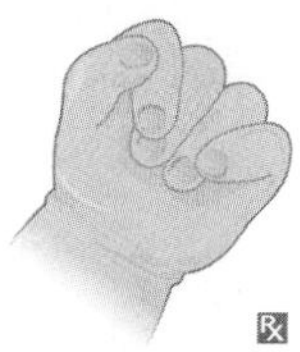

Findings: **PRINCE E**dward—**P**rominent occiput, **R**ocker-bottom feet, **I**ntellectual disability, **N**ondisjunction, **C**lenched fists with overlapping fingers, low-set **E**ars, micrognathia (small jaw), congenital heart disease, omphalocele, myelomeningocele. Death usually occurs by age 1.

Incidence 1:8000.

Election age (**18**).

2nd most common autosomal trisomy resulting in live birth (most common is Down syndrome).

In **E**dwards syndrome, every prenatal screening marker **d**ecreases.

Patau syndrome (trisomy 13)

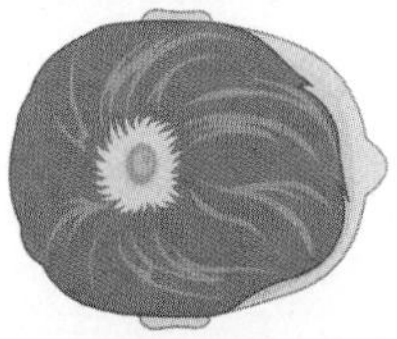

Cutis aplasia

Findings: severe intellectual disability, rocker-bottom feet, microphthalmia, microcephaly, cleft lip/palate, holoprosencephaly, polydactyly, cutis aplasia, congenital heart (pump) disease, polycystic kidney disease, omphalocele. Death usually occurs by age 1.

Incidence 1:15,000.

Puberty at age **13**.

Defect in fusion of prechordal mesoderm → midline defects.

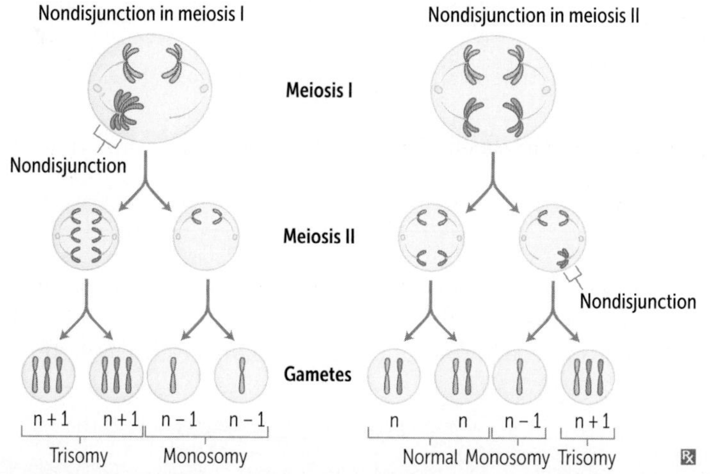

1st trimester screening		
Trisomy	β-hCG	PAPP-A
21	↑	↓
18	↓	↓
13	↓	↓

2nd trimester screening				
Trisomy	β-hCG	Inhibin A	Estriol	AFP
21	↑	↑	↓	↓
18	↓	— or ↓	↓	↓
13	—	—	—	—

Genetic disorders by chromosome

CHROMOSOME	SELECTED EXAMPLES
3	von Hippel-Lindau disease, renal cell carcinoma
4	ADPKD (*PKD2*), achondroplasia, Huntington disease
5	Cri-du-chat syndrome, familial adenomatous polyposis
6	Hemochromatosis (*HFE*)
7	Williams syndrome, cystic fibrosis
9	Friedreich ataxia, tuberous sclerosis (*TSC1*)
11	Wilms tumor, β-globin gene defects (eg, sickle cell disease, β-thalassemia), MEN1
13	Patau syndrome, Wilson disease, retinoblastoma (*RB1*), *BRCA2*
15	Prader-Willi syndrome, Angelman syndrome, Marfan syndrome
16	ADPKD (*PKD1*), α-globin gene defects (eg, α-thalassemia), tuberous sclerosis (*TSC2*)
17	Neurofibromatosis type 1, *BRCA1*, *TP53* (Li-Fraumeni syndrome)
18	Edwards syndrome
21	Down syndrome
22	Neurofibromatosis type 2, DiGeorge syndrome (22q11)
X	Fragile X syndrome, X-linked agammaglobulinemia, Klinefelter syndrome (XXY)

Robertsonian translocation

Chromosomal translocation that commonly involves chromosome pairs 21, 22, 13, 14, and 15. One of the most common types of translocation. Occurs when the long arms of 2 acrocentric chromosomes (chromosomes with centromeres near their ends) fuse at the centromere and the 2 short arms are lost.

Balanced translocations (no gain or loss of significant genetic material) normally do not cause abnormal phenotype. Unbalanced translocations (missing or extra genes) can result in miscarriage, stillbirth, and chromosomal imbalance (eg, Down syndrome, Patau syndrome).

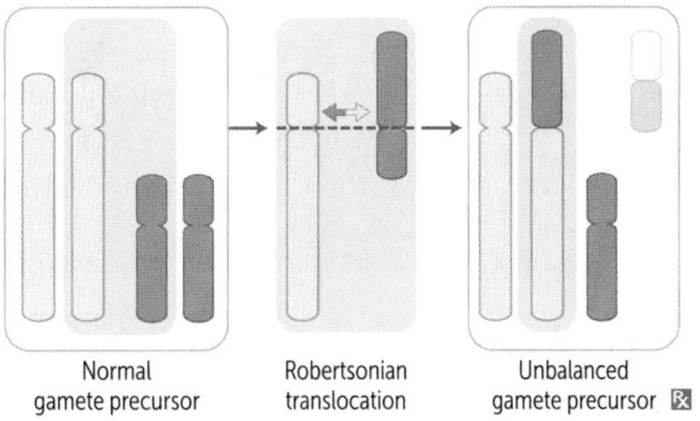
Normal gamete precursor
Robertsonian translocation
Unbalanced gamete precursor

Cri-du-chat syndrome

Cri du chat = cry of the cat. Congenital deletion on short arm of chromosome 5 (46,XX or XY, 5p–).

Findings: microcephaly, moderate to severe intellectual disability, high-pitched crying, epicanthal folds, cardiac abnormalities (VSD).

Williams syndrome

Congenital microdeletion of long arm of chromosome 7 (deleted region includes elastin gene).

Findings: distinctive "elfin" facies, intellectual disability, hypercalcemia, well-developed verbal skills, extreme friendliness with strangers, cardiovascular problems (eg, supravalvular aortic stenosis, renal artery stenosis).

▶ BIOCHEMISTRY—NUTRITION

Essential fatty acids	Polyunsaturated fatty acids that cannot be synthesized in the body and must be provided in the diet (eg, nuts and seeds, plant oils, seafood). Linoleic acid (omega-6) is metabolized to arachidonic acid, which serves as the precursor to leukotrienes and prostaglandins. Linolenic acid (omega-3) and its metabolites have cardioprotective and antihyperlipidemic effects.	
Vitamins: fat soluble	A, D, E, K. Absorption dependent on ileum and pancreas. Toxicity more common than for water-soluble vitamins because fat-soluble vitamins accumulate in fat.	Malabsorption syndromes with steatorrhea (eg, cystic fibrosis and celiac disease) or mineral oil intake can cause fat-soluble vitamin deficiencies.
Vitamins: water soluble	B_1 (thiamine: TPP) B_2 (riboflavin: FAD, FMN) B_3 (niacin: NAD^+) B_5 (pantothenic acid: CoA) B_6 (pyridoxine: PLP) B_7 (biotin) B_9 (folate) B_{12} (cobalamin) C (ascorbic acid)	Wash out easily from body except B_{12} and B_9. B_{12} stored in liver for ~ 3–4 years. B_9 stored in liver for ~ 3–4 months. B-complex deficiencies often result in dermatitis, glossitis, and diarrhea. Can be coenzymes (eg, ascorbic acid) or precursors to coenzymes (eg, FAD, NAD^+).

Vitamin A

Includes retinal, retinol, retinoic acid.

FUNCTION	Antioxidant; constituent of visual pigments (**retinal**); essential for normal differentiation of epithelial cells into specialized tissue (pancreatic cells, mucus-secreting cells); prevents squamous metaplasia.	**Retinol** is vitamin **A**, so think **retin-A** (used topically for wrinkles and **A**cne). Found in liver and leafy vegetables. Supplementation in vitamin A-deficient measles patients may improve outcomes. Use oral isotretinoin to treat severe cystic acne. Use *all*-trans retinoic acid to treat acute promyelocytic leukemia.
DEFICIENCY 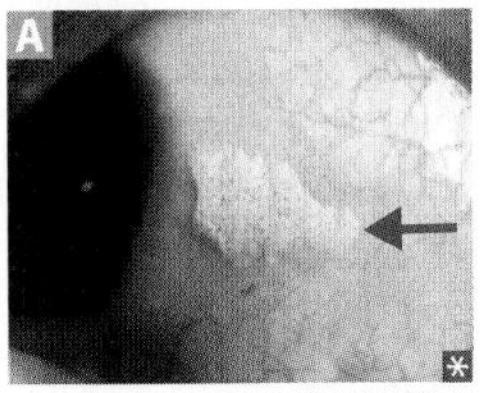	Night blindness (nyctalopia); dry, scaly skin (xerosis cutis); dry eyes (xerophthalmia); corneal squamous metaplasia → Bitot spots (keratin debris; foamy appearance on conjunctiva A); corneal degeneration (keratomalacia); immunosuppression.	
EXCESS	Acute toxicity—nausea, vomiting, ↑ ICP (eg, vertigo, blurred vision). Chronic toxicity—alopecia, dry skin (eg, scaliness), hepatic toxicity and enlargement, arthralgias, and idiopathic intracranial hypertension.	Teratogenic (cleft palate, cardiac abnormalities), therefore a ⊖ pregnancy test and two forms of contraception are required before isotretinoin (vitamin A derivative) is prescribed. **Isotretinoin is teratogenic.**

Vitamin B_1

Also called thiamine.

FUNCTION

In thiamine pyrophosphate (TPP), a cofactor for several dehydrogenase enzyme reactions (**Be APT**):

- **B**ranched-chain ketoacid dehydrogenase
- **α**-Ketoglutarate dehydrogenase (TCA cycle)
- **P**yruvate dehydrogenase (links glycolysis to TCA cycle)
- **T**ransketolase (HMP shunt)

DEFICIENCY

Impaired glucose breakdown → ATP depletion worsened by glucose infusion; highly aerobic tissues (eg, brain, heart) are affected first. In patients with chronic alcohol overuse or malnutrition, give thiamine before dextrose to ↓ risk of precipitating Wernicke encephalopathy.

Diagnosis made by ↑ in RBC transketolase activity following vitamin B_1 administration.

DISORDER	CHARACTERISTICS	
Wernicke encephalopathy	Acute, reversible, life-threatening neurologic condition. Symptoms: **Co**nfusion, **O**phthalmoplegia/**N**ystagmus, **A**taxia (**CorONA** beer).	
Korsakoff syndrome	Amnestic disorder due to chronic alcohol overuse; presents with confabulation, personality changes, memory loss (permanent).	
Wernicke-Korsakoff syndrome	Damage to medial dorsal nucleus of thalamus, mammillary bodies. Presentation is combination of Wernicke encephalopathy and Korsakoff syndrome.	
Dry beriberi	Polyneuropathy, symmetric muscle wasting.	Spell beriberi as Ber1Ber1 to remember vitamin B_1.
Wet beriberi	High-output cardiac failure (dilated cardiomyopathy), edema.	

Vitamin B_2	Also called riboflavin.	
FUNCTION	Component of flavins FAD and FMN, used as cofactors in redox reactions, eg, the succinate dehydrogenase reaction in the TCA cycle.	FAD and FMN are derived from riboFlavin ($B_2 \approx 2$ ATP).
DEFICIENCY	Cheilosis (inflammation of lips, scaling and fissures at the corners of the mouth), "magenta" tongue, corneal vascularization.	The 2 C's of B_2.

Vitamin B_3	Also called niacin, nicotinic acid.	
FUNCTION	Constituent of NAD^+, $NADP^+$ (used in redox reactions and as cofactor by dehydrogenases). Derived from tryptophan. Synthesis requires vitamins B_2 and B_6. Used to treat dyslipidemia (↓ VLDL, ↑ HDL).	NAD derived from Niacin ($B_3 \approx 3$ ATP).
DEFICIENCY 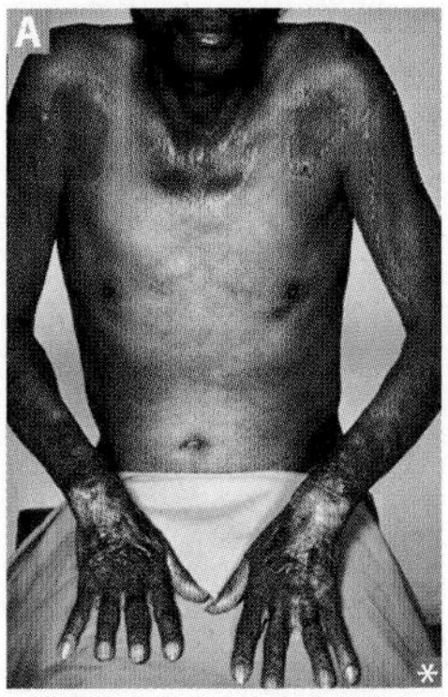	Glossitis. Severe deficiency of B_3 leads to pellagra, which can also be caused by Hartnup disease, malignant carcinoid syndrome (↑ tryptophan metabolism → ↑ serotonin synthesis), and isoniazid (↓ vitamin B_6). Symptoms of B_3 deficiency (pellagra) (the 3 D's): diarrhea, dementia (also hallucinations), dermatitis (C3/C4 dermatome circumferential "broad collar" rash [Casal necklace], hyperpigmentation of sun-exposed limbs A).	**Hartnup disease**—autosomal recessive. Deficiency of neutral amino acid (eg, tryptophan) transporters in proximal renal tubular cells and on enterocytes → neutral aminoaciduria and ↓ absorption from the gut → ↓ tryptophan for conversion to niacin → pellagra-like symptoms. Treat with high-protein diet and nicotinic acid. Deficiency of vitamin B_3 → pellagra. Less B_3.
EXCESS	Facial flushing (induced by prostaglandin, not histamine; can avoid by taking aspirin with niacin), hyperglycemia, hyperuricemia.	Excess of vitamin B_3 → podagra (gout). Overdose (excess) B_3.

Vitamin B_5	Also called pantothenic acid. B_5 is "pento"thenic acid.
FUNCTION	Component of coenzyme A (CoA, a cofactor for acyl transfers) and fatty acid synthase.
DEFICIENCY	Dermatitis, enteritis, alopecia, adrenal insufficiency may lead to burning sensation of feet ("burning feet syndrome"; distal paresthesias, dysesthesia).

Vitamin B_6	Also called pyridoxine.
FUNCTION	Converted to pyridoxal phosphate (PLP), a cofactor used in transamination (eg, ALT and AST), decarboxylation reactions, glycogen phosphorylase. Synthesis of glutathione, cystathionine, heme, niacin, histamine, and neurotransmitters including serotonin, epinephrine, norepinephrine (NE), dopamine, and GABA.
DEFICIENCY	Convulsions, hyperirritability, peripheral neuropathy (deficiency inducible by isoniazid and oral contraceptives), sideroblastic anemia (due to impaired hemoglobin synthesis and iron excess).

Vitamin B_7	Also called biotin.
FUNCTION	Cofactor for carboxylation enzymes (which add a 1-carbon group): ▪ Pyruvate carboxylase (gluconeogenesis): pyruvate (3C) → oxaloacetate (4C) ▪ Acetyl-CoA carboxylase (fatty acid synthesis): acetyl-CoA (2C) → malonyl-CoA (3C) ▪ Propionyl-CoA carboxylase (fatty acid oxidation): propionyl-CoA (3C) → methylmalonyl-CoA (4C)
DEFICIENCY	Relatively rare. Dermatitis, enteritis, alopecia. Caused by long-term antibiotic use or excessive ingestion of raw egg whites. "**Avid**in in egg whites **avid**ly binds biotin."

Vitamin B_9	Also called folate.	
FUNCTION	Converted to tetrahydrofolic acid (THF), a coenzyme for 1-carbon transfer/methylation reactions. Important for the synthesis of nitrogenous bases in DNA and RNA.	Found in leafy green vegetables. Also produced by gut flora. Absorbed in jejunum. **Fol**ate from **fol**iage. Small reserve pool stored primarily in the liver.
DEFICIENCY	Macrocytic, megaloblastic anemia; hypersegmented polymorphonuclear cells (PMNs); glossitis; no neurologic symptoms (as opposed to vitamin B_{12} deficiency). Labs: ↑ homocysteine, normal methylmalonic acid levels. Seen in chronic alcohol overuse and in pregnancy.	Deficiency can be caused by several drugs (eg, phenytoin, sulfonamides, methotrexate). Supplemental folic acid at least 1 month prior to conception and during early pregnancy to ↓ risk of neural tube defects. Give vitamin B_9 for the 9 months of pregnancy.

Vitamin B_{12}

Also called cobalamin.

FUNCTION	Cofactor for methionine synthase (transfers CH_3 groups as methylcobalamin) and methylmalonyl-CoA mutase. Important for DNA synthesis.	Found in animal products. Synthesized only by microorganisms. Very large reserve pool (several years) stored primarily in the liver. Deficiency caused by malabsorption (eg, sprue, enteritis, *Diphyllobothrium latum*, achlorhydria, bacterial overgrowth, alcohol overuse), lack of intrinsic factor (eg, pernicious anemia, gastric bypass surgery), absence of terminal ileum (surgical resection, eg, for Crohn disease), certain drugs (eg, metformin), or insufficient intake (eg, veganism). B_9 supplementation can mask the hematologic symptoms of B_{12} deficiency, but not the neurologic symptoms.
DEFICIENCY	Macrocytic, megaloblastic anemia; hypersegmented PMNs; paresthesias and subacute combined degeneration (degeneration of dorsal columns, lateral corticospinal tracts, and spinocerebellar tracts) due to abnormal myelin. Associated with ↑ serum homocysteine and methylmalonic acid levels, along with 2° folate deficiency. Prolonged deficiency → irreversible nerve damage.	

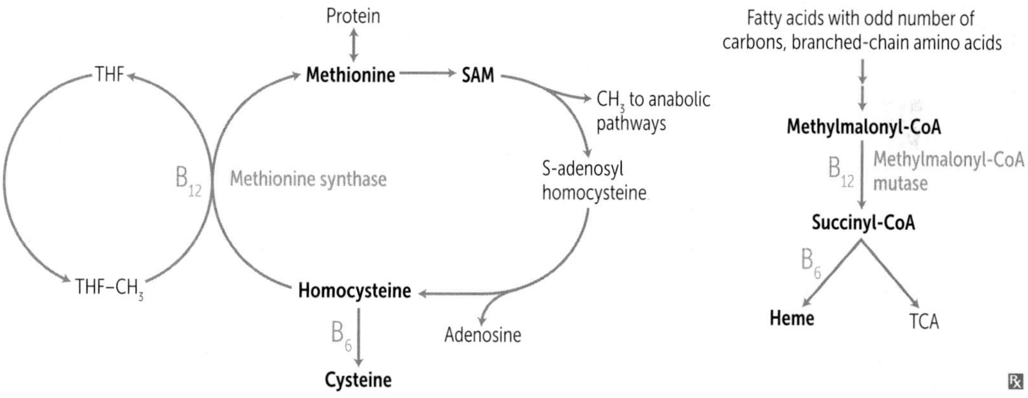

Vitamin C

Also called ascorbic acid.

FUNCTION	Antioxidant; also facilitates iron absorption by reducing it to Fe^{2+} state. Necessary for hydroxylation of proline and lysine in collagen synthesis. Necessary for dopamine β-hydroxylase (converts dopamine to NE).	Found in fruits and vegetables. Pronounce "**absorbic**" acid. Ancillary treatment for methemoglobinemia by reducing Fe^{3+} to Fe^{2+}.
DEFICIENCY	Scurvy—swollen gums, easy bruising, petechiae, hemarthrosis, anemia, poor wound healing, perifollicular and subperiosteal hemorrhages, "corkscrew" hair. Weakened immune response.	Deficiency may be precipitated by tea and toast diet. Vitamin C deficiency causes sCurvy due to a Collagen hydroCylation defect.
EXCESS	Nausea, vomiting, diarrhea, fatigue, calcium oxalate nephrolithiasis. Can ↑ iron toxicity in predisposed individuals by increasing dietary iron absorption (ie, can worsen hemochromatosis or transfusion-related iron overload).	

Vitamin D	D_3 (cholecalciferol) from exposure of skin (stratum basale) to sun, ingestion of fish, milk, plants. D_2 (ergocalciferol) from ingestion of plants, fungi, yeasts. Both converted to 25-OH D_3 (storage form) in liver and to the active form 1,25-$(OH)_2$ D_3 (calcitriol) in kidney.
FUNCTION	↑ intestinal absorption of Ca^{2+} and PO_4^{3-}. ↑ bone mineralization at low levels. ↑ bone resorption at higher levels.
REGULATION	↑ PTH, ↓ Ca^{2+}, ↓ PO_4^{3-} → ↑ 1,25-$(OH)_2D_3$ production. 1,25-$(OH)_2D_3$ feedback inhibits its own production. ↑ PTH → ↑ Ca^{2+} reabsorption and ↓ PO_4^{3-} reabsorption in the kidney.
DEFICIENCY 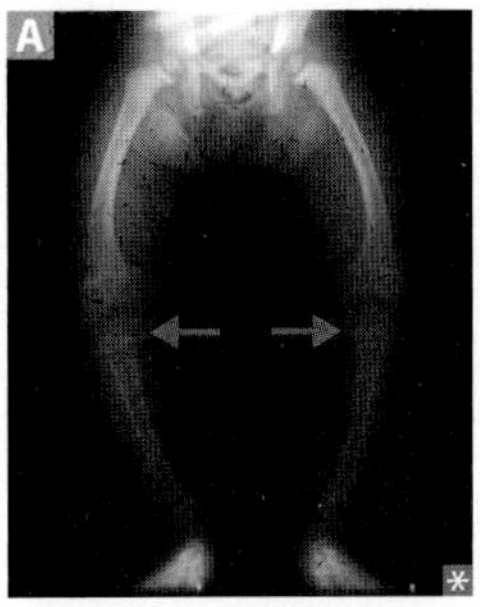	Rickets in children (deformity, such as genu varum "bowlegs" A), osteomalacia in adults (bone pain and muscle weakness), hypocalcemic tetany. Caused by malabsorption, ↓ sun exposure, poor diet, chronic kidney disease (CKD), advanced liver disease. Give oral vitamin D to breastfed infants. Darker skin and prematurity predispose to deficiency.
EXCESS	Hypercalcemia, hypercalciuria, loss of appetite, stupor. Seen in granulomatous diseases (↑ activation of vitamin D by epithelioid macrophages).

Vitamin E	Includes tocopherol, tocotrienol.	
FUNCTION	Antioxidant (protects RBCs and membranes from free radical damage).	
DEFICIENCY	Hemolytic anemia, acanthocytosis, muscle weakness, demyelination of posterior columns (↓ proprioception and vibration sensation) and spinocerebellar tract (ataxia).	Neurologic presentation may appear similar to vitamin B_{12} deficiency, but without megaloblastic anemia, hypersegmented neutrophils, or ↑ serum methylmalonic acid levels.
EXCESS	Risk of enterocolitis in infants.	High-dose supplementation may alter metabolism of vitamin K → enhanced anticoagulant effects of warfarin.

Vitamin K	Includes phytomenadione, phylloquinone, phytonadione, menaquinone.	
FUNCTION	Activated by epoxide reductase to the reduced form, which is a cofactor for the γ-carboxylation of glutamic acid residues on various proteins required for blood clotting. Synthesized by intestinal flora.	K is for Koagulation. Necessary for the maturation of clotting factors II, VII, IX, X, and proteins C and S. Warfarin inhibits vitamin K–dependent synthesis of these factors and proteins.
DEFICIENCY	Neonatal hemorrhage with ↑ PT and ↑ aPTT but normal bleeding time (neonates have sterile intestines and are unable to synthesize vitamin K). Can also occur after prolonged use of broad-spectrum antibiotics.	Not in breast milk; "breast-fed infants Don't Know about vitamins D and K". Neonates are given vitamin K injection at birth to prevent hemorrhagic disease of the newborn.

Zinc	
FUNCTION	Mineral essential for the activity of 100+ enzymes. Important in the formation of zinc fingers (transcription factor motif).
DEFICIENCY 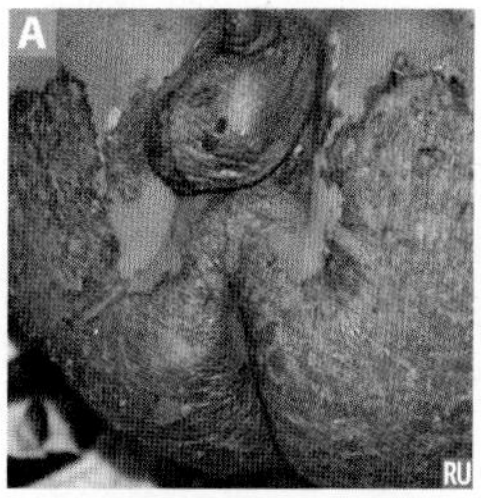	Delayed wound healing, suppressed immunity, male hypogonadism, ↓ adult hair (axillary, facial, pubic), dysgeusia, anosmia. Associated with acrodermatitis enteropathica (A, defect in intestinal zinc absorption). May predispose to alcoholic cirrhosis.

Protein-energy malnutrition

Kwashiorkor	Protein malnutrition resulting in skin lesions, edema due to ↓ plasma oncotic pressure (due to low serum albumin), liver malfunction (fatty change due to ↓ apolipoprotein synthesis and deposition). Clinical picture is small child with swollen abdomen A. Kwashiorkor results from protein-deficient MEALS: Malnutrition Edema Anemia Liver (fatty) Skin lesions (eg, hyperkeratosis, dyspigmentation)	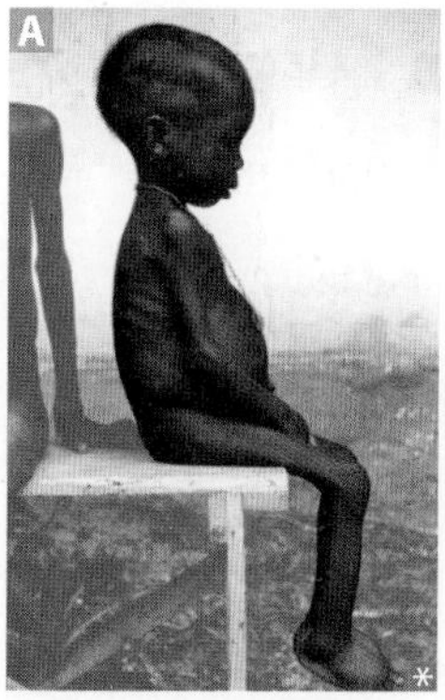 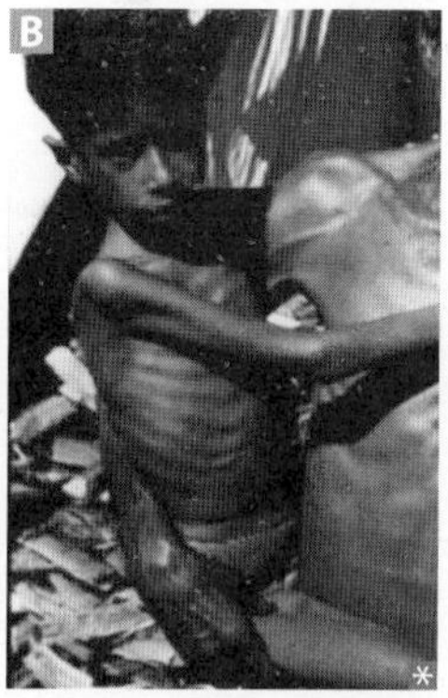
Marasmus	Malnutrition not causing edema. Diet is deficient in calories but no nutrients are entirely absent. Marasmus results in muscle wasting B.	

Ethanol metabolism

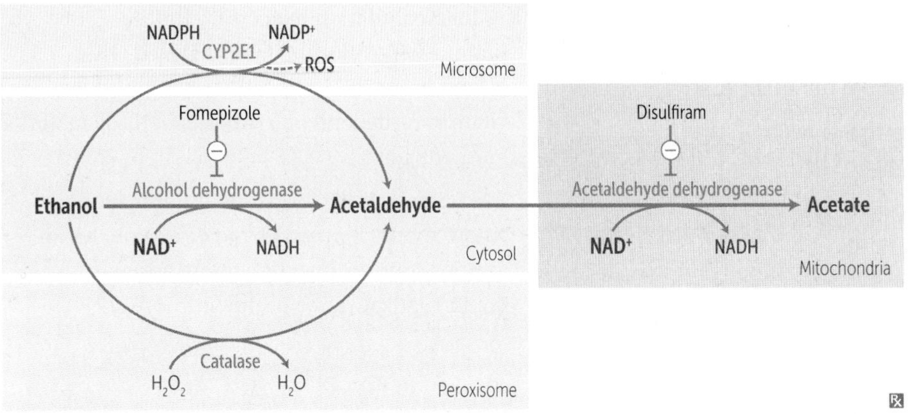

↑ NADH/NAD$^+$ ratio inhibits TCA cycle → ↑ acetyl-CoA used in ketogenesis (→ ketoacidosis), lipogenesis (→ hepatosteatosis).

Females are more susceptible than males to effects of alcohol due to ↓ activity of gastric alcohol dehydrogenase, ↓ body size, ↓ percentage of water in body weight.

NAD$^+$ is the limiting reagent.

Alcohol dehydrogenase operates via zero-order kinetics.

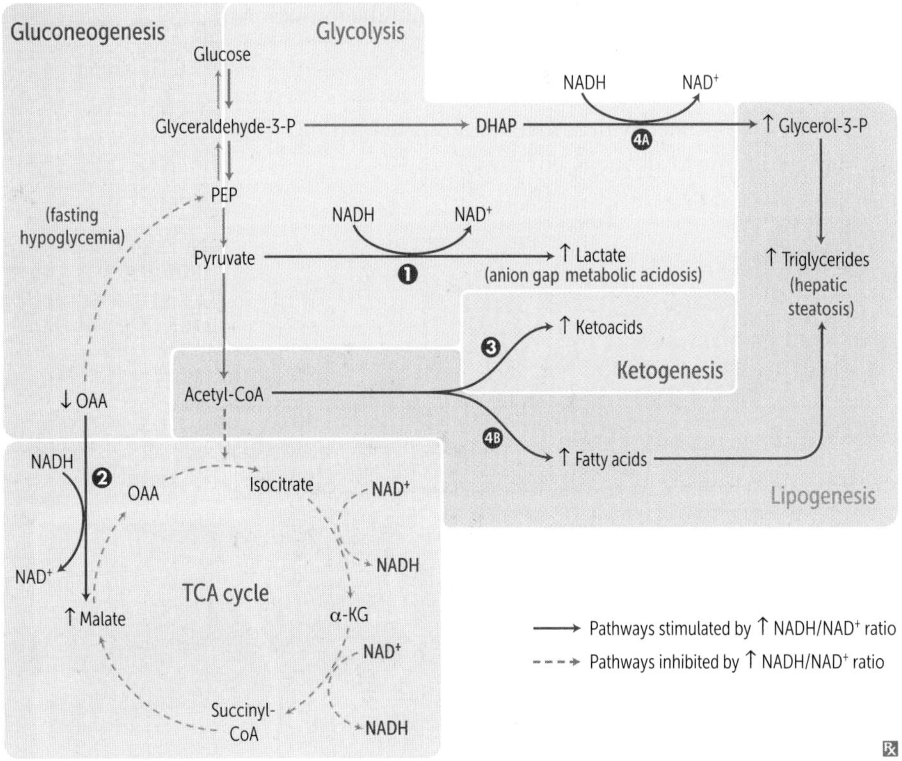

Ethanol metabolism ↑ NADH/NAD$^+$ ratio in liver, causing:

1. Lactic acidosis—↑ pyruvate conversion to lactate
2. Fasting hypoglycemia—↓ gluconeogenesis due to ↑ conversion of OAA to malate
3. Ketoacidosis—diversion of acetyl-CoA into ketogenesis rather than TCA cycle
4. Hepatosteatosis—↑ conversion of DHAP to glycerol-3-P 4A; acetyl-CoA diverges into fatty acid synthesis 4B, which combines with glycerol-3-P to synthesize triglycerides

Fomepizole—blocks alcohol dehydrogenase; preferred antidote for overdoses of methanol or ethylene glycol. Alcohol dehydrogenase has higher affinity for ethanol than for methanol or ethylene glycol → ethanol can be used as competitive inhibitor of alcohol dehydrogenase to treat methanol or ethylene glycol poisoning.

Disulfiram—blocks acetaldehyde dehydrogenase → ↑ acetaldehyde → ↑ hangover symptoms → discouraging drinking.

▸ BIOCHEMISTRY—METABOLISM

Enzyme terminology	An enzyme's name often describes its function. For example, glucokinase is an enzyme that catalyzes the phosphorylation of glucose using a molecule of ATP. The following are commonly used enzyme descriptors.
Kinase	Catalyzes transfer of a phosphate group from a high-energy molecule (usually ATP) to a substrate (eg, phosphofructokinase).
Phosphorylase	Adds inorganic phosphate onto substrate without using ATP (eg, glycogen phosphorylase).
Phosphatase	Removes phosphate group from substrate (eg, fructose-1,6-bisphosphatase 1).
Dehydrogenase	Catalyzes oxidation-reduction reactions (eg, pyruvate dehydrogenase).
Hydroxylase	Adds hydroxyl group (−OH) onto substrate (eg, tyrosine hydroxylase).
Carboxylase	Transfers CO_2 groups with the help of biotin (eg, pyruvate carboxylase).
Mutase	Relocates a functional group within a molecule (eg, vitamin B_{12}–dependent methylmalonyl-CoA mutase).
Synthase/synthetase	Joins two molecules together using a source of energy (eg, ATP, acetyl-CoA, nucleotide sugar).

Rate-determining enzymes of metabolic processes

PROCESS	ENZYME	REGULATORS
Glycolysis	Phosphofructokinase-1 (PFK-1)	AMP ⊕, fructose-2,6-bisphosphate ⊕ ATP ⊖, citrate ⊖
Gluconeogenesis	Fructose-1,6-bisphosphatase 1	AMP ⊖, fructose-2,6-bisphosphate ⊖
TCA cycle	Isocitrate dehydrogenase	ADP ⊕ ATP ⊖, NADH ⊖
Glycogenesis	Glycogen synthase	Glucose-6-phosphate ⊕, insulin ⊕, cortisol ⊕ Epinephrine ⊖, glucagon ⊖
Glycogenolysis	Glycogen phosphorylase	Epinephrine ⊕, glucagon ⊕, AMP ⊕ Glucose-6-phosphate ⊖, insulin ⊖, ATP ⊖
HMP shunt	Glucose-6-phosphate dehydrogenase (G6PD)	$NADP^+$ ⊕ NADPH ⊖
De novo pyrimidine synthesis	Carbamoyl phosphate synthetase II	ATP ⊕, PRPP ⊕ UTP ⊖
De novo purine synthesis	Glutamine-phosphoribosylpyrophosphate (PRPP) amidotransferase	AMP ⊖, inosine monophosphate (IMP) ⊖, GMP ⊖
Urea cycle	Carbamoyl phosphate synthetase I	N-acetylglutamate ⊕
Fatty acid synthesis	Acetyl-CoA carboxylase (ACC)	Insulin ⊕, citrate ⊕ Glucagon ⊖, palmitoyl-CoA ⊖
Fatty acid oxidation	Carnitine acyltransferase I	Malonyl-CoA ⊖
Ketogenesis	HMG-CoA synthase	
Cholesterol synthesis	HMG-CoA reductase	Insulin ⊕, thyroxine ⊕, estrogen ⊕ Glucagon ⊖, cholesterol ⊖

Metabolism sites

Mitochondria	Fatty acid oxidation (β-oxidation), acetyl-CoA production, TCA cycle, oxidative phosphorylation, ketogenesis.
Cytoplasm	Glycolysis, HMP shunt, and synthesis of cholesterol (SER), proteins (ribosomes, RER), fatty acids, and nucleotides.
Both	Heme synthesis, urea cycle, gluconeogenesis. **Hugs take two** (both).

Summary of pathways

1. Galactokinase *(mild galactosemia)*
2. Galactose-1-phosphate uridyltransferase *(severe galactosemia)*
3. Hexokinase/glucokinase
4. Glucose-6-phosphatase *(von Gierke disease)*
5. Glucose-6-phosphate dehydrogenase
6. Transketolase
7. Phosphofructokinase-1
8. Fructose-1,6-bisphosphatase 1
9. Fructokinase *(essential fructosuria)*
10. Aldolase B *(fructose intolerance)*
11. Aldolase B *(liver)*, A *(muscle)*
12. Triose phosphate isomerase
13. Pyruvate kinase
14. Pyruvate dehydrogenase
15. Pyruvate carboxylase
16. PEP carboxykinase
17. Citrate synthase
18. Isocitrate dehydrogenase
19. α-ketoglutarate dehydrogenase
20. Carbamoyl phosphate synthetase I
21. Ornithine transcarbamylase
22. Propionyl-CoA carboxylase
23. HMG-CoA reductase

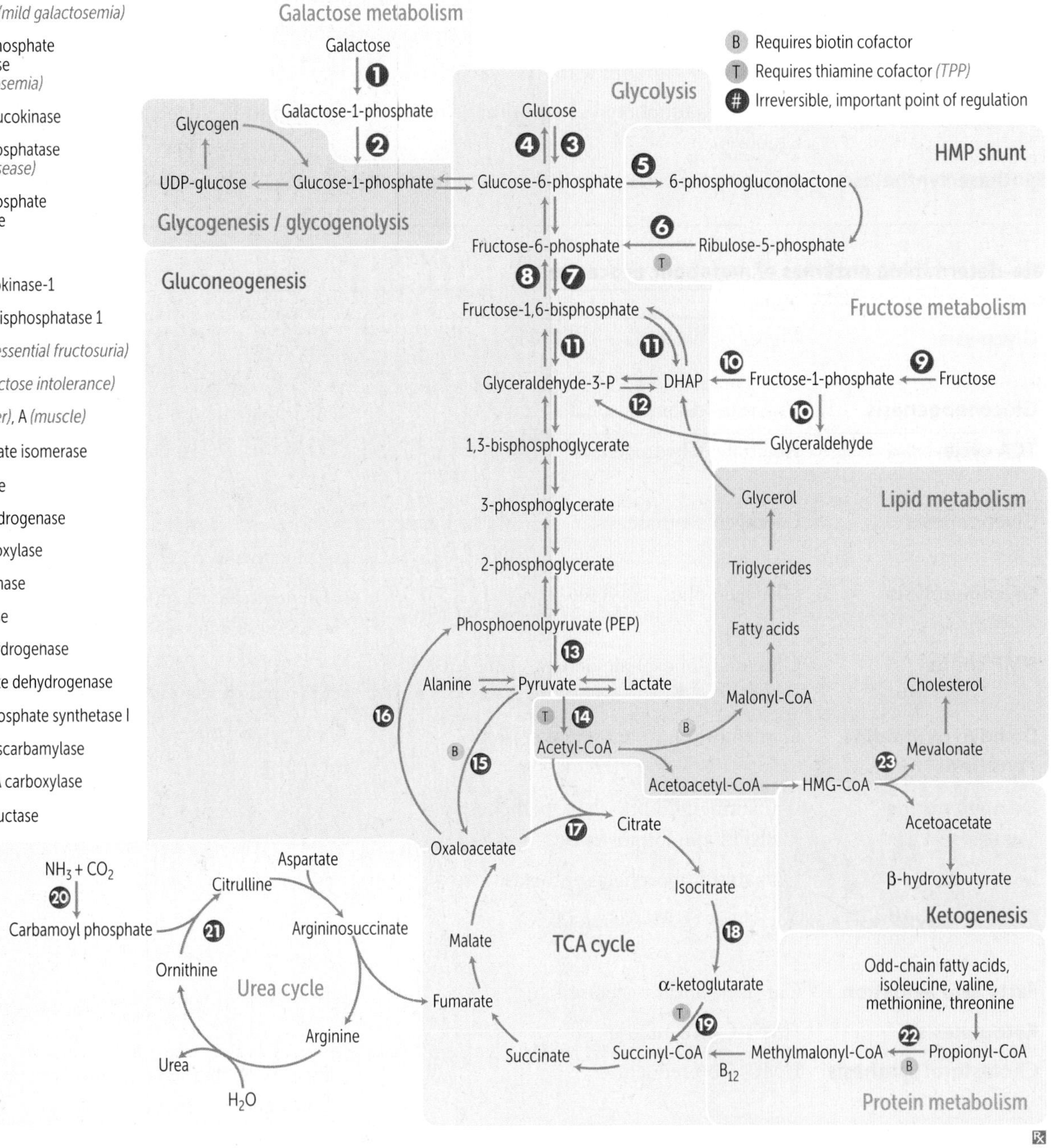

ATP production

Aerobic metabolism of one glucose molecule produces 32 net ATP via malate-aspartate shuttle (heart and liver), 30 net ATP via glycerol-3-phosphate shuttle (muscle).
Anaerobic glycolysis produces only 2 net ATP per glucose molecule.
ATP hydrolysis can be coupled to energetically unfavorable reactions.

Arsenic causes glycolysis to produce zero net ATP.

Activated carriers

CARRIER MOLECULE	CARRIED IN ACTIVATED FORM
ATP	Phosphoryl groups
NADH, NADPH, $FADH_2$	Electrons
CoA, lipoamide	Acyl groups
Biotin	CO_2
Tetrahydrofolates	1-carbon units
S-adenosylmethionine (SAM)	CH_3 groups
TPP	Aldehydes

Universal electron acceptors

Nicotinamides (NAD^+, $NADP^+$ from vitamin B_3) and flavin nucleotides (FAD from vitamin B_2).
NAD^+ is generally used in **catabolic** processes to carry reducing equivalents away as NADH.
NADPH is used in **anabolic** processes (eg, steroid and fatty acid synthesis) as a supply of reducing equivalents.

NADPH is a product of the HMP shunt.
NADPH is used in:
- Anabolic processes
- Respiratory burst
- Cytochrome P-450 system
- Glutathione reductase

Hexokinase vs glucokinase

Phosphorylation of glucose to yield glucose-6-phosphate is catalyzed by glucokinase in the liver and hexokinase in other tissues. Hexokinase sequesters glucose in tissues, where it is used even when glucose concentrations are low. At high glucose concentrations, glucokinase helps to store glucose in liver. Glucokinase deficiency is a cause of maturity onset diabetes of the young (MODY) and gestational diabetes.

	Hexokinase	Glucokinase
Location	Most tissues, except liver and pancreatic β cells	Liver, β cells of pancreas
K_m	Lower (↑ affinity)	Higher (↓ affinity)
V_{max}	Lower (↓ capacity)	Higher (↑ capacity)
Induced by insulin	No	Yes
Feedback inhibition by	Glucose-6-phosphate	Fructose-6-phosphate

Glycolysis regulation, key enzymes

Net glycolysis (cytoplasm):
Glucose + 2 P_i + 2 ADP + 2 NAD^+ → 2 pyruvate + 2 ATP + 2 NADH + 2 H^+ + 2 H_2O.

Equation not balanced chemically, and exact balanced equation depends on ionization state of reactants and products.

REQUIRE ATP	Glucose → Glucose-6-P (Hexokinase/glucokinase)	Glucose-6-P ⊖ hexokinase. Fructose-6-P ⊖ glucokinase.
	Fructose-6-P → Fructose-1,6-BP (Phosphofructokinase-1 (rate-limiting step))	AMP ⊕, fructose-2,6-bisphosphate ⊕. ATP ⊖, citrate ⊖.
PRODUCE ATP	1,3-BPG ⟷ 3-PG (Phosphoglycerate kinase)	
	Phosphoenolpyruvate → Pyruvate (Pyruvate kinase)	Fructose-1,6-bisphosphate ⊕. ATP ⊖, alanine ⊖, glucagon ⊖.

Regulation by fructose-2,6-bisphosphate

Fructose bisphosphatase-2 (FBPase-2) and phosphofructokinase-2 (PFK-2) are the same bifunctional enzyme whose function is reversed by phosphorylation by protein kinase A.

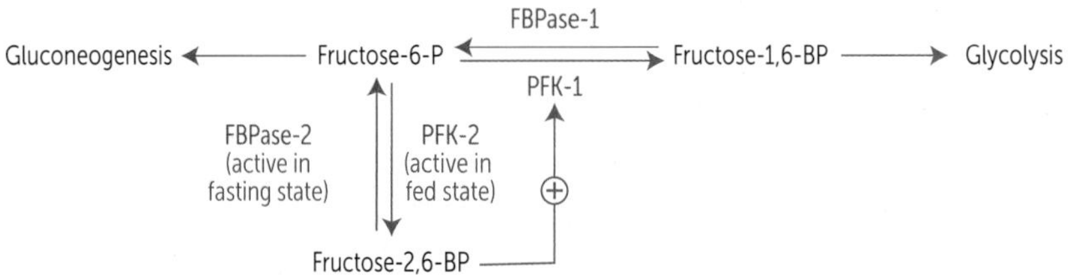

Fasting state: ↑ glucagon → ↑ cAMP → ↑ protein kinase A → ↑ FBPase-2, ↓ PFK-2, less glycolysis, more gluconeogenesis.

FaBian the Peasant (FBP) has to work hard when starving.

Fed state: ↑ insulin → ↓ cAMP → ↓ protein kinase A → ↓ FBPase-2, ↑ PFK-2, more glycolysis, less gluconeogenesis.

Prince FredericK (PFK) works only when fed.

Pyruvate dehydrogenase complex

Mitochondrial enzyme complex linking glycolysis and TCA cycle. Differentially regulated in fed (active)/fasting (inactive) states.
Reaction: pyruvate + NAD^+ + CoA → acetyl-CoA + CO_2 + NADH.
Contains 3 enzymes requiring 5 cofactors:
1. Thiamine pyrophosphate (B_1)
2. Lipoic acid
3. CoA (B_5, pantothenic acid)
4. FAD (B_2, riboflavin)
5. NAD^+ (B_3, niacin)

Activated by: ↑ NAD^+/NADH ratio, ↑ ADP ↑ Ca^{2+}.

The complex is similar to the α-ketoglutarate dehydrogenase complex (same cofactors, similar substrate and action), which converts α-ketoglutarate → succinyl-CoA (TCA cycle).

The lovely coenzymes for nerds.
Arsenic inhibits lipoic acid. Arsenic poisoning clinical findings: imagine a vampire (pigmentary skin changes, skin cancer), vomiting and having diarrhea, running away from a cutie (QT prolongation) with garlic breath.

Pyruvate dehydrogenase complex deficiency	Causes a buildup of pyruvate that gets shunted to lactate (via LDH) and alanine (via ALT). X-linked.
FINDINGS	Neurologic defects, lactic acidosis, ↑ serum alanine starting in infancy.
TREATMENT	↑ intake of ketogenic nutrients (eg, high fat content or ↑ lysine and leucine).

Pyruvate metabolism

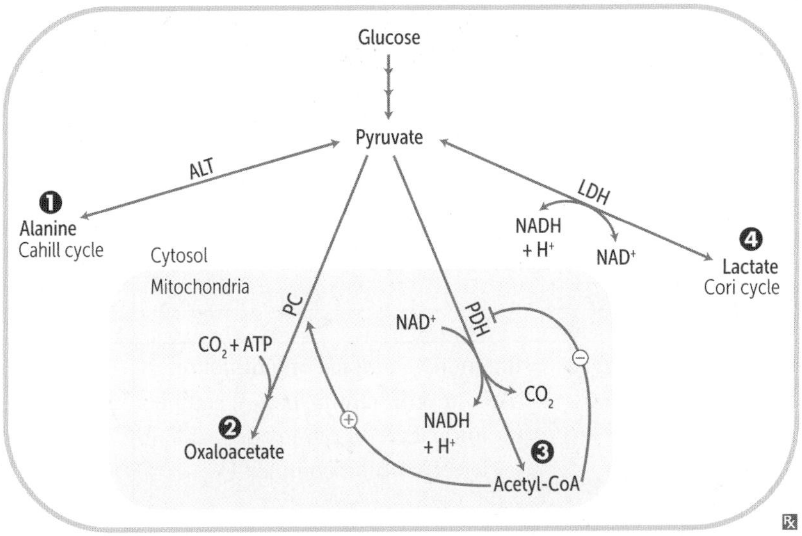
Glucose
Pyruvate
ALT
LDH
❶
Alanine
Cahill cycle
Cytosol
Mitochondria
PC
NADH
+ H+
NAD+
❹
Lactate
Cori cycle
NAD+
PDH
CO2 + ATP
CO2
❷
Oxaloacetate
NADH
+ H+
❸
Acetyl-CoA

Functions of different pyruvate metabolic pathways (and their associated cofactors):

❶ Alanine aminotransferase (B_6): alanine carries amino groups to the liver from muscle

❷ Pyruvate carboxylase (B_7): oxaloacetate can replenish TCA cycle or be used in gluconeogenesis

❸ Pyruvate dehydrogenase (B_1, B_2, B_3, B_5, lipoic acid): transition from glycolysis to the TCA cycle

❹ Lactic acid dehydrogenase (B_3): end of anaerobic glycolysis (major pathway in RBCs, WBCs, kidney medulla, lens, testes, and cornea)

TCA cycle

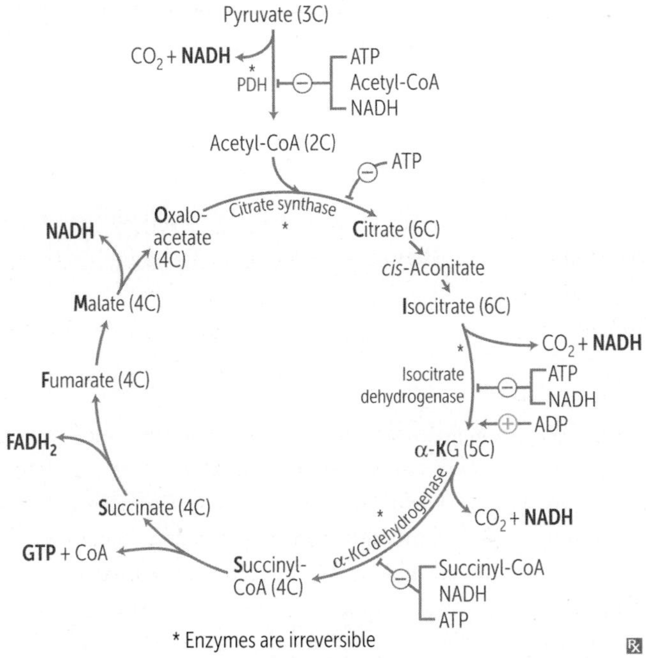
Pyruvate (3C)
CO2 + NADH
PDH
ATP
Acetyl-CoA
NADH
Acetyl-CoA (2C)
ATP
Citrate synthase
Oxalo-
acetate
(4C)
NADH
Citrate (6C)
cis-Aconitate
Malate (4C)
Isocitrate (6C)
CO2 + NADH
Fumarate (4C)
Isocitrate
dehydrogenase
ATP
NADH
ADP
FADH2
α-KG (5C)
Succinate (4C)
α-KG dehydrogenase
CO2 + NADH
GTP + CoA
Succinyl-
CoA (4C)
Succinyl-CoA
NADH
ATP
* Enzymes are irreversible

Also called Krebs cycle. Pyruvate → acetyl-CoA produces 1 NADH, 1 CO_2.

The TCA cycle produces 3 NADH, 1 $FADH_2$, 2 CO_2, 1 GTP per acetyl-CoA = 10 ATP/acetyl-CoA (2× everything per glucose). TCA cycle reactions occur in the mitochondria.

α-ketoglutarate dehydrogenase complex requires the same cofactors as the pyruvate dehydrogenase complex (vitamins B_1, B_2, B_3, B_5, lipoic acid).

Citrate is Krebs' starting substrate for making oxaloacetate.

Electron transport chain and oxidative phosphorylation

NADH electrons from glycolysis enter mitochondria via the malate-aspartate or glycerol-3-phosphate shuttle. $FADH_2$ electrons are transferred to complex II (at a lower energy level than NADH). The passage of electrons results in the formation of a proton gradient that, coupled to oxidative phosphorylation, drives the production of ATP.

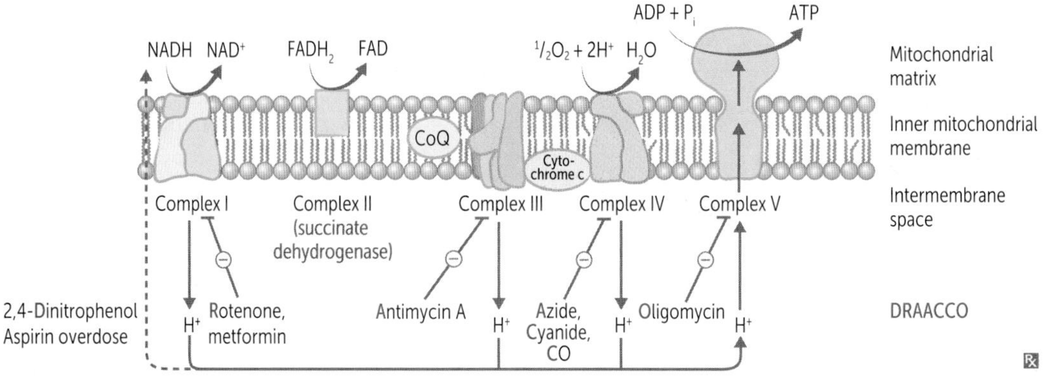

ATP PRODUCED VIA ATP SYNTHASE		
	1 NADH → 2.5 ATP; 1 $FADH_2$ → 1.5 ATP.	

OXIDATIVE PHOSPHORYLATION POISONS		
Electron transport inhibitors	Directly inhibit electron transport, causing a ↓ proton gradient and block of ATP synthesis.	Rotenone: complex one inhibitor. "An-3-mycin" (antimycin) A: complex 3 inhibitor. Cyanide, carbon monoxide, azide (the -ides, 4 letters) inhibit complex IV.
ATP synthase inhibitors	Directly inhibit mitochondrial ATP synthase, causing an ↑ proton gradient. No ATP is produced because electron transport stops.	Oligomycin.
Uncoupling agents	↑ permeability of membrane, causing a ↓ proton gradient and ↑ O_2 consumption. ATP synthesis stops, but electron transport continues. Produces heat.	2,4-Dinitrophenol (used illicitly for weight loss), aspirin (fevers often occur after overdose), thermogenin in brown fat (has more mitochondria than white fat).

Gluconeogenesis, irreversible enzymes		Pathway produces fresh glucose.
Pyruvate carboxylase	In mitochondria. Pyruvate → oxaloacetate.	Requires biotin, ATP. Activated by acetyl-CoA.
Phosphoenolpyruvate carboxykinase	In cytosol. Oxaloacetate → phosphoenolpyruvate (PEP).	Requires GTP.
Fructose-1,6-bisphosphatase 1	In cytosol. Fructose-1,6-bisphosphate → fructose-6-phosphate.	Citrate ⊕, AMP ⊖, fructose 2,6-bisphosphate ⊖.
Glucose-6-phosphatase	In ER. Glucose-6-phosphate → glucose.	

Occurs primarily in liver; serves to maintain euglycemia during fasting. Enzymes also found in kidney, intestinal epithelium. Deficiency of the key gluconeogenic enzymes causes hypoglycemia. (Muscle cannot participate in gluconeogenesis because it lacks glucose-6-phosphatase).

Odd-chain **fatty acids** yield 1 propionyl-CoA during metabolism, which can enter the TCA cycle (as succinyl-CoA), undergo gluconeogenesis, and serve as a **glucose** source (It's **odd** for **fatty acids** to make **glucose**). Even-chain fatty acids cannot produce new glucose, since they yield only acetyl-CoA equivalents.

Pentose phosphate pathway

Also called HMP shunt. Provides a source of NADPH from abundantly available glucose-6-P (NADPH is required for reductive reactions, eg, glutathione reduction inside RBCs, fatty acid and cholesterol biosynthesis). Additionally, this pathway yields ribose for nucleotide synthesis. Two distinct phases (oxidative and nonoxidative), both of which occur in the cytoplasm. No ATP is used or produced.

Sites: lactating mammary glands, liver, adrenal cortex (sites of fatty acid or steroid synthesis), RBCs.

REACTIONS

Oxidative (irreversible)

Nonoxidative (reversible)

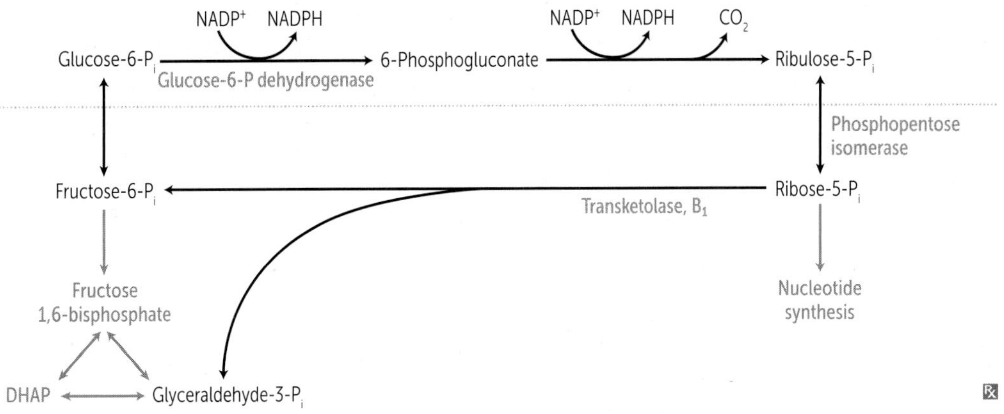

Glucose-6-phosphate dehydrogenase deficiency

NADPH is necessary to keep glutathione reduced, which in turn detoxifies free radicals and peroxides. ↓ NADPH in RBCs leads to hemolytic anemia due to poor RBC defense against oxidizing agents (eg, fava beans, sulfonamides, nitrofurantoin, primaquine/chloroquine, antituberculosis drugs). Infection (most common cause) can also precipitate hemolysis; inflammatory response produces free radicals that diffuse into RBCs, causing oxidative damage.

X-linked recessive disorder; most common human enzyme deficiency; more prevalent among descendants of populations in malaria-endemic regions (eg, sub-Saharan Africa, Southeast Asia).

Heinz bodies—denatured globin chains precipitate within RBCs due to oxidative stress.

Bite cells—result from the phagocytic removal of **Heinz** bodies by splenic macrophages. Think, "**Bite** into some **Heinz** ketchup."

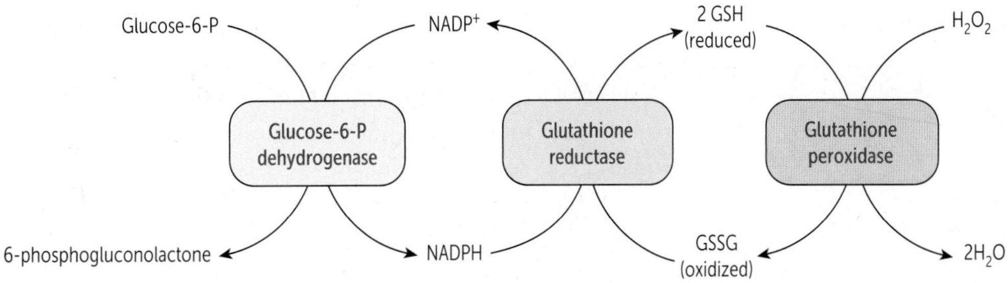

Disorders of fructose metabolism

Essential fructosuria	Involves a defect in **fructokinase**. Autosomal recessive. A benign, asymptomatic condition (fructokinase deficiency is kinder), since fructose is not trapped in cells. Hexokinase becomes 1° pathway for converting fructose to fructose-6-phosphate. Symptoms: fructose appears in blood and urine. Disorders of fructose metabolism cause milder symptoms than analogous disorders of galactose metabolism.
Hereditary fructose intolerance	Hereditary deficiency of **aldolase B**. Autosomal recessive. Fructose-1-phosphate accumulates, causing a ↓ in available phosphate, which results in inhibition of glycogenolysis and gluconeogenesis. Symptoms present following consumption of fruit, juice, or honey. Urine dipstick will be ⊖ (tests for glucose only); reducing sugar can be detected in the urine (nonspecific test for inborn errors of carbohydrate metabolism). Symptoms: hypoglycemia, jaundice, cirrhosis, vomiting. Treatment: ↓ intake of fructose, sucrose (glucose + fructose), and sorbitol (metabolized to fructose).

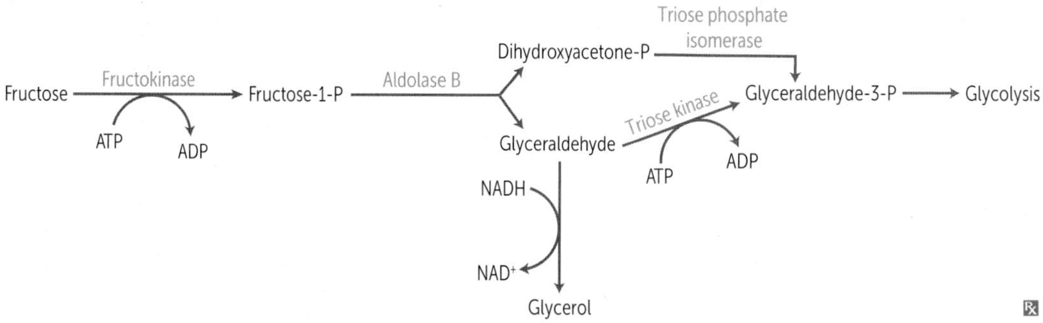

Disorders of galactose metabolism

Galactokinase deficiency	Hereditary deficiency of **galactokinase**. Galactitol accumulates if galactose is present in diet. Relatively mild condition. Autosomal recessive. Symptoms: galactose appears in blood (galactosemia) and urine (galactosuria); infantile cataracts. May present as failure to track objects or to develop a social smile. Galacto**k**inase deficiency is **k**inder (benign condition).
Classic galactosemia	Absence of **galactose-1-phosphate uridyltransferase**. Autosomal recessive. Damage is caused by accumulation of toxic substances (including galactitol, which accumulates in the lens of the eye). Symptoms develop when infant begins feeding (lactose present in breast milk and routine formula) and include failure to thrive, jaundice, hepatomegaly, infantile cataracts, intellectual disability. Can predispose to *E coli* sepsis in neonates. Treatment: exclude galactose and lactose (galactose + glucose) from diet.

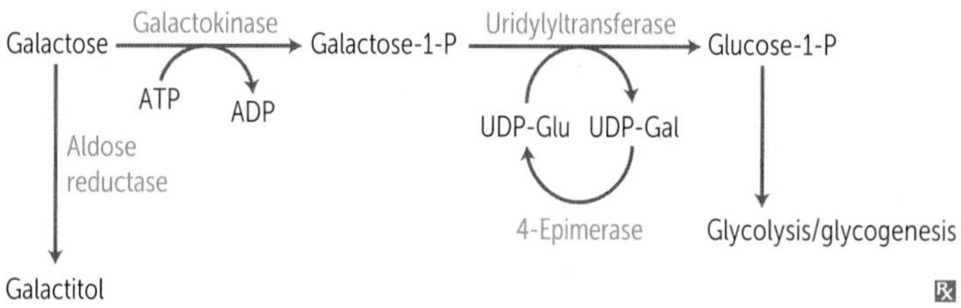

Fructose is to **A**ldolase **B** as **G**alactose is to **U**ridyl**T**ransferase (**FAB GUT**).
The more serious defects lead to PO_4^{3-} depletion.

Sorbitol

An alternative method of trapping glucose in the cell is to convert it to its alcohol counterpart, sorbitol, via aldose reductase. Some tissues then convert sorbitol to fructose using sorbitol dehydrogenase; tissues with an insufficient amount/activity of this enzyme are at risk of intracellular sorbitol accumulation, causing osmotic damage (eg, cataracts, retinopathy, and peripheral neuropathy seen with chronic hyperglycemia in diabetes).

High blood levels of galactose also result in conversion to the osmotically active galactitol via aldose reductase.

Liver, ovaries, and seminal vesicles have both enzymes (they **lose** sorbitol).

$$\text{Glucose} \xrightarrow[\text{NADPH}]{\text{Aldose reductase}} \text{Sorbitol} \xrightarrow[\text{NAD}^+]{\text{Sorbitol dehydrogenase}} \text{Fructose}$$

Lens has primarily **A**ldose reductase. **R**etina, **K**idneys, and **S**chwann cells have only aldose reductase (**LARKS**).

Lactase deficiency

Insufficient lactase enzyme → dietary lactose intolerance. Lactase functions on the intestinal brush border to digest lactose (in milk and milk products) into glucose and galactose.

Primary: age-dependent decline after childhood (absence of lactase-persistent allele), common in people of Asian, African, or Native American descent.

Secondary: loss of intestinal brush border due to gastroenteritis (eg, rotavirus), autoimmune disease.

Congenital lactase deficiency: rare, due to defective gene.

Stool demonstrates ↓ pH and breath shows ↑ hydrogen content with lactose hydrogen breath test (H^+ is produced when colonic bacteria ferment undigested lactose). Intestinal biopsy reveals normal mucosa in patients with hereditary lactose intolerance.

FINDINGS: Bloating, cramps, flatulence, osmotic diarrhea.

TREATMENT: Avoid dairy products or add lactase pills to diet; lactose-free milk.

Amino acids

Only L-amino acids are found in proteins.

Essential

PVT TIM HaLL: **P**henylalanine, **V**aline, **T**ryptophan, **T**hreonine, **I**soleucine, **M**ethionine, **H**istidine, **L**eucine, **L**ysine.

Glucogenic: **Met**hionine, **his**tidine, **val**ine. We **met his val**entine, who is so **sweet** (**gluco**genic).

Glucogenic/ketogenic: Isoleucine, phenylalanine, threonine, tryptophan.

Ketogenic: leucine, lysine. The only purely ketogenic amino acids.

Acidic

Aspartic **acid**, glutamic **acid**.

Negatively charged at body pH.

Basic

Arginine, **his**tidine, **lys**ine.

Arginine is most **basic**. Histidine has no charge at body pH.

Arginine and histidine are required during periods of growth.

Arginine and lysine are ↑ in histones which bind negatively charged DNA.

His lys (lies) **are basic**.

Urea cycle

Amino acid catabolism generates common metabolites (eg, pyruvate, acetyl-CoA), which serve as metabolic fuels. Excess nitrogen is converted to urea and excreted by the kidneys.

Ordinarily, Careless Crappers Are Also Frivolous About Urination.

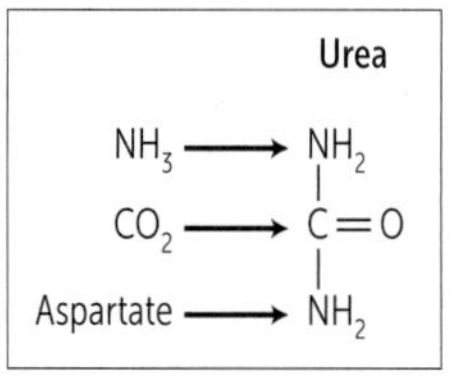

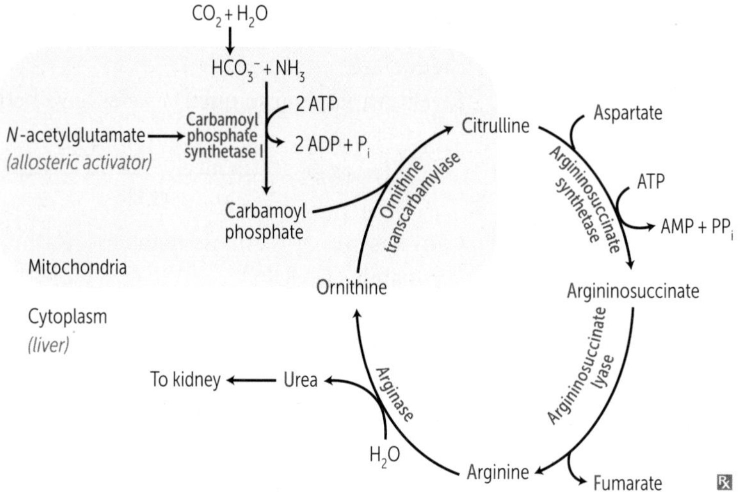

Transport of ammonia by alanine

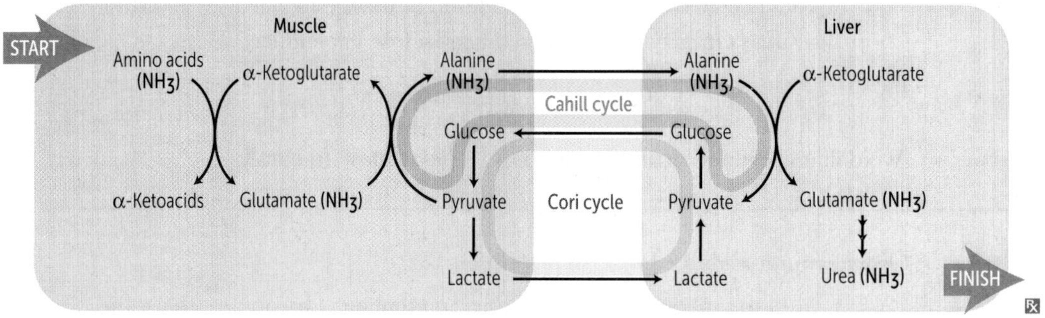

Hyperammonemia

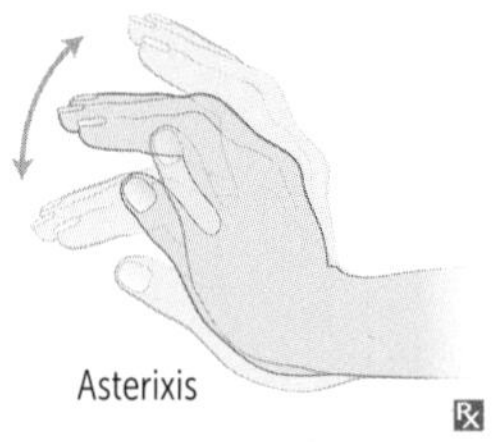

Can be acquired (eg, liver disease) or hereditary (eg, urea cycle enzyme deficiencies).

Presents with flapping tremor (asterixis), slurring of speech, somnolence, vomiting, cerebral edema, blurring of vision.

↑ NH_3 changes relative amounts of α-ketoglutarate, glutamate, GABA, and glutamine to favor ↑ glutamine. CNS toxicity may involve ↓ GABA, ↓ α-ketoglutarate, TCA cycle inhibition, and cerebral edema due to glutamine-induced osmotic shifts.

Treatment: limit protein in diet.

May be given to ↓ ammonia levels:

- Lactulose to acidify GI tract and trap NH_4^+ for excretion.
- Antibiotics (eg, rifaximin, neomycin) to ↓ ammoniagenic bacteria.
- Benzoate, phenylacetate, or phenylbutyrate react with glycine or glutamine, forming products that are excreted renally.

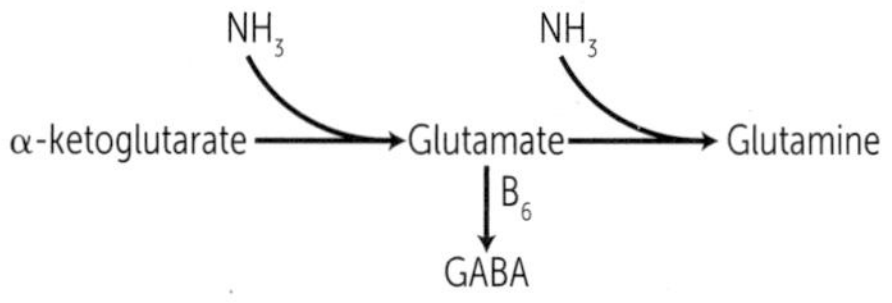

Ornithine transcarbamylase deficiency

Most common urea cycle disorder. X-linked recessive (vs other urea cycle enzyme deficiencies, which are autosomal recessive). Interferes with the body's ability to eliminate ammonia. Often evident in the first few days of life, but may present later. Excess carbamoyl phosphate is converted to orotic acid (part of the pyrimidine synthesis pathway).

Findings: ↑ orotic acid in blood and urine, ↓ BUN, symptoms of hyperammonemia. No megaloblastic anemia (vs orotic aciduria).

Amino acid derivatives

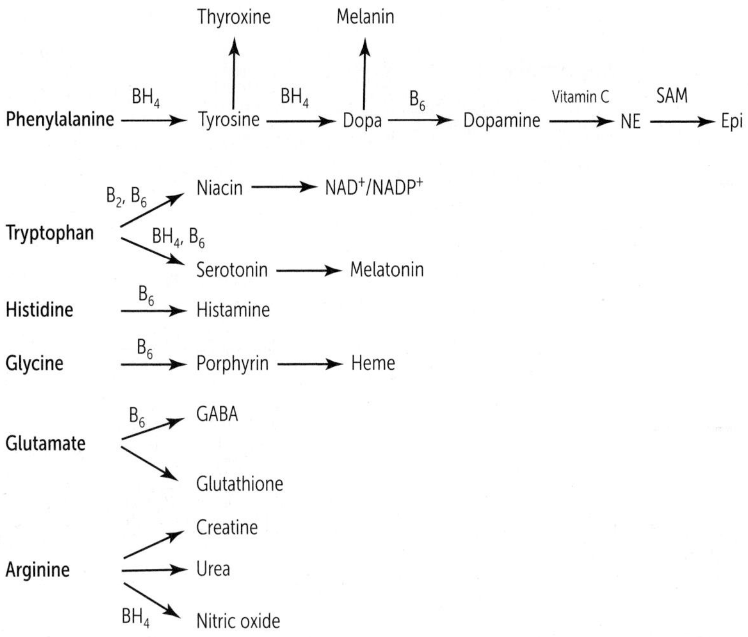

BH_4 = tetrahydrobiopterin

Catecholamine synthesis/tyrosine catabolism

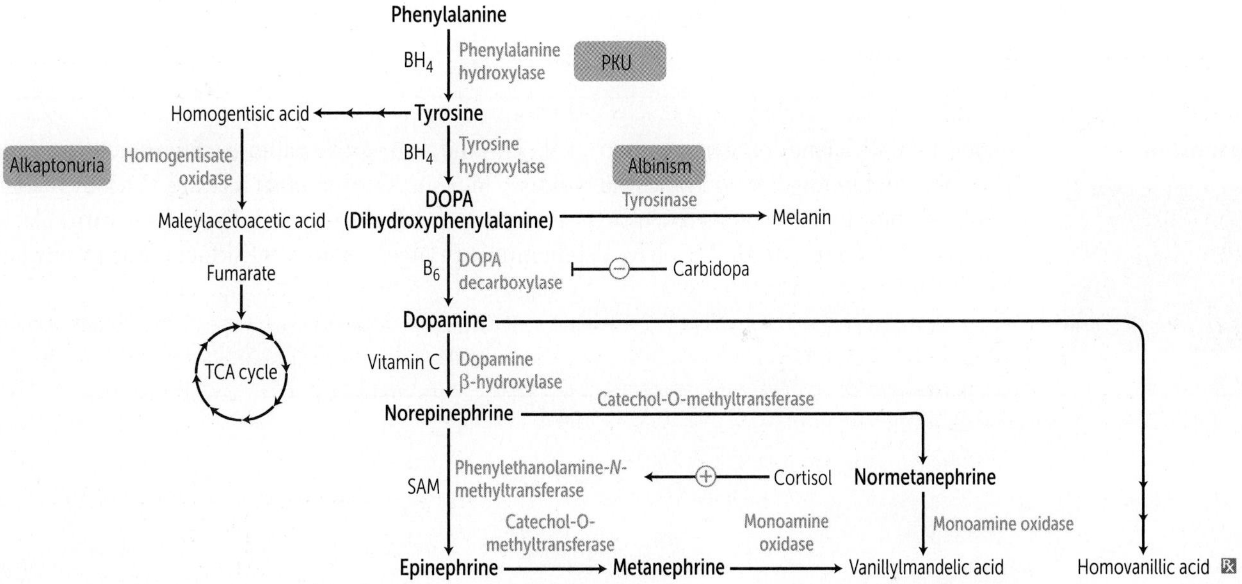

Phenylketonuria

Caused by ↓ phenylalanine hydroxylase or ↓ tetrahydrobiopterin (BH_4) cofactor (malignant PKU). Tyrosine becomes essential. ↑ phenylalanine → ↑ phenyl ketones in urine.

Findings: intellectual disability, microcephaly, seizures, hypopigmented skin, eczema, musty body odor.

Treatment: ↓ phenylalanine and ↑ tyrosine in diet, tetrahydrobiopterin supplementation.

Maternal PKU—due to elevated maternal phenylalanine levels. Can be prevented by dietary intake. Findings in infant: microcephaly, intellectual disability, growth restriction, congenital heart defects.

Autosomal recessive. Incidence ≈ 1:10,000.

Screening occurs 2–3 days after birth (normal at birth because of maternal enzyme during fetal life).

Phenyl ketones—phenylacetate, phenyllactate, and phenylpyruvate.

Disorder of **aromatic** amino acid metabolism → musty body **odor.**

PKU patients must avoid the artificial sweetener aspartame, which contains phenylalanine.

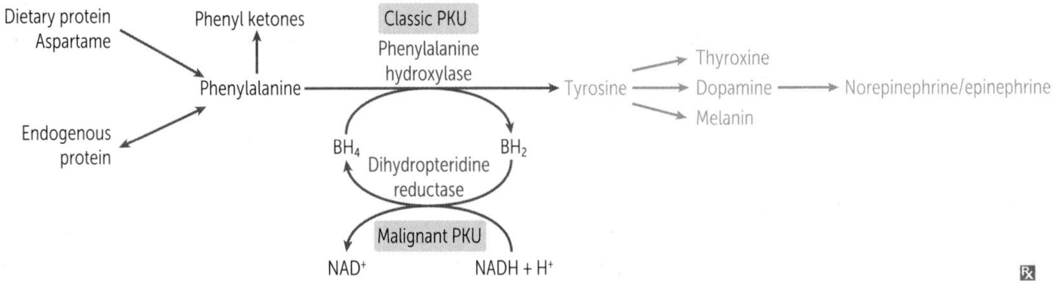

Maple syrup urine disease

Blocked degradation of **branched** amino acids (**I**soleucine, **l**eucine, **v**aline) due to ↓ branched-chain α-ketoacid dehydrogenase (B_1). Causes ↑ α-ketoacids in the blood, especially those of leucine.

Treatment: restriction of isoleucine, leucine, valine in diet, and thiamine supplementation.

Autosomal recessive.

Presentation: vomiting, poor feeding, urine smells like maple syrup/burnt sugar. Causes progressive neurological decline.

I love **V**ermont **maple syrup** from maple trees (with **B**$_1$**ranches**).

Alkaptonuria

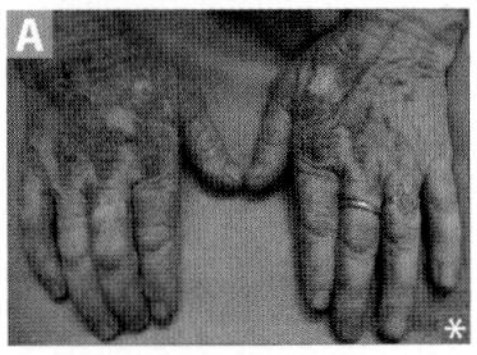

Congenital deficiency of homogentisate oxidase in the degradative pathway of tyrosine to fumarate → pigment-forming homogentisic acid builds up in tissue A. Autosomal recessive. Usually benign.

Findings: bluish-black connective tissue, ear cartilage, and sclerae (ochronosis); urine turns black on prolonged exposure to air. May have debilitating arthralgias (homogentisic acid toxic to cartilage).

Homocystinuria

Causes (all autosomal recessive):
- Cystathionine synthase deficiency (treatment: ↓ methionine, ↑ cysteine, ↑ B_6, B_{12}, and folate in diet)
- ↓ affinity of cystathionine synthase for pyridoxal phosphate (treatment: ↑↑ B_6 and ↑ cysteine in diet)
- Methionine synthase (homocysteine methyltransferase) deficiency (treatment: ↑ methionine in diet)
- Methylenetetrahydrofolate reductase (MTHFR) deficiency (treatment: ↑ folate in diet)

All forms result in excess homocysteine.
HOMOCYstinuria: ↑↑ Homocysteine in urine, Osteoporosis, Marfanoid habitus, Ocular changes (downward and inward lens subluxation), Cardiovascular effects (thrombosis and atherosclerosis → stroke and MI), kYphosis, intellectual disability, hypopigmented skin. In homocystinuria, lens subluxes "down and in" (vs Marfan, "up and fans out").

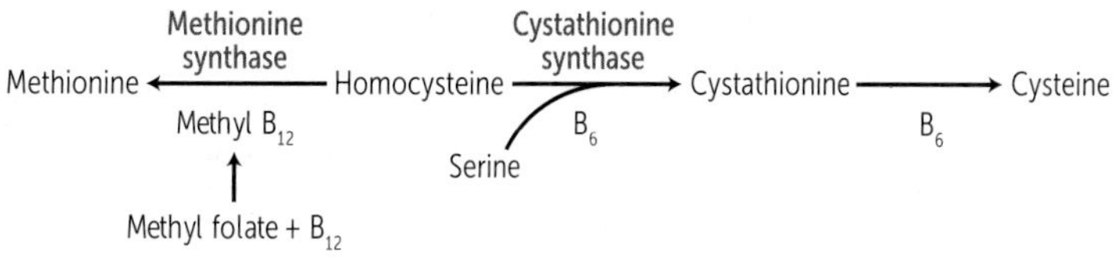

Cystinuria

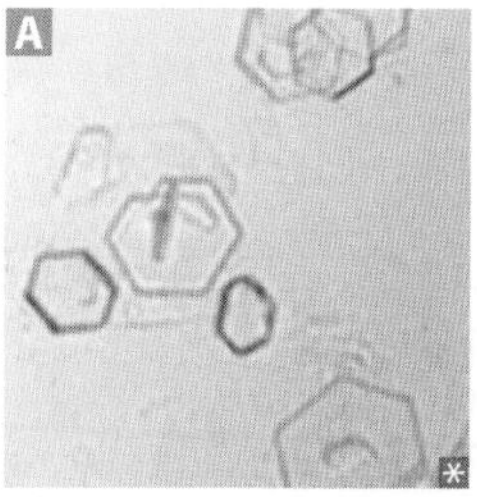

Hereditary defect of renal PCT and intestinal amino acid transporter that prevents reabsorption of Cystine, Ornithine, Lysine, and Arginine (COLA).
Cystine is made of 2 cysteines connected by a disulfide bond.
Excess cystine in the urine can lead to recurrent precipitation of hexagonal cystine stones A.
Treatment: urinary alkalinization (eg, potassium citrate, acetazolamide) and chelating agents (eg, penicillamine) ↑ solubility of cystine stones; good hydration; diet low in methionine.

Autosomal recessive. Common (1:7000).
Cystinuria detected with urinary sodium-cyanide nitroprusside test and proton nuclear magnetic resonance spectroscopy of urine.

Organic acidemias

Most commonly present in infancy with poor feeding, vomiting, hypotonia, high anion gap metabolic acidosis, hepatomegaly, seizures. Organic acid accumulation:
- Inhibits gluconeogenesis → ↓ fasting blood glucose levels, ↑ ketoacidosis → high anion gap metabolic acidosis
- Inhibits urea cycle → hyperammonemia

Propionic acidemia

Deficiency of propionyl-CoA carboxylase → ↑ propionyl-CoA, ↓ methylmalonic acid.

Methylmalonic acidemia

Deficiency of methylmalonyl-CoA mutase or vitamin B_{12}.

Treatment (propionic and methylmalonic acidemia): low-protein diet limited in substances that metabolize into propionyl-CoA: Valine, Odd-chain fatty acids, Methionine, Isoleucine, Threonine (VOMIT).

Glycogen regulation by insulin and glucagon/epinephrine

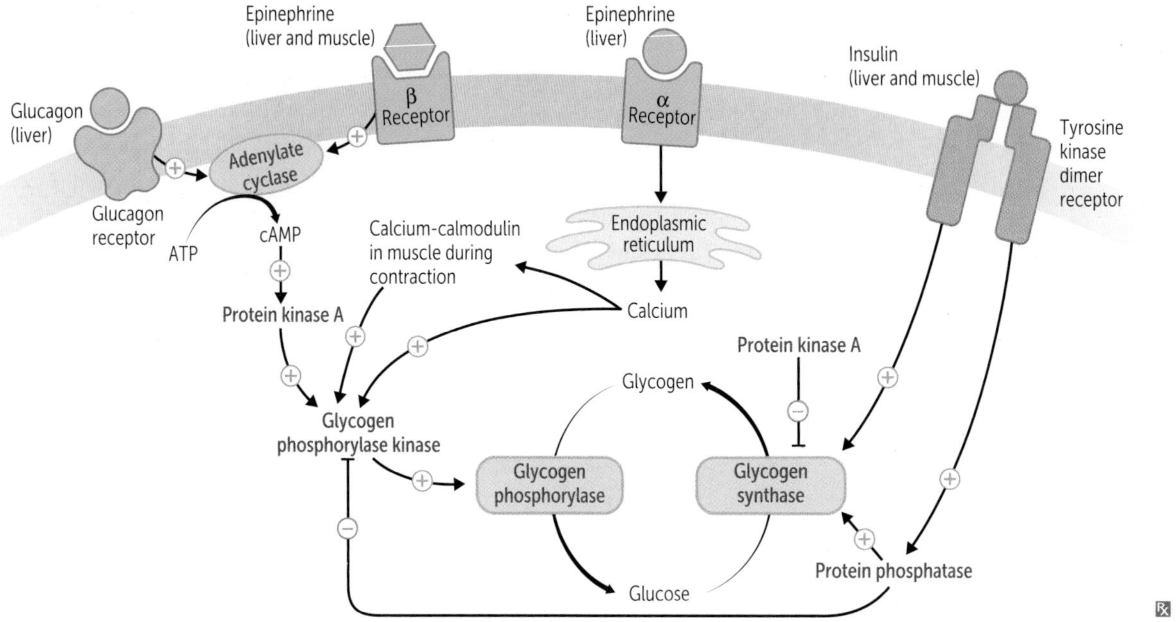

Glycogen	Branches have α-(1,6) bonds; linkages have α-(1,4) bonds.
Skeletal muscle	Glycogen undergoes glycogenolysis → glucose-1-phosphate → glucose-6-phosphate, which is rapidly metabolized during exercise.
Hepatocytes	Glycogen is stored and undergoes glycogenolysis to maintain blood sugar at appropriate levels. Glycogen phosphorylase ❹ liberates glucose-1-phosphate residues off branched glycogen until 4 glucose units remain on a branch. Then 4-α-D-glucanotransferase (debranching enzyme ❺) moves 3 of the 4 glucose units from the branch to the linkage. Then α-1,6-glucosidase (debranching enzyme ❻) cleaves off the last residue, liberating glucose. "Limit dextrin" refers to the two to four residues remaining on a branch after glycogen phosphorylase has already shortened it.

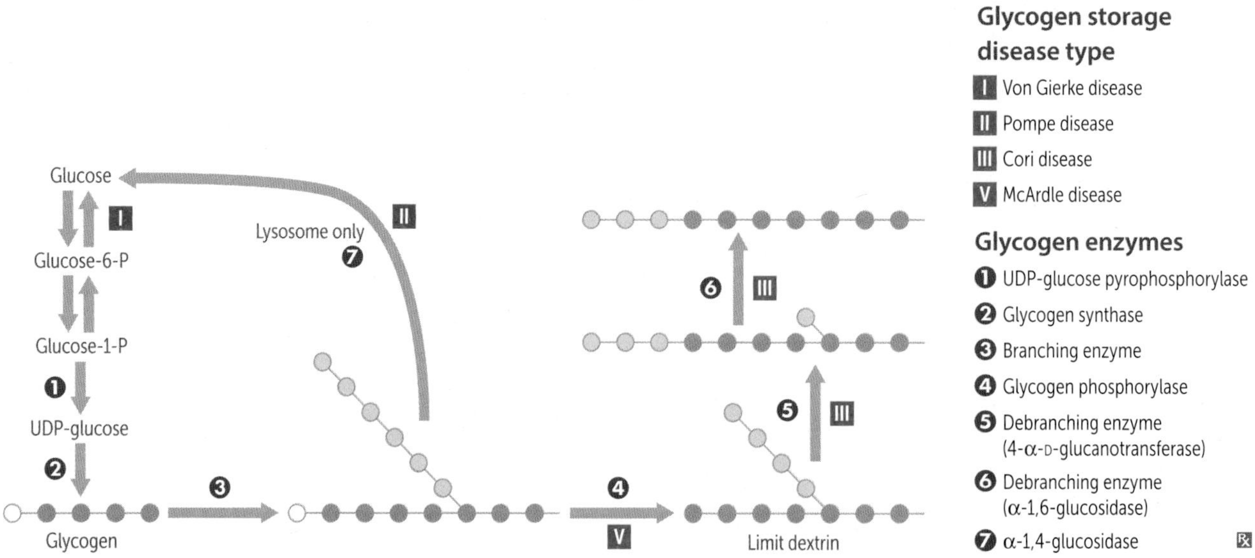

Note: A small amount of glycogen is degraded in lysosomes by ❼ α-1,4-glucosidase (acid maltase).

Glycogen storage diseases

At least 15 types have been identified, all resulting in abnormal glycogen metabolism and an accumulation of glycogen within cells. Periodic acid–Schiff stain identifies glycogen and is useful in identifying these diseases.

Vice president can't accept money.
Types I-V are autosomal recessive.
Andersen: Branching.
Cori: Debranching. (ABCD)

DISEASE	FINDINGS	DEFICIENT ENZYME	COMMENTS
Von Gierke disease (type I)	Severe fasting hypoglycemia, ↑↑ Glycogen in liver and kidneys, ↑ blood lactate, ↑ triglycerides, ↑ uric acid (Gout), and hepatomegaly, renomegaly. Liver does not regulate blood glucose.	Glucose-6-phosphatase.	Treatment: frequent oral glucose/cornstarch; avoidance of fructose and galactose. Impaired gluconeogenesis and glycogenolysis.
Pompe disease (type II)	Cardiomyopathy, hypotonia, exercise intolerance, and systemic findings lead to early death.	Lysosomal acid α-1,4-glucosidase (acid maltase) with α-1,6-glucosidase activity.	Pompe trashes the pump (1st and 4th letter; heart, liver, and muscle).
Cori disease (type III)	Similar to von Gierke disease, but milder symptoms and normal blood lactate levels. Can lead to cardiomyopathy. Limit dextrin–like structures accumulate in cytosol.	Debranching enzymes (α-1,6-glucosidase and 4-α-D-glucanotransferase).	Gluconeogenesis is intact.
Andersen disease (type IV)	Most commonly presents with hepatosplenomegaly and failure to thrive in early infancy. Other findings include infantile cirrhosis, muscular weakness, hypotonia, cardiomyopathy early childhood death.	Branching enzyme. Neuromuscular form can present at any age.	Hypoglycemia occurs late in the disease.
McArdle disease (type V)	↑ glycogen in muscle, but muscle cannot break it down → painful muscle cramps, myoglobinuria (red urine) with strenuous exercise, and arrhythmia from electrolyte abnormalities. Second-wind phenomenon noted during exercise due to ↑ muscular blood flow.	Skeletal muscle glycogen phosphorylase (myophosphorylase). Characterized by a flat venous lactate curve with normal rise in ammonia levels during exercise.	Blood glucose levels typically unaffected. McArdle = muscle.

Lysosomal storage diseases

Lysosomal enzyme deficiency → accumulation of abnormal metabolic products. ↑ incidence of Tay-Sachs, Niemann-Pick, and some forms of Gaucher disease in Ashkenazi Jews.

DISEASE	FINDINGS	DEFICIENT ENZYME	ACCUMULATED SUBSTRATE	INHERITANCE
Sphingolipidoses				
Tay-Sachs disease 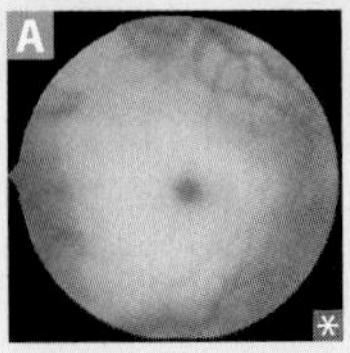	Progressive neurodegeneration, developmental delay, hyperreflexia, hyperacusis, "cherry-red" spot on macula A (lipid accumulation in ganglion cell layer), lysosomes with onion skin, no hepatosplenomegaly (vs Niemann-Pick).	❶ Hexosaminidase A ("TAy-Sax").	GM_2 ganglioside.	AR
Fabry disease 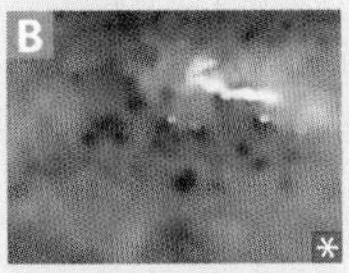	Early: triad of episodic peripheral neuropathy, angiokeratomas B, hypohidrosis. Late: progressive renal failure, cardiovascular disease.	❷ α-galactosidase A.	Ceramide trihexoside (globotriaosylceramide).	XR
Metachromatic leukodystrophy	Central and peripheral demyelination with ataxia, dementia.	❸ Arylsulfatase A.	Cerebroside sulfate.	AR
Krabbe disease	Peripheral neuropathy, destruction of oligodendrocytes, developmental delay, optic atrophy, globoid cells.	❹ Galactocerebrosidase (galactosylceramidase).	Galactocerebroside, psychosine.	AR
Gaucher disease 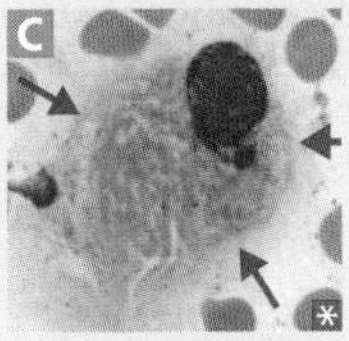	Most common. Hepatosplenomegaly, pancytopenia, osteoporosis, avascular necrosis of femur, bone crises, Gaucher cells C (lipid-laden macrophages resembling crumpled tissue paper).	❺ Glucocerebrosidase (β-glucosidase); treat with recombinant glucocerebrosidase.	Glucocerebroside.	AR
Niemann-Pick disease 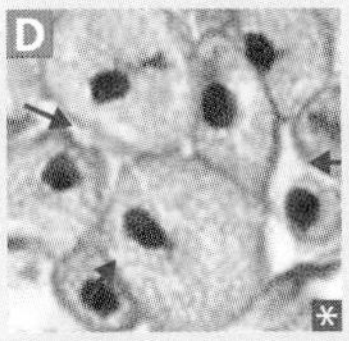	Progressive neurodegeneration, hepatosplenomegaly, foam cells (lipid-laden macrophages) D, "cherry-red" spot on macula A.	❻ Sphingomyelinase.	Sphingomyelin.	AR
Mucopolysaccharidoses				
Hurler syndrome	Developmental delay, skeletal abnormalities, airway obstruction, corneal clouding, hepatosplenomegaly.	α-L-iduronidase.	Heparan sulfate, dermatan sulfate.	AR
Hunter syndrome	Mild Hurler + aggressive behavior, no corneal clouding.	Iduronate-2 (two)-sulfatase.	Heparan sulfate, dermatan sulfate.	XR

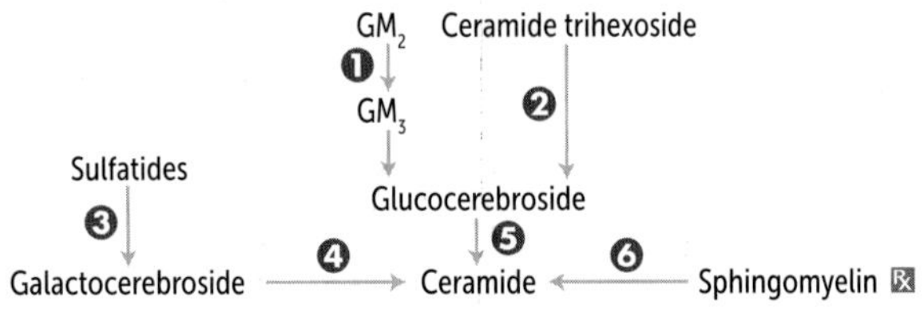

Hunters see clearly (no corneal clouding) and aggressively aim for the **X** (X-linked recessive).

Fatty acid metabolism

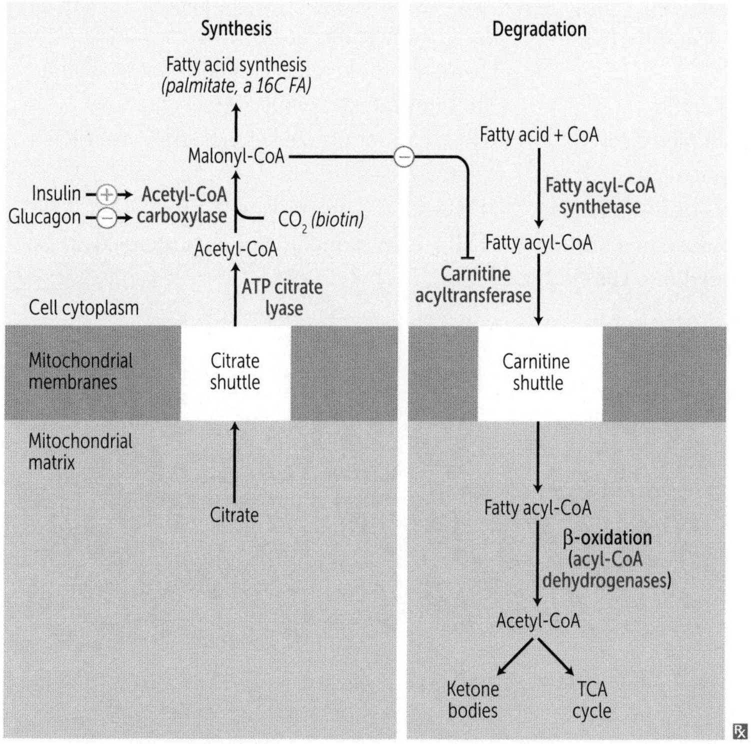

Fatty acid synthesis requires transport of citrate from mitochondria to cytosol. Predominantly occurs in liver, lactating mammary glands, and adipose tissue.

Long-chain fatty acid (LCFA) degradation requires carnitine-dependent transport into the mitochondrial matrix.

"Sytrate" = synthesis.
Carnitine = carnage of fatty acids.

Systemic 1° carnitine deficiency—no cellular uptake of carnitine → no transport of LCFAs into mitochondria → toxic accumulation of LCFAs in the cytosol. Causes weakness, hypotonia, hypoketotic hypoglycemia, dilated cardiomyopathy.

Medium-chain acyl-CoA dehydrogenase deficiency—↓ ability to break down fatty acids into acetyl-CoA → accumulation of fatty acyl carnitines in the blood with hypoketotic hypoglycemia. Causes vomiting, lethargy, seizures, coma, liver dysfunction, hyperammonemia. Can lead to sudden death in infants or children. Treat by avoiding fasting.

Ketone bodies

In the liver, fatty acids and amino acids are metabolized to acetoacetate and β-hydroxybutyrate (to be used in muscle and brain).

In prolonged starvation and diabetic ketoacidosis, oxaloacetate is depleted for gluconeogenesis. With chronic alcohol overuse, excess NADH shunts oxaloacetate to malate. All of these processes lead to a buildup of acetyl-CoA, which is shunted into ketone body synthesis.

Ketone bodies: acetone, acetoacetate, β-hydroxybutyrate.

Breath smells like acetone (fruity odor).

Urine test for ketones can detect acetoacetate, but not β-hydroxybutyrate.

RBCs cannot utilize ketones; they strictly use glucose.

HMG-CoA lyase for ketone production.

HMG-CoA reductase for cholesterol synthesis.

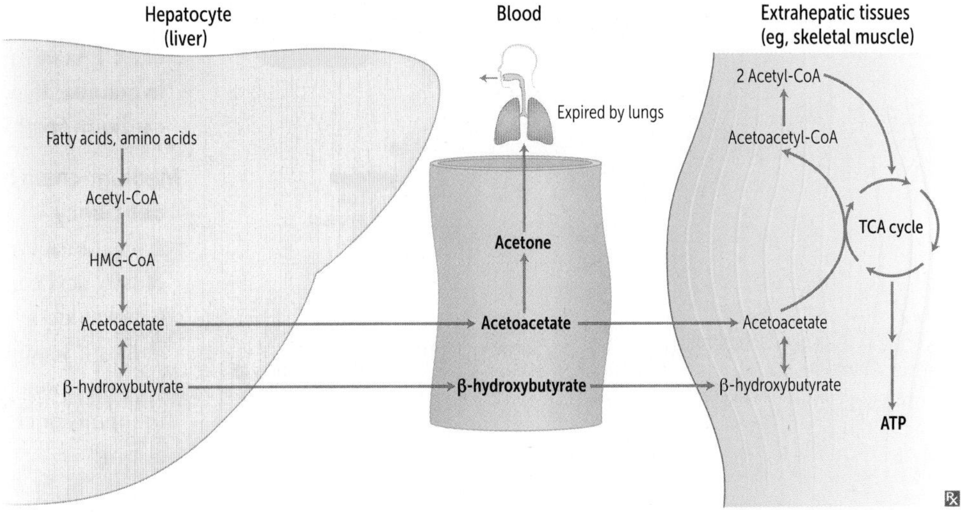

Fasted vs fed state

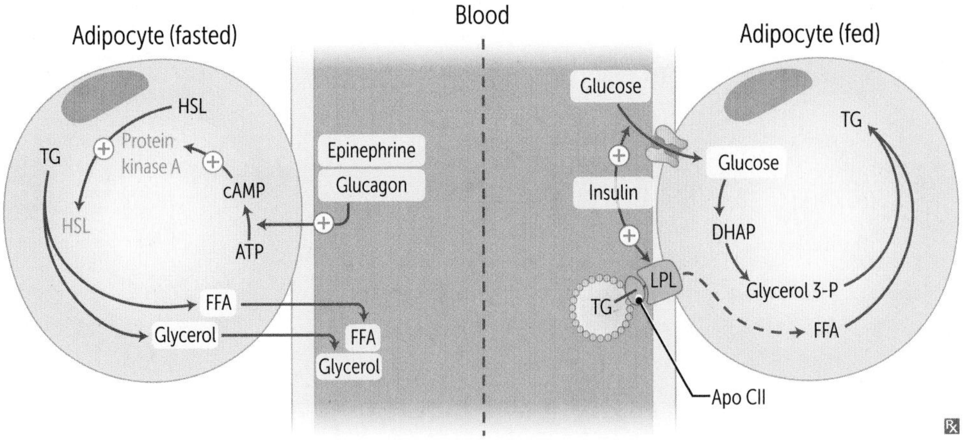

Metabolic fuel use

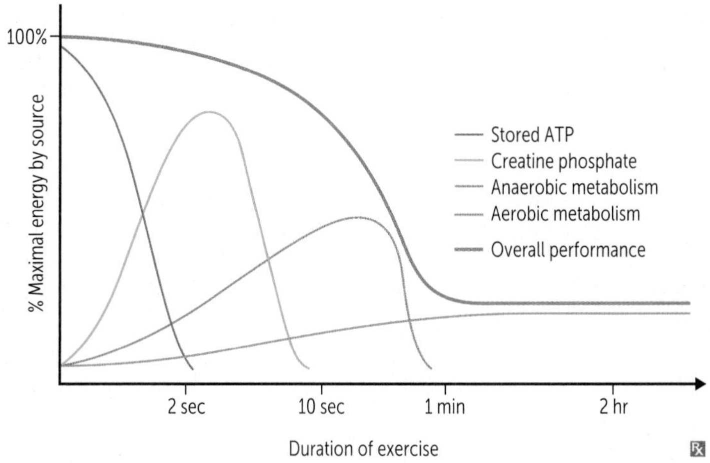

1g carb/protein = 4 kcal
1g alcohol = 7 kcal
1g fatty acid = 9 kcal
(# letters = # kcal)

Fasting and starvation	Priorities are to supply sufficient glucose to the brain and RBCs and to preserve protein.	
Fed state (after a meal)	Glycolysis and aerobic respiration.	Insulin stimulates storage of lipids, proteins, and glycogen.
Fasting (between meals)	Hepatic glycogenolysis (major); hepatic gluconeogenesis, adipose release of FFA (minor).	Glucagon and epinephrine stimulate use of fuel reserves.
Starvation days 1–3	Blood glucose levels maintained by: ▪ Hepatic glycogenolysis ▪ Adipose release of FFA ▪ Muscle and liver, which shift fuel use from glucose to FFA ▪ Hepatic gluconeogenesis from peripheral tissue lactate and alanine, and from adipose tissue glycerol and propionyl-CoA (from odd-chain FFA—the only triacylglycerol components that contribute to gluconeogenesis)	Glycogen reserves depleted after day 1. RBCs lack mitochondria and therefore cannot use ketones. 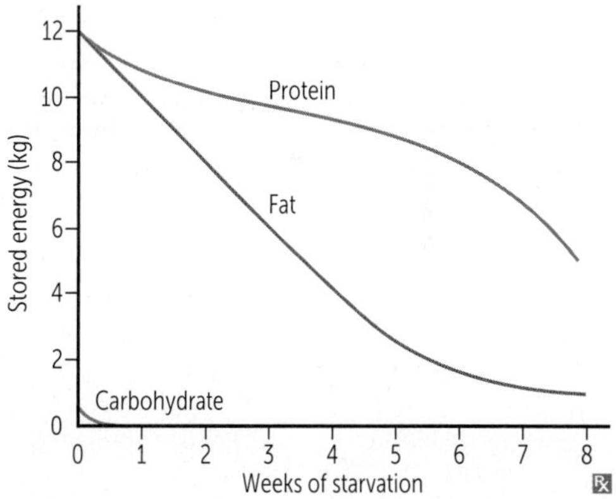
Starvation after day 3	Adipose stores (ketone bodies become the main source of energy for the brain). After these are depleted, vital protein degradation accelerates, leading to organ failure and death. Amount of excess stores determines survival time.	

Lipid transport

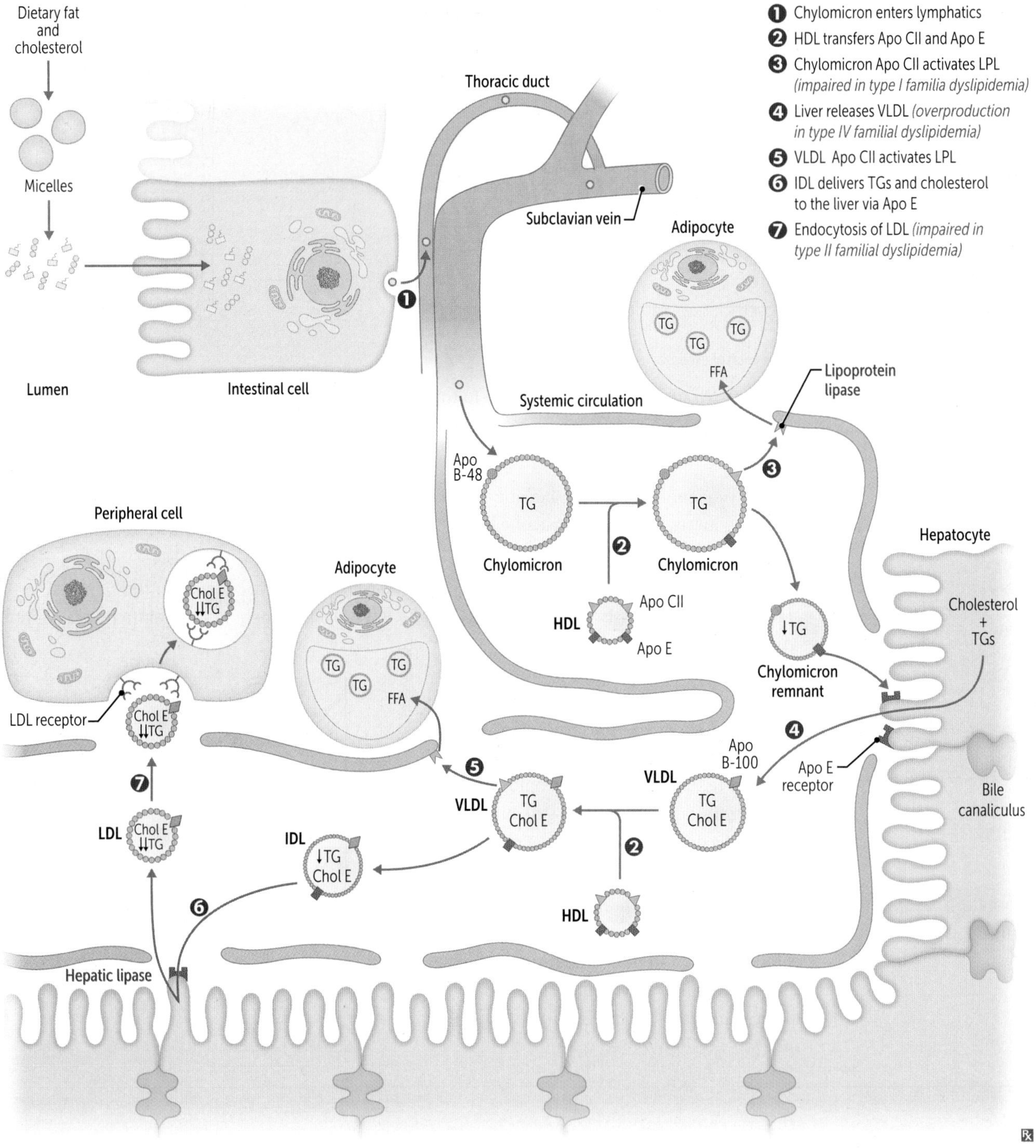
Dietary fat and cholesterol
Micelles
Lumen
Intestinal cell
Thoracic duct
Subclavian vein
Adipocyte
TG
FFA
Lipoprotein lipase
Systemic circulation
Apo B-48
Chylomicron
Chylomicron
HDL
Apo CII
Apo E
↓TG
Chylomicron remnant
Hepatocyte
Cholesterol + TGs
Peripheral cell
Chol E ↓↓TG
LDL receptor
Adipocyte
VLDL
TG Chol E
Apo B-100
Apo E receptor
Bile canaliculus
IDL
↓TG Chol E
LDL
HDL
Hepatic lipase
1 Chylomicron enters lymphatics
2 HDL transfers Apo CII and Apo E
3 Chylomicron Apo CII activates LPL (impaired in type I familia dyslipidemia)
4 Liver releases VLDL (overproduction in type IV familial dyslipidemia)
5 VLDL Apo CII activates LPL
6 IDL delivers TGs and cholesterol to the liver via Apo E
7 Endocytosis of LDL (impaired in type II familial dyslipidemia)

Key enzymes in lipid transport

Cholesteryl ester transfer protein	Mediates transfer of cholesteryl esters to other lipoprotein particles.
Hepatic lipase	Degrades TGs remaining in IDL and chylomicron remnants.
Hormone-sensitive lipase	Degrades TGs stored in adipocytes. Promotes gluconeogenesis by releasing glycerol.
Lecithin-cholesterol acyltransferase	Catalyzes esterification of ⅔ of plasma cholesterol (ie, required for HDL maturation).
Lipoprotein lipase	Degrades TGs in circulating chylomicrons.
Pancreatic lipase	Degrades dietary TGs in small intestine.
PCSK9	Degrades LDL receptor → ↑ serum LDL. Inhibition → ↑ LDL receptor recycling → ↓ serum LDL.

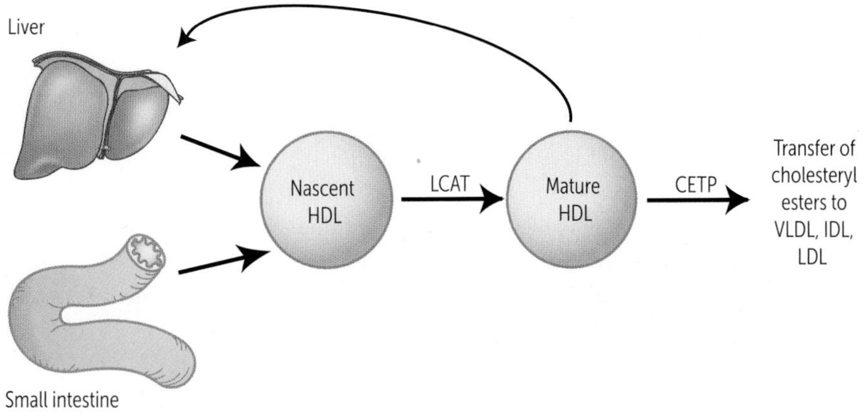

Major apolipoproteins

Apolipoprotein	Function	Chylomicron	Chylomicron remnant	VLDL	IDL	LDL	HDL
E	Mediates remnant uptake (everything except LDL)	✓	✓	✓	✓		✓
A-I	Found only on alpha-lipoproteins (HDL), activates LCAT						✓
C-II	Lipoprotein lipase cofactor that catalyzes cleavage.	✓		✓	✓		✓
B-48	Mediates chylomicron secretion into lymphatics Only on particles originating from the intestines	✓	✓				
B-100	Binds LDL receptor Only on particles originating from the liver			✓	✓	✓	

Lipoprotein functions	Lipoproteins are composed of varying proportions of cholesterol, TGs, and phospholipids. LDL and HDL carry the most cholesterol. Cholesterol is needed to maintain cell membrane integrity and synthesize bile acids, steroids, and vitamin D.
Chylomicron	Delivers dietary TGs to peripheral tissues. Delivers cholesterol to liver in the form of chylomicron remnants, which are mostly depleted of their TGs. Secreted by intestinal epithelial cells.
VLDL	Delivers hepatic TGs to peripheral tissue. Secreted by liver.
IDL	Delivers TGs and cholesterol to liver. Formed from degradation of VLDL.
LDL	Delivers hepatic cholesterol to peripheral tissues. Formed by hepatic lipase modification of IDL in the liver and peripheral tissue. Taken up by target cells via receptor-mediated endocytosis. **L**DL is **L**ethal.
HDL	Mediates reverse cholesterol transport from peripheral tissues to liver. Acts as a repository for apolipoproteins C and E (which are needed for chylomicron and VLDL metabolism). Secreted from both liver and intestine. Alcohol ↑ synthesis. **H**DL is **H**ealthy.

Abetalipoproteinemia

A

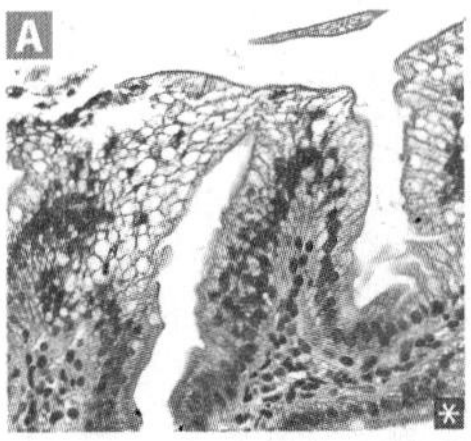

Autosomal recessive. Mutation in gene that encodes microsomal transfer protein (*MTP*). Chylomicrons, VLDL, LDL absent. Deficiency in ApoB-48, ApoB-100. Affected infants present with severe fat malabsorption, steatorrhea, failure to thrive. Later manifestations include retinitis pigmentosa, spinocerebellar degeneration due to vitamin E deficiency, progressive ataxia, acanthocytosis. Intestinal biopsy shows lipid-laden enterocytes A.

Treatment: restriction of long-chain fatty acids, large doses of oral vitamin E.

Familial dyslipidemias

TYPE	INHERITANCE	PATHOGENESIS	↑ BLOOD LEVEL	CLINICAL
I—Hyper-chylomicronemia	AR	Lipoprotein lipase or ApoC-2 deficiency	Chylomicrons, TG, cholesterol	Pancreatitis, hepatosplenomegaly, and eruptive/pruritic xanthomas (no ↑ risk for atherosclerosis). Creamy layer in supernatant.
II—Hyper-cholesterolemia	AD	Absent or defective LDL receptors, or defective ApoB-100	IIa: LDL, cholesterol IIb: LDL, cholesterol, VLDL	Heterozygotes (1:500) have cholesterol ≈ 300 mg/dL; homozygotes (very rare) have cholesterol ≥ 700 mg/dL. Accelerated atherosclerosis (may have MI before age 20), tendon (Achilles) xanthomas, and corneal arcus.
III—Dysbeta-lipoproteinemia	AR	ApoE (defective in type thrEE)	Chylomicrons, VLDL	Premature atherosclerosis, tuberoeruptive and palmar xanthomas. **ApE's palms.**
IV—Hyper-triglyceridemia	AD	Hepatic overproduction of VLDL	VLDL, TG	Hypertriglyceridemia (> 1000 mg/dL) can cause acute pancreatitis. Related to insulin resistance.

HIGH-YIELD PRINCIPLES IN

Immunology

"I hate to disappoint you, but my rubber lips are immune to your charms."

—*Batman & Robin*

"Imagine the action of a vaccine not just in terms of how it affects a single body, but also in terms of how it affects the collective body of a community."

—Eula Biss

"Some people are immune to good advice."

—Saul Goodman, *Breaking Bad*

Learning the components of the immune system and their roles in host defense at the cellular level is essential for both the understanding of disease pathophysiology and clinical practice. Know the immune mechanisms of responses to vaccines. Both congenital and acquired immunodeficiencies are very testable. Cell surface markers are high yield for understanding immune cell interactions and for laboratory diagnosis. Know the roles and functions of major cytokines and chemokines.

▶ IMMUNOLOGY—LYMPHOID STRUCTURES

Immune system organs

1° organs:
- Bone marrow—immune cell production, B cell maturation
- Thymus—T cell maturation

2° organs:
- Spleen, lymph nodes, tonsils, Peyer patches
- Allow immune cells to interact with antigen

Lymph node

A 2° lymphoid organ that has many afferents, 1 or more efferents. Encapsulated, with trabeculae A B. Functions are nonspecific filtration by macrophages, circulation of B and T cells, and immune response activation.

Follicle

Site of B-cell localization and proliferation. In outer cortex. 1° follicles are dense and quiescent. 2° follicles have pale central germinal centers and are active.

Medulla

Consists of medullary cords (closely packed lymphocytes and plasma cells) and medullary sinuses. Medullary sinuses communicate with efferent lymphatics and contain reticular cells and macrophages.

Paracortex

Contains T cells. Region of cortex between follicles and medulla. Contains high endothelial venules through which T and B cells enter from blood. Not well developed in patients with DiGeorge syndrome.

Paracortex enlarges in an extreme cellular immune response (eg, EBV and other viral infections → paracortical hyperplasia → lymphadenopathy).

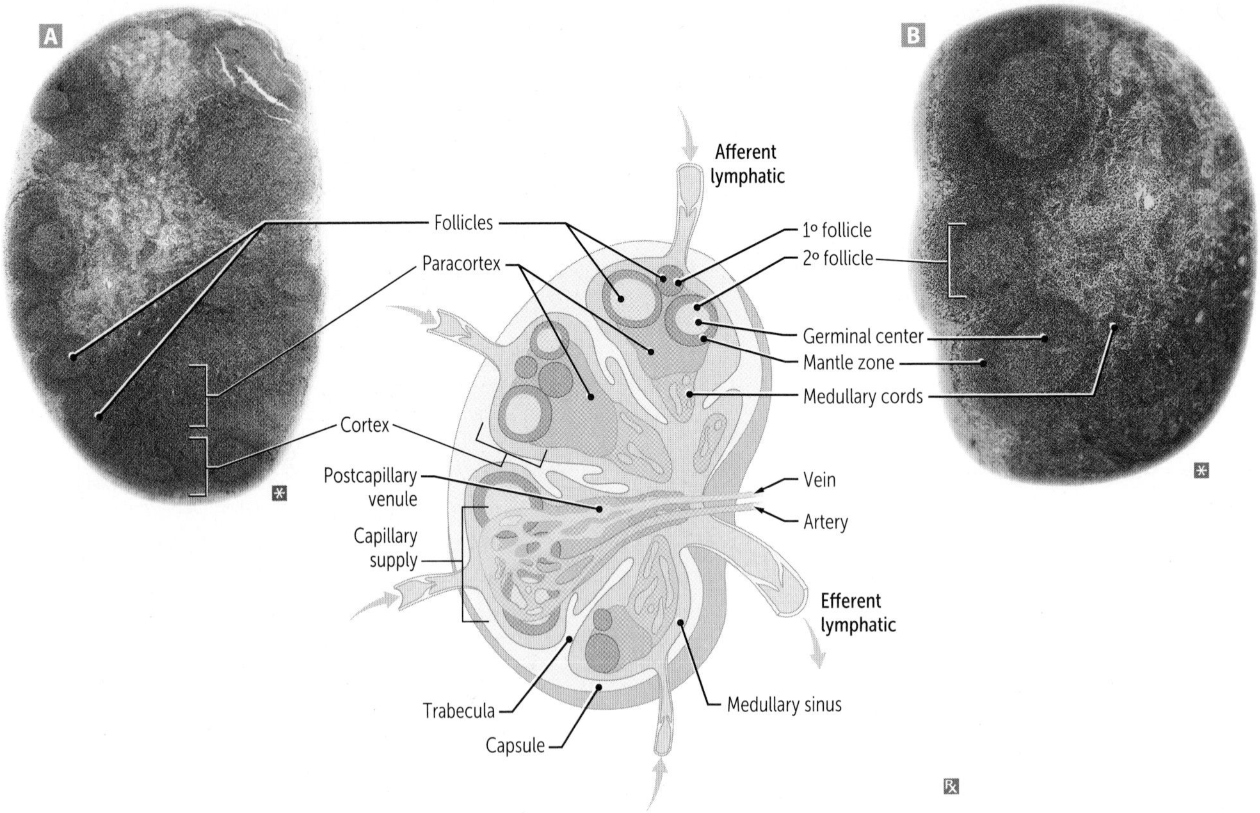

Lymphatic drainage associations

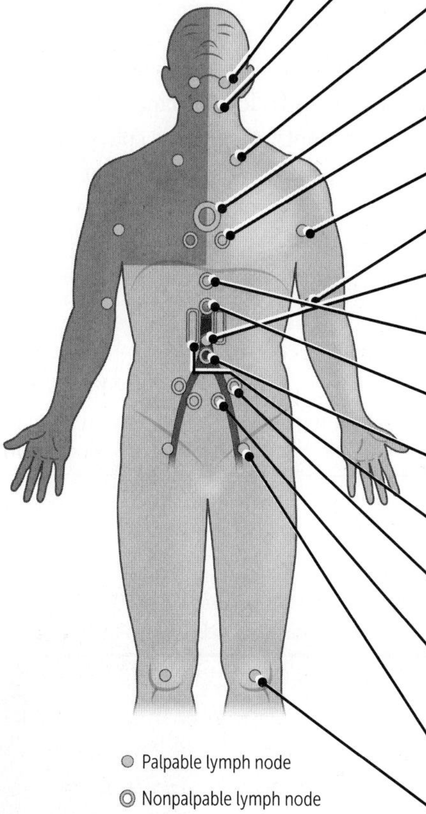

Palpable lymph node
Nonpalpable lymph node

Lymph node cluster	Area of body drained	Associated pathology
Submandibular	Oral cavity	Malignancy of oral cavity
Deep cervical	Head, neck, oropharynx	Upper respiratory tract infection Infectious mononucleosis Kawasaki disease Malignancy of head, neck, oropharynx
Supraclavicular (Virchow node)	Abdomen, pelvis	Malignancy of abdomen, pelvis
Mediastinal	Trachea, esophagus	Pulmonary TB (unilateral hilar) Sarcoidosis (bilateral hilar) Lung cancer Granulomatous disease
Hilar	Lungs	
Axillary	Upper limb, breast, skin above umbilicus	Mastitis Metastasis (especially breast cancer)
Epitrochlear	Hand, forearm	Secondary syphilis
Periumbilical (Sister Mary Joseph node)	Abdomen, pelvis	Gastric cancer
Celiac	Liver, stomach, spleen, pancreas, upper duodenum	Mesenteric lymphadenitis Inflammatory bowel disease Celiac disease
Superior mesenteric	Lower duodenum, jejunum, ileum, colon to splenic flexure	
Inferior mesenteric	Colon from splenic flexure to upper rectum	
Para-aortic	**Pair** of testes, ovaries, kidneys, fallopian tubes (uterus)	Metastasis
External iliac	Cervix, superior bladder, body of uterus	Sexually transmitted infections Medial foot/leg cellulitis (superficial inguinal)
Internal iliac	Lower rectum to anal canal (above pectinate line), bladder, vagina (middle third), cervix, prostate	
Superficial inguinal	Anal canal (below pectinate line), skin below umbilicus (except popliteal area), scrotum, vulva	
Popliteal ("pop-**lateral**")	Dorso**lateral** foot, posterior calf	**Lateral** foot/leg cellulitis

Right lymphatic duct drains right side of body above diaphragm into junction of the right subclavian and internal jugular vein

Thoracic duct drains below the diaphragm and left thorax and upper limb into junction of left subclavian and internal jugular veins (rupture of thoracic duct can cause chylothorax)

Spleen

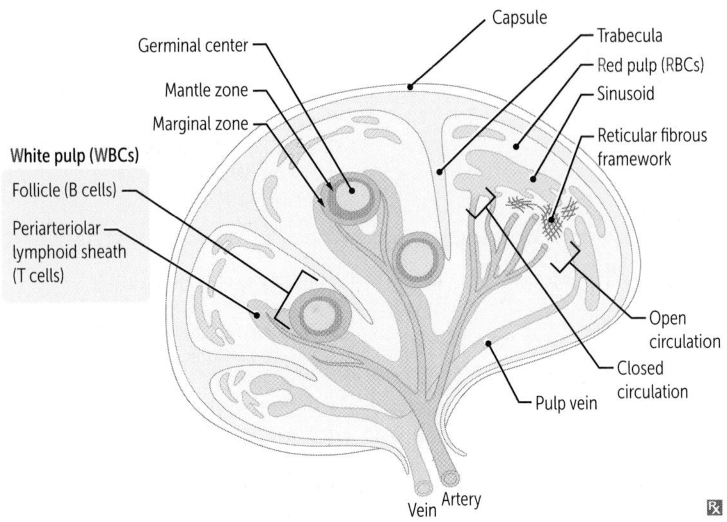
Capsule
Germinal center
Trabecula
Red pulp (RBCs)
Mantle zone
Sinusoid
Marginal zone
Reticular fibrous framework
White pulp (WBCs)
Follicle (B cells)
Periarteriolar lymphoid sheath (T cells)
Open circulation
Closed circulation
Pulp vein
Vein
Artery

Located in LUQ of abdomen, anterolateral to left kidney, protected by 9th-11th ribs.
Splenic dysfunction (eg, postsplenectomy, sickle cell disease autosplenectomy) → ↓ IgM → ↓ complement activation → ↓ C3b opsonization → ↑ susceptibility to encapsulated organisms.

Postsplenectomy findings:

- Howell-Jolly bodies (nuclear remnants)
- Target cells
- Thrombocytosis (loss of sequestration and removal)
- Lymphocytosis (loss of sequestration)

Vaccinate patients undergoing splenectomy or with splenic dysfunction against encapsulated organisms (pneumococci, Hib, meningococci).

Periarteriolar lymphatic sheath	Contains T cells. Located within white pulp.
Follicle	Contains B cells. Located within white pulp.
Marginal zone	Contains macrophages and specialized B cells. Site where antigen-presenting cells (APCs) capture blood-borne antigens for recognition by lymphocytes. Located between red pulp and white pulp.

Thymus

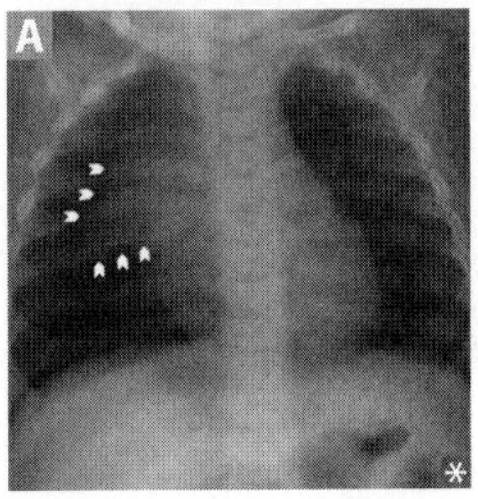

Located in the anterosuperior mediastinum. Site of T-cell differentiation and maturation. Encapsulated. Thymus epithelium is derived from third pharyngeal pouch (endoderm), whereas thymic lymphocytes are of mesodermal origin. Cortex is dense with immature T cells; medulla is pale with mature T cells and Hassall corpuscles containing epithelial reticular cells.
Normal neonatal thymus "sail-shaped" on CXR (asterisks in A), involutes by age 3 years.

T cells = Thymus
B cells = Bone marrow
Absent thymic shadow or hypoplastic thymus seen in some immunodeficiencies (eg, SCID, DiGeorge syndrome).

Thymoma—neoplasm of thymus. Associated with myasthenia gravis, superior vena cava syndrome, pure red cell aplasia, Good syndrome.

▸ IMMUNOLOGY—CELLULAR COMPONENTS

Innate vs adaptive immunity

	Innate immunity	Adaptive immunity
COMPONENTS	Neutrophils, macrophages, monocytes, dendritic cells, natural killer (NK) cells (lymphoid origin), complement, physical epithelial barriers, secreted enzymes	T cells, B cells, circulating antibodies
MECHANISM	Germline encoded	Variation through V(D)J recombination during lymphocyte development
RESPONSE TO PATHOGENS	Nonspecific Occurs rapidly (minutes to hours) No memory response	Highly specific, refined over time Develops over long periods; memory response is faster and more robust
SECRETED PROTEINS	Lysozyme, complement, C-reactive protein (CRP), defensins, cytokines	Immunoglobulins, cytokines
KEY FEATURES IN PATHOGEN RECOGNITION	Toll-like receptors (TLRs): pattern recognition receptors that recognize pathogen-associated molecular patterns (PAMPs) and lead to activation of NF-κB. Examples of PAMPs: LPS (gram ⊖ bacteria), flagellin (bacteria), nucleic acids (viruses)	Memory cells: activated B and T cells; subsequent exposure to a previously encountered antigen → stronger, quicker immune response

Major histocompatibility complex I and II

MHC encoded by HLA genes. Present antigen fragments to T cells and bind T-cell receptors (TCRs).

	MHC I	MHC II
LOCI	HLA-A, HLA-B, HLA-C MHC I loci have 1 letter	HLA-DP, HLA-DQ, HLA-DR MHC II loci have 2 letters
BINDING	TCR and CD8	TCR and CD4
STRUCTURE	1 long chain, 1 short chain	2 equal-length chains (2 α, 2 β)
EXPRESSION	All nucleated cells, APCs, platelets (except RBCs)	APCs
FUNCTION	Present endogenous antigens (eg, viral or cytosolic proteins) to CD8+ cytotoxic T cells	Present exogenous antigens (eg, bacterial proteins) to CD4+ helper T cells
ANTIGEN LOADING	Antigen peptides loaded onto MHC I in RER after delivery via TAP (transporter associated with antigen processing)	Antigen loaded following release of invariant chain in an acidified endosome
ASSOCIATED PROTEINS	β_2-microglobulin	Invariant chain
STRUCTURE	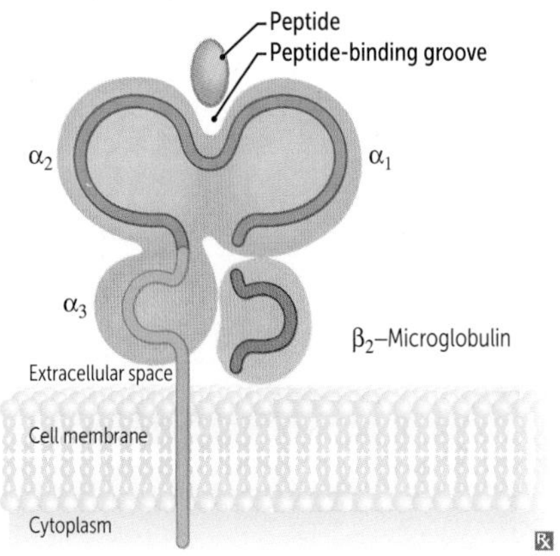	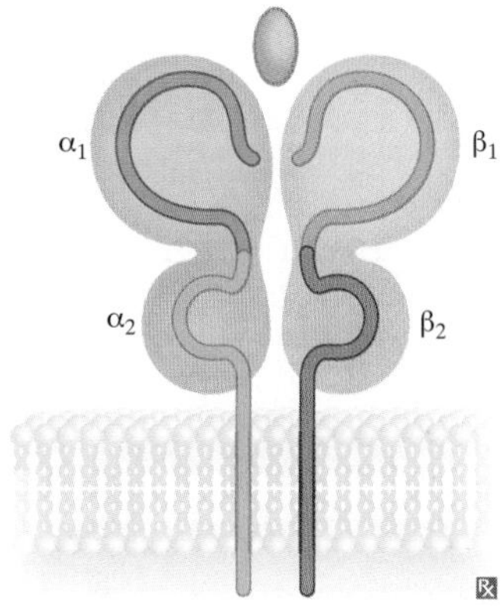

HLA subtypes associated with diseases

HLA SUBTYPE	DISEASE	MNEMONIC
B27	**P**soriatic arthritis, **A**nkylosing spondylitis, **I**BD-associated arthritis, **R**eactive arthritis	**PAIR.** Also called seronegative arthropathies
B57	Abacavir hypersensitivity	
DQ2/DQ8	Celiac disease	I ate (8) too (2) much gluten at Dairy Queen
DR3	DM type 1, **SLE**, Graves disease, Hashimoto thyroiditis, Addison disease	2-3, S-L-E DM type 1: HLA-3 and -4 (1 + 3 = 4)
DR4	**Rheum**atoid arthritis, DM type 1, Addison disease	There are 4 walls in 1 "**rheum**" (room)

Functions of natural killer cells	Lymphocyte member of innate immune system. Use perforin and granzymes to induce apoptosis of virally infected cells and tumor cells. Activity enhanced by IL-2, IL-12, IFN-α, and IFN-β. Induced to kill when exposed to a nonspecific activation signal on target cell and/or to an absence of an inhibitory signal such as MHC I on target cell surface. Also kills via antibody-dependent cell-mediated cytotoxicity (CD16 binds Fc region of bound IgG, activating the NK cell).

Major functions of B and T cells

B cells	Humoral immunity. Recognize and present antigen—undergo somatic hypermutation to optimize antigen specificity. Produce antibody—differentiate into plasma cells to secrete specific immunoglobulins. Maintain immunologic memory—memory B cells persist and accelerate future response to antigen.
T cells	Cell-mediated immunity. CD4+ T cells help B cells make antibodies and produce cytokines to recruit phagocytes and activate other leukocytes. CD8+ T cells directly kill virus-infected and tumor cells via perforin and granzymes (similar to NK cells). Delayed cell-mediated hypersensitivity (type IV). Acute and chronic cellular organ rejection. Rule of 8: MHC II × CD4 = 8; MHC I × CD8 = 8.

Differentiation of T cells

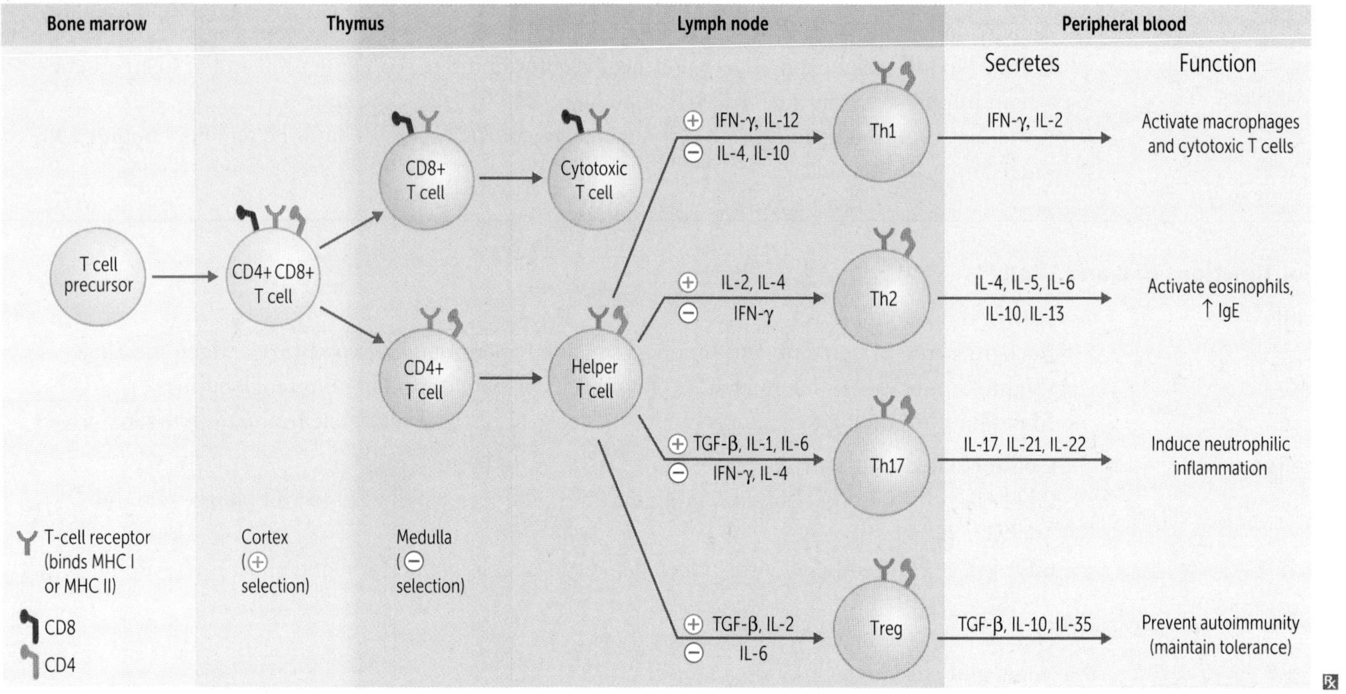

Positive selection — Thymic cortex. T cells expressing TCRs capable of binding self-MHC on cortical epithelial cells survive.

Negative selection — Thymic medulla. T cells expressing TCRs with high affinity for self antigens undergo apoptosis or become regulatory T cells. Tissue-restricted self-antigens are expressed in the thymus due to the action of autoimmune regulator (**AIRE**); deficiency leads to autoimmune polyendocrine syndrome-1 (**C**hronic mucocutaneous candidiasis, **H**ypoparathyroidism, **A**drenal insufficiency, **R**ecurrent *Candida* infections). "Without **AIRE**, your body will **CHAR**".

Macrophage-lymphocyte interaction — Th1 cells secrete IFN-γ, which enhances the ability of monocytes and macrophages to kill microbes they ingest. This function is also enhanced by interaction of T cell CD40L with CD40 on macrophages. Macrophages also activate lymphocytes via antigen presentation.

Cytotoxic T cells — Kill virus-infected, neoplastic, and donor graft cells by inducing apoptosis.
Release cytotoxic granules containing preformed proteins (eg, perforin, granzyme B).
Cytotoxic T cells have CD8, which binds to MHC I on virus-infected cells.

Regulatory T cells — Help maintain specific immune tolerance by suppressing $CD4^+$ and $CD8^+$ T-cell effector functions.
Identified by expression of CD3, CD4, CD25, and FOXP3.
Activated regulatory T cells (Tregs) produce anti-inflammatory cytokines (eg, IL-10, TGF-β).

IPEX (Immune dysregulation, Polyendocrinopathy, Enteropathy, X-linked) syndrome—genetic deficiency of FOXP3 → autoimmunity. Characterized by enteropathy, endocrinopathy, nail dystrophy, dermatitis, and/or other autoimmune dermatologic conditions. Associated with diabetes in male infants.

T- and B-cell activation	APCs: B cells, dendritic cells, Langerhans cells, macrophages. Two signals are required for T-cell activation, B-cell activation, and class switching.
T-cell activation	❶ Dendritic cell (specialized APC) ingests and processes antigen, then migrates to the draining lymph node. ❷ T-cell activation (signal 1): exogenous antigen is presented on MHC II and recognized by TCR on Th (CD4+) cell. Endogenous or cross-presented antigen is presented on MHC I to Tc (CD8+) cell. ❸ Proliferation and survival (signal 2): costimulatory signal via interaction of B7 protein (CD80/86) on dendritic cell and CD28 on naïve T cell. ❹ Activated Th cell produces cytokines. Tc cell able to recognize and kill virus-infected cell.
B-cell activation and class switching	❶ Th-cell activation as above. ❷ B-cell receptor–mediated endocytosis. ❸ Exogenous antigen is presented on MHC II and recognized by TCR on Th cell. ❹ CD40 receptor on B cell binds CD40 ligand (CD40L) on Th cell. ❺ Th cells secrete cytokines that determine Ig class switching of B cells. ❻ B cells are activated and produce IgM. They undergo class switching and affinity maturation.

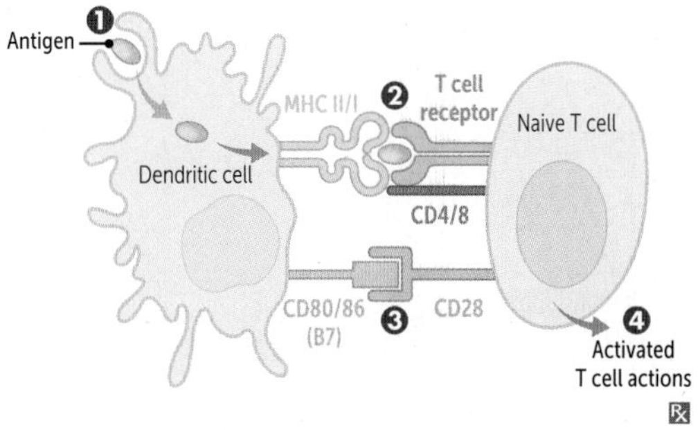

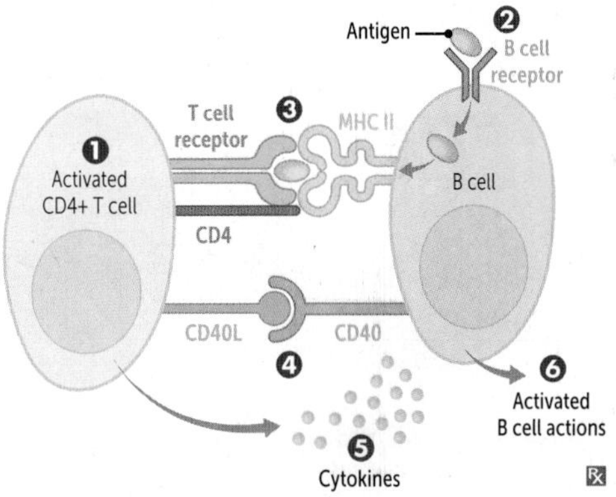

▸ IMMUNOLOGY—IMMUNE RESPONSES

Antibody structure and function

Fab fragment consisting of light (L) and heavy (H) chains recognizes antigens. Fc region of IgM and IgG fixes complement. Heavy chain contributes to Fc and Fab regions. Light chain contributes only to Fab region.

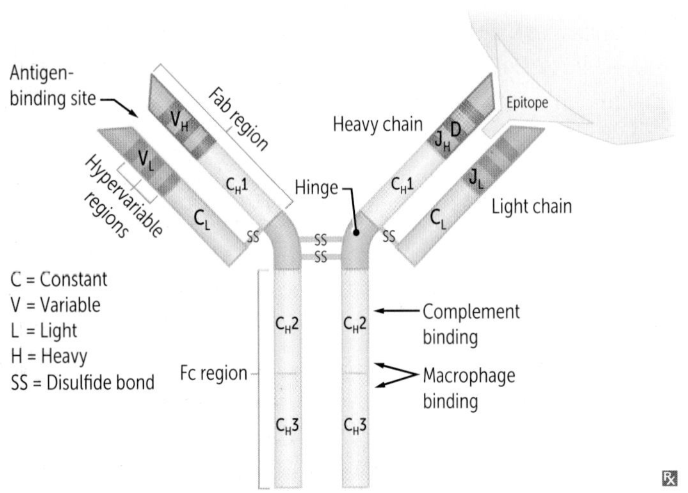
Antigen-binding site
V_H
Fab region
V_L
Hypervariable regions
C_H1
C_L
SS
Heavy chain
J_H D
Epitope
Hinge
C_H1
J_L
C_L
Light chain
SS
SS
SS
C = Constant
V = Variable
L = Light
H = Heavy
SS = Disulfide bond
Fc region
C_H2
C_H2
Complement binding
Macrophage binding
C_H3
C_H3

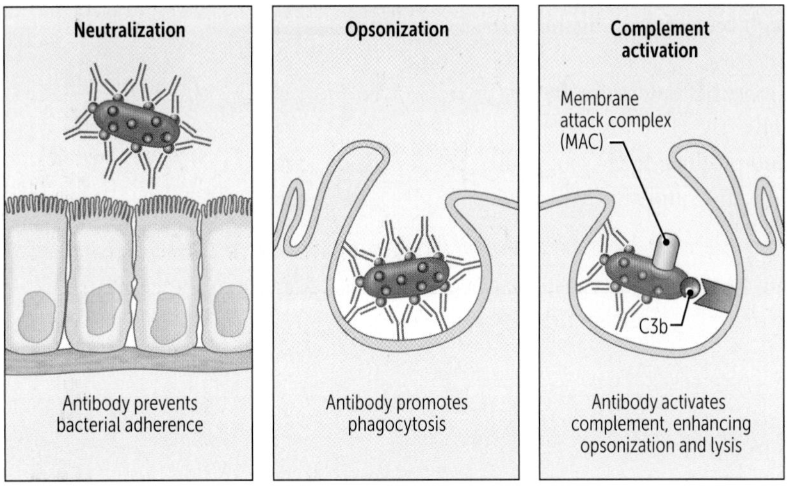
Neutralization
Antibody prevents bacterial adherence
Opsonization
Antibody promotes phagocytosis
Complement activation
Membrane attack complex (MAC)
C3b
Antibody activates complement, enhancing opsonization and lysis

Fab:
- Fragment, antigen binding
- Determines idiotype: unique antigen-binding pocket; only 1 antigenic specificity expressed per B cell

Fc (5 C's):
- Constant
- Carboxy terminal
- Complement binding
- Carbohydrate side chains
- Confers (determines) isotype (IgM, IgD, etc)

Generation of antibody diversity (antigen independent)
1. Random recombination of VJ (light-chain) or V(D)J (heavy-chain) genes
2. Random addition of nucleotides to DNA during recombination by terminal deoxynucleotidyl transferase (TdT)
3. Random combination of heavy chains with light chains

Generation of antibody specificity (antigen dependent)
4. Somatic hypermutation and affinity maturation (variable region)
5. Isotype switching (constant region)

Immunoglobulin isotypes

All isotypes can exist as monomers. Mature, naïve B cells prior to activation express IgM and IgD on their surfaces. They may differentiate in germinal centers of lymph nodes by isotype switching (gene rearrangement; induced by cytokines and CD40L) into plasma cells that secrete IgA, IgE, or IgG.

Affinity refers to the individual antibody-antigen interaction, while avidity describes the cumulative binding strength of all antibody-antigen interactions in a multivalent molecule.

IgG

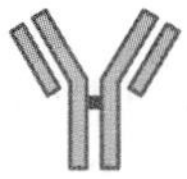

Main antibody in 2° response to an antigen. Most abundant isotype in serum. Fixes complement, opsonizes bacteria, neutralizes bacterial toxins and viruses. Only isotype that crosses the placenta (provides infants with passive immunity that starts to wane after birth). "IgG Greets the Growing fetus." Associated with **warm** autoimmune hemolytic anemia ("**warm** weather is Great!").

IgA

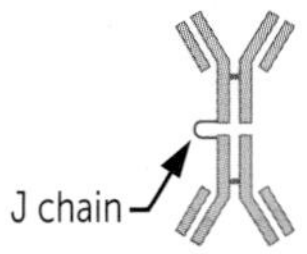

Prevents attachment of bacteria and viruses to mucous membranes; does not fix complement. Monomer (in circulation) or dimer (with J chain when secreted). Crosses epithelial cells by transcytosis. Produced in GI tract (eg, by Peyer patches) and protects against gut infections (eg, *Giardia*). Most produced antibody overall, but has lower serum concentrations. Released into secretions (tears, saliva, mucus) and breast milk. Picks up secretory component from epithelial cells, which protects the Fc portion from luminal proteases.

IgM

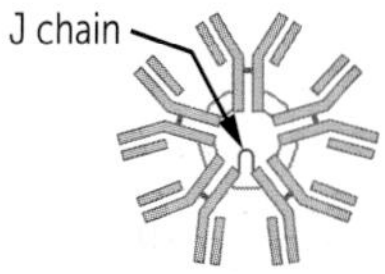

Produced in the 1° (IMmediate) response to an antigen. Fixes complement. Antigen receptor on the surface of B cells. Monomer on B cell, pentamer with J chain when secreted. Pentamer enables avid binding to antigen while humoral response evolves. Associated with cold autoimmune hemolytic anemia.

IgD

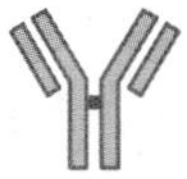

Unclear function. Found on surface of many B cells and in serum.

IgE

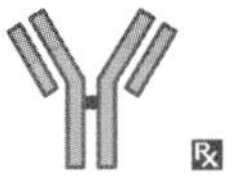

Binds mast cells and basophils; cross-links when exposed to allergen, mediating immediate (type I) hypersensitivity through release of inflammatory mediators such as histamine. Contributes to immunity to parasites by activating Eosinophils.

Antigen type and memory

Thymus-independent antigens

Antigens lacking a peptide component (eg, lipopolysaccharides from gram ⊖ bacteria); cannot be presented by MHC to T cells. Weakly immunogenic; vaccines often require boosters and adjuvants (eg, capsular polysaccharide subunit of *Streptococcus pneumoniae* PPSV23 vaccine).

Thymus-dependent antigens

Antigens containing a protein component (eg, diphtheria toxoid). Class switching and immunologic memory occur as a result of direct contact of B cells with Th cells.

Complement	System of hepatically synthesized plasma proteins that play a role in innate immunity and inflammation. Membrane attack complex (MAC) defends against gram ⊖ bacteria. The CH_{50} test is used to screen for activation of the classical complement pathway.	
ACTIVATION PATHWAYS	**Classic**—**IgG** or **IgM** mediated. Alternative—microbe surface molecules. Lectin—mannose or other sugars on microbe surface.	**GM** makes **classic** cars.
FUNCTIONS	C3b—opsonization. C3a, C4a, C5a—anaphylaxis. C5a—neutrophil chemotaxis. C5b-9 (MAC)—cytolysis.	**C3b** binds to lipopolysaccharides on **bacteria**. **MAC** complex is important for neutralizing *Neisseria* species. Deficiency results in recurrent infection. Get "**Neis**" (nice) Big **MACs** from **5-9** pm.
	Opsonins—C3b and IgG are the two 1° opsonins in bacterial defense; enhance phagocytosis. C3b also helps clear immune complexes.	*Opsonin* (Greek) = to prepare for eating.
	Inhibitors—decay-accelerating factor (DAF, aka CD55) and C1 esterase inhibitor help prevent complement activation on self cells (eg, RBCs).	

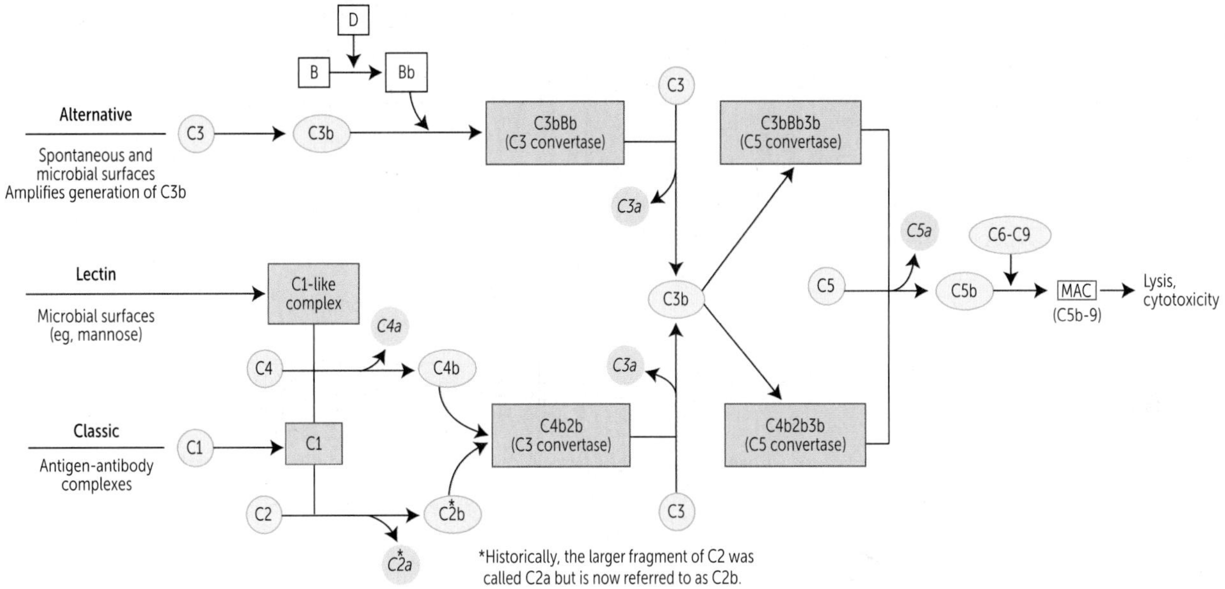

*Historically, the larger fragment of C2 was called C2a but is now referred to as C2b.

Complement disorders

Complement protein deficiencies	
Early complement deficiencies (C1-C4)	↑ risk of severe, recurrent pyogenic sinus and respiratory tract infections. C3b used in clearance of antigen-antibody complexes → ↑ risk of SLE (think SLEarly).
Terminal complement deficiencies (C5–C9)	↑ susceptibility to recurrent *Neisseria* bacteremia.
Complement regulatory protein deficiencies	
C1 esterase inhibitor deficiency	Causes hereditary angioedema due to unregulated activation of kallikrein → ↑ bradykinin. Characterized by ↓ C4 levels. ACE inhibitors are contraindicated (also ↑ bradykinin).
Paroxysmal nocturnal hemoglobinuria 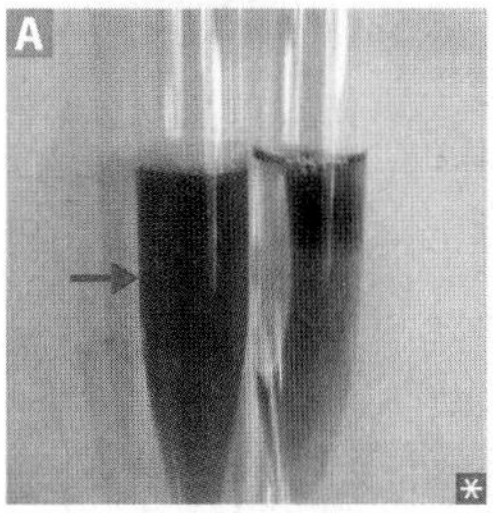	A defect in the *PIGA* gene prevents the formation of glycosylphosphatidylinositol (GPI) anchors for complement inhibitors, such as decay-accelerating factor (DAF/CD55) and membrane inhibitor of reactive lysis (MIRL/CD59). Causes complement-mediated intravascular hemolysis → ↓ haptoglobin, dark urine A. Can cause atypical venous thrombosis (eg, Budd-Chiari syndrome; portal vein, cerebral, or dermal thrombosis).

Important cytokines	Acute (IL-1, IL-6, TNF-α), then recruit (IL-8, IL-12).	
SECRETED BY MACROPHAGES		
Interleukin-1	Causes fever, acute inflammation. Activates endothelium to express adhesion molecules. Induces chemokine secretion to recruit WBCs. Also called osteoclast-activating factor.	"**Hot T-bone stEAK**": IL-1: fever (**hot**). IL-2: stimulates **T** cells. IL-3: stimulates **bone** marrow. IL-4: stimulates Ig**E** production. IL-5: stimulates Ig**A** production. IL-6: stimulates a**K**ute-phase protein production.
Interleukin-6	Causes fever and stimulates production of acute-phase proteins.	
Tumor necrosis factor-α	Activates endothelium. Causes WBC recruitment, vascular leak.	Causes cachexia in malignancy. Maintains granulomas in TB. IL-1, IL-6, TNF-α can mediate fever and sepsis.
Interleukin-8	Major chemotactic factor for neutrophils.	"**Clean up** on **aisle** 8." Neutrophils are recruited by **IL-8** to **clear** infections.
Interleukin-12	Induces differentiation of T cells into Th1 cells. Activates NK cells.	Facilitates granuloma formation in TB.
SECRETED BY T CELLS		
Interleukin-2	Stimulates growth of helper, cytotoxic, and regulatory T cells, and NK cells.	
Interleukin-3	Supports growth and differentiation of bone marrow stem cells. Functions like GM-CSF.	
FROM Th1 CELLS		
Interferon-γ	Secreted by NK cells and T cells in response to antigen or IL-12 from macrophages; stimulates macrophages to kill phagocytosed pathogens. Inhibits differentiation of Th2 cells. Induces IgG isotype switching in B cells.	Also activates NK cells to kill virus-infected cells. Increases MHC expression and antigen presentation by all cells. Activates macrophages to induce granuloma formation.
FROM Th2 CELLS		
Interleukin-4	Induces differentiation of T cells into Th (**helper**) 2 cells. Promotes growth of **B** cells. Enhances class switching to Ig**E** and Ig**G**.	Ain't too proud **2 BEG 4 help**.
Interleukin-5	Promotes growth and differentiation of **B** cells. Enhances class switching to Ig**A**. Stimulates growth and differentiation of **E**osinophils.	I have **5 BAE**s.
Interleukin-10	Attenuates inflammatory response. Decreases expression of MHC class II and Th1 cytokines. Inhibits activated macrophages and dendritic cells. Also secreted by regulatory T cells.	TGF-β and IL-10 both attenuate the immune response.
Interleukin-13	Promotes IgE production by B cells. Induces alternative macrophage activation.	

Respiratory burst

Also called oxidative burst. Involves the activation of the phagocyte NADPH oxidase complex (eg, in neutrophils, monocytes), which utilizes O_2 as a substrate. Plays an important role in the immune response → rapid release of reactive oxygen species (ROS). NADPH plays a role in both the creation and neutralization of ROS. Myeloperoxidase contains a blue-green, heme-containing pigment that gives sputum its color.

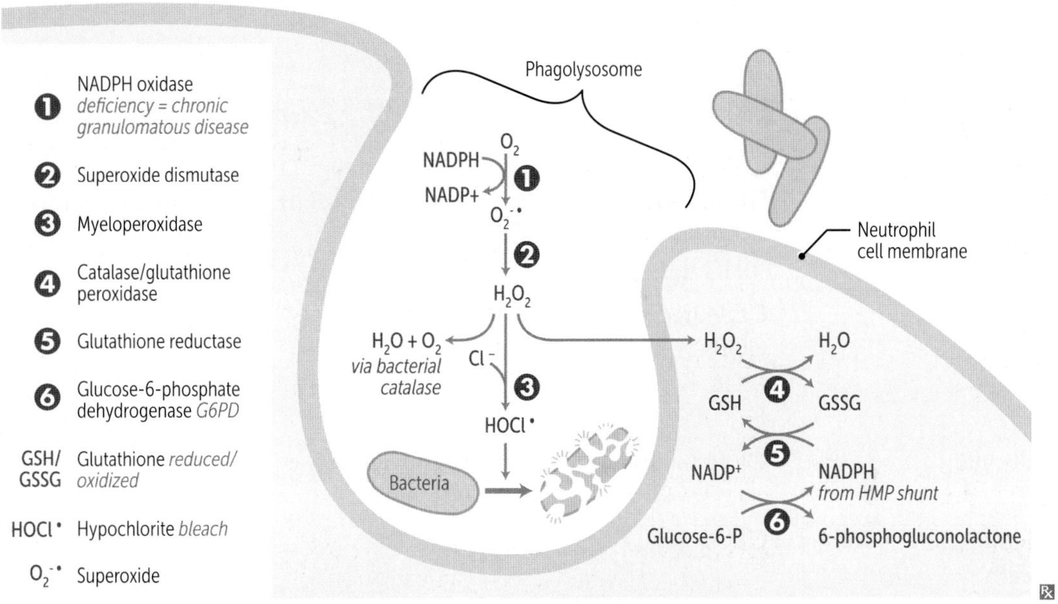

Phagocytes of patients with CGD can utilize H_2O_2 generated by invading organisms and convert it to ROS. Patients are at ↑ risk for infection by catalase ⊕ species (eg, *S aureus*, *Aspergillus*) capable of neutralizing their own H_2O_2, leaving phagocytes without ROS for fighting infections.

Pyocyanin of *P aeruginosa* generates ROS to kill competing pathogens. Oxidative burst also leads to K^+ influx, which releases lysosomal enzymes. Lactoferrin is a protein found in secretory fluids and neutrophils that inhibits microbial growth via iron chelation.

Interferons	IFN-α, IFN-β, IFN-γ
MECHANISM	A part of innate host defense, **interferons interfere** with both RNA and DNA viruses. Cells infected with a virus synthesize these glycoproteins, which act on local cells, priming them for viral defense by downregulating protein synthesis to resist potential viral replication and by upregulating MHC expression to facilitate recognition of infected cells. Also play a major role in activating antitumor immunity.
CLINICAL USE	Chronic HBV, Kaposi sarcoma, hairy cell leukemia, condyloma acuminatum, renal cell carcinoma, malignant melanoma, multiple sclerosis, chronic granulomatous disease.
ADVERSE EFFECTS	Flu-like symptoms, depression, neutropenia, myopathy, interferon-induced autoimmunity.

Cell surface proteins

T cells	TCR (binds antigen-MHC complex) CD3 (associated with TCR for signal transduction) CD28 (binds B7 on APC)	
Helper T cells	CD4, CD40L, CXCR4/CCR5 (co-receptors for HIV)	
Cytotoxic T cells	CD8	
Regulatory T cells	CD4, CD25	
B cells	Ig (binds antigen) CD19, CD20, CD21 (receptor for Epstein-**Barr** virus), CD40 MHC II, B7	Must be **21** to drink **Beer** in a **Barr**
Macrophages	CD14 (receptor for PAMPs, eg, LPS), CD40 CCR5 MHC II, B7 (CD80/86) Fc and C3b receptors (enhanced phagocytosis)	
NK cells	CD16 (binds Fc of IgG), CD56 (suggestive marker for NK)	
Hematopoietic stem cells	CD34	

Anergy State during which a cell cannot become activated by exposure to its antigen. T and B cells become anergic when exposed to their antigen without costimulatory signal (signal 2). Another mechanism of self-tolerance.

Passive vs active immunity

	Passive	Active
MEANS OF ACQUISITION	Receiving preformed antibodies	Exposure to exogenous antigens
ONSET	Rapid	Slow
DURATION	Short span of antibodies (half-life = 3 weeks)	Long-lasting protection (memory)
EXAMPLES	IgA in breast milk, maternal IgG crossing placenta, antitoxin, humanized monoclonal antibody	Natural infection, vaccines, toxoid
NOTES	After exposure to **T**etanus toxin, **H**BV, **V**aricella, **R**abies virus, **B**otulinum toxin, or **D**iphtheria toxin, unvaccinated patients are given preformed antibodies (passive)—"to **H**eal **v**ery **r**apidly **b**efore **d**ying"	Combined passive and active immunizations can be given for hepatitis B or rabies exposure

Vaccination Induces an active immune response (humoral and/or cellular) to specific pathogens.

VACCINE TYPE	DESCRIPTION	PROS/CONS	EXAMPLES
Live attenuated vaccine	Microorganism rendered nonpathogenic but retains capacity for transient growth within inoculated host. Induces **cellular and humoral responses.** MMR and varicella vaccines can be given to people living with HIV without evidence of immunity if CD4 cell count ≥ 200 cells/mm^3.	Pros: induces strong, often lifelong immunity. Cons: may revert to virulent form. Contraindicated in pregnant and immunodeficient patients.	Adenovirus (nonattenuated, given to military recruits), typhoid (Ty21a, oral), polio (Sabin), varicella (chickenpox), **small**pox, BCG, yellow fever, **influenza** (intranasal), **MMR**, rotavirus. "Attention teachers! Please vaccinate **small**, Beautiful young **infants** with **MMR** regularly!"
Killed or inactivated vaccine	Pathogen is inactivated by heat or chemicals. Maintaining epitope structure on surface antigens is important for immune response. Mainly induces a **humoral response.**	Pros: safer than live vaccines. Cons: weaker immune response; booster shots usually required.	Hepatitis A, Typhoid (Vi polysaccharide, intramuscular), Rabies, Influenza, Polio (SalK). A TRIP could Kill you.
Subunit	Includes only the antigens that best stimulate the immune system.	Pros: lower chance of adverse reactions. Cons: expensive, weaker immune response.	HBV (antigen = HBsAg), HPV (types 6, 11, 16, and 18), acellular pertussis (aP), *Neisseria meningitidis* (various strains), *Streptococcus pneumoniae*, *Haemophilus influenzae* type b.
Toxoid	Denatured bacterial toxin with an intact receptor binding site. Stimulates the immune system to make antibodies without potential for causing disease.	Pros: protects against the bacterial toxins. Cons: antitoxin levels decrease with time, may require a booster.	*Clostridium tetani*, *Corynebacterium diphtheriae*.

Hypersensitivity types

Four types (ABCD): Anaphylactic and Atopic (type I), AntiBody-mediated (type II), Immune Complex (type III), Delayed (cell-mediated, type IV). Types I, II, and III are all antibody-mediated.

Type I hypersensitivity

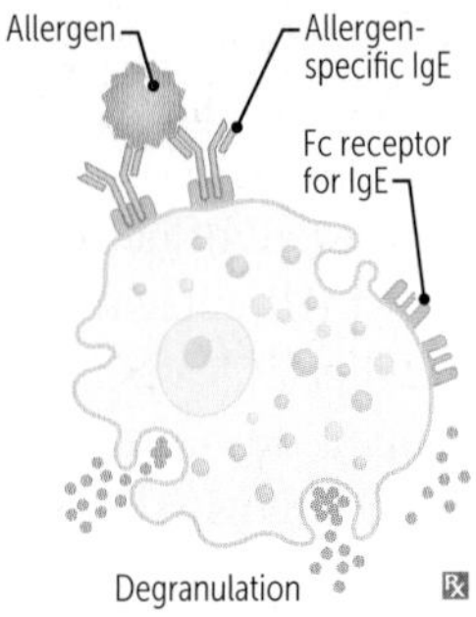
Allergen
Allergen-specific IgE
Fc receptor for IgE
Degranulation

Anaphylactic and atopic—two phases:

- Immediate (minutes): antigen crosslinks preformed IgE on presensitized mast cells → immediate degranulation → release of histamine (a vasoactive amine), tryptase (marker of mast cell activation), and leukotrienes.
- Late (hours): chemokines (attract inflammatory cells, eg, eosinophils) and other mediators from mast cells → inflammation and tissue damage.

First (type) and Fast (anaphylaxis).

Test: skin test or blood test (ELISA) for allergen-specific IgE.

Example:

- Anaphylaxis (eg, food, drug, or bee sting allergies)
- Allergic asthma

Type II hypersensitivity

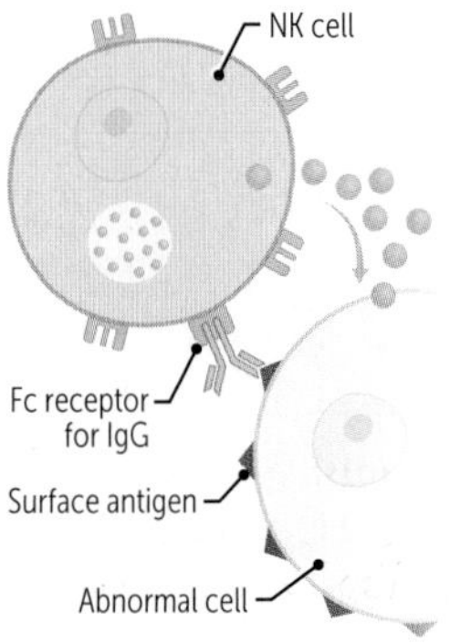
NK cell
Fc receptor for IgG
Surface antigen
Abnormal cell

Antibody-dependent cellular cytotoxicity

Antibodies bind to cell-surface antigens → cellular destruction, inflammation, and cellular dysfunction.

Direct Coombs test—detects antibodies attached **directly** to the RBC surface.
Indirect Coombs test—detects presence of unbound antibodies in the serum.

Cellular destruction—cell is opsonized (coated) by antibodies, leading to either:

- Phagocytosis and/or activation of complement system.
- NK cell killing (antibody-dependent cellular cytotoxicity).

Examples:

- Autoimmune hemolytic anemia (including drug-induced form)
- Immune thrombocytopenia
- Transfusion reactions
- Hemolytic disease of the newborn

Inflammation—binding of antibodies to cell surfaces → activation of complement system and Fc receptor-mediated inflammation.

Examples:

- Goodpasture syndrome
- Rheumatic fever
- Hyperacute transplant rejection

Cellular dysfunction—antibodies bind to cell surface receptors → abnormal blockade or activation of downstream process.

Examples:

- Myasthenia gravis
- Graves disease
- Pemphigus vulgaris

Hypersensitivity types *(continued)*

Type III hypersensitivity	Immune complex—antigen-antibody (mostly IgG) complexes activate complement, which attracts neutrophils; neutrophils release lysosomal enzymes. Can be associated with vasculitis and systemic manifestations.	In type **III** reaction, imagine an immune complex as **3** things stuck together: antigen-antibody-complement. Examples: ▪ SLE ▪ Rheumatoid arthritis ▪ Reactive arthritis ▪ Polyarteritis nodosa ▪ Poststreptococcal glomerulonephritis
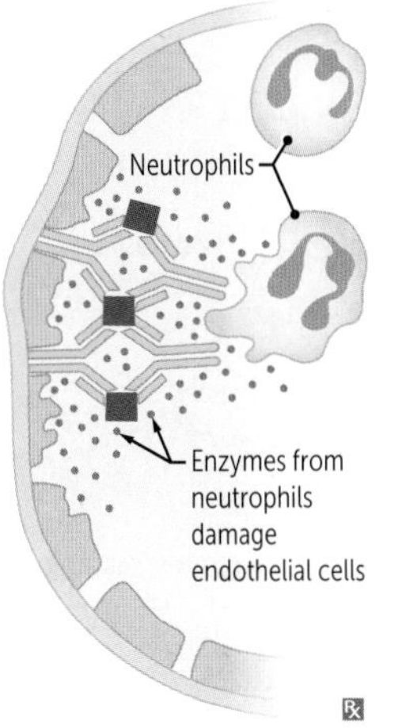Neutrophils Enzymes from neutrophils damage endothelial cells	**Serum sickness**—the prototypic immune complex disease. Antibodies to foreign proteins are produced and 1–2 weeks later, antibody-antigen complexes form and deposit in tissues → complement activation → inflammation and tissue damage (↓ serum C3, C4).	Fever, urticaria, arthralgia, proteinuria, lymphadenopathy occur 1–2 weeks after antigen exposure. Serum sickness-like reactions are associated with some drugs (may act as haptens, eg, penicillin, monoclonal antibodies) and infections (eg, hepatitis B).
	Arthus reaction—a local subacute immune complex-mediated hypersensitivity reaction. Intradermal injection of antigen into a presensitized (has circulating IgG) individual leads to immune complex formation in the skin (eg, enhanced local reaction to a booster vaccination). Characterized by edema, fibrinoid necrosis, activation of complement.	
Type IV hypersensitivity 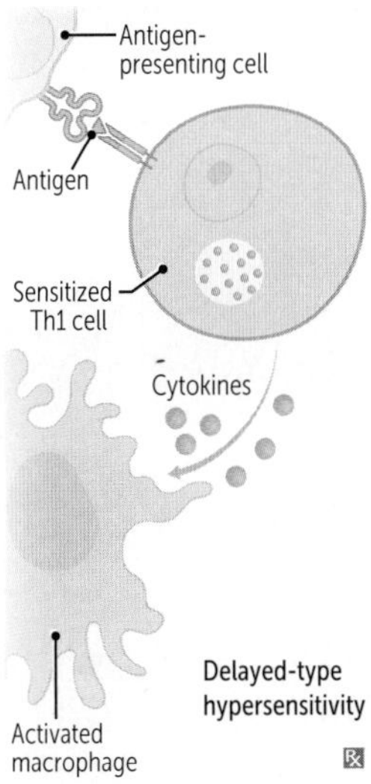Antigen-presenting cell Antigen Sensitized Th1 cell Cytokines Activated macrophage Delayed-type hypersensitivity	Two mechanisms, each involving T cells: 1. Direct cell cytotoxicity: CD8+ cytotoxic T cells kill targeted cells. 2. Inflammatory reaction: effector CD4+ T cells recognize antigen and release inflammation-inducing cytokines (shown in illustration).	Response does not involve antibodies (vs types I, II, and III). Examples: ▪ Contact dermatitis (eg, poison ivy, nickel allergy) ▪ Graft-versus-host disease Tests: PPD for TB infection; patch test for contact dermatitis; *Candida* skin test for T cell immune function. 4T's: T cells, Transplant rejections, TB skin tests, Touching (contact dermatitis). **Fourth** (type) and **last** (delayed).

Blood transfusion reactions

TYPE	PATHOGENESIS	TIMING	CLINICAL PRESENTATION	DONOR BLOOD	HOST BLOOD
Allergic/ anaphylactic reaction	Type I hypersensitivity reaction against plasma proteins in transfused blood IgA-deficient individuals should receive blood products without IgA	Within minutes to 2-3 hr (due to release of preformed inflammatory mediators in degranulating mast cells)	Allergies: urticaria, pruritus Anaphylaxis: wheezing, hypotension, respiratory arrest, shock	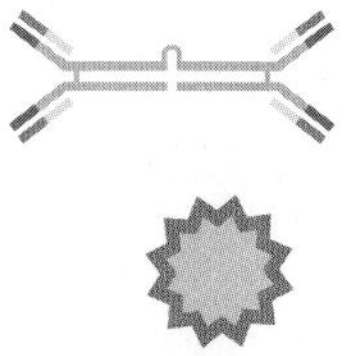 Donor plasma proteins, including IgA	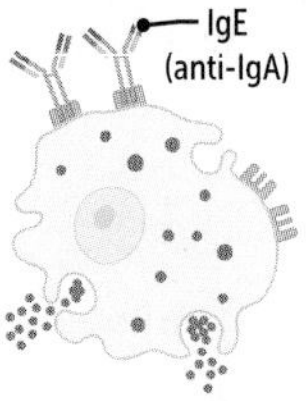 IgE (anti-IgA) Host mast cell
Acute hemolytic transfusion reaction	Type II hypersensitivity reaction Typically causes intravascular hemolysis (ABO blood group incompatibility)	During transfusion or within 24 hr (due to preformed antibodies)	Fever, hypotension, tachypnea, tachycardia, flank pain, hemoglobinuria (intravascular), jaundice (extravascular)	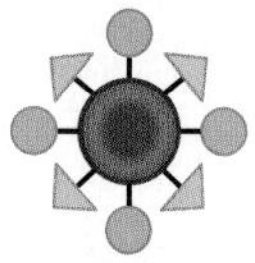 Donor RBC with A and/ or B group antigens	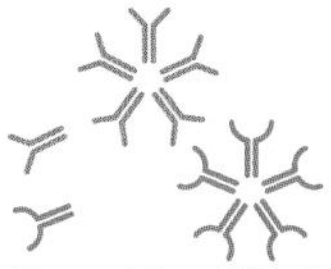 Host anti-A, anti-B IgG, IgM
Febrile nonhemolytic transfusion reaction	Cytokines created by donor WBCs accumulate during storage of blood products Reactions prevented by leukoreduction of blood products	Within 1-6 hr (due to preformed cytokines)	Fever, headaches, chills, flushing More common in children	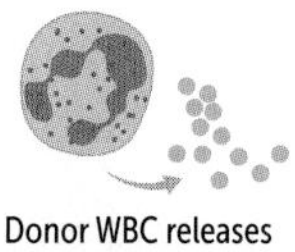 Donor WBC releases preformed cytokines	
Transfusion-related acute lung injury	Two-hit mechanism: ▪ Neutrophils are sequestered and primed in pulmonary vasculature due to recipient risk factors ▪ Neutrophils are activated by a product (eg, antileukocyte antibodies) in the transfused blood and release inflammatory mediators → ↑ capillary permeability → pulmonary edema	Within minutes to 6 hr	Respiratory distress, noncardiogenic pulmonary edema	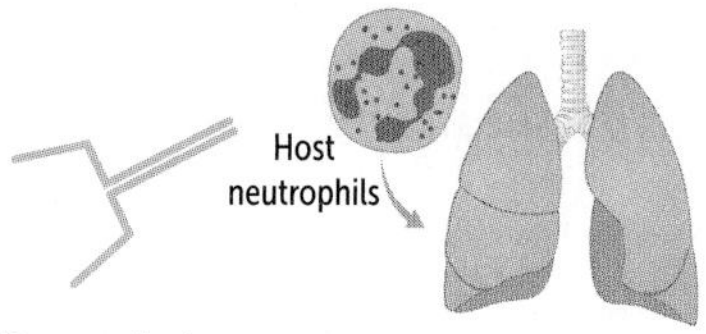 Host neutrophils Donor antileukocyte IgG	
Delayed hemolytic transfusion reaction	Anamnestic response to a foreign antigen on donor RBCs (Rh [D] or other minor blood group antigens) previously encountered by recipient Typically causes extravascular hemolysis	Onset over 24 hr Usually presents within 1-2 wk (due to slow destruction by reticuloendothelial system)	Generally self limited and clinically silent Mild fever, hyperbilirubinemia	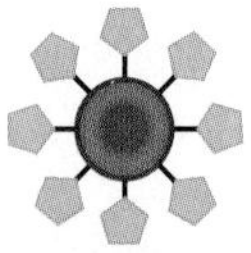 Donor RBC with foreign antigens	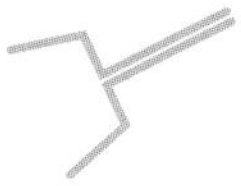 Host IgG

Autoantibodies

AUTOANTIBODY	ASSOCIATED DISORDER
Anti-postsynaptic ACh receptor	Myasthenia gravis
Anti-presynaptic voltage-gated calcium channel	Lambert-Eaton myasthenic syndrome
Anti-β_2 glycoprotein I	Antiphospholipid syndrome
Antinuclear (ANA)	Nonspecific screening antibody, often associated with SLE
Anticardiolipin, lupus anticoagulant	SLE, antiphospholipid syndrome
Anti-dsDNA, anti-Smith	SLE
Antihistone	Drug-induced lupus
Anti-U1 RNP (ribonucleoprotein)	Mixed connective tissue disease
Rheumatoid factor (IgM antibody against IgG Fc region), anti-CCP (more specific)	Rheumatoid arthritis
Anti-Ro/SSA, anti-La/SSB	Sjögren syndrome
Anti-Scl-70 (anti-DNA topoisomerase I)	Scleroderma (diffuse)
Anticentromere	Limited scleroderma (CREST syndrome)
Antisynthetase (eg, anti-Jo-1), anti-SRP, anti-helicase (anti-Mi-2)	Polymyositis, dermatomyositis
Antimitochondrial	1° biliary cholangitis
Anti-smooth muscle, anti-liver/kidney microsomal-1	Autoimmune hepatitis
Myeloperoxidase-antineutrophil cytoplasmic antibody (MPO-ANCA)/perinuclear ANCA (p-ANCA)	Microscopic polyangiitis, eosinophilic granulomatosis with polyangiitis, ulcerative colitis, 1° sclerosing cholangitis
PR3-ANCA/cytoplasmic ANCA (c-ANCA)	Granulomatosis with polyangiitis
Anti-phospholipase A_2 receptor	1° membranous nephropathy
Anti-hemidesmosome	Bullous pemphigoid
Anti-desmoglein (anti-desmosome)	Pemphigus vulgaris
Antithyroglobulin, antithyroid peroxidase (antimicrosomal)	Hashimoto thyroiditis
Anti-TSH receptor	Graves disease
IgA anti-endomysial, IgA anti-tissue transglutaminase, IgA and IgG deamidated gliadin peptide	Celiac disease
Anti-glutamic acid decarboxylase, islet cell cytoplasmic antibodies	Type 1 diabetes mellitus
Antiparietal cell, anti-intrinsic factor	Pernicious anemia
Anti-glomerular basement membrane	Goodpasture syndrome

Immunodeficiencies

DISEASE	DEFECT	PRESENTATION	FINDINGS
B-cell disorders			
X-linked (Bruton) agammaglobulinemia	Defect in *BTK*, a tyrosine kinase gene → no B-cell maturation; X-linked recessive (↑ in Boys)	Recurrent bacterial and enteroviral infections after 6 months (↓ maternal IgG)	Absent B cells in peripheral blood, ↓ Ig of all classes. Absent/scanty lymph nodes and tonsils (1° follicles and germinal centers absent) → live vaccines contraindicated
Selective IgA deficiency	Cause unknown Most common 1° immunodeficiency	Majority Asymptomatic Can see Airway and GI infections, Autoimmune disease, Atopy, Anaphylaxis to IgA in blood products	↓ IgA with normal IgG, IgM levels ↑ susceptibility to giardiasis Can cause false-negative celiac disease test
Common variable immunodeficiency	Defect in B-cell differentiation. Cause unknown in most cases	May present in childhood but usually diagnosed after puberty ↑ risk of autoimmune disease, bronchiectasis, lymphoma, sinopulmonary infections	↓ plasma cells, ↓ immunoglobulins
T-cell disorders			
Thymic aplasia	22q11 microdeletion; failure to develop 3rd and 4th pharyngeal pouches → absent thymus and parathyroids DiGeorge syndrome—thymic, parathyroid, cardiac defects Velocardiofacial syndrome—palate, facial, cardiac defects	**CATCH-22**: **C**ardiac defects (conotruncal abnormalities [eg, tetralogy of Fallot, truncus arteriosus]), **A**bnormal facies, **T**hymic hypoplasia → T-cell deficiency (recurrent viral/fungal infections), **C**left palate, **H**ypocalcemia 2° to parathyroid aplasia → tetany	↓ T cells, ↓ PTH, ↓ Ca^{2+} Thymic shadow absent on CXR
IL-12 receptor deficiency	↓ Th1 response; autosomal recessive	Disseminated mycobacterial and fungal infections; may present after administration of BCG vaccine	↓ IFN-γ Most common cause of Mendelian susceptibility to mycobacterial diseases (MSMD)
Autosomal dominant hyper-IgE syndrome (Job syndrome)	Deficiency of Th17 cells due to *STAT3* mutation → impaired recruitment of neutrophils to sites of infection	Cold (noninflamed) staphylococcal **A**bscesses, retained **B**aby teeth, **C**oarse facies, **D**ermatologic problems (eczema), ↑ Ig**E**, bone **F**ractures from minor trauma	↑ IgE ↑ eosinophils Learn the **ABCDEF**'s to get a **Job**!
Chronic mucocutaneous candidiasis	T-cell dysfunction Impaired cell-mediated immunity against *Candida* sp Classic form caused by defects in *AIRE*	Persistent noninvasive *Candida albicans* infections of skin and mucous membranes	Absent in vitro T-cell proliferation in response to *Candida* antigens Absent cutaneous reaction to *Candida* antigens

Immunodeficiencies *(continued)*

DISEASE	DEFECT	PRESENTATION	FINDINGS
B- and T-cell disorders			
Severe combined immunodeficiency	Several types including defective IL-2R gamma chain (most common, X-linked recessive); adenosine deaminase deficiency (autosomal recessive); *RAG* mutation → VDJ recombination defect	Failure to thrive, chronic diarrhea, thrush Recurrent viral, bacterial, fungal, and protozoal infections	↓ T-cell receptor excision circles (TRECs) Part of newborn screening for SCID Absence of thymic shadow (CXR), germinal centers (lymph node biopsy), and T cells (flow cytometry)
Ataxia-telangiectasia 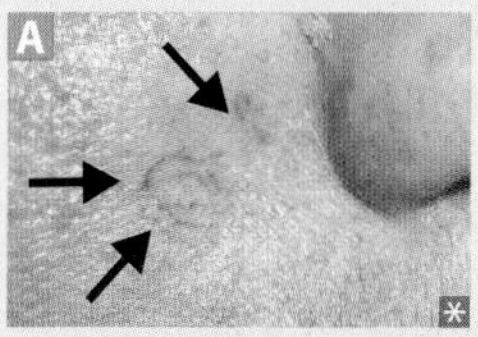	Defects in *ATM* gene → failure to detect DNA damage → failure to halt progression of cell cycle → mutations accumulate; autosomal recessive	Triad: cerebellar defects (Ataxia), spider Angiomas (telangiectasia A), IgA deficiency ↑↑ sensitivity to radiation (limit x-ray exposure)	↑ AFP ↓ IgA, IgG, and IgE Lymphopenia, cerebellar atrophy ↑ risk of lymphoma and leukemia
Hyper-IgM syndrome	Most commonly due to defective CD40L on Th cells → class switching defect; X-linked recessive	Severe pyogenic infections early in life; opportunistic infection with *Pneumocystis*, *Cryptosporidium*, CMV	Normal or ↑ IgM ↓↓ IgG, IgA, IgE Failure to make germinal centers
Wiskott-Aldrich syndrome	Mutation in *WAS* gene; leukocytes and platelets unable to reorganize actin cytoskeleton → defective antigen presentation; X-linked recessive	WATER: Wiskott-Aldrich: Thrombocytopenia, Eczema, Recurrent (pyogenic) infections ↑ risk of autoimmune disease and malignancy	↓ to normal IgG, IgM ↑ IgE, IgA Fewer and smaller platelets
Phagocyte dysfunction			
Leukocyte adhesion deficiency (type 1)	Defect in LFA-1 integrin (CD18) protein on phagocytes; impaired migration and chemotaxis; autosomal recessive	Late separation (>30 days) of umbilical cord, absent pus, dysfunctional neutrophils → recurrent skin and mucosal bacterial infections	↑ neutrophils in blood Absence of neutrophils at infection sites → impaired wound healing
Chédiak-Higashi syndrome 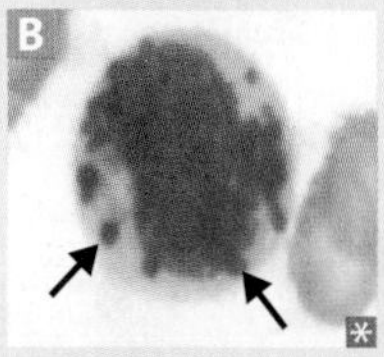	Defect in lysosomal trafficking regulator gene (*LYST*) Microtubule dysfunction in phagosome-lysosome fusion; autosomal recessive	PLAIN: Progressive neurodegeneration, Lymphohistiocytosis, Albinism (partial), recurrent pyogenic Infections, peripheral Neuropathy	Giant granules (B, arrows) in granulocytes and platelets Pancytopenia Mild coagulation defects
Chronic granulomatous disease	Defect of NADPH oxidase → ↓ reactive oxygen species (eg, superoxide) and ↓ respiratory burst in neutrophils; X-linked form most common	↑ susceptibility to catalase ⊕ organisms Recurrent infections and granulomas	Abnormal dihydrorhodamine (flow cytometry) test (↓ green fluorescence) Nitroblue tetrazolium dye reduction test (obsolete) fails to turn blue

Infections in immunodeficiency

PATHOGEN	↓ T CELLS	↓ B CELLS	↓ GRANULOCYTES	↓ COMPLEMENT
Bacteria	Sepsis	Encapsulated (Please SHINE my SKiS): *Pseudomonas aeruginosa*, *Streptococcus pneumoniae*, *Haemophilus Influenzae* type b, *Neisseria meningitidis*, *Escherichia coli*, *Salmonella*, *Klebsiella pneumoniae*, group B *Streptococcus*	Some Bacteria Produce No Serious granules: *Staphylococcus*, *Burkholderia cepacia*, *Pseudomonas aeruginosa*, *Nocardia*, *Serratia*	Encapsulated species with early complement deficiencies *Neisseria* with late complement (C5–C9) deficiencies
Viruses	CMV, EBV, JC virus, VZV, chronic infection with respiratory/GI viruses	Enteroviral encephalitis, poliovirus (live vaccine contraindicated)	N/A	N/A
Fungi/parasites	*Candida* (local), PCP, *Cryptococcus*	GI giardiasis (no IgA)	*Candida* (systemic), *Aspergillus*, *Mucor*	N/A

Note: B-cell deficiencies tend to produce recurrent bacterial infections, whereas T-cell deficiencies produce more fungal and viral infections.

Transplant rejection

TYPE OF REJECTION	ONSET	PATHOGENESIS	FEATURES
Hyperacute 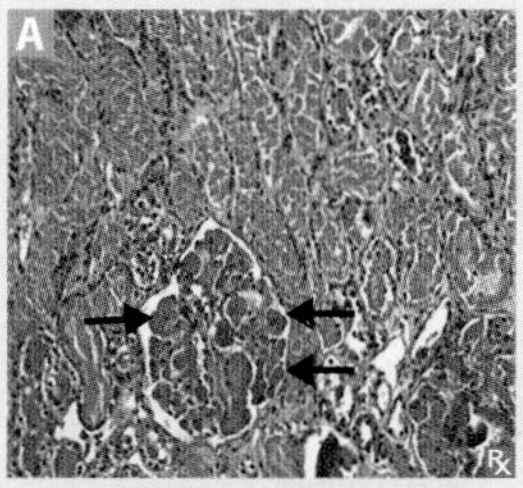	Within minutes	Pre-existing recipient antibodies react to donor antigen (type II hypersensitivity reaction), activate complement	Widespread thrombosis of graft vessels (arrows within glomerulus A) → ischemia and fibrinoid necrosis Graft must be removed
Acute 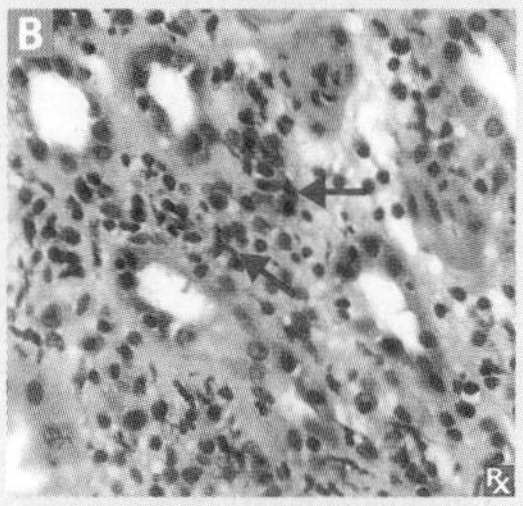	Weeks to months	Cellular: CD8+ T cells and/or CD4+ T cells activated against donor MHCs (type IV hypersensitivity reaction) Humoral: similar to hyperacute, except antibodies develop after transplant (associated with C4d deposition)	Vasculitis of graft vessels with dense interstitial lymphocytic infiltrate B Prevent/reverse with immunosuppressants
Chronic 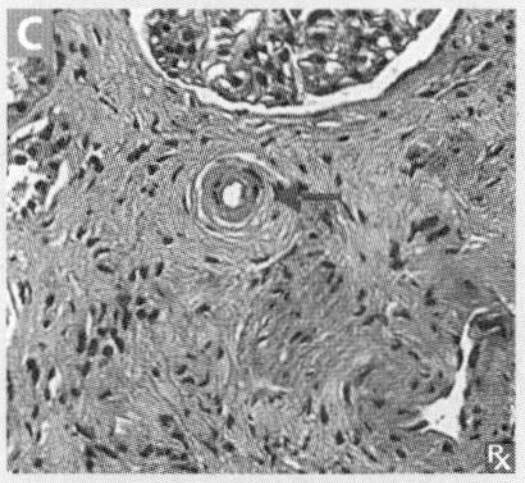	Months to years	CD4+ T cells respond to recipient APCs presenting donor peptides, including allogeneic MHC Both cellular and humoral components (type II and IV hypersensitivity reactions)	Recipient T cells react and secrete cytokines → proliferation of vascular smooth muscle, parenchymal atrophy, interstitial fibrosis Dominated by arteriosclerosis C Organ-specific examples: ▪ Chronic allograft nephropathy ▪ Bronchiolitis obliterans ▪ Accelerated atherosclerosis (heart) ▪ Vanishing bile duct syndrome
Graft-versus-host disease	Varies	Grafted immunocompetent T cells proliferate in the immunocompromised host and reject host cells with "foreign" proteins → severe organ dysfunction Type IV hypersensitivity reaction	Maculopapular rash, jaundice, diarrhea, hepatosplenomegaly Usually in bone marrow and liver transplants (rich in lymphocytes) Potentially beneficial in bone marrow transplant for leukemia (graft-versus-tumor effect) For patients who are immunocompromised, irradiate blood products prior to transfusion to prevent GVHD

▶ IMMUNOLOGY—IMMUNOSUPPRESSANTS

Immunosuppressants Agents that block lymphocyte activation and proliferation. Reduce acute transplant rejection by suppressing cellular immunity (used as prophylaxis). Frequently combined to achieve greater efficacy with ↓ toxicity. Chronic suppression ↑ risk of infection and malignancy.

DRUG	MECHANISM	INDICATIONS	TOXICITY	NOTES
Cyclosporine	Calcineurin inhibitor; binds cyclophilin Blocks T-cell activation by **preventing IL-2 transcription**	Psoriasis, rheumatoid arthritis	**Nephrotoxicity**, hypertension, hyperlipidemia, neurotoxicity, gingival hyperplasia, hirsutism	Both calcineurin inhibitors are highly nephrotoxic, especially in higher doses or in patients with ↓ renal function
Tacrolimus (FK506)	Calcineurin inhibitor; binds FK506 binding protein (FKBP) Blocks T-cell activation by **preventing IL-2 transcription**	Immunosuppression after solid organ transplant	Similar to cyclosporine, ↑ risk of diabetes and neurotoxicity; no gingival hyperplasia or hirsutism	
Sirolimus (Rapamycin)	mTOR inhibitor; binds FKBP Blocks T-cell activation and B-cell differentiation by **preventing response to IL-2**	Kidney transplant rejection prophylaxis specifically **Sir Basil**'s kidney transplant	"Pansirtopenia" (pancytopenia), insulin resistance, hyperlipidemia; **not nephrotoxic**	Kidney "**sir**-vives." Synergistic with cyclosporine Also used in drug-eluting stents
Basiliximab	Monoclonal antibody; blocks IL-2R		Edema, hypertension, tremor	
Azathioprine	Antimetabolite precursor of 6-mercaptopurine Inhibits lymphocyte proliferation by blocking nucleotide synthesis	Rheumatoid arthritis, Crohn disease, glomerulonephritis, other autoimmune conditions	Pancytopenia	6-MP degraded by xanthine oxidase; toxicity ↑ by allopurinol Pronounce "azathio-**purine**"
Mycophenolate Mofetil	Reversibly inhibits IMP dehydrogenase, preventing purine synthesis of B and T cells	Glucocorticoid-sparing agent in rheumatic disease	GI upset, pancytopenia, hypertension, hyperglycemia Less nephrotoxic and neurotoxic	Associated with invasive CMV infection
Glucocorticoids	Inhibit NF-κB Suppress both B- and T-cell function by ↓ transcription of many cytokines Induce T cell apoptosis	Many autoimmune and inflammatory disorders, adrenal insufficiency, asthma, CLL, non-Hodgkin lymphoma	Cushing syndrome, osteoporosis, hyperglycemia, diabetes, amenorrhea, adrenocortical atrophy, peptic ulcers, psychosis, cataracts, avascular necrosis (femoral head)	Demargination of WBCs causes artificial leukocytosis Adrenal insufficiency may develop if drug is stopped abruptly after chronic use

Immunosuppression targets

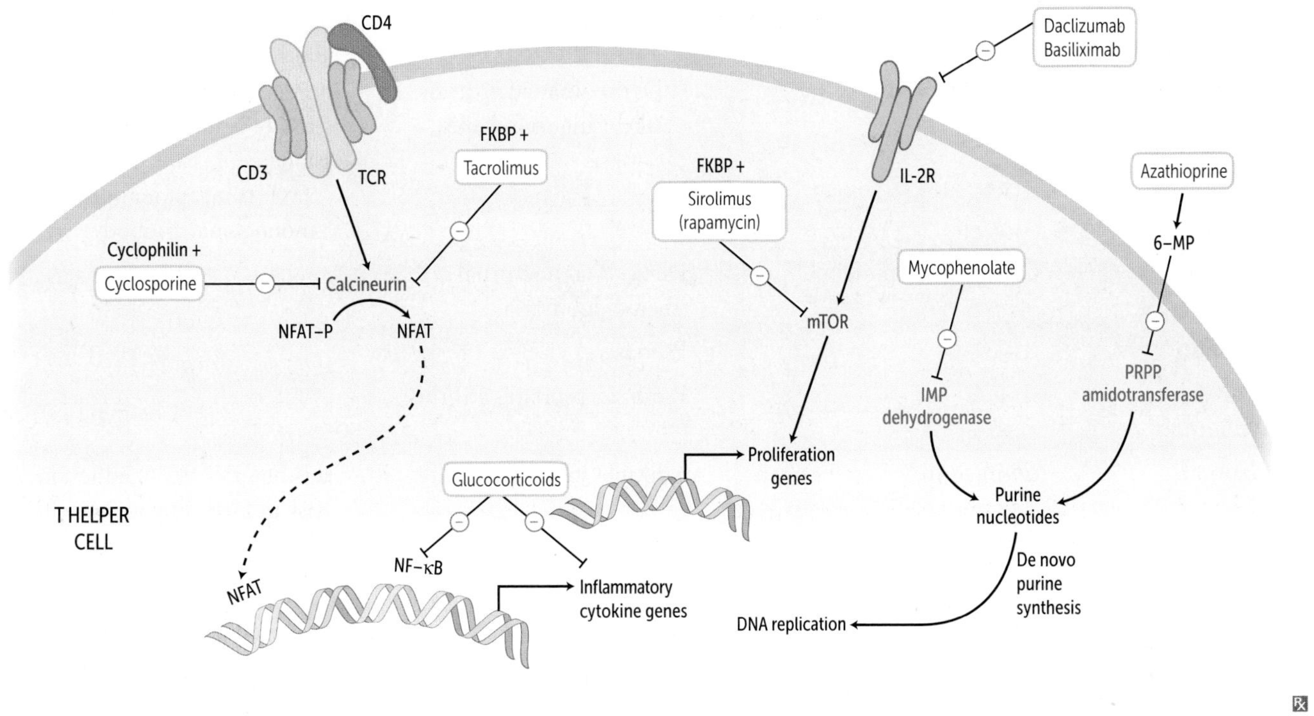

Recombinant cytokines and clinical uses

CYTOKINE	AGENT	CLINICAL USES
Bone marrow stimulation		
Erythropoietin	Epoetin alfa (EPO analog)	Anemias (especially in renal failure) Associated with ↑ risk of hypertension, thromboembolic events
Colony stimulating factors	Filgrastim (G-CSF), Sargramostim (GM-CSF)	Leukopenia; recovery of granulocyte and monocyte counts
Thrombopoietin	Romiplostim (TPO analog), eltrombopag (think "elthrombopag." TPO receptor agonist)	Autoimmune thrombocytopenia Platelet stimulator
Immunotherapy		
Toll-like receptor 7	Imiquimod	Anogenital warts, actinic keratosis
Interleukin-2	Aldesleukin	Renal cell carcinoma, metastatic melanoma
Interferons	IFN-α	Chronic hepatitis C (not preferred) and B, renal cell carcinoma
	IFN-β	Multiple sclerosis
	IFN-γ	Chronic granulomatous disease

Therapeutic antibodies

AGENT	TARGET	CLINICAL USE	NOTES
Autoimmune disease therapy			
Adalimumab, infliximab	Soluble TNF-α	IBD, rheumatoid arthritis, ankylosing spondylitis, psoriasis	Screen patients for TB due to risk of reactivation Etanercept is a decoy TNF-α receptor and not a monoclonal antibody
Eculizumab	Complement protein C5	Paroxysmal nocturnal hemoglobinuria	
Guselkumab	IL-23	Psoriasis	
Ixekizumab, secukinumab	IL-17A	Psoriasis, psoriatic arthritis	
Natalizumab	α4-integrin	Multiple sclerosis, Crohn disease	α4-integrin: WBC adhesion Risk of PML in patients with JC virus
Ustekinumab	IL-12/IL-23	Psoriasis, psoriatic arthritis	
Vedolizumab	α4-integrin	IBD	Gut-specific anti-integrin, preventing migration of leukocytes to the gastrointestinal tract
Other applications			
Denosumab	RANKL	Osteoporosis; inhibits osteoclast maturation (mimics osteoprotegerin)	**Deno**sumab helps make **dense** bones
Emicizumab	Factor IXa and X	Hemophilia A	Bispecific; mimics factor VIII
Omalizumab	IgE	Refractory allergic asthma; prevents IgE binding to FcεRI	
Palivizumab	RSV F protein	RSV prophylaxis for high-risk infants	Palivizumab—virus

HIGH-YIELD PRINCIPLES IN

Microbiology

"Support bacteria. They're the only culture some people have."

—Steven Wright

"What lies behind us and what lies ahead of us are tiny matters compared to what lies within us."

—Henry S. Haskins

"Wise and humane management of the patient is the best safeguard against infection."

—Florence Nightingale

"I sing and play the guitar, and I'm a walking, talking bacterial infection."

—Kurt Cobain

Microbiology questions on the Step 1 exam often require two (or more) steps: Given a certain clinical presentation, you will first need to identify the most likely causative organism, and you will then need to provide an answer regarding some features of that organism or relevant antimicrobial agents. For example, a description of a child with fever and a petechial rash will be followed by a question that reads, "From what site does the responsible organism usually enter the blood?"

This section therefore presents organisms in two major ways: in individual microbial "profiles" and in the context of the systems they infect and the clinical presentations they produce. You should become familiar with both formats. When reviewing the systems approach, remind yourself of the features of each microbe by returning to the individual profiles. Also be sure to memorize the laboratory characteristics that allow you to identify microbes.

▶ MICROBIOLOGY—BASIC BACTERIOLOGY

Bacterial structures

STRUCTURE	CHEMICAL COMPOSITION	FUNCTION
Appendages		
Flagellum	Proteins	Motility
Pilus/fimbria	Glycoprotein	Mediate adherence of bacteria to cell surface; sex pilus forms during conjugation
Specialized structures		
Spore	Keratin-like coat; dipicolinic acid; peptidoglycan, DNA	Gram ⊕ only Survival: resist dehydration, heat, chemicals
Cell envelope		
Capsule	Discrete layer usually made of polysaccharides (and rarely proteins)	Protects against phagocytosis
Slime (S) layer	Loose network of polysaccharides	Mediates adherence to surfaces, plays a role in biofilm formation (eg, indwelling catheters)
Outer membrane	Outer leaflet: contains endotoxin (LPS/LOS) Embedded proteins: porins and other outer membrane proteins (OMPs) Inner leaflet: phospholipids	Gram ⊖ only Endotoxin: lipid A induces TNF and IL-1; antigenic O polysaccharide component Most OMPs are antigenic Porins: transport across outer membrane
Periplasm	Space between cytoplasmic membrane and outer membrane in gram ⊖ bacteria (peptidoglycan in middle)	Accumulates components exiting gram ⊖ cells, including hydrolytic enzymes (eg, β-lactamases)
Cell wall	Peptidoglycan is a sugar backbone with peptide side chains cross-linked by transpeptidase	Net-like structure gives rigid support, protects against osmotic pressure damage
Cytoplasmic membrane	Phospholipid bilayer sac with embedded proteins (eg, penicillin-binding proteins [PBPs]) and other enzymes Lipoteichoic acids (gram positive) only extend from membrane to exterior	Site of oxidative and transport enzymes; PBPs involved in cell wall synthesis Lipoteichoic acids induce TNF-α and IL-1

Cell envelope

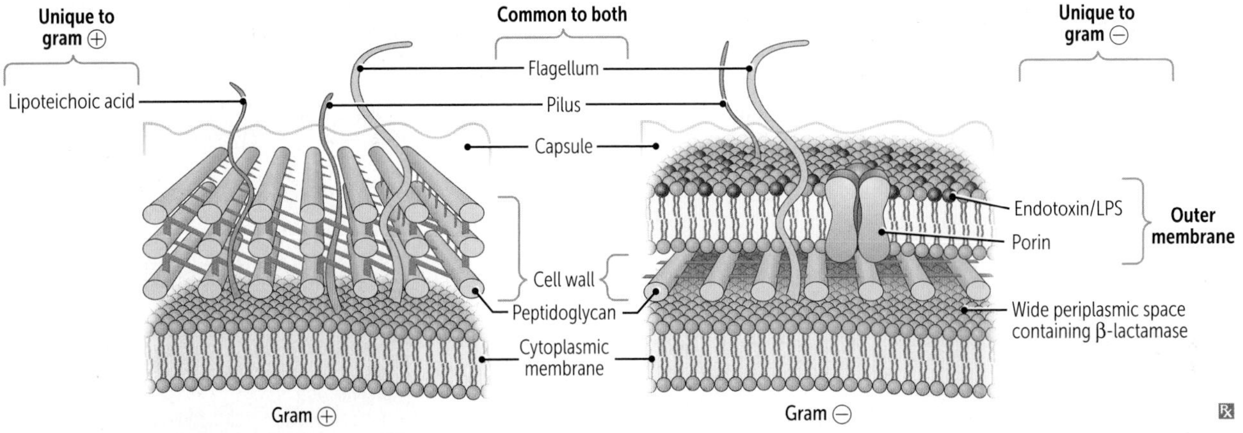

Stains

Gram stain	First-line lab test in bacterial identification. Bacteria with thick peptidoglycan layer retain crystal violet dye (gram ⊕); bacteria with thin peptidoglycan layer turn red or pink (gram ⊖) with counterstain. These bugs do not Gram stain well (These Little Microbes May Unfortunately Lack Real Color But Are Everywhere):	
	Treponema, *Leptospira*	Too thin to be visualized
	Mycobacteria	Cell wall has high lipid content
	Mycoplasma, *Ureaplasma*	No cell wall
	Legionella, *Rickettsia*, *Chlamydia*, *Bartonella*, *Anaplasma*, *Ehrlichia*	Primarily intracellular; also, *Chlamydia* lack classic peptidoglycan because of ↓ muramic acid
Giemsa stain	*Chlamydia*, *Rickettsia*, Trypanosomes A, *Borrelia*, *Helicobacter pylori*, *Plasmodium*	Clumsy Rick Tripped on a Borrowed Helicopter Plastered in Gems
Periodic acid–Schiff stain	Stains glycogen, mucopolysaccharides; used to diagnose Whipple disease (*Tropheryma whipplei* B)	PaSs the sugar
Ziehl-Neelsen stain (carbol fuchsin)	Acid-fast bacteria (eg, *Mycobacteria* C, *Nocardia*; stains mycolic acid in cell wall); protozoa (eg, *Cryptosporidium* oocysts)	Auramine-rhodamine stain is more often used for screening (inexpensive, more sensitive)
India ink stain	*Cryptococcus neoformans* D; mucicarmine can also be used to stain thick polysaccharide capsule red	
Silver stain	Fungi (eg, *Coccidioides* E, *Pneumocystis jirovecii*), *Legionella*, *Helicobacter pylori*	
Fluorescent antibody stain	Used to identify many bacteria, viruses, *Pneumocystis jirovecii*, *Giardia*, and *Cryptosporidium*	Example is FTA-ABS for syphilis

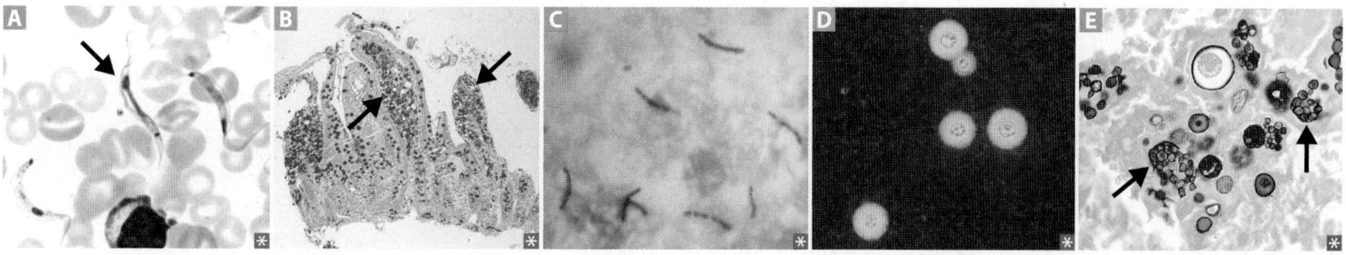

Properties of growth media	The same type of media can possess both (or neither) of these properties.
Selective media	Favors the growth of particular organism while preventing growth of other organisms. Example: Thayer-Martin agar contains antibiotics that allow the selective growth of *Neisseria* by inhibiting the growth of other sensitive organisms.
Indicator (differential) media	Yields a color change in response to the metabolism of certain organisms. Example: MacConkey agar contains a pH indicator; a lactose fermenter like *E coli* will convert lactose to acidic metabolites → color changes to pink.

Special culture requirements

BUG	MEDIA USED FOR ISOLATION	MEDIA CONTENTS/OTHER
H influenzae	Chocolate agar	Factors V (NAD^+) and X (hematin)
N gonorrhoeae, N meningitidis	Thayer-Martin agar	Selectively favors growth of *Neisseria* by inhibiting growth of gram ⊕ organisms with vancomycin, gram ⊖ organisms except *Neisseria* with trimethoprim and colistin, and fungi with nystatin Very typically cultures *Neisseria*
B pertussis	Bordet-Gengou agar (**Bordet** for ***Bordetella***) Regan-Lowe medium	Potato extract Charcoal, blood, and antibiotic
C diphtheriae	Tellurite agar, Löffler medium	
M tuberculosis	Löwenstein-Jensen medium, Middlebrook medium, rapid automated broth cultures	
M pneumoniae	Eaton agar	Requires cholesterol
Lactose-fermenting enterics	MacConkey agar	Fermentation produces acid, causing colonies to turn pink
E coli	Eosin–methylene blue (EMB) agar	Colonies with green metallic sheen
Brucella, Francisella, Legionella, Pasteurella	**Charcoal** yeast extract agar buffered with **cysteine** and **iron**	The **Ella** siblings, **Bruce**, **Francis**, a **legionnaire**, and a **pasteur** (pastor), built the Sistine (**cysteine**) chapel out of **charcoal** and **iron**
Fungi	Sabouraud agar	"**Sab's a fun guy!**"

Aerobes	Use an O_2-dependent system to generate ATP. Examples include *Nocardia, Pseudomonas aeruginosa, Mycobacterium tuberculosis,* and *Bordetella pertussis.* Reactivation of *M tuberculosis* (eg, after immunocompromise or TNF-α inhibitor use) has a predilection for the apices of the lung.

Anaerobes	Examples include *Clostridium*, *Bacteroides*, *Fusobacterium*, and *Actinomyces israelii*. They lack catalase and/or superoxide dismutase and are thus susceptible to oxidative damage. Generally foul smelling (short-chain fatty acids), are difficult to culture, and produce gas in tissue (CO_2 and H_2).	Anaerobes Can't Breathe Fresh Air. Anaerobes are normal flora in GI tract, typically pathogenic elsewhere. AminO_2glycosides are ineffective against anaerobes because these antibiotics require O_2 to enter into bacterial cell.
Facultative anaerobes	May use O_2 as a terminal electron acceptor to generate ATP, but can also use fermentation and other O_2-independent pathways.	Streptococci, staphylococci, and enteric gram ⊖ bacteria.

Intracellular bacteria

Obligate intracellular	*Rickettsia*, *Chlamydia*, *Coxiella* Rely on host ATP	Stay inside (cells) when it is Really Chilly and Cold
Facultative intracellular	*Salmonella*, *Neisseria*, *Brucella*, *Mycobacterium*, *Listeria*, *Francisella*, *Legionella*, *Yersinia pestis*	Some Nasty Bugs May Live FacultativeLY

Encapsulated bacteria 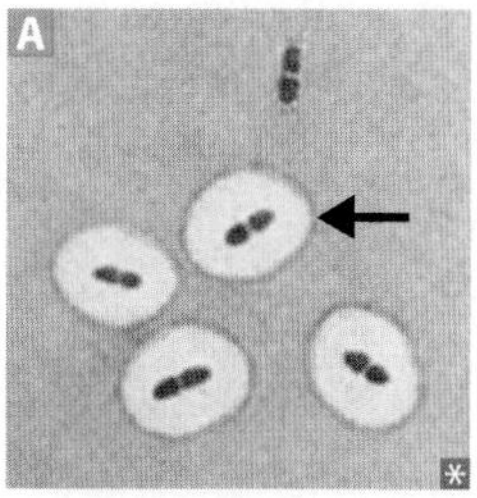	Examples are *Pseudomonas aeruginosa*, *Streptococcus pneumoniae* A, *Haemophilus influenzae* type b, *Neisseria meningitidis*, *Escherichia coli*, *Salmonella*, *Klebsiella pneumoniae*, and group B Strep. Their capsules serve as an antiphagocytic virulence factor. Capsular polysaccharide + protein conjugate serves as an antigen in vaccines.	Please SHiNE my SKiS. Are opsonized, and then cleared by spleen. Asplenics (No Spleen Here) have ↓ opsonizing ability and thus ↑ risk for severe infections; need vaccines to protect against: ▪ *N meningitidis* ▪ *S pneumoniae* ▪ *H influenzae*
Encapsulated bacteria vaccines	Some vaccines containing polysaccharide capsule antigens are conjugated to a carrier protein, enhancing immunogenicity by promoting T-cell activation and subsequent class switching. A polysaccharide antigen alone cannot be presented to T cells.	Pneumococcal vaccines: PCV13 (pneumococcal conjugate vaccine), PPSV23 (pneumococcal polysaccharide vaccine with no conjugated protein). *H influenzae* type b (conjugate vaccine). Meningococcal vaccine (conjugate vaccine).
Urease-positive organisms	*Proteus*, *Cryptococcus*, *H pylori*, *Ureaplasma*, *Nocardia*, *Klebsiella*, *S epidermidis*, *S saprophyticus*. Urease hydrolyzes urea to release ammonia and CO_2 → ↑ pH. Predisposes to struvite (magnesium ammonium phosphate) stones, particularly *Proteus*.	Pee CHUNKSS.

Catalase-positive organisms

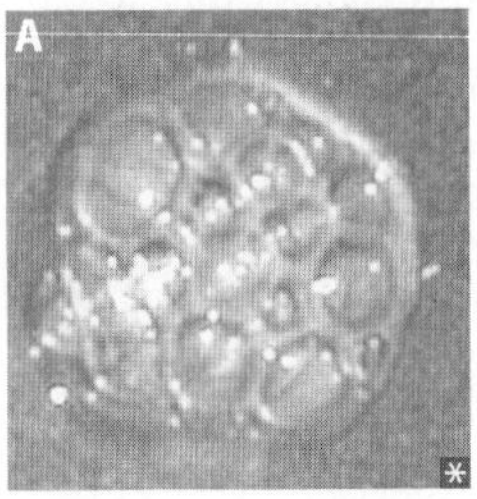

Catalase degrades H_2O_2 into H_2O and bubbles of O_2 A before it can be converted to microbicidal products by the enzyme myeloperoxidase. People with chronic granulomatous disease (NADPH oxidase deficiency) have recurrent infections with certain catalase ⊕ organisms.
Examples: *Nocardia, Staphylococci, Serratia, Candida, Listeria, E coli, Burkholderia cepacia, Pseudomonas, Aspergillus, Helicobacter pylori, Bordetella pertussis.*

Pigment-producing bacteria	*Actinomyces israelii*—yellow "sulfur" granules, which are composed of filaments of bacteria	Israel has yellow sand
	S aureus—golden yellow pigment	*Aureus* (Latin) = gold
	P aeruginosa—blue-green pigment (pyocyanin and pyoverdin)	Aerugula is green
	Serratia marcescens—red pigment	Think red Sriracha hot sauce

In vivo biofilm-producing bacteria	*S epidermidis*	Catheter and prosthetic device infections
	Viridans streptococci (*S mutans, S sanguinis*)	Dental plaques, infective endocarditis
	P aeruginosa	Respiratory tree colonization in patients with cystic fibrosis, ventilator-associated pneumonia Contact lens–associated keratitis
	Nontypeable (unencapsulated) *H influenzae*	Otitis media

Spore-forming bacteria 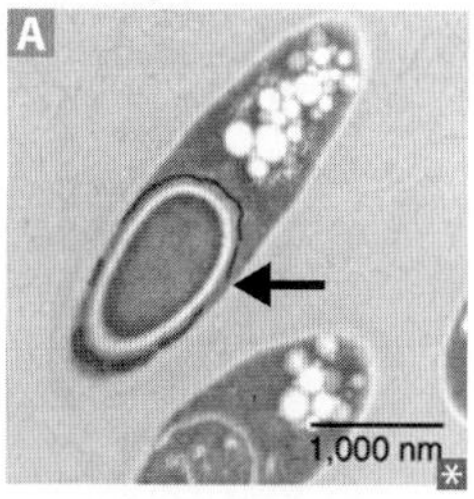	Some gram ⊕ bacteria can form spores A when nutrients are limited. Spores lack metabolic activity and are highly resistant to heat and chemicals. Core contains dipicolinic acid (responsible for heat resistance). Must autoclave to kill spores (as is done to surgical equipment) by steaming at 121°C for 15 minutes. Hydrogen peroxide and iodine-based agents are also sporicidal.	Examples: *B anthracis* (anthrax), *B cereus* (food poisoning), *C botulinum* (botulism), *C difficile* (pseudomembranous colitis), *C perfringens* (gas gangrene), *C tetani* (tetanus).

Bacterial virulence factors	These promote evasion of host immune response.
Protein A	Binds Fc region of IgG. Prevents opsonization and phagocytosis. Expressed by *S aureus*.
IgA protease	Enzyme that cleaves IgA, allowing bacteria to adhere to and colonize mucous membranes. Secreted by *S pneumoniae, H influenzae* type b, and *Neisseria* (SHiN).
M protein	Helps prevent phagocytosis. Expressed by group A streptococci. Sequence homology with human tropomyosin and myosin (molecular mimicry); possibly underlies the autoimmune response seen in acute rheumatic fever.

Bacterial genetics

Transformation

Competent bacteria can bind and import short pieces of environmental naked bacterial chromosomal DNA (from bacterial cell lysis). The transfer and expression of newly transferred genes is called transformation. A feature of many bacteria, especially *S pneumoniae*, *H influenzae* type b, and *Neisseria* (**SHiN**).

Adding deoxyribonuclease degrades naked DNA, preventing transformation.

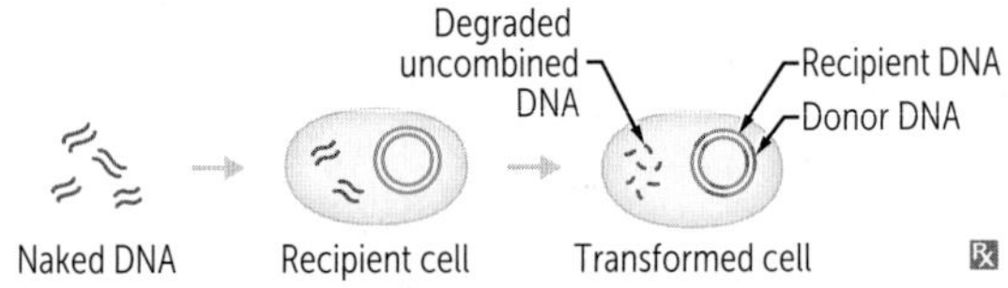

Conjugation

$F^+ \times F^-$

F^+ plasmid contains genes required for sex pilus and conjugation. Bacteria without this plasmid are termed F^-. Sex pilus on F^+ bacterium contacts F^- bacterium. A single strand of plasmid DNA is transferred across the conjugal bridge ("mating bridge"). No transfer of chromosomal DNA.

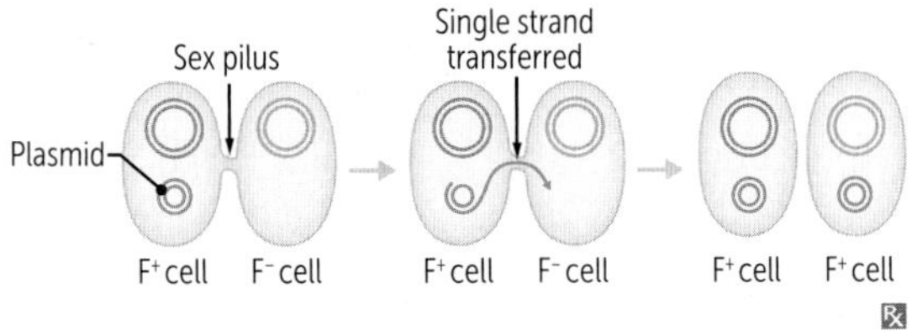

Hfr $\times F^-$

F^+ plasmid can become incorporated into bacterial chromosomal DNA, termed high-frequency recombination (Hfr) cell. Transfer of leading part of plasmid and a few flanking chromosomal genes. High-frequency recombination may integrate some of those bacterial genes. Recipient cell remains F^- but now may have new bacterial genes.

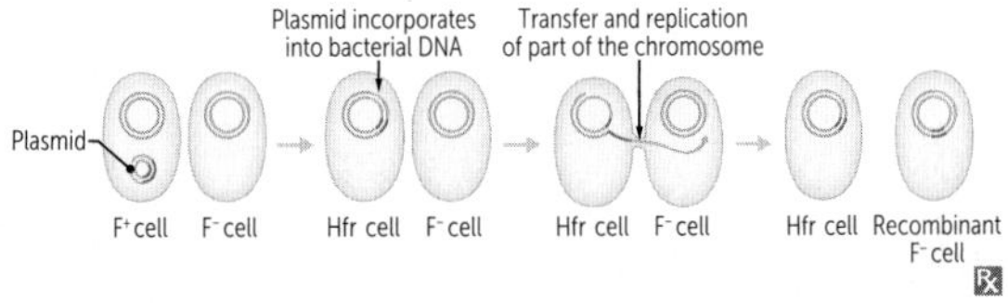

Transduction

Generalized

A "packaging" error. Lytic phage infects bacterium, leading to cleavage of bacterial DNA. Parts of bacterial chromosomal DNA may become packaged in phage capsid. Phage infects another bacterium, transferring these genes.

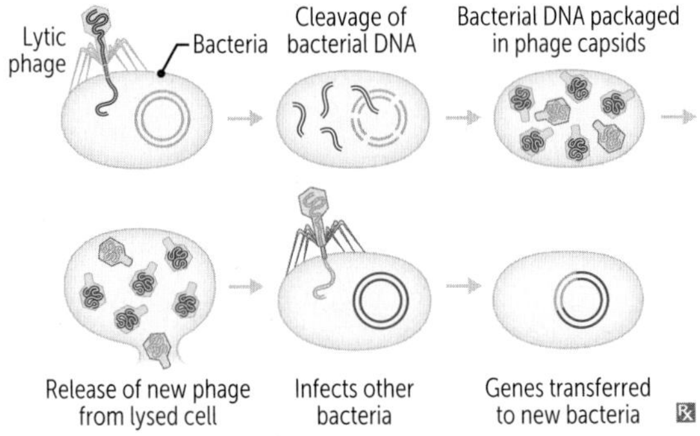

Specialized

An "excision" event. Lysogenic phage infects bacterium; viral DNA incorporates into bacterial chromosome. When phage DNA is excised, flanking bacterial genes may be excised with it. DNA is packaged into phage capsid and can infect another bacterium.

Genes for the following 5 bacterial toxins are encoded in a lysogenic phage (**ABCD'S**): Group **A** strep erythrogenic toxin, **B**otulinum toxin, **C**holera toxin, **D**iphtheria toxin, **S**higa toxin.

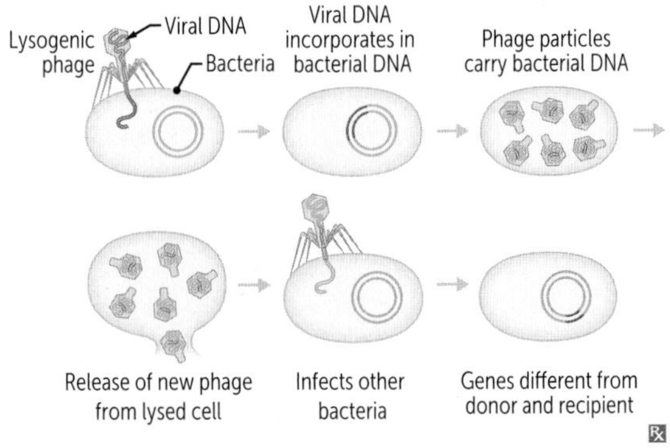

Bacterial genetics *(continued)*

Transposition A "jumping" process involving a transposon (specialized segment of DNA), which can copy and excise itself and then insert into the same DNA molecule or an unrelated DNA (eg, plasmid or chromosome). Critical in creating plasmids with multiple drug resistance and transfer across species lines (eg, Tn*1546* with *van*A from *Enterococcus* to *S aureus*).

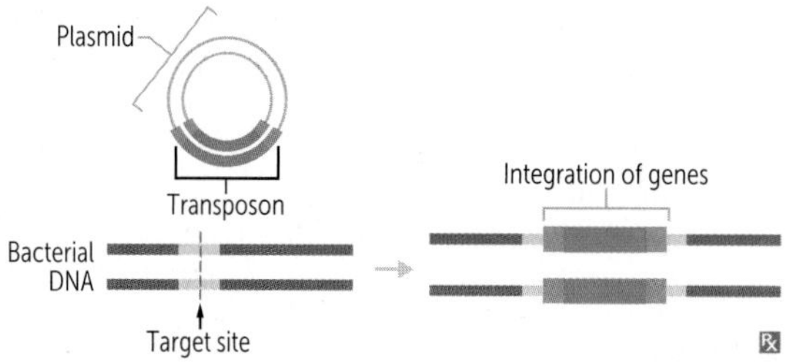

Main features of exotoxins and endotoxins

	Exotoxins	Endotoxins
SOURCE	Certain species of gram ⊕ and gram ⊖ bacteria	Outer cell membrane of most gram ⊖ bacteria
SECRETED FROM CELL	Yes	No
CHEMISTRY	Polypeptide	Lipid A component of LPS (structural part of bacteria; released when lysed)
LOCATION OF GENES	Plasmid or bacteriophage	Bacterial chromosome
TOXICITY	High (fatal dose on the order of 1 µg)	Low (fatal dose on the order of hundreds of micrograms)
CLINICAL EFFECTS	Various effects (see following pages)	Fever, shock (hypotension), DIC
MODE OF ACTION	Various modes (see following pages)	Induces TNF, IL-1, and IL-6
ANTIGENICITY	Induces high-titer antibodies called antitoxins	Poorly antigenic
VACCINES	Toxoids used as vaccines	No toxoids formed and no vaccine available
HEAT STABILITY	Destroyed rapidly at 60°C (except staphylococcal enterotoxin and *E coli* heat-stable toxin)	Stable at 100°C for 1 hr
TYPICAL DISEASES	Tetanus, botulism, diphtheria, cholera	Meningococcemia; sepsis by gram ⊖ rods

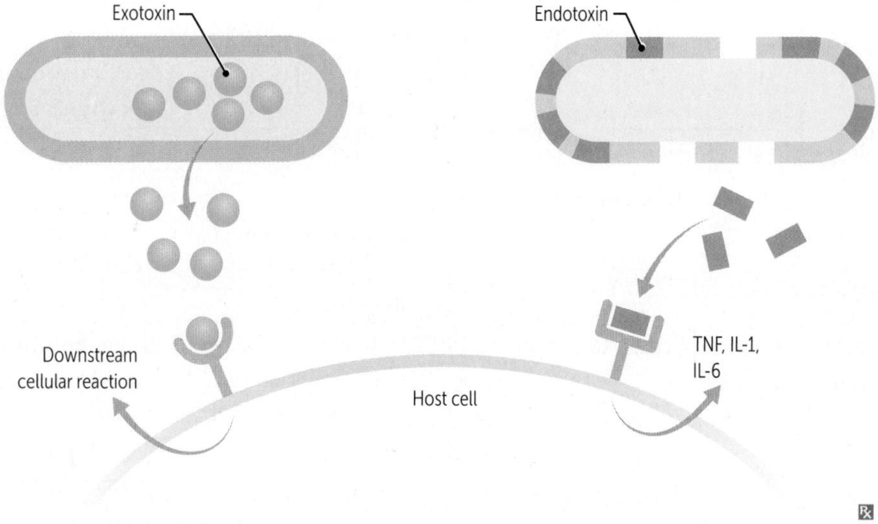

Bacteria with exotoxins

BACTERIA	TOXIN	MECHANISM	MANIFESTATION
Inhibit protein synthesis			
Corynebacterium diphtheriae	Diphtheria toxin[a]	Inactivate elongation factor (EF-2)	Pharyngitis with pseudomembranes in throat and severe lymphadenopathy (bull neck), myocarditis
Pseudomonas aeruginosa	Exotoxin A[a]		Host cell death
Shigella* spp** **Enterohemorrhagic *E coli	Shiga toxin[a]	Inactivate 60S ribosome by removing adenine from rRNA	Damages GI mucosa → dysentery Enhances cytokine release → hemolytic-uremic syndrome (HUS; prototypically in EHEC serotype O157:H7) Unlike *Shigella*, EHEC does not invade host cells
Increase fluid secretion			
Enterotoxigenic *E coli*	Heat-**labile** toxin (LT)[a]	Overactivates adenylate cyclase (↑ cAMP) → ↑ Cl^- secretion in gut and H_2O efflux	Watery diarrhea: "**labile** in the **Air** (**A**denylate cyclase), **stable** on the **G**round (**G**uanylate cyclase)" Bacteria that ↑ **cAMP** include Cholera, Anthracis, Pertussis, *E coli*; "**Increase cAMP** with **CAPE**"
	Heat-**stable** toxin (ST)	Overactivates guanylate cyclase (↑ cGMP) → ↓ resorption of NaCl and H_2O in gut	
Bacillus anthracis	Anthrax toxin[a]	Mimics adenylate cyclase (↑ cAMP)	Likely responsible for characteristic edematous borders of black eschar in cutaneous anthrax
Vibrio cholerae	Cholera toxin[a]	Overactivates adenylate cyclase (↑ cAMP) by permanently activating G_s	Voluminous "rice-water" diarrhea
Inhibit phagocytic ability			
Bordetella pertussis	Pertussis toxin[a]	Inactivates inhibitory G subunit (G_i) → activation of adenylate cyclase → ↑ cAMP	Whooping cough—child coughs on expiration and "whoops" on inspiration; can cause "100-day cough" in adults; associated with posttussive emesis
Inhibit release of neurotransmitter			
Clostridium tetani	Tetanospasmin[a]	Both are proteases that cleave SNARE (soluble NSF attachment protein receptor), a set of proteins required for neurotransmitter release via vesicular fusion	Toxin prevents release of **inhibitory** (GABA and glycine) neurotransmitters from Renshaw cells in spinal cord → spastic paralysis, risus sardonicus, trismus (lockjaw), opisthotonos
Clostridium botulinum	Botulinum toxin[a]		Infant botulism—caused by ingestion of spores (eg, from soil, raw honey). Toxin produced in vivo Foodborne botulism—caused by ingestion of preformed toxin (eg, from canned foods)

[a] An AB toxin (aka, two-component toxin [or three for anthrax]) with **B** enabling **B**inding and triggering uptake (endocytosis) of the Active **A** component. The A components are usually ADP ribosyltransferases; others have enzymatic activities as listed in chart.

Bacteria with exotoxins *(continued)*

BACTERIA	TOXIN	MECHANISM	MANIFESTATION
Lyse cell membranes			
Clostridium perfringens	Alpha toxin	Phospholipase (lecithinase) that degrades tissue and cell membranes	Degradation of phospholipids → myonecrosis ("gas gangrene") and hemolysis ("double zone" of hemolysis on blood agar)
Streptococcus pyogenes	Streptolysin O	Protein that degrades cell membrane	Lyses RBCs; contributes to β-hemolysis; host antibodies against toxin (ASO) used to diagnose rheumatic fever (do not confuse with immune complexes of poststreptococcal glomerulonephritis)
Superantigens causing shock			
Staphylococcus aureus	Toxic shock syndrome toxin (TSST-1)	Cross-links β region of TCR to MHC class II on APCs outside of the antigen binding site → overwhelming release of IL-1, IL-2, IFN-γ, and TNF-α → shock	Toxic shock syndrome: fever, rash, shock; other toxins cause scalded skin syndrome (exfoliative toxin) and food poisoning (heat-stable enterotoxin)
Streptococcus pyogenes	Erythrogenic exotoxin A		Toxic shock–like syndrome: fever, rash, shock; scarlet fever

Endotoxin

LPS found in outer membrane of gram ⊖ bacteria (both cocci and rods). Composed of O-antigen + core polysaccharide + lipid A (the toxic component).

Released upon cell lysis or by living cells by blebs detaching from outer surface membrane (vs exotoxin, which is actively secreted).

Three main effects: macrophage activation (TLR4/CD14), complement activation, and tissue factor activation.

ENDOTOXINS:
- Edema
- Nitric oxide
- DIC/Death
- Outer membrane
- TNF-α
- O-antigen + core polysaccharide + lipid A
- eXtremely heat stable
- IL-1 and IL-6
- Neutrophil chemotaxis
- Shock

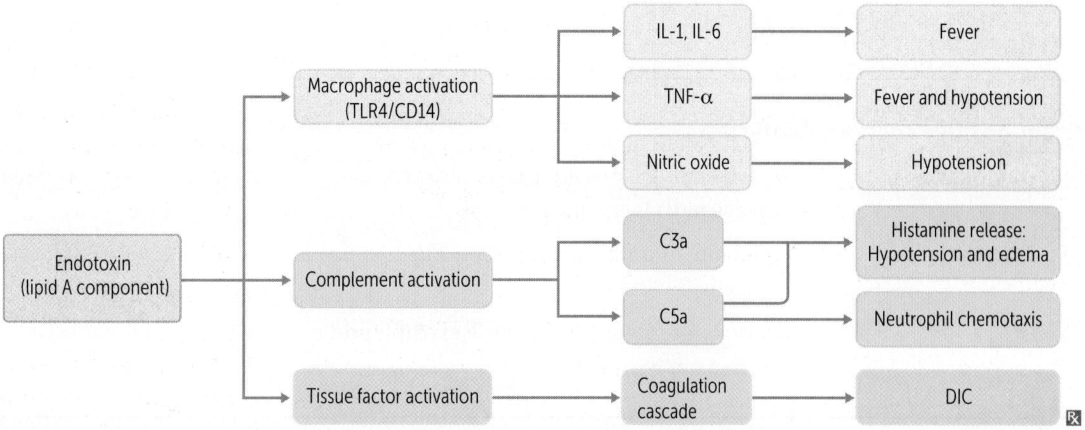

▸ MICROBIOLOGY—CLINICAL BACTERIOLOGY

Gram-positive lab algorithm

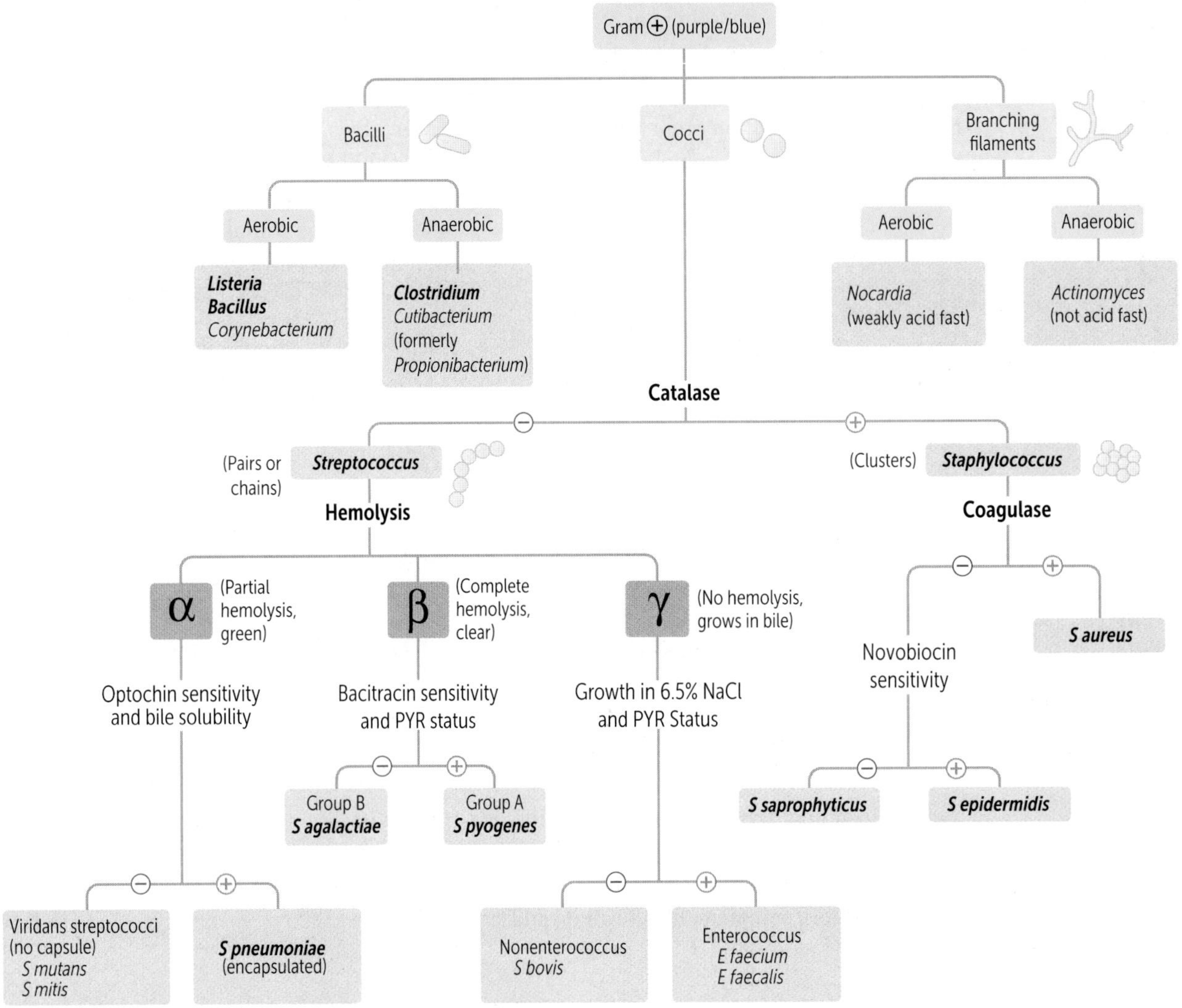

Important **tests** are in **bold.** Important ***pathogens*** are in ***bold italics.***
Note: Enterococcus is either α- or γ-hemolytic.

Gram-positive cocci antibiotic tests

Staphylococci	Novobiocin—Saprophyticus is resistant; epidermidis is sensitive	Sapro is a no-go on Novo
Streptococci	Optochin—*Viridans* is Resistant; *Pneumoniae* is Sensitive	OVRPS (overpass)
	Bacitracin—group B strep are Resistant; group A strep are Sensitive	B-BRAS

α-hemolytic bacteria

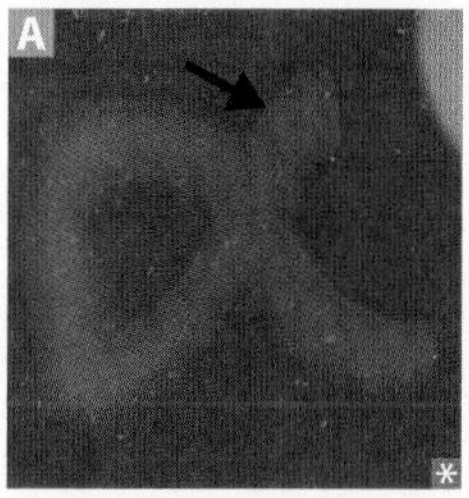

Gram $\oplus$ cocci. Partial oxidation of hemoglobin causes greenish or brownish color without clearing around growth on blood agar A. Include the following organisms:
- *Streptococcus pneumoniae* (catalase $\ominus$ and optochin sensitive)
- Viridans streptococci (catalase $\ominus$ and optochin resistant)

β-hemolytic bacteria

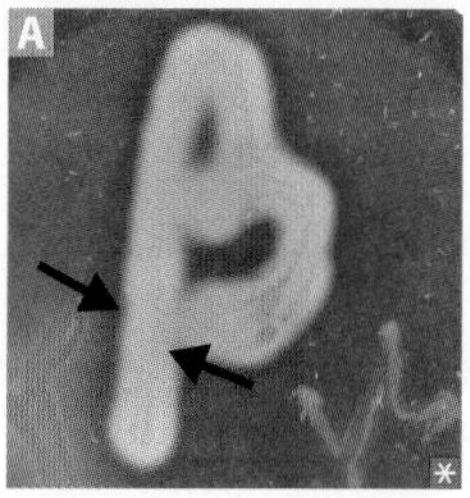

Gram $\oplus$ cocci. Complete lysis of RBCs → pale/clear area surrounding colony on blood agar A. Include the following organisms:
- *Staphylococcus aureus* (catalase and coagulase $\oplus$)
- *Streptococcus pyogenes*—group A strep (catalase $\ominus$ and bacitracin sensitive)
- *Streptococcus agalactiae*—group B strep (catalase $\ominus$ and bacitracin resistant)

Staphylococcus aureus

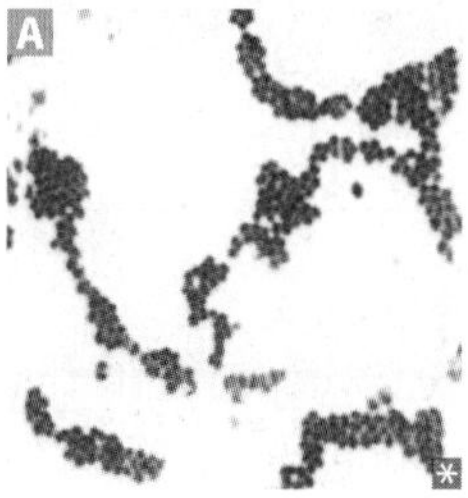

Gram $\oplus$, β-hemolytic, catalase $\oplus$, coagulase $\oplus$ cocci in clusters A. Protein A (virulence factor) binds Fc-IgG, inhibiting complement activation and phagocytosis. Commonly colonizes the nares, ears, axilla, and groin.

Causes:
- Inflammatory disease—skin infections, organ abscesses, pneumonia (often after influenza virus infection), endocarditis, septic arthritis, and osteomyelitis.
- Toxin-mediated disease—toxic shock syndrome (TSST-1), scalded skin syndrome (exfoliative toxin), rapid-onset food poisoning (enterotoxins).

MRSA (methicillin-resistant *S aureus*)—important cause of serious nosocomial and community-acquired infections. Resistance due to altered penicillin-binding proteins (conferred by *mec*A gene). Some strains release Panton-Valentine leukocidin (PVL), which kills leukocytes and causes tissue necrosis.

TSST-1 is a superantigen that binds to MHC II and T-cell receptor, resulting in polyclonal T-cell activation and cytokine release.

Staphylococcal toxic shock syndrome (TSS)—fever, vomiting, diarrhea, rash, desquamation, shock, end-organ failure. TSS results in ↑ AST, ↑ ALT, ↑ bilirubin. Associated with prolonged use of vaginal tampons or nasal packing.

Compare with *Streptococcus pyogenes* TSS (a toxic shock–like syndrome associated with painful skin infection).

S aureus food poisoning due to ingestion of preformed toxin → short incubation period (2–6 hr) followed by nonbloody diarrhea and emesis. Enterotoxin is heat stable → not destroyed by cooking.

S aureus makes coagulase and toxins. Forms fibrin clot around itself → abscess.

Staphylococcus epidermidis

Gram $\oplus$, catalase $\oplus$, coagulase $\ominus$, urease $\oplus$ cocci in clusters. Novobiocin sensitive. Does not ferment mannitol (vs *S aureus*).

Normal flora of skin; contaminates blood cultures.

Infects prosthetic devices (eg, hip implant, heart valve) and IV catheters by producing adherent biofilms.

Staphylococcus saprophyticus

Gram ⊕, catalase ⊕, coagulase ⊖, urease ⊕ cocci in clusters. Novobiocin resistant.
Normal flora of female genital tract and perineum.
Second most common cause of uncomplicated UTI in young females (most common is *E coli*).

Streptococcus pneumoniae

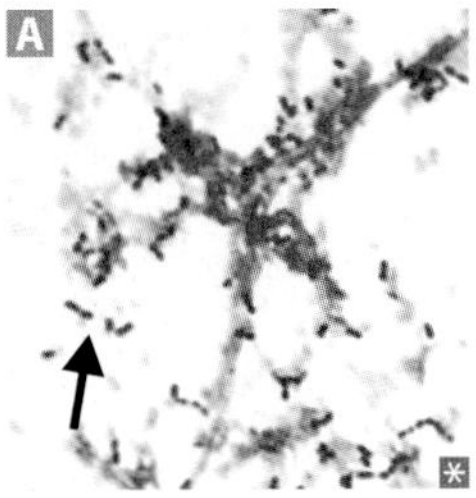

Gram ⊕, α-hemolytic, lancet-shaped diplococci A.
Encapsulated. IgA protease. Optochin sensitive and bile soluble.
Most commonly causes **MOPS**:
- **M**eningitis
- **O**titis media (in children)
- **P**neumonia
- **S**inusitis

Pneumococcus is associated with "rusty" sputum, patients with hyposplenia or asplenia.
No virulence without capsule.

Viridans group streptococci

Gram ⊕, α-hemolytic cocci. Optochin resistant and bile insoluble. Normal flora of the oropharynx.
Streptococcus mutans and *S mitis* cause dental caries.
S sanguinis makes dextrans that bind to fibrin-platelet aggregates on damaged **heart** valves, causing subacute bacterial endocarditis.

Viridans group strep live in the mouth, because they are not afraid **of-the-chin** (**op-to-chin** resistant).
Sanguinis = **blood**. Think, "there is lots of **blood** in the **heart**" (endocarditis).

***Streptococcus pyogenes* (group A streptococci)**

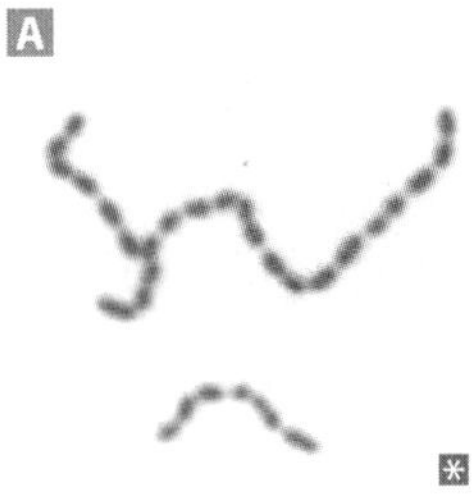

Gram ⊕ cocci in chains A. Group A strep cause:
- Pyogenic—pharyngitis, cellulitis, impetigo ("honey-crusted" lesions), erysipelas
- Toxigenic—scarlet fever, toxic shock–like syndrome, necrotizing fasciitis
- Immunologic—rheumatic fever, glomerulonephritis

Bacitracin sensitive, β-hemolytic, pyrrolidonyl arylamidase (PYR) ⊕. Hyaluronic acid capsule and M protein inhibit phagocytosis. Antibodies to M protein enhance host defenses against *S pyogenes* but can give rise to rheumatic fever.
Diagnose strep pharyngitis via throat swab, which can be tested with an antigen detection assay (rapid, in-office results) or cultured on blood agar (results in 48 hours).

"**Ph**"yogenes **ph**aryngitis can result in rheumatic "**ph**ever" and glomerulone**ph**ritis.
Strains causing impetigo can induce glomerulonephritis.
Key virulence factors include DNase, erythrogenic exotoxin, streptokinase, streptolysin O. ASO titer or anti-DNase B antibodies indicate recent *S pyogenes* infection.
Scarlet fever—blanching, sandpaper-like body rash, strawberry tongue, and circumoral pallor in the setting of group A streptococcal pharyngitis (erythrogenic toxin ⊕).

***Streptococcus agalactiae* (group B streptococci)**	Gram ⊕ cocci, bacitracin resistant, β-hemolytic, colonizes vagina; causes pneumonia, meningitis, and sepsis, mainly in **b**abies. Polysaccharide capsule confers virulence. Produces CAMP factor, which enlarges the area of hemolysis formed by *S aureus*. (Note: CAMP stands for the authors of the test, not cyclic AMP.) Hippurate test ⊕. PYR ⊖. Screen pregnant patients at 35–37 weeks' gestation with rectal and vaginal swabs. Patients with ⊕ culture receive intrapartum penicillin/ampicillin prophylaxis.	Group **B** for **B**abies!
Streptococcus bovis	Gram ⊕ cocci, colonizes the gut. *S gallolyticus* (*S bovis* biotype 1) can cause bacteremia and subacute endocarditis. Patients with *S bovis* endocarditis have ↑ incidence of colon cancer.	Bovis in the blood = cancer in the colon.
Enterococci	Gram ⊕ cocci. Enterococci (*E faecalis* and *E faecium*) are normal colonic flora that are penicillin G resistant and cause UTI, biliary tract infections, and subacute endocarditis (following GI/GU procedures). Catalase ⊖, PYR ⊕, typically nonhemolytic. VRE (vancomycin-resistant enterococci) are an important cause of nosocomial infection.	Enterococci are more resilient than streptococci, can grow in 6.5% NaCl and bile (lab test). *Entero* = intestine, *faecalis* = feces, *strepto* = twisted (chains), *coccus* = berry.

Bacillus anthracis	Gram ⊕, spore-forming rod that produces anthrax toxin (an exotoxin consisting of protective antigen, lethal factor, and edema factor). Has a polypeptide capsule (poly D-glutamate). Colonies show a halo of projections, sometimes referred to as "medusa head" appearance.
Cutaneous anthrax 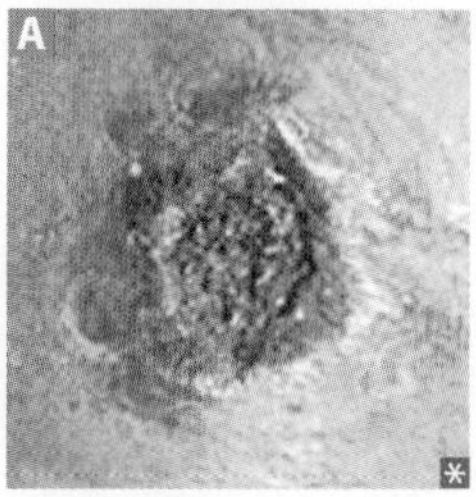	Painless papule surrounded by vesicles → ulcer with black eschar A (painless, necrotic) → uncommonly progresses to bacteremia and death.
Pulmonary anthrax	Inhalation of spores, most commonly from contaminated animals or animal products, although also a potential bioweapon → flu-like symptoms that rapidly progress to fever, pulmonary hemorrhage, mediastinitis (CXR may show widened mediastinum), and shock. Also called woolsorter's disease. Prophylaxis with ciprofloxacin or doxycycline when exposed.

Bacillus cereus	Gram ⊕ rod. Causes food poisoning. Spores survive cooking rice (reheated rice syndrome). Keeping rice warm results in germination of spores and enterotoxin formation. Emetic type causes nausea and vomiting within 1–5 hours. Caused by cereulide, a preformed toxin. Diarrheal type causes watery, nonbloody diarrhea and GI pain within 8–18 hours. Management: supportive care (antibiotics are ineffective against toxins).	
Clostridia	Gram ⊕, spore-forming, obligate anaerobic rods. Tetanus toxin and botulinum toxin are proteases that cleave SNARE proteins involved in neurotransmission.	
Clostridium tetani	Pathogen is noninvasive and remains localized to wound site. Produces tetanospasmin, an exotoxin causing tetanus. Tetanospasmin spreads by retrograde axonal transport to CNS and blocks release of GABA and glycine from Renshaw cells in spinal cord. Causes spastic paralysis, trismus (lockjaw), risus sardonicus (raised eyebrows and open grin), opisthotonos (spasms of spinal extensors).	**Tetanus** is **tetanic** paralysis. Prevent with tetanus vaccine. Treat with antitoxin +/– vaccine booster, antibiotics, diazepam (for muscle spasms), and wound debridement.
Clostridium botulinum	Produces a heat-labile toxin that inhibits ACh release at the neuromuscular junction, causing botulism. In babies, ingestion of spores (eg, in honey) leads to disease (**floppy** baby syndrome). In adults, disease is caused by ingestion of preformed toxin (eg, in canned food). Symptoms of botulism (the 5 D's): **d**iplopia, **d**ysarthria, **d**ysphagia, **d**yspnea, **d**escending **flaccid** paralysis. Does not present with sensory deficits.	***Botulinum*** is from bad **bottles** of food, juice, and honey. Treatment: human botulinum immunoglobulin. Local botulinum toxin A (Botox) injections used to treat focal dystonia, hyperhidrosis, muscle spasms, and cosmetic reduction of facial wrinkles.
Clostridium perfringens 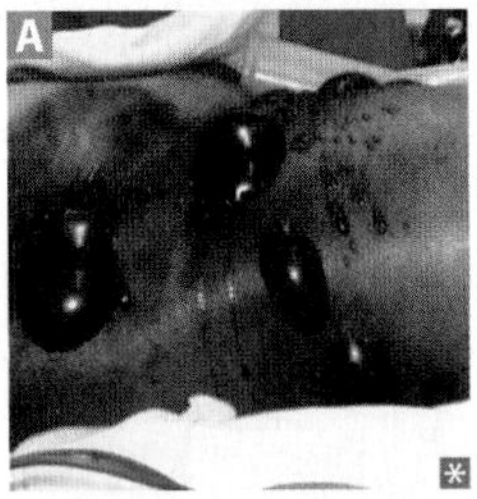	Produces α-toxin (lecithinase, a phospholipase) that can cause myonecrosis (gas gangrene A; presents as soft tissue crepitus) and hemolysis. If heavily spore-contaminated food is cooked but left standing too long at < 60°C, spores germinate → vegetative bacteria → heat-labile enterotoxin → late-onset (10-12 hours) food poisoning symptoms, resolution in 24 hours.	***Perfringens*** **perforates** a gangrenous leg.
Clostridioides difficile 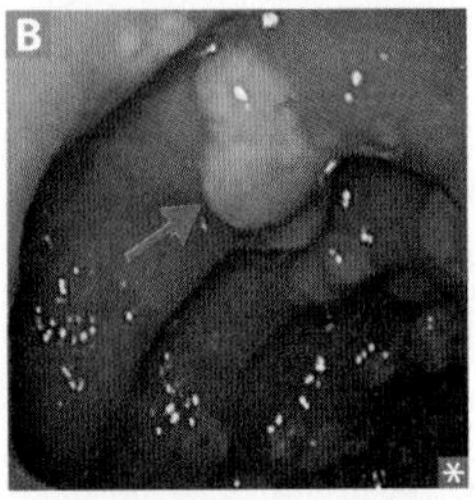	Produces toxins A and B, which damage enterocytes. Both toxins lead to watery diarrhea → pseudomembranous colitis B. Often 2° to antibiotic use, especially clindamycin, ampicillin, cephalosporins, fluoroquinolones; associated with PPIs. Fulminant infection: toxic megacolon, ileus, shock.	***Difficile*** causes **diarrhea**. Diagnosed by PCR or antigen detection of one or both toxins in stool. Treatment: oral vancomycin or fidaxomicin. For recurrent cases, consider repeating prior regimen or fecal microbiota transplant.

Corynebacterium diphtheriae

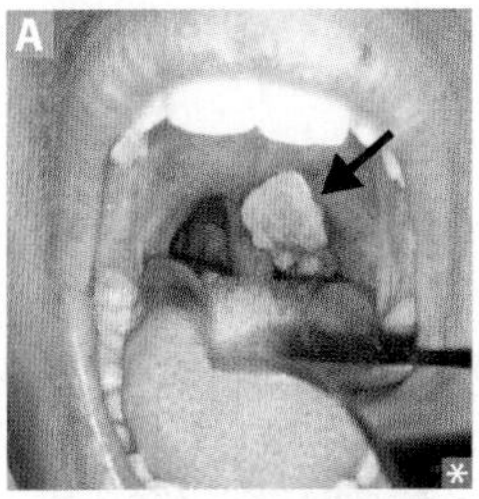

Gram ⊕ rods occurring in angular arrangements; transmitted via respiratory droplets. Causes diphtheria via exotoxin encoded by β-prophage. Potent exotoxin inhibits protein synthesis via ADP-ribosylation of EF-2, leading to possible necrosis in pharynx, cardiac, and CNS tissue.

Symptoms include pseudomembranous pharyngitis (grayish-white membrane A) with lymphadenopathy ("bull's neck" appearance). Toxin dissemination may cause myocarditis, arrhythmias, neuropathies.

Lab diagnosis based on gram ⊕ rods with metachromatic (blue and red) granules and ⊕ Elek test for toxin.

Toxoid vaccine prevents diphtheria.

Coryne = club shaped (metachromatic granules on Löffler media).

Black colonies on cystine-tellurite agar.

ABCDEFG:
- ADP-ribosylation
- β-prophage
- *Corynebacterium*
- *Diphtheriae*
- Elongation Factor 2
- Granules

Treatment: diphtheria antitoxin +/– erythromycin or penicillin.

Listeria monocytogenes

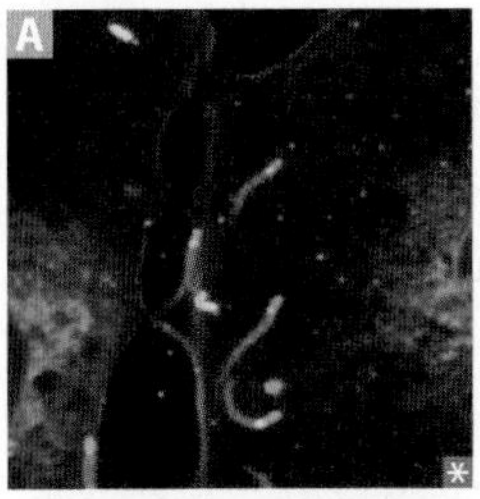

Gram ⊕, facultative intracellular rod; acquired by ingestion of unpasteurized dairy products and cold deli meats, transplacental transmission, by vaginal transmission during birth. Grows well at refrigeration temperatures ("cold enrichment").

Forms "rocket tails" (red in A) via actin polymerization that allow intracellular movement and cell-to-cell spread across cell membranes, thereby avoiding antibody. Characteristic tumbling motility in broth.

Can cause amnionitis, septicemia, and spontaneous abortion in pregnant patients; granulomatosis infantiseptica; meningitis in immunocompromised patients, neonates, and older adults; mild, self-limited gastroenteritis in healthy individuals.

Treatment: ampicillin.

Nocardia* vs *Actinomyces

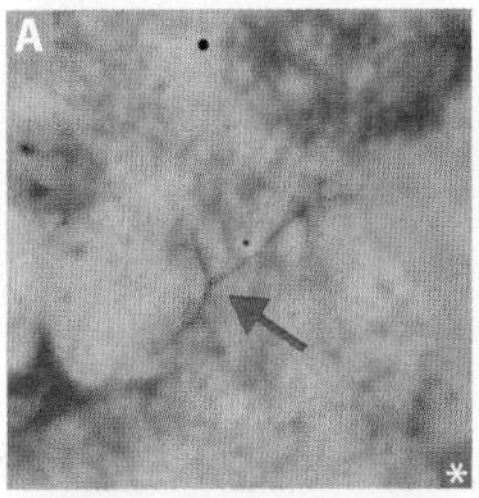

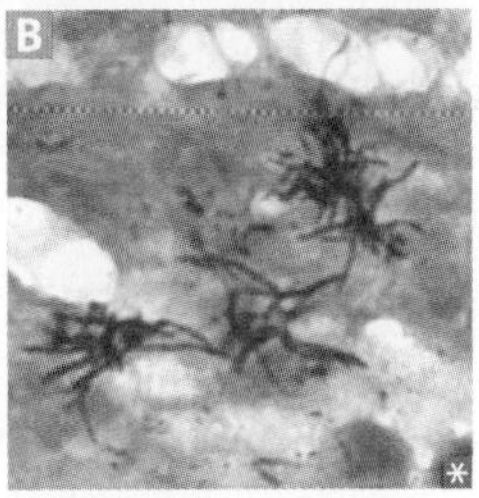

Both are gram ⊕ and form long, branching filaments resembling fungi.

Nocardia	*Actinomyces*
Aerobe	Anaerobe
Acid fast (weak) A	Not acid fast B
Found in soil	Normal oral, reproductive, and GI flora
Causes pulmonary infections in immunocompromised (can mimic TB but with ⊖ PPD); cutaneous infections after trauma in immunocompetent; can spread to CNS → cerebral abscess	Causes oral/facial abscesses that drain through sinus tracts; often associated with dental caries/extraction and other maxillofacial trauma; forms yellow "sulfur granules"; can also cause PID with IUDs
Treat with sulfonamides (TMP-SMX)	Treat with penicillin

Treatment is a SNAP: Sulfonamides—*Nocardia*; *Actinomyces*—Penicillin

Mycobacteria

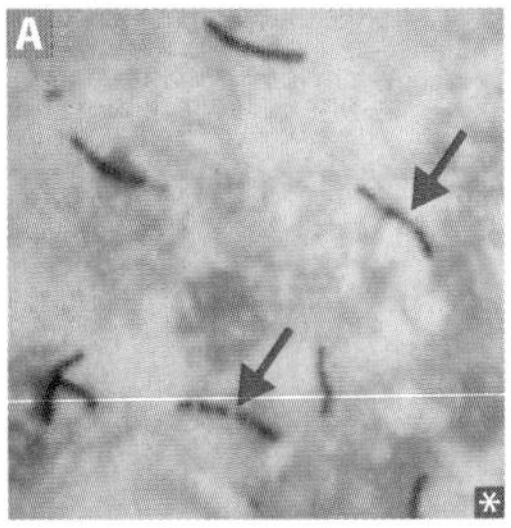

Acid-fast rods (pink rods, arrows in A).

Mycobacterium tuberculosis (TB, often resistant to multiple drugs).

M avium–intracellulare (causes disseminated, non-TB disease in AIDS; often resistant to multiple drugs). Prophylaxis with azithromycin when CD4+ count < 50 cells/mm^3.

M scrofulaceum (cervical lymphadenitis in children).

M marinum (hand infection in aquarium handlers).

TB symptoms include fever, night sweats, weight loss, cough (nonproductive or productive), hemoptysis.

Cord factor creates a "serpentine cord" appearance in virulent *M tuberculosis* strains; activates macrophages (promoting granuloma formation) and induces release of TNF-α. Sulfatides (surface glycolipids) inhibit phagolysosomal fusion.

Tuberculosis

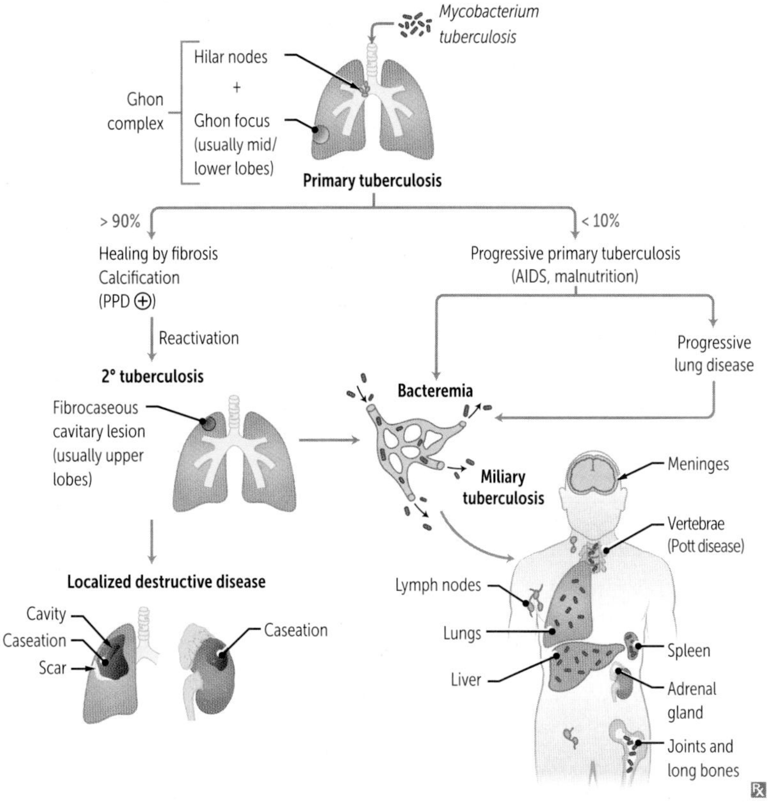

PPD ⊕ if current infection or past exposure.

PPD ⊖ if no infection and in immunocompromised patients (especially with low CD4+ cell count).

Interferon-γ release assay (IGRA) has fewer false positives from BCG vaccination.

Caseating granulomas with central necrosis and Langhans giant cell (single example in A) are characteristic of 2° tuberculosis. Do not confuse Langhans giant cell with Langerhans cell, an APC.

TB reactivation risk highest in immunocompromised individuals (eg, HIV, organ transplant recipients).

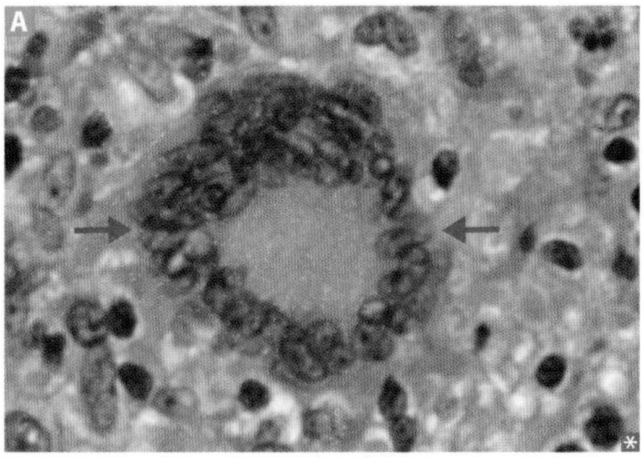

Leprosy

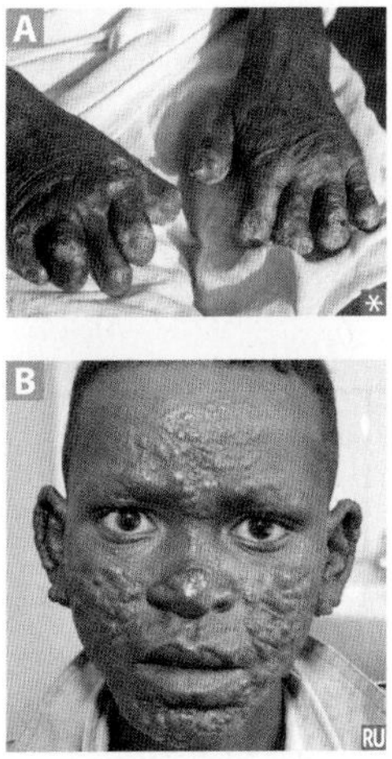

Also called Hansen disease. Caused by *Mycobacterium leprae*, an acid-fast bacillus that likes cool temperatures (infects skin and superficial nerves—"glove and stocking" loss of sensation A) and cannot be grown in vitro. Diagnosed via skin biopsy or tissue PCR. Reservoir in United States: armadillos.

Leprosy has 2 forms (many cases fall temporarily between two extremes):

- Lepromatous—presents diffusely over the skin, with leonine (lion-like) facies B, and is communicable (high bacterial load); characterized by low cell-mediated immunity with a largely Th2 response. Lepromatous form can be lethal.
- Tuberculoid—limited to a few hypoesthetic, hairless skin plaques; characterized by high cell-mediated immunity with a largely Th1-type response and low bacterial load.

Treatment: dapsone and rifampin for tuberculoid form; clofazimine is added for lepromatous form.

Gram-negative lab algorithm

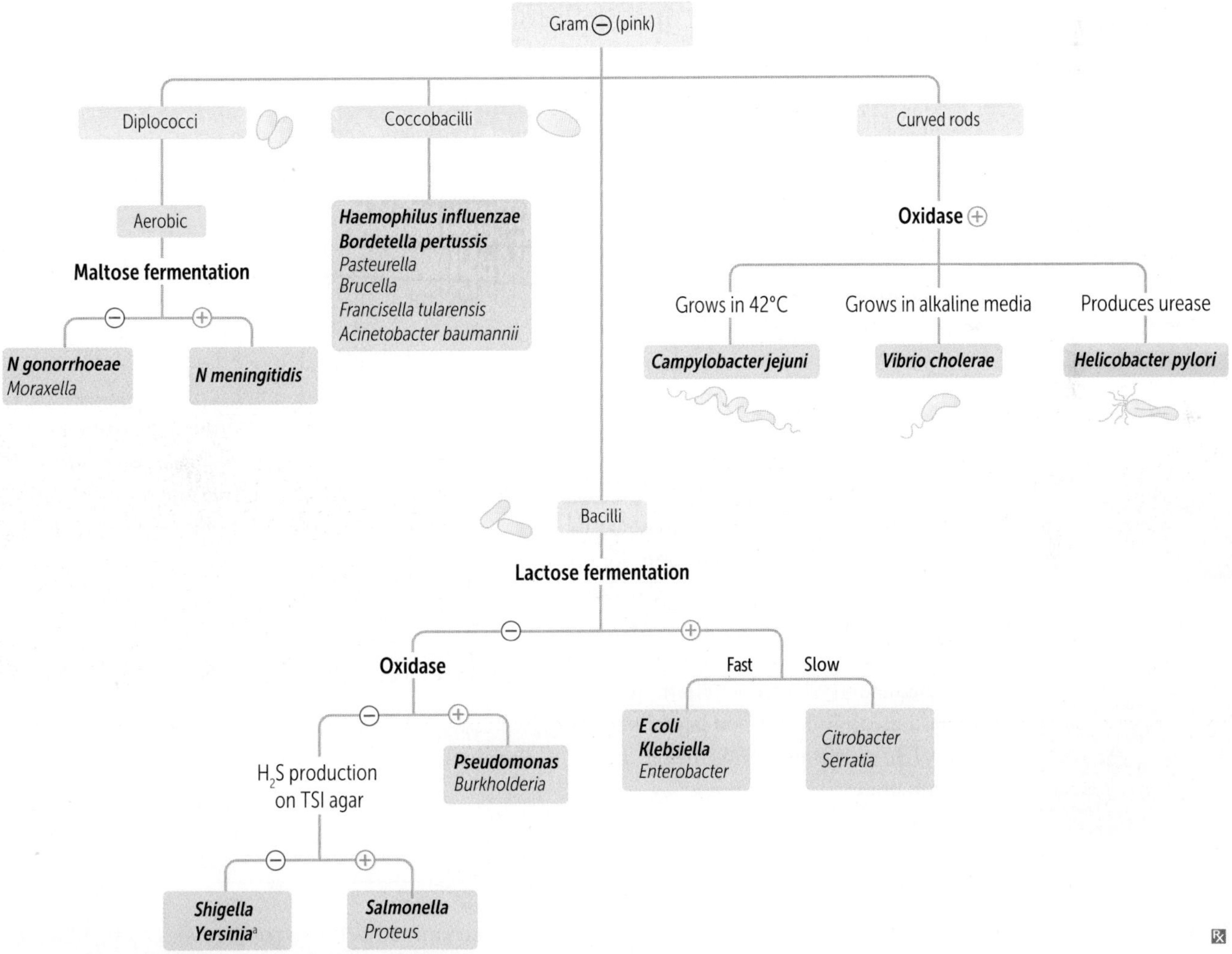

Important **tests** are in **bold.** Important ***pathogens*** are in ***bold italics.***
[a]Pleomorphic rod/coccobacillus

Neisseria

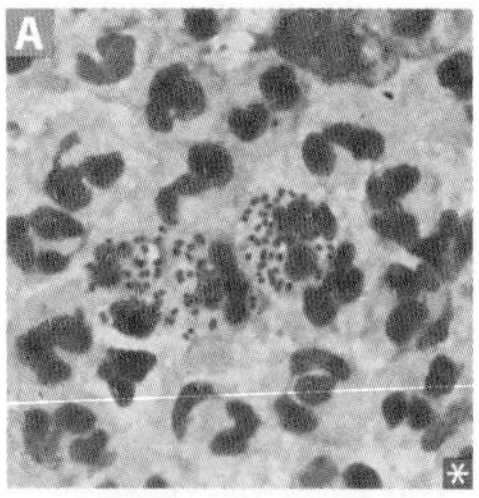

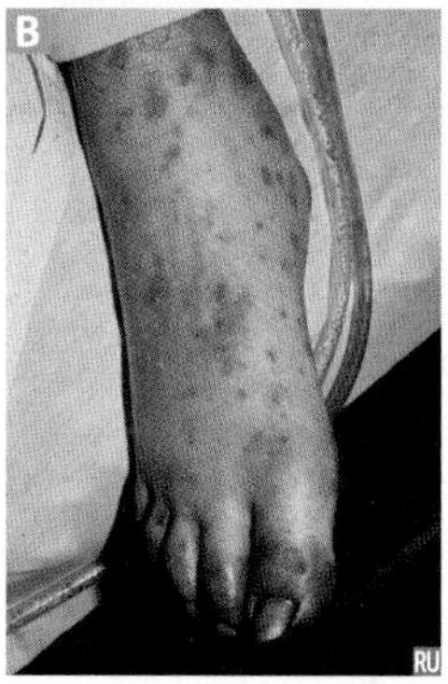

Gram ⊖ diplococci. Metabolize glucose and produce IgA proteases. Contain lipooligosaccharides (LOS) with strong endotoxin activity.

N *gonorrhoeae* is often intracellular (within neutrophils) A.

Acid production: meningococci—maltose and glucose; gonococci—glucose.

Gonococci	Meningococci
No polysaccharide capsule	Polysaccharide capsule
No maltose acid detection	Maltose acid detection
No vaccine due to antigenic variation of pilus proteins	Vaccine (type B vaccine available for at-risk individuals)
Sexually or perinatally transmitted	Transmitted via respiratory and oral secretions. More common among individuals in close quarters (eg, army barracks, college dorms)
Causes gonorrhea, septic arthritis, neonatal conjunctivitis (2–5 days after birth), pelvic inflammatory disease (PID), and Fitz-Hugh–Curtis syndrome	Causes meningococcemia with petechial hemorrhages and gangrene of toes B, meningitis, Waterhouse-Friderichsen syndrome (adrenal insufficiency, fever, DIC)
Diagnosed with NAT	Diagnosed via culture-based tests or PCR
Condoms ↓ sexual transmission, erythromycin eye ointment prevents neonatal blindness	Rifampin, ciprofloxacin, or ceftriaxone prophylaxis in close contacts
Treatment: ceftriaxone + azithromycin (to cover possible chlamydial coinfection, ceftriaxone-resistant strains)	Treatment: ceftriaxone or penicillin G

Haemophilus influenzae

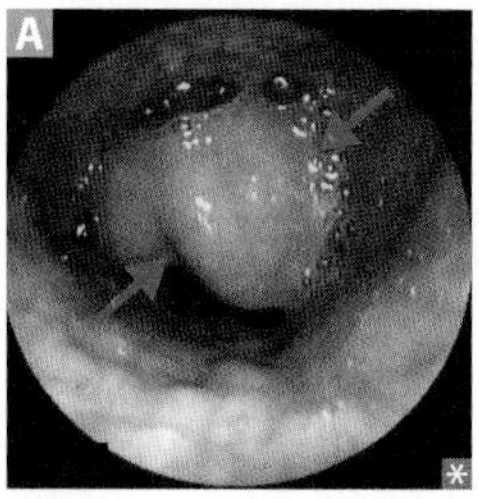

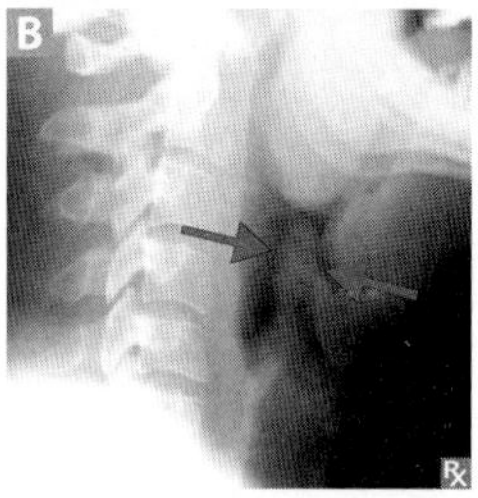

Small gram ⊖ (coccobacillary) rod. Aerosol transmission. Nontypeable (unencapsulated) strains are the most common cause of mucosal infections (otitis media, conjunctivitis, bronchitis) as well as invasive infections since the vaccine for capsular type b was introduced. Produces IgA protease.

Culture on chocolate agar, which contains factors V (NAD^+) and X (hematin) for growth; can also be grown with *S aureus*, which provides factor V via RBC hemolysis.

Haemophilus causes epiglottitis (endoscopic appearance in A, can be "cherry red" in children; "thumb sign" on lateral neck x-ray B), meningitis, otitis media, and pneumonia.

Vaccine contains type b capsular polysaccharide (polyribosylribitol phosphate) conjugated to diphtheria toxoid or other protein. Given between 2 and 18 months of age.

Does not cause the flu (influenza virus does).

Treatment: amoxicillin +/– clavulanate for mucosal infections; ceftriaxone for meningitis; rifampin prophylaxis for close contacts.

Burkholderia cepacia complex

Gram ⊖ bacilli. Causes pneumonia in and can be transmitted between patients with cystic fibrosis. Often multidrug resistant. Infection is a relative contraindication to undergoing lung transplant due to its association with poor outcomes.

Bordetella pertussis

Gram ⊖, aerobic coccobacillus. Virulence factors include pertussis toxin (disables G_i), adenylate cyclase toxin (↑ cAMP), and tracheal cytotoxin. Three clinical stages:

- Catarrhal—low-grade fevers, coryza.
- Paroxysmal—paroxysms of intense cough followed by inspiratory "whoop" ("whooping cough"), posttussive vomiting.
- Convalescent—gradual recovery of chronic cough.

Prevented by Tdap, DTaP vaccines.
Treatment: macrolides; if allergic use TMP-SMX.

Brucella

Gram ⊖, aerobic coccobacillus. Transmitted via ingestion of contaminated animal products (eg, **u**npasteurized milk). Survives in macrophages in the reticuloendothelial system. Can form noncaseating granulomas. Typically presents with **u**ndulant fever, night sweats, and arthralgia.
Treatment: doxycycline + rifampin or streptomycin.

Legionella pneumophila

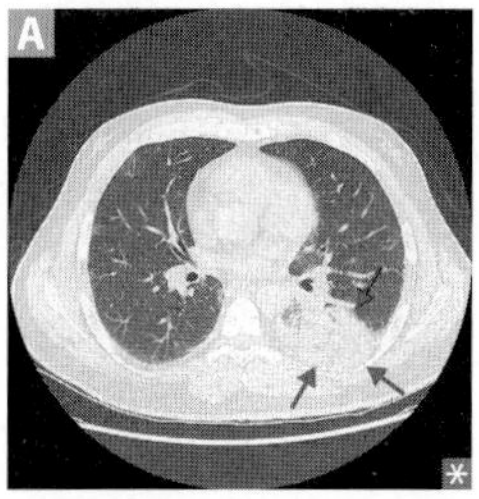

Gram ⊖ rod. Gram stains poorly—use **silver** stain. Grow on **charcoal** yeast extract medium with **iron** and **cysteine**. Detected by presence of antigen in urine. Labs may show hyponatremia.
Aerosol transmission from environmental water source habitat (eg, air conditioning systems, hot water tanks). Outbreaks associated with cruise ships, nursing homes. No person-to-person transmission.
Treatment: macrolide or quinolone.

Think of a French **legionnaire** (soldier) with his **silver** helmet, sitting around a campfire (**charcoal**) with his **iron** dagger—he is missing his **sister** (cysteine).
Legionnaires' disease—severe pneumonia (often unilateral and lobar **A**), fever, GI and CNS symptoms. Risk factors include older age, tobacco smoking, chronic lung disease.
Pontiac fever—mild flu-like symptoms.

Pseudomonas aeruginosa

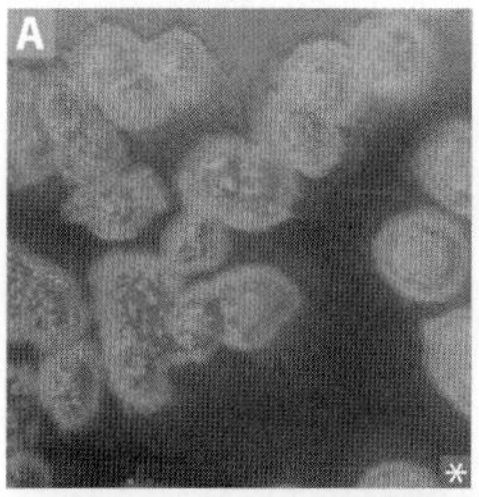

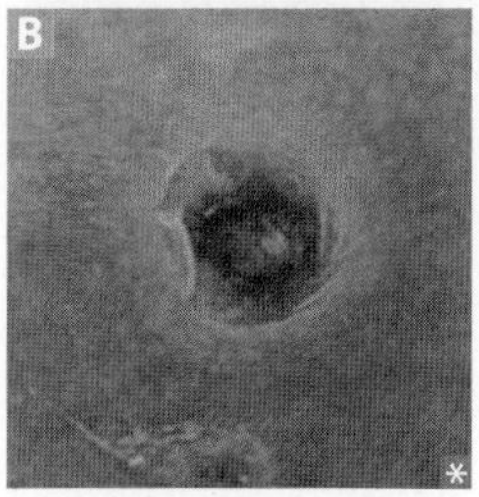

Aeruginosa—**aer**obic; motile, catalase ⊕, gram ⊖ rod. Non-lactose fermenting. Oxidase ⊕. Frequently found in water. Has a grape-like odor.
PSEUDOMONAS is associated with: **P**neumonia, **S**epsis, **E**cthyma gangrenosum, **U**TIs, **D**iabetes, **O**steomyelitis, **M**ucoid polysaccharide capsule, **O**titis externa (swimmer's ear), **N**osocomial infections (eg, catheters, equipment), **A**ddiction (people who inject drugs), **S**kin infections (eg, hot tub folliculitis, wound infection in burn victims).
Mucoid polysaccharide capsule may contribute to chronic pneumonia in patients with cystic fibrosis due to biofilmformation.
Produces **PEEP**: **P**hospholipase C (degrades cell membranes); **E**ndotoxin (fever, shock); **E**xotoxin A (inactivates EF-2); **P**igments: pyoverdine and pyocyanin (blue-green pigment **A**; also generates ROS).

Corneal ulcers/keratitis in contact lens wearers/minor eye trauma.
Ecthyma gangrenosum—rapidly progressive, necrotic cutaneous lesion **B** caused by *Pseudomonas* bacteremia. Typically seen in immunocompromised patients.
Treatments:

- Antipseudomonal penicillins in combination with β-lactamase inhibitor (eg, piperacillin-tazobactam)
- 3rd- and 4th-generation cephalosporins (eg, ceftazidime, cefepime)
- Monobactams
- Fluoroquinolones
- Carbapenems

Salmonella vs _Shigella_

Both *Salmonella* and *Shigella* are gram ⊖ rods, non-lactose fermenters, oxidase ⊖, and can invade the GI tract via M cells of Peyer patches.

	Salmonella typhi **(ty-Vi)**	***Salmonella*** **spp. except** ***S typhi***	***Shigella***
RESERVOIRS	Humans only	Humans and animals	Humans only
SPREAD	Hematogenous spread	Hematogenous spread	Cell to cell; no hematogenous spread
H_2S PRODUCTION	Yes	Yes	No
FLAGELLA	Yes (salmon swim)	Yes (salmon swim)	No
VIRULENCE FACTORS	Endotoxin; Vi capsule (pronounce "tyVi")	Endotoxin	Endotoxin; Shiga toxin (enterotoxin)
INFECTIOUS DOSE (ID_{50})	High—large inoculum required; acid-labile (inactivated by gastric acids)	High	Low—very small inoculum required; acid stable (resistant to gastric acids)
EFFECT OF ANTIBIOTICS ON FECAL EXCRETION	Prolongs duration	Prolongs duration	Shortens duration
IMMUNE RESPONSE	Primarily monocytes	PMNs in disseminated disease	Primarily PMN infiltration
GI MANIFESTATIONS	Constipation, followed by diarrhea	Diarrhea (possibly bloody)	Crampy abdominal pain → tenesmus, bloody mucoid stools (bacillary dysentery)
VACCINE	Oral vaccine contains live attenuated *S typhi* IM vaccine contains Vi capsular polysaccharide	No vaccine	No vaccine
UNIQUE PROPERTIES	▪ Causes typhoid fever (rose spots on abdomen, constipation, abdominal pain, fever [pulse-temperature dissociation]; later GI ulceration and hemorrhage); treat with ceftriaxone or fluoroquinolone ▪ Carrier state with gallbladder colonization	▪ Poultry, eggs, pets, and turtles are common sources ▪ Antibiotics not indicated ▪ Gastroenteritis is usually caused by non-typhoidal *Salmonella*	▪ 4 F's: fingers, flies, food, feces ▪ In order of decreasing severity (less toxin produced): *S dysenteriae*, *S flexneri*, *S boydii*, *S sonnei* ▪ Invasion of M cells is key to pathogenicity: organisms that produce little toxin can cause disease

Yersinia enterocolitica

Gram ⊖ pleomorphic rod/coccobacillus. Usually transmitted from pet feces (eg, cats, dogs), contaminated milk, or pork. Can cause acute bloody diarrhea, pseudoappendicitis (right lower abdominal pain due to mesenteric adenitis and/or terminal ileitis), reactive arthritis in adults.

Lactose-fermenting enteric bacteria

Fermentation of lactose → pink colonies on MacConkey agar. Examples include *Citrobacter*, *E coli*, *Enterobacter*, *Klebsiella*, *Serratia*. *E coli* produces β-galactosidase, which breaks down lactose into glucose and galactose.

McCowkey CEEKS milk.

EMB agar—lactose fermenters grow as purple/black colonies. *E coli* grows colonies with a green sheen.

Escherichia coli

Gram ⊖, indole ⊕ rod. *E coli* virulence factors: fimbriae—cystitis and pyelonephritis (P pili); K capsule—pneumonia, neonatal meningitis; LPS endotoxin—septic shock.

STRAIN	TOXIN AND MECHANISM	PRESENTATION
Enteroinvasive *E coli*	Microbe invades intestinal mucosa and causes necrosis and inflammation.	EIEC is Invasive; dysentery. Clinical manifestations similar to *Shigella*.
Enterotoxigenic *E coli*	Produces heat-labile and heat-stable enteroToxins. No inflammation or invasion.	ETEC; Traveler's diarrhea (watery).
Enteropathogenic *E coli*	No toxin produced. Adheres to apical surface, flattens villi, prevents absorption.	Diarrhea, usually in children (think EPEC and Pediatrics).
Enterohemorrhagic *E coli*	O157:H7 is most common serotype in US. Often transmitted via undercooked meat, raw leafy vegetables. Shiga toxin causes hemolytic-uremic syndrome—triad of anemia, thrombocytopenia, and acute kidney injury due to microthrombi forming on damaged endothelium → mechanical hemolysis (with schistocytes on peripheral blood smear), platelet consumption, and ↓ renal blood flow.	Dysentery (toxin alone causes necrosis and inflammation). Does not ferment sorbitol (vs other *E coli*). EHEC associated with hemorrhage, hamburgers, hemolytic-uremic syndrome.

Klebsiella

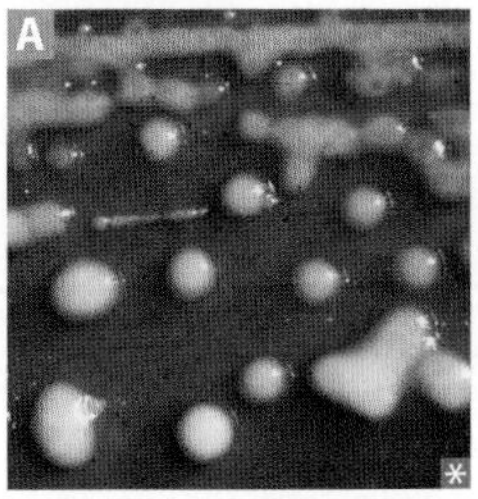

Gram ⊖ rod; intestinal flora that causes lobar pneumonia in patients with alcohol overuse and patients with diabetes when aspirated. Very mucoid colonies **A** caused by abundant polysaccharide capsules. Dark red "currant jelly" sputum (blood/mucus).

Also cause of nosocomial UTIs. Associated with evolution of multidrug resistance (MDR).

ABCDE's of Klebsiella:
- Aspiration pneumonia
- aBscess in lungs and liver
- "Currant jelly" sputum
- Diabetes mellitus
- EtOH overuse

Campylobacter jejuni

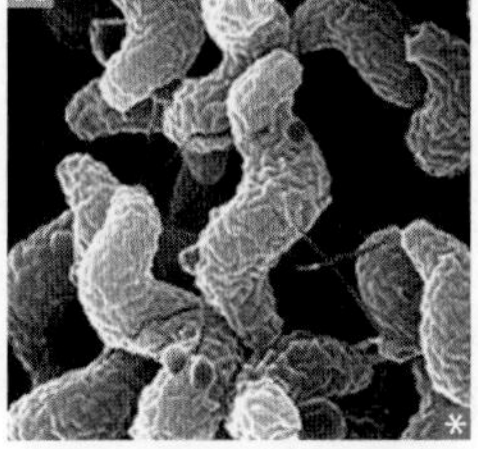

Gram ⊖, comma or S shaped (with polar flagella) **A**, oxidase ⊕, grows at 42°C ("*Campylobacter* likes the **hot campfire**").

Major cause of bloody diarrhea, especially in children. Fecal-oral transmission through person-to-person contact or via ingestion of undercooked contaminated poultry or meat, unpasteurized milk. Contact with infected animals (dogs, cats, pigs) is also a risk factor.

Common antecedent to Guillain-Barré syndrome and reactive arthritis.

Vibrio cholerae

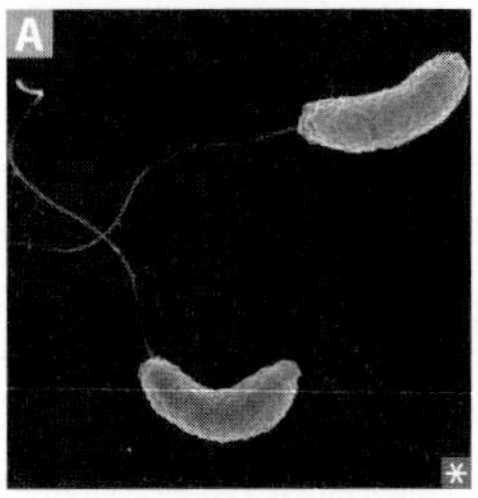

Gram ⊖, flagellated, comma shaped [A], oxidase ⊕, grows in alkaline media. Endemic to developing countries. Produces profuse rice-water diarrhea via enterotoxin that permanently activates G_s, ↑ cAMP. Sensitive to stomach acid (acid labile); requires large inoculum (high ID_{50}) unless host has ↓ gastric acidity. Transmitted via ingestion of contaminated water or uncooked food (eg, raw shellfish). Treat promptly with oral rehydration solution.

Vibrio vulnificus—gram ⊖ bacillus, usually found in marine environments. Causes severe wound infections or septicemia due to exposure to contaminated sea water. Presents as cellulitis that can progress to necrotizing fasciitis in high-risk patients, especially those with liver disease (eg, cirrhosis). Serious wound infection requires surgical debridement.

Helicobacter pylori

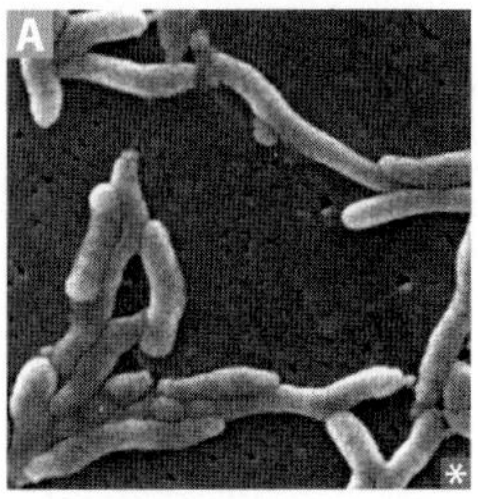

Curved, flagellated (motile), gram ⊖ rod [A] that is **triple** ⊕: catalase ⊕, oxidase ⊕, and urease ⊕ (can use urea breath test or fecal antigen test for diagnosis). Urease produces ammonia, creating an alkaline environment, which helps *H pylori* survive in acidic mucosa. Colonizes mainly antrum of stomach; causes gastritis and peptic ulcers (especially duodenal). Risk factor for peptic ulcer disease, gastric adenocarcinoma, and MALT lymphoma.

Most common initial treatment is **triple** therapy: amoxicillin (metronidazole if penicillin allergy) + clarithromycin + proton pump inhibitor; antibiotics cure *Pylori*. Bismuth-based quadruple therapy if concerned about macrolide resistance.

Spirochetes

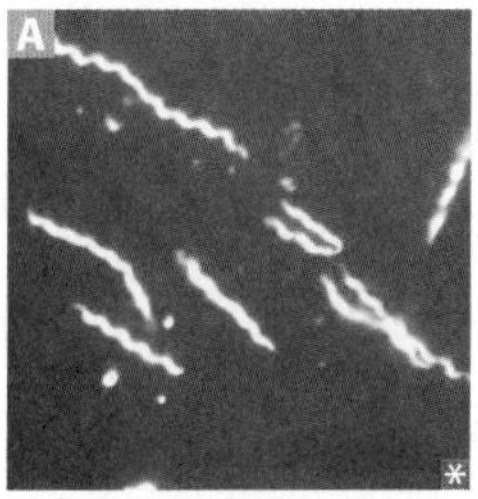

Spiral-shaped bacteria [A] with axial filaments. Includes *Leptospira*, *Treponema*, and *Borrelia*. Only *Borrelia* can be visualized using aniline dyes (Wright or Giemsa stain) in light microscopy due to size. *Treponema* is visualized by dark-field microscopy or direct fluorescent antibody (DFA) microscopy.

Little Twirling Bacteria

Lyme disease

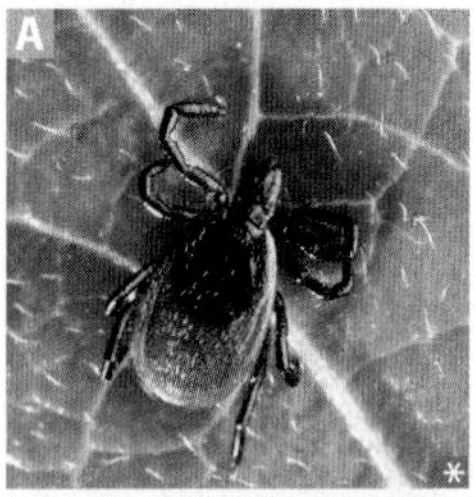

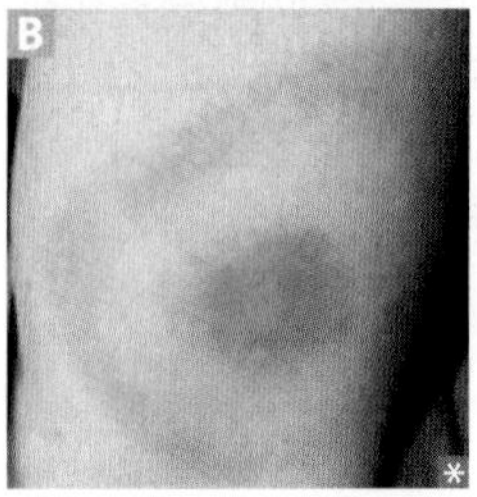

Caused by *Borrelia burgdorferi*, which is transmitted by the *Ixodes* deer tick [A] (also vector for *Anaplasma* spp. and protozoa *Babesia*). Natural reservoir is the mouse; deer are essential to tick life cycle but do not harbor *Borrelia*.

Common in northeastern United States.

Stage 1—early localized: erythema migrans (typical "bulls-eye" configuration [B] is pathognomonic but not always present), flu-like symptoms.

Stage 2—early disseminated: secondary lesions, carditis, AV block, facial nerve (Bell) palsy, migratory myalgias/transient arthritis.

Stage 3—late disseminated: encephalopathy, chronic arthritis, peripheral neuropathy.

A Key Lyme pie to the FACE:
- Facial nerve palsy (typically bilateral)
- Arthritis
- Cardiac block
- Erythema migrans

Treatment: doxycycline (1st line); amoxicillin (pregnant patients, children < 8 years old); ceftriaxone if IV therapy required

---

Leptospira interrogans

Spirochete with hook-shaped ends found in water contaminated with animal urine.

Leptospirosis—flu-like symptoms, myalgias (classically of calves), jaundice, photophobia with conjunctival suffusion (erythema without exudate). Prevalent among surfers and in tropics (eg, Hawaii).

Weil disease (icterohemorrhagic leptospirosis)—severe form with jaundice and azotemia from liver and kidney dysfunction, fever, hemorrhage, and anemia.

Syphilis

Caused by spirochete *Treponema pallidum*. Treatment: penicillin G.

Primary syphilis

Localized disease presenting with **painless** chancre A. Use fluorescent or dark-field microscopy to visualize treponemes in fluid from chancre B. VDRL ⊕ in ~ 80%.

Secondary syphilis

Disseminated disease with constitutional symptoms, maculopapular rash C (including palms D and soles), condylomata lata E (smooth, painless, wart-like white lesions on genitals), lymphadenopathy, patchy hair loss; also confirmable with dark-field microscopy.

Serologic testing: VDRL/RPR (nonspecific), confirm diagnosis with specific test (eg, FTA-ABS).

Secondary syphilis = systemic. Latent syphilis (⊕ serology without symptoms) may follow.

Tertiary syphilis

Gummas F (chronic granulomas), aortitis (vasa vasorum destruction), neurosyphilis (tabes dorsalis, "general paresis"), Argyll Robertson pupil (constricts with accommodation but is not reactive to light).

Signs: broad-based ataxia, ⊕ Romberg, Charcot joint, stroke without hypertension.

For neurosyphilis: test spinal fluid with VDRL, FTA-ABS, and PCR.

Congenital syphilis

Presents with facial abnormalities such as rhagades (linear scars at angle of mouth, black arrow in G), snuffles (nasal discharge, red arrow in G), saddle nose, notched (Hutchinson) teeth H, mulberry molars, and short maxilla; saber shins; CN VIII deafness.

To prevent, treat patient early in pregnancy, as placental transmission typically occurs after first trimester.

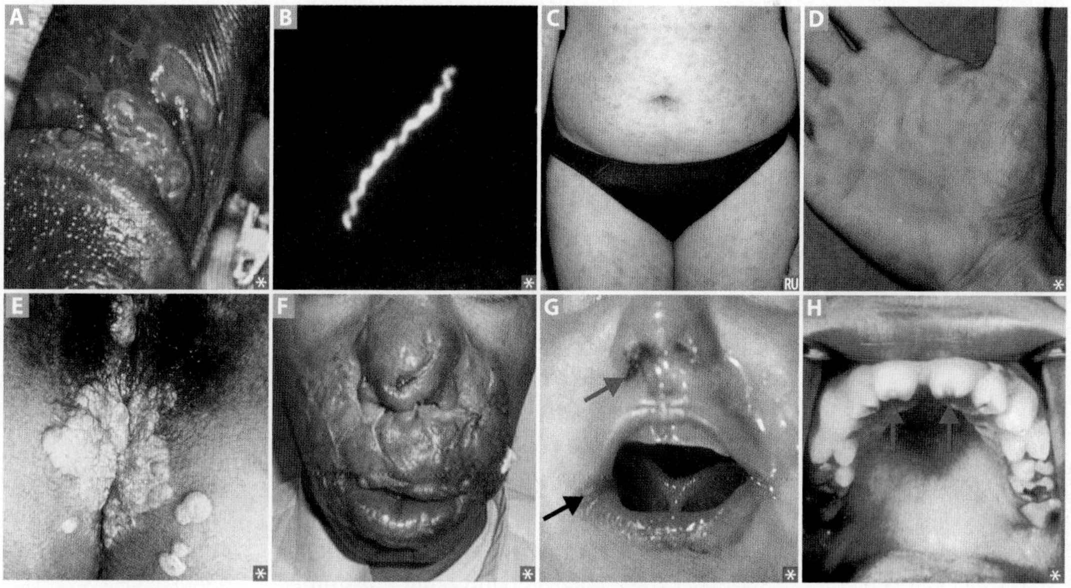

Diagnosing syphilis

VDRL and RPR detects nonspecific antibody that reacts with beef cardiolipin. Quantitative, inexpensive, and widely available test for syphilis (sensitive but not specific).

False-Positive results on VDRL with:
- Pregnancy
- Viral infection (eg, EBV, hepatitis)
- Drugs (eg, chlorpromazine, procainamide)
- Rheumatic fever (rare)
- Lupus (anticardiolipin antibody) and Leprosy

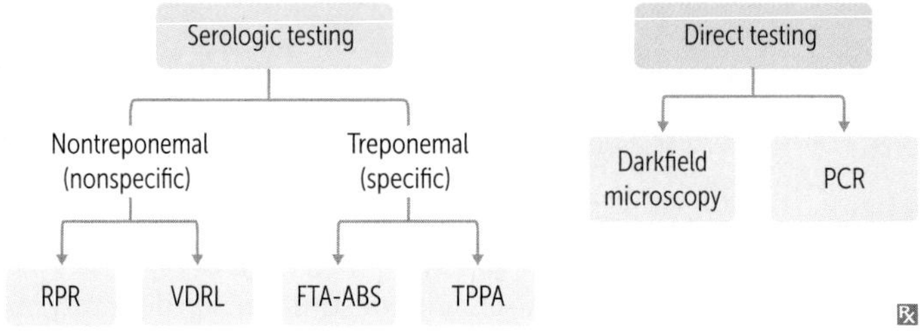

Jarisch-Herxheimer reaction

Flu-like symptoms (fever, chills, headache, myalgia) after antibiotics are started due to host response to sudden release of bacterial antigens.

Gardnerella vaginalis

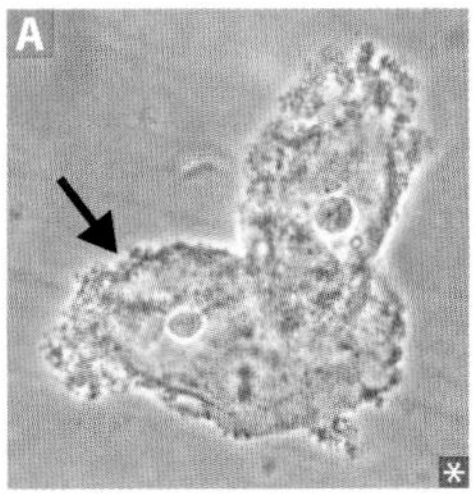

A pleomorphic, gram-variable rod involved in bacterial vaginosis. Presents as a gray vaginal discharge with a fishy smell; nonpainful (vs vaginitis). Associated with sexual activity, but not sexually transmitted. Bacterial vaginosis is also characterized by overgrowth of certain anaerobic bacteria in vagina (due to ↓ lactobacilli). Clue cells (vaginal epithelial cells covered with *Gardnerella*) have stippled appearance along outer margin (arrow in A).

Amine whiff test—mixing discharge with 10% KOH enhances fishy odor.

Vaginal pH >4.5 during infection.

Treatment: metronidazole or clindamycin.

Chlamydiae

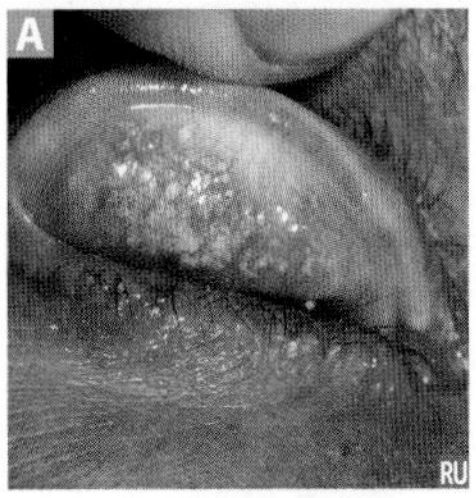

Chlamydiae cannot make their own ATP. They are obligate intracellular organisms that cause mucosal infections. 2 forms:
- Elementary body (small, dense) is "enfectious" and enters cell via endocytosis; transforms into reticulate body.
- Reticulate body replicates in cell by fission; reorganizes into elementary bodies.

Chlamydia trachomatis causes neonatal and follicular adult conjunctivitis A, nongonococcal urethritis, PID, and reactive arthritis.

Chlamydophila pneumoniae and *Chlamydophila psittaci* cause atypical pneumonia; transmitted by aerosol.

Chlamydial cell wall lacks classic peptidoglycan (due to reduced muramic acid), rendering β-lactam antibiotics ineffective.

Chlamys = cloak (intracellular).

C psittaci—has an avian reservoir (parrots), causes atypical pneumonia.

Lab diagnosis: PCR, nucleic acid amplification test. Cytoplasmic inclusions (reticulate bodies) seen on Giemsa or fluorescent antibody–stained smear.

Treatment: azithromycin (favored because one-time treatment) or doxycycline. Add ceftriaxone for possible concomitant gonorrhea.

Chlamydia trachomatis serotypes

Types A, B, and C	Chronic infection, cause blindness due to follicular conjunctivitis in resource-limited areas.	ABC = Africa, Blindness, Chronic infection.
Types D–K	Urethritis/PID, ectopic pregnancy, neonatal pneumonia (staccato cough) with eosinophilia, neonatal conjunctivitis (1–2 weeks after birth).	D–K = everything else. Neonatal disease can be acquired during vaginal birth if pregnant patient is infected.
Types L1, L2, and L3	Lymphogranuloma venereum—small, painless ulcers on genitals → swollen, painful inguinal lymph nodes that ulcerate (buboes). Treat with doxycycline.	

Zoonotic bacteria

Zoonosis—infectious disease transmitted between animals and humans.

SPECIES	DISEASE	TRANSMISSION AND SOURCE
***Anaplasma* spp**	Anaplasmosis	*Ixodes* ticks (live on deer and mice)
***Bartonella* spp**	Cat scratch disease, bacillary angiomatosis	Cat scratch
Borrelia burgdorferi	Lyme disease	*Ixodes* ticks (live on deer and mice)
Borrelia recurrentis	Relapsing fever	Louse (recurrent due to variable surface antigens)
***Brucella* spp**	Brucellosis/undulant fever	Unpasteurized dairy
Campylobacter	Bloody diarrhea	Feces from infected pets/animals; contaminated meats/foods/hands
Chlamydophila psittaci	Psittacosis	Parrots, other birds
Coxiella burnetii	Q fever	Aerosols of cattle/sheep amniotic fluid
Ehrlichia chaffeensis	Ehrlichiosis	*Amblyomma* (Lone Star tick)
Francisella tularensis	Tularemia	Ticks, rabbits, deer flies
***Leptospira* spp**	Leptospirosis	Animal urine in water; recreational water use
Mycobacterium leprae	Leprosy	Humans with lepromatous leprosy; armadillo (rare)
Pasteurella multocida	Cellulitis, osteomyelitis	Animal bite, cats, dogs
Rickettsia prowazekii	Epidemic typhus	Human to human via human body louse
Rickettsia rickettsii	Rocky Mountain spotted fever	*Dermacentor* (dog tick)
Rickettsia typhi	Endemic typhus	Fleas
***Salmonella* spp (except *S typhi*)**	Diarrhea (which may be bloody), vomiting, fever, abdominal cramps	Reptiles and poultry
Yersinia pestis	Plague	Fleas (rats and prairie dogs are reservoirs)

Rickettsial diseases and vector-borne illnesses

Treatment: doxycycline.

RASH COMMON		
Rocky Mountain spotted fever	*Rickettsia rickettsii*, vector is tick. Despite its name, disease occurs primarily in the South Atlantic states, especially North Carolina. Rash typically starts at wrists A and ankles and then spreads to trunk, palms, and soles.	Classic triad—headache, fever, rash (vasculitis). **Palms** and **soles** rash is seen in Coxsackievirus A infection (hand, foot, and mouth disease), Rocky Mountain spotted fever, and 2° Syphilis (you drive **CARS** using your **palms** and **soles**).
Typhus	Endemic (fleas)—*R typhi*. Epidemic (human body louse)—*R prowazekii*. Rash starts centrally and spreads out, sparing palms and soles.	*Rickettsii* on the wrists, typhus on the trunk.
RASH RARE		
Ehrlichiosis	*Ehrlichia*, vector is tick. Monocytes with morulae B (mulberry-like inclusions) in cytoplasm.	MEGA: Monocytes = Ehrlichiosis Granulocytes = Anaplasmosis
Anaplasmosis	*Anaplasma*, vector is tick. Granulocytes with morulae C in cytoplasm.	
Q fever	*Coxiella burnetii*, no arthropod vector. Bacterium inhaled as aerosols from cattle/sheep amniotic fluid. Presents with headache, cough, influenza-like symptoms, pneumonia, possibly in combination with hepatitis. Common cause of culture ⊖ endocarditis.	Q fever is caused by a Quite Complicated bug because it has no rash or vector and its causative organism can survive outside in its endospore form. Not in the *Rickettsia* genus, but closely related.

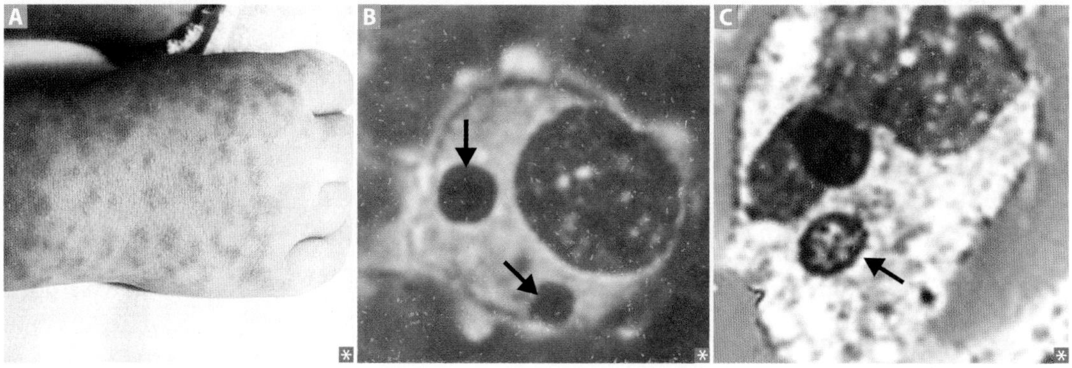

Mycoplasma pneumoniae

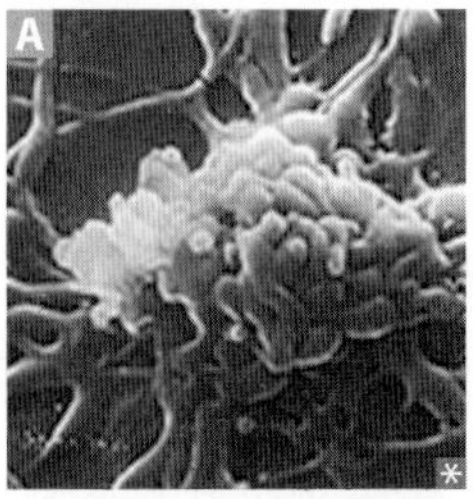

Classic cause of atypical "walking pneumonia" (insidious onset, headache, nonproductive cough, patchy or diffuse interstitial infiltrate, macular rash).

Occurs frequently in those <30 years old; outbreaks in military recruits, prisons, colleges.

Treatment: macrolides, doxycycline, or fluoroquinolone (penicillin ineffective since *Mycoplasma* has no cell wall).

Not seen on Gram stain. Pleomorphic A. Bacterial membrane contains sterols for stability. Grown on Eaton agar.

CXR appears more severe than patient presentation. High titer of **cold** agglutinins (IgM), which can agglutinate RBCs. *Mycoplasma* gets **cold** without a **coat** (no cell wall).

Can cause atypical variant of Stevens-Johnson syndrome, typically in children and adolescents.

▸ MICROBIOLOGY—MYCOLOGY

Systemic mycoses

All of the following can cause pneumonia and can disseminate.
All are caused by dimorphic fungi: **cold** (20°C) = **mold**; **heat** (37°C) = **yeast**. Only exception is *Coccidioides*, which is a spherule (not yeast) in tissue.
Systemic mycoses can form granulomas (like TB); cannot be transmitted person-to-person (unlike TB).
Treatment: fluconazole or itraconazole for **local** infection; amphotericin B for **systemic** infection.

DISEASE	ENDEMIC LOCATION	PATHOLOGIC FEATURES	UNIQUE SIGNS/SYMPTOMS	NOTES
Histoplasmosis 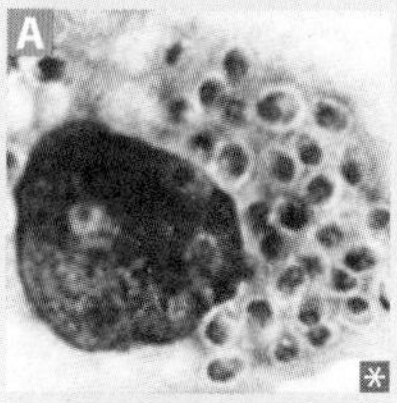	Mississippi and Ohio River Valleys	Macrophage filled with *Histoplasma* (smaller than RBC) A	Palatal/tongue ulcers, splenomegaly, pancytopenia, erythema nodosum	**Histo hides** (within macrophages) Associated with bird or bat droppings (eg, caves) Diagnosis via urine/serum antigen
Blastomycosis 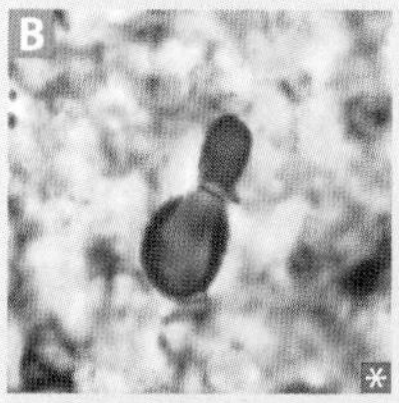	Eastern and Central US, Great Lakes	**Broad**-based budding of *Blastomyces* (same size as RBC) B	Inflammatory lung disease Disseminates to bone/skin (verrucous lesions, may mimic SCC).	**Blasto** buds **broadly**
Coccidioidomycosis 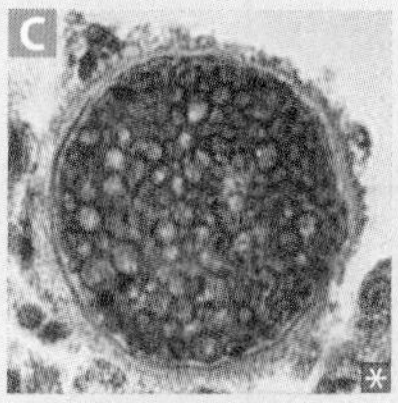	Southwestern US, California	Spherule (much larger than RBC) filled with endospores of *Coccidioides* C	Disseminates to bone/skin Erythema nodosum (desert bumps) or multiforme Arthralgias (desert rheumatism) Can cause meningitis	Associated with dust exposure in endemic areas (eg, archeological excavations, earthquakes)
Para-coccidioidomycosis 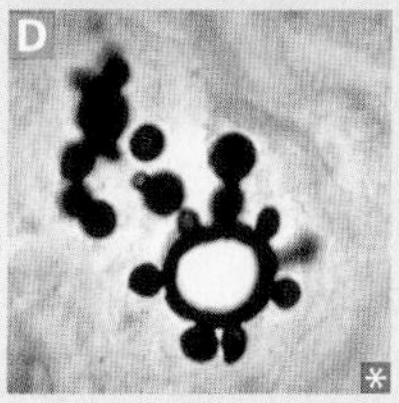	Latin America	Budding yeast of *Paracoccidioides* with **"captain's wheel"** formation (much larger than RBC) D	Similar to blastomycosis, males > females	**Paracoccidio parasails** with the **captain's wheel** all the way to **Latin America**

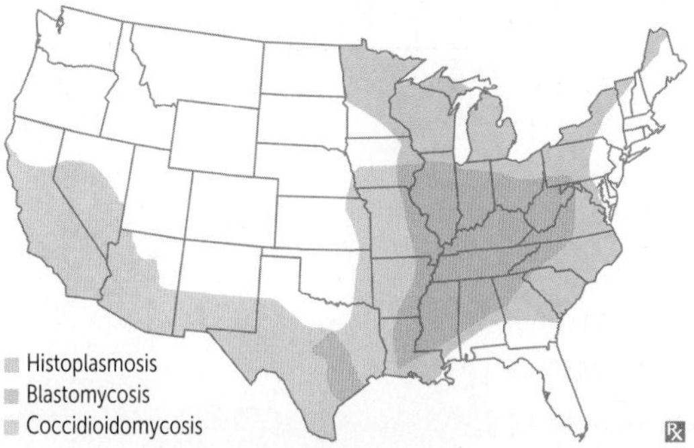
Histoplasmosis
Blastomycosis
Coccidioidomycosis

Cutaneous mycoses

Tinea (dermatophytes)	Clinical name for dermatophyte (cutaneous fungal) infections. Dermatophytes include *Microsporum*, *Trichophyton*, and *Epidermophyton*. Branching septate hyphae visible on KOH preparation with blue fungal stain A. Associated with pruritus.
Tinea capitis	Occurs on head, scalp. Associated with lymphadenopathy, alopecia, scaling B.
Tinea corporis	Occurs on body (usually torso). Characterized by enlarging erythematous, scaly rings ("ringworm") with central clearing C. Can be acquired from contact with infected pets or farm animals.
Tinea cruris	Occurs in inguinal area ("jock itch") D. Often does not show the central clearing seen in tinea corporis.
Tinea pedis	Three varieties ("athlete's foot"): ▪ Interdigital E; most common ▪ Moccasin distribution F ▪ Vesicular type
Tinea unguium	Onychomycosis; occurs on nails.
Tinea (pityriasis) versicolor	Caused by *Malassezia* spp. (*Pityrosporum* spp.), a yeast-like fungus (not a dermatophyte despite being called tinea). Degradation of lipids produces acids that inhibit tyrosinase (involved in melanin synthesis) → hypopigmentation G; hyperpigmentation and/or pink patches can also occur due to inflammatory response. Less pruritic than dermatophytes. Can occur any time of year, but more common in summer (hot, humid weather). "Spaghetti and meatballs" appearance on microscopy H. Treatment: selenium sulfide, topical and/or oral antifungal medications.

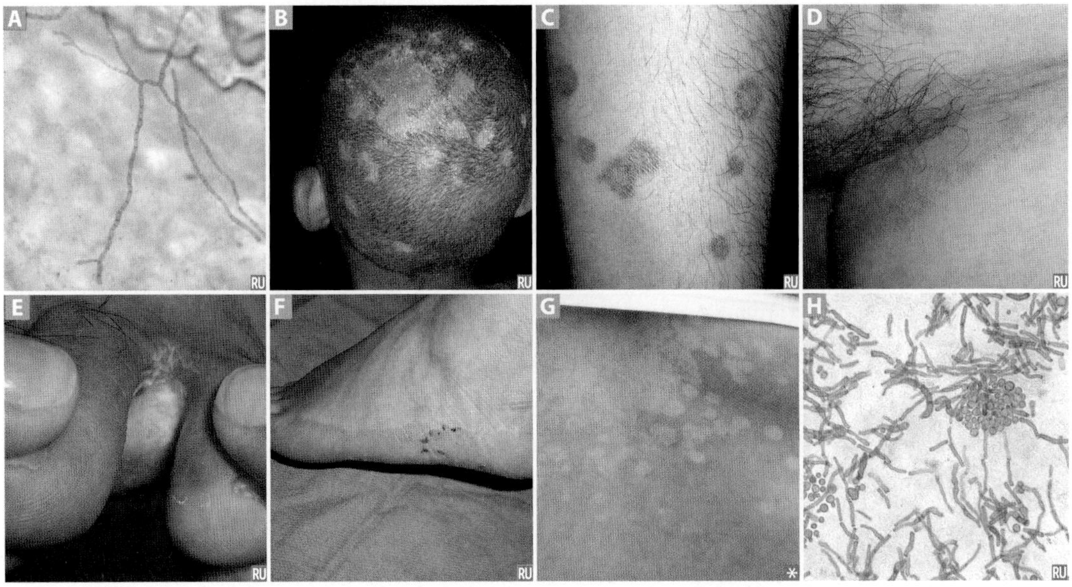

Opportunistic fungal infections

Candida albicans	*alba* = white. Dimorphic; forms pseudohyphae and budding yeasts at 20°C **A**, germ tubes at 37°C **B**. Systemic or superficial fungal infection. Causes oral **C** and esophageal thrush in immunocompromised (neonates, steroids, diabetes, AIDS), vulvovaginitis (diabetes, use of antibiotics), diaper rash, endocarditis (people who inject drugs), disseminated candidiasis (especially in neutropenic patients), chronic mucocutaneous candidiasis. Treatment: oral fluconazole/topical azoles for vaginal; nystatin, azoles, or, rarely, echinocandins for oral; fluconazole, echinocandins, or amphotericin B for esophageal or systemic disease.
Aspergillus fumigatus	Septate hyphae that branch at 45° Acute Angle **D** **E**. Causes invasive aspergillosis in immunocompromised patients, especially those with neutrophil dysfunction (eg, chronic granulomatous disease) because *Aspergillus* is catalase ⊕. Can cause aspergillomas **F** in pre-existing lung cavities, especially after TB infection. Some species of *Aspergillus* produce Aflatoxins (associated with hepatocellular carcinoma). Treatment: voriconazole or echinocandins (2nd-line). Allergic bronchopulmonary aspergillosis (ABPA)—hypersensitivity response to *Aspergillus* growing in lung mucus. Associated with asthma and cystic fibrosis; may cause bronchiectasis and eosinophilia.
Cryptococcus neoformans	5–10 μm with narrow budding. Heavily encapsulated yeast. Not dimorphic. Found in soil, pigeon droppings. Acquired through inhalation with hematogenous dissemination to meninges. Highlighted with India ink (clear halo **G**) and mucicarmine (red inner capsule **H**). Latex agglutination test detects polysaccharide capsular antigen and is more sensitive and specific. Causes cryptococcosis, cryptococcal meningitis, cryptococcal encephalitis ("soap bubble" lesions in brain), primarily in immunocompromised. Treatment: amphotericin B + flucytosine followed by fluconazole for cryptococcal meningitis.
***Mucor* and *Rhizopus* spp**	Irregular, broad, nonseptate hyphae branching at wide angles **I**. Causes mucormycosis, mostly in patients with DKA and/or neutropenia (eg, leukemia). Inhalation of spores → fungi proliferate in blood vessel walls, penetrate cribriform plate, and enter brain. Rhinocerebral, frontal lobe abscess; cavernous sinus thrombosis. Headache, facial pain, black necrotic eschar on face **J**; may have cranial nerve involvement. Treatment: surgical debridement, amphotericin B or isavuconazole.

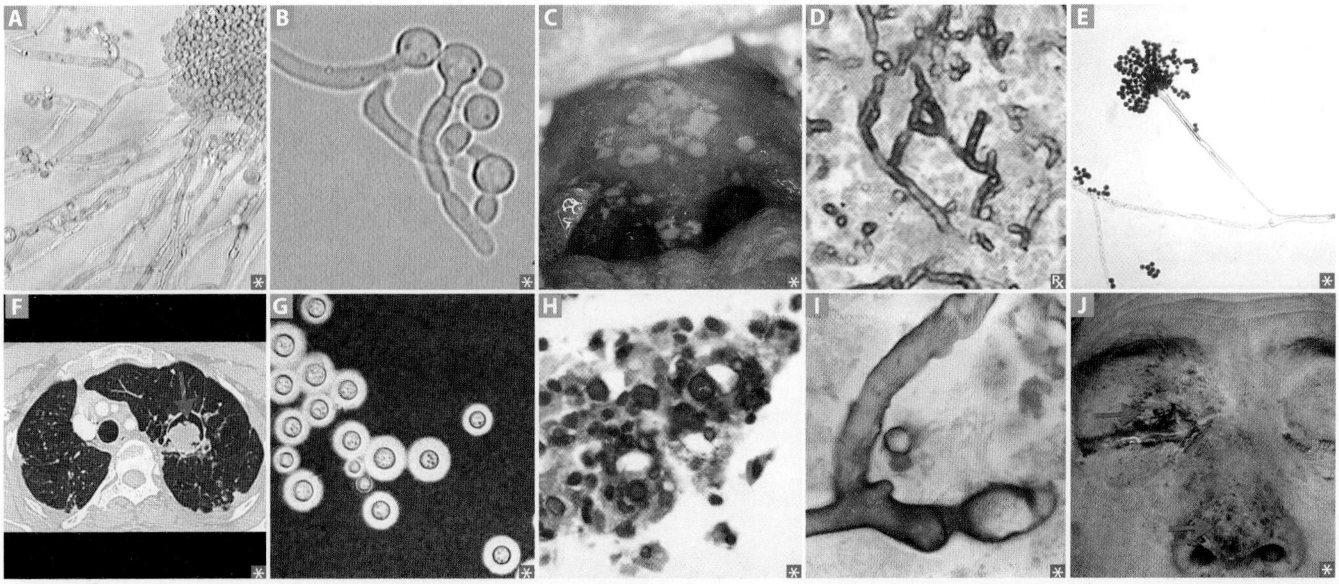

Pneumocystis jirovecii

Causes *Pneumocystis* pneumonia (PCP), a diffuse interstitial pneumonia A. Yeast-like fungus (originally classified as protozoan). Most infections are asymptomatic. Immunosuppression (eg, AIDS) predisposes to disease. Diffuse, bilateral ground-glass opacities on chest imaging, with pneumatoceles B. Diagnosed by bronchoalveolar lavage or lung biopsy. Disc-shaped yeast seen on methenamine silver stain of lung tissue C or with fluorescent antibody.

Treatment/prophylaxis: TMP-SMX, pentamidine, dapsone (prophylaxis as single agent, or treatment in combination with TMP), atovaquone. Start prophylaxis when CD4+ cell count drops to < 200 cells/mm^3 in people living with HIV.

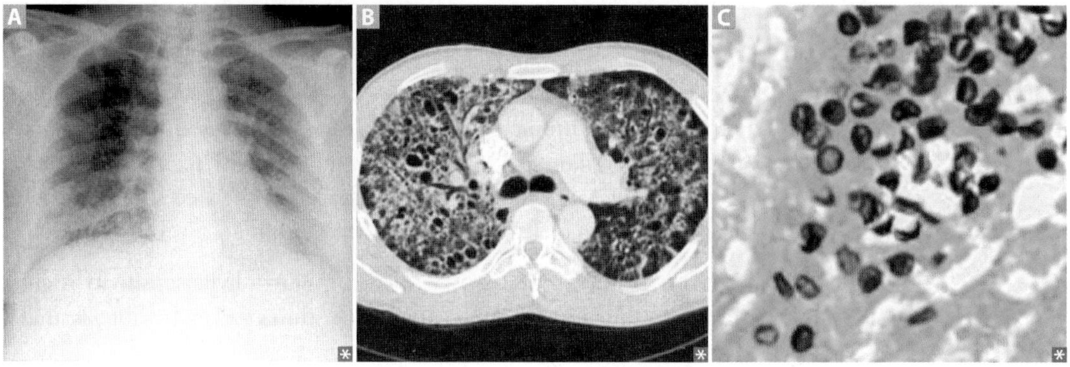

Sporothrix schenckii

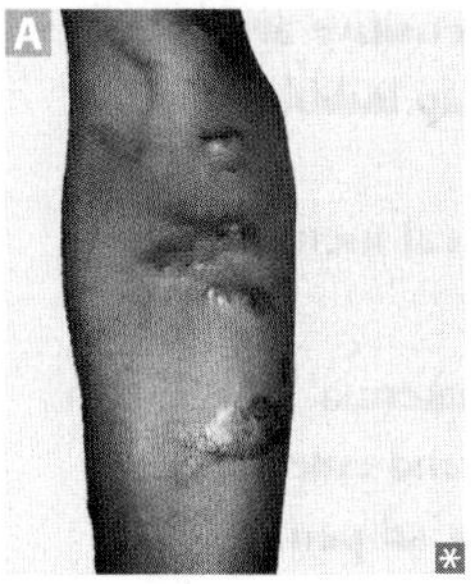

Causes sporotrichosis. Dimorphic fungus. Exists as a **cigar**-shaped yeast at 37 °C in the human body and as hyphae with spores in soil (conidia). Lives on vegetation. When spores are traumatically introduced into the skin, typically by a thorn ("**rose gardener**'s disease"), causes local pustule or ulcer with nodules along draining lymphatics (ascending lymphangitis A). Disseminated disease possible in immunocompromised host.

Treatment: itraconazole or **pot**assium iodide (only for cutaneous/lymphocutaneous).

Think of a **rose gardener** who smokes a **cigar** and **pot**.

▶ MICROBIOLOGY—PARASITOLOGY

Protozoa—gastrointestinal infections

ORGANISM	DISEASE	TRANSMISSION	DIAGNOSIS	TREATMENT
Giardia lamblia	**Giardiasis**—bloating, flatulence, foul-smelling, nonbloody, fatty diarrhea (often seen in campers/hikers)—think fat-rich Ghirardelli chocolates for fatty stools of *Giardia*	Cysts in water	Multinucleated trophozoites A or cysts B in stool, antigen detection, PCR	Metronidazole
Entamoeba histolytica	**Amebiasis**—bloody diarrhea (dysentery), liver abscess ("anchovy paste" exudate), RUQ pain; histology of colon biopsy shows flask-shaped ulcers	Cysts in water	Serology, antigen testing, PCR, and/or trophozoites (with engulfed RBCs C in the cytoplasm) or cysts with up to 4 nuclei in stool D; *Entamoeba* Eats Erythrocytes	Metronidazole; paromomycin or iodoquinol for asymptomatic cyst passers
Cryptosporidium	Severe diarrhea in AIDS Mild disease (watery diarrhea) in immunocompetent hosts	Oocysts in water	Oocysts on acid-fast stain E, antigen detection, PCR	Prevention (by filtering city water supplies); nitazoxanide in immunocompetent hosts

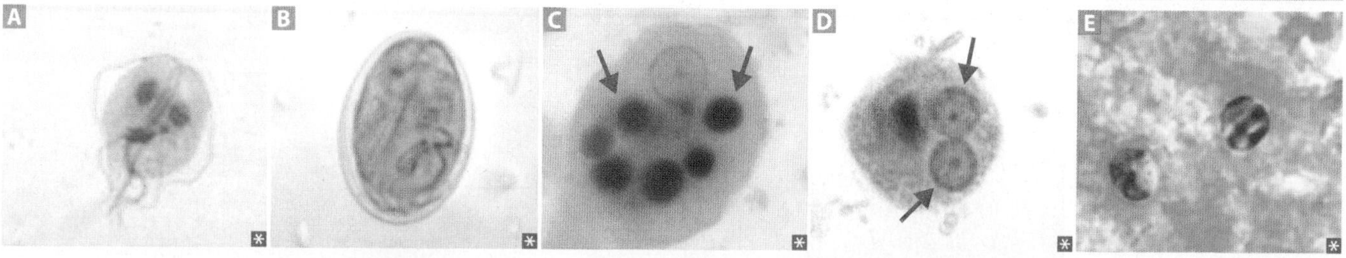

Protozoa—CNS infections

ORGANISM	DISEASE	TRANSMISSION	DIAGNOSIS	TREATMENT
Toxoplasma gondii	Immunocompetent: mononucleosis-like symptoms, ⊖ heterophile antibody test Reactivation in AIDS → brain abscesses usually seen as multiple ring-enhancing lesions on MRI A Congenital toxoplasmosis: classic triad of chorioretinitis, hydrocephalus, and intracranial calcifications	Cysts in meat (most common); oocysts in cat feces; crosses placenta (pregnant patients should avoid cats)	Serology, biopsy (tachyzoite) B; PCR of amniotic fluid for possible intrauterine disease	Sulfadiazine + pyrimethamine Prophylaxis with TMP-SMX when CD4+ cell count < 100 cells/mm^3
Naegleria fowleri	Rapidly fatal meningoencephalitis	Swimming in warm freshwater; enters via cribriform plate	Amoebas in CSF C	Amphotericin B has been effective for a few survivors
Trypanosoma brucei	**African sleeping sickness**—enlarged lymph nodes, recurring fever (due to antigenic variation), somnolence, coma	Tsetse fly, a painful bite	Trypomastigote in blood smear D	**Suramin** for blood-borne disease or **melarsoprol** for CNS penetration (“**I sure am mellow** when I’m **sleeping**”)

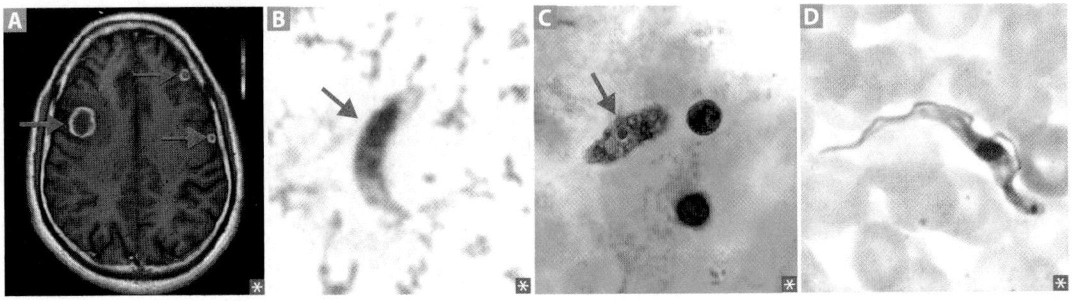

Protozoa—hematologic infections

ORGANISM	DISEASE	TRANSMISSION	DIAGNOSIS	TREATMENT
Plasmodium ***P vivax/ovale*** ***P falciparum*** ***P malariae*** 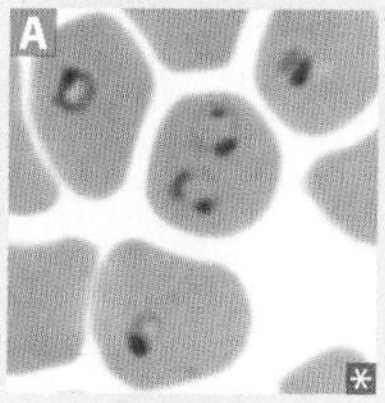 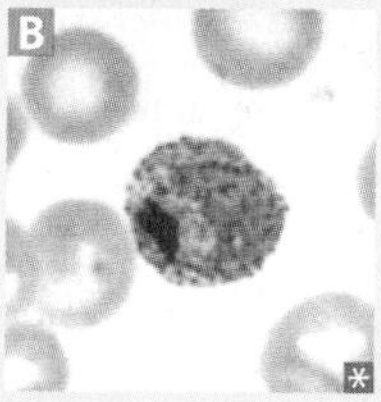	**Malaria**—fever, headache, anemia, splenomegaly; hypoglycemia in severe disease *P vivax/ovale*—48-hr cycle (tertian; includes fever on first day and third day, thus fevers are actually 48 hr apart); dormant form (hypnozoite) in liver *P falciparum*—severe; irregular fever patterns; parasitized RBCs occlude capillaries in brain (cerebral malaria), kidneys, lungs *P malariae*—72-hr cycle (quartan)	*Anopheles* mosquito	Blood smear: trophozoite ring form within RBC A, schizont containing merozoites; red granules (Schüffner stippling) B throughout RBC cytoplasm seen with *P vivax/ovale*	Chloroquine (for sensitive species); if resistant, use mefloquine or atovaquone/proguanil If life-threatening, use intravenous quinidine or artesunate (test for G6PD deficiency) For *P vivax/ovale*, add primaquine for hypnozoite (test for G6PD deficiency)
Babesia 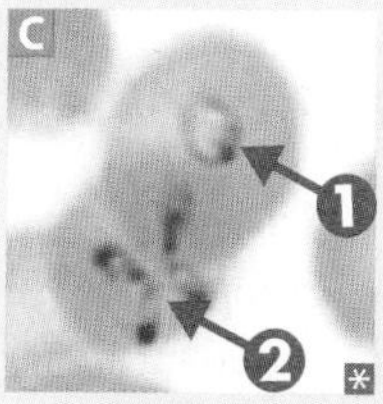	**Babesiosis**—fever and hemolytic anemia; predominantly in northeastern and north central United States; asplenia ↑ risk of severe disease due to inability to clear infected RBCs	*Ixodes* tick (also vector for *Borrelia burgdorferi* and *Anaplasma* spp)	Blood smear: ring form C1, "Maltese cross" C2; PCR	Atovaquone + azithromycin

Protozoa—others

ORGANISM	DISEASE	TRANSMISSION	DIAGNOSIS	TREATMENT
Visceral infections				
Trypanosoma cruzi	**Chagas disease**—dilated cardiomyopathy with apical atrophy, megacolon, megaesophagus; predominantly in South America Unilateral periorbital swelling (Romaña sign) characteristic of acute stage	Triatomine insect (kissing bug) bites and defecates around the mouth or eyes → fecal transmission into bite site or mucosa	Trypomastigote in blood smear A	**Benz**nidazole or nifur**t**imox; **cruz**ing in my **Benz**, with a **fur** coat on
***Leishmania* spp**	**Visceral leishmaniasis (kala-azar)**—spiking fevers, hepatosplenomegaly, pancytopenia **Cutaneous leishmaniasis**—skin ulcers B	Sandfly	Macrophages containing amastigotes C	Amphotericin B, sodium stibogluconate
Sexually transmitted infections				
Trichomonas vaginalis	**Vaginitis**—foul-smelling, greenish discharge; itching and burning; do not confuse with *Gardnerella vaginalis*, a gram-variable bacterium associated with bacterial vaginosis	Sexual (cannot exist outside human because it cannot form cysts)	Trophozoites (motile) D on wet mount; punctate cervical hemorrhages ("strawberry cervix")	Metronidazole for patient and partner(s) (prophylaxis; check for STI)

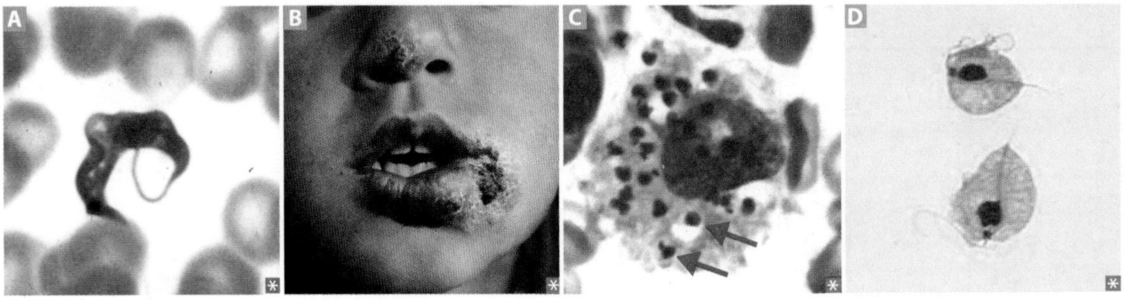

Nematode routes of infection

Nematode routes of infection	Ingested—*Enterobius, Ascaris, Toxocara, Trichinella, Trichuris*	You'll get sick if you EATTT these!
	Cutaneous—*Strongyloides, Ancylostoma, Necator*	These get into your feet from the SANd
	Bites—*Loa loa, Onchocerca volvulus, Wuchereria bancrofti*	Lay LOW to avoid getting bitten

Nematodes (roundworms)

ORGANISM	DISEASE	TRANSMISSION	TREATMENT
Intestinal			
Enterobius vermicularis **(pinworm)**	Causes anal pruritus (diagnosed by seeing egg A via the tape test).	Fecal-oral.	Bendazoles, pyrantel pamoate.
Ascaris lumbricoides **(giant roundworm)**	May cause obstruction at ileocecal valve, biliary obstruction, intestinal perforation, migrates from nose/mouth. Migration of larvae to alveoli → Löeffler syndrome (pulmonary eosinophilia).	Fecal-oral; knobby-coated, oval eggs seen in feces under microscope B.	Bendazoles.
Strongyloides stercoralis **(threadworm)**	GI (eg, duodenitis), pulmonary (eg, dry cough, hemoptysis), and cutaneous (eg, pruritus) symptoms. Hyperinfection syndrome caused by autoinfection (larvae enter bloodstream).	Larvae in soil penetrate skin; rhabditiform larvae seen in feces under microscope.	Ivermectin or bendazoles.
Ancylostoma **spp,** ***Necator americanus*** **(hookworms)**	Cause microcytic anemia by sucking blood from intestinal wall. Cutaneous larva migrans—pruritic, serpiginous rash C.	Larvae penetrate skin from walking barefoot on contaminated beach/soil.	Bendazoles or pyrantel pamoate.
Trichinella spiralis	Larvae enter bloodstream, encyst in striated muscle D → myositis. Trichinosis—fever, vomiting, nausea, periorbital edema, myalgia.	Undercooked meat (especially pork); fecal-oral (less likely).	Bendazoles.
Trichuris trichiura **(whipworm)**	Often asymptomatic; loose stools, anemia, rectal prolapse in children.	Fecal-oral.	Bendazoles.
Tissue			
Toxocara canis	Visceral larva migrans—migration into blood → inflammation of liver, eyes (visual impairment, blindness), CNS (seizures, coma), heart (myocarditis). Patients often asymptomatic.	Fecal-oral.	Bendazoles.
Onchocerca volvulus	Skin changes, loss of elastic fibers, river blindness (**black** skin nodules, "**black** sight"); allergic reaction possible.	Female **black** fly.	Ivermectin (**iver**mectin for **river** blindness).
Loa loa	Swelling in skin, worm in conjunctiva.	Deer fly, horse fly, mango fly.	Diethylcarbamazine.
Wuchereria bancrofti, Brugia malayi	Lymphatic filariasis (elephantiasis)—worms invade lymph nodes. → inflammation → lymphedema E; symptom onset after 9 mo–1 yr.	Female mosquito.	Diethylcarbamazine.

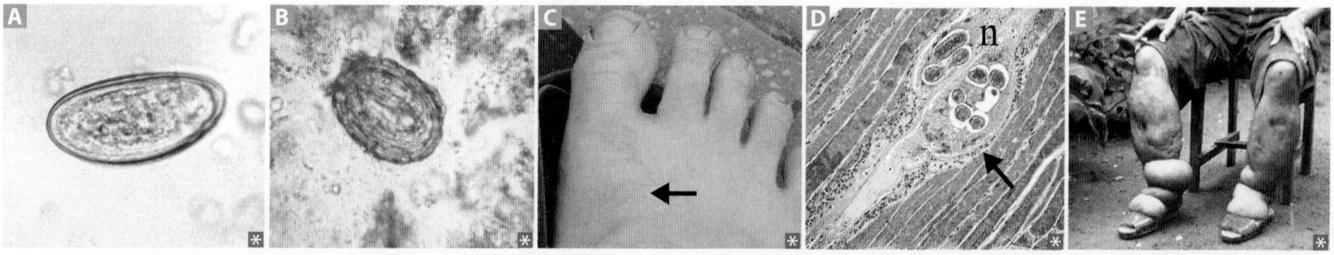

Cestodes (tapeworms)

ORGANISM	DISEASE	TRANSMISSION	TREATMENT
Taenia solium A	Intestinal tapeworm	Ingestion of larvae encysted in undercooked pork	Praziquantel
	Cysticercosis, neurocysticercosis (cystic CNS lesions, seizures) B	Ingestion of eggs in food contaminated with human feces	Praziquantel; albendazole for neurocysticercosis
Diphyllobothrium latum	Vitamin B_{12} deficiency (tapeworm competes for B_{12} in intestine) → megaloblastic anemia	Ingestion of larvae in raw freshwater fish	Praziquantel, niclosamide
Echinococcus granulosus C	Hydatid cysts D ("eggshell calcification") in liver E; cyst rupture can cause anaphylaxis	Ingestion of eggs in food contaminated with dog feces Sheep are an intermediate host	Albendazole; surgery for complicated cysts

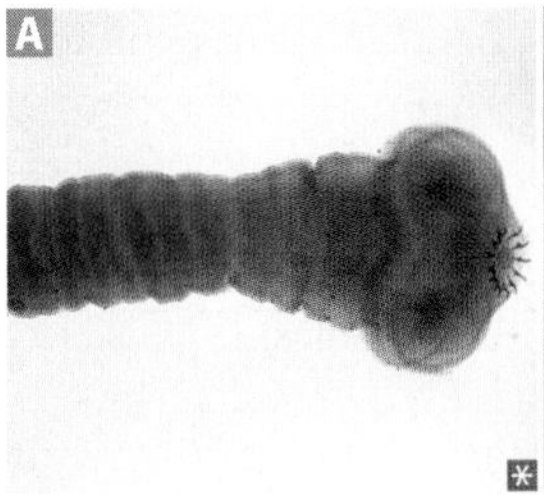
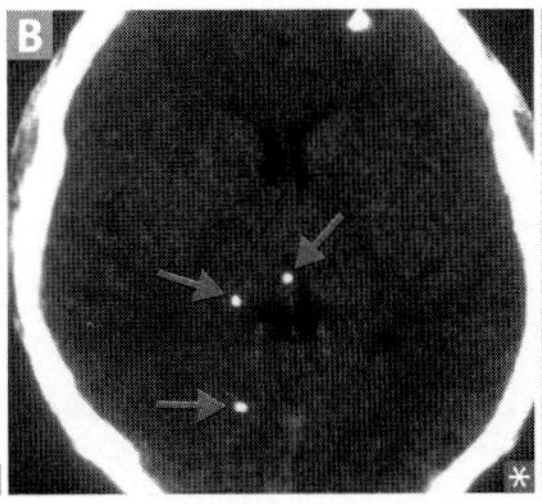
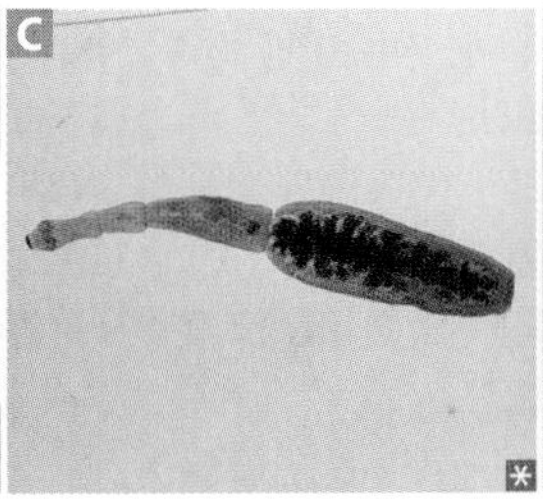
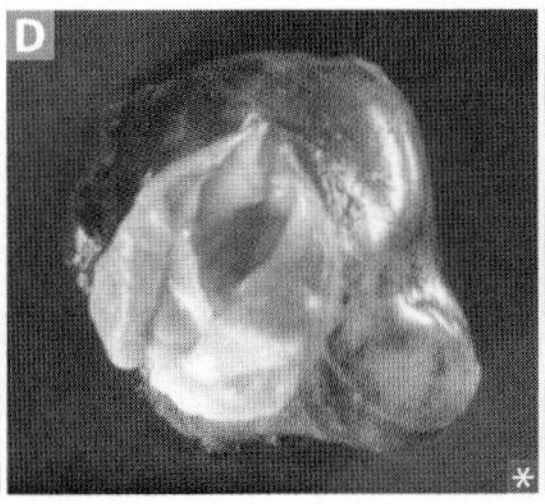
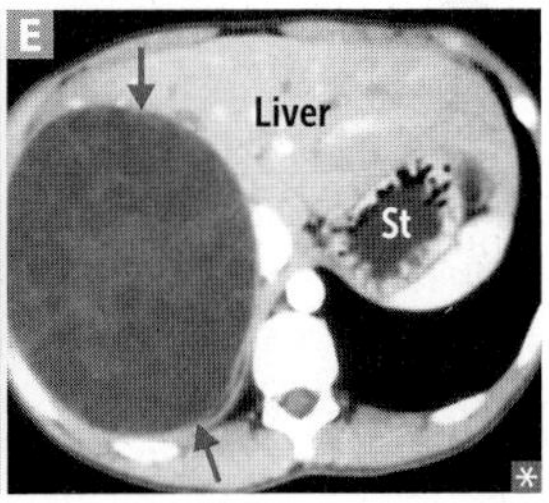

Trematodes (flukes)

ORGANISM	DISEASE	TRANSMISSION	TREATMENT
Schistosoma A 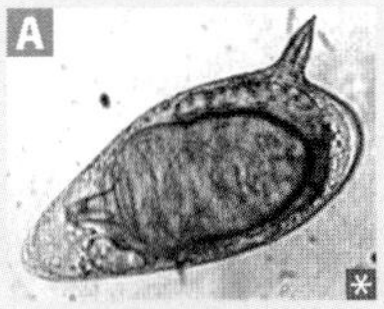 B 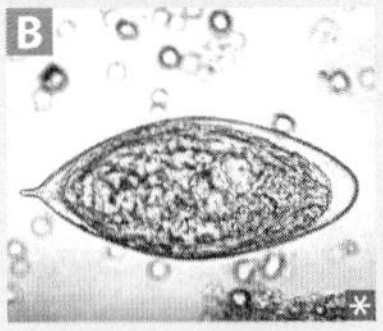	Liver and spleen enlargement (A shows *S mansoni* egg with lateral spine), fibrosis, inflammation, portal hypertension Chronic infection with *S haematobium* (egg with terminal spine B) can lead to squamous cell carcinoma of the bladder (painless hematuria) and pulmonary hypertension	Snails are intermediate host; cercariae penetrate skin of humans in contact with contaminated fresh water (eg, swimming or bathing)	Praziquantel
Clonorchis sinensis	Biliary tract inflammation → pigmented gallstones Associated with cholangiocarcinoma	Undercooked fish	Praziquantel

Ectoparasites

Sarcoptes scabiei 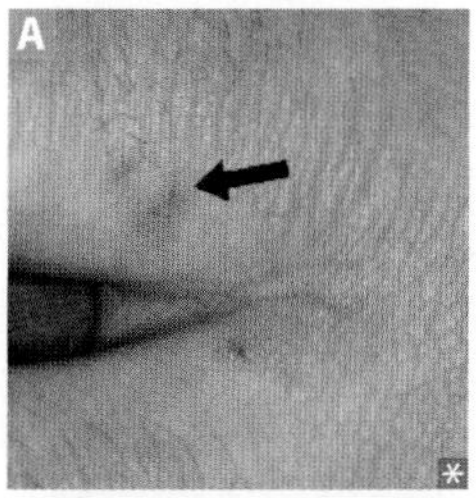	Mites burrow into stratum corneum and cause **scabies**—pruritus (worse at night) and serpiginous burrows (lines) often between fingers and toes A.	Common in children, crowded populations (jails, nursing homes); transmission through skin-to-skin contact (most common) or via fomites. Treatment: permethrin cream, oral ivermectin, washing/drying all clothing/bedding, treat close contacts.
Pediculus humanus/ Phthirus pubis 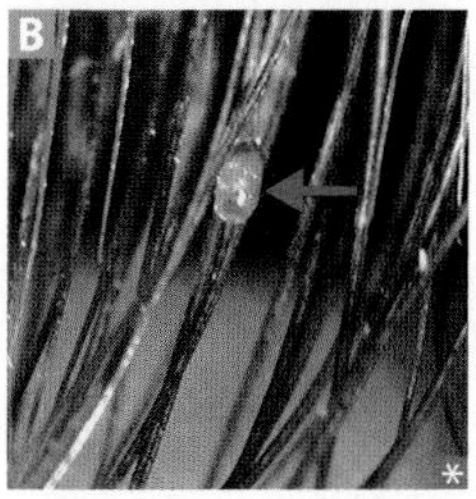	Blood-sucking lice that cause intense pruritus with associated excoriations, commonly on scalp and neck (head lice), waistband and axilla (body lice), or pubic and perianal regions (pubic lice).	Body lice can transmit *Rickettsia prowazekii* (epidemic typhus), *Borrelia recurrentis* (relapsing fever), *Bartonella quintana* (trench fever). Treatment: pyrethroids, malathion, or ivermectin lotion, and nit B combing. Children with head lice can be treated at home without interrupting school attendance.

Parasite hints

ASSOCIATIONS	ORGANISM
Biliary tract disease, cholangiocarcinoma	*Clonorchis sinensis*
Brain cysts, seizures	*Taenia solium* (neurocysticercosis)
Hematuria, squamous cell bladder cancer	*Schistosoma haematobium*
Liver (hydatid) cysts, exposure to infected dogs	*Echinococcus granulosus*
Iron deficiency anemia	*Ancylostoma*, *Necator*
Myalgias, periorbital edema	*Trichinella spiralis*
Nocturnal perianal pruritus	*Enterobius*
Portal hypertension	*Schistosoma mansoni*, *Schistosoma japonicum*
Vitamin B_{12} deficiency	*Diphyllobothrium latum*

▸ MICROBIOLOGY—VIROLOGY

Viral structure—general features

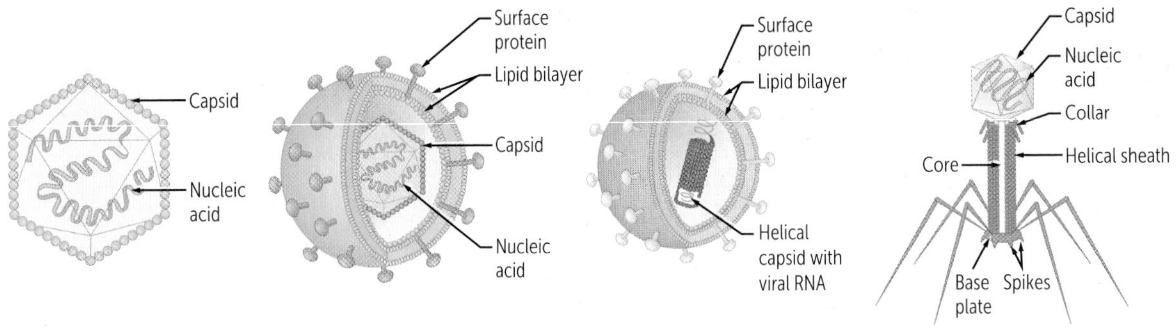

Naked virus with icosahedral capsid | Enveloped virus with icosahedral capsid | Enveloped virus with helical capsid | Bacteriophage

Viral genetics

Recombination

Exchange of genes between 2 chromosomes by crossing over within regions of significant base sequence homology.

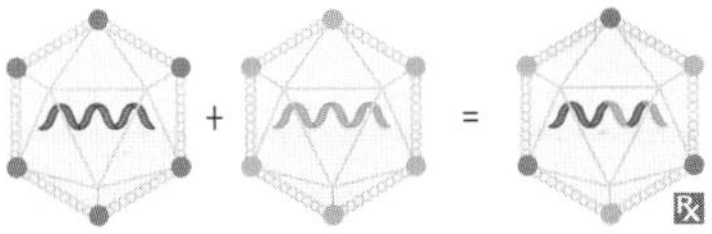

Reassortment

When viruses with segmented genomes (eg, influenza virus) exchange genetic material. For example, the 2009 novel H1N1 influenza A pandemic emerged via complex viral reassortment of genes from human, swine, and avian viruses. Has potential to cause antigenic shift.

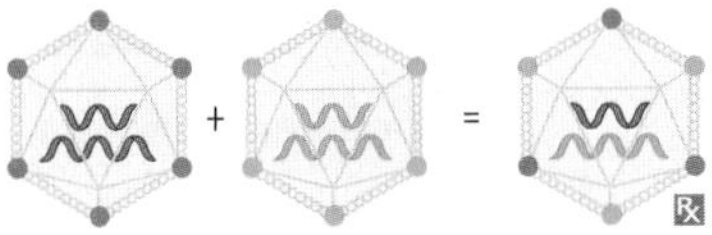

Complementation

When 1 of 2 viruses that infect the cell has a mutation that results in a nonfunctional protein, the nonmutated virus "complements" the mutated one by making a functional protein that serves both viruses. For example, hepatitis D virus requires the presence of replicating hepatitis B virus to supply HBsAg, the envelope protein for HDV.

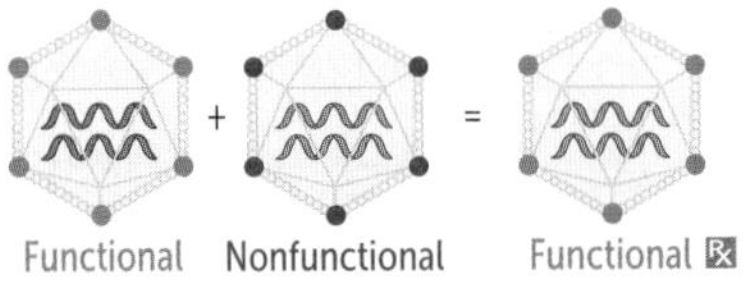

Phenotypic mixing

Occurs with simultaneous infection of a cell with 2 viruses. For progeny 1, genome of virus A can be partially or completely coated (forming pseudovirion) with the surface proteins of virus B. Type B protein coat determines the tropism (infectivity) of the hybrid virus. Progeny from subsequent infection of a cell by progeny 1 will have a type A coat that is encoded by its type A genetic material.

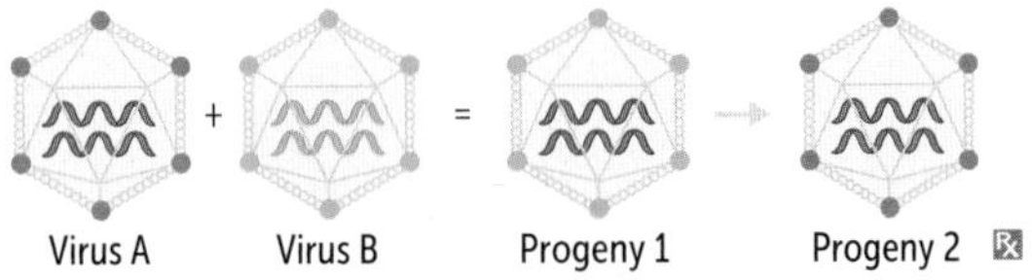

DNA viral genomes	All DNA viruses have dsDNA genomes except Parvoviridae (ssDNA). All are linear except papilloma-, polyoma-, and hepadnaviruses (circular).	All are dsDNA (like our cells), except "**part-of-a-virus**" (**parvovirus**) is ssDNA. *Parvus* = small.
RNA viral genomes	All RNA viruses have ssRNA genomes except Reoviridae (dsRNA). ⊕ stranded RNA viruses: I went to a **retro** (**retrovirus**) **toga** (**togavirus**) party, where I drank **flavored** (**flavivirus**) **Corona** (**coronavirus**) and ate **hippie** (**hepevirus**) **California** (**calicivirus**) **pickles** (**picornavirus**).	All are ssRNA, except "**repeato-virus**" (**reovirus**) is dsRNA.
Naked viral genome infectivity	Purified nucleic acids of most dsDNA viruses (except poxviruses and HBV) and ⊕ strand ssRNA (≈ mRNA) viruses are infectious. Naked nucleic acids of ⊖ strand ssRNA and dsRNA viruses are not infectious. They require polymerases contained in the complete virion.	
Viral envelopes	Generally, enveloped viruses acquire their envelopes from plasma membrane when they exit from cell. Exceptions include herpesviruses, which acquire envelopes from nuclear membrane. Naked (nonenveloped) viruses include papillomavirus, adenovirus, parvovirus, polyomavirus, calicivirus, picornavirus, reovirus, and hepevirus.	Enveloped DNA viruses (**herpesvirus**, **hepadnavirus**, **poxvirus**) have **helpful protection**.

DNA virus characteristics

Some general rules—all DNA viruses:

GENERAL RULE	COMMENTS
Are **HHAPPPPy** viruses	**H**epadna, **H**erpes, **A**deno, **P**ox, **P**arvo, **P**apilloma, **P**olyoma.
Are double stranded	Except parvo (single stranded).
Have linear genomes	Except papilloma and polyoma (circular, supercoiled) and hepadna (circular, incomplete).
Are icosahedral	Except pox (complex).
Replicate in the nucleus	Except pox (carries own DNA-dependent RNA polymerase).

DNA viruses All replicate in the nucleus (except poxvirus). "Pox is out of the box (nucleus)."

VIRAL FAMILY	ENVELOPE	DNA STRUCTURE	MEDICAL IMPORTANCE
Herpesviruses	Yes	DS and linear	See Herpesviruses entry
Poxvirus	Yes	DS and linear (largest DNA virus)	Smallpox eradicated world wide by use of the live-attenuated vaccine Cowpox ("milkmaid blisters") **Molluscum contagiosum**—flesh-colored papule with central umbilication
Hepadnavirus	Yes	Partially DS and circular	HBV: ▪ Acute or chronic hepatitis ▪ Not a retrovirus but has reverse transcriptase
Adenovirus A 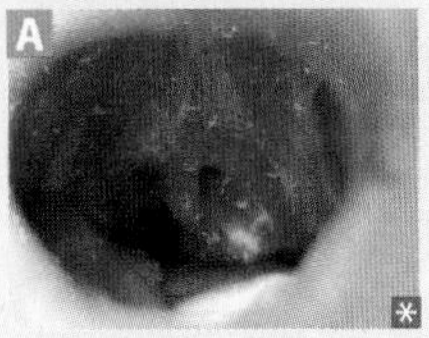	No	DS and linear	Febrile pharyngitis A—sore throat Acute hemorrhagic cystitis Pneumonia Conjunctivitis—"pink eye" Gastroenteritis Myocarditis
Papillomavirus	No	DS and circular	HPV—warts, cancer (cervical, anal, penile, or oropharyngeal); serotypes 1, 2, 6, 11 associated with warts; serotypes 16, 18 associated with cancer
Polyomavirus	No	DS and circular	JC virus—progressive multifocal leukoencephalopathy (PML) in HIV BK virus—transplant patients, commonly targets kidney **JC**: **J**unky **C**erebrum; **BK**: **B**ad **K**idney
Parvovirus	No	SS and linear (smallest DNA virus)	B19 virus—aplastic crises in sickle cell disease, "slapped cheek" rash in children (erythema infectiosum, or fifth disease); infects RBC precursors and endothelial cells → RBC destruction → hydrops fetalis and death in fetus, pure RBC aplasia and rheumatoid arthritis–like symptoms in adults

Herpesviruses Enveloped, DS, and linear viruses

VIRUS	ROUTE OF TRANSMISSION	CLINICAL SIGNIFICANCE	NOTES
Herpes simplex virus-1	Respiratory secretions, saliva	Gingivostomatitis, keratoconjunctivitis A, herpes labialis (cold sores) B, herpetic whitlow on finger, temporal lobe encephalitis, esophagitis, erythema multiforme	Most commonly latent in trigeminal ganglia Most common cause of sporadic encephalitis, can present as altered mental status, seizures, and/or aphasia
Herpes simplex virus-2	Sexual contact, perinatal	Herpes genitalis C, neonatal herpes	Most commonly latent in sacral ganglia Viral meningitis more common with HSV-2 than with HSV-1

Herpesviruses *(continued)*

VIRUS	ROUTE OF TRANSMISSION	CLINICAL SIGNIFICANCE	NOTES
Varicella-Zoster virus (HHV-3)	Respiratory secretions, contact with fluid from vesicles	Varicella-zoster (chickenpox D, shingles E), encephalitis, pneumonia Most common complication of shingles is post-herpetic neuralgia	Latent in dorsal root or trigeminal ganglia; CN V_1 branch involvement can cause herpes zoster ophthalmicus
Epstein-Barr virus (HHV-4)	Respiratory secretions, saliva; aka "kissing disease," (common in teens, young adults)	**Mononucleosis**—fever, hepatosplenomegaly F, pharyngitis, and lymphadenopathy (especially posterior cervical nodes); avoid contact sports until resolution due to risk of splenic rupture Associated with lymphomas (eg, endemic Burkitt lymphoma), nasopharyngeal carcinoma (especially Asian adults), lymphoproliferative disease in transplant patients	Infects **B** cells through CD**21**, "Must be **21** to drink **Beer** in a **Barr**" Atypical lymphocytes on peripheral blood smear G—not infected B cells but reactive cytotoxic T cells ⊕ Monospot test—heterophile antibodies detected by agglutination of sheep or horse RBCs Use of amoxicillin (eg, for presumed strep pharyngitis) can cause maculopapular rash
Cytomegalovirus (HHV-5)	Congenital, transfusion, sexual contact, saliva, urine, transplant	Mononucleosis (⊖ Monospot) in immunocompetent patients; infection in immunocompromised, especially pneumonia in transplant patients; esophagitis; AIDS **retinitis** ("**sight**omegalovirus"): hemorrhage, cotton-wool exudates, vision loss Congenital CMV	Infected cells have characteristic "owl eye" intranuclear inclusions H Latent in mononuclear cells
Human herpes-viruses 6 and 7	Saliva	Roseola infantum (exanthem subitum): high fevers for several days that can cause seizures, followed by diffuse macular rash (starts on trunk then spreads to extremities) I; usually seen in children <2 years old	**Ros**eola: fever first, **Ros**y (rash) later Self-limited illness HHV-7—less common cause of roseola
Human herpesvirus 8	Sexual contact	Kaposi sarcoma (neoplasm of endothelial cells). Seen in HIV/AIDS and transplant patients. Dark/violaceous plaques or nodules J representing vascular proliferations	Can also affect GI tract and lungs

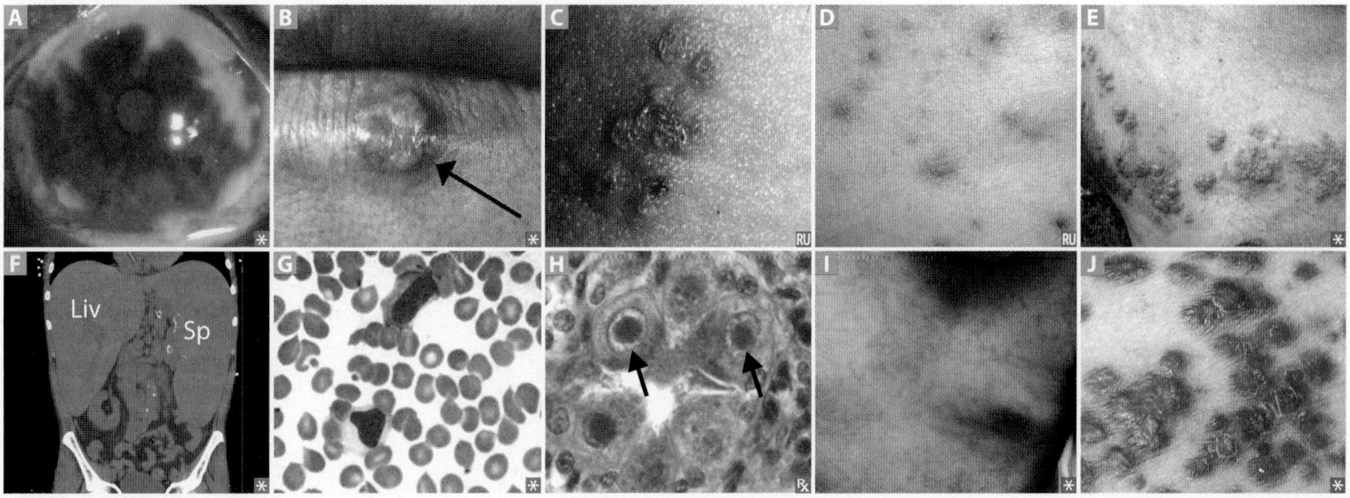

HSV identification

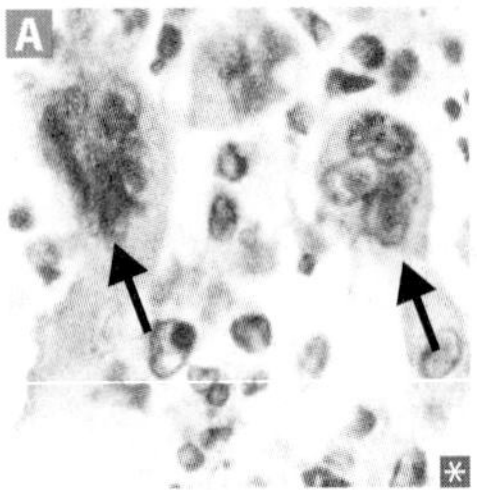

PCR of skin lesions is test of choice.
CSF PCR for herpes encephalitis.
Tzanck test (outdated)—a smear of an opened skin vesicle to detect multinucleated giant cells A commonly seen in HSV-1, HSV-2, and VZV infection.
Intranuclear eosinophilic Cowdry A inclusions also seen with HSV-1, HSV-2, VZV.

Receptors used by viruses

VIRUS	RECEPTORS
CMV	Integrins (heparan sulfate)
EBV	CD21
HIV	CD4, CXCR4, CCR5
Parvovirus B19	P antigen on RBCs
Rabies	Nicotinic AChR
Rhinovirus	ICAM-1 (I CAMe to see the rhino)

RNA viruses All replicate in the cytoplasm (except retrovirus and influenza virus). "Retro flu is outta cyt (sight)."

VIRAL FAMILY	ENVELOPE	RNA STRUCTURE	CAPSID SYMMETRY	MEDICAL IMPORTANCE
Reoviruses	No	DS linear Multisegmented	Icosahedral (double)	Coltivirus[a]—Colorado tick fever Rotavirus—cause of fatal diarrhea in children
Picornaviruses	No	SS ⊕ linear	Icosahedral	Poliovirus—polio-Salk/Sabin vaccines—IPV/OPV Echovirus—aseptic meningitis Rhinovirus—"common cold" Coxsackievirus—aseptic meningitis; herpangina (mouth blisters, fever); hand, foot, and mouth disease; myocarditis; pericarditis HAV—acute viral hepatitis PERCH
Hepevirus	No	SS ⊕ linear	Icosahedral	HEV
Caliciviruses	No	SS ⊕ linear	Icosahedral	Norovirus—viral gastroenteritis
Flaviviruses	Yes	SS ⊕ linear	Icosahedral	HCV Yellow fever[a] Dengue[a] St. Louis encephalitis[a] West Nile virus[a]—meningoencephalitis, flaccid paralysis Zika virus[a]
Togaviruses	Yes	SS ⊕ linear	Icosahedral	Toga CREW—Chikungunya virus[a] (co-infection with dengue virus can occur), Rubella, Eastern and Western equine encephalitis
Retroviruses	Yes	SS ⊕ linear 2 copies	Icosahedral (HTLV), complex and conical (HIV)	Have reverse transcriptase HTLV—T-cell leukemia HIV—AIDS
Coronaviruses	Yes	SS ⊕ linear	Helical	"Common cold," SARS, MERS, COVID-19
Orthomyxoviruses	Yes	SS ⊖ linear 8 segments	Helical	Influenza virus
Paramyxoviruses	Yes	SS ⊖ linear Nonsegmented	Helical	PaRaMyxovirus: Parainfluenza—croup RSV—bronchiolitis in babies Measles, Mumps
Rhabdoviruses	Yes	SS ⊖ linear	Helical	Rabies
Filoviruses	Yes	SS ⊖ linear	Helical	Ebola/Marburg hemorrhagic fever—often fatal.
Arenaviruses	Yes	SS ⊕ and ⊖ circular 2 segments	Helical	LCMV—lymphocytic choriomeningitis virus Lassa fever encephalitis—spread by rodents
Bunyaviruses	Yes	SS ⊖ circular 3 segments	Helical	California encephalitis[a] Sandfly/Rift Valley fevers[a] Crimean-Congo hemorrhagic fever[a] Hantavirus—hemorrhagic fever, pneumonia
Delta virus	Yes	SS ⊖ circular	Uncertain	HDV is a "Defective" virus that requires the presence of HBV to replicate

SS, single-stranded; DS, double-stranded; ⊕, positive sense; ⊖, negative sense; [a]= arbovirus, arthropod borne (mosquitoes, ticks).

Negative-stranded viruses	Must transcribe ⊖ strand to ⊕. Virion brings its own RNA-dependent RNA polymerase. They include arenaviruses, bunyaviruses, paramyxoviruses, orthomyxoviruses, filoviruses, and rhabdoviruses.	Always bring polymerase or fail replication.
Segmented viruses	All are RNA viruses. They include Bunyaviruses (3 segments), Orthomyxoviruses (influenza viruses) (8 segments), Arenaviruses (2 segments), and Reoviruses (10–12 segments).	BOARding flight 382 in 10–12 minutes.
Picornavirus	Includes Poliovirus, Echovirus, Rhinovirus, Coxsackievirus, and HAV. RNA is translated into 1 large polypeptide that is cleaved by virus-encoded proteases into functional viral proteins. Poliovirus, echovirus, and coxsackievirus are enteroviruses and can cause aseptic (viral) meningitis.	PicoRNAvirus = small RNA virus. PERCH on a "peak" (pico).
Rhinovirus	A picornavirus. Nonenveloped RNA virus. Cause of common cold; > 100 serologic types. Acid labile—destroyed by stomach acid; therefore, does not infect the GI tract (unlike the other picornaviruses).	Rhino has a runny nose.
Rotavirus 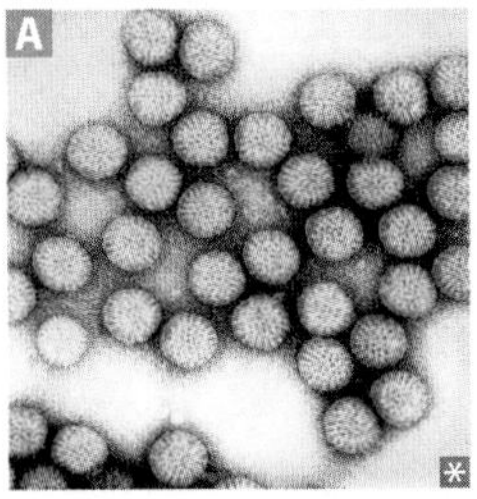	Segmented dsRNA virus (a reovirus) A. Most important global cause of infantile gastroenteritis. Major cause of acute diarrhea in the United States during winter, especially in day care centers, kindergartens. Villous destruction with atrophy leads to ↓ absorption of Na^+ and loss of K^+.	Rotavirus = right out the anus. CDC recommends routine vaccination of all infants except those with a history of intussusception (rare adverse effect of rotavirus vaccination) or SCID.

Influenza viruses

Orthomyxoviruses. Enveloped, ⊖ ssRNA viruses with segmented genome. Contain hemagglutinin (binds sialic acid and promotes viral entry) and neuraminidase (promotes progeny virion release) antigens. Patients at risk for fatal bacterial superinfection, most commonly *S aureus*, *S pneumoniae*, and *H influenzae*.

Treatment: supportive +/– neuraminidase inhibitor (eg, oseltamivir, zanamivir).

Hemagglutinin: lets the virus in

Neuraminidaways: sends the virus away

Reformulated vaccine ("the flu shot") contains viral strains most likely to appear during the flu season, due to the virus' rapid genetic change.

Killed viral vaccine is most frequently used.

Live attenuated vaccine contains temperature-sensitive mutant that replicates in the nose but not in the lung; administered intranasally.

Sudden shift is more deadly than gradual drift.

Genetic/antigenic shift

Infection of 1 cell by 2 different segmented viruses (eg, swine influenza and human influenza viruses) → RNA segment reassortment → dramatically different virus (genetic shift) → major global outbreaks (pandemics).

Genetic/antigenic drift

Random mutation in hemagglutinin (HA) or neuraminidase (NA) genes → minor changes in HA or NA protein (drift) occur frequently → major global outbreaks (pandemics).

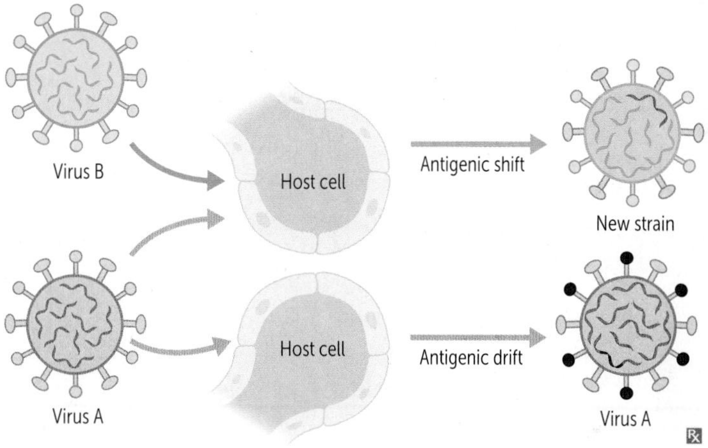

Rubella virus

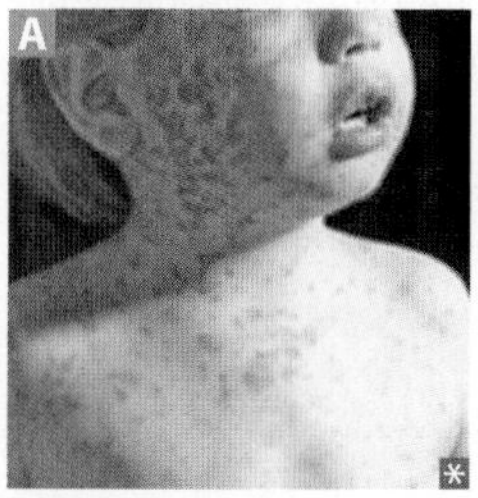

A togavirus. Causes rubella, once known as German (3-day) measles. Fever, postauricular and other lymphadenopathy, arthralgias, and fine, maculopapular rash that starts on face and spreads centrifugally to involve trunk and extremities A.

Causes mild disease in children but serious congenital disease (a TORCH infection). Congenital rubella findings include classic triad of sensorineural deafness, cataracts, and patent ductus arteriosus. "Blueberry muffin" appearance may be seen due to dermal extramedullary hematopoiesis.

Paramyxoviruses

Paramyxoviruses cause disease in children. They include those that cause parainfluenza (croup), mumps, measles, RSV, and human metapneumovirus. All subtypes can cause respiratory tract infection (bronchiolitis, pneumonia) in infants. All contain surface F (fusion) protein, which causes respiratory epithelial cells to fuse and form multinucleated cells. Palivizumab (monoclonal antibody against F protein) prevents pneumonia caused by RSV infection in premature infants.

Palivizumab for paramyxovirus (RSV) prophylaxis in preemies.

Acute laryngotracheobronchitis

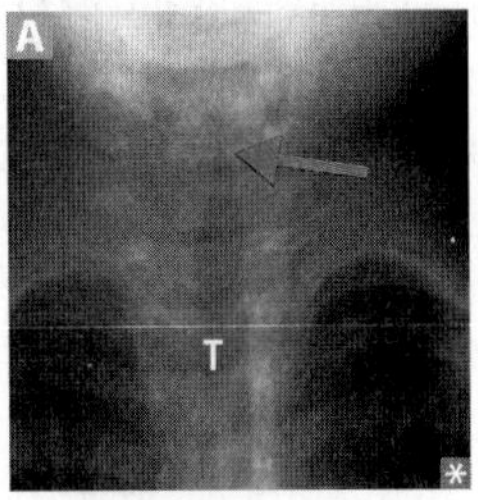

Also called croup. Caused by parainfluenza viruses. Virus membrane contains hemagglutinin (binds sialic acid and promotes viral entry) and neuraminidase (promotes progeny virion release) antigens. Results in a "seal-like" barking cough and inspiratory stridor. Narrowing of upper trachea and subglottis leads to characteristic steeple sign on x-ray A.

Measles (rubeola) virus

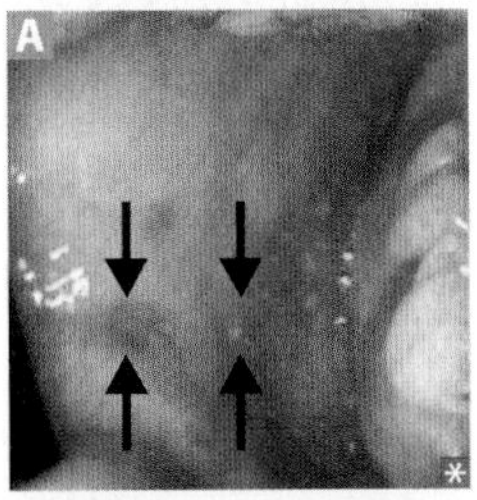

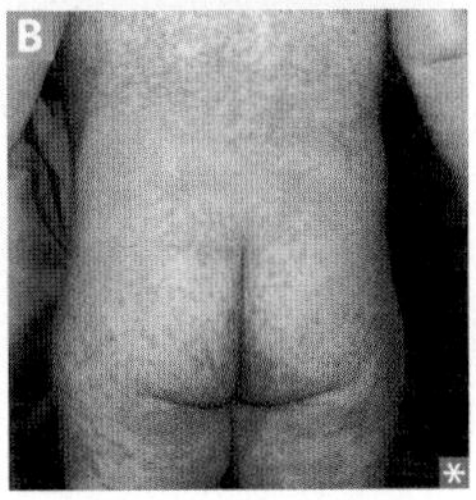

Usual presentation involves prodromal fever with cough, coryza, and conjunctivitis, then eventually Koplik spots (bright red spots with blue-white center on buccal mucosa A), followed 1–2 days later by a maculopapular rash B that starts at the head/neck and spreads downward.

Lymphadenitis with Warthin-Finkeldey giant cells (fused lymphocytes) in a background of paracortical hyperplasia. Possible sequelae:

- Subacute sclerosing panencephalitis (SSPE): personality changes, dementia, autonomic dysfunction, death (occurs years later)
- Encephalitis (1:1000): symptoms appear within few days of rash
- Giant cell pneumonia (rare except in immunosuppressed)

4 C's of measles:
Cough
Coryza
Conjunctivitis
"C"oplik spots

Vitamin A supplementation can reduce morbidity and mortality from measles, particularly in malnourished children.

Pneumonia is the most common cause of measles-associated death in children.

Mumps virus

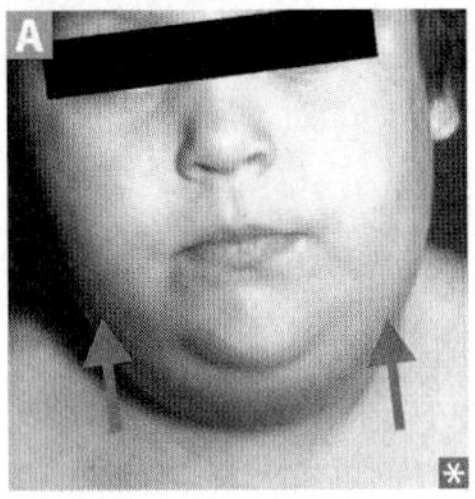

Uncommon due to effectiveness of MMR vaccine.

Symptoms: Parotitis A, Orchitis (inflammation of testes), aseptic Meningitis, and Pancreatitis. Can cause sterility (especially after puberty).

Mumps makes your parotid glands and testes as big as POM-Poms.

Chikungunya virus

An alphavirus member of togavirus family, transmitted by *Aedes* mosquito. Systemic infection that produces inflammatory polyarthritis that can become chronic. Other symptoms include high fever, maculopapular rash, headache, lymphadenopathy. Hemorrhagic manifestations are uncommon (vs dengue fever). Diagnosed with RT-PCR or serology. No antiviral therapy and no vaccine.

Dengue virus

A flavivirus, transmitted by *Aedes* mosquito; most common mosquito-borne viral disease in the world. Can present as dengue fever (fever, rash, headache, myalgias, arthralgias, neutropenia), dengue hemorrhagic fever (dengue fever + bleeding and plasma leakage due to thrombocytopenia and extremely high or low hematocrit), or dengue shock syndrome (plasma leakage leading to circulatory collapse). Diagnosed by PCR or serology.

Dengue hemorrhagic fever is most common in patients infected with a different serotype after their initial infection due to antibody-dependent enhancement of disease.

Presents similarly to Chikungunya virus and is transmitted by the same mosquito vector; coinfections can occur. Dengue virus is more likely to cause neutropenia, thrombocytopenia, hemorrhage, shock, and death.

Live, recombinant vaccine uses yellow fever virus as a backbone into which the genes for the envelope and premembrane proteins of dengue virus have been inserted.

Rabies virus

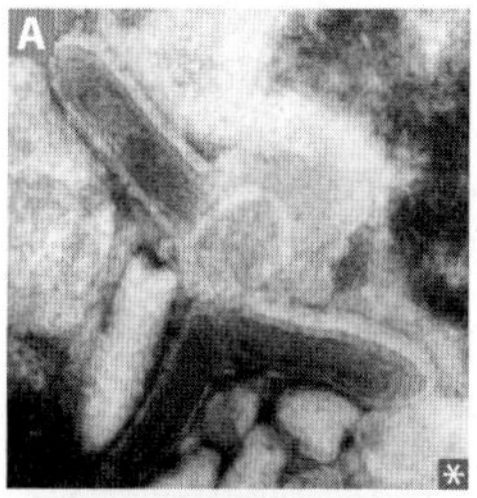

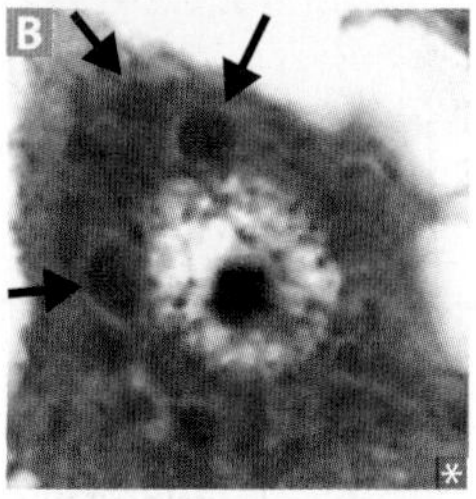

Bullet-shaped virus A. Negri bodies (cytoplasmic inclusions B) commonly found in Purkinje cells of cerebellum and in hippocampal neurons. Rabies has long incubation period (weeks to months) before symptom onset. Postexposure prophylaxis is wound cleaning plus immunization with killed vaccine and rabies immunoglobulin. Example of passive-active immunity.

Travels to the CNS by migrating in a retrograde fashion (via dynein motors) up nerve axons after binding to ACh receptors.

Progression of disease: fever, malaise → agitation, photophobia, hydrophobia, hypersalivation → paralysis, coma → death.

Infection more commonly from bat, raccoon, and skunk bites than from dog bites in the United States; aerosol transmission (eg, bat caves) also possible.

Yellow fever virus

A flavivirus (also an arbovirus) transmitted by *Aedes* mosquitoes. Virus has a monkey or human reservoir.

Symptoms: high fever, black vomitus, jaundice, hemorrhage, backache. May see Councilman bodies (eosinophilic apoptotic globules) on liver biopsy.

Flavi = yellow, jaundice.

Ebola virus

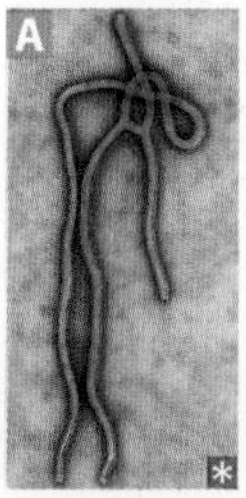

A filovirus A. Following an incubation period of up to 21 days, presents with abrupt onset of flu-like symptoms, diarrhea/vomiting, high fever, myalgia. Can progress to DIC, diffuse hemorrhage, shock.

Diagnosed with RT-PCR within 48 hr of symptom onset. High mortality rate.

Transmission requires direct contact with bodily fluids, fomites (including dead bodies), infected bats or primates (apes/monkeys); high incidence of nosocomial infection.

Supportive care, no definitive treatment. Vaccination of contacts, strict isolation of infected individuals, and barrier practices for health care workers are key to preventing transmission.

Zika virus

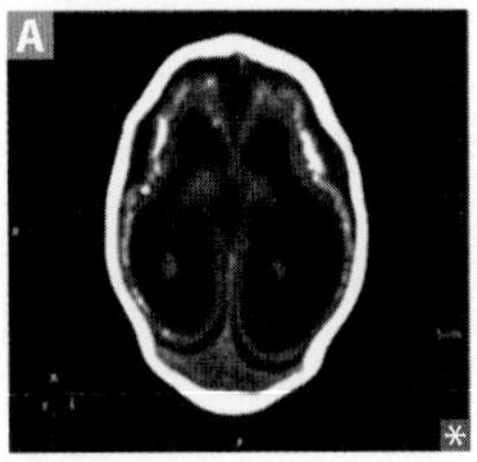
A

A flavivirus most commonly transmitted by *Aedes* mosquito bites.

Causes conjunctivitis, low-grade pyrexia, and itchy rash in 20% of cases. Outbreaks more common in tropical and subtropical climates. Supportive care, no definitive treatment.

Diagnose with RT-PCR or serology.

Sexual and vertical transmission occurs.

Can lead to miscarriage or congenital Zika syndrome: brain imaging A shows ventriculomegaly, subcortical calcifications. Clinical features include:

- Microcephaly
- Ocular anomalies
- Motor abnormalities (spasticity, seizures)

Severe acute respiratory syndrome coronavirus 2

SARS-CoV-2 is a novel ⊕ ssRNA coronavirus and the cause of the ongoing COVID-19 pandemic. Spreads primarily through respiratory droplets and aerosols. Host cell entry occurs by attachment of viral spike protein to angiotensin-converting enzyme 2 receptor on cell membranes.

Clinical course varies; often asymptomatic. Symptoms include

- Common: fever, dry cough, shortness of breath, fatigue.
- More specific: anosmia (loss of smell), dysgeusia (altered taste).

Potential complications include respiratory failure, hypercoagulability, shock, organ failure, death.

Risk factors for severe illness or death include increasing age, obesity, diabetes, hypertension, chronic kidney disease, and severe cardiopulmonary illness.

Diagnosed by RT-PCR (most common); antigen and antibody tests are available.

Treatment options for hospitalized adults include remdesivir (nucleoside analog), convalescent plasma, and dexamethasone (to treat cytokine release syndrome).

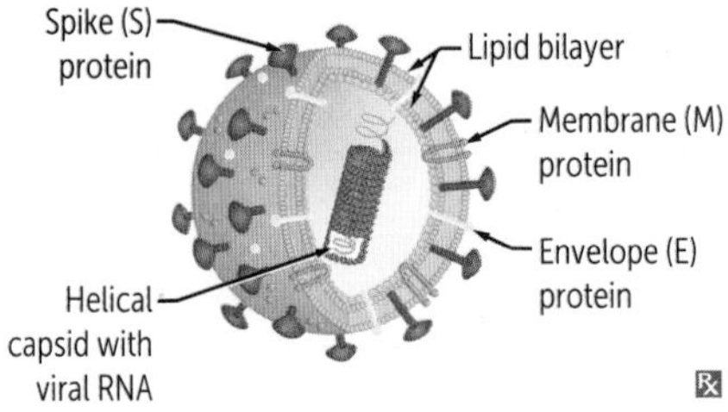
Spike (S) protein
Lipid bilayer
Membrane (M) protein
Envelope (E) protein
Helical capsid with viral RNA

Hepatitis viruses

Signs and symptoms of all hepatitis viruses: episodes of fever, jaundice, ↑ ALT and AST. Naked viruses (HAV and HEV) lack an envelope and are not destroyed by the gut: the **vowels** hit your **bowels**.

HBV DNA polymerase has DNA- and RNA-dependent activities. Upon entry into nucleus, the polymerase completes the partial dsDNA. Host RNA polymerase transcribes mRNA from viral DNA to make viral proteins. The DNA polymerase then reverse transcribes viral RNA to DNA, which is the genome of the progeny virus.

HCV lacks 3′-5′ exonuclease activity → no proofreading ability → antigenic variation of HCV envelope proteins. Host antibody production lags behind production of new mutant strains of HCV.

Virus	HAV	HBV	HCV	HDV	HEV
FAMILY	RNA picornavirus	DNA hepadnavirus	RNA flavivirus	RNA deltavirus	RNA hepevirus
TRANSMISSION	Fecal-oral (shellfish, travelers, day care)	Parenteral (**B**lood), sexual (**B**edroom), perinatal (**B**irthing)	Primarily blood (IV drugs, posttransfusion)	Parenteral, sexual, perinatal	Fecal-oral, especially waterborne
INCUBATION	Short (weeks)	Long (months)	Long	Superinfection (HDV after HBV) = short Coinfection (HDV with HBV) = long	Short
CLINICAL COURSE	**A**cute and self limiting (adults), **A**symptomatic (children)	Initially like serum sickness (fever, arthralgias, rash); may progress to carcinoma	May progress to **C**irrhosis or **C**arcinoma	Similar to HBV	Fulminant hepatitis in **E**xpectant (pregnant) patients
PROGNOSIS	Good	Adults → mostly full resolution; neonates → worse prognosis	Majority develop stable, **C**hronic hepatitis **C**	Superinfection → worse prognosis	High mortality in pregnant patients
HCC RISK	No	Yes	Yes	Yes	No
LIVER BIOPSY	Hepatocyte swelling, monocyte infiltration, Councilman bodies	Granular eosinophilic "ground glass" appearance due to accumulation of surface antigen within infected hepatocytes; cytotoxic T cells mediate damage	Lymphoid aggregates with focal areas of macrovesicular steatosis	Similar to HBV	Patchy necrosis
NOTES	No carrier state	Carrier state common	Carrier state very common	**D**efective virus, **D**epends on HBV HBsAg coat for entry into hepatocytes	**E**nteric, **E**pidemic (eg, in parts of Asia, Africa, Middle East), no carrier state

Extrahepatic manifestations of hepatitis B and C

	Hepatitis B	Hepatitis C
HEMATOLOGIC	Aplastic anemia	Essential mixed cryoglobulinemia, ↑ risk B-cell NHL, ITP, autoimmune hemolytic anemia
RENAL	Membranous GN > membranoproliferative GN	Membranoproliferative GN > membranous GN
VASCULAR	Polyarteritis nodosa	Leukocytoclastic vasculitis
DERMATOLOGIC		Sporadic porphyria cutanea tarda, lichen planus
ENDOCRINE		↑ risk of diabetes mellitus, autoimmune hypothyroidism

Hepatitis serologic markers

Anti-HAV (IgM)	IgM antibody to HAV; best test to detect acute hepatitis A.
Anti-HAV (IgG)	IgG antibody indicates prior HAV infection and/or prior vaccination; protects against reinfection.
HBsAg	Antigen found on surface of HBV; indicates hepatitis B infection.
Anti-HBs	Antibody to HBsAg; indicates immunity to hepatitis B due to vaccination or recovery from infection.
HBcAg	Antigen associated with core of HBV.
Anti-HBc	Antibody to HBcAg; IgM = acute/recent infection; IgG = prior exposure or chronic infection. IgM anti-HBc may be the sole ⊕ marker of infection during window period.
HBeAg	Secreted by infected hepatocyte into circulation. Not part of mature HBV virion. Indicates active viral replication and therefore high transmissibility and poorer prognosis.
Anti-HBe	Antibody to HBeAg; indicates low transmissibility.

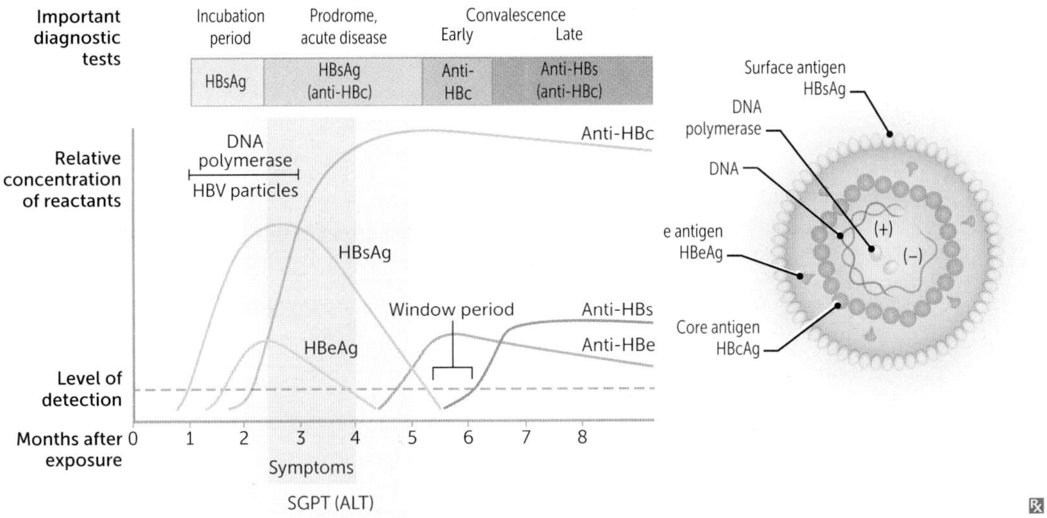

	HBsAg	Anti-HBs	HBeAg	Anti-HBe	Anti-HBc
Acute HBV	✓		✓		IgM
Window				✓	IgM
Chronic HBV (high infectivity)	✓		✓		IgG
Chronic HBV (low infectivity)	✓			✓	IgG
Recovery		✓		✓	IgG
Immunized		✓			

HIV

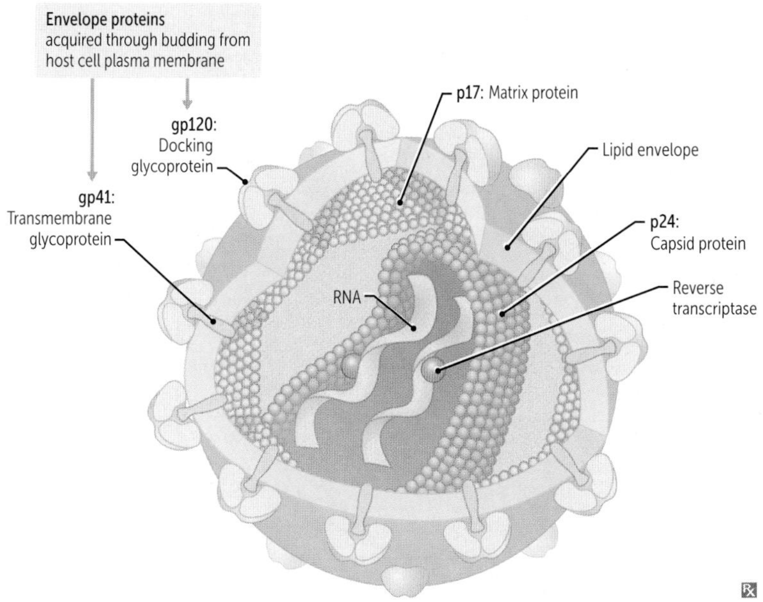
Envelope proteins
acquired through budding from host cell plasma membrane
gp120: Docking glycoprotein
gp41: Transmembrane glycoprotein
p17: Matrix protein
Lipid envelope
p24: Capsid protein
RNA
Reverse transcriptase

Diploid genome (2 molecules of RNA).
The 3 structural genes (protein coded for):
- *env* (gp120 and gp41):
  - Formed from cleavage of gp160 to form envelope glycoproteins.
  - gp120—attachment to host CD4+ T cell.
  - gp41—fusion and entry.
- *gag* (p24 and p17)—capsid and matrix proteins, respectively.
- *pol*—Reverse transcriptase, Integrase, Protease; **RIP "Pol"** (Paul)

Reverse transcriptase synthesizes dsDNA from genomic RNA; dsDNA integrates into host genome.

Virus binds CD4 as well as a coreceptor, either CCR5 on macrophages (early infection) or CXCR4 on T cells (late infection).

Homozygous CCR5 mutation = immunity.

Heterozygous CCR5 mutation = slower course.

HIV diagnosis

Diagnosis made with HIV-1/2 Ag/Ab immunoassays. These immunoassays detect viral p24 Ag capsid protein and IgG Abs to HIV-1/2. Very high sensitivity/specificity.

Viral load tests determine the amount of viral RNA in the plasma. Use viral load to monitor effect of drug therapy. Use HIV genotyping to determine appropriate therapy.

AIDS diagnosis: ≤ 200 CD4+ cells/mm^3 (normal: 500–1500 cells/mm^3) or HIV ⊕ with AIDS-defining condition (eg, *Pneumocystis* pneumonia).

Western blot tests are no longer recommended by the CDC for confirmatory testing.

HIV-1/2 Ag/Ab testing is not recommended in babies with suspected HIV due to maternally transferred antibody. Use HIV viral load instead.

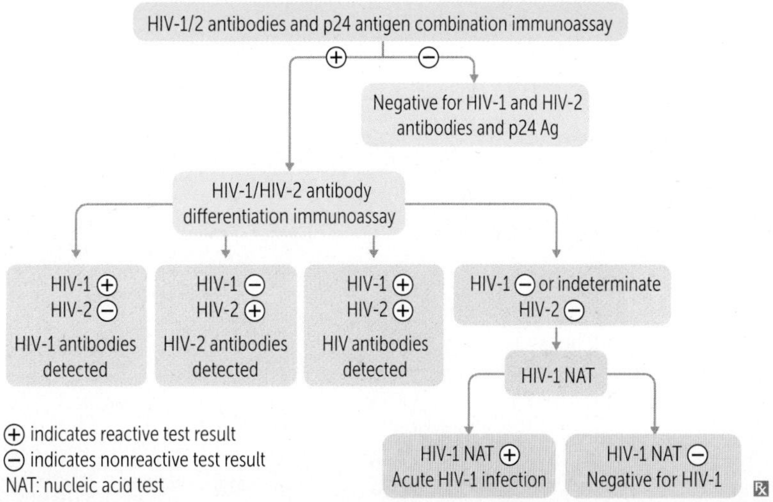
HIV-1/2 antibodies and p24 antigen combination immunoassay
⊕
⊖
Negative for HIV-1 and HIV-2 antibodies and p24 Ag
HIV-1/HIV-2 antibody differentiation immunoassay
HIV-1 ⊕ HIV-2 ⊖ HIV-1 antibodies detected
HIV-1 ⊖ HIV-2 ⊕ HIV-2 antibodies detected
HIV-1 ⊕ HIV-2 ⊕ HIV antibodies detected
HIV-1 ⊖ or indeterminate HIV-2 ⊖
HIV-1 NAT
HIV-1 NAT ⊕ Acute HIV-1 infection
HIV-1 NAT ⊖ Negative for HIV-1
⊕ indicates reactive test result
⊖ indicates nonreactive test result
NAT: nucleic acid test

Time course of untreated HIV infection

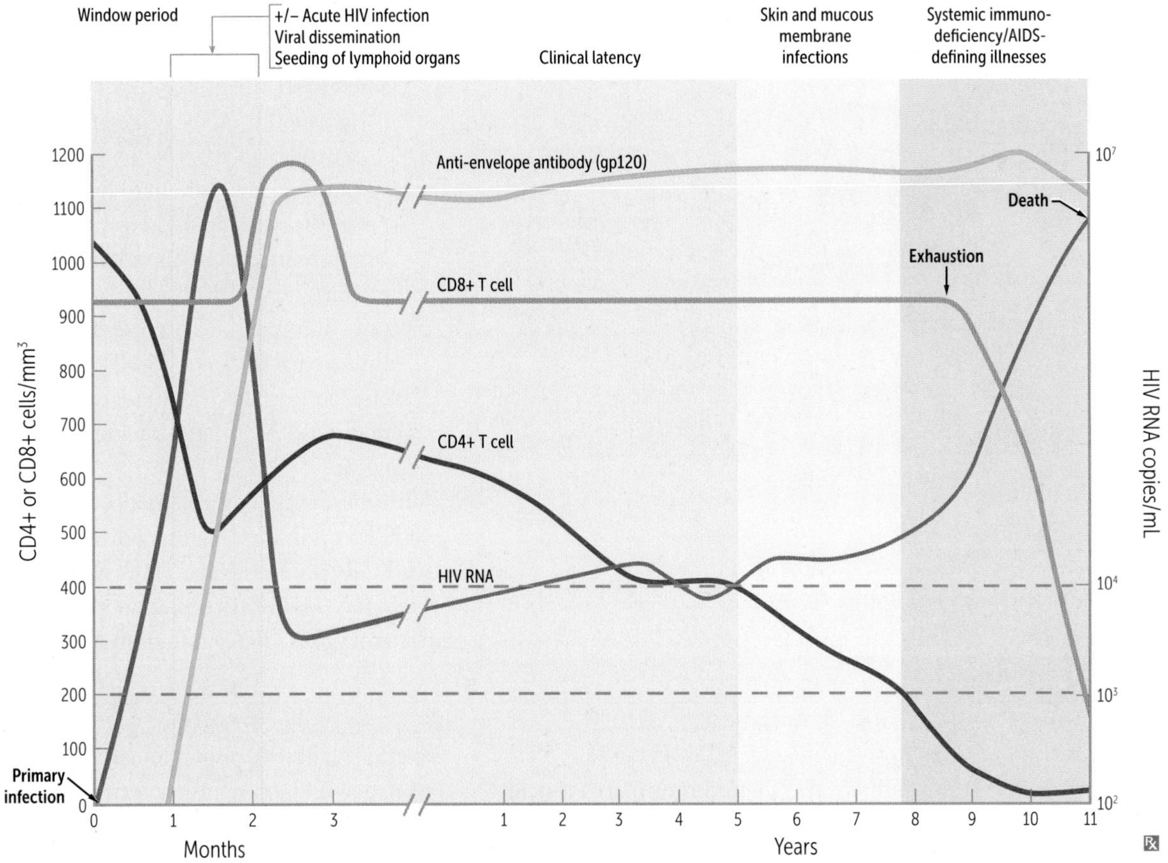

Dashed lines on CD4+ cell count axis indicate moderate immunocompromise (< 400 CD4+ cells/mm^3) and when AIDS-defining illnesses emerge (< 200 CD4+ cells/mm^3).

Most patients who do not receive treatment eventually die of complications of HIV infection.

Four stages of untreated infection:

1. Flu-like (acute)
2. Feeling fine (latent)
3. Falling count
4. Final crisis

During clinical latency phase, virus replicates in lymph nodes

Common diseases of HIV-positive adults

↓ CD4+ cell count → reactivation of past infections (eg, TB, HSV, shingles), dissemination of bacterial infections and fungal infections (eg, coccidioidomycosis), and non-Hodgkin lymphomas.

PATHOGEN	PRESENTATION	FINDINGS
CD4+ cell count < 500/mm³		
Candida albicans	Oral thrush	Scrapable white plaque, pseudohyphae on microscopy
EBV	Oral hairy leukoplakia	Unscrapable white plaque on lateral tongue
HHV-8	Kaposi sarcoma	Perivascular spindle cells invading and forming vascular tumors on histology
HPV	Squamous cell carcinoma at site(s) of sexual contact (most commonly anus, cervix, oropharynx)	
CD4+ cell count < 200/mm³		
Histoplasma capsulatum	Fever, weight loss, fatigue, cough, dyspnea, nausea, vomiting, diarrhea	Oval yeast cells within macrophages
HIV	Dementia	Cerebral atrophy on neuroimaging
JC virus (reactivation)	Progressive multifocal leukoencephalopathy	Nonenhancing areas of demyelination on MRI
Pneumocystis jirovecii	*Pneumocystis* pneumonia	"Ground-glass" opacities on chest imaging
CD4+ cell count < 100/mm³		
Aspergillus fumigatus	Hemoptysis, pleuritic pain	Cavitation or infiltrates on chest imaging
Bartonella spp	Bacillary angiomatosis	Multiple red to purple papules or nodules Biopsy with neutrophilic inflammation
Candida albicans	Esophagitis	White plaques on endoscopy; yeast and pseudohyphae on biopsy
CMV	Colitis, Retinitis, Esophagitis, Encephalitis, Pneumonitis (CREEP)	Linear ulcers on endoscopy, cotton-wool spots on fundoscopy Biopsy reveals cells with intranuclear (owl eye) inclusion bodies
Cryptococcus neoformans	Meningitis	Encapsulated yeast on India ink stain or capsular antigen ⊕
Cryptosporidium spp	Chronic, watery diarrhea	Acid-fast oocysts in stool
EBV	B-cell lymphoma (eg, non-Hodgkin lymphoma, CNS lymphoma)	CNS lymphoma—ring enhancing, may be solitary (vs *Toxoplasma*)
Mycobacterium avium–intracellulare, Mycobacterium avium complex	Nonspecific systemic symptoms (fever, night sweats, weight loss) or focal lymphadenitis	Most common if CD4+ cell count < 50/mm³
Toxoplasma gondii	Brain abscesses	Multiple ring enhancing lesions on MRI

Prions

Prion diseases are caused by the conversion of a normal (predominantly α-helical) protein termed prion protein (PrP^{c}) to a β-pleated form (PrP^{sc}), which is transmissible via CNS-related tissue (iatrogenic CJD) or food contaminated by BSE-infected animal products (variant CJD). PrP^{sc} resists protease degradation and facilitates the conversion of still more PrP^{c} to PrP^{sc}. Resistant to standard sterilizing procedures, including standard autoclaving. Accumulation of PrP^{sc} results in spongiform encephalopathy and dementia, ataxia, startle myoclonus, and death.

Creutzfeldt-Jakob disease—rapidly progressive dementia, typically sporadic (some familial forms).

Bovine spongiform encephalopathy—also called "mad cow disease."

Kuru—acquired prion disease noted in tribal populations practicing human cannibalism.

▶ MICROBIOLOGY—SYSTEMS

Normal flora: dominant

Neonates delivered by C-section have no flora but are rapidly colonized after birth.

LOCATION	MICROORGANISM
Skin	*S epidermidis*
Nose	*S epidermidis*; colonized by *S aureus*
Oropharynx	Viridans group streptococci
Dental plaque	*S mutans*
Colon	*B fragilis* > *E coli*
Vagina	*Lactobacillus*; colonized by *E coli* and group B strep

Bugs causing food-borne illness

S aureus and *B cereus* food poisoning starts quickly and ends quickly.

MICROORGANISM	SOURCE OF INFECTION
B cereus	Reheated rice. "Food poisoning from reheated rice? Be serious!" (*B cereus*)
C botulinum	Improperly canned foods (toxins), raw honey (spores)
C perfringens	Reheated meat
E coli O157:H7	Undercooked meat
L monocytogenes	Deli meats, soft cheeses
Salmonella	Poultry, meat, and eggs
S aureus	Meats, mayonnaise, custard; preformed toxin
V parahaemolyticus and *V vulnificus*[a]	Raw/undercooked seafood

[a] *V vulnificus* predominantly causes wound infections from contact with contaminated water or shellfish.

Bugs causing diarrhea

Bloody diarrhea	
Campylobacter	Comma- or S-shaped organisms; growth at 42°C
E histolytica	Protozoan; amebic dysentery; liver abscess
Enterohemorrhagic *E coli*	O157:H7; can cause HUS; makes Shiga toxin
Enteroinvasive *E coli*	Invades colonic mucosa
Salmonella (non-typhoidal)	Lactose ⊖; flagellar motility; has animal reservoir, especially poultry and eggs
Shigella	Lactose ⊖; very low ID_{50}; produces Shiga toxin; human reservoir only; bacillary dysentery
Y enterocolitica	Day care outbreaks; pseudoappendicitis
Watery diarrhea	
C difficile	Pseudomembranous colitis; associated with antibiotics and PPIs; occasionally bloody diarrhea
C perfringens	Also causes gas gangrene
Enterotoxigenic *E coli*	Travelers' diarrhea; produces heat-labile (LT) and heat-stable (ST) toxins
Protozoa	*Giardia*, *Cryptosporidium*
V cholerae	Comma-shaped organisms; rice-water diarrhea; often from infected seafood
Viruses	Norovirus (most common cause in developed countries), rotavirus (↓ incidence in developed countries due to vaccination), enteric adenovirus

Common causes of pneumonia

NEONATES (< 4 WK)	CHILDREN (4 WK–18 YR)	ADULTS (18–40 YR)	ADULTS (40–65 YR)	ELDERLY
Group B streptococci *E coli*	Viruses (RSV) *Mycoplasma* *C trachomatis* (infants–3 yr) *C pneumoniae* (school-aged children) *S pneumoniae* Runts May Cough Chunky Sputum	*Mycoplasma* *C pneumoniae* *S pneumoniae* Viruses (eg, influenza)	*S pneumoniae* *H influenzae* Anaerobes Viruses *Mycoplasma*	*S pneumoniae* Influenza virus Anaerobes *H influenzae* Gram ⊖ rods

Special groups	
Alcohol overuse	*Klebsiella*, anaerobes usually due to aspiration (eg, *Peptostreptococcus*, *Fusobacterium*, *Prevotella*, *Bacteroides*)
IV drug use	*S pneumoniae*, *S aureus*
Aspiration	Anaerobes
Atypical	*Mycoplasma*, *Chlamydophila*, *Legionella*, viruses (RSV, CMV, influenza, adenovirus)
Cystic fibrosis	*Pseudomonas*, *S aureus*, *S pneumoniae*, *Burkholderia cepacia*
Immunocompromised	*S aureus*, enteric gram ⊖ rods, fungi, viruses, *P jirovecii* (with HIV)
Nosocomial	*S aureus*, *Pseudomonas*, other enteric gram ⊖ rods
Postviral	*S pneumoniae*, *S aureus*, *H influenzae*
COPD	*S pneumoniae*, *H influenzae*, *M catarrhalis*, *Pseudomonas*

Common causes of meningitis

NEWBORN (0–6 MO)	CHILDREN (6 MO–6 YR)	6–60 YR	60 YR +
Group B *Streptococcus* *E coli* *Listeria*	*S pneumoniae* *N meningitidis* *H influenzae* type b Group B *Streptococcus* Enteroviruses	*S pneumoniae* *N meningitidis* Enteroviruses HSV	*S pneumoniae* *N meningitidis* *H influenzae* type b Group B *Streptococcus* *Listeria*

Give ceftriaxone and vancomycin empirically (add ampicillin if *Listeria* is suspected).

Viral causes of meningitis: enteroviruses (especially coxsackievirus), HSV-2 (HSV-1 = encephalitis), HIV, West Nile virus (also causes encephalitis), VZV.

In HIV: *Cryptococcus* spp.

Note: Incidence of Group B streptococcal meningitis in neonates has ↓ greatly due to screening and antibiotic prophylaxis in pregnancy. Incidence of *H influenzae* meningitis has ↓ greatly due to conjugate *H influenzae* vaccinations. Today, cases are usually seen in unimmunized children.

Cerebrospinal fluid findings in meningitis

	OPENING PRESSURE	CELL TYPE	PROTEIN	GLUCOSE
Bacterial	↑	↑ PMNs	↑	↓
Fungal/TB	↑	↑ lymphocytes	↑	↓
Viral	Normal/↑	↑ lymphocytes	Normal/↑	Normal

Infections causing brain abscess

Most commonly viridans streptococci and *Staphylococcus aureus*. If dental infection or extraction precedes abscess, oral anaerobes commonly involved.

Multiple abscesses are usually from bacteremia; single lesions from contiguous sites: otitis media and mastoiditis → temporal lobe and cerebellum; sinusitis or dental infection → frontal lobe.

Toxoplasma reactivation in AIDS.

Osteomyelitis

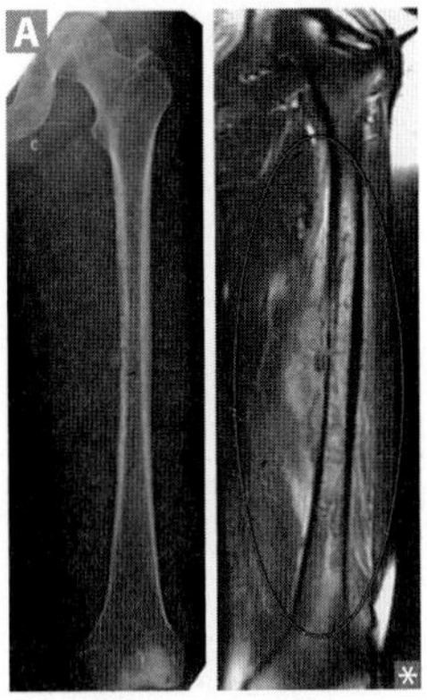

RISK FACTOR	ASSOCIATED INFECTION
Assume if no other information is available	*S aureus* (most common overall)
Sexually active	*Neisseria gonorrhoeae* (rare), septic arthritis more common
Sickle cell disease	*Salmonella* and *S aureus*
Prosthetic joint replacement	*S aureus* and *S epidermidis*
Vertebral involvement	*S aureus*, *M tuberculosis* (Pott disease)
Cat and dog bites	*Pasteurella multocida*
IV drug use	*S aureus*; also *Pseudomonas*, *Candida*

Elevated ESR and CRP sensitive but not specific.

Radiographs are insensitive early but can be useful in chronic osteomyelitis (A, left). MRI is best for detecting acute infection and detailing anatomic involvement (A, right). Biopsy or aspiration with culture necessary to identify organism.

Urinary tract infections

Cystitis presents with dysuria, frequency, urgency, suprapubic pain, and WBCs (but not WBC casts) in urine. Primarily caused by ascension of microbes from urethra to bladder. Ascension to kidney results in pyelonephritis, which presents with fever, chills, flank pain, costovertebral angle tenderness, hematuria, and WBC casts.

Ten times more common in females (shorter urethras colonized by fecal flora).

Risk factors: obstruction (eg, kidney stones, enlarged prostate), kidney surgery, catheterization, congenital GU malformation (eg, vesicoureteral reflux), diabetes, pregnancy.

SPECIES	FEATURES	COMMENTS
Escherichia coli	Leading cause of UTI. Colonies show strong pink lactose-fermentation on MacConkey agar.	Diagnostic markers: ⊕ Leukocyte esterase = evidence of WBC activity. ⊕ Nitrite test = reduction of urinary nitrates by gram ⊖ bacterial species (eg, *E coli*).
Staphylococcus saprophyticus	2nd leading cause of UTI, particularly in young, sexually active females.	
Klebsiella pneumoniae	3rd leading cause of UTI. Large mucoid capsule and viscous colonies.	
Serratia marcescens	Some strains produce a red pigment; often nosocomial and drug resistant.	
Enterococcus	Often nosocomial and drug resistant.	
Proteus mirabilis	Motility causes "swarming" on agar; associated with struvite stones. Produces urease.	
Pseudomonas aeruginosa	Blue-green pigment and fruity odor; usually nosocomial and drug resistant.	

Common vaginal infections

	Bacterial vaginosis	*Trichomonas* vaginitis	*Candida* vulvovaginitis
SIGNS AND SYMPTOMS	No inflammation Thin, white discharge A with fishy odor	Inflammation ("strawberry cervix") Frothy, yellow-green, foul-smelling discharge	Inflammation Thick, white, "cottage cheese" discharge C
LAB FINDINGS	Clue cells pH > 4.5 ⊕ KOH whiff test	Motile pear-shaped trichomonads B pH > 4.5	Pseudohyphae pH normal (4.0–4.5)
TREATMENT	Metronidazole or clindamycin	Metronidazole Treat sexual partner(s)	Azoles

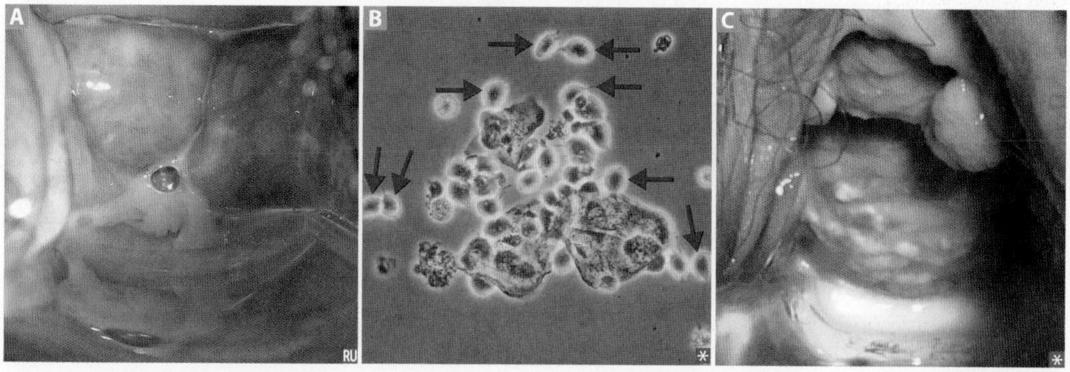

TORCH infections

Microbes that may pass from mother to fetus. Transmission is transplacental in most cases, or via vaginal delivery (especially HSV-2). Nonspecific signs common to many **ToRCHHeS** infections include hepatosplenomegaly, jaundice, thrombocytopenia, and growth restriction.

Other important infectious agents include *Streptococcus agalactiae* (group B streptococci), *E coli*, and *Listeria monocytogenes*—all causes of meningitis in neonates. Parvovirus B19 causes hydrops fetalis.

AGENT	MATERNAL ACQUISITION	MATERNAL MANIFESTATIONS	NEONATAL MANIFESTATIONS
Toxoplasma gondii	Cat feces or ingestion of undercooked meat	Usually asymptomatic; lymphadenopathy (rarely)	Classic triad: chorioretinitis, hydrocephalus, and intracranial calcifications, +/– "blueberry muffin" rash A
Rubella	Respiratory droplets	Rash, lymphadenopathy, polyarthritis, polyarthralgia	Classic triad: abnormalities of **eye** (cataracts B) and **ear** (deafness) and congenital **heart** disease (PDA); +/– "blueberry muffin" rash. "**I** (eye) ♥ **ruby** (**rub**ella) **ear**rings"
Cytomegalovirus	Sexual contact, organ transplants	Usually asymptomatic; mononucleosis-like illness	Hearing loss, seizures, petechial rash, "blueberry muffin" rash, chorioretinitis, periventricular calcifications C
HIV	Sexual contact, needlestick	Variable presentation depending on CD4+ cell count	Recurrent infections, chronic diarrhea
Herpes simplex virus-2	Skin or mucous membrane contact	Usually asymptomatic; herpetic (vesicular) lesions	Meningoencephalitis, herpetic (vesicular) lesions
Syphilis	Sexual contact	Chancre (1°) and disseminated rash (2°) are the two stages likely to result in fetal infection	Often results in stillbirth, hydrops fetalis; if child survives, presents with facial abnormalities (eg, notched teeth, saddle nose, short maxilla), saber shins, CN VIII deafness

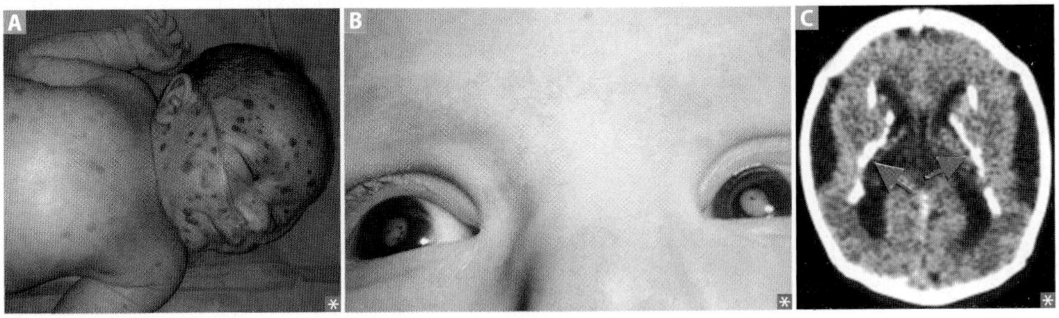

Red rashes of childhood

AGENT	ASSOCIATED SYNDROME/DISEASE	CLINICAL PRESENTATION
Coxsackievirus type A	Hand-foot-mouth disease	Oval-shaped vesicles on palms and soles A; vesicles and ulcers in oral mucosa (herpangina)
Human herpesvirus 6	Roseola (exanthem subitum)	Asymptomatic rose-colored macules appear on body after several days of high fever; can present with febrile seizures; usually affects infants
Measles virus	Measles (rubeola)	Confluent rash beginning at head and moving down; preceded by cough, coryza, conjunctivitis, and blue-white (Koplik) spots on buccal mucosa
Parvovirus B19	Erythema infectiosum (fifth disease)	"Slapped cheek" rash on face B (can cause hydrops fetalis in pregnant patients)
Rubella virus	Rubella	Pink macules and papules begin at head and move down, remain discrete → fine desquamating truncal rash; postauricular lymphadenopathy
Streptococcus pyogenes	Scarlet fever	**S**ore throat, **C**ircumoral pallor C, group **A** strep, **R**ash (sandpaper-like, from neck to trunk and extremities), **L**ymphadenopathy, **E**rythrogenic toxin, strawberry **T**ongue (**SCARLET**)
Varicella-Zoster virus	Chickenpox	Vesicular rash begins on trunk; spreads to face D and extremities with lesions of different stages

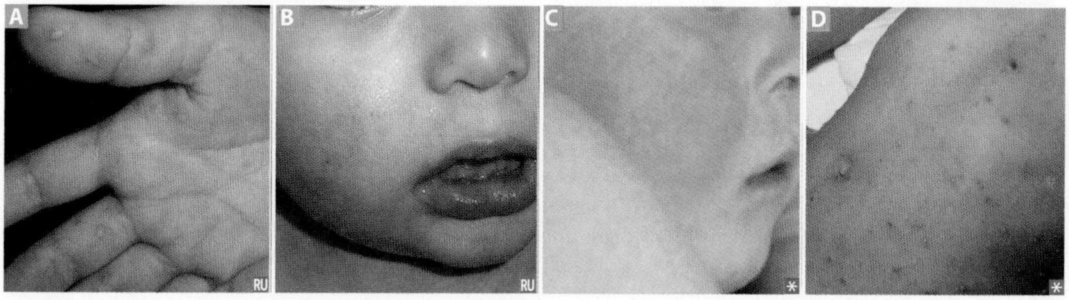

Sexually transmitted infections

DISEASE	CLINICAL FEATURES	PATHOGEN
AIDS	Opportunistic infections, Kaposi sarcoma, lymphoma	HIV
Chancroid 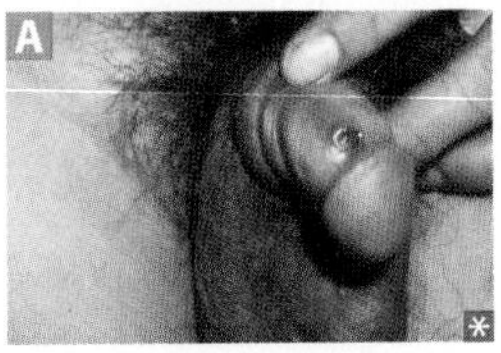	Painful genital ulcer with exudate, inguinal adenopathy A	*Haemophilus ducreyi* (it's so painful, you "do cry")
Chlamydia	Urethritis, cervicitis, epididymitis, conjunctivitis, reactive arthritis, PID	*Chlamydia trachomatis* (D–K)
Condylomata acuminata	Genital warts, koilocytes	HPV-6 and -11
Genital herpes	Painful penile, vulvar, or cervical vesicles and ulcers; can cause systemic symptoms such as fever, headache, myalgia	HSV-2, less commonly HSV-1
Gonorrhea	Urethritis, cervicitis, PID, prostatitis, epididymitis, arthritis, creamy purulent discharge	*Neisseria gonorrhoeae*
Granuloma inguinale (Donovanosis) 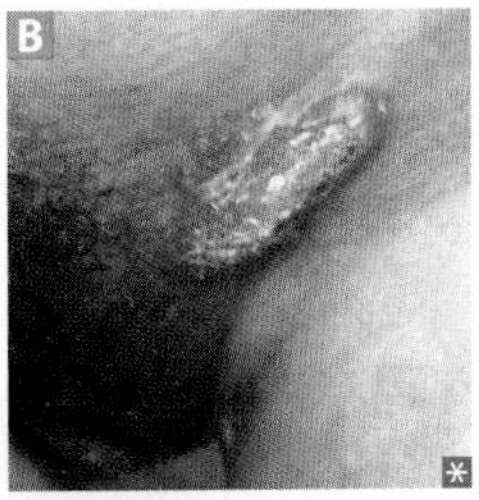	Painless, beefy red ulcer that bleeds readily on contact B Uncommon in US	*Klebsiella (Calymmatobacterium) granulomatis*; cytoplasmic Donovan bodies (bipolar staining) seen on microscopy
Hepatitis B	Jaundice	HBV
Lymphogranuloma venereum	Infection of lymphatics; painless genital ulcers, painful lymphadenopathy (ie, buboes)	*C trachomatis* (L1–L3)
Primary syphilis	Painless chancre	*Treponema pallidum*
Secondary syphilis	Fever, lymphadenopathy, skin rashes, condylomata lata	
Tertiary syphilis	Gummas, tabes dorsalis, general paresis, aortitis, Argyll Robertson pupil	
Trichomoniasis	Vaginitis, strawberry cervix, motile in wet prep	*Trichomonas vaginalis*

Pelvic inflammatory disease

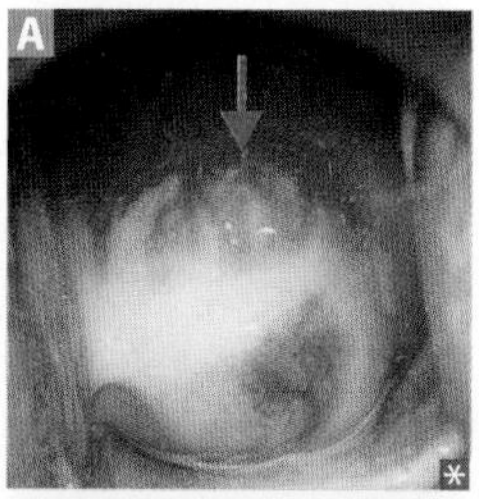

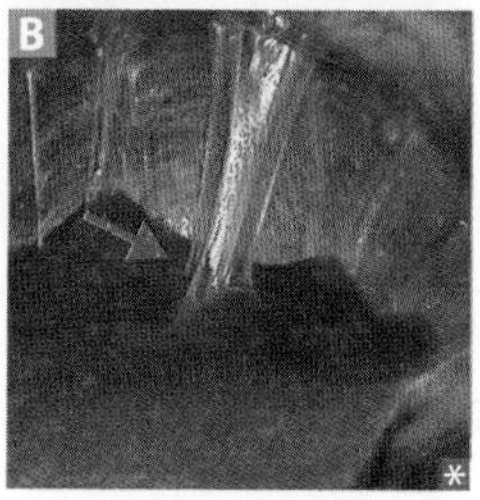

Top bugs—*Chlamydia trachomatis* (subacute, often undiagnosed), *Neisseria gonorrhoeae* (acute).

C trachomatis—most common bacterial STI in the United States.

Signs include cervical motion tenderness, adnexal tenderness, purulent cervical discharge A.

PID may include salpingitis, endometritis, hydrosalpinx, and tubo-ovarian abscess.

Salpingitis is a risk factor for ectopic pregnancy, infertility, chronic pelvic pain, and adhesions.

Can lead to perihepatitis (**Fitz-Hugh–Curtis syndrome**)—infection and inflammation of liver capsule and "violin string" adhesions of peritoneum to liver B.

Nosocomial infections *E coli* (UTI) and *S aureus* (wound infection) are the two most common causes.

RISK FACTOR	PATHOGEN	UNIQUE SIGNS/SYMPTOMS
Antibiotic use	*Clostridium difficile*	Watery diarrhea, leukocytosis
Aspiration (2° to altered mental status, old age)	Polymicrobial, gram ⊖ bacteria, often anaerobes	Right lower lobe infiltrate or right upper/middle lobe (patient recumbent); purulent malodorous sputum
Decubitus ulcers, surgical wounds, drains	*S aureus* (including MRSA), gram ⊖ anaerobes (*Bacteroides, Prevotella, Fusobacterium*)	Erythema, tenderness, induration, drainage from surgical wound sites
Intravascular catheters	*S aureus* (including MRSA), *S epidermidis* (long term)	Erythema, induration, tenderness, drainage from access sites
Mechanical ventilation, endotracheal intubation	Late onset: *P aeruginosa, Klebsiella, Acinetobacter, S aureus*	New infiltrate on CXR, ↑ sputum production; sweet odor (*Pseudomonas*)
Renal dialysis unit, needlestick	HBV, HCV	
Urinary catheterization	*Proteus* spp, *E coli, Klebsiella* (PEcK)	Dysuria, leukocytosis, flank pain or costovertebral angle tenderness
Water aerosols	*Legionella*	Signs of pneumonia, GI symptoms (diarrhea, nausea, vomiting), neurologic abnormalities

Bugs affecting unvaccinated children

CLINICAL PRESENTATION	FINDINGS/LABS	PATHOGEN
Dermatologic		
Rash	Beginning at head and moving down with postauricular lymphadenopathy	Rubella virus
	Beginning at head and moving down; preceded by cough, coryza, conjunctivitis, and Koplik spots	Measles virus
Neurologic		
Meningitis	Microbe colonizes nasopharynx	*H influenzae* type b
	Can also lead to myalgia and paralysis	Poliovirus
Tetanus	Muscle spasms and spastic paralysis (eg, lockjaw, opisthotonus)	*Clostridium tetani*
Respiratory		
Epiglottitis	Fever with dysphagia, drooling, and difficulty breathing due to edema	*H influenzae* type b (also capable of causing epiglottitis in fully immunized children)
Pertussis	Low-grade fevers, coryza → whooping cough, posttussive vomiting → gradual recovery	*Bordetella pertussis*
Pharyngitis	Grayish pseudomembranes (may obstruct airways)	*Corynebacterium diphtheriae*

▶ MICROBIOLOGY—ANTIMICROBIALS

Antimicrobial therapy

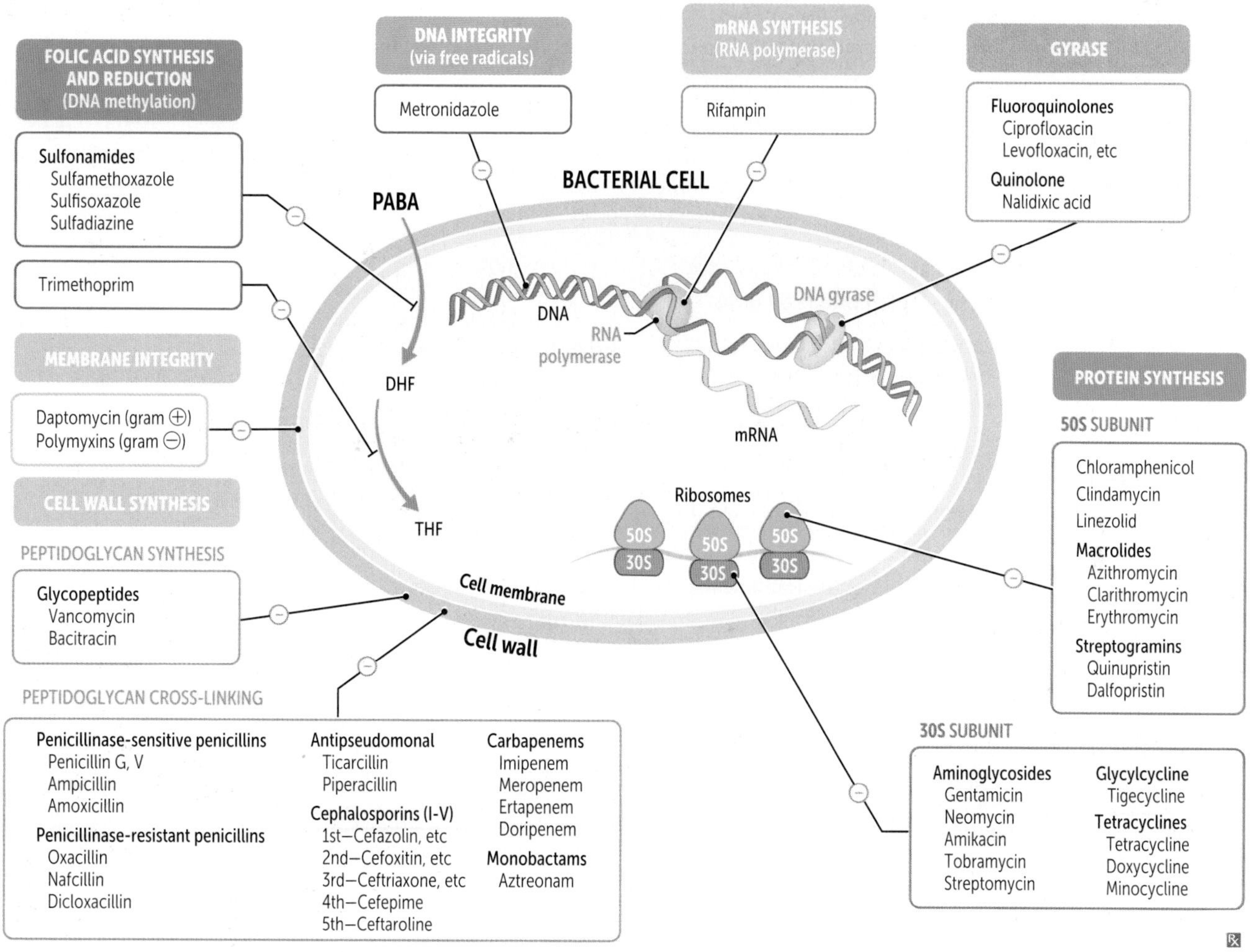

Penicillin G, V	Penicillin G (IV and IM form), penicillin V (oral). Prototype β-lactam antibiotics.
MECHANISM	D-Ala-D-Ala structural analog. Bind penicillin-binding proteins (transpeptidases). Block transpeptidase cross-linking of peptidoglycan in cell wall. Activate autolytic enzymes.
CLINICAL USE	Mostly used for gram ⊕ organisms (*S pneumoniae, S pyogenes, Actinomyces*). Also used for gram ⊖ cocci (mainly *N meningitidis*) and spirochetes (mainly *T pallidum*). Bactericidal for gram ⊕ cocci, gram ⊕ rods, gram ⊖ cocci, and spirochetes. β-lactamase sensitive.
ADVERSE EFFECTS	Hypersensitivity reactions, direct Coombs ⊕ hemolytic anemia, drug-induced interstitial nephritis.
RESISTANCE	β-lactamase cleaves the β-lactam ring. Mutations in PBPs.

Penicillinase-sensitive penicillins	Amoxicillin, ampicillin; aminopenicillins.	
MECHANISM	Same as penicillin. Wider spectrum; penicillinase sensitive. Also combine with clavulanic acid to protect against destruction by β-lactamase.	**A**minopenicillins are **amp**ed-up penicillin. Am**o**xicillin has greater **o**ral bioavailability than ampicillin.
CLINICAL USE	Extended-spectrum penicillin—*H influenzae, H pylori, E coli,* Enterococci, *Listeria monocytogenes, Proteus mirabilis, Salmonella, Shigella.*	Coverage: ampicillin/amoxicillin **HHEELPSS** kill enterococci.
ADVERSE EFFECTS	Hypersensitivity reactions, rash, pseudomembranous colitis.	
MECHANISM OF RESISTANCE	Penicillinase (a type of β-lactamase) cleaves β-lactam ring.	

Penicillinase-resistant penicillins	Dicloxacillin, nafcillin, oxacillin.	
MECHANISM	Same as penicillin. Narrow spectrum; penicillinase resistant because bulky R group blocks access of β-lactamase to β-lactam ring.	
CLINICAL USE	*S aureus* (except MRSA).	"Use **naf** (nafcillin) for **staph**."
ADVERSE EFFECTS	Hypersensitivity reactions, interstitial nephritis.	
MECHANISM OF RESISTANCE	MRSA has altered penicillin-binding protein target site.	

Antipseudomonal penicillins	Piperacillin, ticarcillin.
MECHANISM	Same as penicillin. Extended spectrum. Penicillinase sensitive; use with β-lactamase inhibitors.
CLINICAL USE	*Pseudomonas* spp. and gram ⊖ rods.
ADVERSE EFFECTS	Hypersensitivity reactions.

Cephalosporins

MECHANISM	β-lactam drugs that inhibit cell wall synthesis but are less susceptible to penicillinases. Bactericidal.	Organisms typically not covered by 1st–4th generation cephalosporins are **LAME**: *Listeria*, Atypicals (*Chlamydia*, *Mycoplasma*), MRSA, and Enterococci.
CLINICAL USE	1st generation (cefazolin, cephalexin)—gram ⊕ cocci, *Proteus mirabilis*, *E coli*, *Klebsiella pneumoniae*. Cefazolin used prior to surgery to prevent *S aureus* wound infections.	1st generation—⊕ **PEcK**.
	2nd generation (cefaclor, cefoxitin, cefuroxime, cefotetan)—gram ⊕ cocci, *H influenzae*, *Enterobacter aerogenes*, *Neisseria* spp., *Serratia marcescens*, *Proteus mirabilis*, *E coli*, *Klebsiella pneumoniae*.	**2nd** graders wear **fake fox fur** to **tea** parties. 2nd generation—⊕ **HENS PEcK**.
	3rd generation (ceftriaxone, cefotaxime, cefpodoxime, ceftazidime, cefixime)—serious gram ⊖ infections resistant to other β-lactams.	Can cross blood-brain barrier. Ceftriaxone—meningitis, gonorrhea, disseminated Lyme disease. Ceftazidime—*Pseudomonas*.
	4th generation (cefepime)—gram ⊖ organisms, with ↑ activity against *Pseudomonas* and gram ⊕ organisms.	
	5th generation (ceftaroline)—broad gram ⊕ and gram ⊖ organism coverage; unlike 1st–4th generation cephalosporins, ceftaroline covers MRSA, and *Enterococcus faecalis*—does not cover *Pseudomonas*.	
ADVERSE EFFECTS	Hypersensitivity reactions, autoimmune hemolytic anemia, disulfiram-like reaction, vitamin K deficiency. Low rate of cross-reactivity even in penicillin-allergic patients. ↑ nephrotoxicity of aminoglycosides.	
MECHANISM OF RESISTANCE	Inactivated by cephalosporinases (a type of β-lactamase). Structural change in penicillin-binding proteins (transpeptidases).	

β-lactamase inhibitors	Include Clavulanic acid, Avibactam, Sulbactam, Tazobactam. Often added to penicillin antibiotics to protect the antibiotic from destruction by β-lactamase.	**CAST** (eg, amoxicillin-clavulanate, ceftazidime-avibactam, ampicillin-sulbactam, piperacillin-tazobactam).

Carbapenems

Doripenem, imipenem, meropenem, ertapenem.

"**Pens**" (carbapenems) cost a **dime**."

MECHANISM	Imipenem is a broad-spectrum, β-lactamase–resistant carbapenem. Always administered with cilastatin (inhibitor of renal dehydropeptidase I) to ↓ inactivation of drug in renal tubules.	With imipenem, "the kill is **lastin'** with **cilastatin**." Newer carbapenems include ertapenem (limited *Pseudomonas* coverage) and doripenem.
CLINICAL USE	Gram ⊕ cocci, gram ⊖ rods, and anaerobes. Wide spectrum and significant side effects limit use to life-threatening infections or after other drugs have failed. Meropenem has a ↓ risk of seizures and is stable to dehydropeptidase I.	
ADVERSE EFFECTS	GI distress, rash, and CNS toxicity (seizures) at high plasma levels.	
MECHANISM OF RESISTANCE	Inactivated by carbapenemases produced by, eg, *K pneumoniae, E coli, E aerogenes.*	

Aztreonam

MECHANISM	Less susceptible to β-lactamases. Prevents peptidoglycan cross-linking by binding to penicillin-binding protein 3. Synergistic with aminoglycosides. No cross-allergenicity with penicillins.
CLINICAL USE	Gram ⊖ rods only—no activity against gram ⊕ rods or anaerobes. For penicillin-allergic patients and those with renal insufficiency who cannot tolerate aminoglycosides.
ADVERSE EFFECTS	Usually nontoxic; occasional GI upset.

Vancomycin

MECHANISM	Inhibits cell wall peptidoglycan formation by binding D-Ala-D-Ala portion of cell wall precursors. Bactericidal against most bacteria (bacteriostatic against *C difficile*). Not susceptible to β-lactamases.
CLINICAL USE	Gram ⊕ bugs only—for serious, multidrug-resistant organisms, including MRSA, *S epidermidis*, sensitive *Enterococcus* species, and *Clostridium difficile* (oral route).
ADVERSE EFFECTS 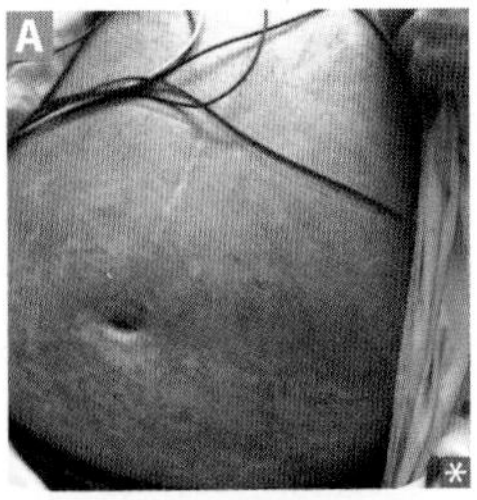	Well tolerated in general but **not** trouble free: nephrotoxicity, ototoxicity, thrombophlebitis, diffuse flushing (red man syndrome A idiopathic reaction largely preventable by pretreatment with antihistamines), DRESS syndrome.
MECHANISM OF RESISTANCE	Occurs in bacteria (eg, *Enterococcus*) via amino acid modification of D-Ala-D-Ala to **D-Ala-D-Lac**. "If you **Lack** a **D-Ala** (dollar), you can't ride the **van** (vancomycin)."

Protein synthesis inhibitors

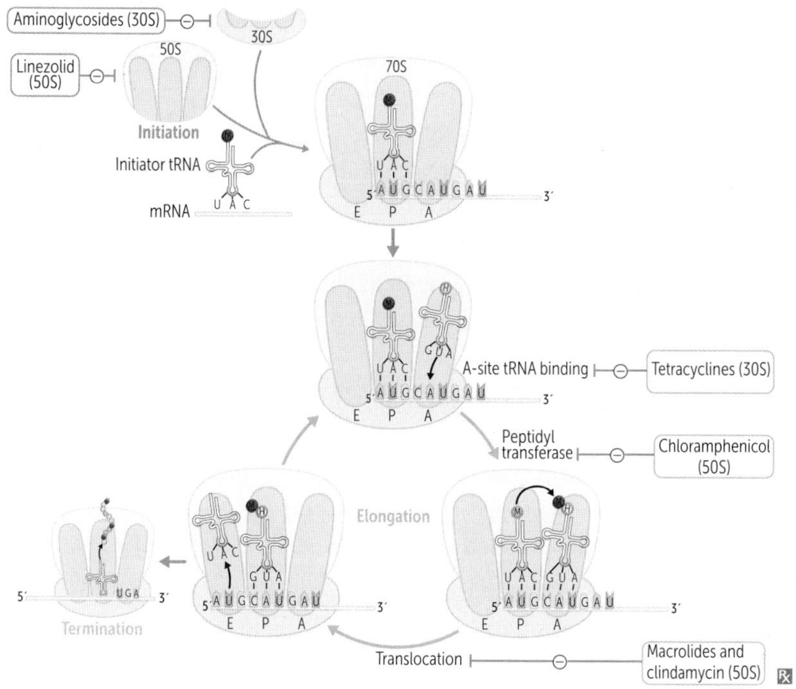

Specifically target smaller bacterial ribosome (70S, made of 30S and 50S subunits), leaving human ribosome (80S) unaffected.

All are bacteriostatic, except aminoglycosides (bactericidal) and linezolid (variable).

30S inhibitors
Aminoglycosides Tetracyclines
50S inhibitors
Chloramphenicol, clindamycin erythromycin (macrolides) linezolid

"Buy at 30, ccel (sell) at 50."

Aminoglycosides	Gentamicin, Neomycin, Amikacin, Tobramycin, Streptomycin.	"Mean" (aminoglycoside) GNATS cannot kill anaerobes.
MECHANISM	Bactericidal; irreversible inhibition of initiation complex through binding of the 30S subunit. Can cause misreading of mRNA. Also block translocation. Require O_2 for uptake; therefore ineffective against anaerobes.	
CLINICAL USE	Severe gram ⊖ rod infections. Synergistic with β-lactam antibiotics. Neomycin for bowel surgery.	
ADVERSE EFFECTS	Nephrotoxicity, neuromuscular blockade (absolute contraindication with myasthenia gravis), ototoxicity (especially with loop diuretics), teratogenicity.	
MECHANISM OF RESISTANCE	Bacterial transferase enzymes inactivate the drug by acetylation, phosphorylation, or adenylation.	

Tetracyclines

Tetracycline, doxycycline, minocycline.

MECHANISM	Bacteriostatic; bind to 30S and prevent attachment of aminoacyl-tRNA. Limited CNS penetration. Doxycycline is fecally eliminated and can be used in patients with renal failure. Do not take tetracyclines with milk (Ca^{2+}), antacids (eg, Ca^{2+} or Mg^{2+}), or iron-containing preparations because divalent cations inhibit drugs' absorption in the gut.
CLINICAL USE	*Borrelia burgdorferi*, *M pneumoniae*. Drugs' ability to accumulate intracellularly makes them very effective against *Rickettsia* and *Chlamydia*. Also used to treat acne. Doxycycline effective against community-acquired MRSA.
ADVERSE EFFECTS	GI distress, discoloration of teeth and inhibition of bone growth in children, photosensitivity. "**Terato**cylines" are **terato**genic; generally avoided in pregnancy and in children (except doxycycline).
MECHANISM OF RESISTANCE	↓ uptake or ↑ efflux out of bacterial cells by plasmid-encoded transport pumps.

Tigecycline

MECHANISM	Tetracycline derivative. Binds to 30S, inhibiting protein synthesis. Generally bacteriostatic.
CLINICAL USE	Broad-spectrum anaerobic, gram ⊖, and gram ⊕ coverage. Multidrug-resistant organisms (MRSA, VRE) or infections requiring deep tissue penetration.
ADVERSE EFFECTS	Nausea, vomiting.

Chloramphenicol

MECHANISM	Blocks peptidyltransferase at 50S ribosomal subunit. Bacteriostatic.
CLINICAL USE	Meningitis (*Haemophilus influenzae, Neisseria meningitidis, Streptococcus pneumoniae*) and rickettsial diseases (eg, Rocky Mountain spotted fever [*Rickettsia rickettsii*]). Limited use due to toxicity but often still used in developing countries because of low cost.
ADVERSE EFFECTS	Anemia (dose dependent), aplastic anemia (dose independent), gray baby syndrome (in premature infants because they lack liver UDP-glucuronosyltransferase).
MECHANISM OF RESISTANCE	Plasmid-encoded acetyltransferase inactivates the drug.

Clindamycin

MECHANISM	Blocks peptide transfer (translocation) at 50S ribosomal subunit. Bacteriostatic.
CLINICAL USE	Anaerobic infections (eg, *Bacteroides* spp., *Clostridium perfringens*) in aspiration pneumonia, lung abscesses, and oral infections. Also effective against invasive group A streptococcal infection. Treats anaerobic infections above the diaphragm vs metronidazole (anaerobic infections below diaphragm).
ADVERSE EFFECTS	Pseudomembranous colitis (*C difficile* overgrowth), fever, diarrhea.

Linezolid

MECHANISM	Inhibits protein synthesis by binding to 50S subunit and preventing formation of the initiation complex.
CLINICAL USE	Gram ⊕ species including MRSA and VRE.
ADVERSE EFFECTS	Bone marrow suppression (especially thrombocytopenia), peripheral neuropathy, serotonin syndrome (due to partial MAO inhibition).
MECHANISM OF RESISTANCE	Point mutation of ribosomal RNA.

Macrolides

Azithromycin, clarithromycin, erythromycin.

MECHANISM	Inhibit protein synthesis by blocking **trans**location ("macro**slides**"); bind to the 23S rRNA of the 50S ribosomal subunit. Bacteriostatic.
CLINICAL USE	Atypical pneumonias (*Mycoplasma*, *Chlamydia*, *Legionella*), STIs (*Chlamydia*), gram ⊕ cocci (streptococcal infections in patients allergic to penicillin), and *B pertussis*.
ADVERSE EFFECTS	**MACRO**: Gastrointestinal **M**otility issues, **A**rrhythmia caused by prolonged QT interval, acute **C**holestatic hepatitis, **R**ash, e**O**sinophilia. Increases serum concentration of theophylline, oral anticoagulants. Clarithromycin and erythromycin inhibit cytochrome P-450.
MECHANISM OF RESISTANCE	Methylation of 23S rRNA-binding site prevents binding of drug.

Polymyxins

Colistin (polymyxin E), polymyxin B.

MECHANISM	Cation polypeptides that bind to phospholipids on cell membrane of gram ⊖ bacteria. Disrupt cell membrane integrity → leakage of cellular components → cell death.
CLINICAL USE	Salvage therapy for multidrug-resistant gram ⊖ bacteria (eg, *P aeruginosa*, *E coli*, *K pneumoniae*). Polymyxin B is a component of a triple antibiotic ointment used for superficial skin infections.
ADVERSE EFFECTS	Nephrotoxicity, neurotoxicity (eg, slurred speech, weakness, paresthesias), respiratory failure.

Sulfonamides	Sulfamethoxazole (SMX), sulfisoxazole, sulfadiazine.
MECHANISM	Inhibit dihydropteroate synthase, thus inhibiting folate synthesis. Bacteriostatic (bactericidal when combined with trimethoprim).
CLINICAL USE	Gram ⊕, gram ⊖, *Nocardia*. TMP-SMX for simple UTI.
ADVERSE EFFECTS	Hypersensitivity reactions, hemolysis if G6PD deficient, nephrotoxicity (tubulointerstitial nephritis), photosensitivity, Stevens-Johnson syndrome, kernicterus in infants, displace other drugs from albumin (eg, warfarin).
MECHANISM OF RESISTANCE	Altered enzyme (bacterial dihydropteroate synthase), ↓ uptake, or ↑ PABA synthesis.

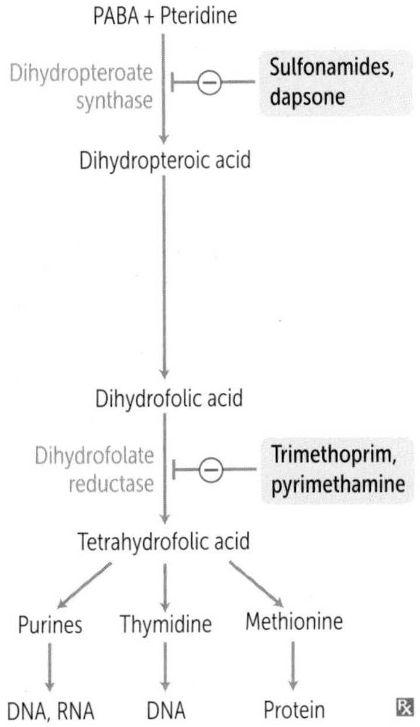
PABA + Pteridine
Dihydropteroate synthase
Sulfonamides, dapsone
Dihydropteroic acid
Dihydrofolic acid
Dihydrofolate reductase
Trimethoprim, pyrimethamine
Tetrahydrofolic acid
Purines
Thymidine
Methionine
DNA, RNA
DNA
Protein

Dapsone	
MECHANISM	Similar to sulfonamides, but structurally distinct agent.
CLINICAL USE	Leprosy (lepromatous and tuberculoid), *Pneumocystis jirovecii* prophylaxis, or treatment when used in combination with TMP.
ADVERSE EFFECTS	Hemolysis if G6PD deficient, methemoglobinemia, agranulocytosis.

Trimethoprim	
MECHANISM	Inhibits bacterial dihydrofolate reductase. Bacteriostatic.
CLINICAL USE	Used in combination with sulfonamides (trimethoprim-sulfamethoxazole [TMP-SMX]), causing sequential block of folate synthesis. Combination used for UTIs, *Shigella*, *Salmonella*, *Pneumocystis jirovecii* pneumonia treatment and prophylaxis, toxoplasmosis prophylaxis.
ADVERSE EFFECTS	Hyperkalemia (high doses), megaloblastic anemia, leukopenia, granulocytopenia, which may be avoided with coadministration of leucovorin (folinic acid). TMP Treats Marrow Poorly.

Fluoroquinolones

Ciprofloxacin, enoxacin, norfloxacin, ofloxacin; respiratory fluoroquinolones: gemifloxacin, levofloxacin, moxifloxacin.

MECHANISM	Inhibit prokaryotic enzymes topoisomerase II (DNA gyrase) and topoisomerase IV. Bactericidal. Must not be taken with antacids.	
CLINICAL USE	Gram ⊖ rods of urinary and GI tracts (including *Pseudomonas*), some gram ⊕ organisms, otitis externa.	
ADVERSE EFFECTS	GI upset, superinfections, skin rashes, headache, dizziness. Less commonly, can cause leg cramps and myalgias. Contraindicated during pregnancy or breastfeeding and in children < 18 years old due to possible damage to cartilage. Some may prolong QT interval.	May cause tendonitis or tendon rupture in people > 60 years old and in patients taking prednisone. Ciprofloxacin inhibits cytochrome P-450. Fluoroquinolones hurt attachments to your bones.
MECHANISM OF RESISTANCE	Chromosome-encoded mutation in DNA gyrase, plasmid-mediated resistance, efflux pumps.	

Daptomycin

MECHANISM	Lipopeptide that disrupts cell membranes of gram ⊕ cocci by creating transmembrane channels.	
CLINICAL USE	*S aureus* skin infections (especially MRSA), bacteremia, endocarditis, VRE.	Not used for pneumonia (avidly binds to and is inactivated by surfactant). "Dapto-**myo**-**skin**" is used for **skin** infections but can cause **myo**pathy.
ADVERSE EFFECTS	Myopathy, rhabdomyolysis.	

Metronidazole

MECHANISM	Forms toxic free radical metabolites in the bacterial cell that damage DNA. Bactericidal, antiprotozoal.	
CLINICAL USE	Treats *Giardia*, *Entamoeba*, *Trichomonas*, *Gardnerella vaginalis*, Anaerobes (*Bacteroides*, *C difficile*). Can be used in place of amoxicillin in *H pylori* "triple therapy" in case of penicillin allergy.	**GET GAP** on the **Metro** with **metro**nidazole! Treats anaerobic infection **below** the diaphragm vs clindamycin (anaerobic infections **above** diaphragm).
ADVERSE EFFECTS	Disulfiram-like reaction (severe flushing, tachycardia, hypotension) with alcohol; headache, metallic taste.	

Antimycobacterial therapy

BACTERIUM	PROPHYLAXIS	TREATMENT
M tuberculosis	Isoniazid	Rifampin, Isoniazid, Pyrazinamide, Ethambutol (**RIPE** for treatment)
M avium–intracellulare	Azithromycin, rifabutin	Azithromycin or clarithromycin + ethambutol Can add rifabutin or ciprofloxacin
M leprae	N/A	Long-term treatment with dapsone and rifampin for tuberculoid form Add clofazimine for lepromatous form

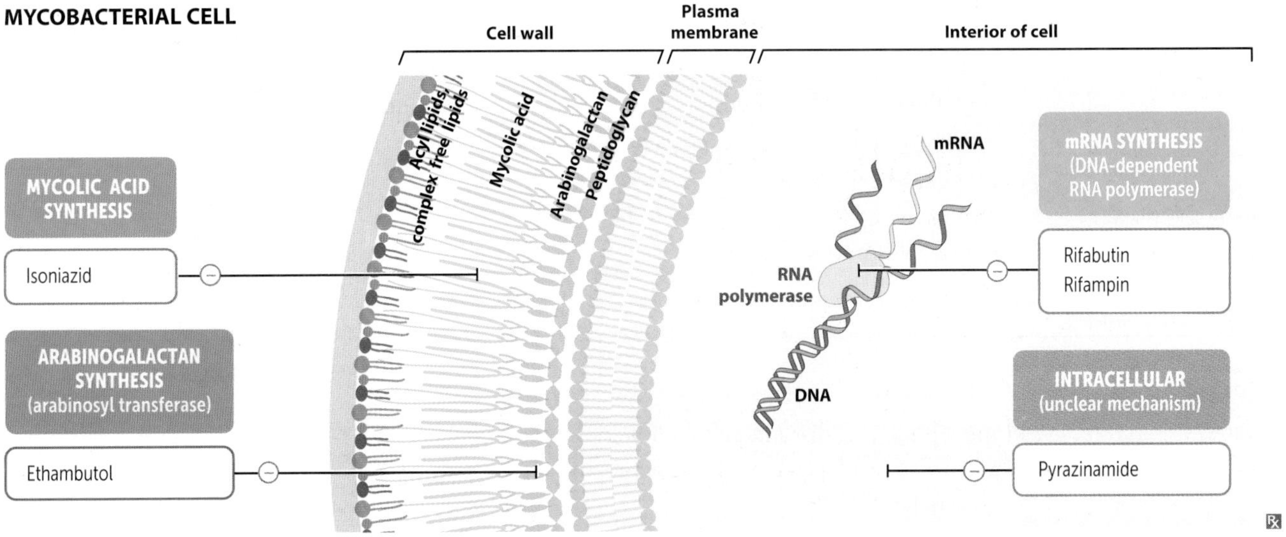

Rifamycins

Rifampin, rifabutin, rifapentine.

MECHANISM	Inhibit DNA-dependent RNA polymerase.	Rifampin's 4 R's: RNA polymerase inhibitor Ramps up microsomal cytochrome P-450 Red/orange body fluids Rapid resistance if used alone **Rifampin ramps** up cytochrome P-450, **but** rifa**b**utin does not.
CLINICAL USE	*Mycobacterium tuberculosis*; delay resistance to dapsone when used for leprosy. Used for meningococcal prophylaxis and chemoprophylaxis in contacts of children with *H influenzae* type b.	
ADVERSE EFFECTS	Minor hepatotoxicity and drug interactions (↑ cytochrome P-450); orange body fluids (nonhazardous side effect). Rifabutin favored over rifampin in patients with HIV infection due to less cytochrome P-450 stimulation.	
MECHANISM OF RESISTANCE	Mutations reduce drug binding to RNA polymerase. Monotherapy rapidly leads to resistance.	

Isoniazid

MECHANISM	↓ synthesis of mycolic acids. Bacterial catalase-peroxidase (encoded by KatG) needed to convert INH to active metabolite.	
CLINICAL USE	*Mycobacterium tuberculosis*. The only agent used as solo prophylaxis against TB. Also used as monotherapy for latent TB.	Different INH half-lives in fast vs slow acetylators.
ADVERSE EFFECTS	Hepatotoxicity, cytochrome P-450 inhibition, drug-induced SLE, anion gap metabolic acidosis, vitamin B_6 deficiency (peripheral neuropathy, sideroblastic anemia), seizures (in high doses, refractory to benzodiazepines). Administer with pyridoxine (B_6).	**I**NH **I**njures **N**eurons and **H**epatocytes.
MECHANISM OF RESISTANCE	Mutations leading to underexpression of KatG.	

Pyrazinamide

MECHANISM	Mechanism uncertain. Pyrazinamide is a prodrug that is converted to the active compound pyrazinoic acid. Works best at acidic pH (eg, in host phagolysosomes).
CLINICAL USE	*Mycobacterium tuberculosis*.
ADVERSE EFFECTS	Hyperuricemia, hepatotoxicity.

Ethambutol

MECHANISM	↓ carbohydrate polymerization of mycobacterium cell wall by blocking arabinosyltransferase.
CLINICAL USE	*Mycobacterium tuberculosis*.
ADVERSE EFFECTS	**Optic** neuropathy (red-green color blindness, usually reversible). Pronounce "eyethambutol."

Streptomycin

MECHANISM	Interferes with 30S component of ribosome.
CLINICAL USE	*Mycobacterium tuberculosis* (2nd line).
ADVERSE EFFECTS	Tinnitus, vertigo, ataxia, nephrotoxicity.

Antimicrobial prophylaxis

CLINICAL SCENARIO	MEDICATION
Exposure to meningococcal infection	Ceftriaxone, ciprofloxacin, or rifampin
High risk for endocarditis and undergoing surgical or dental procedures	Amoxicillin
History of recurrent UTIs	TMP-SMX
Malaria prophylaxis for travelers	Atovaquone-proguanil, mefloquine, doxycycline, primaquine, or chloroquine (for areas with sensitive species)
Pregnant patients carrying group B strep	Intrapartum penicillin G or ampicillin
Prevention of gonococcal conjunctivitis in newborn	Erythromycin ointment on eyes
Prevention of postsurgical infection due to *S aureus*	Cefazolin; vancomycin if ⊕ for MRSA
Prophylaxis of strep pharyngitis in child with prior rheumatic fever	Benzathine penicillin G or oral penicillin V

Prophylaxis in HIV infection/AIDS

CELL COUNT	PROPHYLAXIS	INFECTION
CD4 < 200 cells/mm^3	TMP-SMX	*Pneumocystis* pneumonia
CD4 < 100 cells/mm^3	TMP-SMX	*Pneumocystis* pneumonia and toxoplasmosis

Treatment of highly resistant bacteria

MRSA: vancomycin, daptomycin, linezolid, tigecycline, ceftaroline, doxycycline.

VRE: daptomycin, linezolid, tigecycline, and streptogramins (quinupristin, dalfopristin).

Multidrug-resistant *P aeruginosa*, multidrug-resistant *Acinetobacter baumannii*: polymyxins B and E (colistin).

Antifungal therapy

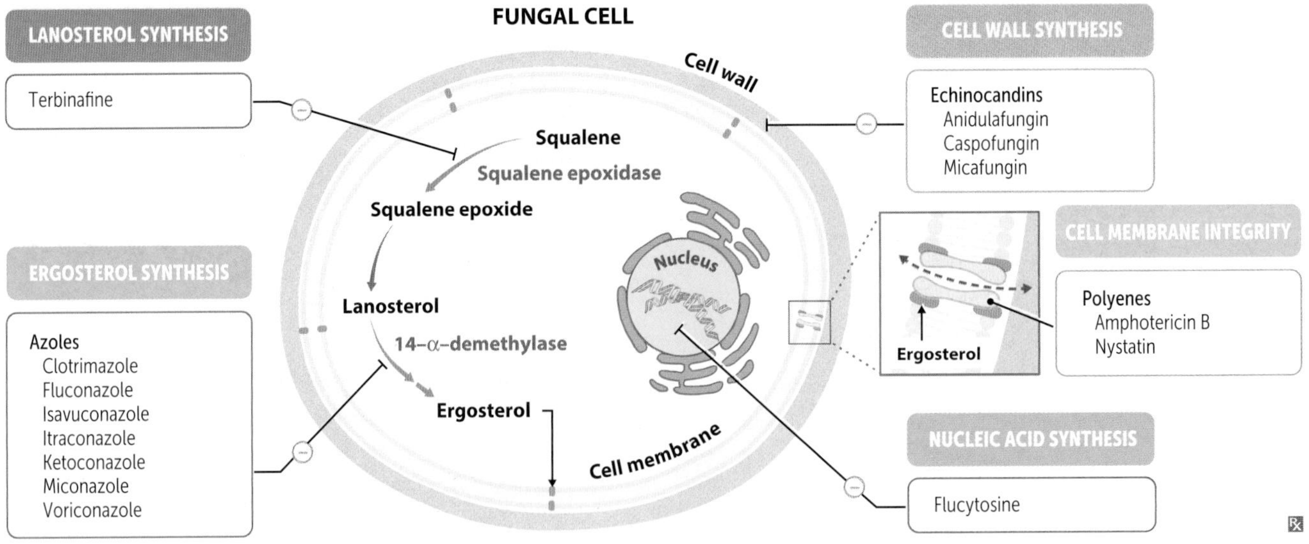

Amphotericin B

MECHANISM	Binds ergosterol (unique to fungi); forms membrane pores that allow leakage of electrolytes.	Amphotericin "**tears**" holes in the fungal membrane by forming pores.
CLINICAL USE	Serious, systemic mycoses. *Cryptococcus* (amphotericin B +/– flucytosine for cryptococcal meningitis), *Blastomyces*, *Coccidioides*, *Histoplasma*, *Candida*, *Mucor*. Intrathecally for coccidioidal meningitis.	Supplement K^+ and Mg^{2+} because of altered renal tubule permeability.
ADVERSE EFFECTS	Fever/chills ("shake and bake"), hypotension, nephrotoxicity, arrhythmias, anemia, IV phlebitis ("**amphoterrible**").	Hydration ↓ nephrotoxicity. Liposomal amphotericin ↓ toxicity.

Nystatin

MECHANISM	Same as amphotericin B. Topical use only as too toxic for systemic use.
CLINICAL USE	"Swish and swallow" for oral candidiasis (thrush); topical for diaper rash or vaginal candidiasis.

Flucytosine

MECHANISM	Inhibits DNA and RNA biosynthesis by conversion to 5-fluorouracil by cytosine deaminase.
CLINICAL USE	Systemic fungal infections (especially meningitis caused by *Cryptococcus*) in combination with amphotericin B.
ADVERSE EFFECTS	Bone marrow suppression.

Azoles

	Clotrimazole, fluconazole, isavuconazole, itraconazole, ketoconazole, miconazole, voriconazole.
MECHANISM	Inhibit fungal sterol (ergosterol) synthesis by inhibiting the cytochrome P-450 enzyme that converts lanosterol to ergosterol.
CLINICAL USE	Local and less serious systemic mycoses. Fluconazole for chronic suppression of cryptococcal meningitis in people living with HIV and candidal infections of all types. Itraconazole may be used for *Blastomyces*, *Coccidioides*, *Histoplasma*, *Sporothrix schenckii*. Clotrimazole and miconazole for topical fungal infections. Voriconazole for *Aspergillus* and some *Candida*. Isavuconazole for serious *Aspergillus* and *Mucor* infections.
ADVERSE EFFECTS	Testosterone synthesis inhibition (gynecomastia, especially with ketoconazole), liver dysfunction (inhibits cytochrome P-450).

Terbinafine

MECHANISM	Inhibits the fungal enzyme squalene epoxidase.
CLINICAL USE	Dermatophytoses (especially onychomycosis—fungal infection of finger or toe nails).
ADVERSE EFFECTS	GI upset, headaches, hepatotoxicity, taste disturbance.

Echinocandins	Anidulafungin, caspofungin, micafungin.
MECHANISM	Inhibit cell wall synthesis by inhibiting synthesis of β-glucan.
CLINICAL USE	Invasive aspergillosis, *Candida*.
ADVERSE EFFECTS	GI upset, flushing (by histamine release).

Griseofulvin	
MECHANISM	Interferes with microtubule function; disrupts mitosis. Deposits in keratin-containing tissues (eg, nails).
CLINICAL USE	Oral treatment of superficial infections; inhibits growth of dermatophytes (tinea, ringworm).
ADVERSE EFFECTS	Teratogenic, carcinogenic, confusion, headaches, disulfiram-like reaction, ↑ cytochrome P-450 and warfarin metabolism.

Antiprotozoal therapy	Pyrimethamine (toxoplasmosis), suramin and melarsoprol (*Trypanosoma brucei*), nifurtimox (*T cruzi*), sodium stibogluconate (leishmaniasis).

Anti-mite/louse therapy	Permethrin, malathion (acetylcholinesterase inhibitor), topical or oral ivermectin. Used to treat scabies (*Sarcoptes scabiei*) and lice (*Pediculus* and *Pthirus*).

Chloroquine	
MECHANISM	Blocks detoxification of heme into hemozoin. Heme accumulates and is toxic to plasmodia.
CLINICAL USE	Treatment of plasmodial species other than *P falciparum* (frequency of resistance in *P falciparum* is too high). Resistance due to membrane pump that ↓ intracellular concentration of drug. Treat *P falciparum* with artemether/lumefantrine or atovaquone/proguanil. For life-threatening malaria, use quinidine in US (quinine elsewhere) or artesunate.
ADVERSE EFFECTS	Retinopathy; pruritus (especially in dark-skinned individuals).

Antihelminthic therapy	Pyrantel pamoate, ivermectin, me**bend**azole (microtubule inhibitor to treat "**bend**y worms"), praziquantel (↑ Ca^{2+} permeability, ↑ vacuolization), diethylcarbamazine.

Antiviral therapy

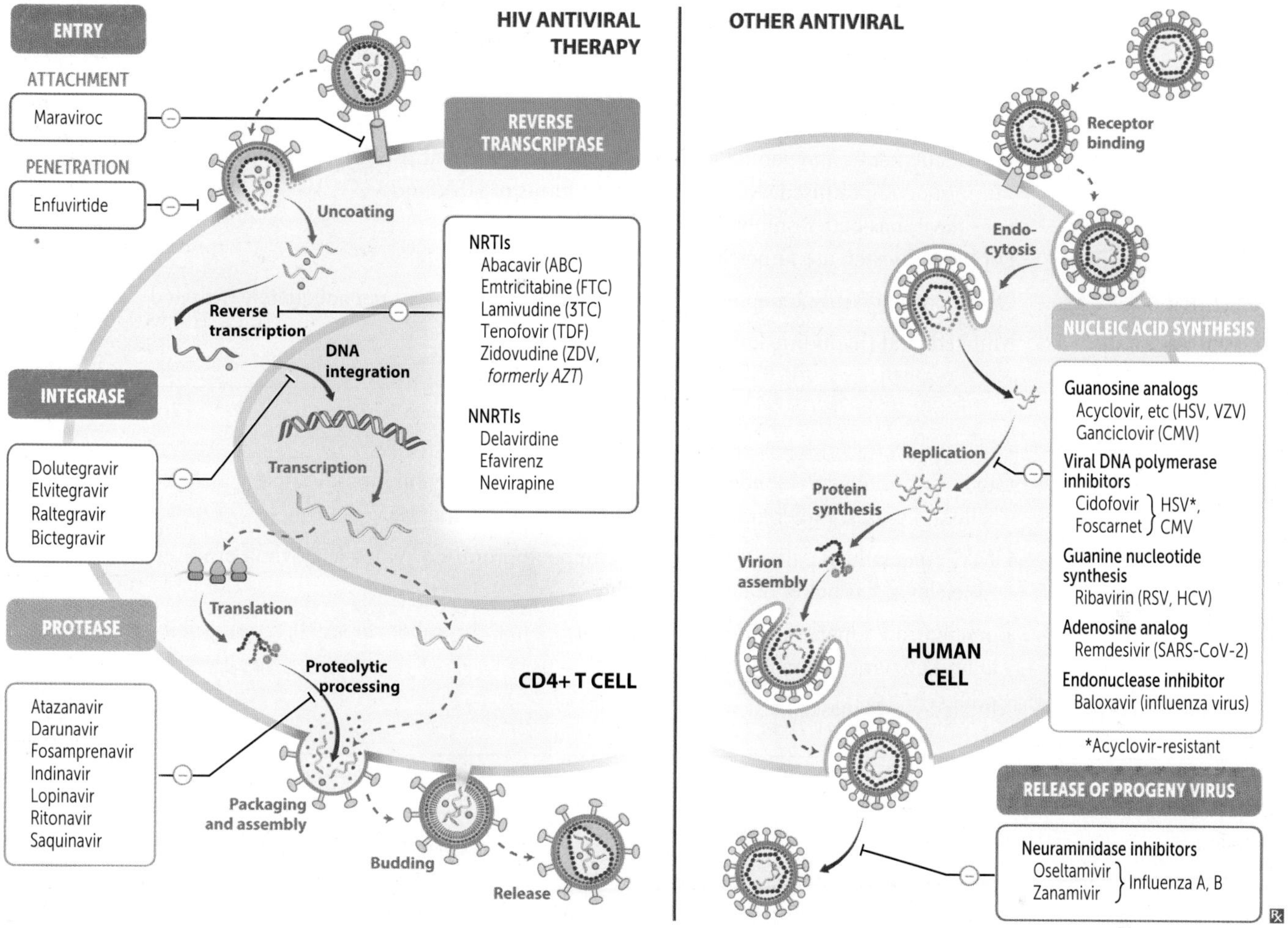
HIV ANTIVIRAL THERAPY
ENTRY
ATTACHMENT
Maraviroc
PENETRATION
Enfuvirtide
Uncoating
REVERSE TRANSCRIPTASE
NRTIs
Abacavir (ABC)
Emtricitabine (FTC)
Lamivudine (3TC)
Tenofovir (TDF)
Zidovudine (ZDV, formerly AZT)
NNRTIs
Delavirdine
Efavirenz
Nevirapine
Reverse transcription
DNA integration
INTEGRASE
Dolutegravir
Elvitegravir
Raltegravir
Bictegravir
Transcription
Translation
PROTEASE
Atazanavir
Darunavir
Fosamprenavir
Indinavir
Lopinavir
Ritonavir
Saquinavir
Proteolytic processing
CD4+ T CELL
Packaging and assembly
Budding
Release
OTHER ANTIVIRAL
Receptor binding
Endo-cytosis
NUCLEIC ACID SYNTHESIS
Guanosine analogs
Acyclovir, etc (HSV, VZV)
Ganciclovir (CMV)
Viral DNA polymerase inhibitors
Cidofovir } HSV*,
Foscarnet } CMV
Guanine nucleotide synthesis
Ribavirin (RSV, HCV)
Adenosine analog
Remdesivir (SARS-CoV-2)
Endonuclease inhibitor
Baloxavir (influenza virus)
*Acyclovir-resistant
Replication
Protein synthesis
Virion assembly
HUMAN CELL
RELEASE OF PROGENY VIRUS
Neuraminidase inhibitors
Oseltamivir } Influenza A, B
Zanamivir

Oseltamivir, zanamivir

MECHANISM	Inhibit influenza neuraminidase → ↓ release of progeny virus.
CLINICAL USE	Treatment and prevention of influenza A and B. Beginning therapy within 48 hours of symptom onset may shorten duration of illness.

Baloxavir

MECHANISM	Inhibits the "cap snatching" endonuclease activity of the influenza virus RNA polymerase → ↓ viral replication.
CLINICAL USE	Treatment within 48 hours of symptom onset shortens duration of illness.

Remdesivir

MECHANISM	Prodrug of an ATP analog. The active metabolite inhibits viral RNA-dependent RNA polymerase and evades proofreading by viral exoribonuclease (ExoN) → ↓ viral RNA production.
CLINICAL USE	Recently approved for treatment of COVID-19 requiring hospitalization.

Acyclovir, famciclovir, valacyclovir

MECHANISM	Guanosine analogs. Monophosphorylated by HSV/VZV thymidine kinase and not phosphorylated in uninfected cells → few adverse effects. Triphosphate formed by cellular enzymes. Preferentially inhibit viral DNA polymerase by chain termination.
CLINICAL USE	HSV and VZV. Weak activity against EBV. No activity against CMV. Used for HSV-induced mucocutaneous and genital lesions as well as for encephalitis. Prophylaxis in patients who are immunocompromised. No effect on latent forms of HSV and VZV. Valacyclovir, a prodrug of acyclovir, has better oral bioavailability. For herpes zoster, use famciclovir.
ADVERSE EFFECTS	Obstructive crystalline nephropathy and acute kidney injury if not adequately hydrated.
MECHANISM OF RESISTANCE	Mutated viral thymidine kinase.

Ganciclovir

MECHANISM	Guanosine analog. 5′-monophosphate formed by a CMV viral kinase. Triphosphate formed by cellular kinases. Preferentially inhibits viral DNA polymerase.
CLINICAL USE	CMV, especially in patients who are immunocompromised. Valganciclovir, a prodrug of ganciclovir, has better oral bioavailability.
ADVERSE EFFECTS	Bone marrow suppression (leukopenia, neutropenia, thrombocytopenia), renal toxicity. More toxic to host enzymes than acyclovir.
MECHANISM OF RESISTANCE	Mutated viral kinase.

Foscarnet

MECHANISM	Viral DNA/RNA polymerase inhibitor and HIV reverse transcriptase inhibitor. Binds to pyrophosphate-binding site of enzyme. Does not require any kinase activation.	**Fos**carnet = pyro**fos**phate analog.
CLINICAL USE	CMV retinitis in immunocompromised patients when ganciclovir fails; acyclovir-resistant HSV.	
ADVERSE EFFECTS	Nephrotoxicity, electrolyte abnormalities (hypo- or hypercalcemia, hypo- or hyperphosphatemia, hypokalemia, hypomagnesemia) can lead to seizures.	
MECHANISM OF RESISTANCE	Mutated DNA polymerase.	

Cidofovir

MECHANISM	Preferentially inhibits viral DNA polymerase. Does not require phosphorylation by viral kinase.
CLINICAL USE	CMV retinitis in immunocompromised patients; acyclovir-resistant HSV. Long half-life.
ADVERSE EFFECTS	Nephrotoxicity (coadminister with probenecid and IV saline to ↓ toxicity).

HIV therapy

Antiretroviral therapy (ART): often initiated at the time of HIV diagnosis.

Strongest indication for use with patients presenting with AIDS-defining illness, low CD4+ cell counts (< 500 cells/mm^3), or high viral load. Regimen consists of 3 drugs to prevent resistance: 2 NRTIs and preferably an integrase inhibitor.

Most ARTs are active against both HIV-1 and HIV-2 (exceptions: NNRTIs and enfuvirtide not effective against HIV-2).

DRUG	MECHANISM	TOXICITY
NRTIs		
Abacavir (ABC) Emtricitabine (FTC) Lamivudine (3TC) Tenofovir (TDF) Zidovudine (ZDV, formerly AZT)	Competitively inhibit nucleotide binding to reverse transcriptase and terminate the DNA chain (lack a 3′ OH group). Tenofovir is a nucleoTide; the others are nucleosides. All need to be phosphorylated to be active. ZDV can be used for general prophylaxis and during pregnancy to ↓ risk of fetal transmission. Have **you dined** (**vudine**) with my **nuclear** (**nucleosides**) family?	Bone marrow suppression (can be reversed with granulocyte colony-stimulating factor [G-CSF] and erythropoietin), peripheral neuropathy, lactic acidosis (nucleosides), anemia (ZDV). Abacavir contraindicated if patient has HLA-B*5701 mutation due to ↑ risk of hypersensitivity.
NNRTIs		
Delavirdine Efavirenz Nevirapine	Bind to reverse transcriptase at site different from NRTIs. Do not require phosphorylation to be active or compete with nucleotides.	Rash and hepatotoxicity are common to all NNRTIs. Vivid dreams and CNS symptoms are common with efavirenz.
Integrase inhibitors		
Bictegravir Dolutegravir Elvitegravir Raltegravir	Inhibits HIV genome integration into host cell chromosome by reversibly inhibiting HIV integrase.	↑ creatine kinase.
Protease inhibitors		
Atazanavir Darunavir Lopinavir Ritonavir	Assembly of virions depends on HIV-1 protease (*pol* gene), which cleaves the polypeptide products of HIV mRNA into their functional parts. Thus, protease inhibitors prevent maturation of new viruses. Ritonavir can "boost" other drug concentrations by inhibiting cytochrome P-450. **Navir** (never) **tease** a **protease**.	Hyperglycemia, GI intolerance (nausea, diarrhea), lipodystrophy (Cushing-like syndrome). Rifampin (potent CYP/UGT inducer) reduces protease inhibitor concentrations; use rifabutin instead.
Entry inhibitors		
Enfuvirtide	Binds gp41, inhibiting viral entry.	Skin reaction at injection sites. Enfuvirtide inhibits **fusion**.
Maraviroc	Binds CCR-5 on surface of T cells/monocytes, inhibiting interaction with gp120.	Maraviroc inhibits **docking**.

Hepatitis C therapy

Chronic HCV infection treated with multidrug therapy that targets specific steps within HCV replication cycle (HCV-encoded proteins). Examples of drugs are provided.

DRUG	MECHANISM	TOXICITY
NS5A inhibitors		
Ledipasvir Ombitasvir Velpatasvir	Inhibits NS5A, a viral phosphoprotein that plays a key role in RNA replication Exact mechanism unknown	Headache, diarrhea
NS5B inhibitors		
Sofosbuvir Dasabuvir	Inhibits NS5B, an RNA-dependent RNA polymerase acting as a chain terminator Prevents viral RNA replication	Fatigue, headache
NS3/4A inhibitors		
Grazoprevir Simeprevir	Inhibits NS3/4A, a viral protease, preventing viral replication	Grazoprevir: headache, fatigue Simeprevir: photosensitivity reactions, rash
Alternative drugs		
Ribavirin	Inhibits synthesis of guanine nucleotides by competitively inhibiting IMP dehydrogenase Used as adjunct in cases refractory to newer medications	Hemolytic anemia, severe teratogen

Disinfection and sterilization

Goals include the reduction of pathogenic organism counts to safe levels (disinfection) and the inactivation of all microbes including spores (sterilization).
Chlorine and **heat** are sporicidal.

Autoclave	Pressurized steam at > 120°C. Sporicidal. May not reliably inactivate prions.
Alcohols	Denature proteins and disrupt cell membranes. Not sporicidal.
Chlorhexidine	Disrupts cell membranes and coagulates intracellular components.
Chlorine	Oxidizes and denatures proteins. Sporicidal.
Ethylene oxide	Alkylating agent. Sporicidal.
Hydrogen peroxide	Free radical oxidation. Sporicidal.
Iodine and iodophors	Halogenation of DNA, RNA, and proteins. May be sporicidal.
Quaternary amines	Impair permeability of cell membranes. Not sporicidal.

Antimicrobials to avoid in pregnancy

ANTIMICROBIAL	ADVERSE EFFECT
Sulfonamides	Kernicterus
Aminoglycosides	Ototoxicity
Fluoroquinolones	Cartilage damage
Clarithromycin	Embryotoxic
Tetracyclines	Discolored teeth, inhibition of bone growth
Ribavirin	Teratogenic
Griseofulvin	Teratogenic
Chloramphenicol	Gray baby syndrome

Safe **c**hildren **t**ake **r**eally **g**ood **c**are.

HIGH-YIELD PRINCIPLES IN

Pathology

"Digressions, objections, delight in mockery, carefree mistrust are signs of health; everything unconditional belongs in pathology."

—Friedrich Nietzsche

"You cannot separate passion from pathology any more than you can separate a person's spirit from his body."

—Richard Selzer

"My business is not prognosis, but diagnosis. I am not engaged in therapeutics, but in pathology."

—H.L. Mencken

The fundamental principles of pathology are key to understanding diseases in all organ systems. Major topics such as inflammation and neoplasia appear frequently in questions across different organ systems, and such topics are definitely high yield. For example, the concepts of cell injury and inflammation are key to understanding the inflammatory response that follows myocardial infarction, a very common subject of board questions. Similarly, a familiarity with the early cellular changes that culminate in the development of neoplasias—for example, esophageal or colon cancer—is critical. Finally, make sure you recognize the major tumor-associated genes and are comfortable with key cancer concepts such as tumor staging and metastasis.

▶ PATHOLOGY—CELLULAR INJURY

Cellular adaptations	Reversible changes that can be physiologic (eg, uterine enlargement during pregnancy) or pathologic (eg, myocardial hypertrophy 2° to systemic HTN). If stress is excessive or persistent, adaptations can progress to cell injury (eg, significant LV hypertrophy → injury to myofibrils → HF).
Hypertrophy	↑ structural proteins and organelles → ↑ in size of cells. Example: cardiac hypertrophy.
Hyperplasia	Controlled proliferation of stem cells and differentiated cells → ↑ in number of cells (eg, benign prostatic hyperplasia). Excessive stimulation → pathologic hyperplasia (eg, endometrial hyperplasia), which may progress to dysplasia and cancer.
Atrophy	↓ in tissue mass due to ↓ in size (↑ cytoskeleton degradation via ubiquitin-proteasome pathway and autophagy; ↓ protein synthesis) and/or number of cells (apoptosis). Causes include disuse, denervation, loss of blood supply, loss of hormonal stimulation, poor nutrition.
Metaplasia	Reprogramming of stem cells → replacement of one cell type by another that can adapt to a new stress. Usually due to exposure to an irritant, such as gastric acid (→ Barrett esophagus) or tobacco smoke (→ respiratory ciliated columnar epithelium replaced by stratified squamous epithelium). May progress to dysplasia → malignant transformation with persistent insult (eg, Barrett esophagus → esophageal adenocarcinoma). Metaplasia of connective tissue can also occur (eg, myositis ossificans, the formation of bone within muscle after trauma).
Dysplasia	Disordered, precancerous epithelial cell growth; not considered a true adaptive response. Characterized by loss of uniformity of cell size and shape (pleomorphism); loss of tissue orientation; nuclear changes (eg, ↑ nuclear:cytoplasmic ratio and clumped chromatin). Mild and moderate dysplasias (ie, do not involve entire thickness of epithelium) may regress with alleviation of inciting cause. Severe dysplasia often becomes irreversible and progresses to carcinoma in situ. Usually preceded by persistent metaplasia or pathologic hyperplasia.

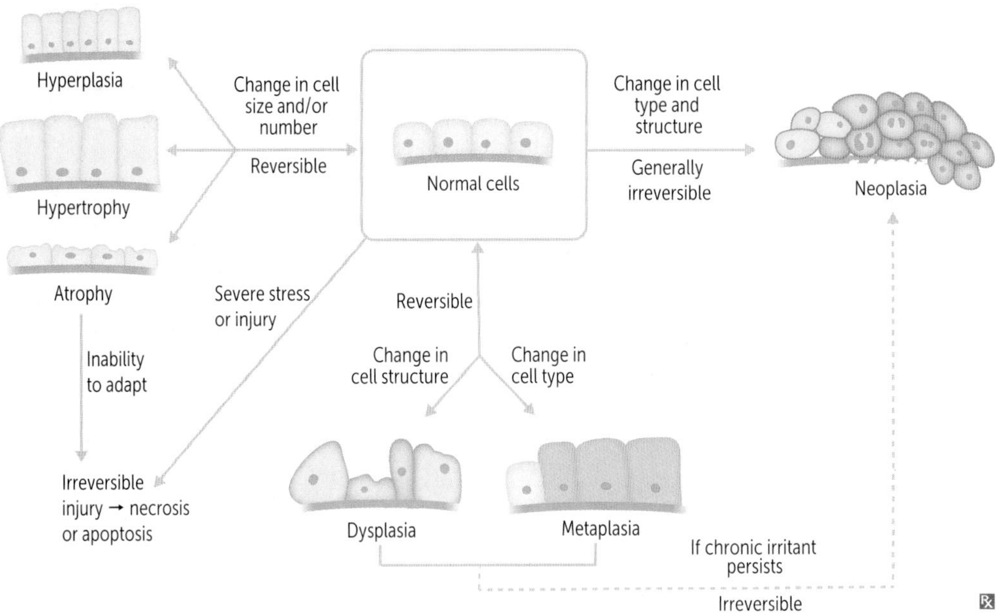

Cell injury

Reversible cell injury	▪ ↓ ATP → ↓ activity of Ca^{2+} and Na^+/K^+ pumps → cellular swelling (earliest morphologic manifestation), mitochondrial swelling ▪ Ribosomal/polysomal detachment → ↓ protein synthesis ▪ Plasma membrane changes (eg, blebbing) ▪ Nuclear changes (eg, chromatin clumping) ▪ Rapid loss of function (eg, myocardial cells are noncontractile after 1-2 minutes of ischemia) ▪ Myelin figures (aggregation of peroxidized lipids)
Irreversible cell injury	▪ Breakdown of plasma membrane → cytosolic enzymes (eg, troponin) leak outside of cell, influx of Ca^{2+} → activation of degradative enzymes ▪ Mitochondrial damage/dysfunction → loss of electron transport chain → ↓ ATP ▪ Rupture of lysosomes → autolysis ▪ Nuclear degradation: pyknosis (nuclear condensation) → karyorrhexis (nuclear fragmentation caused by endonuclease-mediated cleavage) → karyolysis (nuclear dissolution) ▪ Amorphous densities/inclusions in mitochondria

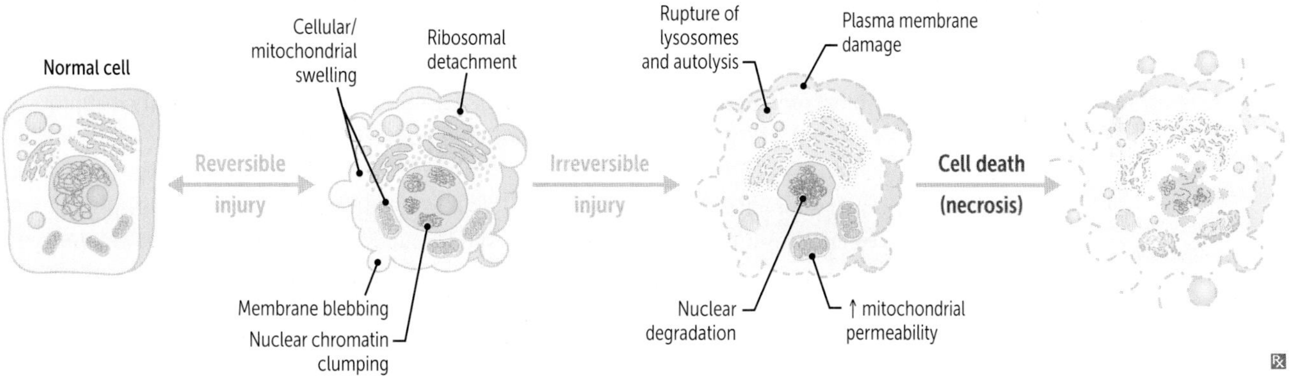

Apoptosis

ATP-dependent programmed cell death.

Intrinsic and extrinsic pathways; both pathways activate caspases (cytosolic proteases) → cellular breakdown including cell shrinkage, chromatin condensation, membrane blebbing, and formation of apoptotic bodies, which are then phagocytosed.

Characterized by deeply eosinophilic cytoplasm and basophilic nucleus, pyknosis, and karyorrhexis.

Cell membrane typically remains intact without significant inflammation (unlike necrosis).

DNA laddering (fragments in multiples of 180 bp) is a sensitive indicator of apoptosis.

Intrinsic (mitochondrial) pathway

Involved in tissue remodeling in embryogenesis. Occurs when a regulating factor is withdrawn from a proliferating cell population (eg, ↓ IL-2 after a completed immunologic reaction → apoptosis of proliferating effector cells). Also occurs after exposure to injurious stimuli (eg, radiation, toxins, hypoxia).

Regulated by Bcl-2 family of proteins. **BAX** and **BAK** are proapoptotic (**BA**d for survivial), while **B**c**l**-2 and **B**c**l**-xL are antiapoptotic (**Be** c**l**ever, live).

BAX and BAK form pores in the mitochondrial membrane → release of cytochrome C from inner mitochondrial membrane into the cytoplasm → activation of caspases.

Bcl-2 keeps the mitochondrial membrane impermeable, thereby preventing cytochrome C release. Bcl-2 overexpression (eg, follicular lymphoma t[14;18]) → ↓ caspase activation → tumorigenesis.

Extrinsic (death receptor) pathway

2 pathways:

- Ligand receptor interactions (FasL binding to Fas [CD95] or TNF-α binding to its receptor)
- Immune cell (cytotoxic T-cell release of perforin and granzyme B)

Fas-FasL interaction is necessary in thymic medullary negative selection.

Defective Fas-FasL interactions → failure of clonal deletion → ↑ numbers of self-reacting lymphocytes → autoimmune lymphoproliferative syndrome.

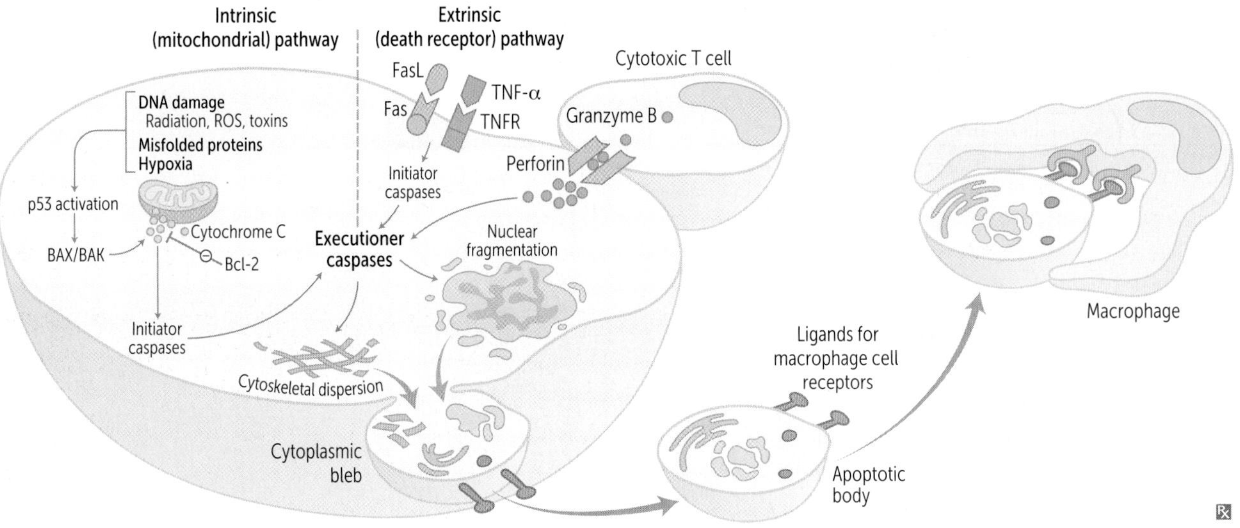

Necrosis Exogenous injury → plasma membrane damage → cell undergoes enzymatic degradation and protein denaturation, intracellular components leak → local inflammatory reaction (unlike apoptosis).

TYPE	SEEN IN	DUE TO	HISTOLOGY
Coagulative	Ischemia/infarcts in most tissues (except brain)	Ischemia or infarction; injury denatures enzymes → proteolysis blocked	Preserved cellular architecture (cell outlines seen), but nuclei disappear; ↑ cytoplasmic binding of eosin stain (→ ↑ eosinophilia; red/pink color) A
Liquefactive	Bacterial abscesses, brain infarcts	Neutrophils release lysosomal enzymes that digest the tissue B	Early: cellular debris and macrophages Late: cystic spaces and cavitation (brain) Neutrophils and cell debris seen with bacterial infection
Caseous	TB, systemic fungi (eg, *Histoplasma capsulatum*), *Nocardia*	Macrophages wall off the infecting microorganism → granular debris	Cheese-like gross appearance C Fragmented cells and debris surrounded by lymphocytes and macrophages (granuloma)
Fat	Enzymatic: acute pancreatitis (saponification of peripancreatic fat) Nonenzymatic: traumatic (eg, injury to breast tissue)	Damaged pancreatic cells release lipase, which breaks down triglycerides; liberated fatty acids bind calcium → saponification (chalky-white appearance)	Outlines of dead fat cells without peripheral nuclei; saponification of fat (combined with Ca^{2+}) appears dark blue on H&E stain D
Fibrinoid	Immune vascular reactions (eg, PAN) Nonimmune vascular reactions (eg, hypertensive emergency, preeclampsia)	Immune complex deposition (type III hypersensitivity reaction) and/or plasma protein (eg, fibrin) leakage from damaged vessel	Vessel walls contain eosinophilic layer of proteinaceous material E
Gangrenous	Distal extremity and GI tract, after chronic ischemia	Dry: ischemia F	Coagulative
		Wet: superinfection	Liquefactive superimposed on coagulative

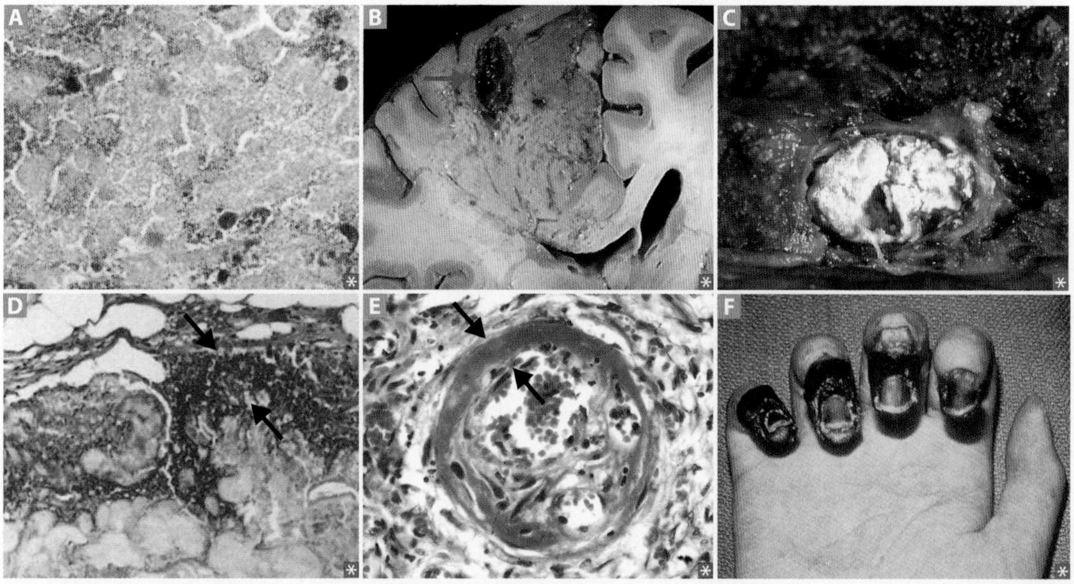

Ischemia

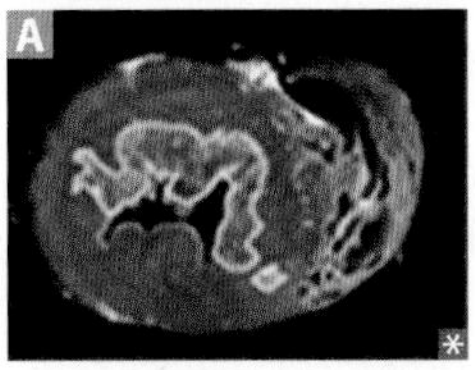

Inadequate blood supply to meet demand. Mechanisms include ↓ arterial perfusion (eg, atherosclerosis), ↓ venous drainage (eg, testicular torsion, Budd-Chiari syndrome), shock.
Regions most vulnerable to hypoxia/ischemia and subsequent infarction:

ORGAN	REGION
Brain	ACA/MCA/PCA boundary areas[a,b]
Heart	Subendocardium of LV (yellow lines in A outline a subendocardial infarction)
Kidney	Straight segment of proximal tubule (medulla) Thick ascending limb (medulla)
Liver	Area around central vein (zone III)
Colon	Splenic flexure (Griffith point),[a] rectosigmoid junction (Sudeck point)[a]

[a]Watershed areas (border zones) receive blood supply from most distal branches of 2 arteries with limited collateral vascularity. These areas are susceptible to ischemia from hypoperfusion.
[b]Neurons most vulnerable to hypoxic-ischemic insults include Purkinje cells of the cerebellum and pyramidal cells of the hippocampus and neocortex (zones 3, 5, 6).

Types of infarcts

Red infarct

Occurs in venous occlusion and tissues with multiple blood supplies (eg, liver, lung A, intestine, testes), and with reperfusion (eg, after angioplasty). Reperfusion injury is due to damage by free radicals.

Pale infarct

Occurs in solid organs with a single (end-arterial) blood supply (eg, heart, kidney B).

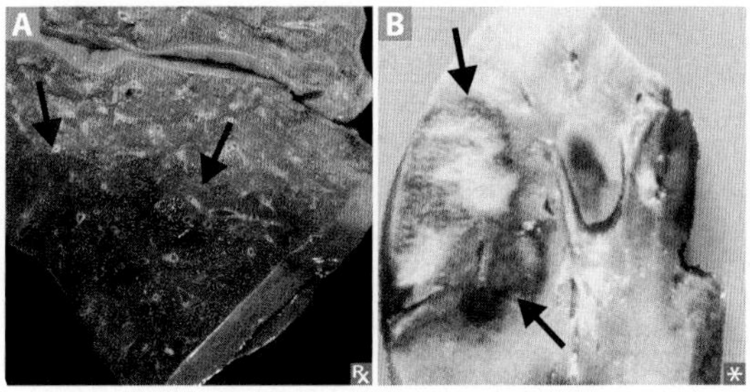

Free radical injury

Free radicals damage cells via membrane lipid peroxidation, protein modification, DNA breakage. Initiated via radiation exposure (eg, cancer therapy), metabolism of drugs (phase I), redox reactions, nitric oxide (eg, inflammation), transition metals, WBC (eg, neutrophils, macrophages) oxidative burst.
Free radicals can be eliminated by scavenging enzymes (eg, catalase, superoxide dismutase, glutathione peroxidase), spontaneous decay, antioxidants (eg, vitamins A, C, E), and certain metal carrier proteins (eg, transferrin, ceruloplasmin).
Examples:

- Oxygen toxicity: retinopathy of prematurity (abnormal vascularization), bronchopulmonary dysplasia, reperfusion injury after thrombolytic therapy
- Drug/chemical toxicity: acetaminophen overdose (hepatotoxicity), carbon tetrachloride (converted by cytochrome P-450 into CCl_3 free radical → fatty liver [cell injury → ↓ apolipoprotein synthesis → fatty change], centrilobular necrosis)
- Metal storage diseases: hemochromatosis (iron) and Wilson disease (copper)

Ionizing radiation toxicity

Ionization radiation induces cellular and DNA damage directly (via photons or particles) and indirectly (via generation of reactive oxygen species) → progressive inflammation and tissue damage. Rapidly regenerating tissues (eg, skin epithelia, bone marrow, GI tract, GU tract, gonads) more susceptible to injury. Can cause both acute and delayed (late) toxicities.

RADIATION TOXICITY	SYSTEM	DISEASE/CLINICAL MANIFESTATION
Full exposure		
Acute radiation syndrome	Skin	Hair loss, erythema, desquamation, ulcers/necrosis
	Hematopoietic	Myelosuppression
	Gastrointestinal	Mucosal denudation, inflammation, edema → abdominal pain, diarrhea, GI bleeding, nausea, vomiting, stomatitis
	Neurovascular	Papilledema, seizures, ataxia, impaired reflexes, cognitive deficits
Partial exposure		
Acute local toxicity	Skin, gonads, eye	Blisters, sterility, ↓ spermatogenesis, cataracts
Late complication		
Radiation-induced fibrosis	Skin, subcutaneous tissue	Induration, thickening, loss of elasticity, shrinkage, lymphedema
	Lung	Pulmonary fibrosis
	Head and neck	Trismus, mucosal fibrosis, ulceration, fistulae
	Gastrointestinal	Obstruction, ulcerations, fistulae
	Genitourinary	Ureteral and urethral stenosis, fibrotic bladder constriction → obstructive uropathy; fibrosis of ovaries, vulva, vagina; azoospermia
Radiation-related malignancies	Thyroid	Papillary thyroid carcinoma
	Hematopoietic	Myelodysplastic syndromes, lymphomas, leukemias (eg, CML, AML, ALL)
	Skin	Angiosarcoma
	Bone	Osteosarcoma
	Others	Solid tumors (eg, breast, ovarian, lung)

Types of calcification Calcium deposits appear deeply basophilic (arrow in A) on H&E stain.

	Dystrophic calcification	Metastatic calcification
Ca^{2+} DEPOSITION	In abnormal (**d**iseased) tissues	In normal tissues
EXTENT	Tends to be localized (eg, calcific aortic stenosis)	Widespread (ie, diffuse, metastatic)
ASSOCIATED CONDITIONS 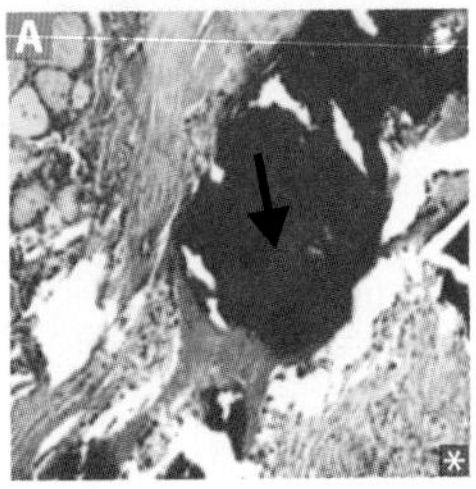	TB (lung and pericardium) and other granulomatous infections, liquefactive necrosis of chronic abscesses, fat necrosis, infarcts, thrombi, schistosomiasis, congenital CMV, toxoplasmosis, rubella, psammoma bodies, CREST syndrome, atherosclerotic plaques can become calcified	Predominantly in interstitial tissues of kidney, lung, and gastric mucosa (these tissues lose acid quickly; ↑ pH favors Ca^{2+} deposition) Nephrocalcinosis of collecting ducts may lead to nephrogenic diabetes insipidus and renal failure
ETIOLOGY	2° to injury or necrosis	2° to hypercalcemia (eg, 1° hyperparathyroidism, sarcoidosis, hypervitaminosis D) or high calcium-phosphate product levels (eg, chronic kidney disease with 2° hyperparathyroidism, long-term dialysis, calciphylaxis, multiple myeloma)
SERUM Ca^{2+} LEVELS	Normal	Usually abnormal

Lipofuscin

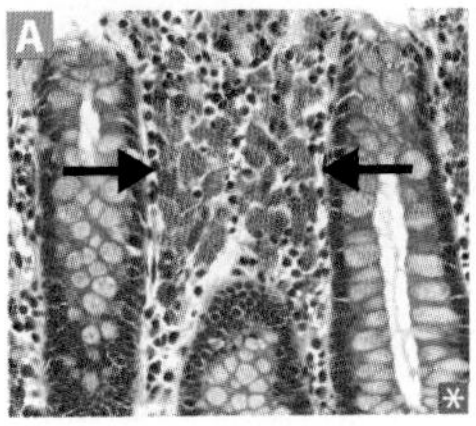

A yellow-brown "wear and tear" pigment A associated with normal aging.

Composed of polymers of lipids and phospholipids complexed with protein. May be derived through lipid peroxidation of polyunsaturated lipids of subcellular membranes.

Autopsy of elderly person will reveal deposits in heart, colon, liver, kidney, eye, and other organs.

Amyloidosis

Abnormal aggregation of proteins (or their fragments) into β-pleated linear sheets → insoluble fibrils → cellular damage and apoptosis. Amyloid deposits visualized by Congo red stain (red/orange on nonpolarized light [arrows in A]), (apple-green birefringence on polarized light [arrows in B]), and H&E stain (shows deposits in glomerular mesangial areas). Tubular basement membranes are enlarged on light microscopy.

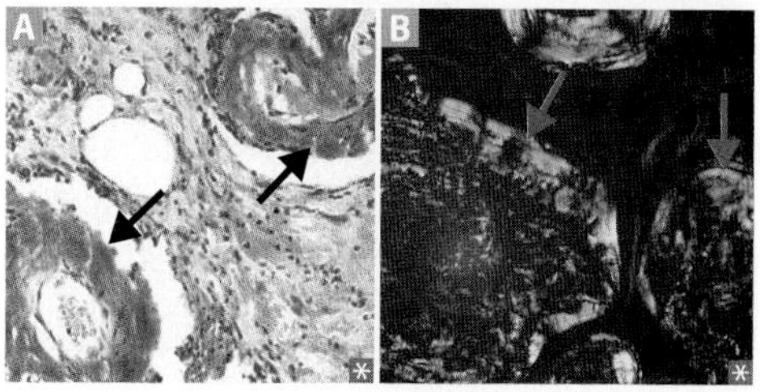

COMMON TYPES	FIBRIL PROTEIN	DESCRIPTION	
Systemic			
Primary amyloidosis	AL (from Ig Light chains)	Seen in plasma cell disorders (eg, multiple myeloma)	Manifestations include: ▪ Cardiac (eg, restrictive cardiomyopathy) ▪ GI (eg, macroglossia, hepatomegaly) ▪ Renal (eg, nephrotic syndrome) ▪ Hematologic (eg, easy bruising, splenomegaly) ▪ Neurologic (eg, neuropathy) ▪ Musculoskeletal (eg, carpal tunnel syndrome)
Secondary amyloidosis	Serum Amyloid A (AA)	Seen in chronic inflammatory conditions, (eg, rheumatoid arthritis, IBD, familial Mediterranean fever, protracted infection)	
Dialysis-related amyloidosis	β_2-microglobulin	Seen in patients with ESRD and/or on long-term dialysis	
Localized			
Alzheimer disease	β-amyloid protein	Cleaved from amyloid precursor protein (APP)	
Type 2 diabetes mellitus	Islet amyloid polypeptide (IAPP)	Caused by deposition of amylin in pancreatic islets	
Medullary thyroid cancer	Calcitonin		
Isolated atrial amyloidosis	ANP	Common in normal aging ↑ risk of atrial fibrillation	
Systemic senile (age-related) amyloidosis	Normal (wild-type) transthyretin (TTR)	Seen predominantly in cardiac ventricles	Cardiac dysfunction more insidious than in AL amyloidosis
Hereditary			
Familial amyloid cardiomyopathy	Mutated transthyretin (ATTR)	Ventricular endomyocardium deposition → restrictive cardiomyopathy, arrhythmias	3–4% of African-Americans are carriers of a mutated allele
Familial amyloid polyneuropathies	Mutated transthyretin (ATTR)	Due to transthyretin gene mutation	

▸ PATHOLOGY—INFLAMMATION

Inflammation Response to eliminate initial cause of cell injury, to remove necrotic cells resulting from the original insult, and to initiate tissue repair. Divided into acute and chronic. The inflammatory response itself can be harmful to the host if the reaction is excessive (eg, septic shock), prolonged (eg, persistent infections such as TB), or inappropriate (eg, autoimmune diseases such as SLE).

SIGN	MECHANISM	MEDIATORS
Cardinal signs		
Rubor and calor	Redness and warmth. Vasodilation (relaxation of arteriolar smooth muscle) → ↑ blood flow.	Histamine, prostaglandins, bradykinin, NO.
Tumor	Swelling. Endothelial contraction/disruption (eg, from tissue damage) → ↑ vascular permeability → leakage of protein-rich fluid from postcapillary venules into interstitial space (exudate) → ↑ interstitial oncotic pressure.	Endothelial contraction: leukotrienes (C_4, D_4, E_4), histamine, serotonin.
Dolor	Pain. Sensitization of sensory nerve endings.	Bradykinin, PGE_2, histamine.
Functio laesa	Loss of function. Inflammation impairs function (eg, inability to make fist due to hand cellulitis).	
Systemic manifestations (acute-phase reaction)		
Fever	Pyrogens (eg, LPS) induce macrophages to release IL-1 and TNF → ↑ COX activity in perivascular cells of anterior hypothalamus → ↑ PGE_2 → ↑ temperature set point.	
Leukocytosis	↑ WBC count; type of predominant cell depends on inciting agent or injury (eg, bacteria → ↑ neutrophils).	
↑ plasma acute-phase reactants	Serum concentrations significantly change in response to acute and chronic inflammation. Produced by liver.	Notably induced by IL-6.

Acute phase reactants More FFiSHH Pee in the C (sea).

POSITIVE (UPREGULATED)	
Ferritin	Binds and sequesters iron to inhibit microbial iron scavenging.
Fibrinogen	Coagulation factor; promotes endothelial repair; correlates with ESR.
Serum amyloid A	Prolonged elevation can lead to amyloidosis.
Hepcidin	↓ iron absorption (by degrading ferroportin) and ↓ iron release (from macrophages) → anemia of chronic disease.
Haptoglobin	Binds extracellular hemoglobin, protects against oxidative stress.
Procalcitonin	Rises in bacterial infections.
C-reactive protein	Opsonin; fixes complement and facilitates phagocytosis. Measured clinically as a nonspecific sign of ongoing inflammation.
NEGATIVE (DOWNREGULATED)	
Albumin	Reduction conserves amino acids for positive reactants.
Transferrin	Internalized by macrophages to sequester iron.

Erythrocyte sedimentation rate

RBCs normally remain separated via ⊖ charges. Products of inflammation (eg, fibrinogen) coat RBCs → ↓ ⊖ charge → ↑ RBC aggregation. Denser RBC aggregates fall at a faster rate within a pipette tube → ↑ ESR. Often co-tested with CRP (more specific marker of inflammation).

↑ ESR	↓ ESR
Most anemias	Sickle cell anemia (altered shape)
Infections	Polycythemia (↑ RBCs "dilute" aggregation factors)
Inflammation (eg, giant cell [temporal] arteritis, polymyalgia rheumatica)	HF
Cancer (eg, metastases, multiple myeloma)	Microcytosis
Renal disease (end-stage or nephrotic syndrome)	Hypofibrinogenemia
Pregnancy	

Acute inflammation

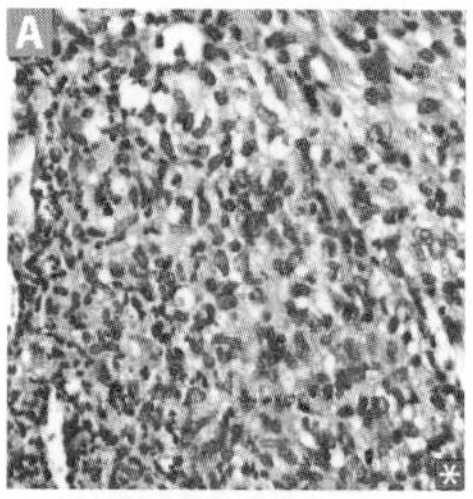

Transient and early response to injury or infection. Characterized by neutrophils in tissue A, often with associated edema. Rapid onset (seconds to minutes) and short duration (minutes to days). Represents a reaction of the innate immune system (ie, less specific response than chronic inflammation).

STIMULI

Infections, trauma, necrosis, foreign bodies.

MEDIATORS

Toll-like receptors, arachidonic acid metabolites, neutrophils, eosinophils, antibodies (pre-existing), mast cells, basophils, complement, Hageman factor (factor XII).

Inflammasome—Cytoplasmic protein complex that recognizes products of dead cells, microbial products, and crystals (eg, uric acid crystals) → activation of IL-1 and inflammatory response.

COMPONENTS

- Vascular: vasodilation (→ ↑ blood flow and stasis) and ↑ endothelial permeability (contraction of endothelial cells opens interendothelial junctions)
- Cellular: extravasation of leukocytes (mainly neutrophils) from postcapillary venules and accumulation in the focus of injury followed by leukocyte activation

To bring cells and proteins to site of injury or infection.

Leukocyte extravasation has 4 steps: margination and rolling, adhesion, transmigration, and migration (chemoattraction).

OUTCOMES

- Resolution and healing (IL-10, TGF-β)
- Persistent acute inflammation (IL-8)
- Abscess (acute inflammation walled off by fibrosis)
- Chronic inflammation (antigen presentation by macrophages and other APCs → activation of $CD4^+$ Th cells)
- Scarring

Macrophages predominate in the late stages of acute inflammation (peak 2–3 days after onset) and influence outcome by secreting cytokines.

Leukocyte extravasation

Extravasation predominantly occurs at postcapillary venules.

STEP	VASCULATURE/STROMA	LEUKOCYTE
❶ Margination and rolling—defective in leukocyte adhesion deficiency type 2 (↓ Sialyl Lewis^X)	E-selectin (upregulated by TNF and IL-1) P-selectin (released from Weibel-palade bodies) GlyCAM-1, CD34	Sialyl Lewis^X Sialyl Lewis^X L-selectin
❷ Tight binding (adhesion)—defective in leukocyte adhesion deficiency type 1 (↓ CD18 integrin subunit)	ICAM-1 (CD54) VCAM-1 (CD106)	CD11/18 integrins (LFA-1, Mac-1) VLA-4 integrin
❸ DiaPEdesis (transmigration)—WBC travels between endothelial cells and exits blood vessel	PECAM-1 (CD31)	PECAM-1 (CD31)
❹ Migration—WBC travels through interstitium to site of injury or infection guided by chemotactic signals	Chemotactic factors: C5a, IL-8, LTB_4, kallikrein, platelet-activating factor, N-formylmethionyl peptides	Various

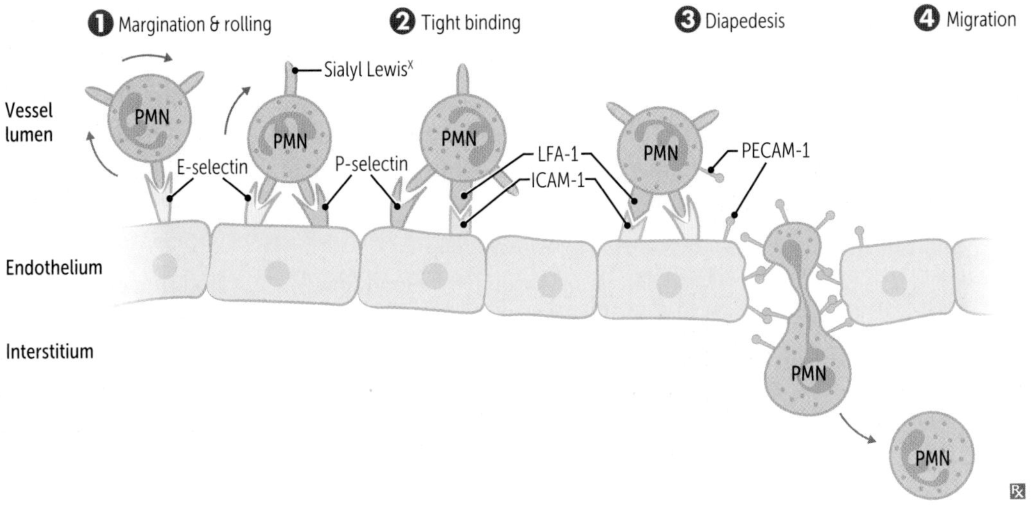

Chronic inflammation	Prolonged inflammation characterized by mononuclear infiltration (macrophages, lymphocytes, plasma cells), which leads to simultaneous tissue destruction and repair (including angiogenesis and fibrosis). May be preceded by acute inflammation.
STIMULI	Persistent infections (eg, TB, *T pallidum*, certain fungi and viruses) → type IV hypersensitivity, autoimmune diseases, prolonged exposure to toxic agents (eg, silica) and foreign material.
MEDIATORS	Macrophages are the dominant cells. Interaction of macrophages and T lymphocytes → chronic inflammation. ▪ Th1 cells secrete IFN-γ → macrophage classical activation (proinflammatory) ▪ Th2 cells secrete IL-4 and IL-13 → macrophage alternative activation (repair and anti-inflammatory)
OUTCOMES	Scarring, amyloidosis, and neoplastic transformation (eg, chronic HCV infection → chronic inflammation → hepatocellular carcinoma; *Helicobacter pylori* infection → chronic gastritis → gastric adenocarcinoma).

Wound healing

Tissue mediators	MEDIATOR	ROLE
	FGF	Stimulates angiogenesis
	TGF-β	Angiogenesis, fibrosis
	VEGF	Stimulates angiogenesis
	PDGF	Secreted by activated platelets and macrophages Induces vascular remodeling and smooth muscle cell migration Stimulates fibroblast growth for collagen synthesis
	Metalloproteinases	Tissue remodeling
	EGF	Stimulates cell growth via tyrosine kinases (eg, EGFR/*ErbB1*)

PHASE OF WOUND HEALING	EFFECTOR CELLS	CHARACTERISTICS
Inflammatory (up to 3 days after wound)	Platelets, neutrophils, macrophages	Clot formation, ↑ vessel permeability and neutrophil migration into tissue; macrophages clear debris 2 days later
Proliferative (day 3–weeks after wound)	Fibroblasts, myofibroblasts, endothelial cells, keratinocytes, macrophages	Deposition of granulation tissue and type III collagen, angiogenesis, epithelial cell proliferation, dissolution of clot, and wound contraction (mediated by myofibroblasts) Delayed second phase of wound healing in vitamin C and copper deficiency
Remodeling (1 week–6+ months after wound)	Fibroblasts	Type III collagen replaced by type I collagen, ↑ tensile strength of tissue Collagenases (require zinc to function) break down type III collagen Zinc deficiency → delayed wound healing

Granulomatous inflammation

A pattern of chronic inflammation. Can be induced by persistent T-cell response to certain infections (eg, TB), immune-mediated diseases, and foreign bodies. Granulomas "wall off" a resistant stimulus without completely eradicating or degrading it → persistent inflammation→ fibrosis, organ damage.

HISTOLOGY

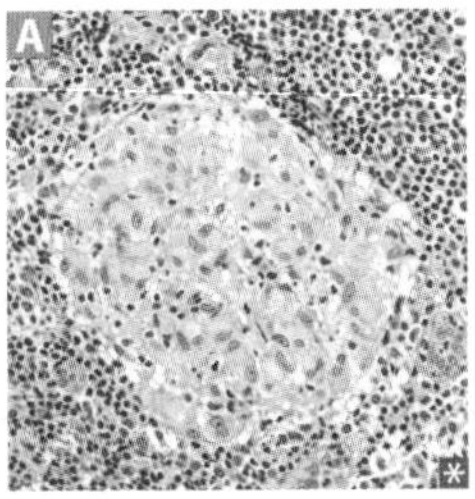

Focus of epithelioid cells (activated macrophages with abundant pink cytoplasm) surrounded by lymphocytes and multinucleated giant cells (formed by fusion of several activated macrophages). Two types:

Caseating: associated with central necrosis. Seen with infectious etiologies (eg, TB, fungal).

Noncaseating A: no central necrosis. Seen with autoimmune diseases (eg, sarcoidosis, Crohn disease).

MECHANISM

❶ APCs present antigens to CD4+ Th cells and secrete IL-12 → CD4+ Th cells differentiate into Th1 cells

❷ Th1 secretes IFN-γ → macrophage activation

❸ Macrophages ↑ cytokine secretion (eg, TNF) → formation of epithelioid macrophages and giant cells

Anti-TNF therapy can cause sequestering granulomas to break down → disseminated disease. Always test for latent TB before starting anti-TNF therapy.

Associated with hypercalcemia due to ↑ 1α-hydroxylase activity in activated macrophages, resulting in ↑ vitamin D activity.

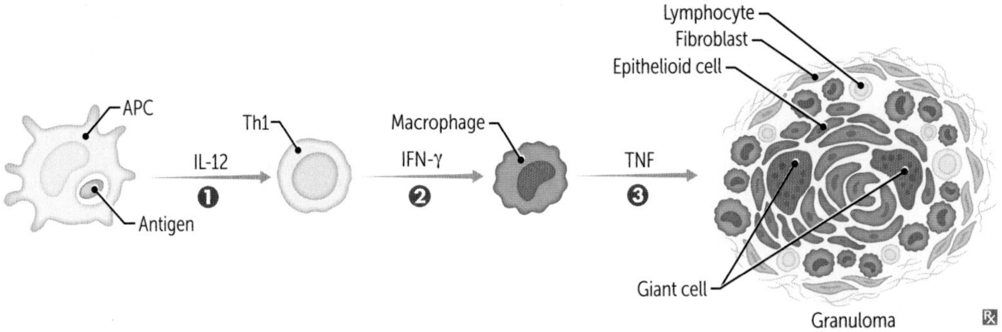

ETIOLOGIES

INFECTIOUS	NONINFECTIOUS
Bacterial: *Mycobacteria* (tuberculosis, leprosy), *Bartonella henselae* (cat scratch disease; stellate necrotizing granulomas), *Listeria monocytogenes* (granulomatosis infantiseptica), *Treponema pallidum* (3° syphilis) Fungal: endemic mycoses (eg, histoplasmosis) Parasitic: schistosomiasis	Immune-mediated: sarcoidosis, Crohn disease, 1° biliary cholangitis, subacute (de Quervain/granulomatous) thyroiditis Vasculitis: granulomatosis with polyangiitis, eosinophilic granulomatosis with polyangiitis, giant cell (temporal) arteritis, Takayasu arteritis Foreign bodies: berylliosis, talcosis, hypersensitivity pneumonitis Chronic granulomatous disease

Scar formation

Occurs when repair cannot be accomplished by cell regeneration alone. Nonregenerated cells (2° to severe acute or chronic injury) are replaced by connective tissue. 70–80% of tensile strength regained at 3 months; little tensile strength regained thereafter. Associated with excess TGF-β.

SCAR TYPE	Hypertrophic A	Keloid B
COLLAGEN SYNTHESIS	↑ (type III collagen)	↑↑↑ (types I and III collagen)
COLLAGEN ORGANIZATION	Parallel	Disorganized
EXTENT OF SCAR	Confined to borders of original wound	Extends beyond borders of original wound with "claw-like" projections typically on earlobes, face, upper extremities
RECURRENCE	Infrequent	Frequent
PREDISPOSITION	None	↑ incidence in people with darker skin

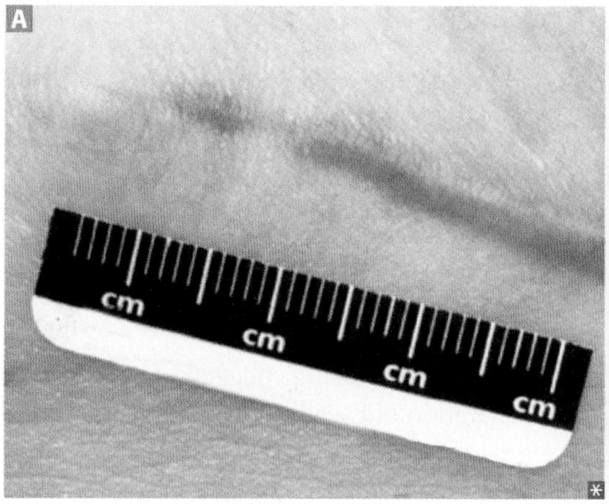

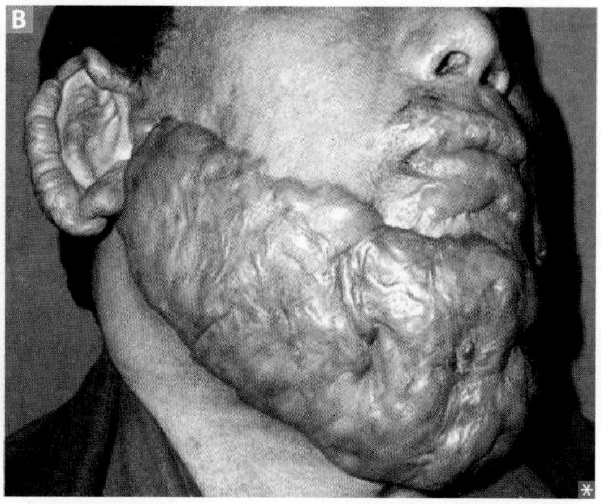

▸ PATHOLOGY—NEOPLASIA

Neoplasia and neoplastic progression

Uncontrolled, monoclonal proliferation of cells. Can be benign or malignant. Any neoplastic growth has two components: parenchyma (neoplastic cells) and supporting stroma (non-neoplastic; eg, blood vessels, connective tissue).

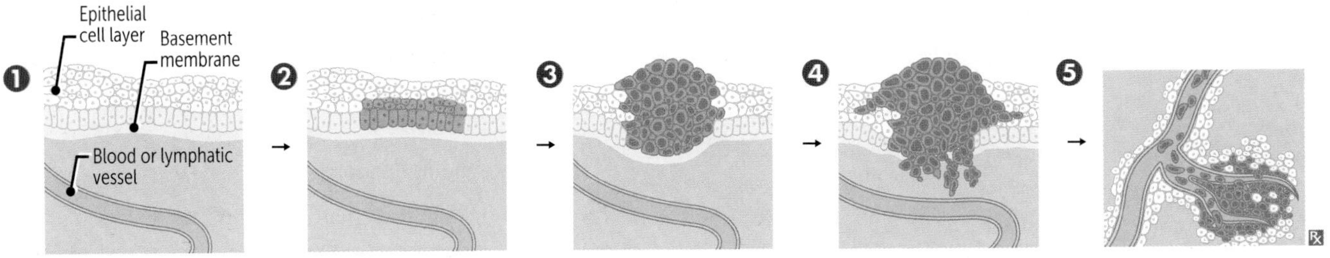

Epithelial cell layer
Basement membrane
Blood or lymphatic vessel

Normal cells	❶ Normal cells with basal → apical polarity. See cervical example A, which shows normal cells and spectrum of dysplasia, as discussed below.
Dysplasia	❷ Loss of uniformity in cell size and shape (pleomorphism); loss of tissue orientation; nuclear changes (eg, ↑ nuclear:cytoplasmic ratio) A; often reversible.
Carcinoma in situ/ preinvasive	❸ Irreversible severe dysplasia that involves the entire thickness of epithelium but does not penetrate the intact basement membrane A.
Invasive carcinoma	❹ Cells have invaded basement membrane using collagenases and hydrolases (metalloproteinases). Cell-cell contacts lost by inactivation of E-cadherin.
Metastasis	❺ Spread to distant organ(s) via lymphatics or blood.

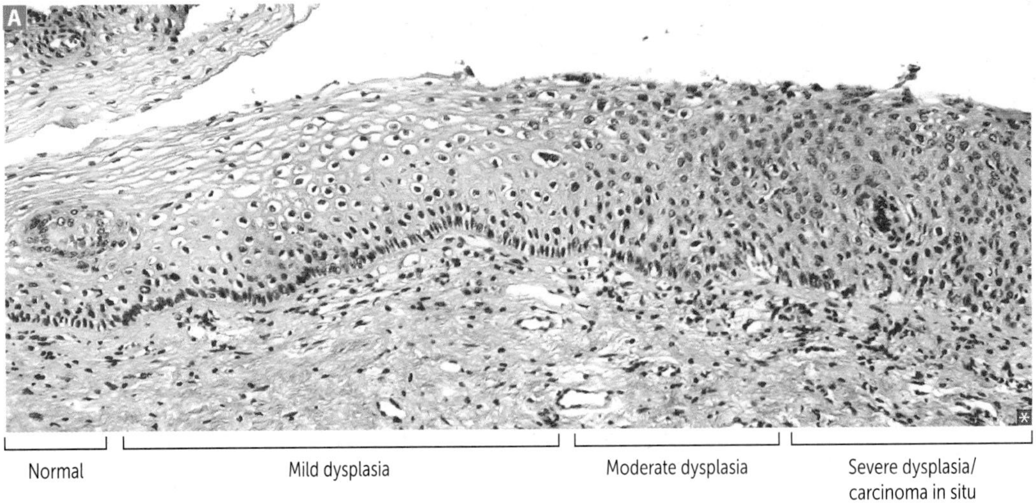

A
Normal
Mild dysplasia
Moderate dysplasia
Severe dysplasia/ carcinoma in situ

Tumor nomenclature

Carcinoma implies epithelial origin, whereas **sarcoma** denotes mesenchymal origin. Both terms generally imply malignancy.

Benign tumors are usually well-differentiated and well-demarcated, with low mitotic activity, no metastases, and no necrosis.

Malignant tumors (cancers) may show poor differentiation, erratic growth, local invasion, metastasis, and ↓ apoptosis.

Terms for non-neoplastic malformations include hamartoma (disorganized overgrowth of tissues in their native location, eg, Peutz-Jeghers polyps) and choristoma (normal tissue in a foreign location, eg, gastric tissue located in distal ileum in Meckel diverticulum).

CELL TYPE	BENIGN	MALIGNANT
Epithelium	Adenoma, papilloma	Adenocarcinoma, papillary carcinoma
Mesenchyme		
Blood cells		Leukemia, lymphoma
Blood vessels	Hemangioma	Angiosarcoma
Smooth muscle	Leiomyoma	Leiomyosarcoma
Striated muscle	Rhabdomyoma	Rhabdomyosarcoma
Connective tissue	Fibroma	Fibrosarcoma
Bone	Osteoma	Osteosarcoma
Fat	Lipoma	Liposarcoma
Melanocyte	Nevus/mole	Melanoma

Tumor grade vs stage

Differentiation—degree to which a tumor resembles its tissue of origin. Well-differentiated tumors (often less aggressive) closely resemble their tissue of origin, whereas poorly differentiated tumors (often more aggressive) do not.

Anaplasia—complete lack of differentiation of cells in a malignant neoplasm.

Grade

Degree of cellular differentiation and mitotic activity on histology. Ranges from low grade (well-differentiated) to high grade (poorly differentiated, undifferentiated, or anaplastic).

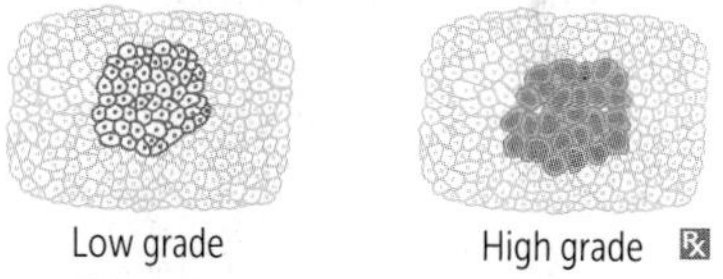
Low grade
High grade

Stage

Degree of localization/spread based on site and size of 1° lesion, spread to regional lymph nodes, presence of metastases. Based on clinical (c) or pathologic (p) findings. Stage generally has more prognostic value than grade (eg, a high-stage yet low-grade tumor is usually worse than a low-stage yet high-grade tumor). Stage determines Survival.

TNM staging system (Stage = Spread): T = Tumor size/invasiveness, N = Node involvement, M = Metastases, eg, cT3N1M0. Each TNM factor has independent prognostic value; N and M are often most important.

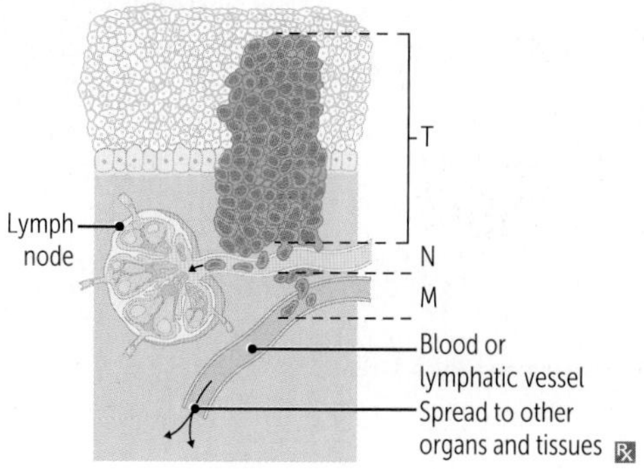
T
Lymph node
N
M
Blood or lymphatic vessel
Spread to other organs and tissues

Hallmarks of cancer Cancer is caused by (mostly acquired) DNA mutations that affect fundamental cellular processes (eg, growth, DNA repair, survival).

HALLMARK	MECHANISM
Growth signal self-sufficiency	Mutations in genes encoding: ▪ Proto-oncogenes → ↑ growth factors → autocrine loop (eg, ↑ PDGF in brain tumors) ▪ Growth factor receptors → constitutive signaling (eg, *HER2/neu* in breast cancer) ▪ Signaling molecules (eg, *RAS*) ▪ Transcription factors (eg, *MYC*) ▪ Cell cycle regulators (eg, cyclins, CDKs)
Anti-growth signal insensitivity	▪ Mutations in tumor suppressor genes (eg, *Rb*) ▪ Loss of E-cadherin function → loss of contact inhibition (eg, *NF2* mutations)
Evasion of apoptosis	Mutations in genes that regulate apoptosis (eg, *TP53*, *BCL2* → follicular B cell lymphoma).
Limitless replicative potential	Reactivation of telomerase → maintenance and lengthening of telomeres → prevention of chromosome shortening and cell aging.
Sustained angiogenesis	↑ pro-angiogenic factors (eg, VEGF) or ↓ inhibitory factors. Factors may be produced by tumor or stromal cells. Vessels can sprout from existing capillaries (neoangiogenesis) or endothelial cells are recruited from bone marrow (vasculogenesis). Vessels may be leaky and/or dilated.
Tissue invasion	Loss of E-cadherin function → loosening of intercellular junctions → metalloproteinases degrade basement membrane and ECM → cells attach to ECM proteins (eg, laminin, fibronectin) → cells migrate through degraded ECM ("locomotion") → vascular dissemination.
Metastasis	Tumor cells or emboli spread via lymphatics or blood → adhesion to endothelium → extravasation and homing. Site of metastasis can be predicted by site of 1° tumor, as the target organ is often the first-encountered capillary bed. Some cancers show organ tropism (eg, lung cancers commonly metastasize to adrenals).
Warburg effect	Shift of glucose metabolism away from mitochondrial oxidative phosphorylation toward glycolysis. Glycolysis provides rapidly dividing cancer cells with the carbon needed for synthesis of cellular structures.
Immune evasion in cancer	Normally, immune cells can recognize and attack tumor cells. For successful tumorigenesis, tumor cells must evade the immune system. Multiple escape mechanisms exist: ▪ ↓ MHC class I expression by tumor cells → cytotoxic T cells are unable to recognize tumor cells. ▪ Tumor cells secrete immunosuppressive factors (eg, TGF-β) and recruit regulatory T cells to down regulate immune response. ▪ Tumor cells up regulate immune checkpoint molecules, which inhibit immune response.

Immune checkpoint interactions

Signals that modulate T cell activation and function → ↓ immune response against tumor cells. Targeted by several cancer immunotherapies. Examples:

- Interaction between PD-1 (on T cells) and PD-L1/2 (on tumor cells or immune cells in tumor microenvironment) → T cell dysfunction (exhaustion). Inhibited by antibodies against PD-1 (eg, pembrolizumab, nivolumab, cemiplimab) or PD-L1 (eg, atezolizumab, durvalumab, avelumab).
- CTLA-4 on T cells outcompetes CD28 for B7 on APCs → loss of T cell costimulatory signal. Inhibited by ipilimumab (anti-CTLA-4 antibody).

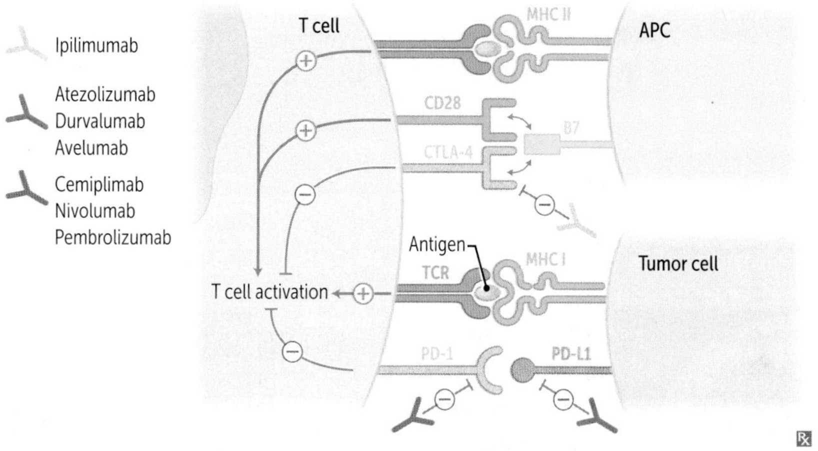

Cancer epidemiology

Skin cancer (basal > squamous >> melanoma) is the most common cancer (not included below).

	MALES	FEMALES	CHILDREN (AGE 0–14)	NOTES
Cancer incidence	1. Prostate 2. Lung 3. Colon/rectum	1. Breast 2. Lung 3. Colon/rectum	1. Leukemia 2. CNS 3. Neuroblastoma	Lung cancer incidence has ↓ in males, but has not changed significantly in females.
Cancer mortality	1. Lung 2. Prostate 3. Colon/rectum	1. Lung 2. Breast 3. Colon/rectum	1. Leukemia 2. CNS 3. Neuroblastoma	Cancer is the 2nd leading cause of death in the United States (heart disease is 1st).

Common metastases Most sarcomas spread hematogenously; most carcinomas spread via lymphatics. However, four carcinomas route hematogenously: follicular thyroid carcinoma, choriocarcinoma, renal cell carcinoma, and hepatocellular carcinoma.

SITE OF METASTASIS	1° TUMOR	NOTES
Brain	Lung > breast > melanoma, colon, kidney (lots of brain metastases can kill)	50% of brain tumors are from metastases Commonly seen as multiple well-circumscribed tumors at gray/white matter junction A B
Liver	Colon >> stomach > pancreas (cancer sometimes penetrates liver)	Liver C D and lung are the most common sites of metastasis after the regional lymph nodes
Bone	Prostate, breast > kidney, thyroid, lung (painful bones kill the lungs)	Bone metastasis E F >> 1° bone tumors (eg, multiple myeloma) Predilection for axial skeleton G Bone metastasis can be: ▪ Lytic (eg, thyroid, kidney, non-small cell lung cancer) ▪ Blastic (eg, prostate, small cell lung cancer) ▪ Mixed (eg, breast cancer)

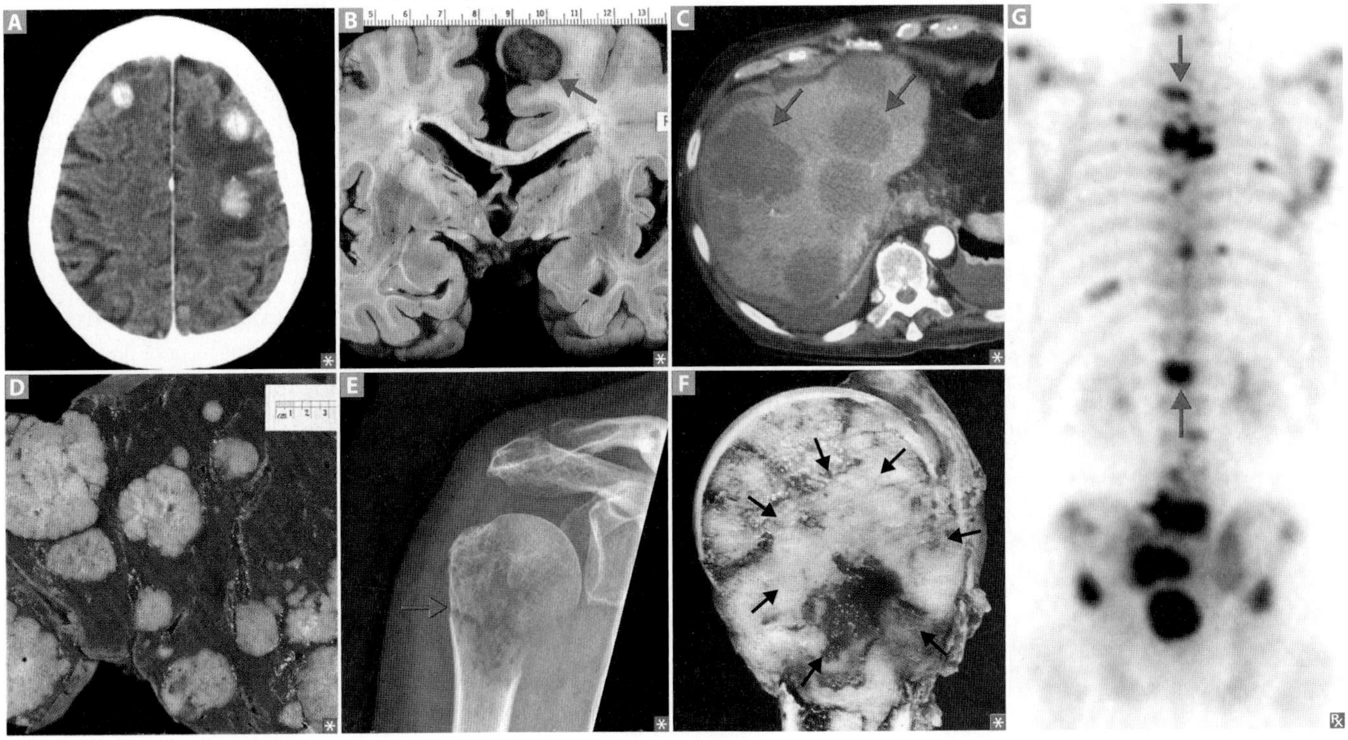

Oncogenes

Gain of function mutation converts proto-oncogene (normal gene) to oncogene → ↑ cancer risk. Requires damage to only **one** allele of a proto-**onc**ogene.

GENE	GENE PRODUCT	ASSOCIATED NEOPLASM
ALK	Receptor tyrosine kinase	Lung adenocarcinoma
HER2/neu (ERBB2)	Receptor tyrosine kinase	Breast and gastric carcinomas
RET	**RE**ceptor **T**yrosine kinase	MEN 2A and 2B, medullary and papillary thyroid carcinoma, pheochromocytoma
BCR-ABL	Non-receptor tyrosine kinase	CML, ALL
JAK2	Non-receptor tyrosine kinase	Myeloproliferative neoplasms
BRAF	Serine/threonine kinase	Melanoma, non-Hodgkin lymphoma, colorectal carcinoma, papillary thyroid carcinoma, hairy cell leukemia
c-KIT	Cyto**KI**ne receptor	Gastrointestinal stromal tumor (GIST), mastocytosis
c-MYC	Transcription factor	Burkitt lymphoma
MYCL1	Transcription factor	Lung cancer
MYCN (N-myc)	Transcription factor	Neuroblastoma
KRAS	RAS GTPase	Colorectal, lung, pancreatic cancers
BCL-2	Antiapoptotic molecule (inhibits apoptosis)	Follicular and diffuse large **B-C**ell **L**ymphomas

Tumor suppressor genes

Loss of function → ↑ cancer risk; both (**two**) alleles of a **tu**mor suppressor gene must be lost for expression of disease (Knudson's 2-hit hypothesis).

GENE	GENE PRODUCT	ASSOCIATED CONDITION
APC	Negative regulator of β-catenin/WNT pathway	Colorectal cancer (associated with FAP)
BRCA1/BRCA2	BRCA1/BRCA2 proteins	**BR**east, ovarian, prostate, pancreatic **CA**ncers
CDKN2A	p16, blocks G_1 → S phase	Many cancers (eg, melanoma, lung)
DCC	**DCC**—**D**eleted in **C**olorecta **C**ancer	Colorectal cancer
SMAD4 (DPC4)	**DPC**—**D**eleted in **P**ancreatic **C**ancer	Pancreatic cancer, colorectal cancer
MEN1	**MEN**in	**M**ultiple **E**ndocrine **N**eoplasia type 1
NF1	Neurofibromin (Ras GTPase activating protein)	**N**euro**F**ibromatosis type **1**
NF2	Merlin (schwannomin) protein	**N**euro**F**ibromatosis type **2**
PTEN	Negative regulator of PI3k/AKT pathway	**P**rostate, breas**T**, and **EN**dometrial cancers
RB1	Inhibits E2F; blocks G_1 → S phase	**R**etino**b**lastoma, osteosarcoma (**b**one cancer)
TP53	p53, activates p21, blocks G_1 → S phase	Most cancers, Li-Fraumeni syndrome (multiple malignancies at early age, aka, **SBLA** syndrome: **S**arcoma, **B**reast, **L**eukemia, **A**drenal gland)
TSC1	Hamartin protein	Tuberous sclerosis
TSC2	Tuberin ("2berin")	Tuberous sclerosis
VHL	Inhibits hypoxia-inducible factor 1a	von Hippel-Lindau disease
WT1	Urogenital development transcription factor	**W**ilms **T**umor (nephroblastoma)

Carcinogens

TOXIN	EXPOSURE	ORGAN	IMPACT
Aflatoxins (*Aspergillus*)	Stored grains and nuts	Liver	Hepatocellular carcinoma
Alkylating agents	Oncologic chemotherapy	Blood	Leukemia/lymphoma
Aromatic amines (eg, benzidine, 2-naphthylamine)	Textile industry (dyes), tobacco smoke (2-naphthylamine)	Bladder	Transitional cell carcinoma
Arsenic	Herbicides (vineyard workers), metal smelting, wood preservation	Liver Lung Skin	Hepatic angiosarcoma Lung cancer Squamous cell carcinoma
Asbestos	Old roofing material, shipyard workers	Lung	Bronchogenic carcinoma > mesothelioma
Tobacco smoke		Bladder Cervix Esophagus Kidney Larynx Lung Oropharynx Pancreas	Transitional cell carcinoma Squamous cell carcinoma Squamous cell carcinoma/adenocarcinoma Renal cell carcinoma Squamous cell carcinoma Squamous cell and small cell carcinoma Oropharyngeal cancer Pancreatic adenocarcinoma
Ethanol		Esophagus Liver Breast	Squamous cell carcinoma Hepatocellular carcinoma Breast cancer
Ionizing radiation		Thyroid	Papillary thyroid carcinoma, leukemias
Nickel, chromium, beryllium, silica	Occupational exposure	Lung	Lung cancer
Nitrosamines	Smoked foods	Stomach	Gastric cancer (intestinal type)
Radon	Byproduct of uranium decay, accumulates in basements	Lung	Lung cancer (2nd leading cause after tobacco smoke)
Vinyl chloride	Used to make PVC pipes (plumbers)	LiVer	Hepatic angiosarcoma

Oncogenic microbes

Microbe	Associated cancer
EBV	Burkitt lymphoma, Hodgkin lymphoma, nasopharyngeal carcinoma, 1° CNS lymphoma (in immunocompromised patients)
HBV, HCV	Hepatocellular carcinoma
HHV-8	Kaposi sarcoma
HPV (usually types 16, 18)	Cervical and penile/anal carcinoma, head and neck cancer
H pylori	Gastric adenocarcinoma and MALT lymphoma
HTLV-1	Adult T-cell Leukemia/Lymphoma
Liver fluke (*Clonorchis sinensis*)	Cholangiocarcinoma
Schistosoma haematobium	Squamous cell bladder cancer

Serum tumor markers

Tumor markers should not be used as the 1° tool for cancer diagnosis or screening. They may be used to monitor tumor recurrence and response to therapy, but definitive diagnosis is made via biopsy. Some can be associated with non-neoplastic conditions.

MARKER	IMPORTANT ASSOCIATIONS	NOTES
Alkaline phosphatase	Metastases to bone or liver, Paget disease of bone, seminoma (placental ALP).	Exclude hepatic origin by checking LFTs and GGT levels.
α-fetoprotein	Hepatocellular carcinoma, endodermal sinus (yolk sac) tumor, mixed germ cell tumor, ataxia-telangiectasia, neural tube defects.	Normally made by fetus. Transiently elevated in pregnancy. High levels associated with neural tube and abdominal wall defects, low levels associated with Down syndrome.
hCG	Hydatidiform moles and Choriocarcinomas (Gestational trophoblastic disease), testicular cancer, mixed germ cell tumor.	Produced by syncytiotrophoblasts of the placenta.
CA 15-3/CA 27-29	Breast cancer.	
CA 19-9	Pancreatic adenocarcinoma.	
CA 125	Ovarian cancer.	
Calcitonin	Medullary thyroid carcinoma (alone and in MEN2A, MEN2B).	Calci2nin.
CEA	Colorectal and pancreatic cancers. Minor associations: gastric, breast, and medullary thyroid carcinomas.	CarcinoEmbryonic Antigen. Very nonspecific.
Chromogranin	Neuroendocrine tumors.	
LDH	Testicular germ cell tumors, ovarian dysgerminoma, other cancers.	Can be used as an indicator of tumor burden.
Neuron-specific enolase	Neuroendocrine tumors (eg, small cell lung cancer, carcinoid tumor, neuroblastoma).	
PSA	Prostate cancer.	Prostate-Specific Antigen. Also elevated in BPH and prostatitis. Questionable risk/benefit for screening. Marker for recurrence after treatment.

Important immunohistochemical stains

Determine primary site of origin for metastatic tumors and characterize tumors that are difficult to classify. Can have prognostic and predictive value.

STAIN	TARGET	TUMORS IDENTIFIED
Chromogranin and synaptophysin	Neuroendocrine cells	Small cell carcinoma of the lung, carcinoid tumor, neuroblastoma
Cytokeratin	Epithelial cells	Epithelial tumors (eg, squamous cell carcinoma)
Desmin	Muscle	Muscle tumors (eg, rhabdomyosarcoma)
GFAP	NeuroGlia (eg, astrocytes, Schwann cells, oligodendrocytes)	Astrocytoma, Glioblastoma
Neurofilament	Neurons	Neuronal tumors (eg, neuroblastoma)
PSA	Prostatic epithelium	Prostate cancer
S-100	Neural crest cells	Melanoma, schwannoma, Langerhans cell histiocytosis
TRAP	Tartrate-resistant acid phosphatase	Hairy cell leukemia
Vimentin	Mesenchymal tissue (eg, fibroblasts, endothelial cells, macrophages)	Mesenchymal tumors (eg, sarcoma), but also many other tumors (eg, endometrial carcinoma, renal cell carcinoma, meningioma)

P-glycoprotein

ATP-dependent efflux pump also known as multidrug resistance protein 1 (MDR1). Classically seen in adrenocortical carcinoma but also expressed by other cancer cells (eg, colon, liver). Used to pump out toxins, including chemotherapeutic agents (one mechanism of ↓ responsiveness or resistance to chemotherapy over time).

Psammoma bodies

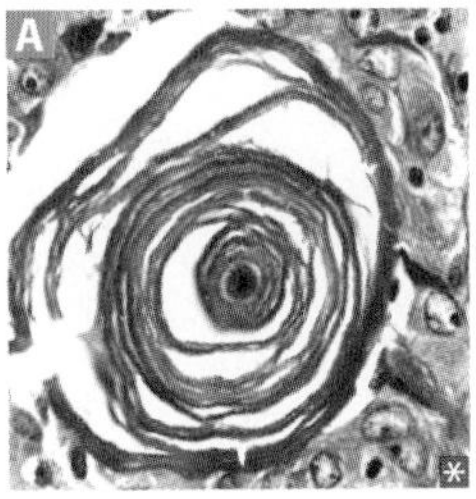

Laminated, concentric spherules with dystrophic calcification A, PSAMMOMaS bodies are seen in:

- Papillary carcinoma of thyroid
- Somatostatinoma
- Adrenals (calcifying fibrous pseudotumor)
- Meningioma
- Malignant Mesothelioma
- Ovarian serous carcinoma
- Prolactinoma (Milk)
- Serous endometrial carcinoma

Cachexia

Weight loss, muscle atrophy, and fatigue that occur in chronic disease (eg, cancer, AIDS, heart failure, COPD). Mediated by TNF-α, IFN-γ, IL-1, and IL-6.

Paraneoplastic syndromes

MANIFESTATION	DESCRIPTION/MECHANISM	MOST COMMONLY ASSOCIATED TUMOR(S)
Musculoskeletal and cutaneous		
Dermatomyositis	Progressive proximal muscle weakness, Gottron papules, heliotrope rash	Adenocarcinomas, especially ovarian
Acanthosis nigricans	Hyperpigmented velvety plaques in axilla and neck	Gastric adenocarcinoma and other visceral malignancies
Sign of Leser-Trélat	Sudden onset of multiple seborrheic keratoses	GI adenocarcinomas and other visceral malignancies
Hypertrophic osteoarthropathy	Abnormal proliferation of skin and bone at distal extremities → clubbing, arthralgia, joint effusions, periostosis of tubular bones	Adenocarcinoma of the lung
Endocrine		
Hypercalcemia	PTHrP	SCa^{2+}mous cell carcinomas of lung, head, and neck; renal, bladder, breast, and ovarian carcinomas
	↑ 1,25-$(OH)_2$ vitamin D_3 (calcitriol)	Lymphoma
Cushing syndrome	↑ ACTH	Small cell lung cancer
Hyponatremia (SIADH)	↑ ADH	
Hematologic		
Polycythemia	↑ Erythropoietin Paraneoplastic rise to High hematocrit levels	Pheochromocytoma, renal cell carcinoma, HCC, hemangioblastoma, leiomyoma
Pure red cell aplasia	Anemia with low reticulocytes	Thymoma
Good syndrome	Hypogammaglobulinemia	
Trousseau syndrome	Migratory superficial thrombophlebitis	Adenocarcinomas, especially pancreatic
Nonbacterial thrombotic (marantic) endocarditis	Deposition of sterile platelet thrombi on heart valves	
Neuromuscular		
Anti-NMDA receptor encephalitis	Psychiatric disturbance, memory deficits, seizures, dyskinesias, autonomic instability, language dysfunction	Ovarian teratoma
Opsoclonus-myoclonus ataxia syndrome	"Dancing eyes, dancing feet"	Neuroblastoma (children), small cell lung cancer (adults)
Paraneoplastic cerebellar degeneration	Antibodies against antigens in Purkinje cells	Small cell lung cancer (anti-Hu), gynecologic and breast cancers (anti-Yo), and Hodgkin lymphoma (anti-Tr)
Paraneoplastic encephalomyelitis	Antibodies against Hu antigens in neurons	Small cell lung cancer
Lambert-Eaton myasthenic syndrome	Antibodies against presynaptic (P/Q-type) Ca^{2+} channels at NMJ	
Myasthenia gravis	Antibodies against postsynaptic ACh receptors at NMJ	Thymoma

▶ NOTES

HIGH-YIELD PRINCIPLES IN

Pharmacology

"Cure sometimes, treat often, and comfort always."

—Hippocrates

"One pill makes you larger, and one pill makes you small."

—Jefferson Airplane, *White Rabbit*

"For the chemistry that works on one patient may not work for the next, because even medicine has its own conditions."

—Suzy Kassem

"I wondher why ye can always read a doctor's bill an' ye niver can read his purscription."

—Finley Peter Dunne

"Love is the drug I'm thinking of."

—The Bryan Ferry Orchestra

Preparation for pharmacology questions is not as straightforward as in years past. The big change is that the USMLE Step 1 is moving away from pharmacotherapeutics. That means you will generally not be required to identify medications indicated for a specific condition. You still need to know all the mechanisms and important adverse effects of key drugs and their major variants. Obscure derivatives are low-yield. Learn their classic and distinguishing toxicities as well as major drug-drug interactions.

Reviewing associated biochemistry, physiology, and microbiology concepts can be useful while studying pharmacology. The exam has a strong emphasis on ANS, CNS, antimicrobial, and cardiovascular agents as well as on NSAIDs, which are covered throughout the text. Specific drug dosages or trade names are generally not testable. The exam may use graphs to test various pharmacology content, so make sure you are comfortable interpreting them.

▶ PHARMACOLOGY—PHARMACOKINETICS AND PHARMACODYNAMICS

Enzyme kinetics

Michaelis-Menten kinetics

K_m is inversely related to the affinity of the enzyme for its substrate.

V_{max} is directly proportional to the enzyme concentration.

Most enzymatic reactions follow a hyperbolic curve (ie, Michaelis-Menten kinetics); however, enzymatic reactions that exhibit a sigmoid curve usually indicate cooperative kinetics (eg, hemoglobin).

[S] = concentration of substrate; V = velocity.

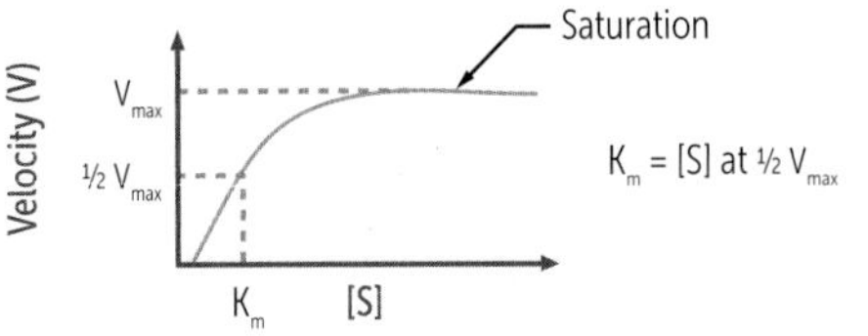

Effects of enzyme inhibition

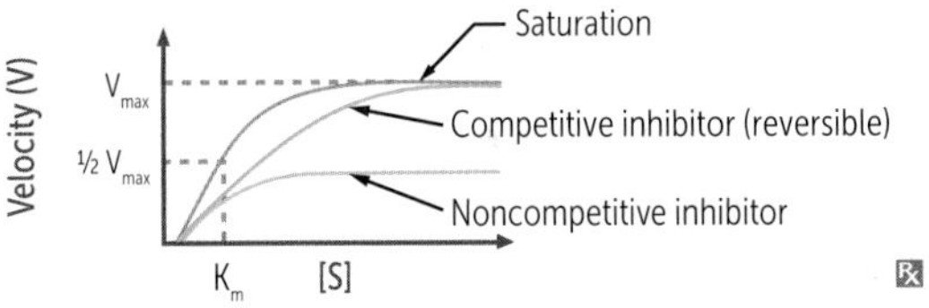

Lineweaver-Burk plot

The closer to 0 on the Y-axis, the higher the V_{max}.

The closer to 0 on the X-axis, the higher the K_m.

The higher the K_m, the lower the affinity.

Competitive inhibitors cross each other, whereas noncompetitive inhibitors do not.

Kompetitive inhibitors increase K_m.

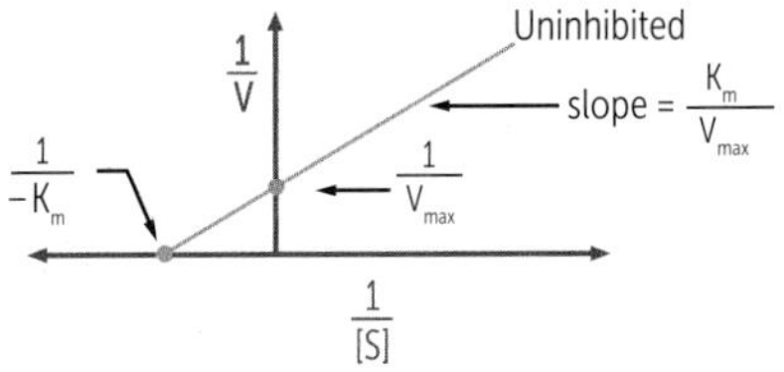

Effects of enzyme inhibition

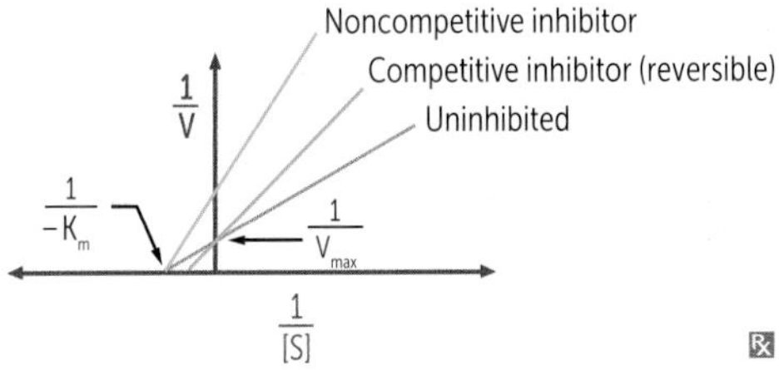

	Competitive inhibitors, reversible	Competitive inhibitors, irreversible	Noncompetitive inhibitors
Resemble substrate	Yes	Yes	No
Overcome by ↑ [S]	Yes	No	No
Bind active site	Yes	Yes	No
Effect on V_{max}	Unchanged	↓	↓
Effect on K_m	↑	Unchanged	Unchanged
Pharmacodynamics	↓ potency	↓ efficacy	↓ efficacy

Pharmacokinetics

Bioavailability (F)

Fraction of administered drug reaching systemic circulation unchanged. For an IV dose, F = 100%.

Orally: F typically < 100% due to incomplete absorption and first-pass metabolism. Can be calculated from the area under the curve in a plot of plasma concentration over time.

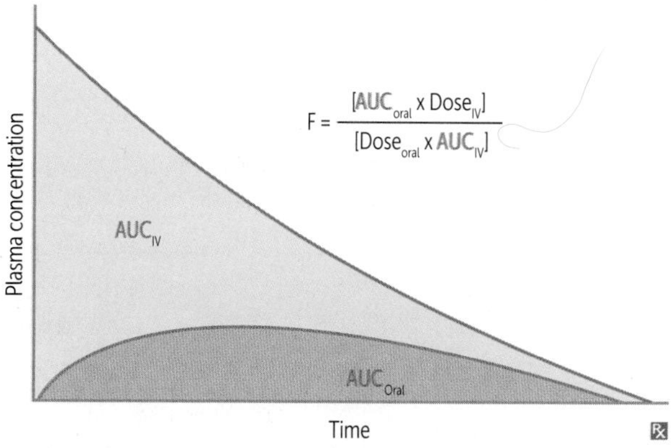
F = [AUC_oral x Dose_IV] / [Dose_oral x AUC_IV]
Plasma concentration
AUC_IV
AUC_Oral
Time

Volume of distribution (V_d)

Theoretical volume occupied by the total amount of drug in the body relative to its plasma concentration. Apparent V_d of plasma protein–bound drugs can be altered by liver and kidney disease (↓ protein binding, ↑ V_d). Drugs may distribute in more than one compartment. Hemodialysis is most effective for drugs with a low V_d.

$$V_d = \frac{\text{amount of drug in the body}}{\text{plasma drug concentration}}$$

V_d	COMPARTMENT	DRUG TYPES
Low	Intravascular	Large/charged molecules; plasma protein bound
Medium	ECF	Small hydrophilic molecules
High	All tissues including fat	Small lipophilic molecules, especially if bound to tissue protein

Clearance (CL)

The volume of plasma cleared of drug per unit time. Clearance may be impaired with defects in cardiac, hepatic, or renal function.

$$CL = \frac{\text{rate of elimination of drug}}{\text{plasma drug concentration}} = V_d \times K_e \text{ (elimination constant)}$$

Half-life ($t_{1/2}$)

The time required to change the amount of drug in the body by ½ during elimination.

Steady state is a dynamic equilibrium in which drug concentration stays constant (ie, rate of drug elimination = rate of drug ingestion).

In first-order kinetics, a drug infused at a constant rate takes 4–5 half-lives to reach steady state. It takes 3.3 half-lives to reach 90% of the steady-state level.

$$t_{1/2} = \frac{0.7 \times V_d}{CL} \text{ in first-order elimination}$$

# of half-lives	1	2	3	4
% remaining	50%	25%	12.5%	6.25%

Dosage calculations

$$\text{Loading dose} = \frac{C_p \times V_d}{F}$$

$$\text{Maintenance dose} = \frac{C_p \times CL \times \tau}{F}$$

C_{ss} = target plasma concentration at steady state

τ = dosage interval (time between doses), if not administered continuously

In renal or liver disease, maintenance dose ↓ and loading dose is usually unchanged.

Time to steady state depends primarily on $t_{1/2}$ and is independent of dose and dosing frequency.

Drug metabolism Geriatric patients lose phase I first. Patients who are slow acetylators have ↑ side effects from certain drugs because of ↓ rate of metabolism (eg, isoniazid).

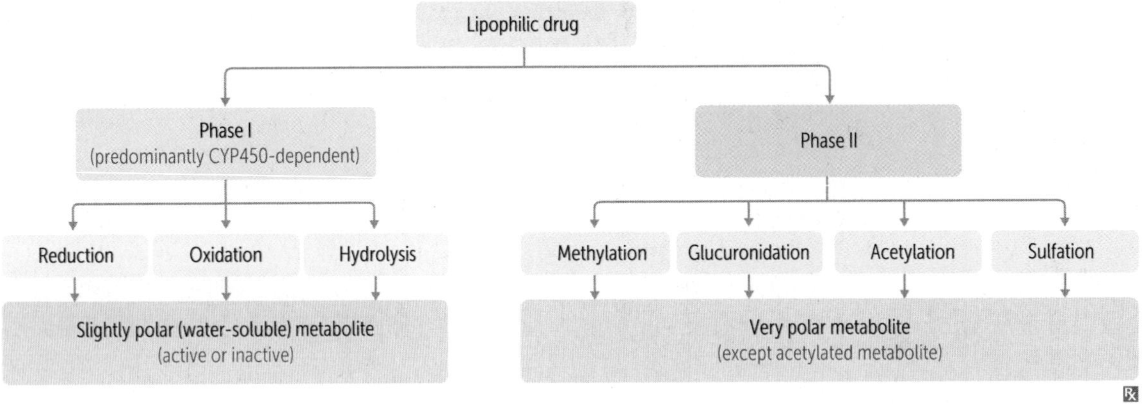

Elimination of drugs

Zero-order elimination	Rate of elimination is constant regardless of C_p (ie, constant **amount** of drug eliminated per unit time). C_p ↓ linearly with time. Examples of drugs—**P**henytoin, **E**thanol, and **A**spirin (at high or toxic concentrations).	Capacity-limited elimination. **PEA** (a pea is round, shaped like the "0" in **zero**-order).
First-order elimination	Rate of first-order elimination is directly proportional to the drug concentration (ie, constant **fraction** of drug eliminated per unit time). C_p ↓ exponentially with time. Applies to most drugs.	**F**low-dependent elimination.

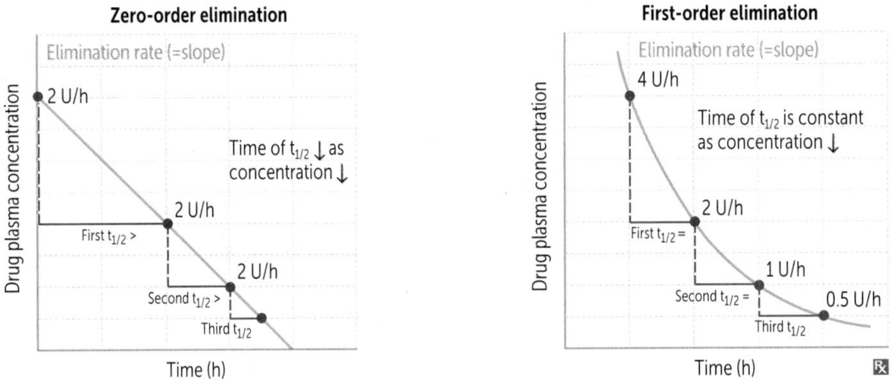

Urine pH and drug elimination

Ionized species are trapped in urine and cleared quickly. Neutral forms can be reabsorbed.

Weak acids

Examples: phenobarbital, methotrexate, aspirin (salicylates). Trapped in basic environments. Treat overdose with sodium bicarbonate to alkalinize urine.

$$\underset{\text{(lipid soluble)}}{RCOOH} \rightleftharpoons \underset{\text{(trapped)}}{RCOO^- + H^+}$$

Weak bases

Examples: TCAs, amphetamines. Trapped in acidic environments. Treat overdose with ammonium chloride to acidify urine.

$$\underset{\text{(trapped)}}{RNH_3^+} \rightleftharpoons \underset{\text{(lipid soluble)}}{RNH_2 + H^+}$$

TCA toxicity is generally treated with sodium bicarbonate to overcome the sodium channel-blocking activity of TCAs, but not for accelerating drug elimination.

pKa

pH at which drugs (weak acid or base) are 50% ionized and 50% nonionized. The pKa represents the strength of the weak acid or base.

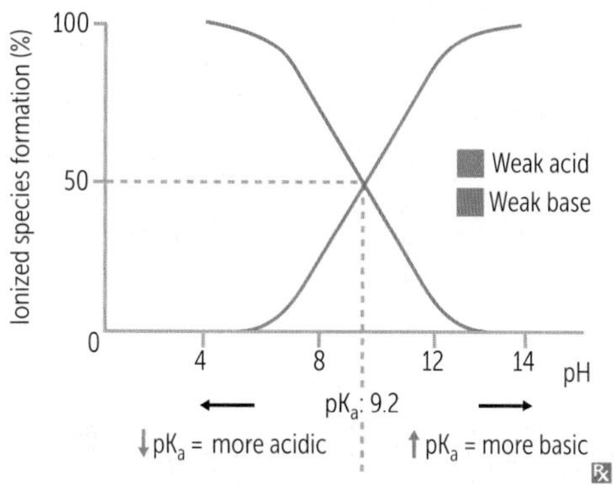

Efficacy vs potency

Efficacy

Maximal effect a drug can produce. Represented by the y-value (V_{max}). ↑ y-value = ↑ V_{max} = ↑ efficacy. Unrelated to potency (ie, efficacious drugs can have high or low potency). Partial agonists have less efficacy than full agonists.

RELATIVE EFFICACY

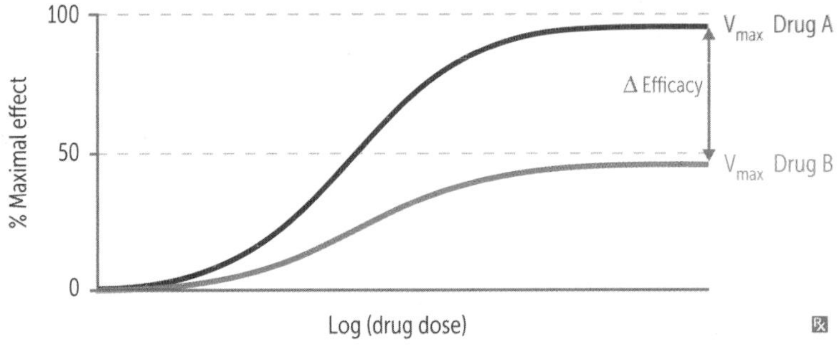

Potency

Amount of drug needed for a given effect. Represented by the x-value (EC_{50}). Left shifting = ↓ EC_{50} = ↑ potency = ↓ drug needed. Unrelated to efficacy (ie, potent drugs can have high or low efficacy).

RELATIVE POTENCY

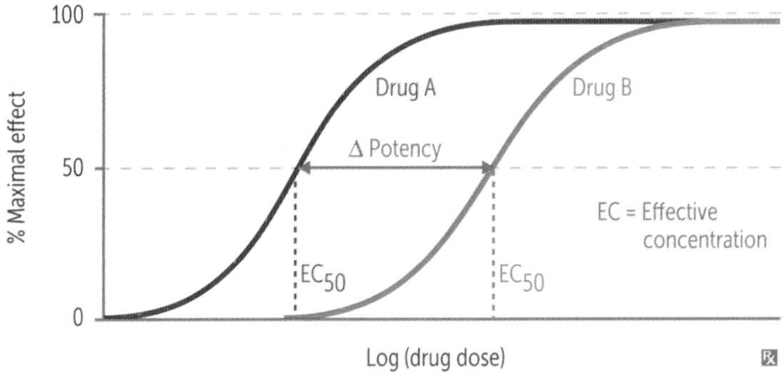

Receptor binding

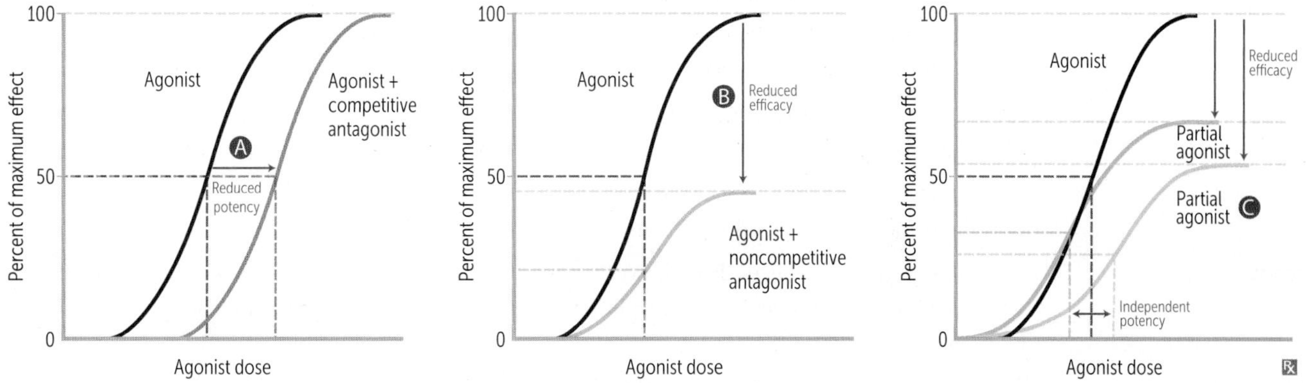

AGONIST WITH	POTENCY	EFFICACY	REMARKS	EXAMPLE
A Competitive antagonist	↓	No change	**Can** be overcome by ↑ agonist concentration	Diazepam (agonist) + flumazenil (competitive antagonist) on $GABA_A$ receptor.
B Noncompetitive antagonist	No change	↓	**Cannot** be overcome by ↑ agonist concentration	Norepinephrine (agonist) + phenoxybenzamine (noncompetitive antagonist) on α-receptors.
C Partial agonist (alone)	Independent	↓	Acts at same site as full agonist	Morphine (full agonist) vs buprenorphine (partial agonist) at opioid μ-receptors.

Therapeutic index

Measurement of drug safety.

$$\frac{TD_{50}}{ED_{50}} = \frac{\text{median toxic dose}}{\text{median effective dose}}$$

Therapeutic window—range of drug concentrations that can safely and effectively treat disease.

TITE: Therapeutic Index = TD_{50} / ED_{50}.

Safer drugs have higher TI values. Drugs with lower TI values frequently require monitoring (eg, warfarin, theophylline, digoxin, antiepileptic drugs, lithium; Warning! These drugs are lethal!).

LD_{50} (lethal median dose) often replaces TD_{50} in animal studies.

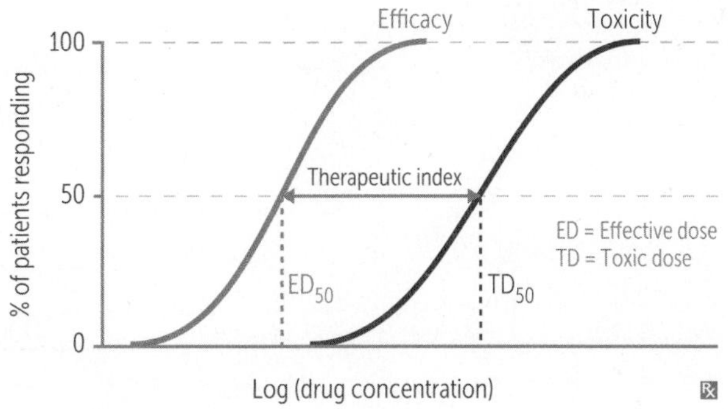

Drug effect modifications

TERM	DEFINITION	EXAMPLE
Additive	Effect of substances A and B together is equal to the sum of their individual effects	Aspirin and acetaminophen "2 + 2 = 4"
Permissive	Presence of substance A is required for the full effects of substance B	Cortisol on catecholamine responsiveness
Synergistic	Effect of substances A and B together is greater than the sum of their individual effects	Clopidogrel with aspirin "2 + 2 > 4"
Potentiation	Similar to synergism, but drug B with no therapeutic action enhances the therapeutic action of drug A	Carbidopa only blocks enzyme to prevent peripheral conversion of levodopa "2 + 0 > 2"
Antagonistic	Effect of substances A and B together is less than the sum of their individual effects	Ethanol antidote for methanol toxicity "2 + 2 < 4"
Tachyphylactic	Acute decrease in response to a drug after initial/repeated administration	Hydralazine, nitrates, niacin, phenylephrine, LSD, MDMA

▶ PHARMACOLOGY—AUTONOMIC DRUGS

Autonomic receptors

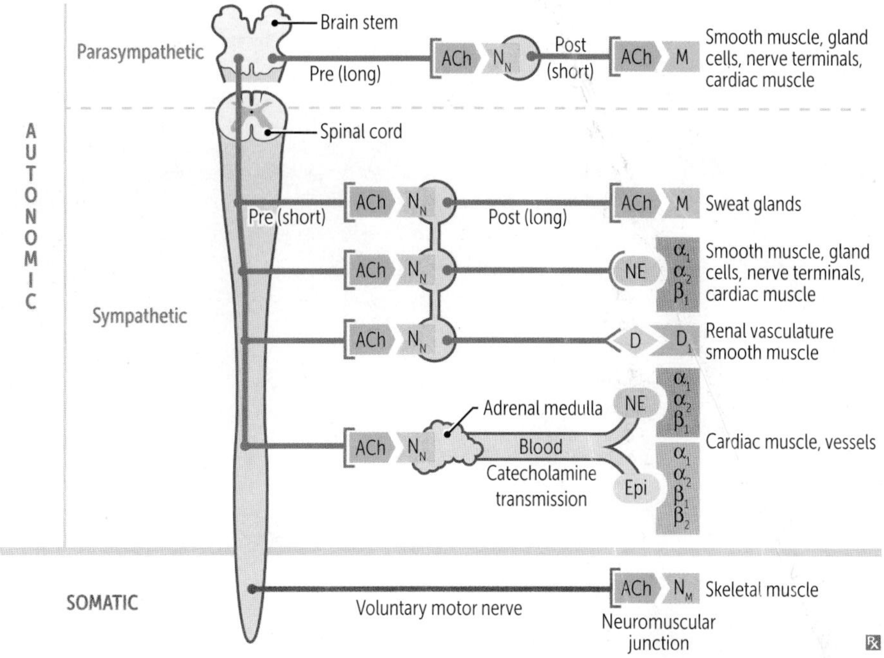

Pelvic splanchnic nerves and CNs III, VII, IX and X are part of the parasympathetic nervous system.
Adrenal medulla is directly innervated by preganglionic sympathetic fibers.
Sweat glands are part of the sympathetic pathway but are innervated by cholinergic fibers (sympathetic nervous system results in a "chold" sweat).

Acetylcholine receptors

Nicotinic ACh receptors are ligand-gated channels allowing efflux of K^+ and influx of Na^+ and in some cases Ca^{2+}. Two subtypes: N_N (found in autonomic ganglia, adrenal medulla) and N_M (found in neuromuscular junction of skeletal muscle).
Muscarinic ACh receptors are G-protein–coupled receptors that usually act through 2nd messengers. 5 subtypes: M_{1-5} found in heart, smooth muscle, brain, exocrine glands, and on sweat glands (cholinergic sympathetic).

Micturition control

Micturition center in pons regulates involuntary bladder function via coordination of sympathetic and parasympathetic nervous systems.

- ⊕ sympathetic → ↑ urinary retention.
- ⊕ parasympathetic → ↑ urine voiding. Some autonomic drugs act on smooth muscle receptors to treat bladder dysfunction.

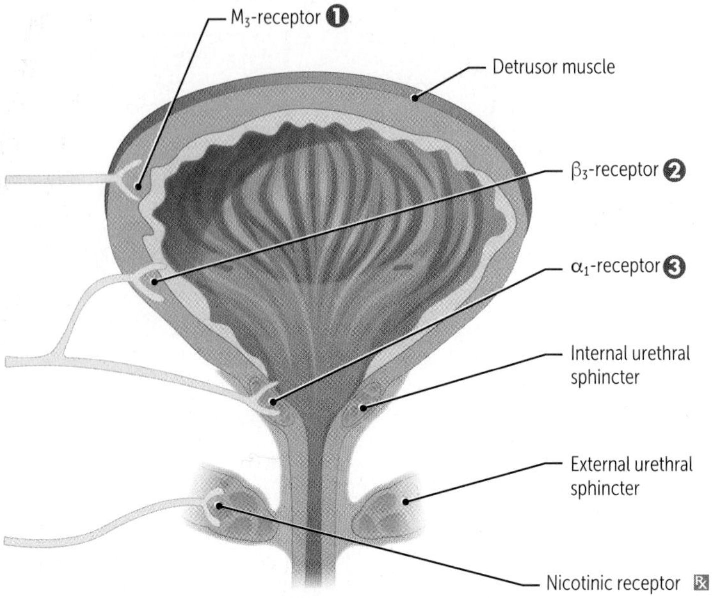

DRUGS	MECHANISM	APPLICATIONS
❶ **Muscarinic antagonists** (eg, oxybutynin)	⊖ M_3 receptor → relaxation of detrusor smooth muscle → ↓ detrusor overactivity	Urgency incontinence
❶ **Muscarinic agonists** (eg, bethanechol)	⊕ M_3 receptor → contraction of detrusor smooth muscle → ↑ bladder emptying	Urinary retention
❷ **Sympathomimetics** (eg, mirabegron)	⊕ β_3 receptor → relaxation of detrusor smooth muscle → ↑ bladder capacity	Urgency incontinence
❸ **α_1-blockers** (eg, tamsulosin)	⊖ α_1-receptor → relaxation of smooth muscle (bladder neck, prostate) → ↓ urinary obstruction	BPH

Tissue distribution of adrenergic receptors

	α_1 receptors	α_2 receptors	β_1 receptors	β_2 receptors	β_3 receptors
Cardiac muscle	–	–	+++	+	+
Skeletal muscle	–	–	–	++	–
Vascular smooth muscle	+++	+	–	++	+
Bronchial smooth muscle	–	–	–	++	–
Liver	+	–	–	+++	–
Adipose tissue	+	+	+	–	++
CNS	++	++	++	++	–
Bladder neck/prostate	+++	+	–	–	+++

G-protein–linked second messengers

RECEPTOR	G-PROTEIN CLASS	MAJOR FUNCTIONS
Adrenergic		
α_1	q	↑ vascular smooth muscle contraction, ↑ pupillary dilator muscle contraction (mydriasis), ↑ intestinal and bladder sphincter muscle contraction
α_2	i	↓ sympathetic (adrenergic) outflow, ↓ insulin release, ↓ lipolysis, ↑ platelet aggregation, ↓ aqueous humor production
β_1	s	↑ heart rate, ↑ contractility (**one** heart), ↑ renin release, ↑ lipolysis
β_2	s	Vasodilation, bronchodilation (**two** lungs), ↑ lipolysis, ↑ insulin release, ↑ glycogenolysis, ↓ uterine tone (tocolysis), ↑ aqueous humor production, ↑ cellular K^+ uptake
β_3	s	↑ lipolysis, ↑ thermogenesis in skeletal muscle, ↑ bladder relaxation
Cholinergic		
M_1	q	Mediates higher cognitive functions, stimulates enteric nervous system
M_2	i	↓ heart rate and contractility of atria
M_3	q	↑ exocrine gland secretions (eg, lacrimal, sweat, salivary, gastric acid), ↑ gut peristalsis, ↑ bladder contraction, bronchoconstriction, ↑ pupillary sphincter muscle contraction (miosis), ciliary muscle contraction (accommodation), ↑ insulin release, endothelium-mediated vasodilation
Dopamine		
D_1	s	Relaxes renal vascular smooth muscle, activates direct pathway of striatum
D_2	i	Modulates transmitter release, especially in brain, inhibits indirect pathway of striatum
Histamine		
H_1	q	↑ nasal and bronchial mucus production, ↑ vascular permeability, bronchoconstriction, pruritus, pain
H_2	s	↑ gastric acid secretion
Vasopressin		
V_1	q	↑ vascular smooth muscle contraction
V_2	s	↑ H_2O permeability and reabsorption via upregulating aquaporin-2 in collecting **two**bules (tubules) of kidney, ↑ release of vWF

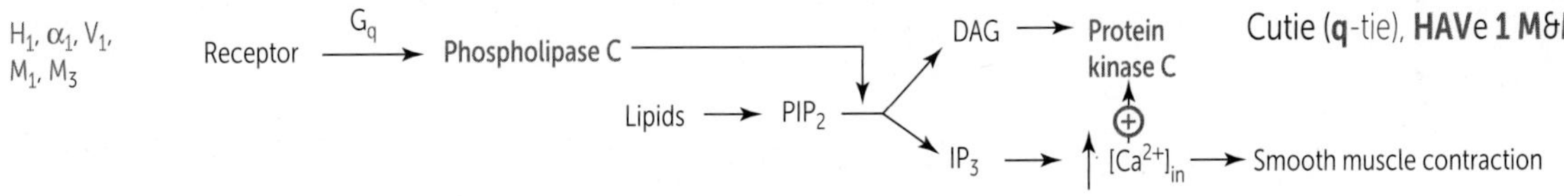
H_1, α_1, V_1, M_1, M_3
Receptor
G_q
Phospholipase C
Lipids
PIP_2
DAG
Protein kinase C
IP_3
↑ $[Ca^{2+}]_{in}$
Smooth muscle contraction

Cutie (**q**-tie), **HAVe 1 M&M!**

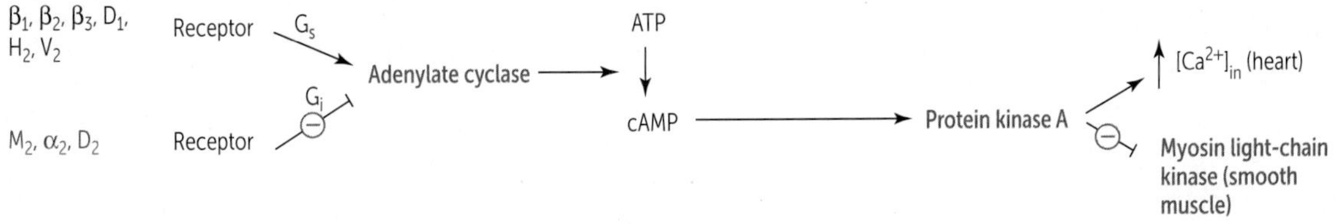
β_1, β_2, β_3, D_1, H_2, V_2
Receptor
G_s
M_2, α_2, D_2
Receptor
G_i
Adenylate cyclase
ATP
cAMP
Protein kinase A
↑ $[Ca^{2+}]_{in}$ (heart)
Myosin light-chain kinase (smooth muscle)

People who are **too (2) MAD** inhibit themselves.

Autonomic drugs

Release of norepinephrine from a sympathetic nerve ending is modulated by NE itself, acting on presynaptic α_2-autoreceptors → negative feedback.

Amphetamines use the NE transporter (NET) to enter the presynaptic terminal, where they utilize the vesicular monoamine transporter (VMAT) to enter neurosecretory vesicles. This displaces NE from the vesicles. Once NE reaches a concentration threshold within the presynaptic terminal, the action of NET is reversed, and NE is expelled into the synaptic cleft, contributing to the characteristics and effects of ↑ NE observed in patients taking amphetamines.

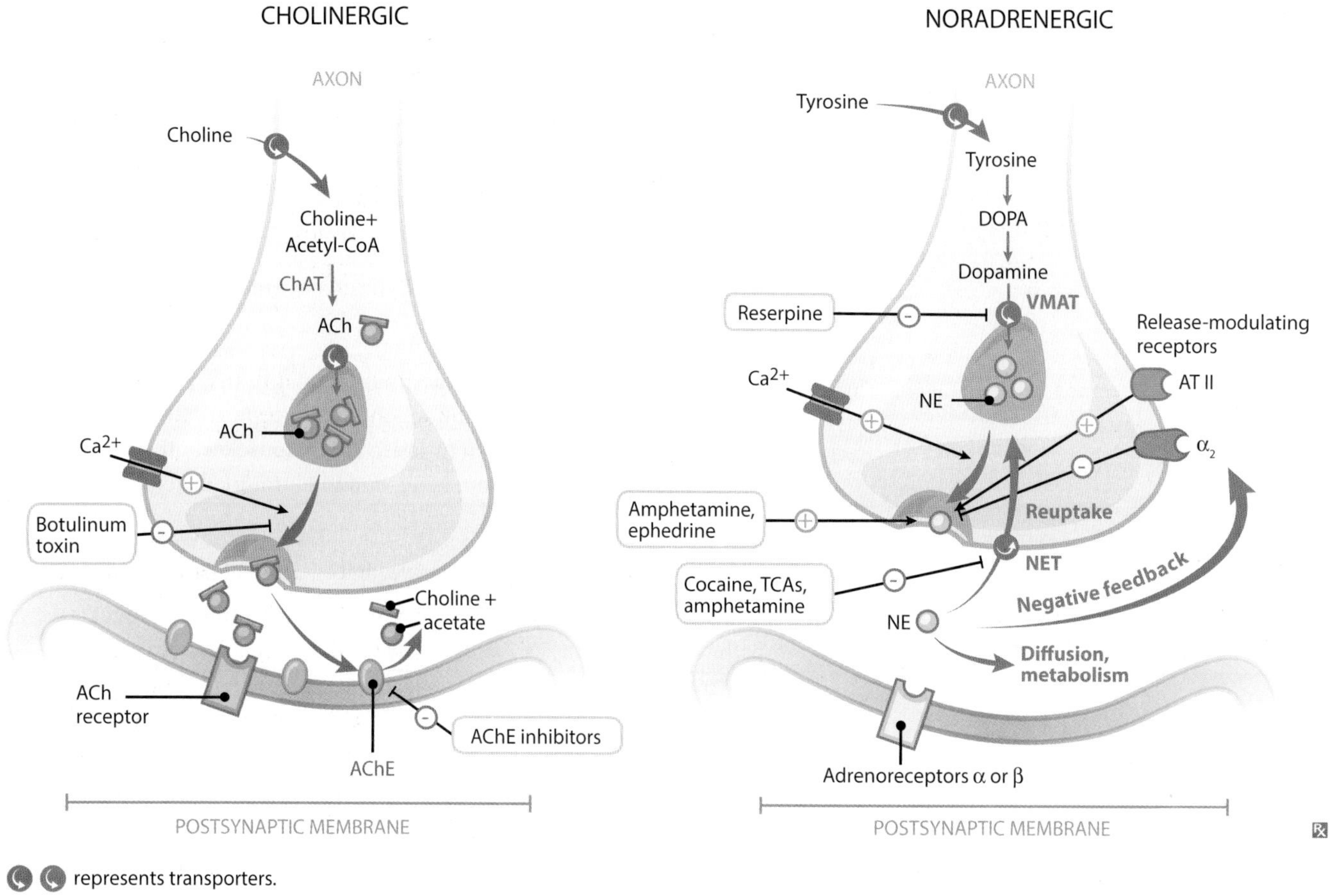

Cholinomimetic agents Watch for exacerbation of COPD, asthma, and peptic ulcers in susceptible patients.

DRUG	ACTION	APPLICATIONS
Direct agonists		
Bethanechol	Activates bladder smooth muscle; resistant to AChE. No nicotinic activity. "**Bethan**y, **call** me to activate your bladder."	Urinary retention.
Carbachol	**Carb**on copy of acetyl**chol**ine (but resistant to AChE).	Constricts pupil and relieves intraocular pressure in open-angle glaucoma.
Methacholine	Stimulates muscarinic receptors in airway when inhaled.	Challenge test for diagnosis of asthma.
Pilocarpine	Contracts ciliary muscle of eye (open-angle glaucoma), pupillary sphincter (closed-angle glaucoma); resistant to AChE, can cross blood-brain barrier (tertiary amine). "You cry, drool, and sweat on your '**pilo**w.'"	Potent stimulator of sweat, tears, and saliva Open-angle and closed-angle glaucoma, xerostomia (Sjögren syndrome).
Indirect agonists (anticholinesterases)		
Donepezil, rivastigmine, galantamine	↑ ACh.	1st line for Alzheimer disease (**Dona Riva** forgot to dance at the **gala**).
Edrophonium	↑ ACh.	Historically used to diagnose myasthenia gravis; replaced by anti-AChR Ab (anti-acetylcholine receptor antibody) test.
Neostigmine	↑ ACh. **Neo** CNS = **no** CNS penetration due to positive charge (quaternary amine).	Postoperative and neurogenic ileus and urinary retention, myasthenia gravis, reversal of neuromuscular junction blockade (postoperative).
Pyridostigmine	↑ ACh; ↑ muscle strength. Used with glycopyrrolate, hyoscyamine, or propantheline to control pyridostigmine side effects. **Pyrid**ostigmine gets **rid** of **m**yasthenia **g**ravis.	Myasthenia gravis (long acting); does not penetrate CNS (quaternary amine).
Physostigmine	↑ ACh. **Ph**reely (freely) crosses blood-brain barrier as not charged → CNS (tertiary amine).	Antidote for anticholinergic toxicity; **phy**sostigmine "**phy**xes" atropine overdose.

Anticholinesterase poisoning Often due to organophosphates (eg, parathion) that irreversibly inhibit AChE. Organophosphates commonly used as insecticides; poisoning usually seen in farmers.

Muscarinic effects	**D**iarrhea, **U**rination, **M**iosis, **B**ronchospasm, **B**radycardia, **E**mesis, **L**acrimation, **S**weating, **S**alivation.	DUMBBELSS. Reversed by atropine, a competitive inhibitor. Atropine can cross BBB to relieve CNS symptoms.
Nicotinic effects	Neuromuscular blockade (mechanism similar to succinylcholine).	Reversed by pralidoxime, regenerates AChE via dephosphorylation if given early. Pralidoxime (quaternary amine) does not readily cross BBB.
CNS effects	Respiratory depression, lethargy, seizures, coma.	

Muscarinic antagonists

DRUGS	ORGAN SYSTEMS	APPLICATIONS
Atropine, homatropine, tropicamide	Eye	Produce mydriasis and cycloplegia
Benztropine, trihexyphenidyl	CNS	**Park**inson disease ("**park** my **Benz**") Acute dystonia
Glycopyrrolate	GI, respiratory	Parenteral: preoperative use to reduce airway secretions Oral: reduces drooling, peptic ulcer
Hyoscyamine, dicyclomine	GI	Antispasmodics for irritable bowel syndrome
Ipratropium, tiotropium	Respiratory	COPD, asthma Duration: tiotropium > ipratropium
Solifenacin, Oxybutynin, Flavoxate, Tolterodine	Genitourinary	Reduce bladder spasms and urge urinary incontinence (overactive bladder) Make bladder **SOFT**
Scopolamine	CNS	Motion sickness

Atropine Muscarinic antagonist. Used to treat bradycardia and for ophthalmic applications.

ORGAN SYSTEM	ACTION	NOTES
Eye	↑ pupil dilation, cycloplegia	Blocks muscarinic effects (**DUMBBELSS**) of anticholinesterases, but not the nicotinic effects
Airway	Bronchodilation, ↓ secretions	
Stomach	↓ acid secretion	
Gut	↓ motility	
Bladder	↓ urgency in cystitis	
ADVERSE EFFECTS	↑ body **temperature** (due to ↓ sweating); ↑ **HR**; dry mouth; **dry, flushed skin**; **cycloplegia**; constipation; **disorientation** Can cause acute angle-closure glaucoma in elderly (due to mydriasis), **urinary retention** in men with prostatic hyperplasia, and hyperthermia in infants	Side effects: **Hot** as a hare **Fast** as a fiddle **Dry** as a bone **Red** as a beet **Blind** as a bat **Mad** as a hatter **Full** as a flask Jimson weed (*Datura*) → gardener's pupil (mydriasis due to plant alkaloids)

Sympathomimetics

DRUG	ACTION	HEMODYNAMIC CHANGES	APPLICATIONS
Direct sympathomimetics			
Albuterol, salmeterol, terbutaline	$\beta_2 > \beta_1$	↑ HR (little effect)	Albuterol for acute asthma/COPD. Salmeterol for serial (long-term) asthma/COPD. Terbutaline for acute bronchospasm in asthma and tocolysis.
Dobutamine	$\beta_1 > \beta_2, \alpha$	—/↓ BP, ↑ HR, ↑ CO	Cardiac stress testing, acute decompensated heart failure (HF) with cardiogenic shock (inotrope)
Dopamine	$D_1 = D_2 > \beta > \alpha$	↑ BP (high dose), ↑ HR, ↑ CO	Unstable bradycardia, shock; inotropic and chronotropic effects at lower doses via β effects; vasoconstriction at high doses via α effects.
Epinephrine	$\beta > \alpha$	↑ BP (high dose), ↑ HR, ↑ CO	Anaphylaxis, asthma, shock, open-angle glaucoma; α effects predominate at high doses. Stronger effect at β_2-receptor than norepinephrine.
Fenoldopam	D_1	↓ BP (vasodilation), ↑ HR, ↑ CO	Postoperative hypertension, hypertensive crisis. Vasodilator (coronary, peripheral, renal, and splanchnic). Promotes natriuresis. Can cause hypotension, tachycardia, flushing, headache.
Isoproterenol	$\beta_1 = \beta_2$	↓ BP (vasodilation), ↑ HR, ↑ CO	Electrophysiologic evaluation of tachyarrhythmias. Can worsen ischemia. Has negligible α effect.
Midodrine	α_1	↑ BP (vasoconstriction), ↓ HR, ↔/↓ CO	Autonomic insufficiency and postural hypotension. May exacerbate supine hypertension.
Mirabegron	β_3		Urinary urgency or incontinence or overactive bladder. Think "mirab3gron."
Norepinephrine	$\alpha_1 > \alpha_2 > \beta_1$	↑ BP, ↓ HR (reflex bradycardia from ↑ BP due to α_1 agonism outweighs direct β_1 chronotropic effect), —/↑ CO	Hypotension, septic shock.
Phenylephrine	$\alpha_1 > \alpha_2$	↑ BP (vasoconstriction), ↓ HR, —/↓ CO	Hypotension (vasoconstrictor), ocular procedures (mydriatic), rhinitis (decongestant), ischemic priapism.
Indirect sympathomimetics			
Amphetamine	Indirect general agonist, reuptake inhibitor, also releases stored catecholamines.		Narcolepsy, obesity, ADHD.
Cocaine	Indirect general agonist, reuptake inhibitor. Causes vasoconstriction and local anesthesia. Caution when giving β-blockers if cocaine intoxication is suspected (unopposed α_1 activation → ↑↑↑ BP, coronary vasospasm).		Causes mydriasis in eyes with intact sympathetic innervation → used to confirm Horner syndrome.
Ephedrine	Indirect general agonist, releases stored catecholamines.		Nasal decongestion (pseudoephedrine), urinary incontinence, hypotension.

Physiologic effects of sympathomimetics

NE ↑ systolic and diastolic pressures as a result of α_1-mediated vasoconstriction → ↑ mean arterial pressure → reflex bradycardia. However, isoproterenol (rarely used) has little α effect but causes β_2-mediated vasodilation, resulting in ↓ mean arterial pressure and ↑ heart rate through β_1 and reflex activity.

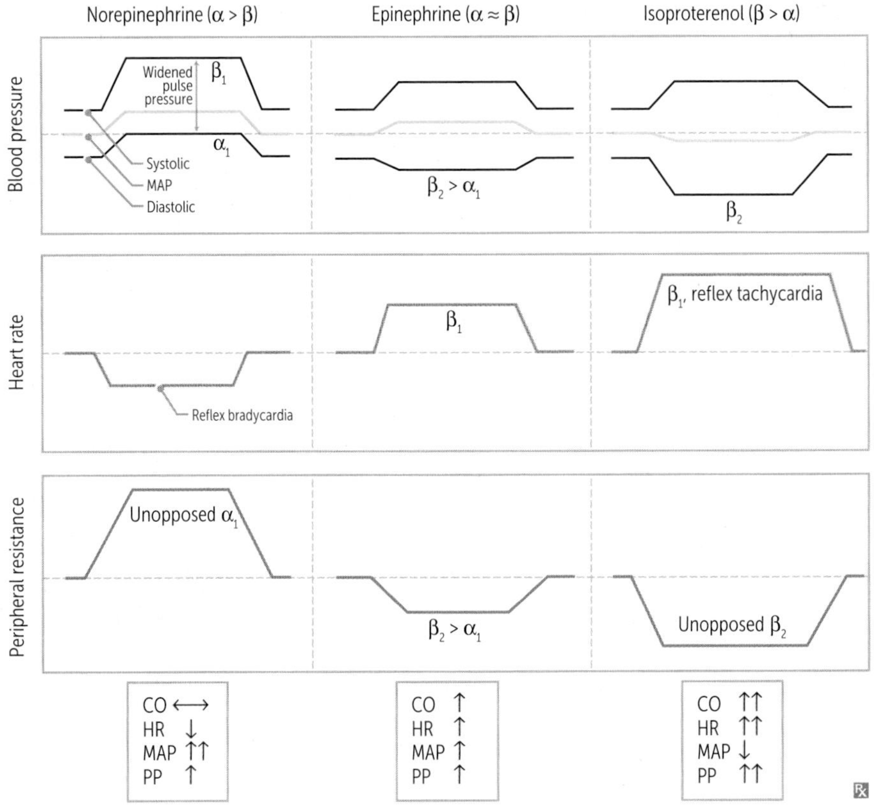

Sympatholytics (α_2-agonists)

DRUG	APPLICATIONS	ADVERSE EFFECTS
Clonidine, guanfacine	Hypertensive urgency (limited situations), ADHD, Tourette syndrome, symptom control in opioid withdrawal	CNS depression, bradycardia, hypotension, respiratory depression, miosis, rebound hypertension with abrupt cessation
α-methyldopa	Hypertension in pregnancy	Direct Coombs ⊕ hemolysis, drug-induced lupus, hyperprolactinemia
Tizanidine	Relief of spasticity	Hypotension, weakness, xerostomia

α-blockers

DRUG	APPLICATIONS	ADVERSE EFFECTS
Nonselective		
Phenoxybenzamine	Irreversible. Pheochromocytoma (used preoperatively) to prevent catecholamine (hypertensive) crisis.	Orthostatic hypotension, reflex tachycardia.
Phentolamine	Reversible. Given to patients on MAO inhibitors who eat tyramine-containing foods and for severe cocaine-induced hypertension (2nd line). Also used to treat norepinephrine extravasation.	
α_1 selective (-osin ending)		
Prazosin, terazosin, doxazosin, tamsulosin	Urinary symptoms of BPH; PTSD (prazosin); hypertension (except tamsulosin).	1st-dose orthostatic hypotension, dizziness, headache.
α_2 selective		
Mirtazapine	Depression.	Sedation, ↑ serum cholesterol, ↑ appetite.

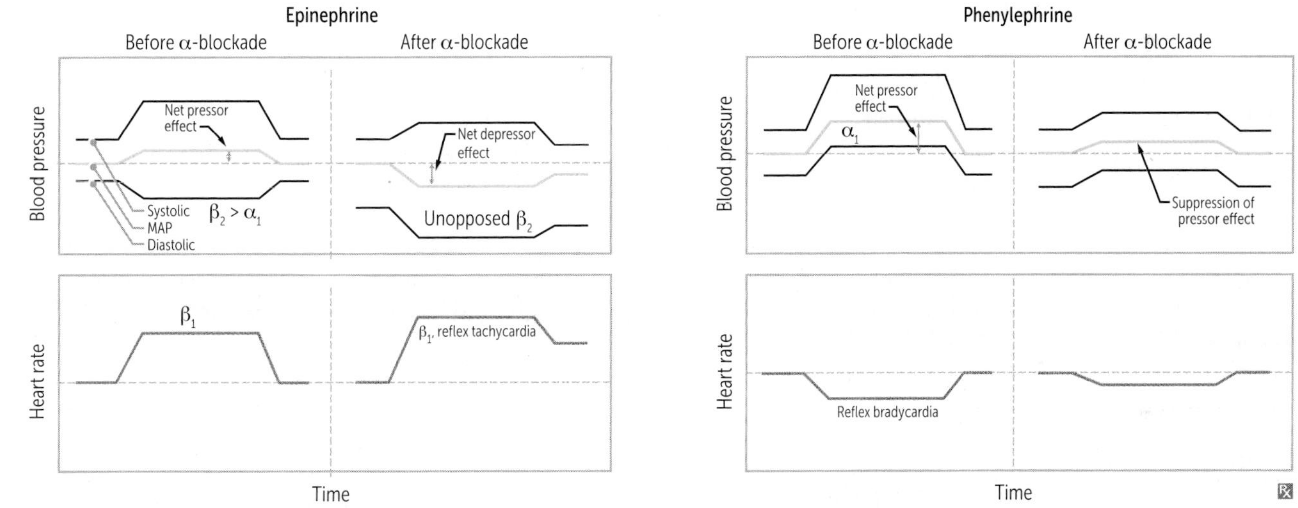

Epinephrine response exhibits reversal of mean arterial pressure from a net increase (the α response) to a net decrease (the β_2 response).

Phenylephrine response is suppressed but not reversed because it is a "pure" α-agonist (lacks β-agonist properties).

β-blockers Acebutolol, atenolol, betaxolol, bisoprolol, carvedilol, esmolol, labetalol, metoprolol, nadolol, nebivolol, pindolol, propranolol, timolol.

APPLICATION	ACTIONS	NOTES/EXAMPLES
Angina pectoris	↓ heart rate and contractility → ↓ O_2 consumption	
Glaucoma	↓ production of aqueous humor	Timolol
Heart failure	Blockade of neurohormonal stress → prevention of deleterious cardiac remodeling → ↓ mortality	Bisoprolol, carvedilol, metoprolol (β-blockers curb mortality)
Hypertension	↓ cardiac output, ↓ renin secretion (due to β_1-receptor blockade on JG cells)	
Hyperthyroidism/ thyroid storm	Symptom control (↓ heart rate, ↓ tremor)	Propranolol
Hypertrophic cardiomyopathy	↓ heart rate → ↑ filling time, relieving obstruction	
Myocardial infarction	↓ O_2 demand (short-term), ↓ mortality (long-term)	
Supraventricular tachycardia	↓ AV conduction velocity (class II antiarrhythmic)	Metoprolol, esmolol
Variceal bleeding	↓ hepatic venous pressure gradient and portal hypertension (prophylactic use)	Nadolol, propranolol, carvedilol
ADVERSE EFFECTS	Erectile dysfunction, cardiovascular (bradycardia, AV block, HF), CNS (seizures, sleep alterations), dyslipidemia (metoprolol), masked hypoglycemia, asthma/COPD exacerbations	Use of β-blockers for acute cocaine-associated chest pain remains controversial due to unsubstantiated concern for unopposed α-adrenergic stimulation
SELECTIVITY	β_1-selective antagonists ($\beta_1 > \beta_2$)—acebutolol (partial agonist), atenolol, betaxolol, bisoprolol, esmolol, metoprolol	Selective antagonists mostly go from **A** to **M** (β_1 with 1st half of alphabet)
	Nonselective antagonists ($\beta_1 = \beta_2$)—nadolol, pindolol (partial agonist), propranolol, timolol	Non**Z**elective antagonists mostly go from **N** to **Z** (β_2 with 2nd half of alphabet)
	Nonselective α- and β-antagonists—carvedi**lol**, labet**alol**	Nonselective α- and β-antagonists have **modified suffixes** (instead of "-olol")
	Nebivolol combines cardiac-selective β_1-adrenergic blockade with stimulation of β_3-receptors (activate NO synthase in the vasculature and ↓ SVR)	NebivOlol increases **NO**

Phosphodiesterase inhibitors

Phosphodiesterase (PDE) inhibitors inhibit PDE, which catalyzes the hydrolysis of cAMP and/or cGMP, and thereby increase cAMP and/or cGMP. These inhibitors have varying specificity for PDE isoforms and thus have different clinical uses.

TYPE OF INHIBITOR	MECHANISM OF ACTION	CLINICAL USES	ADVERSE EFFECTS
Nonspecific PDE inhibitor Theophylline	↓ cAMP hydrolysis → ↑ cAMP → bronchial smooth muscle relaxation → bronchodilation	COPD/asthma (rarely used)	Cardiotoxicity (eg, tachycardia, arrhythmia), neurotoxicity (eg, seizures, headache), abdominal pain
PDE-5 inhibitors Sildena**fil**, vardena**fil**, tadala**fil**, avana**fil**	↓ hydrolysis of cGMP → ↑ cGMP → ↑ smooth muscle relaxation by enhancing NO activity → pulmonary vasodilation and ↑ blood flow in corpus cavernosum **fil**ls the penis	Erectile dysfunction Pulmonary hypertension Benign prostatic hyperplasia (tadalafil only)	Facial flushing, headache, dyspepsia, hypotension in patients taking nitrates; "**h**ot and sweaty," then **h**eadache, **h**eartburn, **h**ypotension Sildenafil only: cyanopia (blue-tinted vision) via inhibition of PDE-6 (six) in retina
PDE-4 inhibitor Roflumilast	↑ cAMP in neutrophils, granulocytes, and bronchial epithelium	Severe COPD	Abdominal pain, weight loss, depression, anxiety, insomnia
PDE-3 inhibitor Milrinone	In cardiomyocytes: ↑ cAMP → ↑ Ca^{2+} influx → ↑ ionotropy and chronotropy In vascular smooth muscle: ↑ cAMP → MLCK inhibition → vasodilation → ↓ preload and afterload	Acute decompensated HF with cardiogenic shock (inotrope)	Tachycardia, ventricular arrhythmias, hypotension
"Platelet inhibitors" Cilostazol[a] Dipyridamole[b]	In platelets: ↑ cAMP → inhibition of platelet aggregation	Intermittent claudication Stroke or TIA prevention (with aspirin) Cardiac stress testing (dipyridamole only, due to coronary vasodilation) Prevention of coronary stent restenosis	Nausea, headache, facial flushing, hypotension, abdominal pain

[a]Cilostazol is a PDE-3 inhibitor, but due to its indications is categorized as a platelet inhibitor together with dipyridamole.
[b]Dipyridamole is a nonspecific PDE inhibitor, leading to inhibition of platelet aggregation. It also prevents adenosine reuptake by platelets → ↑ extracellular adenosine → ↑ vasodilation.

▶ PHARMACOLOGY—TOXICITIES AND SIDE EFFECTS

Ingested seafood toxins

Toxin actions include histamine release, total block of Na^+ channels, or opening of Na^+ channels to cause depolarization.

TOXIN	SOURCE	ACTION	SYMPTOMS	TREATMENT
Histamine (scombroid poisoning)	Spoiled dark-meat fish such as tuna, mahi-mahi, mackerel, and bonito	Bacterial histidine decarboxylase converts histidine to histamine Frequently misdiagnosed as fish allergy	Mimics anaphylaxis: oral burning sensation, facial flushing, erythema, urticaria, itching; may progress to bronchospasm, angioedema, hypotension	Antihistamines Albuterol +/– epinephrine
Tetrodotoxin	Pufferfish	Binds fast voltage-gated Na^+ channels in nerve tissue, preventing depolarization	Nausea, diarrhea, paresthesias, weakness, dizziness, loss of reflexes	Supportive
Ciguatoxin	Reef fish such as barracuda, snapper, and moray eel	Opens Na^+ channels, causing depolarization	Nausea, vomiting, diarrhea; perioral numbness; reversal of hot and cold sensations; bradycardia, heart block, hypotension	Supportive

Age-related changes in pharmacokinetics

It's how aging bodies are MADE.

Metabolism	↓ hepatic mass, ↓ hepatic blood flow and ↓ drug metabolism. Phase I metabolism lost first with aging. Drugs metabolized during phase II (eg, lorazepam, acetaminophen) are safer than drugs metabolized during phase I (eg, diazepam). Thus ↓ therapeutic doses may suffice in elderly.
Absorption	↑ gastric pH, ↓ gastric emptying. Drug absorption influenced via drug-drug/food interactions.
Distribution	↑ body fat content (↑ V_d for lipophilic drugs, eg, propofol). ↓ albumin (↓ binding of acidic drugs). ↓ total body water (↓ V_d for hydrophilic drugs, eg, digoxin).
Elimination	↓ GFR and ↓ tubular secretion. ↑ plasma concentration of renally excreted drugs; thus ↓ therapeutic doses may suffice in elderly.

Beers criteria

Widely used criteria developed to reduce potentially inappropriate prescribing and harmful polypharmacy in the geriatric population. Includes > 50 medications that should be avoided in elderly patients due to ↓ efficacy and/or ↑ risk of adverse events. Examples:

- α-blockers (↑ risk of hypotension)
- Anticholinergics, antidepressants, antihistamines, opioids (↑ risk of delirium, sedation, falls, constipation, urinary retention)
- Benzodiazepines (↑ risk of delirium, sedation, falls)
- NSAIDs (↑ risk of GI bleeding, especially with concomitant anticoagulation)
- PPIs (↑ risk of C *difficile* infection)

Specific toxicity treatments

TOXIN	TREATMENT
Acetaminophen	N-acetylcysteine (replenishes glutathione)
AChE inhibitors, organophosphates	Atropine > pralidoxime
Antimuscarinic, anticholinergic agents	Physostigmine (crosses BBB), control hyperthermia
Arsenic	Dimercaprol, succimer
Benzodiazepines	Flumazenil
β-blockers	Atropine, glucagon, saline
Carbon monoxide	100% O_2, hyperbaric O_2
Copper	"Penny"cillamine (penicillamine), trientine (3 copper pennies)
Cyanide	Hydroxocobalamin, nitrites + sodium thiosulfate
Dabigatran	Idarucizumab
Digoxin	Digoxin-specific antibody fragments
Direct factor Xa inhibitors (eg, apixaban)	Andexanet alfa
Heparin	Protamine sulfate
Iron (Fe)	Deferoxamine, deferasirox, deferiprone
Lead	Calcium disodium EDTA, dimercaprol, succimer, penicillamine
Mercury	Dimercaprol, succimer
Methanol, ethylene glycol (antifreeze)	Fomepizole > ethanol, dialysis
Methemoglobin	Methylene blue, vitamin C (reducing agent)
Methotrexate	Leucovorin
Opioids	Naloxone
Salicylates	$NaHCO_3$ (alkalinize urine), dialysis
TCAs	$NaHCO_3$ (stabilizes cardiac cell membrane)
Warfarin	Vitamin K (delayed effect), PCC (prothrombin complex concentrate)/FFP (immediate effect)

Drug reactions—cardiovascular

DRUG REACTION	CAUSAL AGENTS
Coronary vasospasm	Cocaine, Amphetamines, Sumatriptan, Ergot alkaloids (CASE)
Cutaneous flushing	Vancomycin, Adenosine, Niacin, Ca^{2+} channel blockers, Echinocandins, Nitrates (flushed from VANCEN [dancing]) Red man syndrome—rate-dependent infusion reaction to vancomycin causing widespread pruritic erythema due to histamine release. Manage with diphenhydramine, slower infusion rate.
Dilated cardiomyopathy	Alcohol, anthracycline (eg, doxorubicin, daunorubicin; prevent with dexrazoxane), trastuzumab
Torsades de pointes	Agents that prolong QT interval: antiArrhythmics (class IA, III), antiBiotics (eg, macrolides, fluoroquinolones), anti"C"ychotics (eg, ziprasidone), antiDepressants (eg, TCAs), antiEmetics (eg, ondansetron), antiFungals (eg, fluconazole) (ABCDEF)

Drug reactions—endocrine/reproductive

DRUG REACTION	CAUSAL AGENTS	NOTES
Adrenocortical insufficiency	HPA suppression 2° to glucocorticoid withdrawal	
Diabetes insipidus	Lithium, demeclocycline	
Gynecomastia	Ketoconazole, cimetidine, spironolactone, GnRH analogs/antagonists, androgen receptor inhibitors, 5α-reductase inhibitors	
Hot flashes	SERMs (eg, tamoxifen, clomiphene, raloxifene)	
Hyperglycemia	**T**acrolimus, **p**rotease inhibitors, **n**iacin, **H**CTZ, **c**orticosteroids	**T**he **p**eople **n**eed **h**ard **c**andies
Hyperprolactinemia	Typical antipsychotics (eg, haloperidol), atypical antipsychotics (eg, risperidone), metoclopramide, methyldopa, reserpine	Presents with hypogonadism (eg, infertility, amenorrhea, erectile dysfunction) and galactorrhea
Hyperthyroidism	Amiodarone, iodine, lithium	
Hypothyroidism	**Am**iodarone, **l**ithium	**I am l**ethargic
SIADH	**C**arbamazepine, **C**yclophosphamide, **SS**RIs	**C**an't **C**oncentrate **S**erum **S**odium

Drug reactions—gastrointestinal

DRUG REACTION	CAUSAL AGENTS	NOTES
Acute cholestatic hepatitis, jaundice	Macrolides (eg, erythromycin)	
Diarrhea	Acamprosate, antidiabetic agents (acarbose, metformin, pramlintide), colchicine, cholinesterase inhibitors, lipid-lowering agents (eg, ezetimibe, orlistat), macrolides (eg, erythromycin), SSRIs, chemotherapy (eg, irinotecan)	
Focal to massive hepatic necrosis	**H**alothane, ***A**manita phalloides* (death cap mushroom), **v**alproic acid, **a**cetaminophen	Liver "**hAvac**"
Hepatitis	Rifampin, isoniazid, pyrazinamide, statins, fibrates	
Pancreatitis	**D**idanosine, **c**orticosteroids, **a**lcohol, **v**alproic acid, **a**zathioprine, **d**iuretics (eg, furosemide, HCTZ)	**D**rugs **c**ausing **a** **v**iolent **a**bdominal **d**istress
Pill-induced esophagitis	Bisphosphonates, ferrous sulfate, NSAIDs, potassium chloride, tetracyclines	Usually occurs at anatomic sites of esophageal narrowing (eg, near level of aortic arch); caustic effect minimized with upright posture and adequate water ingestion
Pseudomembranous colitis	Ampicillin, cephalosporins, clindamycin, fluoroquinolones, PPIs	Antibiotics predispose to superinfection by resistant *C difficile*

Drug reactions—hematologic

DRUG REACTION	CAUSAL AGENTS	NOTES
Agranulocytosis	Dapsone, clozapine, carbamazepine, propylthiouracil, methimazole, colchicine, ticlopidine, ganciclovir	Drugs can cause pretty major collapse to granulocytes
Aplastic anemia	Carbamazepine, methimazole, NSAIDs, benzene, chloramphenicol, propylthiouracil	Can't make New blood cells properly
Direct Coombs ⊕ hemolytic anemia	Penicillin, methylDopa, Cephalosporins	P Diddy Coombs
Drug reaction with eosinophilia and systemic symptoms[a]	Allopurinol, antiBiotics, antiConvulsants, sulfa drugs	ABCs
Gray baby syndrome	Chloramphenicol	
Hemolysis in G6PD deficiency	Isoniazid, sulfonamides, dapsone, primaquine, aspirin, ibuprofen, nitrofurantoin	Hemolysis is d pain
Megaloblastic anemia	Hydroxyurea, Phenytoin, Methotrexate, Sulfa drugs	You're having a mega blast with PMS
Thrombocytopenia	Indinavir, heparin, quinidine, ganciclovir, vancomycin, linezolid, abciximab	I have quickly gotten very low amounts
Thrombotic complications	Combined oral contraceptives, hormone replacement therapy, SERMs, epoetin alfa	Estrogen-mediated adverse effect

[a]DRESS is a delayed hypersensitivity reaction associated with latent herpesvirus reactivation. Latency period (2–8 weeks), then fever, morbilliform skin rash, multiorgan involvement. Treatment: withdrawal of offending drug, corticosteroids

Drug reactions—musculoskeletal/skin/connective tissue

DRUG REACTION	CAUSAL AGENTS	NOTES
Drug-induced lupus	Methyldopa, minocycline, hydralazine, isoniazid, phenytoin, sulfa drugs, etanercept, procainamide	Lupus makes my hips extremely painful
Fat redistribution	Protease inhibitors, glucocorticoids	Fat protects glutes
Gingival hyperplasia	Cyclosporine, Ca^{2+} channel blockers, phenytoin	Can Cause puffy gums
Hyperuricemia (gout)	Pyrazinamide, thiazides, furosemide, niacin, cyclosporine	Painful tophi and feet need care
Myopathy	Statins, fibrates, niacin, colchicine, daptomycin, hydroxychloroquine, interferon-α, penicillamine, glucocorticoids	
Osteoporosis	Corticosteroids, depot medroxyprogesterone acetate, GnRH agonists, aromatase inhibitors, anticonvulsants, heparin, PPIs	
Photosensitivity	Sulfonamides, amiodarone, tetracyclines, 5-FU	Sat For photo
Rash (Stevens-Johnson syndrome)	Anti-epileptic drugs (especially lamotrigine), allopurinol, sulfa drugs, penicillin	Steven Johnson has epileptic allergy to sulfa drugs and penicillin
Teeth discoloration	Tetracyclines	Teethracyclines
Tendon/cartilage damage	Fluoroquinolones	

Drug reactions—neurologic

DRUG REACTION	CAUSAL AGENTS	NOTES
Cinchonism	Quinidine, quinine	Can present with tinnitus, hearing/vision loss, psychosis, and cognitive impairment
Parkinson-like syndrome	Antipsychotics, reserpine, metoclopramide	Cogwheel rigidity of arm
Peripheral neuropathy	Isoniazid, phenytoin, platinum agents (eg, cisplatin), paclitaxel, vincristine	
Idiopathic intracranial hypertension	Vitamin A, growth hormones, tetracyclines	Always grow head tension
Seizures	Isoniazid, bupropion, imipenem/cilastatin, tramadol, enflurane	With seizures, I bite my tongue
Tardive dyskinesia	Antipsychotics, metoclopramide	
Visual disturbance	Topiramate (blurred vision/diplopia, haloes), hydroxychloroquine (↓ visual acuity, visual field defects), digoxin (yellow-tinged vision), isoniazid (optic neuritis), vigabatrin (visual field defects), PDE-5 inhibitors (blue-tinged vision), ethambutol (color vision changes)	These horrible drugs irritate very Precious eyes

Drug reactions—renal/genitourinary

DRUG REACTION	CAUSAL AGENTS	NOTES
Fanconi syndrome	Cisplatin, ifosfamide, expired tetracyclines, tenofovir	
Hemorrhagic cystitis	Cyclophosphamide, ifosfamide	Prevent by coadministering with mesna
Interstitial nephritis	Diuretics (Pee), NSAIDs (Pain-free), Penicillins and cephalosporins, PPIs, rifamPin, sulfa drugs	Remember the 5 P's

Drug reactions—respiratory

DRUG REACTION	CAUSAL AGENTS	NOTES
Dry cough	ACE inhibitors	
Pulmonary fibrosis	Methotrexate, nitrofurantoin, carmustine, bleomycin, busulfan, amiodarone	My nose cannot breathe bad air

Drug reactions—multiorgan

DRUG REACTION	CAUSAL AGENTS	NOTES
Antimuscarinic	Atropine, TCAs, H_1-blockers, antipsychotics	
Disulfiram-like reaction	1st-generation sulfonylureas, procarbazine, certain cephalosporins, griseofulvin, metronidazole	Sorry pals, can't go mingle
Nephrotoxicity/ototoxicity	Loop diuretics, cisplatin, aminoglycosides, amphotericin, vancomycin	Listen Cis! Always adjust vancomycin in CKD. Cisplatin toxicity may respond to amifostine

Drugs affecting pupil size

↑ pupil size (mydriasis)	↓ pupil size (miosis)
Anticholinergics (eg, atropine, TCAs, tropicamide, scopolamine, antihistamines)	Sympatholytics (eg, α_2-agonists)
Indirect sympathomimetics (eg, amphetamines, cocaine, LSD), meperidine	Opioids (except meperidine)
Direct sympathomimetics	Parasympathomimetics (eg, pilocarpine), organophosphates

Cytochrome P-450 interactions (selected)

Inducers (+)	Substrates	Inhibitors (–)
St. John's wort Griseofulvin Carbamazepine Chronic alcohol overuse Rifampin Modafinil Nevirapine Phenytoin Phenobarbital	Theophylline OCPs Anti-epileptics Warfarin	Sodium valproate Isoniazid Cimetidine Ketoconazole Fluconazole Acute alcohol overuse Chloramphenicol Erythromycin/clarithromycin Sulfonamides Ciprofloxacin Omeprazole Metronidazole Amiodarone Ritonavir Grapefruit juice
St. John grimaced at the carbs in chronic alcohol overuse, refused more, and never again forgot his phen-phen	The OCPs are anti-war	SICKFACES.COM (when I am really drinking grapefruit juice)

Sulfa drugs

Sulfonamide antibiotics, Sulfasalazine, Probenecid, Furosemide, Acetazolamide, Celecoxib, Thiazides, Sulfonylureas.

Patients with sulfa allergies may develop fever, urinary tract infection, Stevens-Johnson syndrome, hemolytic anemia, thrombocytopenia, agranulocytosis, acute interstitial nephritis, and urticaria (hives).

Scary Sulfa Pharm FACTS

▶ PHARMACOLOGY—MISCELLANEOUS

Drug names

ENDING	CATEGORY	EXAMPLE
Antimicrobial		
-asvir	NS5A inhibitor	Ledipasvir
-bendazole	Antiparasitic/antihelminthic	Mebendazole
-buvir	NS5B inhibitor	Sofosbuvir
-cillin	Transpeptidase inhibitor	Ampicillin
-conazole	Ergosterol synthesis inhibitor	Ketoconazole
-cycline	Protein synthesis inhibitor	Tetracycline
-floxacin	Fluoroquinolone	Ciprofloxacin
-mivir	Neuraminidase inhibitor	Oseltamivir
-navir	Protease inhibitor	Ritonavir
-ovir	Viral DNA polymerase inhibitor	Acyclovir
-previr	NS3/4A inhibitor	Simeprevir
-tegravir	Integrase inhibitor	Elvitegravir
-thromycin	Macrolide	Azithromycin
Antineoplastic		
-case	Recombinant uricase	Rasburicase
-mustine	Nitrosourea	Carmustine
-platin	Platinum compound	Cisplatin
-poside	Topoisomerase II inhibitor	Etoposide
-rubicin	Anthracycline	Doxorubicin
-taxel	Taxane	Paclitaxel
-tecan	Topoisomerase I inhibitor	Irinotecan
CNS		
-ane	Inhaled anesthetic	Halothane
-apine, -idone	Atypical antipsychotic	Quetiapine, risperidone
-azine	Typical antipsychotic	Thioridazine
-barbital	Barbiturate	Phenobarbital
-benazine	VMAT inhibitor	Tetrabenazine
-caine	Local anesthetic	Lidocaine
-capone	COMT inhibitor	Entacapone
-curium, -curonium	Nondepolarizing neuromuscular blocker	Atracurium, pancuronium
-giline	MAO-B inhibitor	Selegiline
-ipramine, -triptyline	TCA	Imipramine, amitriptyline
-triptan	$5\text{-HT}_{1B/1D}$ agonist	Sumatriptan
-zepam, -zolam	Benzodiazepine	Diazepam, alprazolam

Drug names *(continued)*

ENDING	CATEGORY	EXAMPLE
Autonomic		
-chol	Cholinergic agonist	Bethanechol
-olol	β-blocker	Propranolol
-stigmine	AChE inhibitor	Neostigmine
-terol	β_2-agonist	Albuterol
-zosin	α_1-blocker	Prazosin
Cardiovascular		
-afil	PDE-5 inhibitor	Sildenafil
-dipine	Dihydropyridine Ca^{2+} channel blocker	Amlodipine
-parin	Low-molecular-weight heparin	Enoxaparin
-plase	Thrombolytic	Alteplase
-pril	ACE inhibitor	Captopril
-sartan	Angiotensin-II receptor blocker	Losartan
-xaban	Direct factor Xa inhibitor	Apixaban
Metabolic		
-gliflozin	SGLT-2 inhibitor	Dapagliflozin
-glinide	Meglitinide	Repaglinide
-gliptin	DPP-4 inhibitor	Sitagliptin
-glitazone	PPAR-γ activator	Rosiglitazone
-glutide	GLP-1 analog	Liraglutide
-statin	HMG-CoA reductase inhibitor	Lovastatin
Other		
-caftor	CFTR modulator	Lumacaftor
-dronate	Bisphosphonate	Alendronate
-lukast	CysLT1 receptor blocker	Montelukast
-lutamide	Androgen receptor inhibitor	Flutamide
-pitant	NK_1 blocker	Aprepitant
-prazole	Proton pump inhibitor	Omeprazole
-prost	Prostaglandin analog	Latanoprost
-sentan	Endothelin receptor antagonist	Bosentan
-setron	5-HT_3 blocker	Ondansetron
-steride	5α-reductase inhibitor	Finasteride
-tadine	H_1-antagonist	Loratadine
-tidine	H_2-antagonist	Cimetidine
-trozole	Aromatase inhibitor	Anastrozole
-vaptan	ADH antagonist	Tolvaptan

Biologic agents

ENDING	CATEGORY	EXAMPLE
Monoclonal antibodies (-mab)—target overexpressed cell surface receptors		
-ximab	Chimeric human-mouse monoclonal antibody	Rituximab
-zumab	Humanized monoclonal antibody	Bevacizumab
-umab	Human monoclonal antibody	Denosumab
Small molecule inhibitors (-ib)—target intracellular molecules		
-ciclib	Cyclin-dependent kinase inhibitor	Palbociclib
-coxib	COX-2 inhibitor	Celecoxib
-parib	Poly(ADP-ribose) polymerase inhibitor	Olaparib
-rafenib	BRAF inhibitor	Vemurafenib
-tinib	Tyrosine kinase inhibitor	Imatinib
-zomib	Proteasome inhibitor	Bortezomib
Receptor fusion proteins (-cept)		
-cept	TNF-α antagonist	Etanercept
Interleukin receptor modulators (-kin)—agonists and antagonists of interleukin receptors		
-leukin	Interleukin-2 agonist/analog	Aldesleukin
-kinra	Interleukin receptor antagonist	Anakinra

HIGH-YIELD PRINCIPLES IN

Public Health Sciences

"Medicine is a science of uncertainty and an art of probability."

—Sir William Osler

"Whenever a doctor cannot do good, he must be kept from doing harm."

—Hippocrates

"On a long enough timeline, the survival rate for everyone drops to zero."

—Chuck Palahniuk, *Fight Club*

"Of all forms of discrimination and inequalities, injustice in health is the most shocking and inhuman."

—Martin Luther King, Jr.

A heterogenous mix of epidemiology, biostatistics, ethics, law, healthcare delivery, patient safety, quality improvement, and more falls under the heading of public health sciences. Biostatistics and epidemiology are the foundations of evidence-based medicine and are very high yield. Make sure you can quickly apply biostatistical equations such as sensitivity, specificity, and predictive values in a problem-solving format. Also, know how to set up your own 2 × 2 tables, and beware questions that switch the columns. Quality improvement and patient safety topics were introduced a few years ago on the exam and represent trends in health system science. Medical ethics questions often require application of principles. Typically, you are presented with a patient scenario and then asked how you would respond. For this edition, we have added a section on communication skills given their growing emphasis on the exam. Effective communication is essential to the physician-patient partnership. Physicians must seek opportunities to connect with patients, understand their perspectives, express empathy, and form shared decisions and realistic goals.

▶ PUBLIC HEALTH SCIENCES—EPIDEMIOLOGY AND BIOSTATISTICS

Observational studies

STUDY TYPE	DESIGN	MEASURES/EXAMPLE
Case series	Describes several individual patients with the same diagnosis, treatment, or outcome.	Description of clinical findings and symptoms. Has no comparison group, thus cannot show risk factor association with disease.
Cross-sectional study	Frequency of disease and frequency of risk-related factors are assessed in the present. Asks, "What is happening?"	Disease prevalence. Can show risk factor association with disease, but does not establish causality.
Case-control study	Retrospectively compares a group of people with disease to a group without disease. Looks to see if odds of prior exposure or risk factor differ by disease state. Asks, "What happened?"	Odds ratio (**OR**). **Control** the case in the **OR**. Patients with COPD had higher odds of a smoking history than those without COPD.
Cohort study	Compares a group with a given exposure or risk factor to a group without such exposure. Looks to see if exposure or risk factor is associated with later development of disease. Can be prospective or retrospective.	Disease incidence. Relative risk (RR). People who smoke had a higher risk of developing COPD than people who do not. Cohort = **relative** risk.
Twin concordance study	Compares the frequency with which both monozygotic twins vs both dizygotic twins develop the same disease.	Measures heritability and influence of environmental factors ("nature vs nurture").
Adoption study	Compares siblings raised by biological vs adoptive parents.	Measures heritability and influence of environmental factors.
Ecological study	Compares frequency of disease and frequency of risk-related factors across populations. Measures population data not necessarily applicable to individuals (ecological fallacy).	Used to monitor population health. COPD prevalence was higher in more polluted cities.

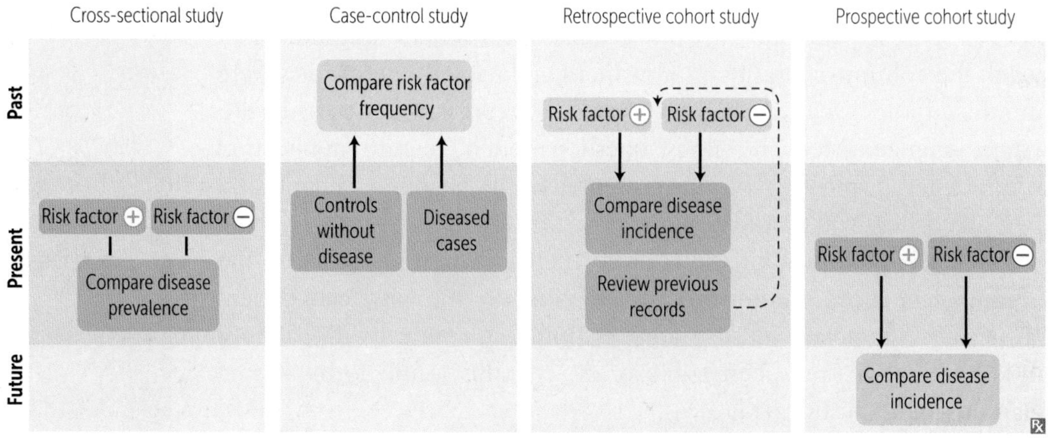

Clinical trial	Experimental study involving humans. Compares therapeutic benefits of ≥2 treatments, or of treatment and placebo. Study quality improves when study is randomized, controlled, and double-blinded (ie, neither patient nor researcher knows whether the patient is in the treatment or control group). Triple-blind refers to the additional blinding of the researchers analyzing the data. Five phases ("Can I SWIM?").
Crossover study	Compares the effect of a series of ≥2 treatments on a participant. Order in which participants receive treatments is randomized. Washout period occurs between treatments. Allows participants to serve as own controls. Intention-to-treat analysis: All patients are analyzed according to their original, randomly assigned treatment. No patients are excluded. Attempts to avoid misleading bias from patients dropping out. Per protocol analysis: Only patients who complete the study "per protocol" are included in analysis. Patients who fail to complete treatment as originally, randomly assigned are excluded. Risk of bias from non-random noncompliance.

DRUG TRIALS	TYPICAL STUDY SAMPLE	PURPOSE
Phase 0	Very small number of either healthy volunteers or patients with disease of interest.	Initial pharmocokinetic and pharmacodynamic assessment. Uses <1% of therapeutic dose. No safety or toxicity assessment.
Phase I	Small number of either healthy volunteers or patients with disease of interest; more than Phase 0.	"Is it Safe?" Assesses safety, toxicity, dosage, pharmacokinetics, and pharmacodynamics.
Phase II	Moderate number of patients with disease of interest.	"Does it Work?" Assesses treatment efficacy, and adverse effects.
Phase III	Large number of patients with disease of interest randomly assigned either to the treatment under investigation or to the standard of care (or placebo).	"Is it as good or better?" Compares the new treatment to the current standard of care (any Improvement?).
Phase IV	Postmarketing surveillance of patients after treatment is approved.	"Can it stay on the Market?" Detects rare or long-term adverse effects and evaluates cost-effectiveness.

Bradford Hill criteria	A group of principles that provide limited support for establishing evidence of a causal relationship between presumed cause and effect.
Strength	Association does not imply causation, but the stronger the association, the more evidence for causation.
Consistency	Repeated observations of the findings in multiple distinct samples.
Specificity	The more specific the presumed cause is to the effect, the stronger the evidence for causation.
Temporality	The presumed cause precedes the effect by an expected amount of time.
Biological gradient	Greater effect observed with greater exposure to the presumed cause (dose-response relationship).
Plausibility	A conceivable mechanism exists by which the cause may lead to the effect.
Coherence	The presumed cause and effect do not conflict with existing scientific consensus.
Experiment	Empirical evidence supporting the presumed cause and effect (eg, animal studies, in vitro studies).
Analogy	The presumed cause and effect are comparable to a similar, established cause and effect.

Quantifying risk

Definitions and formulas are based on the classic 2 × 2 or contingency table.

Exposure or intervention		Disease or outcome ⊕	Disease or outcome ⊖
	⊕	a	b
	⊖	c	d

TERM	DEFINITION	EXAMPLE	FORMULA
Odds ratio	Typically used in case-control studies. Represents the odds of exposure among cases (a/c) vs odds of exposure among controls (b/d). OR = 1 → odds of exposure are equal in cases and controls. OR > 1 → odds of exposure are greater in cases. OR < 1 → odds of exposure are greater in controls.	If in a case-control study, 20/30 patients with lung cancer and 5/25 healthy individuals report smoking, the OR is 8; so the patients with lung cancer are 8 times more likely to have a history of smoking.	$OR = \frac{a/c}{b/d} = \frac{ad}{bc}$ $\begin{array}{\|l\|l\|} \hline a\ \ 20 & b\ \ 5 \\ \hline c\ \ 10 & d\ \ 20 \\ \hline \end{array}$
Relative risk	Typically used in cohort studies. Risk of developing disease in the exposed group divided by risk in the unexposed group. RR = 1 → no association between exposure and disease. RR > 1 → exposure associated with ↑ disease occurrence. RR < 1 → exposure associated with ↓ disease occurrence.	If 5/10 people exposed to radiation are diagnosed with cancer, and 1/10 people not exposed to radiation are diagnosed with cancer, the RR is 5; so people exposed to radiation have a 5 times greater risk of developing cancer. For rare diseases (low prevalence), OR approximates RR.	$RR = \frac{a/(a+b)}{c/(c+d)}$ $\begin{array}{\|l\|l\|} \hline a\ \ 5 & b\ \ 5 \\ \hline c\ \ 1 & d\ \ 9 \\ \hline \end{array}$
Relative risk reduction	The proportion of risk reduction attributable to the intervention as compared to a control.	If 2% of patients who receive a flu shot develop the flu, while 8% of unvaccinated patients develop the flu, then RR = 2/8 = 0.25, and RRR = 0.75.	$RRR = 1 - RR$
Attributable risk	The difference in risk between exposed and unexposed groups.	If risk of lung cancer in people who smoke is 21% and risk in people who don't smoke is 1%, then the attributable risk is 20%.	$AR = \frac{a}{a+b} - \frac{c}{c+d}$ $AR\% = \frac{RR-1}{RR} \times 100$
Absolute risk reduction	The difference in risk (not the proportion) attributable to the intervention as compared to a control.	If 8% of people who receive a placebo vaccine develop the flu vs 2% of people who receive a flu vaccine, then ARR = 8%–2% = 6% = 0.06.	$ARR = \frac{c}{c+d} - \frac{a}{a+b}$
Number needed to treat	Number of patients who need to be treated for 1 patient to benefit. Lower number = better treatment.		NNT = 1/ARR
Number needed to harm	Number of patients who need to be exposed to a risk factor for 1 patient to be harmed. Higher number = safer exposure.		NNH = 1/AR
Case fatality rate	Percentage of deaths occurring among those with disease.	If 4 patients die among 10 cases of meningitis, case fatality rate is 40%.	$CFR\% = \frac{deaths}{cases} \times 100$

Quantifying risk *(continued)*

TERM	DEFINITION	EXAMPLE	FORMULA
Mortality rate	Number of deaths (in general or due to specific cause) within a population over a period, typically scaled to deaths per 1000 people per year.	If 80 people in a town of 10,000 die over 2 years, mortality rate is 4 per 1000 per year.	
Attack rate	Proportion of exposed people who become ill.	If 80 people in a town are exposed and 60 people become ill, attack rate is 75%.	$\frac{\text{People who become ill}}{\text{Total people exposed}}$

Likelihood ratio

$$LR^+ = \frac{\text{probability of positive result in patient with disorder}}{\text{probability of positive result in patient without disorder}} = \frac{\text{sensitivity}}{1 - \text{specificity}} = \frac{\text{TP rate}}{\text{FP rate}}$$

$$LR^- = \frac{\text{probability of negative result in patient with disorder}}{\text{probability of negative result in patient without disorder}} = \frac{1 - \text{sensitivity}}{\text{specificity}} = \frac{\text{FN rate}}{\text{TN rate}}$$

$LR^+ > 10$ indicates a highly specific test, while $LR^- < 0.1$ indicates a highly sensitive test.

Evaluation of diagnostic tests

Sensitivity and specificity are fixed properties of a test. PPV and NPV vary depending on disease prevalence in population being tested.

Test \ Disease	⊕	⊖	
⊕	TP	FP	PPV = TP/(TP + FP)
⊖	FN	TN	NPV = TN/(TN + FN)
	Sensitivity = TP/(TP + FN)	Specificity = TN/(TN + FP)	Prevalence $\frac{TP + FN}{TP + FN + FP + TN}$

Sensitivity (true-positive rate)	Proportion of all people with disease who test positive, or the ability of a test to correctly identify those with the disease. Value approaching 100% is desirable for **ruling out** disease and indicates a **low false-negative rate**.	= TP / (TP + FN) = 1 – FN rate **SN-N-OUT** = highly **S**e**N**sitive test, when **N**egative, rules **OUT** disease High sensitivity test used for screening
Specificity (true-negative rate)	Proportion of all people without disease who test negative, or the ability of a test to correctly identify those without the disease. Value approaching 100% is desirable for **ruling in** disease and indicates a **low false-positive rate**.	= TN / (TN + FP) = 1 – FP rate **SP-P-IN** = highly **SP**ecific test, when **P**ositive, rules **IN** disease High specificity test used for confirmation after a positive screening test
Positive predictive value	Probability that a person who has a positive test result actually has the disease.	PPV = TP / (TP + FP) PPV varies directly with pretest probability (baseline risk, such as prevalence of disease): high pretest probability → high PPV
Negative predictive value	Probability that a person with a negative test result actually does not have the disease.	NPV = TN / (TN + FN) NPV varies inversely with prevalence or pretest probability

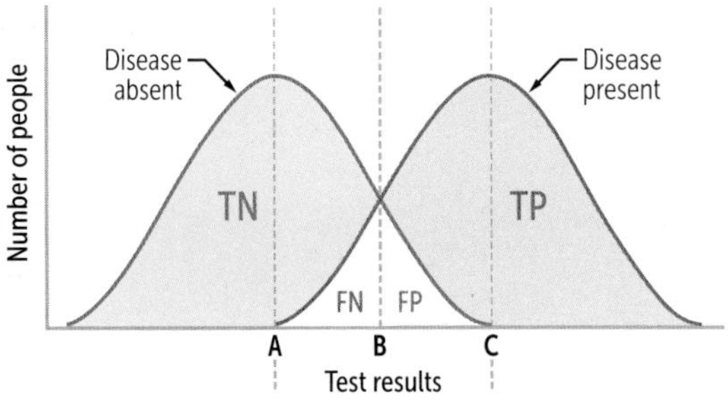

Possible cutoff values for ⊕ vs ⊖ test result
A = 100% sensitivity cutoff value
B = practical compromise between specificity and sensitivity
C = 100% specificity cutoff value

Lowering the cutoff value: B → A (↑ FP ↓ FN)	↑ Sensitivity ↑ NPV ↓ Specificity ↓ PPV
Raising the cutoff value: B → C (↑ FN ↓ FP)	↑ Specificity ↑ PPV ↓ Sensitivity ↓ NPV

Receiver operating characteristic curve

ROC curve demonstrates how well a diagnostic test can distinguish between 2 groups (eg, disease vs healthy). Plots the true-positive rate (sensitivity) against the false-positive rate (1 – specificity).

The better performing test will have a higher area under the curve (AUC), with the curve closer to the upper left corner.

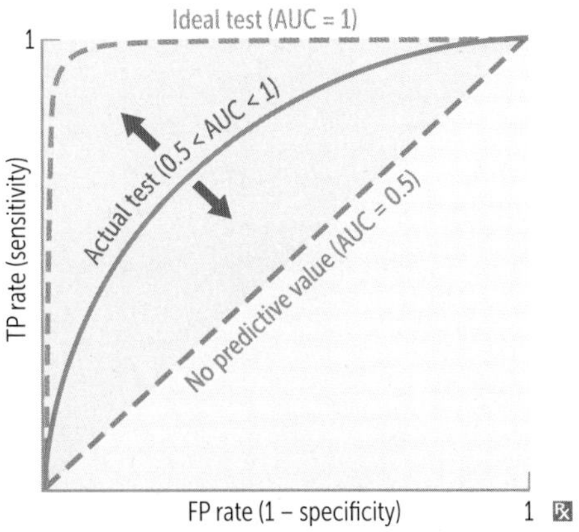

Precision vs accuracy

Precision (reliability)	The consistency and reproducibility of a test. The absence of random variation in a test.	Random error ↓ precision in a test. ↑ precision → ↓ standard deviation. ↑ precision → ↑ statistical power ($1 - \beta$).
Accuracy (validity)	The closeness of test results to the true values. The absence of systematic error or bias in a test.	Systematic error ↓ accuracy in a test.

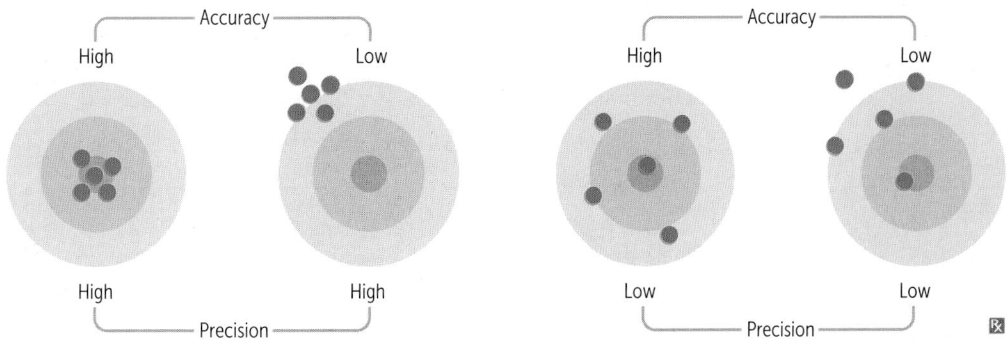

Incidence vs prevalence

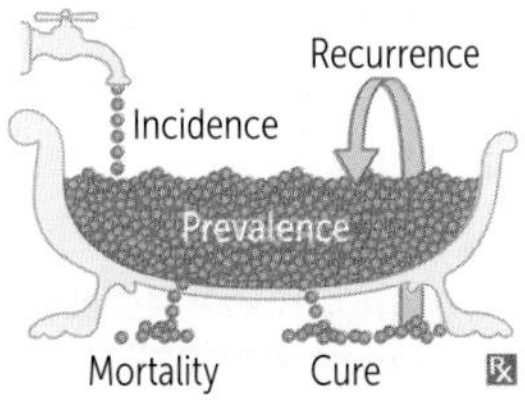

$$\text{Incidence} = \frac{\#\text{ of new cases}}{\#\text{ of people at risk}}$$ (per unit of time)

Incidence looks at new cases (**incidents**).

$$\text{Prevalence} = \frac{\#\text{ of existing cases}}{\text{Total }\#\text{ of people in a population}}$$ (at a point in time)

Prevalence looks at **all** current cases.

$$\frac{\text{Prevalence}}{1 - \text{prevalence}} = \text{Incidence rate} \times \text{average duration of disease}$$

Prevalence ≈ incidence for short duration disease (eg, common cold).

Prevalence > incidence for chronic diseases, due to large # of existing cases (eg, diabetes).

Prevalence ~ pretest probability.

↑ prevalence → ↑ PPV and ↓ NPV.

SITUATION	INCIDENCE	PREVALENCE
↑ survival time	—	↑
↑ mortality	—	↓
Faster recovery time	—	↓
Extensive vaccine administration	↓	↓
↓ risk factors	↓	↓
↑ diagnostic sensitivity	↑	↑

Bias and study errors

TYPE	DEFINITION	EXAMPLES	STRATEGIES TO REDUCE BIAS
Recruiting participants			
Selection bias	Nonrandom sampling or treatment allocation of subjects such that study population is not representative of target population Most commonly a sampling bias	Berkson bias—cases and/or controls selected from hospitals (**bedside bias**) are less healthy and have different exposures Attrition bias—participants lost to follow up have a different prognosis than those who complete the study	Randomization (creates groups with similar distributions of known and unknown variables) Ensure the choice of the right comparison/reference group
Performing study			
Recall bias	Awareness of disorder alters recall by subjects; common in retrospective studies	Patients with disease recall exposure after learning of similar cases	Decrease time from exposure to follow-up
Measurement bias	Information is gathered in a systemically distorted manner	Using a faulty automatic sphygmomanometer Hawthorne effect—participants change behavior upon awareness of being observed	Use objective, standardized, and previously tested methods of data collection that are planned ahead of time Use placebo group
Procedure bias	Subjects in different groups are not treated the same	Patients in treatment group spend more time in highly specialized hospital units	Blinding (masking) and use of placebo reduce influence of participants and researchers on procedures and interpretation of outcomes as neither are aware of group assignments
Observer-expectancy bias	Researcher's belief in the efficacy of a treatment changes the outcome of that treatment (aka, Pygmalion effect)	An observer expecting treatment group to show signs of recovery is more likely to document positive outcomes	
Interpreting results			
Confounding bias	Factor related to both exposure and outcome (but not on causal path) distorts effect of exposure on outcome (vs effect modification, in which the exposure leads to different outcomes in subgroups stratified by the factor)	An uncontrolled study shows an association between drinking coffee and lung cancer; however, people who drink coffee may smoke more, which could account for the association	Multiple/repeated studies Crossover studies (subjects act as their own controls) Matching (patients with similar characteristics in both treatment and control groups)
Lead-time bias	Early detection interpreted as ↑ survival, but the disease course has not changed	Breast cancer diagnosed early by mammography may appear to exaggerate survival time because patients are known to have the cancer for longer	Measure "back-end" survival (adjust survival according to the severity of disease at the time of diagnosis)
Length-time bias	Screening test detects diseases with long latency period, while those with shorter latency period become symptomatic earlier	A slowly progressive cancer is more likely detected by a screening test than a rapidly progressive cancer	A randomized controlled trial assigning subjects to the screening program or to no screening

Statistical distribution

Measures of central tendency	Mean = (sum of values)/(total number of values).	Most affected by outliers (extreme values).
	Median = middle value of a list of data sorted from least to greatest.	If there is an even number of values, the median will be the average of the middle two values.
	Mode = most common value.	Least affected by outliers.
Measures of dispersion	Standard deviation = how much variability exists in a set of values, around the mean of these values. Standard error = an estimate of how much variability exists in a (theoretical) set of sample means around the true population mean.	σ = SD; n = sample size. Variance = $(SD)^2$. SE = $\sigma/\sqrt{n}$. SE ↓ as n ↑.
Normal distribution	Gaussian, also called bell-shaped. Mean = median = mode. For normal distribution, mean is the best measure of central tendency.	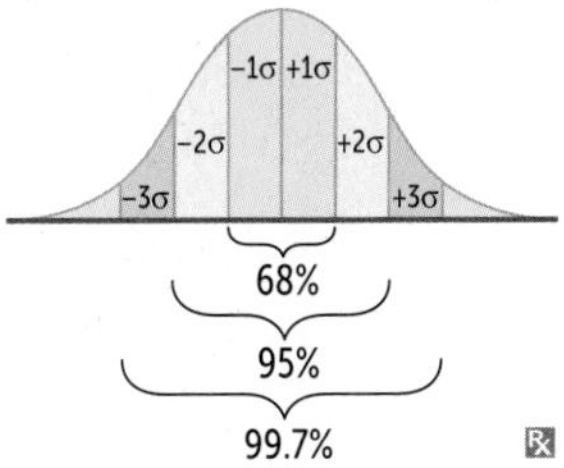
Nonnormal distributions		
Bimodal	Suggests two different populations (eg, metabolic polymorphism such as fast vs slow acetylators; age at onset of Hodgkin lymphoma; suicide rate by age).	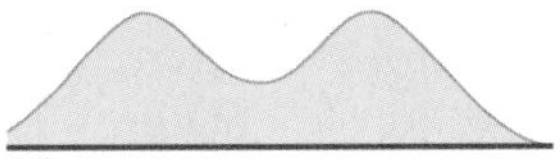
Positive skew	Typically, mean > median > mode. Asymmetry with longer tail on right.	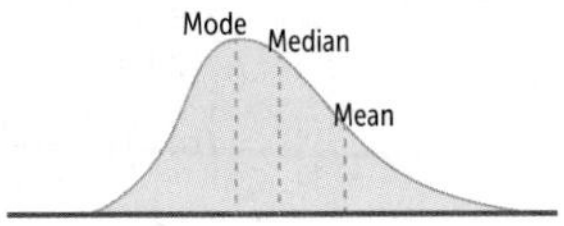
Negative skew	Typically, mean < median < mode. Asymmetry with longer tail on left.	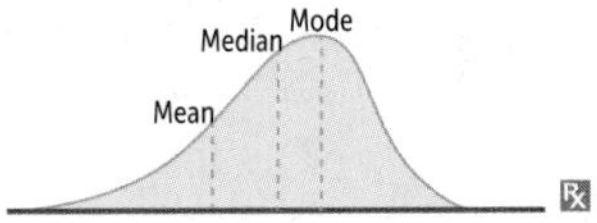

Statistical hypothesis testing

Null hypothesis (H_0) Hypothesis of no difference or relationship (eg, there is no association between the disease and the risk factor in the population).

Alternative hypothesis (H_1) Hypothesis of some difference or relationship (eg, there is some association between the disease and the risk factor in the population).

***p*-value** The probability of obtaining test results at least as extreme as those observed during the test, assuming that H_0 is correct.

Outcomes of statistical hypothesis testing

Correct result

Stating that there is an effect or difference when one exists (H_0 rejected in favor of H_1).

Stating that there is no effect or difference when none exists (H_0 not rejected).

	Reality: H_1	Reality: H_0
Study rejects H_0	Power $(1 - \beta)$	α Type I error
Study does not reject H_0	β Type II error	

Blue shading = correct result.

Testing errors

Type I error (α)

Stating that there is an effect or difference when none exists (H_0 incorrectly rejected in favor of H_1).

α is the probability of making a type I error (usually 0.05 is chosen). If $p < \alpha$, then assuming H_0 is true, the probability of obtaining the test results would be less than the probability of making a type I error. H_0 is therefore rejected as false.

Statistical significance ≠ clinical significance.

Also called false-positive error.

1st time boy cries wolf, the town believes there is a wolf, but there is not (false positive).

You can never "prove" H_1, but you can reject the H_0 as being very unlikely.

Type II error (β)

Stating that there is not an effect or difference when one exists (H_0 is not rejected when it is in fact false).

β is the probability of making a type II error. β is related to statistical power $(1 - \beta)$, which is the probability of rejecting H_0 when it is false.

↑ power and ↓ β by:

- ↑ sample size
- ↑ expected effect size
- ↑ precision of measurement

Also called false-negative error.

2nd time boy cries wolf, the town believes there is no wolf, but there is one.

If you ↑ sample size, you ↑ power. There is **power in numbers**.

Confidence interval	Range of values within which the true mean of the population is expected to fall, with a specified probability. CI = 1 – α. The 95% CI (corresponding to α = 0.05) is often used. As sample size increases, CI narrows. CI for sample mean = $\bar{x} \pm Z(SE)$ For the 95% CI, Z = 1.96. For the 99% CI, Z = 2.58.	H_0 is rejected (and results are significant) when: ▪ 95% CI for mean difference excludes 0 ▪ 95% CI OR or RR excludes 1 ▪ CIs between two groups do not overlap H_0 is accepted (and results are significant) when:. ▪ 95% CI for mean difference includes 0 ▪ 95% CI OR or RR includes 1 ▪ CIs between two groups do overlap

Meta-analysis

A method of statistical analysis that pools summary data (eg, means, RRs) from multiple studies for a more precise estimate of the size of an effect. Also estimates heterogeneity of effect sizes between studies.

Improves power, strength of evidence, and generalizability (external validity) of study findings. Limited by quality of individual studies and bias in study selection.

Common statistical tests

t-test	Checks differences between **means** of **2** groups.	Tea is **meant** for **2**. Example: comparing the mean blood pressure between men and women.
ANOVA	Checks differences between means of 3 or more groups.	3 words: **AN**alysis **O**f **VA**riance. Example: comparing the mean blood pressure between members of 3 different ethnic groups.
Fisher's exact test	Checks differences between 2 percentages or proportions of categorical, nominal outcomes. Use instead of chi-square test with small populations.	Example: comparing the percentage of 20 men and 20 women with hypertension.
Chi-square (χ^2)	Checks differences between 2 or more percentages or proportions of **categorical** outcomes (not mean values).	Pronounce **chi-tegorical**. Example: comparing the proportion of members of 3 age groups who have essential hypertension.

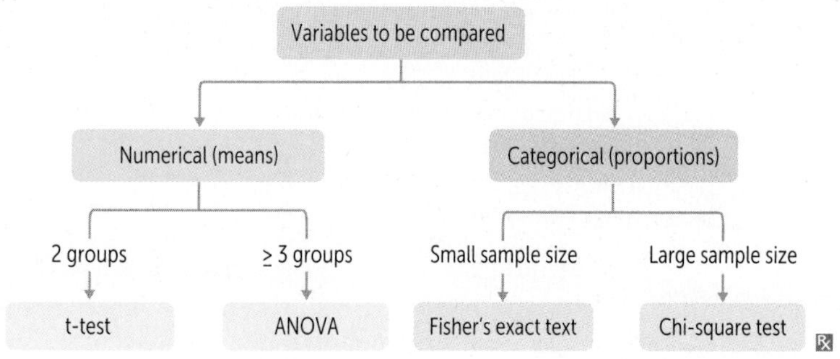

Pearson correlation coefficient

A measure of the linear correlation between two variables. r is always between −1 and +1. The closer the absolute value of r is to 1, the stronger the linear correlation between the 2 variables. Variance is how much the measured values differ from the average value in a data set.

Positive r value → positive correlation (as one variable ↑, the other variable ↑).

Negative r value → negative correlation (as one variable ↑, the other variable ↓).

Coefficient of determination = r^2 (amount of variance in one variable that can be explained by variance in another variable).

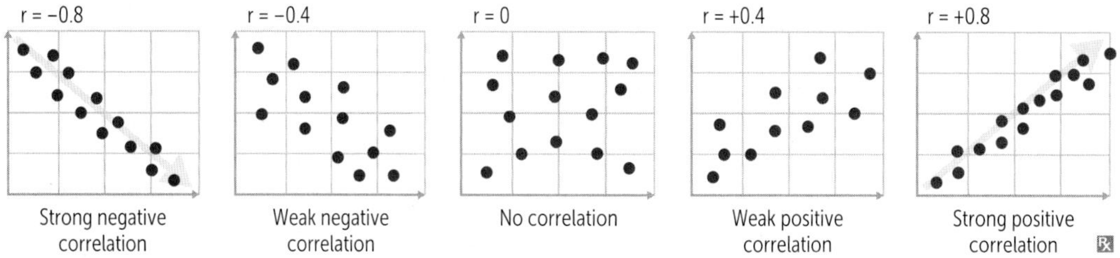

▶ PUBLIC HEALTH SCIENCES—ETHICS

Core ethical principles

Autonomy	Obligation to respect patients as individuals (truth-telling, confidentiality), to create conditions necessary for autonomous choice (informed consent), and to honor their preference in accepting or not accepting medical care.
Beneficence	Physicians have a special ethical (fiduciary) duty to act in the patient's best interest. May conflict with autonomy (an informed patient has the right to decide) or what is best for society (eg, mandatory TB treatment). Traditionally, patient interest supersedes.
Nonmaleficence	"Do no harm." Must be balanced against beneficence; if the benefits outweigh the risks, a patient may make an informed decision to proceed (most surgeries and medications fall into this category).
Justice	To treat persons fairly and equitably. This does not always imply equally (eg, triage).

Decision-making capacity

Physician must determine whether the patient is psychologically and legally capable of making a particular healthcare decision. Note that decisions made with capacity cannot be revoked simply if the patient later loses capacity. Intellectual disabilities and mental illnesses are not exclusion criteria for informed decision-making unless their condition presently impairs their ability to make healthcare decisions.

Capacity is determined by a physician for a specific healthcare-related decision (eg, to refuse medical care). Competency is determined by a judge and usually refers to more global categories of decision making (eg, legally unable to make any healthcare-related decision).

Components (assessing capacity is of **MASSIVE** importance):

- Decision is not a result of **M**ental illness exacerbation
- Patient is ≥ 18 years of **A**ge or otherwise legally emancipated
- Decision is not a result of altered mental **S**tatus (eg, delirium, intoxication)
- Decision remains **S**table over time
- Patient is **I**nformed and understands
- Decision is consistent with patient's **V**alues and goals
- Patient **E**xpresses preferences

Informed consent

A process (not just a document/signature) that requires:

- Disclosure: discussion of pertinent information (using medical interpreter, if needed)
- Understanding: ability to comprehend
- Capacity: ability to reason and make one's own decisions (distinct from competence, a legal determination)
- Voluntariness: freedom from coercion and manipulation

Patients must have a comprehensive understanding of their diagnosis and the risks/benefits of proposed treatment and alternative options, including no treatment.

Patient must be informed of their right to revoke written consent at any time, even orally.

Exceptions to informed consent (**WIPE** it away):

- **W**aiver—patient explicitly relinquishes the right of informed consent
- Legally **I**ncompetent—patient lacks decision-making capacity (obtain consent from legal surrogate)
- Therapeutic **P**rivilege—withholding information when disclosure would severely harm the patient or undermine informed decision-making capacity
- **E**mergency situation—implied consent may apply

Consent for minors	A minor is generally any person < 18 years old. Parental consent laws in relation to healthcare vary by state. In general, parental consent should be obtained, but exceptions exist for emergency treatment (eg, blood transfusions) or if minor is legally emancipated (eg, married, self-supporting, or in the military).	Situations in which parental consent is usually not required: ▪ **Sex** (contraception, STIs, prenatal care—usually not abortion) ▪ **Drugs** (substance use disorder treatment) ▪ **Rock and roll** (emergency/trauma) Physicians should always encourage healthy minor-guardian communication. Physician should seek a minor's assent (agreement of someone unable to legally consent) even if their consent is not required.

Advance directives	Instructions given by a patient in anticipation of the need for a medical decision. Details vary per state law.
Oral advance directive	Incapacitated patient's prior oral statements commonly used as guide. Problems arise from variance in interpretation. If patient was informed, directive was specific, patient made a choice, and decision was repeated over time to multiple people, then the oral directive is more valid.
Written advance directive	Delineates specific healthcare interventions that patient anticipates accepting or rejecting during treatment for a critical or life-threatening illness. A living will is an example.
Medical power of attorney	Patient designates an agent to make medical decisions in the event that the patient loses decision-making capacity. Patient may also specify decisions in clinical situations. Can be revoked by patient if decision-making capacity is intact. More flexible than a living will.
Do not resuscitate order	DNR order prohibits cardiopulmonary resuscitation (CPR). Patient may still consider other life-sustaining measures (eg, intubation, feeding tube, chemotherapy).

Surrogate decision-maker	If a patient loses decision-making capacity and has not prepared an advance directive, individuals (surrogates) who know the patient must determine what the patient would have done. Priority of surrogates: **spouse** → adult **chi**ldren → **p**arents → **s**iblings → other relatives (the **spouse ChiPS** in).

Confidentiality	Confidentiality respects patient privacy and autonomy. If the patient is incapacitated or the situation is emergent, disclosing information to family and friends should be guided by professional judgment of patient's best interest. The patient may voluntarily waive the right to confidentiality (eg, insurance company request). General principles for exceptions to confidentiality: ▪ Potential physical harm to self or others is serious and imminent ▪ Alternative means to warn or protect those at risk is not possible ▪ Steps can be taken to prevent harm Examples of exceptions to patient confidentiality (many are state specific) include the following ("The physician's good judgment **SAVED** the day"): ▪ Patients with **S**uicidal/homicidal ideation ▪ **A**buse (children, elderly, and/or prisoners) ▪ Duty to protect—state-specific laws that sometimes allow physician to inform or somehow protect potential **V**ictim from harm ▪ Patients with **E**pilepsy and other impaired automobile drivers ▪ Reportable **D**iseases (eg, STIs, hepatitis, food poisoning); physicians may have a duty to warn public officials, who will then notify people at risk. Dangerous communicable diseases, such as TB or Ebola, may require involuntary treatment.

▸ PUBLIC HEALTH SCIENCES—COMMUNICATION SKILLS

Patient-centered interviewing techniques

Introduction	Introduce yourself and address the patient by preferred name. Sit at eye-level near the patient.
Agenda setting	Identify concerns and set goals by developing joint agenda between the physician and the patient.
Reflection	Actively listen and synthesize information offered by the patient, particularly with respect to primary concern(s).
Validation	Legitimize or affirm the patient's perspectives.
Recapitulation	Summarize what the patient has said so far to ensure correct interpretation.
Facilitation	Encourage the patient to speak freely without guiding responses or leading questions. Allow the patient to ask questions throughout the encounter.

Expressing empathy	PEARLS
Partnership	Reassure the patient that you will work together through difficult times, and offer appropriate resources.
Empathy	Acknowledge the emotions displayed and demonstrate understanding of why the patient is feeling that way.
Apology	Take personal responsibility when appropriate, or offer condolences for the patient's situation.
Respect	Commend the patient for coming in to discuss a problem, pushing through challenging circumstances, keeping a positive attitude, or other constructive behaviors.
Legitimization	Assure the patient that emotional responses are understandable or common.
Support	Offer to help the patient through difficult times.

Delivering bad news	SPIKES
Setting	Offer in advance for the patient to bring support. Eliminate distractions, ensure privacy, and sit down with the patient to talk.
Perception	Determine the patient's understanding and expectations of the situation.
Invitation	Obtain the patient's permission to disclose the news and what level of detail is desired.
Knowledge	Share the information in small pieces without medical jargon, allowing time to process. Assess the patient's understanding.
Emotions	Acknowledge the patient's emotions, and provide opportunity to express them. Listen and offer empathetic responses.
Strategy	If the patient feels ready, discuss treatment options and goals of care. Offer an agenda for the next appointment.

Gender- and sexuality-inclusive history taking

Avoid making assumptions about sexual orientation, gender identity, gender expression, and behavior (eg, a patient who identifies as heterosexual may engage in same-sex sexual activity).
Use gender-neutral terms (eg, refer to a patient's "partner" rather than assuming a spouse's gender).
A patient's sex assigned at birth and gender identity may differ.
Consider stating what pronouns you use when you introduce yourself (eg, "I'm Dr. Smith, and I use she/her pronouns") and asking patients how they would like to be addressed.
Reassure them about the confidentiality of their appointments and be sensitive to the fact that patients may not be open about their sexual orientation or gender identity to others in their life.
Do not bring up gender or sexuality if it is not relevant to the visit (eg, a gender-nonconforming patient seeking care for a hand laceration).

Trauma-informed communication

Patients with a history of a traumatic experience should receive thorough behavioral health screenings. Regularly assess mood, substance use, social supports, and suicide risk.
Focus assessments on trauma-related symptoms that interfere with social and occupational function.
Do not ask invasive questions requiring the patient to describe trauma in detail.
Before the physical exam, reassure patients that they may signal to end it immediately if they experience too much physical or emotional discomfort. Offer the presence of additional staff for support.

Motivational interviewing	Counseling technique to facilitate behavior modification by helping patients resolve ambivalence about change. Useful for many conditions (eg, nicotine dependence, obesity). Helpful when patient has some desire to change, but it does not require that the patient be committed to making the change. May involve asking patients to examine how their behavior interferes with their life or why they might want to change it. Assess barriers (eg, food access, untreated trauma) that may make behavior change difficult. Assessing a patient's readiness for change is also important for guiding physician-suggested goals. These goals should be Specific, Measurable, Achievable, Relevant, and Time bound (SMART).
Communicating with patients with disabilities	Use "person-first" language, which refers to "a person with a disability" rather than "a disabled person." Consider asking patients what terms they use to describe themselves. Under most circumstances, talk directly to the patient. Do not assume that nonverbal patients do not understand. Accompanying caregivers can add information to any discussion as needed. Ask if assistance is desired rather than assuming the patient cannot do something alone. Most people, including people with disabilities, value their independence. For patients with speech difficulties, provide extra time for the interview. If their speech is difficult to understand, consider asking them to write down a few words or ask them to rephrase their sentence. Repeat what they said to ensure you understood it correctly. For patients with a cognitive impairment, use concrete, specific language. Ask simple, direct questions. Eliminate background noise and distractions. Do not assume the patient can read. Adjust to how the patient understands best (eg, use hand gestures or ask them to demonstrate a task). Ask patients who are deaf or hard of hearing their preferred mode of communication. Use light touch or waving to get their attention. For patients who prefer to speak and lipread, eliminate background noise, face the patient, and do not change your mode of speaking. As with other parts of a medical history, do not bring up a disability if it is not relevant to a visit (eg, a patient in a wheelchair with an ear infection). Do not skip relevant parts of the physical exam even if the disability makes the exam challenging.
Use of interpreters	Visits with a patient who speaks little English should utilize a professionally trained medical interpreter unless the physician is also fluent in the patient's preferred language. Interpretation services may be provided in person, by telephone, or by video call. If the patient prefers to utilize a family member, this should be recorded in the chart. Do not assume that a patient is a poor English speaker because of name, skin tone, or accent. Ask the patient what language is preferred. The physician should make eye contact with the patient and speak to them normally, without use of third-person statements such as "tell him." Allow extra time for the interview, and ask one question at a time. For in-person spoken language interpretation, the interpreter should ideally be next to or slightly behind the patient. For sign language interpretation, the interpreter should be next to or slightly behind the physician.

Challenging patient and ethical scenarios

The most appropriate response is usually one that is open ended, empathetic, and patient centered. It often honors one or more of the principles of autonomy, beneficence, nonmaleficence, and justice. Appropriate responses are respectful of patients and other members of the healthcare team.

SITUATION	APPROPRIATE RESPONSE
Patient is not adherent.	Determine whether there are financial, logistical, or other obstacles preventing the patient's adherence. Do not coerce the patient into adhering or refer the patient to another physician.
Patient desires an unnecessary procedure.	Attempt to understand why the patient wants the procedure and address underlying concerns. Do not refuse to see the patient or refer to another physician. Avoid performing unnecessary procedures.
Patient has difficulty taking medications.	Determine what factors are involved in the patient's difficulties. If comprehension or memory are issues, use techniques such as providing written instructions, using the teach-back method, or simplifying treatment regimens.
Family members ask for information about patient's prognosis.	Avoid discussing issues with relatives without the patient's permission.
A patient's family member asks you not to disclose the results of a test if the prognosis is poor because the patient will be "unable to handle it."	Explore why the family member believes this would be detrimental, including possible cultural factors. Explain that if the patient would like to know information concerning care, it will not be withheld. However, if you believe the patient might seriously harm self or others if informed, you may invoke therapeutic privilege and withhold the information.
A 17-year-old is pregnant and requests an abortion.	Many states require parental notification or consent for minors for an abortion. Unless there are specific medical risks associated with pregnancy, a physician should not sway the patient's decision for, or against, an elective abortion (regardless of patient's age or fetal condition). Discuss options for terminating the pregnancy and refer to abortion care, if needed.
A 15-year-old is pregnant and wants to raise the child. Her parents want you to tell her to give the child up for adoption.	The patient retains the right to make decisions regarding her child, even if her parents disagree. Provide information to the teenager about the practical aspects of caring for a baby. Discuss options for terminating the pregnancy, if requested. Encourage discussion between the teenager and her parents to reach the best decision.
A terminally ill patient requests physician-assisted dying.	The overwhelming majority of states prohibit most forms of physician-assisted dying. Physicians may, however, prescribe medically appropriate analgesics even if they potentially shorten the patient's life.
Patient is suicidal.	Assess the seriousness of the threat. If patient is actively suicidal with a plan, suggest remaining in the hospital voluntarily; patient may be hospitalized involuntarily if needed.
Patient states that you are attractive and asks if you would go on a date.	Use a chaperone if necessary. Romantic relationships with patients are never appropriate. It may be necessary to transition care to another physician.
A woman who had a mastectomy says she now feels "ugly."	Find out why the patient feels this way. Do not offer falsely reassuring statements (eg, "You still look good").
Patient is angry about the long time spent in the waiting room.	Acknowledge the patient's anger, but do not take a patient's anger personally. Thank the patient for being patient and apologize for any inconvenience. Stay away from efforts to explain the delay.
Patient is upset with treatment received from another physician.	Suggest that the patient speak directly to that physician regarding the concern. If the problem is with a member of the office staff, tell the patient you will speak to that person.
An invasive test is performed on the wrong patient.	Regardless of the outcome, a physician is ethically obligated to inform a patient that a mistake has been made.

Challenging patient and ethical scenarios *(continued)*

SITUATION	APPROPRIATE RESPONSE
A patient requires a treatment not covered by insurance.	Discuss all treatment options with patients, even if some are not covered by their insurance companies. Inform patient of financial assistance programs.
A 7-year-old boy loses a sister to cancer and now feels responsible.	At ages 5–7, children begin to understand that death is permanent, that all life functions end completely at death, and that everything that is alive eventually dies. Provide a direct, concrete description of his sister's death. Avoid clichés and euphemisms. Reassure the boy that he is not responsible. Identify and normalize fears and feelings. Encourage play and healthy coping behaviors (eg, remembering her in his own way).
Patient is victim of intimate partner violence.	Ask if patient is safe and help devise an emergency plan if there isn't one. Educate patient on intimate partner violence resources. Do not necessarily pressure patient to leave a partner or disclose the incident to the authorities (unless required by state law).
Patient wants to try alternative or holistic medicine.	Explore any underlying reasons with the patient in a supportive, nonjudgmental manner. Advise the patient of known benefits and risks of treatment, including adverse effects, contraindications, and medication interactions.
Physician colleague presents to work impaired.	This presents a potential risk to patient safety. You have an ethical and usually a legal obligation to report impaired colleagues so they can cease patient care and receive appropriate assistance in a timely manner. Seek guidance in reporting as procedures and applicable law vary by institution and state.
Patient is officially determined to suffer brain death. Patient's family insists on maintaining life support indefinitely because patient is still moving when touched.	Gently explain to family that there is no chance of recovery, and that brain death is equivalent to death. Movement is due to spinal arc reflex and is not voluntary. Bring case to appropriate ethics board regarding futility of care and withdrawal of life support.
A pharmaceutical company offers you a sponsorship in exchange for advertising its new drug.	Reject this offer. Generally, decline gifts and sponsorships to avoid any conflict of interest. The AMA Code of Ethics does make exceptions for gifts directly benefitting patients; special funding for medical education of students, residents, fellows; grants whose recipients are chosen by independent institutional criteria; and funds that are distributed without attribution to sponsors.
Patient requests a nonemergent procedure that is against your personal or religious beliefs.	Provide accurate and unbiased information so patients can make an informed decision. In a neutral, nonjudgmental manner, explain to the patient that you do not perform the procedure but offer to refer to another physician.
Mother and 15-year-old daughter are unresponsive following a car accident and are bleeding internally. Father says do not transfuse because they are Jehovah's Witnesses.	Transfuse daughter, but do not transfuse mother. Emergent care can be refused by the healthcare proxy for an adult, particularly when patient preferences are known or reasonably inferred, but not for a minor based solely on faith.
A dependent patient presents with injuries inconsistent with caretaker's story.	Document detailed history and physical. If possible and appropriate, interview the patient alone. Provide any necessary medical care. If suspicion remains, contact the appropriate agencies or authorities (eg, child or adult protective services) for an evaluation. Inform the caretaker of your obligation to report. Physicians are required by law to report any reasonable suspicion of abuse, neglect, or endangerment.
A pediatrician recommends standard vaccinations for a patient, but the child's parent refuses.	Address any concerns the parent has. Explain the risks and benefits of vaccinations and why they are recommended. Do not administer routine vaccinations without the parent's consent.

▶ PUBLIC HEALTH SCIENCES—HEALTHCARE DELIVERY

Disease prevention

Primary disease prevention	Prevent disease before it occurs (eg, HPV vaccination)
Secondary disease prevention	Screen early for and manage existing but asymptomatic disease (eg, Pap smear for cervical cancer)
Tertiary disease prevention	Treatment to reduce complications from disease that is ongoing or has long-term effects (eg, chemotherapy)
Quaternary disease prevention	Quit (avoid) unnecessary medical interventions to minimize incidental harm (eg, imaging studies, optimizing medications to reduce polypharmacy)

Major medical insurance plans

PLAN	PROVIDERS	PAYMENTS	SPECIALIST CARE
Exclusive provider organization	Restricted to limited panel (except emergencies)		No referral required
Health maintenance organization	Restricted to limited panel (except emergencies)	Most affordable	Requires referral from primary care provider
Point of service	Patient can see providers outside network	Higher copays and deductibles for out-of-network services	Requires referral from primary care provider
Preferred provider organization	Patient can see providers outside network	Higher copays and deductibles for all services	No referral required
Accountable care organization	Providers voluntarily enroll	Medicare	Specialists voluntarily enroll

Healthcare payment models

Bundled payment	Healthcare organization receives a set amount per service, regardless of ultimate cost, to be divided among all providers and facilities involved.
Capitation	Physicians receive a set amount per patient assigned to them per period of time, regardless of how much the patient uses the healthcare system. Used by some HMOs.
Discounted fee-for-service	Insurer and/or patient pays for each individual service at a discounted rate predetermined by providers and payers (eg, PPOs).
Fee-for-service	Insurer and/or patient pays for each individual service.
Global payment	Insurer and/or patient pays for all expenses associated with a single incident of care with a single payment. Most commonly used during elective surgeries, as it covers the cost of surgery as well as the necessary pre- and postoperative visits.

Medicare and Medicaid

Medicare and Medicaid—federal social healthcare programs that originated from amendments to the Social Security Act.
Medicare is available to patients ≥ 65 years old, < 65 with certain disabilities, and those with end-stage renal disease.
Medicaid is joint federal and state health assistance for people with limited income and/or resources.

MedicarE is for Elderly.
MedicaiD is for Disadvantaged.

The 4 parts of Medicare:
- Part A: hospital Admissions, including hospice, skilled nursing
- Part B: Basic medical bills (eg, physician fees, diagnostic testing)
- Part C: (parts A + B = Combo) delivered by approved private companies
- Part D: prescription Drugs

Hospice care

Medical care focused on providing comfort and palliation instead of definitive cure. Available to patients on Medicare or Medicaid and in most private insurance plans whose life expectancy is < 6 months.
During end-of-life care, priority is given to improving the patient's comfort and relieving pain (often includes opioid, sedative, or anxiolytic medications). Facilitating comfort is prioritized over potential side effects (eg, respiratory depression). This prioritization of positive effects over negative effects is called the principle of double effect.

Common causes of death (US) by age

	< 1 YR	1–14 YR	15–34 YR	35–44 YR	45–64 YR	65+ YR
#1	Congenital malformations	Unintentional injury	Unintentional injury	Unintentional injury	Cancer	Heart disease
#2	Preterm birth	Cancer	Suicide	Cancer	Heart disease	Cancer
#3	Pregnancy complications	Congenital malformations	Homicide	Heart disease	Unintentional injury	Chronic respiratory disease

▸ PUBLIC HEALTH SCIENCES—QUALITY AND SAFETY

Safety culture

Organizational environment in which everyone can freely bring up safety concerns without fear of penalty. Facilitates error identification.

Event reporting systems collect data on errors for internal and external monitoring.

Human factors design

Forcing functions (those that prevent undesirable actions [eg, connecting feeding syringe to IV tubing]) are the most effective.
Standardization improves process reliability (eg, clinical pathways, guidelines, checklists).
Simplification reduces wasteful activities (eg, consolidating electronic medical records).

Deficient designs hinder workflow and lead to staff workarounds that bypass safety features (eg, patient ID barcodes affixed to computers due to unreadable wristbands).

PDSA cycle

Process improvement model to test changes in real clinical setting. Impact on patients:

- Plan—define problem and solution
- Do—test new process
- Study—measure and analyze data
- Act—integrate new process into workflow

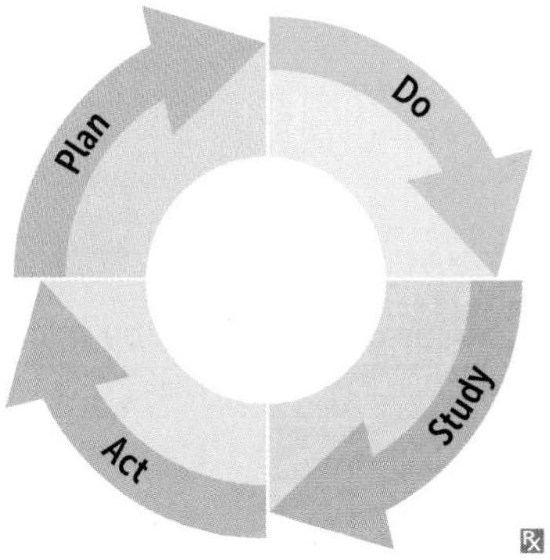

Quality measurements

	MEASURE	EXAMPLE
Structural	Physical equipment, resources, facilities	Number of diabetes educators
Process	Performance of system as planned	Percentage of patients with diabetes whose HbA_{1c} was measured in the past 6 months
Outcome	Impact on patients	Average HbA_{1c} of patients with diabetes
Balancing	Impact on other systems/outcomes	Incidence of hypoglycemia among patients who tried an intervention to lower HbA_{1c}

Swiss cheese model

Focuses on systems and conditions rather than an individual's error. The risk of a threat becoming a reality is mitigated by differing layers and types of defenses. Patient harm can occur despite multiple safeguards when "the holes in the cheese line up."

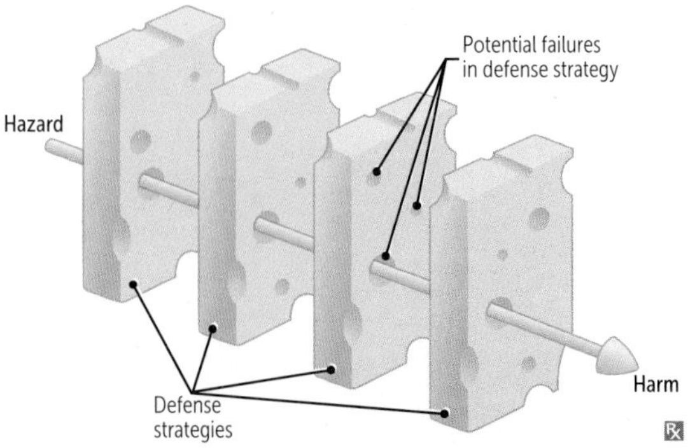

Types of medical errors	May involve patient identification, diagnosis, monitoring, nosocomial infection, medications, procedures, devices, documentation, handoffs. Medical errors should be disclosed to patients, independent of immediate outcome (harmful or not).	
Active error	Occurs at level of frontline operator (eg, wrong IV pump dose programmed).	Immediate impact.
Latent error	Occurs in processes indirect from operator but impacts patient care (eg, different types of IV pumps used within same hospital).	Accident waiting to happen.
Never event	Adverse event that is identifiable, serious, and usually preventable (eg, scalpel retained in a surgical patient's abdomen).	Major error that should never occur.
Near miss	Unplanned event that does not result in harm but has the potential to do so (eg, pharmacist recognizes a medication interaction and cancels the order).	Narrow prevention of harm that exposes dangers.

Burnout vs fatigue

Burnout	Prolonged, excessive stress → cynicism, detachment, ↓ motivation and interest, sense of failure and helplessness, ↓ immunity. Medical errors due to reduced professional efficacy.
Fatigue	Sleep deprivation → ↓ energy and motivation, cognitive impairment. Medical errors due to compromised intellectual function.

Medical error analysis

	DESIGN	METHODS
Root cause analysis	Retrospective approach. Applied after failure event to prevent recurrence.	Uses records and participant interviews to identify all the underlying problems (eg, process, people, environment, equipment, materials, management) that led to an error.
Failure mode and effects analysis	Forward-looking approach. Applied before process implementation to prevent failure occurrence.	Uses inductive reasoning to identify all the ways a process might fail and prioritizes them by their probability of occurrence and impact on patients.

▶ NOTES

SECTION III

High-Yield Organ Systems

"Symptoms, then, are in reality nothing but the cry from suffering organs."
—Jean-Martin Charcot

"Man is an intelligence in servitude to his organs."
—Aldous Huxley

"When every part of the machine is correctly adjusted and in perfect harmony, health will hold dominion over the human organism by laws as natural and immutable as the laws of gravity."
—Andrew T. Still

▶ APPROACHING THE ORGAN SYSTEMS

In this section, we have divided the High-Yield Facts into the major **Organ Systems.** Within each Organ System are several subsections, including **Embryology, Anatomy, Physiology, Pathology,** and **Pharmacology.** As you progress through each Organ System, refer back to information in the previous subsections to organize these basic science subsections into a "vertically integrated" framework for learning. Below is some general advice for studying the organ systems by these subsections.

Embryology

Relevant embryology is included in each organ system subsection. Embryology tends to correspond well with the relevant anatomy, especially with regard to congenital malformations.

Anatomy

Several topics fall under this heading, including gross anatomy, histology, and neuroanatomy. Do not memorize all the small details; however, do not ignore anatomy altogether. Review what you have already learned and what you wish you had learned. Many questions require two or more steps. The first step is to identify a structure on anatomic cross section, electron micrograph, or photomicrograph. The second step may require an understanding of the clinical significance of the structure.

While studying, emphasize clinically important material. For example, be familiar with gross anatomy and radiologic anatomy related to specific diseases (eg, Pancoast tumor, Horner syndrome), traumatic injuries (eg, fractures, sensory and motor nerve deficits), procedures (eg, lumbar puncture), and common surgeries (eg, cholecystectomy). There are also many questions on the exam involving x-rays, CT scans, and neuro MRI scans. Many students suggest browsing through a general radiology atlas, pathology atlas, and histology atlas. Focus on learning basic anatomy at key levels in the body (eg, sagittal brain MRI; axial CT of the midthorax, abdomen, and pelvis). Basic neuroanatomy (especially pathways, blood supply, and functional anatomy), associated neuropathology, and neurophysiology have good yield. Please note that many of the photographic images in this book are for illustrative purposes and are not necessarily reflective of Step 1 emphasis.

Physiology

The portion of the examination dealing with physiology is broad and concept oriented and thus does not lend itself as well to fact-based review. Diagrams are often the best study aids, especially given the increasing number of questions requiring the interpretation of diagrams. Learn to apply basic physiologic relationships in a variety of ways (eg, the Fick equation, clearance equations). You are seldom asked to perform complex calculations. Hormones are the focus of many questions; learn where and how they are synthesized, their regulatory mechanisms and sites of action.

A large portion of the physiology tested on the USMLE Step 1 is clinically relevant and involves understanding physiologic changes associated with pathologic processes (eg, changes in pulmonary function with COPD). Thus, it is worthwhile to review the physiologic changes that are found with common pathologies of the major organ systems (eg, heart, lungs, kidneys, GI tract) and endocrine glands.

Pathology

Questions dealing with this discipline are difficult to prepare for because of the sheer volume of material involved. Review the basic principles and hallmark characteristics of the key diseases. Given the clinical orientation of Step 1, it is no longer sufficient to know only the "buzzword" associations of certain diseases (eg, café-au-lait macules and neurofibromatosis); you must also recognize the clinical descriptions of these high-yield physical exam findings.

Given the clinical slant of the USMLE Step 1, it is also important to review the classic presenting signs and symptoms of diseases as well as their associated laboratory findings. Delve into the signs, symptoms, and pathophysiology of major diseases that have a high prevalence in the United States (eg, alcohol use disorder, diabetes, hypertension, heart failure, ischemic heart disease, infectious disease). Be prepared to think one step beyond the simple diagnosis to treatment or complications.

The examination includes a number of color photomicrographs and photographs of gross specimens that are presented in the setting of a brief clinical history. However, read the question and the choices carefully before looking at the illustration, because the history will help you identify the pathologic process. Flip through an illustrated pathology textbook, color atlases, and appropriate Web sites in order to look at the pictures in the days before the exam. Pay attention to potential clues such as age, sex, ethnicity, occupation, recent activities and exposures, and specialized lab tests.

Pharmacology

Preparation for questions on pharmacology is straightforward. Learning all the key drugs and their characteristics (eg, mechanisms, clinical use, and important side effects) is high yield. Focus on understanding the prototype drugs in each class. Avoid memorizing obscure derivatives. Learn the "classic" and distinguishing toxicities of the major drugs. Do not bother with drug dosages or brand names. Reviewing associated biochemistry, physiology, and microbiology can be useful while studying pharmacology. There is a strong emphasis on ANS, CNS, antimicrobial, and cardiovascular agents as well as NSAIDs. Much of the material is clinically relevant. Newer drugs on the market are also fair game.

▶ NOTES

HIGH-YIELD SYSTEMS

Cardiovascular

"As for me, except for an occasional heart attack, I feel as young as I ever did."

—Robert Benchley

"Hearts will never be practical until they are made unbreakable."

—*The Wizard of Oz*

"As the arteries grow hard, the heart grows soft."

—H. L. Mencken

"Nobody has ever measured, not even poets, how much the heart can hold."

—Zelda Fitzgerald

"The art of medicine has its roots in the heart."

—Paracelsus

"It is not the size of the man but the size of his heart that matters."

—Evander Holyfield

The cardiovascular system is one of the highest yield areas for the boards and, for some students, may be the most challenging. Focusing on understanding the mechanisms instead of memorizing the details can make a big difference, especially for this topic. Pathophysiology of atherosclerosis and heart failure, MOA of drugs (particular physiology interactions) and their adverse effects, ECGs of heart blocks, the cardiac cycle, and the Starling curve are some of the more high-yield topics. Differentiating between systolic and diastolic dysfunction is also very important. Heart murmurs and maneuvers that affect these murmurs have also been high yield and may be asked in a multimedia format.

▶ CARDIOVASCULAR—EMBRYOLOGY

Heart morphogenesis	First functional organ in vertebrate embryos; beats spontaneously by week 4 of development.	
Cardiac looping	Primary heart tube loops to establish left-right polarity; begins in week 4 of development.	Defect in left-right dynein (involved in left-right asymmetry) can lead to dextrocardia, as seen in Kartagener syndrome.
Septation of the chambers		
Atria	❶ Septum primum grows toward endocardial cushions, narrowing ostium primum. ❷ Ostium secundum forms in septum primum due to cell death (ostium primum regresses). ❸ Septum secundum develops on the right side of septum primum, as ostium secundum maintains right-to-left shunt. ❹ Septum secundum expands and covers most of ostium secundum. The residual foramen is the foramen ovale. ❺ Remaining portion of septum primum forms the one-way valve of the foramen ovale.	6. Septum primum closes against septum secundum, sealing the foramen ovale soon after birth because of ↑ LA pressure and ↓ RA pressure. 7. Septum secundum and septum primum fuse during infancy/early childhood, forming the atrial septum. **Patent foramen ovale**—caused by failure of septum primum and septum secundum to fuse after birth; most are left untreated. Can lead to paradoxical emboli (venous thromboemboli entering the systemic arterial circulation through right-to-left shunt) as can occur in atrial septal defect (ASD).

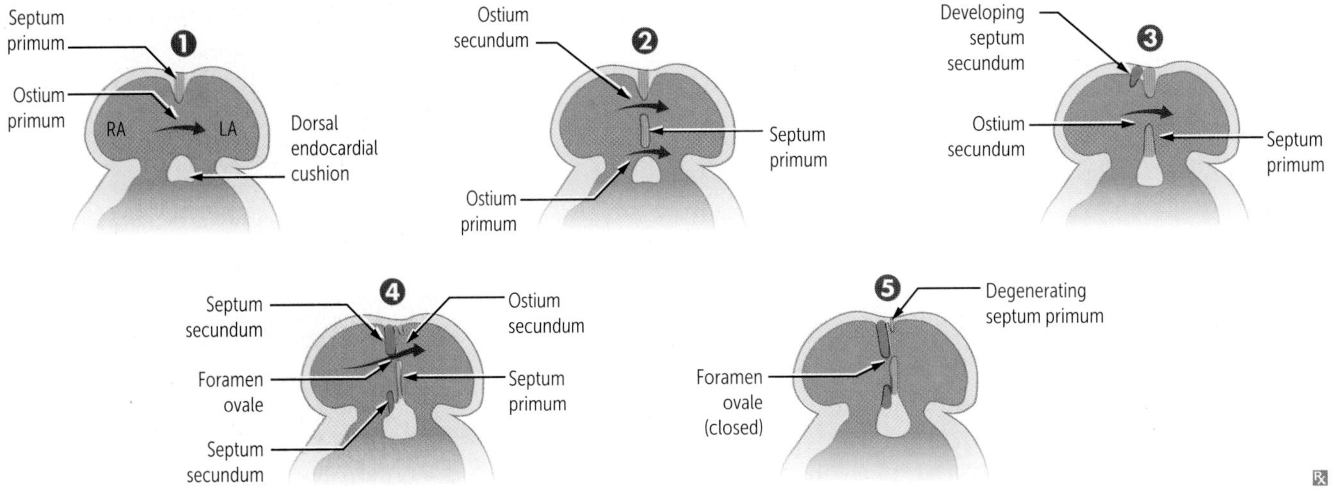

Heart morphogenesis *(continued)*

Ventricles	❶ Muscular interventricular septum forms. Opening is called interventricular foramen. ❷ Aorticopulmonary septum rotates and fuses with muscular ventricular septum to form membranous interventricular septum, closing interventricular foramen. ❸ Growth of endocardial cushions separates atria from ventricles and contributes to both atrial septation and membranous portion of the interventricular septum.	**Ventricular septal defect**—most common congenital cardiac anomaly, usually occurs in membranous septum.

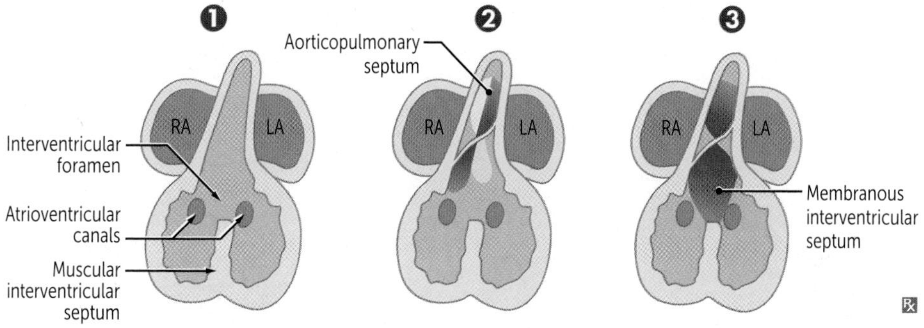
❶
❷
❸
Aorticopulmonary septum
Interventricular foramen
Atrioventricular canals
Muscular interventricular septum
RA
LA
Membranous interventricular septum

Outflow tract formation	Neural crest cell migrations → truncal and bulbar ridges that spiral and fuse to form aorticopulmonary septum → ascending aorta and pulmonary trunk.	Conotruncal abnormalities associated with failure of neural crest cells to migrate: ▪ Transposition of great vessels. ▪ Tetralogy of Fallot. ▪ Persistent truncus arteriosus.
Valve development	Aortic/pulmonary: derived from endocardial cushions of outflow tract. Mitral/tricuspid: derived from fused endocardial cushions of the AV canal.	Valvular anomalies may be stenotic, regurgitant, atretic (eg, tricuspid atresia), or displaced (eg, Ebstein anomaly).

Aortic arch derivatives	Develop into arterial system.
1st	Part of **max**illary artery (branch of external carotid). 1st arch is **max**imal.
2nd	**S**tapedial artery and hyoid artery. **S**econd = **s**tapedial.
3rd	**C**ommon **c**arotid artery and proximal part of internal **c**arotid artery. **C** is **3**rd letter of alphabet.
4th	On left, aortic arch; on right, proximal part of right subclavian artery. **4**th arch (**4** limbs) = systemic.
6th	Proximal part of pulmonary arteries and (on left only) ductus arteriosus. **6**th arch = **p**ulmonary and the **p**ulmonary-to-systemic shunt (ductus arteriosus).

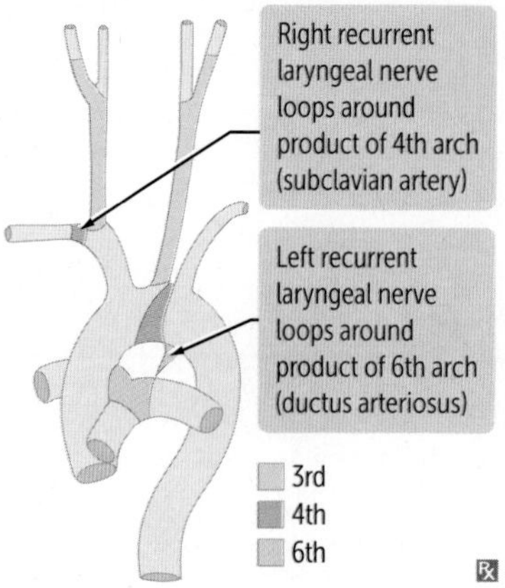
Right recurrent laryngeal nerve loops around product of 4th arch (subclavian artery)
Left recurrent laryngeal nerve loops around product of 6th arch (ductus arteriosus)
3rd
4th
6th

Heart embryology

EMBRYONIC STRUCTURE	GIVES RISE TO
Truncus arteriosus	Ascending aorta and pulmonary trunk
Bulbus cordis	Smooth parts (outflow tract) of left and right ventricles
Primitive ventricle	Trabeculated part of left and right ventricles
Primitive atrium	Trabeculated part of left and right atria
Left horn of sinus venosus	Coronary sinus
Right horn of sinus venosus	Smooth part of right atrium (sinus venarum)
Endocardial cushion	Atrial septum, membranous interventricular septum; AV and semilunar valves
Right common cardinal vein and right anterior cardinal vein	Superior vena cava (SVC)
Posterior, subcardinal, and supracardinal veins	Inferior vena cava (IVC)
Primitive pulmonary vein	Smooth part of left atrium

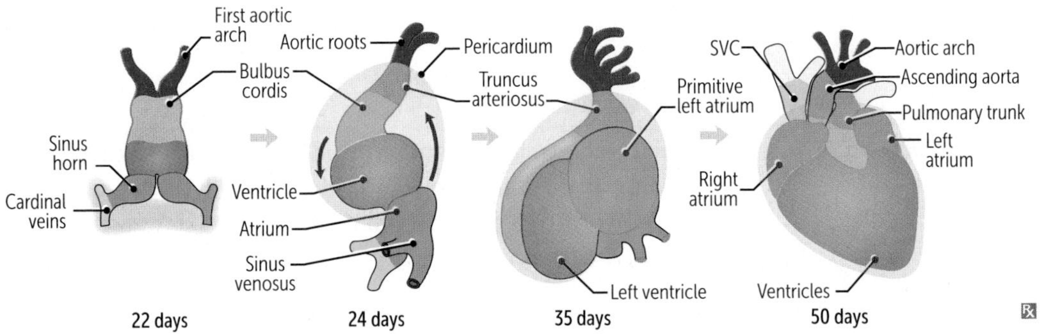

Fetal circulation

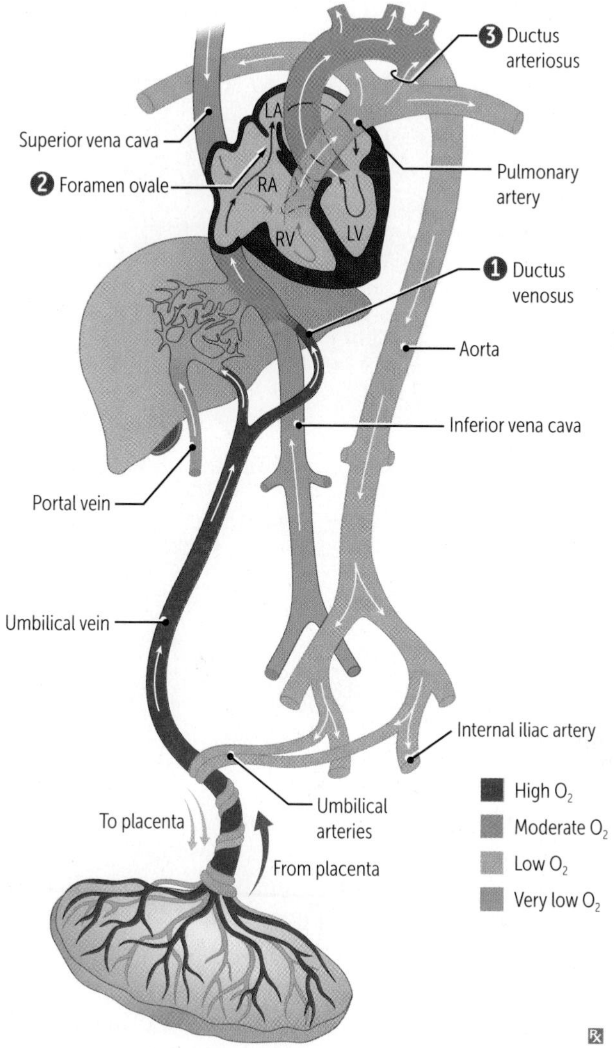

3 Ductus arteriosus
Superior vena cava
2 Foramen ovale
LA
RA
RV
LV
Pulmonary artery
1 Ductus venosus
Aorta
Inferior vena cava
Portal vein
Umbilical vein
Internal iliac artery
To placenta
Umbilical arteries
From placenta
High O_2
Moderate O_2
Low O_2
Very low O_2

Blood in umbilical vein has a Po_2 of ≈ 30 mm Hg and is ≈ 80% saturated with O_2. Umbilical arteries have low O_2 saturation.

3 important shunts:

1. Blood entering fetus through the umbilical vein is conducted via the **ductus venosus** into the IVC, bypassing hepatic circulation.
2. Most of the highly oxygenated blood reaching the heart via the IVC is directed through the **foramen ovale** into the left atrium.
3. Deoxygenated blood from the SVC passes through the RA → RV → main pulmonary artery → **ductus arteriosus** → descending aorta; shunt is due to high fetal pulmonary artery resistance.

At birth, infant takes a breath → ↓ resistance in pulmonary vasculature → ↑ left atrial pressure vs right atrial pressure→ foramen ovale closes (now called fossa ovalis); ↑ in O_2 (from respiration) and ↓ in prostaglandins (from placental separation) → closure of ductus arteriosus.

Indomethacin helps close the patent ductus arteriosus → ligamentum arteriosum (remnant of ductus arteriosus). "**Endomethacin**" **ends** the PDA.

Prostaglandins E_1 and E_2 kEEp PDA open.

Fetal-postnatal derivatives

FETAL STRUCTURE	POSTNATAL DERIVATIVE	NOTES
Ductus arteriosus	Ligamentum arteriosum	Near the left recurrent laryngeal nerve
Ductus venosus	Ligamentum venosum	
Foramen ovale	Fossa ovalis	
Allantois → urachus	Median umbilical ligament	Urachus is part of allantois between bladder and umbilicus
Umbilical arteries	Medial umbilical ligaments	
Umbilical vein	Ligamentum teres hepatis (round ligament)	Contained in falciform ligament

▶ CARDIOVASCULAR—ANATOMY

Anatomy of the heart

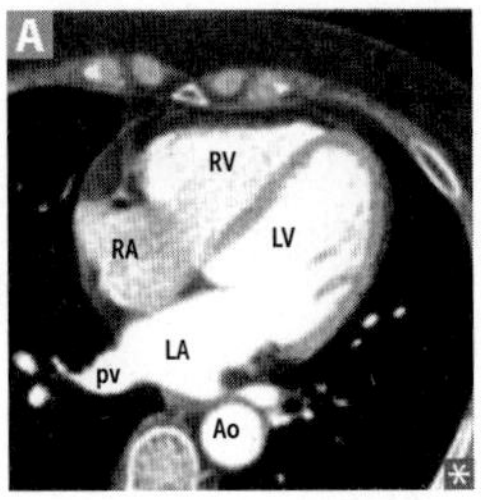

LA is the most posterior part of the heart A B; enlargement of the LA (eg, in mitral stenosis) can lead to compression of the esophagus (dysphagia) and/or the left recurrent laryngeal nerve, a branch of the vagus nerve, causing hoarseness (**Ortner syndrome**).

RV is the most anterior part of the heart and most commonly injured in trauma.

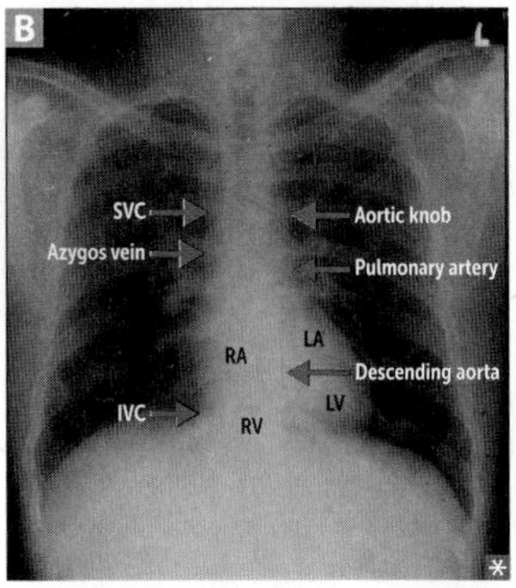

Pericardium

Consists of 3 layers (from outer to inner):
- Fibrous pericardium
- Parietal pericardium
- Epicardium (visceral pericardium)

Pericardial space lies between parietal pericardium and epicardium.

Pericardium innervated by phrenic nerve.

Pericarditis can cause referred pain to the neck, arms, or one or both shoulders (often left).

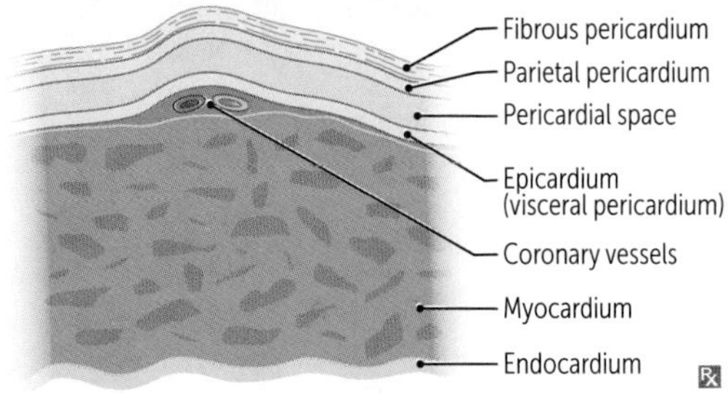

Coronary blood supply

LAD and its branches supply anterior 2/3 of interventricular septum, anterolateral papillary muscle, and anterior surface of LV. Most commonly occluded.

PDA supplies posterior 1/3 of interventricular septum, posterior 2/3 walls of ventricles, and posteromedial papillary muscle.

RCA supplies AV node and SA node. Infarct may cause nodal dysfunction (bradycardia or heart block). Right (acute) marginal artery supplies RV.

Dominance:
- Right-dominant circulation (most common) = PDA arises from RCA
- Left-dominant circulation = PDA arises from LCX
- Codominant circulation = PDA arises from both LCX and RCA

Coronary blood flow to LV and interventricular septum peaks in early diastole.

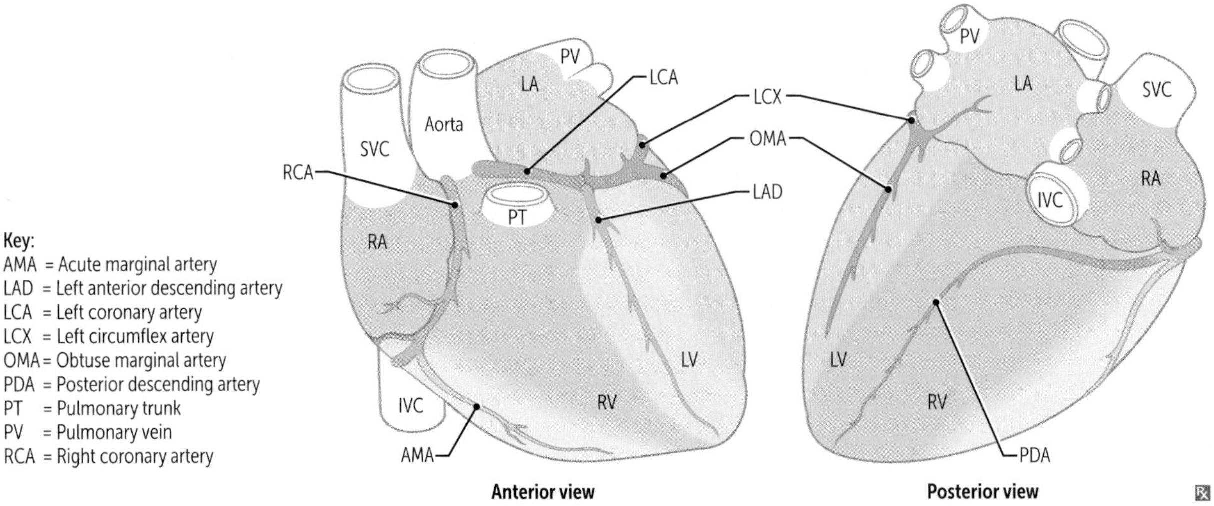

▶ CARDIOVASCULAR—PHYSIOLOGY

Cardiac output variables

Stroke volume	Stroke Volume affected by Contractility, Afterload, and Preload. ↑ SV with: ▪ ↑ Contractility (eg, anxiety, exercise) ▪ ↑ Preload (eg, early pregnancy) ▪ ↓ Afterload	SV CAP. A failing heart has ↓ SV (systolic and/or diastolic dysfunction).

Contractility	Contractility (and SV) ↑ with:
	▪ Catecholamine stimulation via β_1 receptor:
	  ▪ Activated protein kinase A → phospholamban phosphorylation → active Ca^{2+} ATPase → ↑ Ca^{2+} storage in sarcoplasmic reticulum
	  ▪ Activated protein kinase A → Ca^{2+} channel phosphorylation → ↑ Ca^{2+} entry → ↑ Ca^{2+}-induced Ca^{2+} release
	▪ ↑ intracellular Ca^{2+}
	▪ ↓ extracellular Na^+ (↓ activity of Na^+/Ca^{2+} exchanger)
	▪ Digoxin (blocks Na^+/K^+ pump → ↑ intracellular Na^+ → ↓ Na^+/Ca^{2+} exchanger activity → ↑ intracellular Ca^{2+})
		Contractility (and SV) ↓ with:
		▪ β_1-blockade (↓ cAMP)
		▪ HF with systolic dysfunction
		▪ Acidosis
		▪ Hypoxia/hypercapnia (↓ P_{O_2}/↑ P_{CO_2})
		▪ Nondihydropyridine Ca^{2+} channel blockers

Preload	Preload approximated by ventricular end-diastolic volume (EDV); depends on venous tone and circulating blood volume.	Vasodilators (eg, nitroglycerin) ↓ preload.
Afterload	Afterload approximated by MAP. ↑ wall tension per Laplace's law → ↑ pressure → ↑ afterload. LV compensates for ↑ afterload by thickening (hypertrophy) in order to ↓ wall stress.	Arterial vasodilators (eg, hydralazine) ↓ afterload. ACE inhibitors and ARBs ↓ both preload and afterload. Chronic hypertension (↑ MAP) → LV hypertrophy.
Myocardial oxygen demand	Myocardial O_2 demand is ↑ by: ▪ ↑ contractility ▪ ↑ afterload (proportional to arterial pressure) ▪ ↑ heart rate ▪ ↑ diameter of ventricle (↑ wall tension)	Wall tension follows Laplace's law: Wall tension = pressure × radius Wall stress $\propto \frac{\text{pressure} \times \text{radius}}{2 \times \text{wall thickness}}$

Cardiac output equations

	EQUATION	NOTES
Stroke volume	$SV = EDV - ESV$	ESV = end-systolic volume.
Ejection fraction	$EF = \frac{SV}{EDV} = \frac{EDV - ESV}{EDV}$	EF is an index of ventricular contractility (↓ in systolic HF; usually normal in diastolic HF).
Cardiac output	$CO = SV \times HR$ Fick principle: $CO = \frac{\text{rate of } O_2 \text{ consumption}}{(\text{arterial } O_2 \text{ content} - \text{venous } O_2 \text{ content})}$	In early stages of exercise, CO maintained by ↑ HR and ↑ SV. In later stages, CO maintained by ↑ HR only (SV plateaus). Diastole is shortened with ↑↑ HR (eg, ventricular tachycardia) → ↓ diastolic filling time → ↓ SV → ↓ CO.
Pulse pressure	PP = systolic blood pressure (SBP) – diastolic blood pressure (DBP)	PP directly proportional to SV and inversely proportional to arterial compliance. ↑ PP in hyperthyroidism, aortic regurgitation, aortic stiffening (isolated systolic hypertension in elderly), obstructive sleep apnea (↑ sympathetic tone), anemia, exercise (transient). ↓ PP in aortic stenosis, cardiogenic shock, cardiac tamponade, advanced HF.
Mean arterial pressure	MAP = CO × total peripheral resistance (TPR)	MAP (at resting HR) = 2/3 DBP + 1/3 SBP = DBP + 1/3 PP.

Starling curves

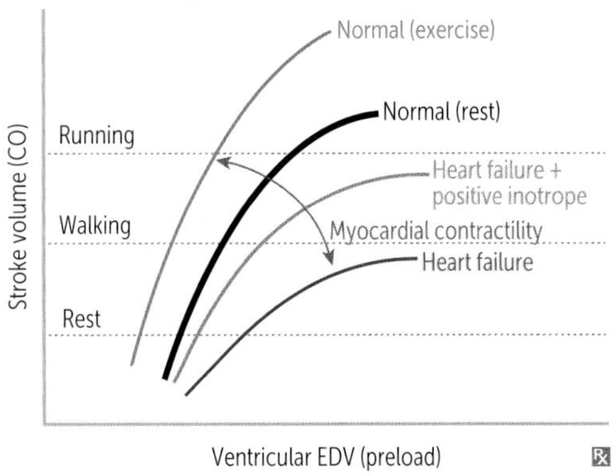

Force of contraction is proportional to end-diastolic length of cardiac muscle fiber (preload).

↑ contractility with catecholamines, positive inotropes (eg, dobutamine, milrinone, digoxin).

↓ contractility with loss of functional myocardium (eg, MI), β-blockers (acutely), nondihydropyridine Ca^{2+} channel blockers, HF.

Resistance, pressure, flow

Volumetric flow rate (Q) = flow velocity (v) × cross-sectional area (A)

Resistance

$$= \frac{\text{driving pressure } (\Delta P)}{Q} = \frac{8\eta \text{ (viscosity)} \times \text{length}}{\pi r^4}$$

Total resistance of vessels in series:

$R_T = R_1 + R_2 + R_3 \ldots$

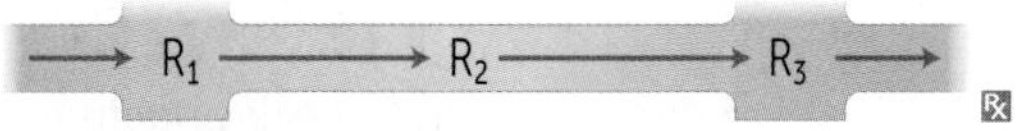

Total resistance of vessels in parallel:

$$\frac{1}{R_T} = \frac{1}{R_1} + \frac{1}{R_2} + \frac{1}{R_3} \ldots$$

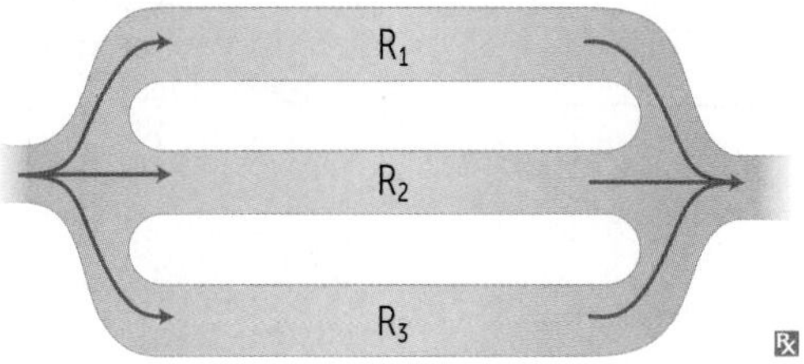

$Q \propto r^4$

$R \propto 1/r^4$

Capillaries have highest total cross-sectional area and lowest flow velocity.

Pressure gradient drives flow from high pressure to low pressure.

Arterioles account for most of TPR. Veins provide most of blood storage capacity.

Viscosity depends mostly on hematocrit.

Viscosity ↑ in hyperproteinemic states (eg, multiple myeloma), polycythemia.

Viscosity ↓ in anemia.

Cardiac and vascular function curves

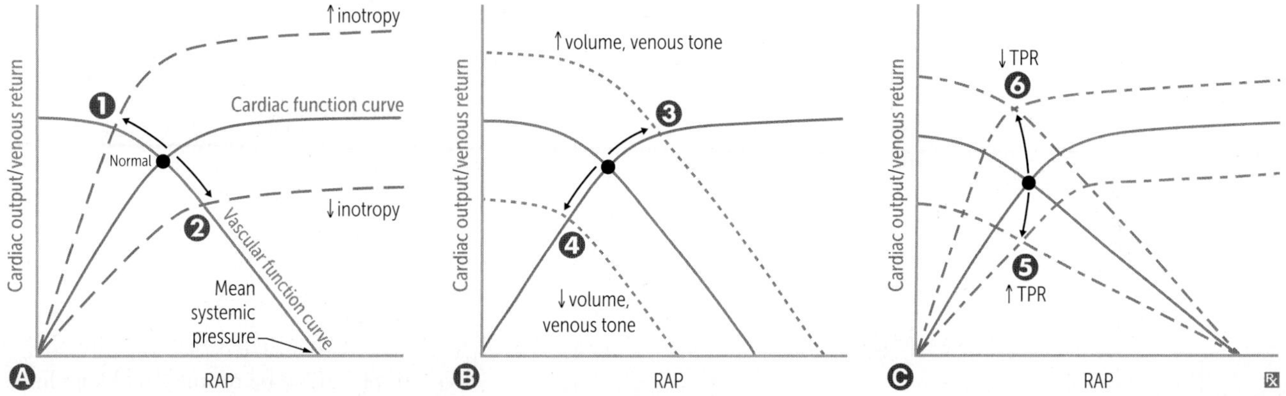

Intersection of curves = operating point of heart (ie, venous return and CO are equal, as circulatory system is a closed system).

GRAPH	EFFECT	EXAMPLES
Ⓐ Inotropy	Changes in contractility → altered SV → altered CO/VR and RA pressure (RAP)	❶ Catecholamines, dobutamine, milrinone, digoxin, exercise ⊕ ❷ HF with reduced EF, narcotic overdose, sympathetic inhibition ⊖
Ⓑ Venous return	Changes in circulating volume → altered RAP → altered SV → change in CO	❸ Fluid infusion, sympathetic activity ⊕ ❹ Acute hemorrhage, spinal anesthesia ⊖
Ⓒ Total peripheral resistance	Changes in TPR → altered CO Change in RAP unpredictable	❺ Vasopressors ⊕ ❻ Exercise, arteriovenous shunt ⊖

Changes often occur in tandem, and may be reinforcing (eg, exercise ↑ inotropy and ↓ TPR to maximize CO) or compensatory (eg, HF ↓ inotropy → fluid retention to ↑ preload to maintain CO).

Pressure-volume loops and cardiac cycle

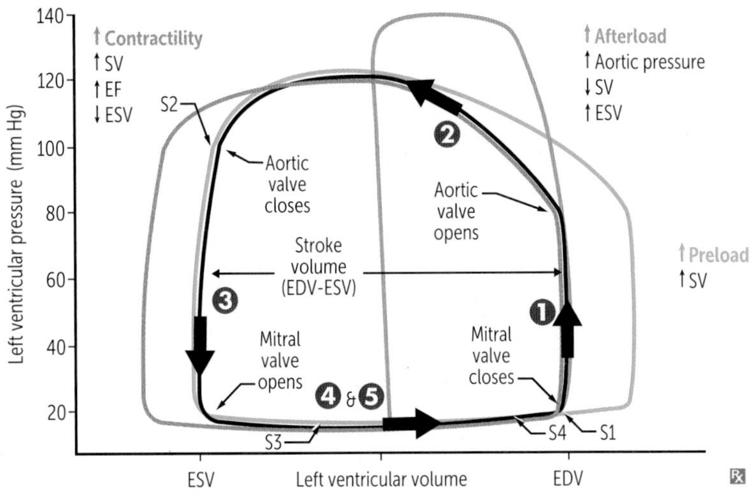

The black loop represents normal cardiac physiology.

Phases—left ventricle:

❶ Isovolumetric contraction—period between mitral valve closing and aortic valve opening; period of highest O_2 consumption

❷ Systolic ejection—period between aortic valve opening and closing

❸ Isovolumetric relaxation—period between aortic valve closing and mitral valve opening

❹ Rapid filling—period just after mitral valve opening

❺ Reduced filling—period just before mitral valve closing

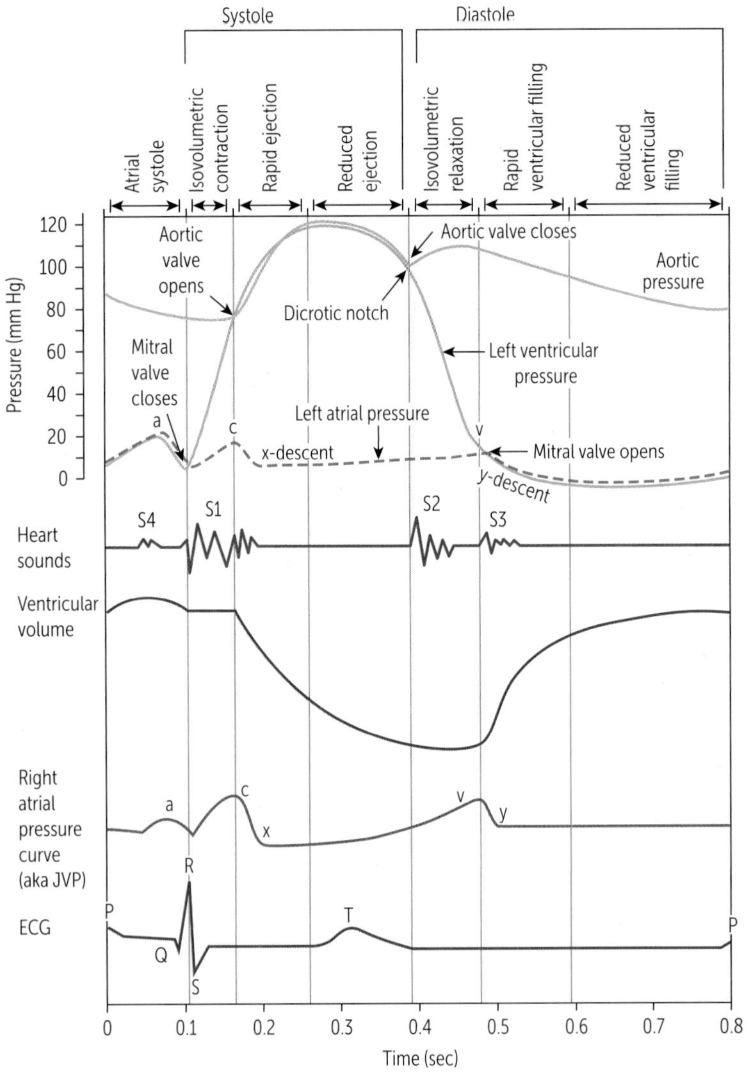

Heart sounds:

S1—mitral and tricuspid valve closure. Loudest at mitral area.

S2—aortic and pulmonary valve closure. Loudest at left upper sternal border.

S3—in early diastole during rapid ventricular filling phase. Best heard at apex with patient in left lateral decubitus position. Associated with ↑ filling pressures (eg, MR, AR, HF, thyrotoxicosis) and more common in dilated ventricles (but can be normal in children, young adults, athletes, and pregnancy). Turbulence caused by blood from LA mixing with ↑ ESV.

S4—in late diastole ("atrial kick"). Turbulence caused by blood entering stiffened LV. Best heard at apex with patient in left lateral decubitus position. High atrial pressure. Associated with ventricular noncompliance (eg, hypertrophy). Can be normal in older adults. Considered abnormal if palpable.

Jugular venous pulse (JVP):

a wave—atrial contraction. Absent in atrial fibrillation.

c wave—RV contraction (closed tricuspid valve bulging into atrium).

x descent—atrial relaxation and downward displacement of closed tricuspid valve during rapid ventricular ejection phase. Reduced or absent in tricuspid regurgitation and right HF because pressure gradients are reduced.

v wave—↑ RA pressure due to ↑ volume against closed tricuspid valve.

y descent—RA emptying into RV. Prominent in constrictive pericarditis, absent in cardiac tamponade.

Pressure-volume loops and valvular disease

Aortic stenosis

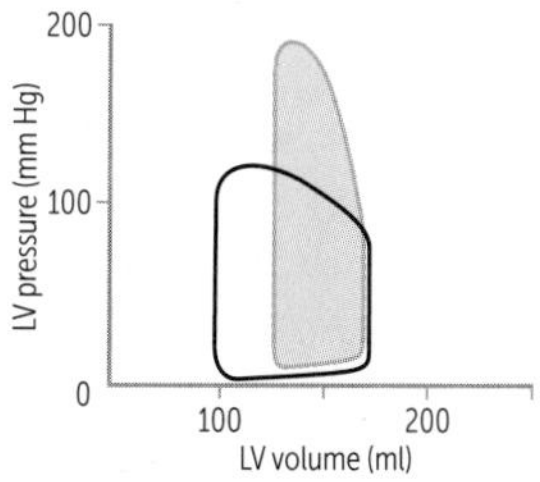

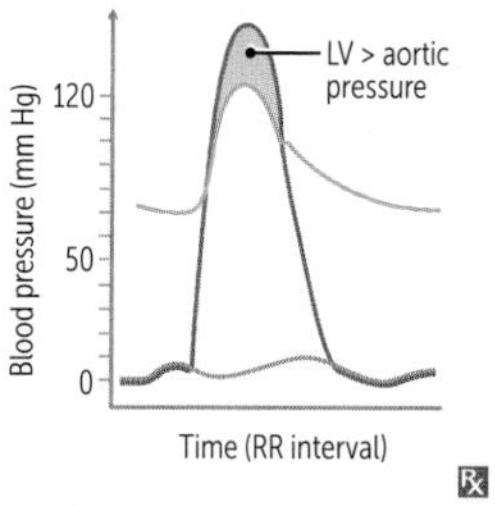

↑ LV pressure
↑ ESV
No change in EDV (if mild)
↓ SV

Ventricular hypertrophy → ↓ ventricular compliance → ↑ EDP for given EDV

Aortic regurgitation

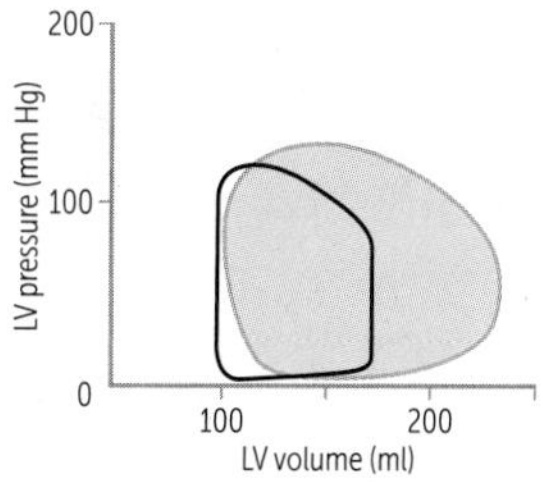

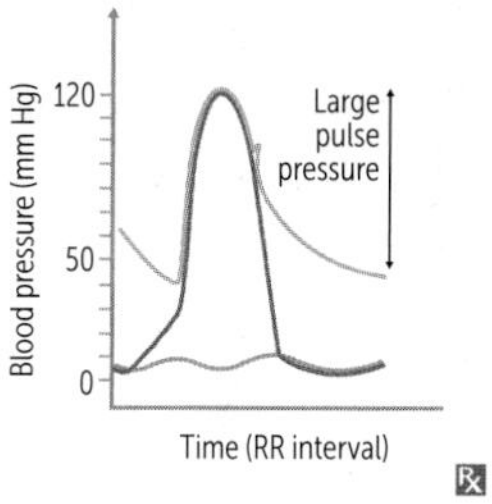

No true isovolumetric phase
↑ EDV
↑ SV
Loss of dichrotic notch

Mitral stenosis

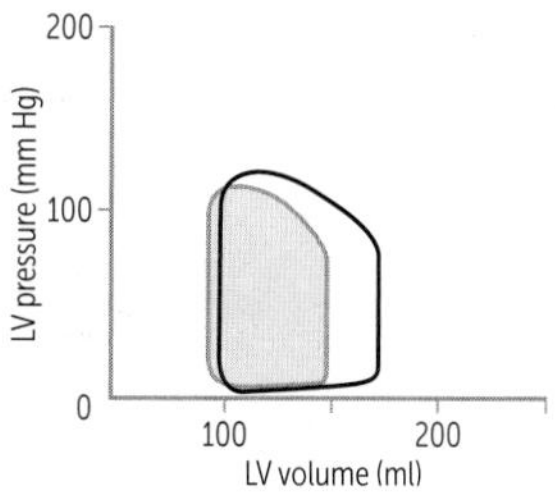

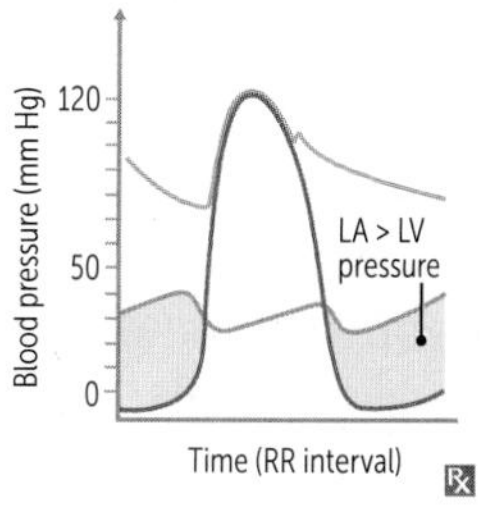

↑ LA pressure
↓ EDV because of impaired ventricular filling
↓ ESV
↓ SV

Mitral regurgitation

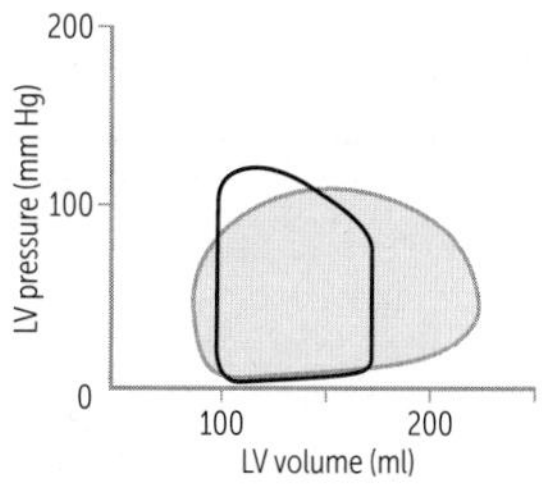

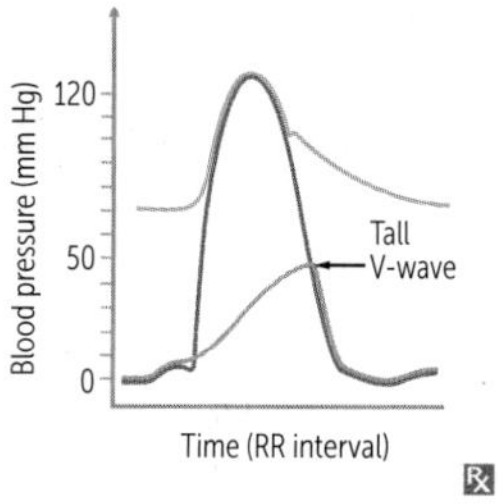

No true isovolumetric phase
↓ ESV due to ↓ resistance and ↑ regurgitation into LA during systole
↑ EDV due to ↑ LA volume/pressure from regurgitation → ↑ ventricular filling
↑ SV (forward flow into systemic circulation plus backflow into LA)

Splitting of S2

Physiologic splitting

Inspiration → drop in intrathoracic pressure → ↑ venous return → ↑ RV filling → ↑ RV stroke volume → ↑ RV ejection time → delayed closure of pulmonic valve. ↓ pulmonary impedance (↑ capacity of the pulmonary circulation) also occurs during inspiration, which contributes to delayed closure of pulmonic valve.

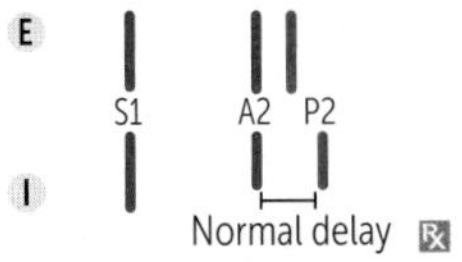
E
I
S1
A2 P2
Normal delay

E = Expiration
I = Inspiration

Wide splitting

Seen in conditions that delay RV emptying (eg, pulmonic stenosis, right bundle branch block). Causes delayed pulmonic sound (especially on inspiration). An exaggeration of normal splitting.

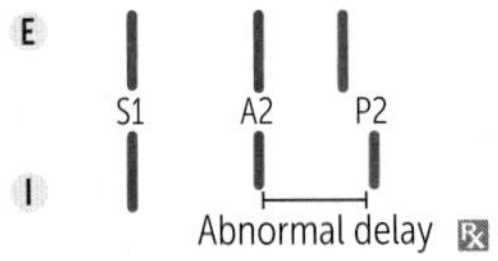
E
I
S1
A2
P2
Abnormal delay

Fixed splitting

Heard in ASD. ASD → left-to-right shunt → ↑ RA and RV volumes → ↑ flow through pulmonic valve → delayed pulmonic valve closure (independent of respiration).

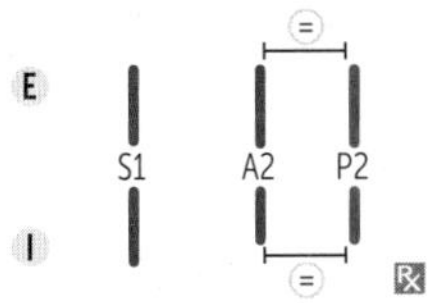
E
I
S1
A2
P2
=
=

Paradoxical splitting

Heard in conditions that delay aortic valve closure (eg, aortic stenosis, left bundle branch block). Normal order of semilunar valve closure is reversed: in paradoxical splitting **P2** occurs before **A2**. On inspiration, P2 closes later and moves closer to A2, "paradoxically" eliminating the split. On expiration, the split can be heard (opposite to physiologic splitting).

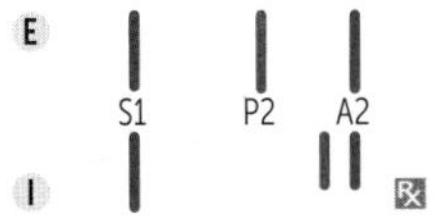
E
I
S1
P2
A2

Auscultation of the heart

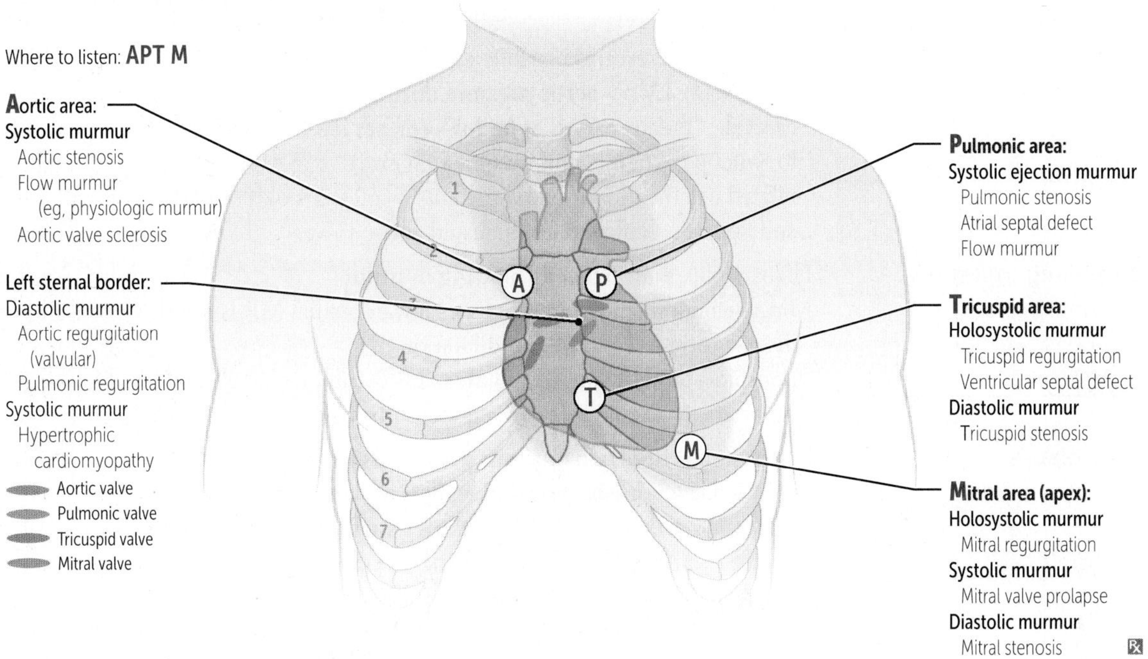
Where to listen: APT M
Aortic area:
Systolic murmur
Aortic stenosis
Flow murmur
(eg, physiologic murmur)
Aortic valve sclerosis
Left sternal border:
Diastolic murmur
Aortic regurgitation
(valvular)
Pulmonic regurgitation
Systolic murmur
Hypertrophic
cardiomyopathy
Aortic valve
Pulmonic valve
Tricuspid valve
Mitral valve
Pulmonic area:
Systolic ejection murmur
Pulmonic stenosis
Atrial septal defect
Flow murmur
Tricuspid area:
Holosystolic murmur
Tricuspid regurgitation
Ventricular septal defect
Diastolic murmur
Tricuspid stenosis
Mitral area (apex):
Holosystolic murmur
Mitral regurgitation
Systolic murmur
Mitral valve prolapse
Diastolic murmur
Mitral stenosis
A
P
T
M
1
2
3
4
5
6
7

MANEUVER	CARDIOVASCULAR CHANGES	MURMURS THAT INCREASE WITH MANEUVER	MURMURS THAT DECREASE WITH MANEUVER
Standing Valsalva (strain phase)	↓ preload (↓ LV volume)	MVP (↓ LV volume) with earlier midsystolic click HCM (↓ LV volume)	Most murmurs (↓ flow through stenotic or regurgitant valve)
Passive leg raise	↑ preload (↑ LV volume)	Most murmurs (↑ flow through stenotic or regurgitant valve)	MVP (↑ LV volume) with later midsystolic click HCM (↑ LV volume)
Squatting	↑ preload, ↑ afterload (↑ LV volume)		
Hand grip	↑↑ afterload → ↑ reverse flow across aortic valve (↑ LV volume)	Most other left-sided murmurs (AR, MR, VSD)	AS (↓ transaortic valve pressure gradient) HCM (↑ LV volume)
Inspiration	↑ venous return to right heart, ↓ venous return to left heart	Most right-sided murmurs	Most left-sided murmurs

Heart murmurs

Systolic

Aortic stenosis

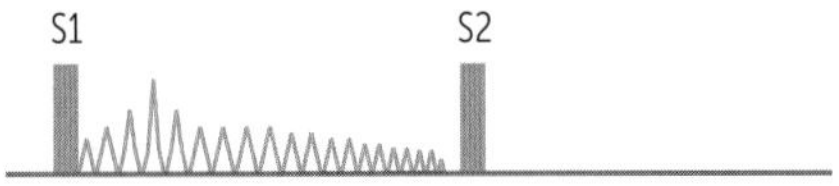

Crescendo-decrescendo systolic ejection murmur and soft S2 (ejection click may be present). LV >> aortic pressure during systole. Loudest at heart base; radiates to carotids. "Pulsus parvus et tardus"—pulses are weak with a delayed peak. Can lead to Syncope, Angina, and Dyspnea on exertion (**SAD**). Most commonly due to age-related calcification in older patients (> 60 years old) or in younger patients with early-onset calcification of bicuspid aortic valve.

Mitral/tricuspid regurgitation

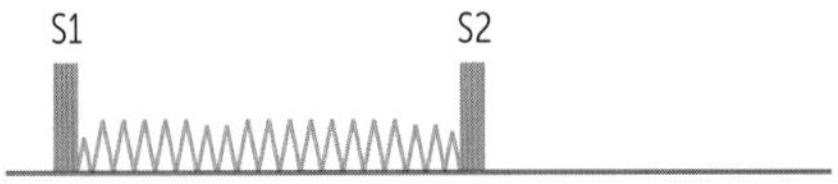

Holosystolic, high-pitched "blowing murmur."

Mitral—loudest at apex and radiates toward axilla. MR is often due to ischemic heart disease (post-MI), MVP, LV dilatation.

Tricuspid—loudest at tricuspid area. TR commonly caused by RV dilatation.

Rheumatic fever and infective endocarditis can cause either MR or TR.

Mitral valve prolapse

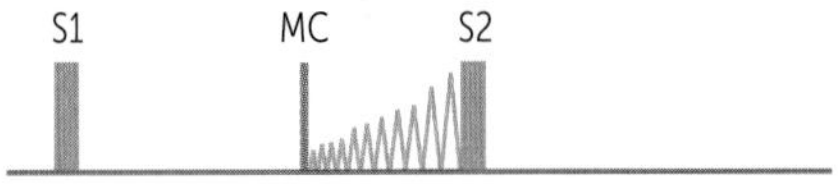

Late systolic crescendo murmur with midsystolic click (MC) due to sudden tensing of chordae tendineae as mitral leaflets prolapse into the LA (chordae cause crescendo with click). Best heard over apex. Loudest just before S2. Usually benign. Can predispose to infective endocarditis. Can be caused by myxomatous degeneration (1° or 2° to connective tissue disease such as Marfan or Ehlers-Danlos syndrome), rheumatic fever (particularly in developing countries), chordae rupture.

Ventricular septal defect

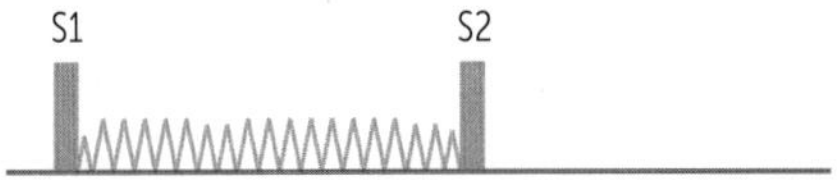

Holosystolic, harsh-sounding murmur. Loudest at tricuspid area. Larger VSDs have a lower intensity murmur than smaller VSDs.

Diastolic

Aortic regurgitation

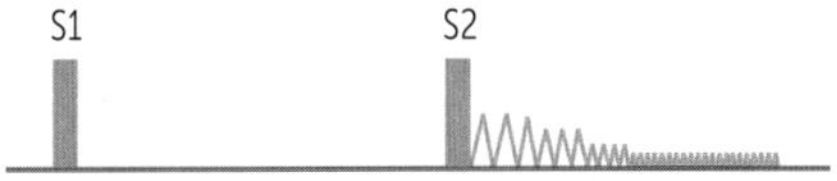

High-pitched "blowing" early diastolic decrescendo murmur. Best heard at base (aortic root dilation) or left sternal border (valvular disease). Long diastolic murmur, hyperdynamic pulse, and head bobbing when severe and chronic. Wide pulse pressure. Causes include **B**icuspid aortic valve, **E**ndocarditis, **A**ortic root dilation, **R**heumatic fever (**BEAR**). Progresses to left HF.

Mitral stenosis

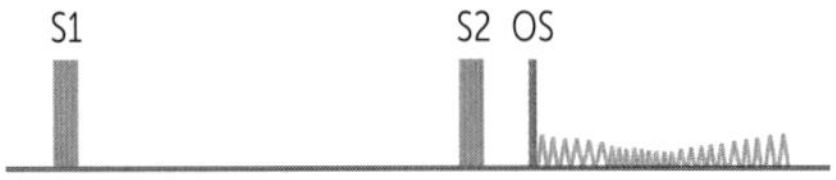

Follows opening snap (OS; due to abrupt halt in leaflet motion in diastole, after rapid opening due to fusion at leaflet tips). Delayed rumbling mid-to-late diastolic murmur (↓ interval between S2 and OS correlates with ↑ severity). LA >> LV pressure during diastole.

Often a late (and highly specific) sequela of rheumatic fever. Chronic MS can result in pulmonary congestion/hypertension and LA dilation → atrial fibrillation and Ortner syndrome.

Continuous

Patent ductus arteriosus

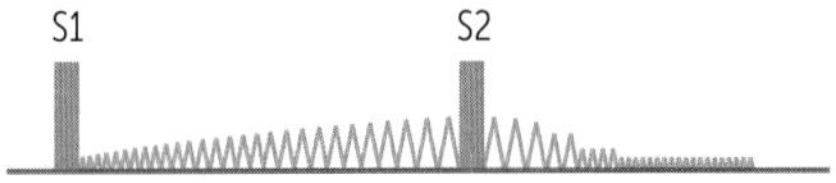

Continuous **machine**-like murmur. Best heard at left infraclavicular area. Loudest at S2. Often due to congenital rubella or prematurity.

You need a **patent** for that **machine**.

Myocardial action potential

Phase 0 = rapid upstroke and depolarization—voltage-gated Na^+ channels open.

Phase 1 = initial repolarization—inactivation of voltage-gated Na^+ channels. Voltage-gated K^+ channels begin to open.

Phase 2 = plateau—Ca^{2+} influx through voltage-gated Ca^{2+} channels balances K^+ efflux. Ca^{2+} influx triggers Ca^{2+} release from sarcoplasmic reticulum and myocyte contraction (excitation-contraction coupling).

Phase 3 = rapid repolarization—massive K^+ efflux due to opening of voltage-gated slow delayed-rectifier K^+ channels and closure of voltage-gated Ca^{2+} channels.

Phase 4 = resting potential—high K^+ permeability through K^+ channels.

In contrast to skeletal muscle:

- Cardiac muscle action potential has a plateau due to Ca^{2+} influx and K^+ efflux.
- Cardiac muscle contraction requires Ca^{2+} influx from ECF to induce Ca^{2+} release from sarcoplasmic reticulum (Ca^{2+}-induced Ca^{2+} release).
- Cardiac myocytes are electrically coupled to each other by gap junctions.

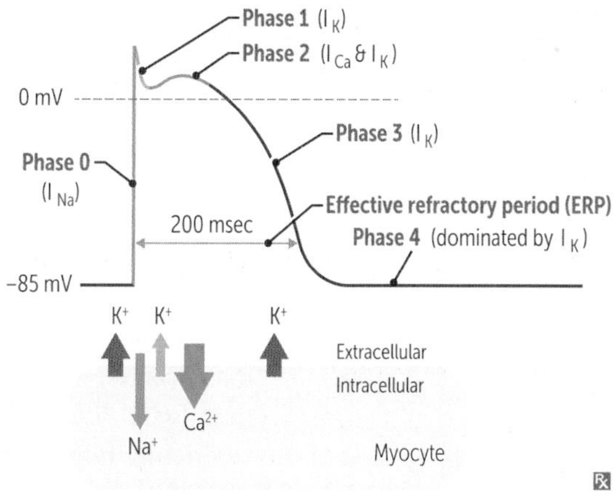

Occurs in all cardiac myocytes except for those in the SA and AV nodes.

Pacemaker action potential

Occurs in the SA and AV nodes. Key differences from the ventricular action potential include:

Phase 0 = upstroke—opening of voltage-gated Ca^{2+} channels. Fast voltage-gated Na^+ channels are permanently inactivated because of the less negative resting potential of these cells. Results in a slow conduction velocity that is used by the AV node to prolong transmission from the atria to ventricles.

Phases 1 and 2 are absent.

Phase 3 = repolarization—inactivation of the Ca^{2+} channels and ↑ activation of K^+ channels → ↑ K^+ efflux.

Phase 4 = slow spontaneous diastolic depolarization due to I_f ("funny current"). I_f channels responsible for a slow, mixed Na^+/K^+ inward current; different from I_{Na} in phase 0 of ventricular action potential. Accounts for automaticity of SA and AV nodes. The slope of phase 4 in the SA node determines HR. ACh/adenosine ↓ the rate of diastolic depolarization and ↓ HR, while catecholamines ↑ depolarization and ↑ HR. Sympathetic stimulation ↑ the chance that I_f channels are open and thus ↑ HR.

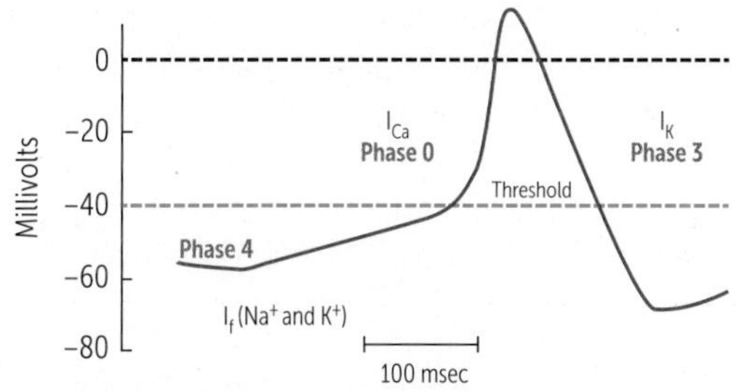

Electrocardiogram

Conduction pathway: SA node → atria → AV node → bundle of His → right and left bundle branches → Purkinje fibers → ventricles; left bundle branch divides into left anterior and posterior fascicles.

SA node—located at junction of RA and SVC; "pacemaker" inherent dominance with slow phase of upstroke.

AV node—located in posteroinferior part of interatrial septum. Blood supply usually from RCA. 100-msec delay allows time for ventricular filling.

Pacemaker rates: SA > AV > bundle of His/ Purkinje/ventricles.

Speed of conduction: **His-Purkinje** > **Atria** > **Ventricles** > **AV** node. **He Parks At Ventura AV**enue.

P wave—atrial depolarization.

PR interval—time from start of atrial depolarization to start of ventricular depolarization (normally 120-200 msec).

QRS complex—ventricular depolarization (normally < 100 msec).

QT interval—ventricular depolarization, mechanical contraction of the ventricles, ventricular repolarization.

T wave—ventricular repolarization. T-wave inversion may indicate ischemia or recent MI.

J point—junction between end of QRS complex and start of ST segment.

ST segment—isoelectric, ventricles depolarized.

U wave—prominent in hypokalemia (think hyp"U"kalemia), bradycardia.

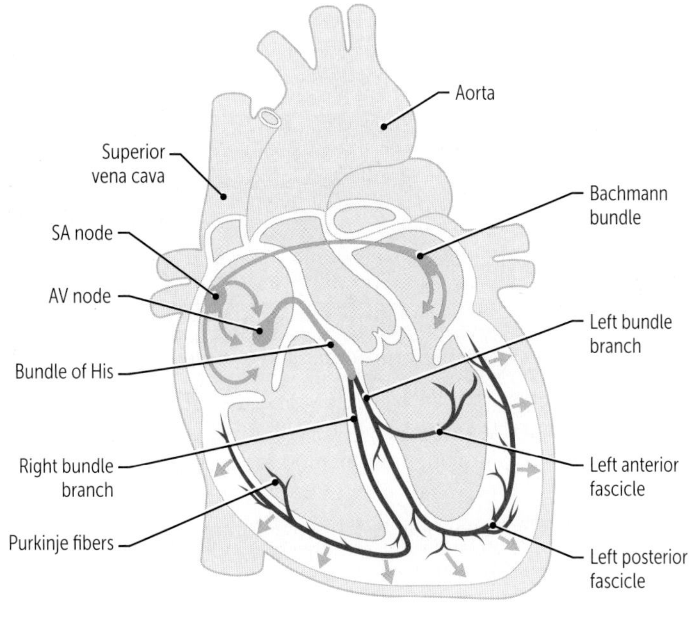

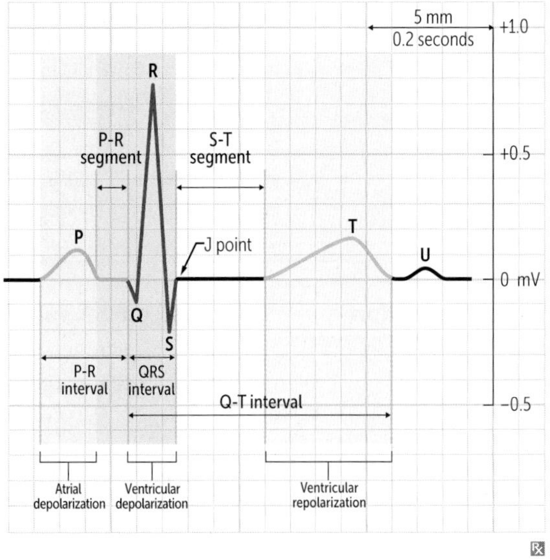

Atrial natriuretic peptide

Released from **atrial myocytes** in response to ↑ blood volume and atrial pressure. Acts via cGMP. Causes vasodilation and ↓ Na^+ reabsorption at the renal collecting tubule. Dilates afferent renal arterioles and constricts efferent arterioles, promoting diuresis and contributing to "aldosterone escape" mechanism.

B-type (brain) natriuretic peptide

Released from **ventricular myocytes** in response to ↑ tension. Similar physiologic action to ANP, with longer half-life. BNP blood test used for diagnosing HF (very good negative predictive value). Available in recombinant form (nesiritide) for treatment of HF.

Baroreceptors and chemoreceptors

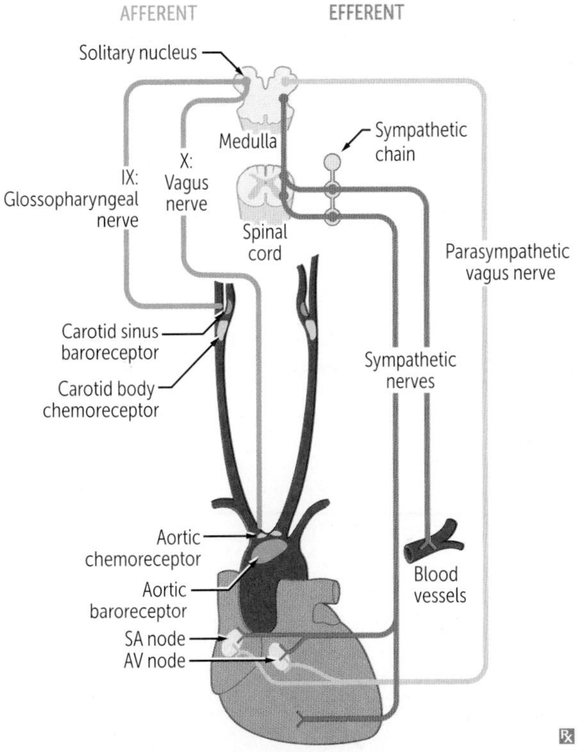

Receptors:
- Aortic arch transmits via vagus nerve to solitary nucleus of medulla (responds to changes in BP).
- Carotid sinus (dilated region superior to bifurcation of carotid arteries) transmits via glossopharyngeal nerve to solitary nucleus of medulla (responds to changes in BP).

Chemoreceptors:
- Peripheral—carotid and aortic bodies are stimulated by ↑ P_{CO_2}, ↓ pH of blood, and ↓ P_{O_2} (< 60 mm Hg).
- Central—are stimulated by changes in pH and P_{CO_2} of brain interstitial fluid, which in turn are influenced by arterial CO_2 as H^+ cannot cross the blood-brain barrier. Do not directly respond to P_{O_2}. Central chemoreceptors become less responsive with chronically ↑ P_{CO_2} (eg, COPD) → ↑ dependence on peripheral chemoreceptors to detect ↓ O_2 to drive respiration.

Baroreceptors:
- Hypotension—↓ arterial pressure → ↓ stretch → ↓ afferent baroreceptor firing → ↑ efferent sympathetic firing and ↓ efferent parasympathetic stimulation → vasoconstriction, ↑ HR, ↑ contractility, ↑ BP. Important in the response to severe hemorrhage.
- Carotid massage—↑ pressure on carotid sinus → ↑ stretch → ↑ afferent baroreceptor firing → ↑ AV node refractory period → ↓ HR.
- Component of Cushing reflex (triad of hypertension, bradycardia, and respiratory depression)—↑ intracranial pressure constricts arterioles → cerebral ischemia → ↑ pCO_2 and ↓ pH → central reflex sympathetic ↑ in perfusion pressure (hypertension) → ↑ stretch → peripheral reflex baroreceptor–induced bradycardia.

Normal cardiac pressures

Pulmonary capillary wedge pressure (PCWP; in mm Hg) is a good approximation of left atrial pressure. In mitral stenosis, PCWP > LV end diastolic pressure. PCWP is measured with pulmonary artery catheter (Swan-Ganz catheter).

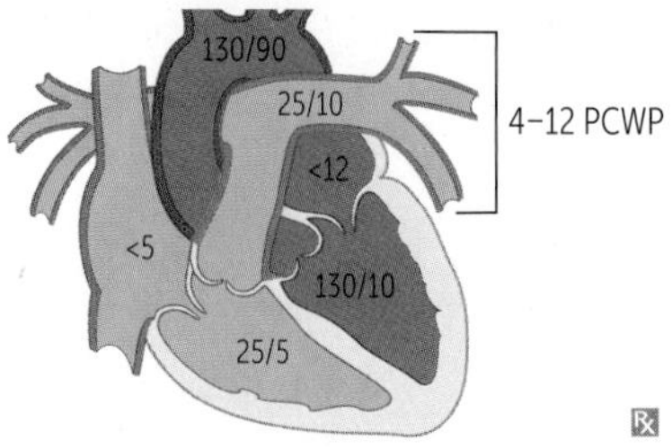

Autoregulation

How blood flow to an organ remains constant over a wide range of perfusion pressures.

ORGAN	FACTORS DETERMINING AUTOREGULATION	
Lungs	Hypoxia causes vasoconstriction	The pulmonary vasculature is unique in that alveolar hypoxia causes vasoconstriction so that only well-ventilated areas are perfused. In other organs, hypoxia causes vasodilation
Heart	Local metabolites (vasodilatory): NO, CO_2, ↓ O_2	
Brain	Local metabolites (vasodilatory): CO_2 (pH)	
Kidneys	Myogenic and tubuloglomerular feedback	
Skeletal muscle	Local metabolites during exercise (vasodilatory): CO_2, H^+, Adenosine, Lactate, K^+ At rest: sympathetic tone in arteries	CHALK
Skin	Sympathetic vasoconstriction most important mechanism for temperature control	

Capillary fluid exchange

Starling forces determine fluid movement through capillary membranes:

- P_c = capillary hydrostatic pressure—pushes fluid out of capillary
- P_i = interstitial hydrostatic pressure—pushes fluid into capillary
- π_c = plasma oncotic pressure—pulls fluid into capillary
- π_i = interstitial fluid oncotic pressure—pulls fluid out of capillary

J_v = net fluid flow = $K_f [(P_c - P_i) - \sigma(\pi_c - \pi_i)]$

K_f = capillary permeability to fluid

σ = reflection coefficient (measure of capillary permeability to protein)

Edema—excess fluid outflow into interstitium commonly caused by:

- ↑ capillary pressure (↑ P_c; eg, HF)
- ↑ capillary permeability (↑ K_f; eg, toxins, infections, burns)
- ↑ interstitial fluid oncotic pressure (↑ π_i; eg, lymphatic blockage)
- ↓ plasma proteins (↓ π_c; eg, nephrotic syndrome, liver failure, protein malnutrition)

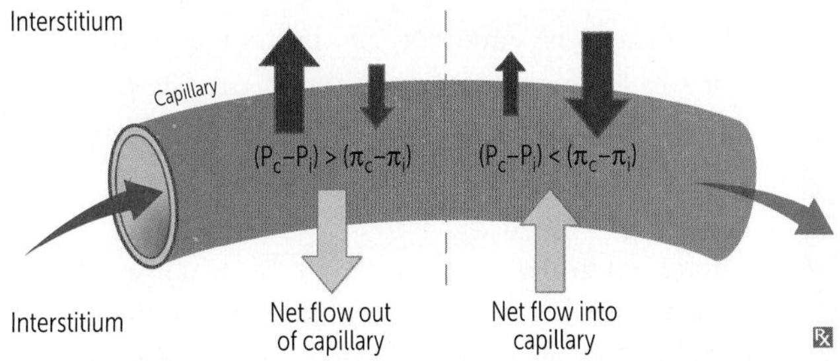
Interstitium
Capillary
$(P_c-P_i) > (\pi_c-\pi_i)$
$(P_c-P_i) < (\pi_c-\pi_i)$
Interstitium
Net flow out of capillary
Net flow into capillary

▶ CARDIOVASCULAR—PATHOLOGY

Congenital heart diseases

RIGHT-TO-LEFT SHUNTS	Early cyanosis—"blue babies." Often diagnosed prenatally or become evident immediately after birth. Usually require urgent surgical treatment and/or maintenance of a PDA.	The 5 T's: 1. Truncus arteriosus (1 vessel) 2. Transposition (2 switched vessels) 3. Tricuspid atresia (3 = Tri) 4. Tetralogy of Fallot (4 = Tetra) 5. TAPVR (5 letters in the name)
Persistent truncus arteriosus	Truncus arteriosus fails to divide into pulmonary trunk and aorta due to failure of aorticopulmonary septum formation; most patients have accompanying VSD.	
D-transposition of great vessels 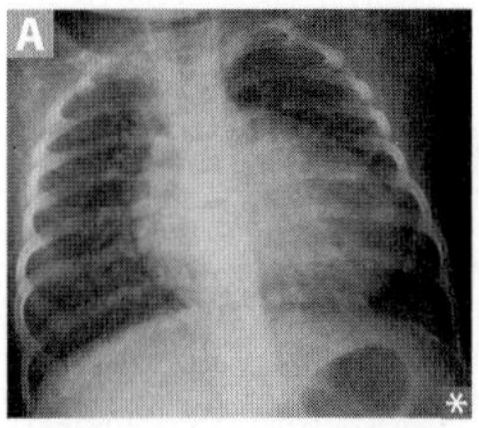 A	Aorta leaves RV (anterior) and pulmonary trunk leaves LV (posterior) → separation of systemic and pulmonary circulations. Not compatible with life unless a shunt is present to allow mixing of blood (eg, VSD, PDA, or patent foramen ovale). Due to failure of the aorticopulmonary septum to spiral ("egg on a string" appearance on CXR) A. Without surgical intervention, most infants die within the first few months of life.	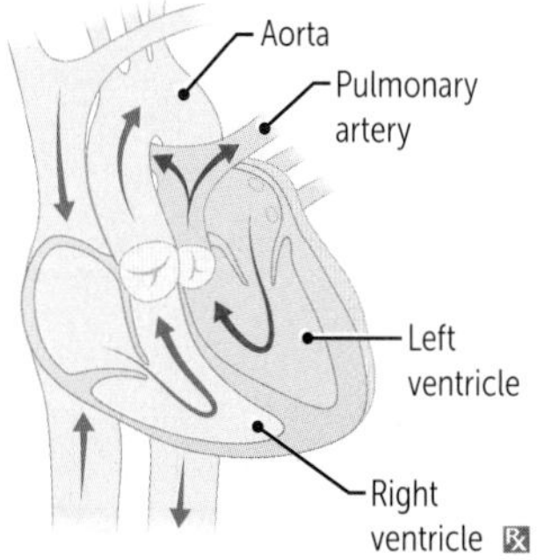
Tricuspid atresia	Absence of tricuspid valve and hypoplastic RV; requires both ASD and VSD for viability.	
Tetralogy of Fallot 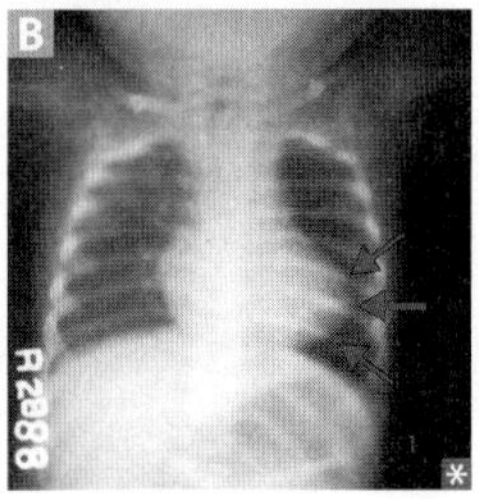 B	Caused by anterosuperior displacement of the infundibular septum. Most common cause of early childhood cyanosis. ❶ Pulmonary infundibular stenosis (most important determinant for prognosis) ❷ Right ventricular hypertrophy (RVH)—boot-shaped heart on CXR B ❸ Overriding aorta ❹ VSD Pulmonary stenosis forces right-to-left flow across VSD → RVH, "tet spells" (often caused by crying, fever, and exercise due to exacerbation of RV outflow obstruction).	PROVe. Squatting: ↑ SVR, ↓ right-to-left shunt, improves cyanosis. Associated with 22q11 syndromes. 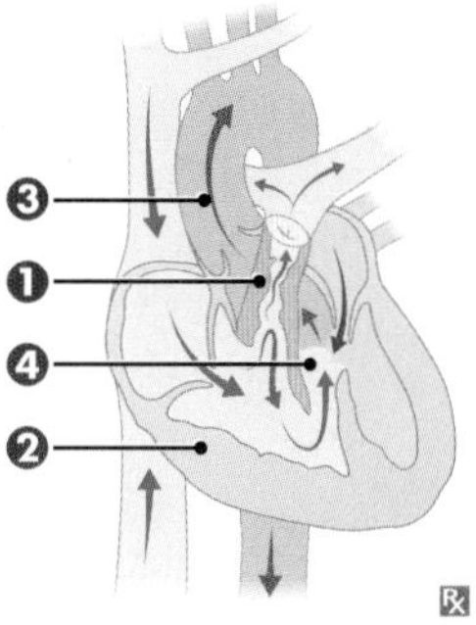
Total anomalous pulmonary venous return	Pulmonary veins drain into right heart circulation (SVC, coronary sinus, etc); associated with ASD and sometimes PDA to allow for right-to-left shunting to maintain CO.	
Ebstein anomaly	Displacement of tricuspid valve leaflets downward into RV, artificially "atrializing" the ventricle. Associated with tricuspid regurgitation, accessory conduction pathways, right-sided HF.	Can be caused by lithium exposure in utero.

Congenital heart diseases *(continued)*

LEFT-TO-RIGHT SHUNTS	Acyanotic at presentation; cyanosis may occur years later. Frequency: VSD > ASD > PDA.	Right-to-left shunts: early cyanosis. Left-to-right shunts: "later" cyanosis.
Ventricular septal defect 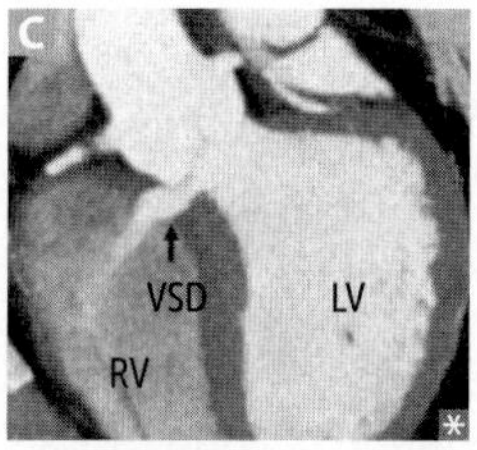	Asymptomatic at birth, may manifest weeks later or remain asymptomatic throughout life. Most self resolve; larger lesions C may lead to LV overload and HF.	O_2 saturation ↑ in RV and pulmonary artery.
Atrial septal defect 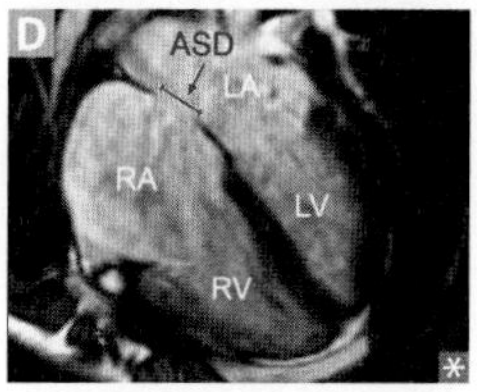	Defect in interatrial septum D; wide, fixed split S2. Ostium secundum defects most common and usually an isolated finding; ostium primum defects rarer and usually occur with other cardiac anomalies. Symptoms range from none to HF. Distinct from patent foramen ovale in that septa are missing tissue rather than unfused.	O_2 saturation ↑ in RA, RV, and pulmonary artery. May lead to paradoxical emboli (systemic venous emboli use ASD to bypass lungs and become systemic arterial emboli). Associated with Down syndrome.
Patent ductus arteriosus 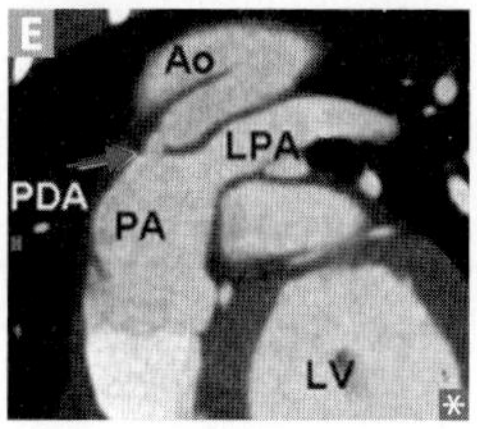	In fetal period, shunt is right to left (normal). In neonatal period, ↓ pulmonary vascular resistance → shunt becomes left to right → progressive RVH and/or LVH and HF. Associated with a continuous, "machine-like" murmur. Patency is maintained by PGE synthesis and low O_2 tension. Uncorrected PDA E can eventually result in late cyanosis in the lower extremities (differential cyanosis).	PDA is normal in utero and normally closes only after birth.
Eisenmenger syndrome	Uncorrected left-to-right shunt (VSD, ASD, PDA) → ↑ pulmonary blood flow → pathologic remodeling of vasculature → pulmonary arterial hypertension. RVH occurs to compensate → shunt becomes right to left. Causes late cyanosis, clubbing, and polycythemia. Age of onset varies depending on size and severity of initial left-to-right shunt.	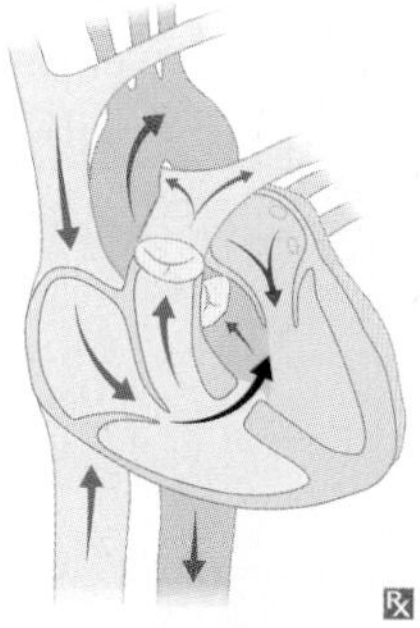
OTHER ANOMALIES		
Coarctation of the aorta 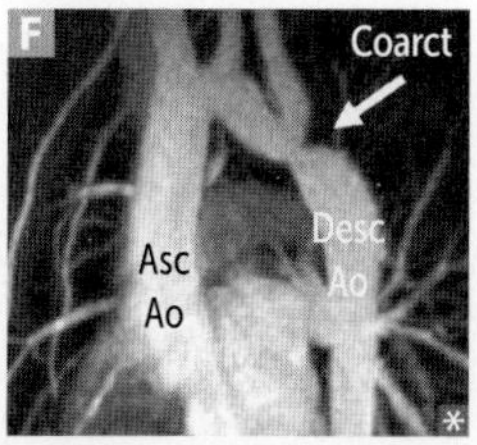	Aortic narrowing F near insertion of ductus arteriosus ("juxtaductal"). Associated with bicuspid aortic valve, other heart defects, and Turner syndrome. Hypertension in upper extremities and weak, delayed pulse in lower extremities (brachial-femoral delay). With age, intercostal arteries enlarge due to collateral circulation; arteries erode ribs → notched appearance on CXR. Complications include HF, ↑ risk of cerebral hemorrhage (berry aneurysms), aortic rupture, and possible endocarditis.	

Congenital cardiac defect associations

ASSOCIATION	DEFECT
Prenatal alcohol exposure (fetal alcohol syndrome)	VSD, PDA, ASD, tetralogy of Fallot
Congenital rubella	PDA, pulmonary artery stenosis, septal defects
Down syndrome	AV septal defect (endocardial cushion defect), VSD, ASD
Infant of patient with diabetes during pregnancy	Transposition of great vessels, VSD
Marfan syndrome	MVP, thoracic aortic aneurysm and dissection, aortic regurgitation
Prenatal lithium exposure	Ebstein anomaly
Turner syndrome	Bicuspid aortic valve, coarctation of aorta
Williams syndrome	Supravalvular aortic stenosis
22q11 syndromes	Truncus arteriosus, tetralogy of Fallot

Hypertension

Persistent systolic BP ≥ 130 mm Hg and/or diastolic BP ≥ 80 mm Hg.

RISK FACTORS

↑ age, obesity, diabetes, physical inactivity, high-sodium diet, excess alcohol intake, tobacco smoking, family history; incidence greatest in Black > White > Asian populations.

FEATURES

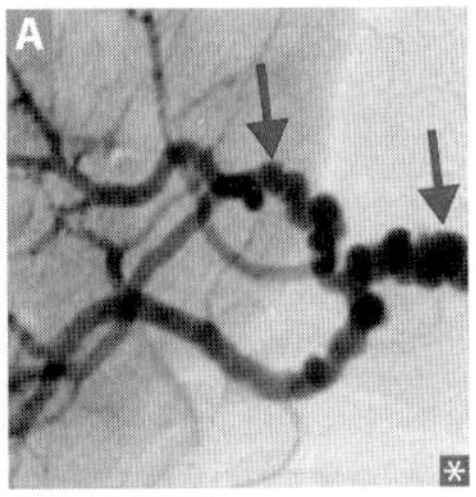

90% of hypertension is 1° (essential) and related to ↑ CO or ↑ TPR. Remaining 10% mostly 2° to renal/renovascular diseases such as fibromuscular dysplasia (characteristic "string of beads" appearance of renal artery A, usually seen in adult females) and atherosclerotic renal artery stenosis or to 1° hyperaldosteronism.

Hypertensive urgency—severe (≥ 180/≥ 120 mm Hg) hypertension without acute end-organ damage.

Hypertensive emergency—severe hypertension with evidence of acute end-organ damage (eg, encephalopathy, stroke, retinal hemorrhages and exudates, papilledema, MI, HF, aortic dissection, kidney injury, microangiopathic hemolytic anemia, eclampsia).

PREDISPOSES TO

CAD, LVH, HF, atrial fibrillation; aortic dissection, aortic aneurysm; stroke; CKD (hypertensive nephropathy); retinopathy.

Hyperlipidemia signs	
Xanthomas	Plaques or nodules composed of lipid-laden histiocytes in skin A, especially the eyelids (xanthelasma B).
Tendinous xanthoma	Lipid deposit in tendon C, especially Achilles tendon and finger extensors.
Corneal arcus	Lipid deposit in cornea. Common in elderly (arcus senilis D), but appears earlier in life with hypercholesterolemia.

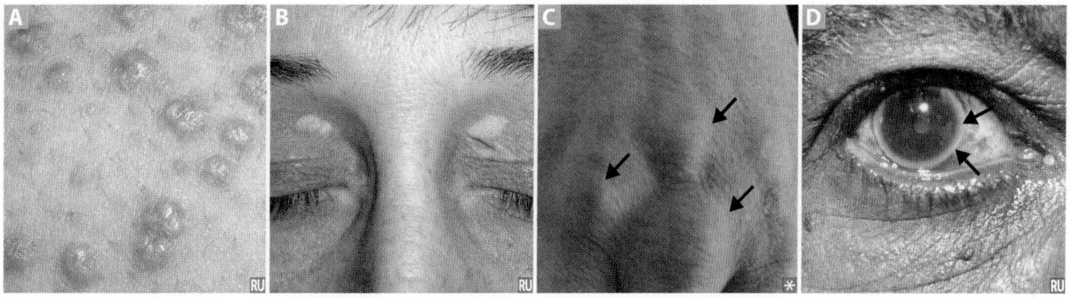

Arteriosclerosis	Hardening of arteries, with arterial wall thickening and loss of elasticity.
Arteriolosclerosis	Common. Affects small arteries and arterioles. Two types: ▪ Hyaline—thickening of vessel walls 2° to plasma protein leak into endothelium in essential hypertension or diabetes mellitus A. ▪ Hyperplastic—"onion skinning" B in severe hypertension with proliferation of smooth muscle cells.
Mönckeberg sclerosis	Also called medial calcific sclerosis. Uncommon. Affects medium-sized arteries. Calcification of internal elastic lamina and media of arteries → vascular stiffening without obstruction. "Pipestem" appearance on x-ray C. Does not obstruct blood flow; intima not involved.

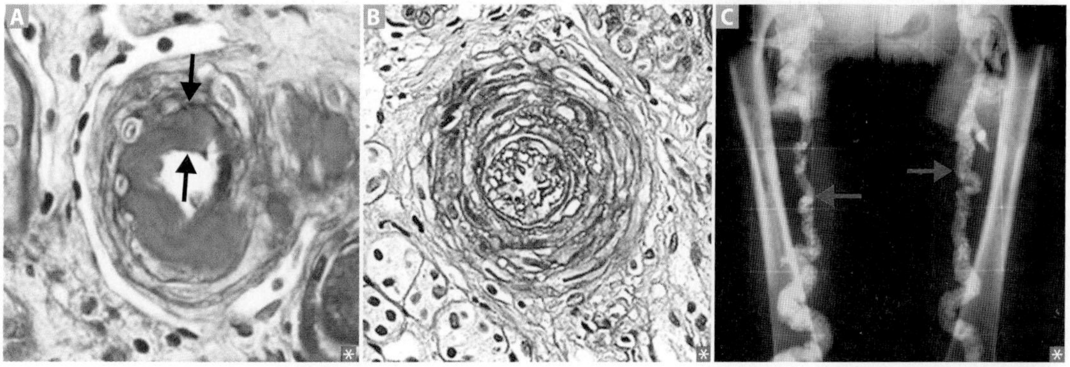

Atherosclerosis	Very common. Disease of elastic arteries and large- and medium-sized muscular arteries; a form of arteriosclerosis caused by buildup of cholesterol plaques in intima.
LOCATION	Abdominal aorta > **co**ronary artery > **p**opliteal artery > **ca**rotid artery > circle of **Willis**. **A co**py **ca**t named **Willis**.
RISK FACTORS	Modifiable: hypertension, tobacco smoking, dyslipidemia (↑ LDL, ↓ HDL), diabetes. Non-modifiable: age, male sex, postmenopausal status, family history.
SYMPTOMS	Angina, claudication, but can be asymptomatic.
PROGRESSION	Inflammation important in pathogenesis: endothelial cell dysfunction → macrophage and LDL accumulation → foam cell formation → fatty streaks → smooth muscle cell migration (involves PDGF and FGF), proliferation, and extracellular matrix deposition → fibrous plaque → complex atheromas A → calcification (calcium content correlates with risk of complications).
COMPLICATIONS	Aneurysms, ischemia, infarcts, peripheral vascular disease, thrombus, emboli.

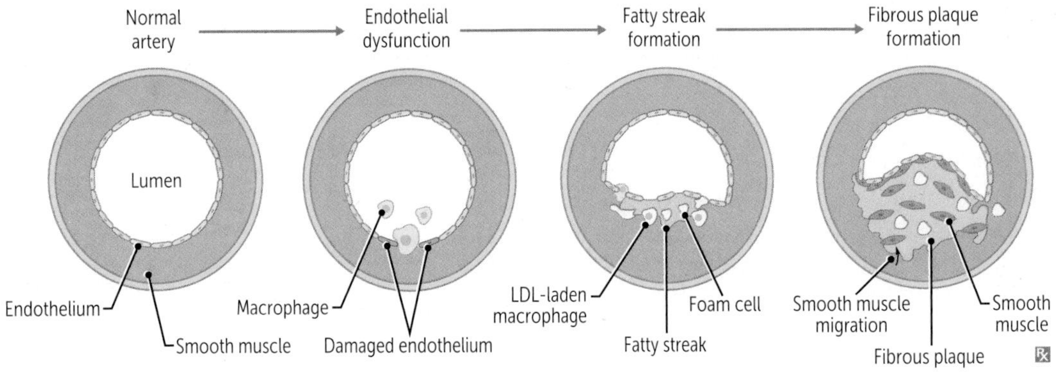
Normal artery
Endothelial dysfunction
Fatty streak formation
Fibrous plaque formation
Lumen
Endothelium
Smooth muscle
Macrophage
Damaged endothelium
LDL-laden macrophage
Fatty streak
Foam cell
Smooth muscle migration
Fibrous plaque
Smooth muscle

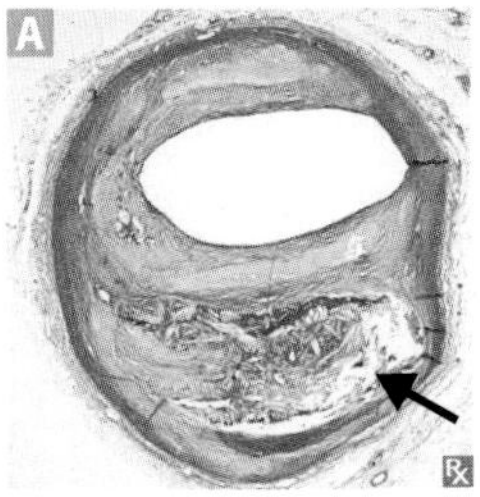
A

Aortic aneurysm	Localized pathologic dilation of the aorta. May cause abdominal and/or back pain, which is a sign of leaking, dissection, or imminent rupture.
Abdominal aortic aneurysm 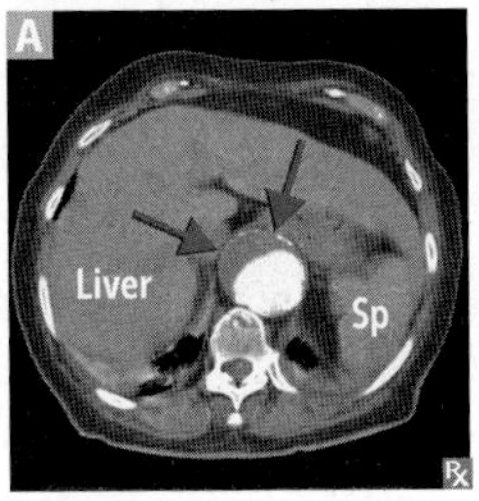	Usually associated with atherosclerosis. Risk factors include history of tobacco use, ↑ age, male sex, family history. May present as palpable pulsatile abdominal mass (arrows in A point to outer dilated calcified aortic wall, with partial crescent-shaped nonopacification of aorta due to flap/clot). Most often infrarenal (distal to origin of renal arteries).
Thoracic aortic aneurysm	Associated with cystic medial degeneration. Risk factors include hypertension, bicuspid aortic valve, connective tissue disease (eg, Marfan syndrome). Also associated with 3° syphilis (obliterative endarteritis of the vasa vasorum). Aortic root dilatation may lead to aortic valve regurgitation.

A
Liver
Sp

Traumatic aortic rupture

Due to trauma and/or deceleration injury, most commonly at aortic isthmus (proximal descending aorta just distal to origin of left subclavian artery). X-ray may reveal widened mediastinum.

Aortic dissection

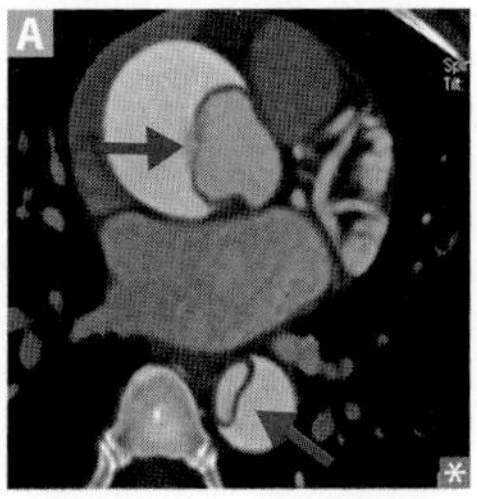

Longitudinal intimal tear forming a false lumen. Associated with hypertension, bicuspid aortic valve, inherited connective tissue disorders (eg, Marfan syndrome). Can present with tearing, sudden-onset chest pain radiating to the back +/– markedly unequal BP in arms. CXR can show mediastinal widening. Can result in organ ischemia, aortic rupture, death.

Stanford type **A** (proximal): involves **A**scending aorta (red arrow in A). May extend to aortic arch or descending aorta (blue arrow in A). May result in acute aortic regurgitation or cardiac tamponade. Treatment: surgery.

Stanford type **B** (distal): involves only descending aorta (**B**elow left subclavian artery). Treatment: β-blockers, then vasodilators.

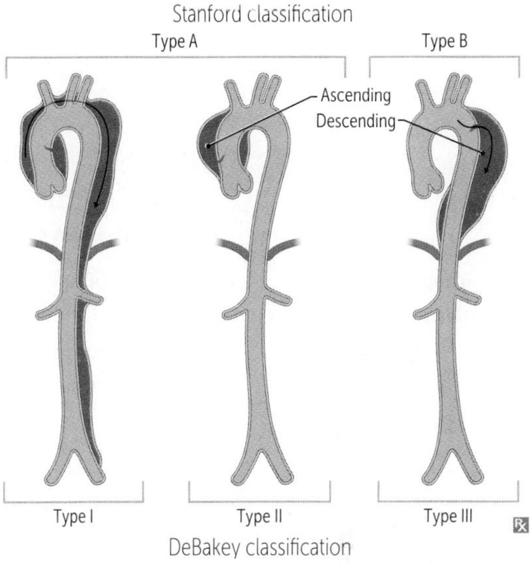

Subclavian steal syndrome

Stenosis of subclavian artery proximal to origin of vertebral artery → hypoperfusion distal to stenosis → reversed blood flow in ipsilateral vertebral artery → reduced cerebral perfusion on exertion of affected arm. Causes arm ischemia, pain, paresthesia, vertebrobasilar insufficiency (dizziness, vertigo). >15 mm Hg difference in systolic BP between arms. Associated with arteriosclerosis, Takayasu arteritis, heart surgery.

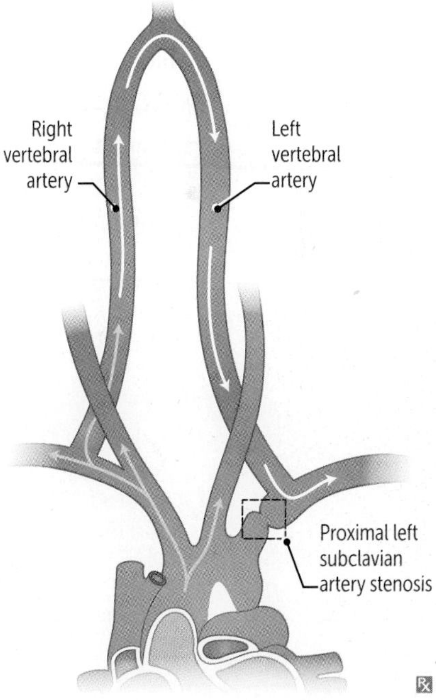

Ischemic heart disease manifestations

Angina

Chest pain due to ischemic myocardium 2° to coronary artery narrowing or spasm; no necrosis.

- Stable—usually 2° to atherosclerosis (≥ 70% occlusion); exertional chest pain in classic distribution (usually with ST depression on ECG), resolving with rest or nitroglycerin.
- Vasospastic (also called Prinzmetal or Variant)—occurs at rest 2° to coronary artery spasm; transient ST elevation on ECG. Tobacco smoking is a risk factor; hypertension and hypercholesterolemia are not. Triggers include cocaine, alcohol, and triptans. Treat with Ca^{2+} channel blockers, nitrates, and smoking cessation (if applicable).
- Unstable—thrombosis with incomplete coronary artery occlusion; +/– ST depression and/or T-wave inversion on ECG but no cardiac biomarker elevation (unlike NSTEMI); ↑ in frequency or intensity of chest pain or any chest pain at rest.

Coronary steal syndrome

Distal to coronary stenosis, vessels are maximally dilated at baseline. Administration of vasodilators (eg, dipyridamole, regadenoson) dilates normal vessels → blood is shunted toward well-perfused areas → ischemia in myocardium perfused by stenosed vessels. Principle behind pharmacologic stress tests with coronary vasodilators.

Sudden cardiac death

Death occurs within 1 hour of symptoms, most commonly due to lethal arrhythmia (eg, ventricular fibrillation). Associated with CAD (up to 70% of cases), cardiomyopathy (hypertrophic, dilated), and hereditary ion channelopathies (eg, long QT syndrome, Brugada syndrome). Prevent with ICD.

Chronic ischemic heart disease

Progressive onset of HF over many years due to chronic ischemic myocardial damage.

Myocardial hibernation—potentially reversible LV systolic dysfunction in the setting of chronic ischemia. Contrast with myocardial stunning, a transient LV systolic dysfunction after a brief episode of acute ischemia.

Myocardial infarction

Most often due to rupture of coronary artery atherosclerotic plaque → acute thrombosis. ↑ cardiac biomarkers (CK-MB, troponins) are diagnostic.

Non–ST-segment elevation MI (NSTEMI)	ST-segment elevation MI (STEMI)
Subendocardial infarcts	Transmural infarcts
Subendocardium (inner 1/3) especially vulnerable to ischemia	Full thickness of myocardial wall involved
ST depression on ECG	ST elevation, pathologic Q waves on ECG

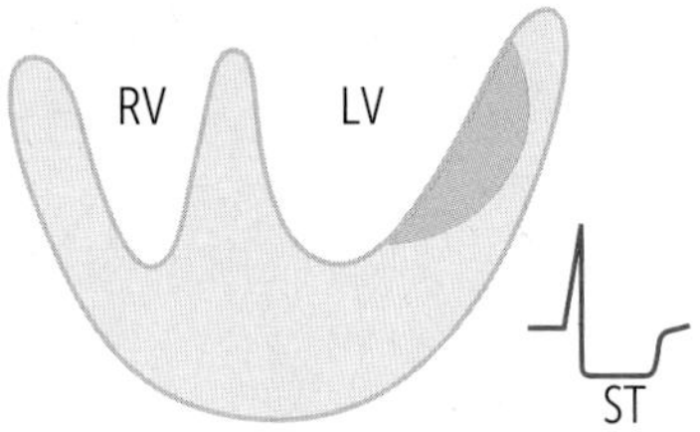

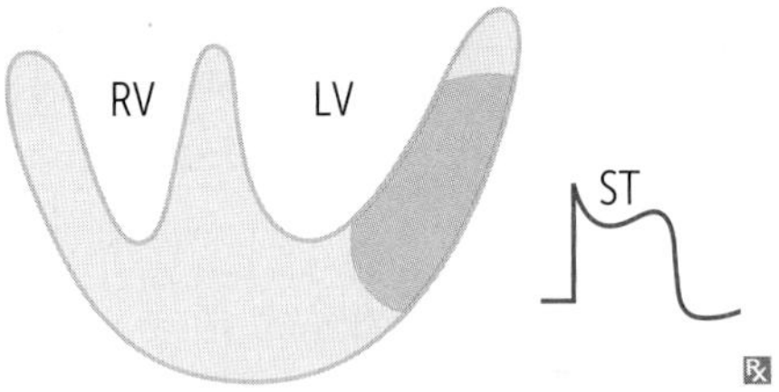

Evolution of myocardial infarction

Commonly occluded coronary arteries: LAD > RCA > circumflex.
Symptoms: diaphoresis, nausea, vomiting, severe retrosternal pain, pain in left arm and/or jaw, shortness of breath, fatigue.

TIME	GROSS	LIGHT MICROSCOPE	COMPLICATIONS
0–24 hours	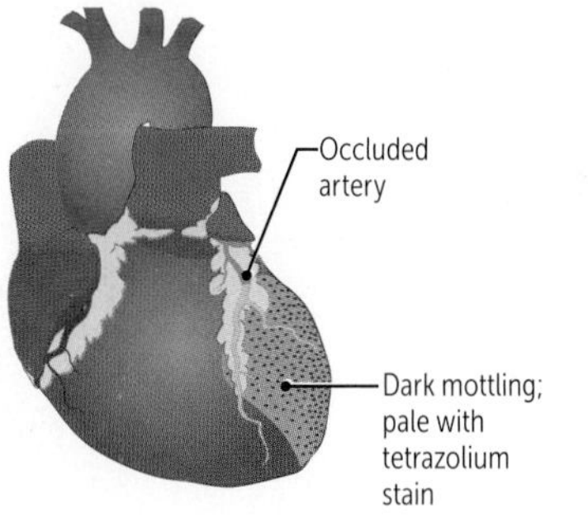Occluded artery Dark mottling; pale with tetrazolium stain	Wavy fibers (0–4 hr), early coagulative necrosis (4–24 hr) A → cell content released into blood; edema, hemorrhage Reperfusion injury → free radicals and ↑ Ca^{2+} influx → hypercontraction of myofibrils (dark eosinophilic stripes) 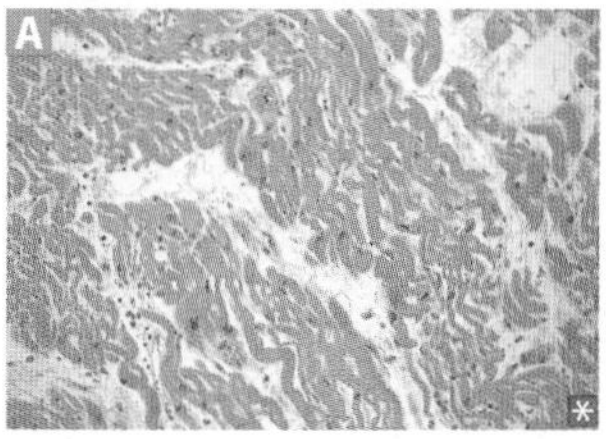	Ventricular arrhythmia, HF, cardiogenic shock
1–3 days	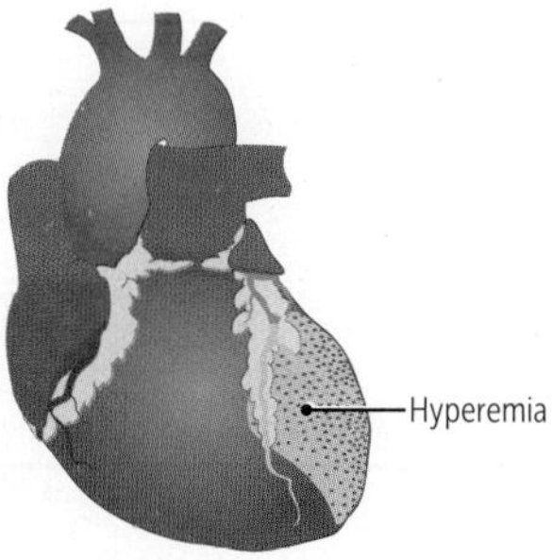Hyperemia	Extensive coagulative necrosis Tissue surrounding infarct shows acute inflammation with neutrophils B 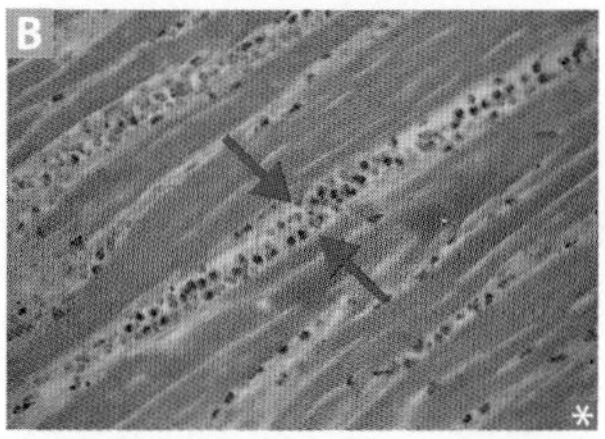	Postinfarction fibrinous pericarditis
3–14 days	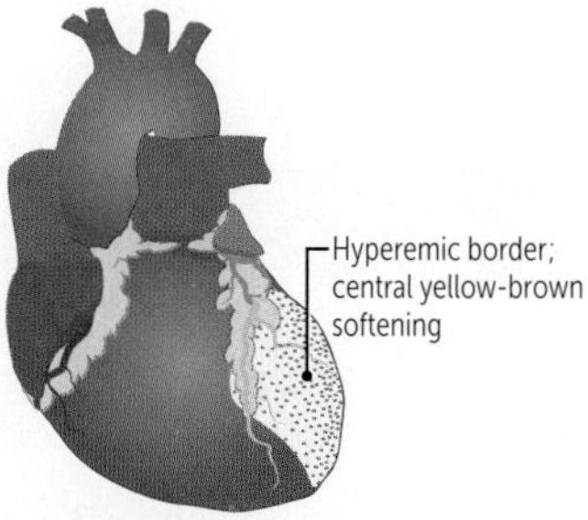Hyperemic border; central yellow-brown softening	Macrophages, then granulation tissue at margins C 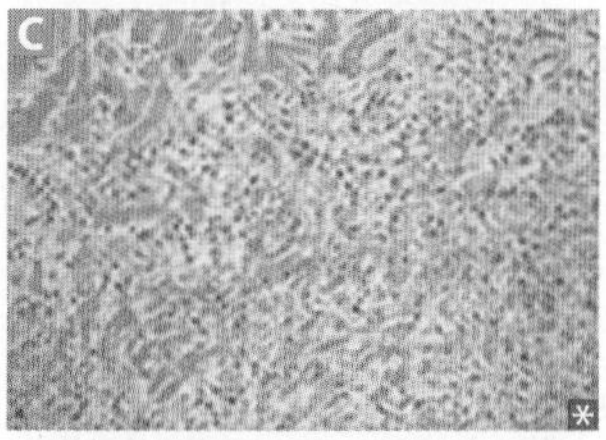	Free wall rupture → tamponade; papillary muscle rupture → mitral regurgitation; interventricular septal rupture due to macrophage-mediated structural degradation → left-to-right shunt LV pseudoaneurysm (risk of rupture)
2 weeks to several months	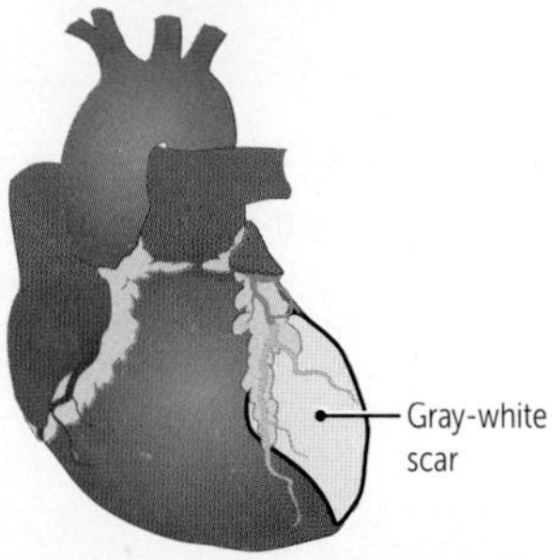Gray-white scar	Contracted scar complete D 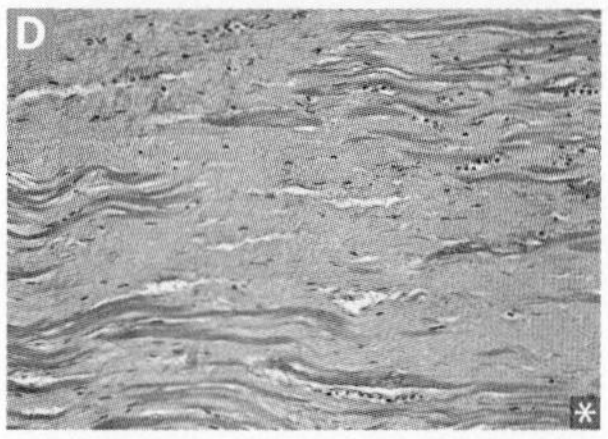	Dressler syndrome, HF, arrhythmias, true ventricular aneurysm (risk of mural thrombus)

Diagnosis of myocardial infarction

In the first 6 hours, ECG is the gold standard.

Cardiac troponin I rises after 4 hours (peaks at 24 hr) and is ↑ for 7–10 days; more specific than other protein markers.

CK-MB rises after 6–12 hours (peaks at 16–24 hr) and is predominantly found in myocardium but can also be released from skeletal muscle. Useful in diagnosing reinfarction following acute MI because levels return to normal after 48 hours.

Large MIs lead to greater elevations in troponin I and CK-MB. Exact curves vary with testing procedure.

ECG changes can include ST elevation (STEMI, transmural infarct), ST depression (NSTEMI, subendocardial infarct), hyperacute (peaked) T waves, T-wave inversion, new left bundle branch block, and pathologic Q waves or poor R wave progression (evolving or old transmural infarct).

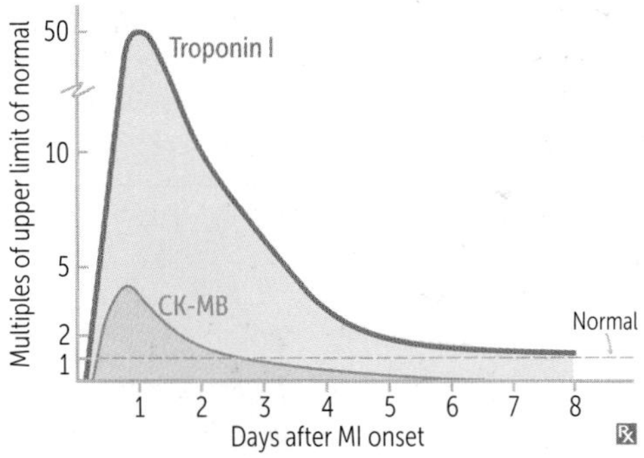

ECG localization of STEMI

INFARCT LOCATION	LEADS WITH ST-SEGMENT ELEVATIONS OR Q WAVES
Anteroseptal (LAD)	V_1–V_2
Anteroapical (distal LAD)	V_3–V_4
Anterolateral (LAD or LCX)	V_5–V_6
Lateral (LCX)	I, aVL
InFerior (RCA)	II, III, aVF
Posterior (PDA)	V_7–V_9, ST depression in V_1–V_3 with tall R waves

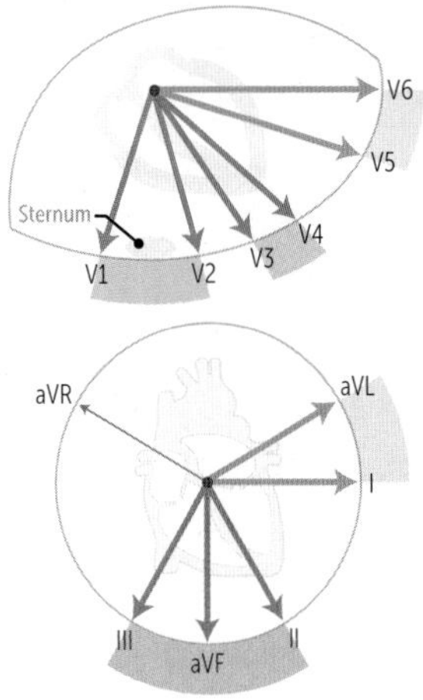

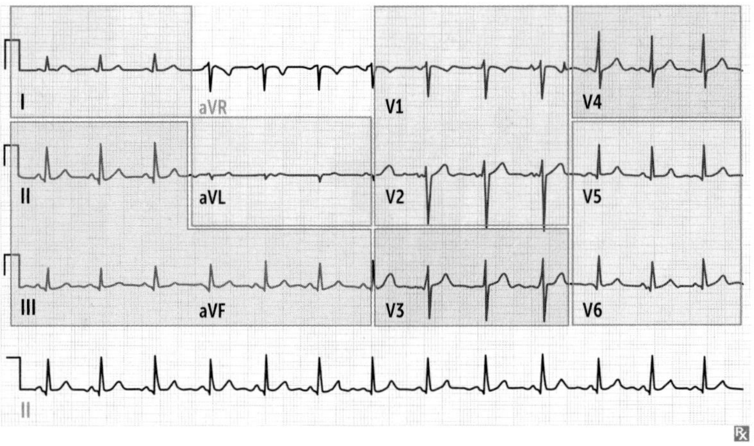

Paroxysmal supraventricular tachycardia

A narrow QRS complex tachycardia. Most often due to atrioventricular nodal reentrant tachycardia. Commonly presents with sudden-onset palpitations, diaphoresis, lightheadedness. Treatment: terminate re-entry by slowing AV node conduction (eg, vagal maneuvers, IV adenosine). Electrical cardioversion if hemodynamically unstable. Definitive treatment is catheter ablation of re-entry tract.

Torsades de pointes

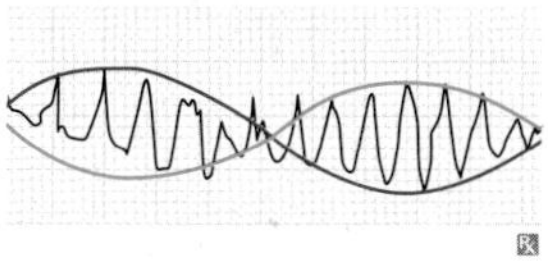

Polymorphic ventricular tachycardia, characterized by shifting sinusoidal waveforms on ECG; can progress to ventricular fibrillation. Long QT interval predisposes to torsades de pointes. Caused by drugs, ↓ K^+, ↓ Mg^{2+}, ↓ Ca^{2+}, congenital abnormalities. Treatment includes magnesium sulfate.

Drug-induced long QT (**ABCDEF**):
- Anti**A**rrhythmics (class IA, III)
- Anti**B**iotics (eg, macrolides, fluoroquinolones)
- Anti"**C**"ychotics (eg, haloperidol, ziprasidone)
- Anti**D**epressants (eg, TCAs)
- Anti**E**metics (eg, ondansetron)
- Anti**F**ungals (eg, azoles)

Torsades de pointes = twisting of the points

Hereditary channelopathies

Inherited mutations of cardiac ion channels → abnormal myocardial action potential → ↑ risk of ventricular tachyarrhythmias and sudden cardiac death (SCD).

Brugada syndrome

Autosomal dominant; most commonly due to loss of function mutation of Na^+ channels. ↑ prevalence in Asian males. ECG pattern of pseudo-right bundle branch block and ST-segment elevations in leads V_1-V_2. Prevent SCD with implantable cardioverter-defibrillator (ICD).

Congenital long QT syndrome

Most commonly due to loss of function mutation of K^+ channels (affects repolarization). Includes:
- Romano-Ward syndrome—autosomal dominant, pure cardiac phenotype (no deafness).
- Jervell and Lange-Nielsen syndrome—autosomal recessive, sensorineural deafness.

Wolff-Parkinson-White syndrome

Most common type of ventricular pre-excitation syndrome. Abnormal fast accessory conduction pathway from atria to ventricle (bundle of Kent) bypasses the rate-slowing AV node → ventricles begin to partially depolarize earlier → characteristic delta wave with widened QRS complex and shortened PR interval on ECG. May result in reentry circuit → supraventricular tachycardia.

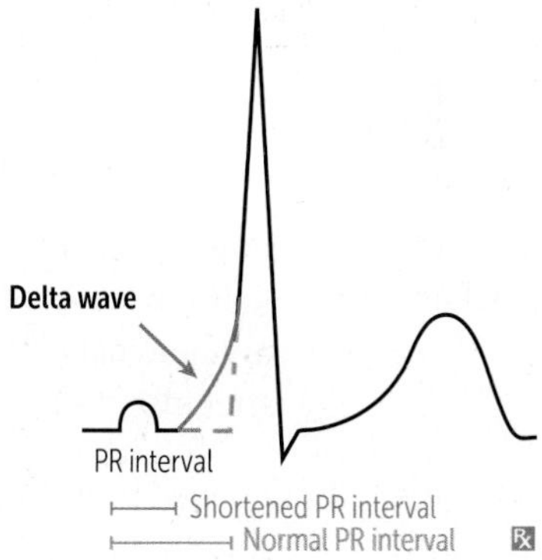
Delta wave
PR interval
Shortened PR interval
Normal PR interval

ECG tracings If the R is far from P, then you have a first degree.
Longer, longer, longer, drop! Then you have a Wenckebach.
If some P's don't get through, then you have a Mobitz II.
If P's and Q's don't agree, then you have a third degree.

RHYTHM	DESCRIPTION	EXAMPLE
Atrial fibrillation	Chaotic and erratic baseline with no discrete P waves in between irregularly spaced QRS complexes. Irregularly irregular heartbeat. Most common risk factors include hypertension and coronary artery disease (CAD). Occasionally seen after episodes of excessive alcohol consumption ("holiday heart syndrome"). Can lead to thromboembolic events, particularly stroke. Treatment: anticoagulation, rate and rhythm control, cardioversion. Definitive treatment is catheter ablation.	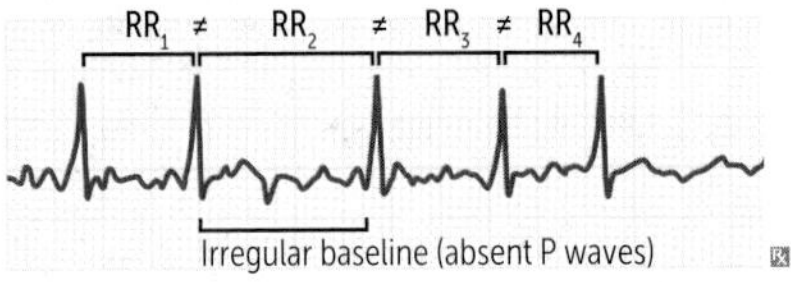$RR_1 \neq RR_2 \neq RR_3 \neq RR_4$ Irregular baseline (absent P waves)
Atrial flutter	A rapid succession of identical, back-to-back atrial depolarization waves. The identical appearance accounts for the "sawtooth" appearance of the flutter waves. Treat like atrial fibrillation +/– catheter ablation of region between tricuspid annulus and IVC.	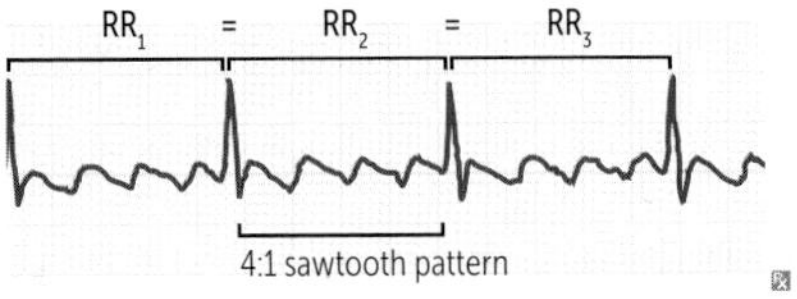$RR_1 = RR_2 = RR_3$ 4:1 sawtooth pattern
Ventricular fibrillation	A completely erratic rhythm with no identifiable waves. Fatal arrhythmia without immediate CPR and defibrillation.	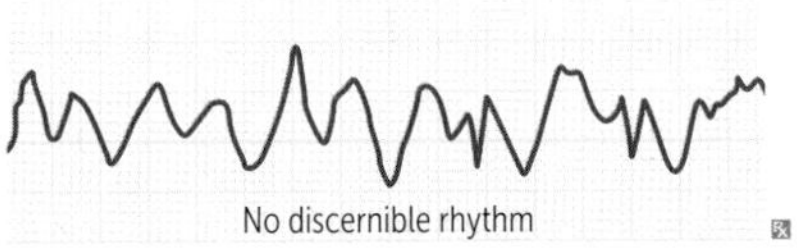No discernible rhythm
AV block		
First-degree AV block	The PR interval is prolonged (> 200 msec). Benign and asymptomatic. No treatment required.	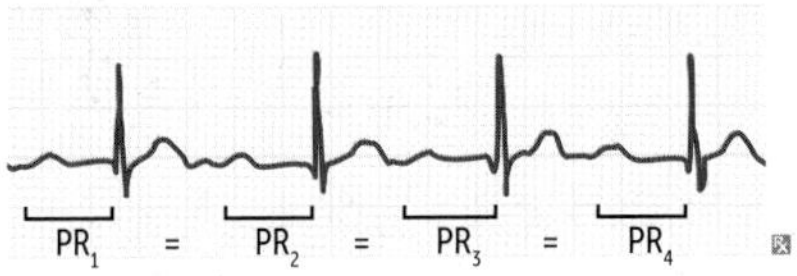$PR_1 = PR_2 = PR_3 = PR_4$
Second-degree AV block		
Mobitz type I (Wenckebach)	Progressive lengthening of PR interval until a beat is "dropped" (a P wave not followed by a QRS complex). Usually asymptomatic. Variable RR interval with a pattern (regularly irregular).	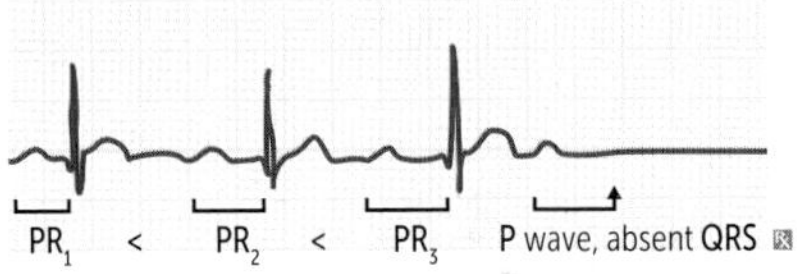$PR_1 < PR_2 < PR_3$ P wave, absent QRS
Mobitz type II	Dropped beats that are not preceded by a change in the length of the PR interval (as in type I). May progress to 3rd-degree block. Often treated with pacemaker.	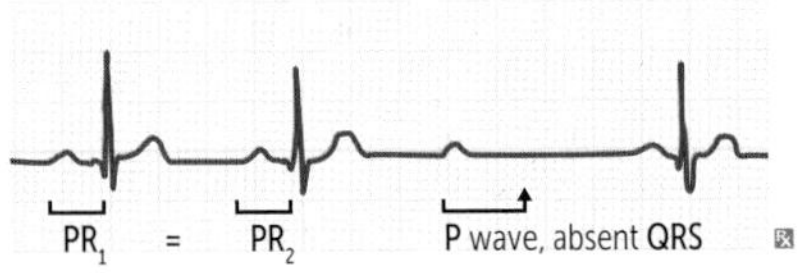$PR_1 = PR_2$ P wave, absent QRS
Third-degree (complete) AV block	The atria and ventricles beat independently of each other. P waves and QRS complexes not rhythmically associated. Atrial rate > ventricular rate. Usually treated with pacemaker. Can be caused by Lym3 disease.	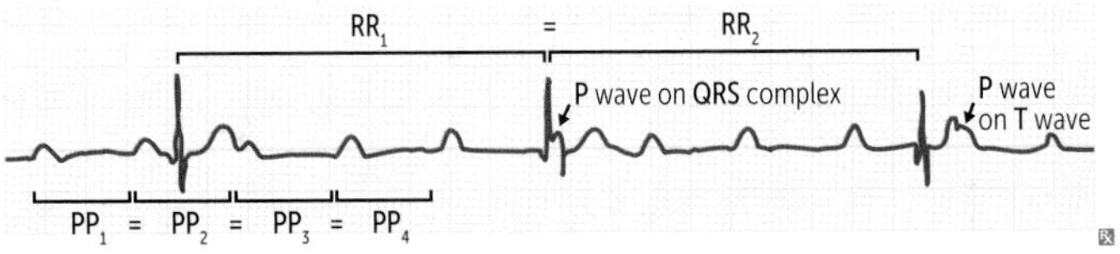$RR_1 = RR_2$ P wave on QRS complex P wave on T wave $PP_1 = PP_2 = PP_3 = PP_4$

Myocardial infarction complications

Cardiac arrhythmia	Occurs within the first few days after MI. Important cause of death before reaching the hospital and within the first 24 hours post-MI.
Postinfarction fibrinous pericarditis	1–3 days: friction rub.
Papillary muscle rupture	2–7 days: posteromedial papillary muscle rupture A ↑ risk due to single blood supply from posterior descending artery. Can result in severe mitral regurgitation.
Interventricular septal rupture	3–5 days: macrophage-mediated degradation → VSD → ↑ O_2 saturation and pressure in RV.
Ventricular pseudoaneurysm formation	3–14 days: free wall rupture contained by adherent pericardium or scar tissue B; ↓ CO, risk of arrhythmia, embolus from mural thrombus.
Ventricular free wall rupture	5–14 days: free wall rupture C → cardiac tamponade. LV hypertrophy and previous MI protect against free wall rupture. Acute form usually leads to sudden death.
True ventricular aneurysm	2 weeks to several months: outward bulge with contraction ("dyskinesia"), associated with fibrosis.
Dressler syndrome	Several weeks: autoimmune phenomenon resulting in fibrinous pericarditis.
LV failure and pulmonary edema	Can occur 2° to LV infarction, VSD, free wall rupture, papillary muscle rupture with mitral regurgitation.

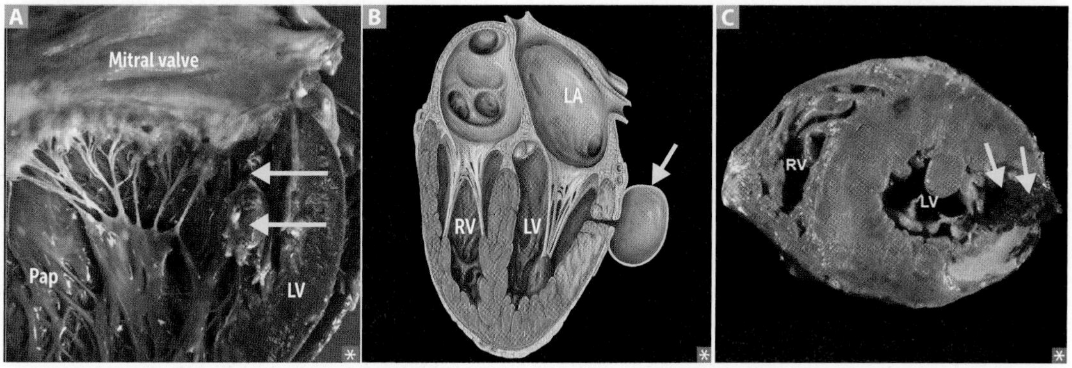

Acute coronary syndrome treatments

Unstable angina/NSTEMI—Anticoagulation (eg, heparin), antiplatelet therapy (eg, aspirin) + ADP receptor inhibitors (eg, clopidogrel), β-blockers, ACE inhibitors, statins. Symptom control with nitroglycerin +/– morphine.

STEMI—In addition to above, reperfusion therapy most important (percutaneous coronary intervention preferred over fibrinolysis). If RV affected (eg, RCA occlusion), support venous return/preload to maintain cardiac output (eg, IV fluids, avoiding nitroglycerin).

Cardiomyopathies

Dilated cardiomyopathy A 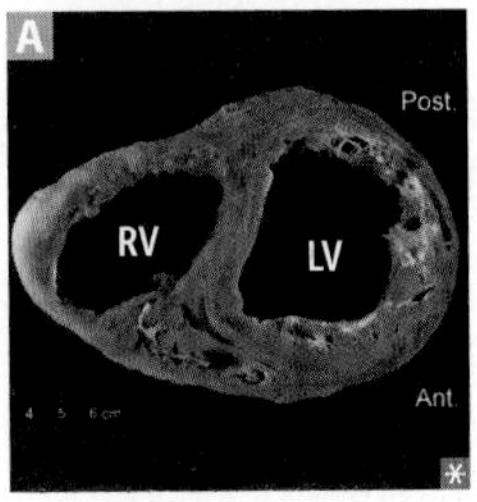	Most common cardiomyopathy (90% of cases). Often idiopathic or familial (eg, due to mutation of *TTN* gene encoding the sarcomeric protein titin). Other etiologies include drugs (eg, alcohol, cocaine, doxorubicin), infection (eg, coxsackie B virus, Chagas disease), ischemia (eg, CAD), systemic conditions (eg, hemochromatosis, sarcoidosis, thyrotoxicosis, wet beriberi), peripartum cardiomyopathy. Findings: HF, S3, systolic regurgitant murmur, dilated heart on echocardiogram, balloon appearance of heart on CXR. Treatment: Na^+ restriction, ACE inhibitors, β-blockers, sacubitril, diuretics, mineralocorticoid receptor blockers (eg, spironolactone), digoxin, ICD, heart transplant.	Leads to systolic dysfunction. Dilated cardiomyopathy A displays eccentric hypertrophy (sarcomeres added in series). Takotsubo cardiomyopathy: broken heart syndrome—ventricular apical ballooning likely due to increased sympathetic stimulation (eg, stressful situations).
Hypertrophic cardiomyopathy B 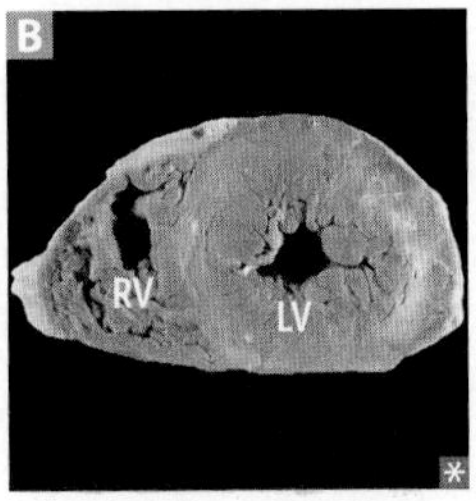	60–70% of cases are familial, autosomal dominant (most commonly due to mutations in genes encoding sarcomeric proteins, such as myosin binding protein C and β-myosin heavy chain). Causes syncope during exercise and may lead to sudden death (eg, in young athletes) due to ventricular arrhythmia. Findings: S4, systolic murmur. May see mitral regurgitation due to impaired mitral valve closure. Treatment: cessation of high-intensity athletics, use of β-blocker or nondihydropyridine Ca^{2+} channel blockers (eg, verapamil). ICD if syncope occurs. Avoid drugs that decrease preload (eg, diuretics, vasodilators).	Diastolic dysfunction ensues. Marked ventricular concentric hypertrophy (sarcomeres added in parallel) B, often septal predominance. Myofibrillar disarray and fibrosis. Classified as hypertrophic obstructive cardiomyopathy when outflow from LV is obstructed. Asymmetric septal hypertrophy and systolic anterior motion of mitral valve → outflow obstruction → dyspnea, possible syncope. Other causes of concentric LV hypertrophy: chronic HTN, Friedreich ataxia.
Restrictive/infiltrative cardiomyopathy	Postradiation fibrosis, Löffler endocarditis, Endocardial fibroelastosis (thick fibroelastic tissue in endocardium of young children), Amyloidosis, Sarcoidosis, Hemochromatosis (PLEASe Help!).	Diastolic dysfunction ensues. Can have low-voltage ECG despite thick myocardium (especially in amyloidosis). Löffler endocarditis—associated with hypereosinophilic syndrome; histology shows eosinophilic infiltrates in myocardium.

Heart failure

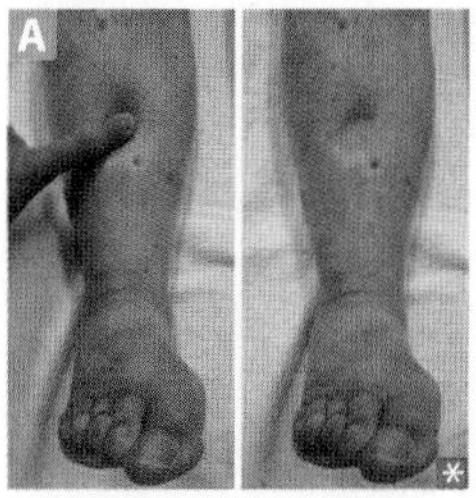

Clinical syndrome of cardiac pump dysfunction → congestion and low perfusion. Symptoms include dyspnea, orthopnea, fatigue; signs include S3 heart sound, rales, jugular venous distention (JVD), pitting edema A.

Systolic dysfunction—reduced EF, ↑ EDV; ↓ contractility often 2° to ischemia/MI or dilated cardiomyopathy.

Diastolic dysfunction—preserved EF, normal EDV; ↓ compliance (↑ EDP) often 2° to myocardial hypertrophy.

Right HF most often results from left HF. Cor pulmonale refers to isolated right HF due to pulmonary cause.

ACE inhibitors or angiotensin II receptor blockers, β-blockers (except in acute decompensated HF), and spironolactone ↓ mortality. Loop and thiazide diuretics are used mainly for symptomatic relief. Hydralazine with nitrate therapy improves both symptoms and mortality in select patients.

Left heart failure	
Orthopnea	Shortness of breath when supine: ↑ venous return from redistribution of blood (immediate gravity effect) exacerbates pulmonary vascular congestion.
Paroxysmal nocturnal dyspnea	Breathless awakening from sleep: ↑ venous return from redistribution of blood, reabsorption of peripheral edema, etc.
Pulmonary edema	↑ pulmonary venous pressure → pulmonary venous distention and transudation of fluid. Presence of hemosiderin-laden macrophages ("HF" cells) in lungs.

Right heart failure	
Hepatomegaly	↑ central venous pressure → ↑ resistance to portal flow. Rarely, leads to "cardiac cirrhosis." Associated with nutmeg liver (mottled appearance) on gross exam.
Jugular venous distention	↑ venous pressure.
Peripheral edema	↑ venous pressure → fluid transudation.

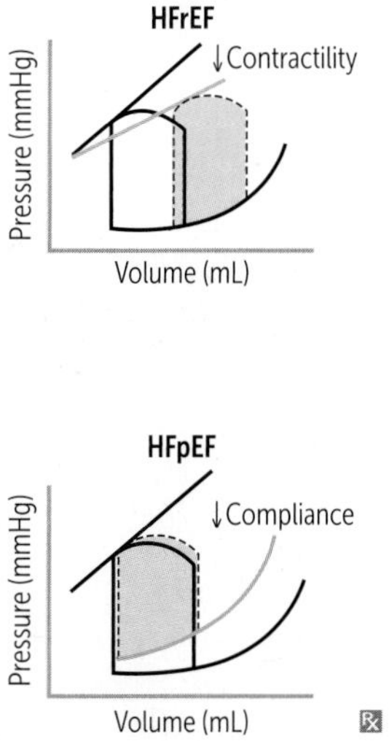

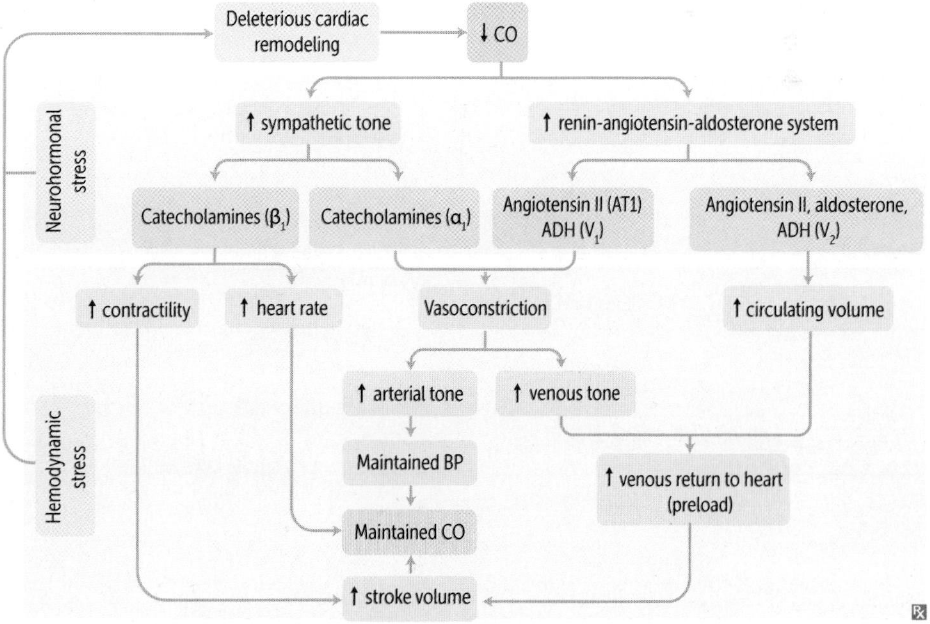

Shock

Inadequate organ perfusion and delivery of nutrients necessary for normal tissue and cellular function. Initially may be reversible but life threatening if not treated promptly.

<table>
<tr><th></th><th>CAUSED BY</th><th>SKIN</th><th>PCWP (PRELOAD)</th><th>CO</th><th>SVR (AFTERLOAD)</th><th>TREATMENT</th></tr>
<tr><td>Hypovolemic shock</td><td>Hemorrhage, dehydration, burns</td><td>Cold, clammy</td><td>↓↓</td><td>↓</td><td>↑</td><td>IV fluids</td></tr>
<tr><td>Cardiogenic shock</td><td>Acute MI, HF, valvular dysfunction, arrhythmia</td><td rowspan="2">Cold, clammy</td><td rowspan="2">↑ or ↓</td><td rowspan="2">↓↓</td><td rowspan="2">↑</td><td>Inotropes, diuresis</td></tr>
<tr><td>Obstructive shock</td><td>Cardiac tamponade, pulmonary embolism, tension pneumothorax</td><td>Relieve obstruction</td></tr>
<tr><td>Distributive shock</td><td>Sepsis, anaphylaxis
CNS injury</td><td>Warm
Dry</td><td>↓
↓</td><td>↑
↓</td><td>↓↓
↓↓</td><td>IV fluids, pressors, epinephrine (anaphylaxis)</td></tr>
</table>

Cardiac tamponade

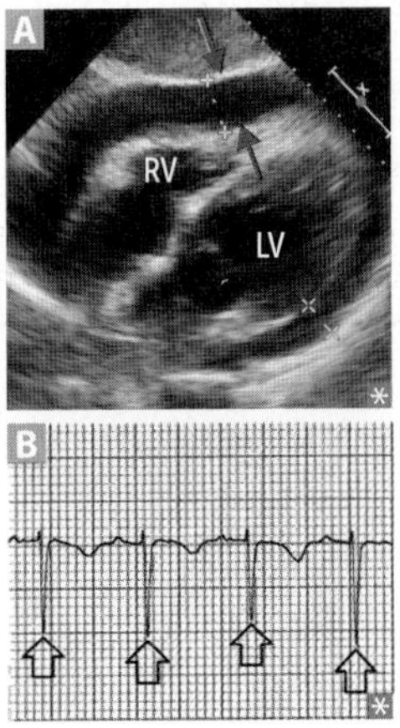

Compression of the heart by fluid (eg, blood, effusions [arrows in A] in pericardial space) → ↓ CO. Equilibration of diastolic pressures in all 4 chambers.

Findings: Beck triad (hypotension, distended neck veins, distant heart sounds), ↑ HR, pulsus paradoxus. ECG shows low-voltage QRS and electrical alternans B (due to "swinging" movement of heart in large effusion).

Treatment: pericardiocentesis or surgical drainage.

Pulsus paradoxus—↓ in amplitude of systolic BP by > 10 mm Hg during inspiration. Seen in constrictive pericarditis, obstructive pulmonary disease (eg, **C**roup, **O**SA, **A**sthma, COPD), cardiac **T**amponade (pea **COAT**).

Bacterial endocarditis

Acute—*S aureus* (high virulence). Large vegetations on previously normal valves A. Rapid onset.

Subacute—viridans streptococci (low virulence). Smaller vegetations on congenitally abnormal or diseased valves. Sequela of dental procedures. Gradual onset.

Symptoms: fever (most common), new murmur, **R**oth spots (**R**ound white spots on **R**etina surrounded by hemorrhage B), **O**sler nodes (**O**uchy raised lesions on finger or toe pads C due to immune complex deposition), Janeway lesions (small, painless, erythematous lesions on palm or sole) D, splinter hemorrhages E on nail bed.

Associated with glomerulonephritis, septic arterial or pulmonary emboli.

May be nonbacterial (marantic/thrombotic) 2° to malignancy, hypercoagulable state, or lupus.

FROM JANE with ♥:
- **F**ever
- **R**oth spots
- **O**sler nodes
- **M**urmur
- **J**aneway lesions
- **A**nemia
- **N**ail-bed hemorrhage
- **E**mboli

Requires multiple blood cultures for diagnosis.

If culture ⊖, most likely *Coxiella burnetii*, *Bartonella* spp.

Mitral valve is most frequently involved.

Tricuspid valve endocarditis is associated with IV **drug** use (don't "**tri**" **drugs**). Associated with *S aureus*, *Pseudomonas*, and *Candida*.

S bovis (gallolyticus) is present in colon cancer, *S epidermidis* on prosthetic valves.

Native valve endocarditis may be due to **HACEK** organisms (***H**aemophilus*, ***A**ggregatibacter* [formerly *Actinobacillus*], ***C**ardiobacterium*, ***E**ikenella*, ***K**ingella*).

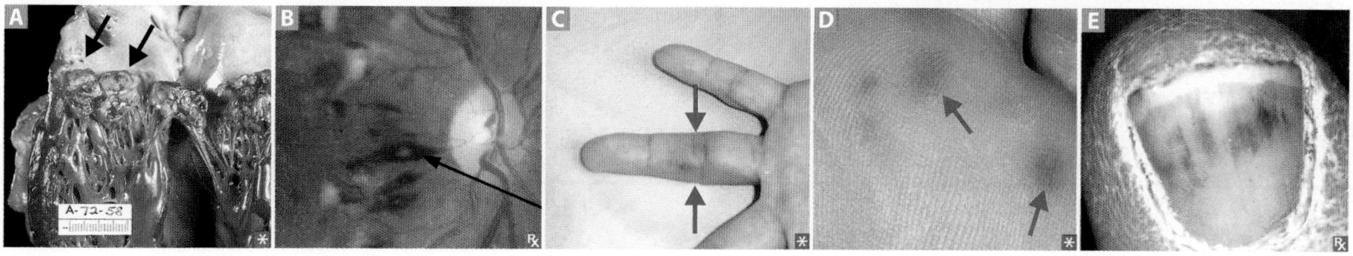

Rheumatic fever

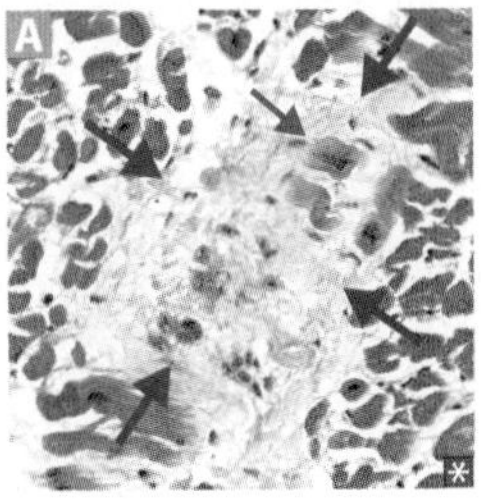

A consequence of pharyngeal infection with group A β-hemolytic streptococci. Late sequelae include rheumatic heart disease, which affects heart valves—mitral > aortic >> tricuspid (high-pressure valves affected most). Early lesion is mitral valve regurgitation; late lesion is mitral stenosis.

Associated with Aschoff bodies (granuloma with giant cells [blue arrows in A]), Anitschkow cells (enlarged macrophages with ovoid, wavy, rod-like nucleus [red arrow in A]), ↑ anti-streptolysin O (ASO) and ↑ anti-DNase B titers.

Immune mediated (type II hypersensitivity); not a direct effect of bacteria. Antibodies to M protein cross-react with self antigens, often myosin (molecular mimicry).

Treatment/prophylaxis: penicillin.

J♥NES (major criteria):
- Joint (migratory polyarthritis)
- ♥ (carditis)
- Nodules in skin (subcutaneous)
- Erythema marginatum (evanescent rash with ring margin)
- Sydenham chorea (involuntary irregular movements of limbs and face)

Syphilitic heart disease

3° syphilis disrupts the vasa vasorum of the aorta with consequent atrophy of vessel wall and dilation of aorta and valve ring.

May see calcification of aortic root, ascending aortic arch, and thoracic aorta. Leads to "tree bark" appearance of aorta.

Can result in aneurysm of ascending aorta or aortic arch, aortic insufficiency.

Acute pericarditis

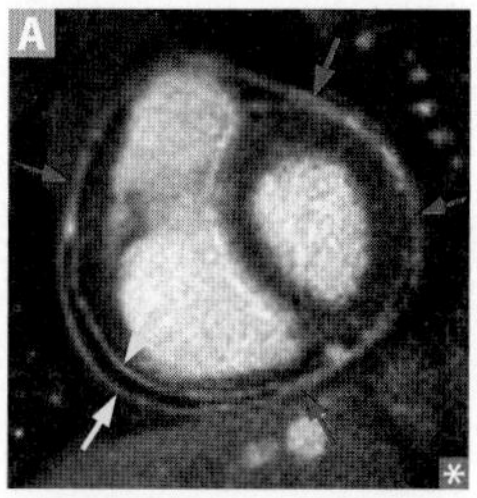

Inflammation of the pericardium (red arrows in A). Commonly presents with sharp pain, aggravated by inspiration, and relieved by sitting up and leaning forward. Often complicated by pericardial effusion [between yellow arrows in A]. Presents with friction rub. ECG changes include widespread ST-segment elevation and/or PR depression.

Causes include idiopathic (most common; presumed viral), confirmed infection (eg, coxsackievirus B), neoplasia, autoimmune (eg, SLE, rheumatoid arthritis), uremia, cardiovascular (acute STEMI or Dressler syndrome), radiation therapy.

Treatment: NSAIDs, colchicine, glucocorticoids, dialysis (uremia).

Myocarditis

Inflammation of myocardium → global enlargement of heart and dilation of all chambers. Major cause of SCD in adults < 40 years old.

Presentation highly variable, can include dyspnea, chest pain, fever, arrhythmias (persistent tachycardia out of proportion to fever is characteristic).

Multiple causes:

- Viral (eg, adenovirus, coxsackie B, parvovirus B19, HIV, HHV-6); lymphocytic infiltrate with focal necrosis highly indicative of viral myocarditis
- Parasitic (eg, *Trypanosoma cruzi*, *Toxoplasma gondii*)
- Bacterial (eg, *Borrelia burgdorferi*, *Mycoplasma pneumoniae*, *Corynebacterium diphtheriae*)
- Toxins (eg, carbon monoxide, black widow venom)
- Rheumatic fever
- Drugs (eg, doxorubicin, cocaine)
- Autoimmune (eg, Kawasaki disease, sarcoidosis, SLE, polymyositis/dermatomyositis)

Complications include sudden death, arrhythmias, heart block, dilated cardiomyopathy, HF, mural thrombus with systemic emboli.

Cardiac tumors	Most common cardiac tumor is a metastasis (eg, melanoma).
Myxomas 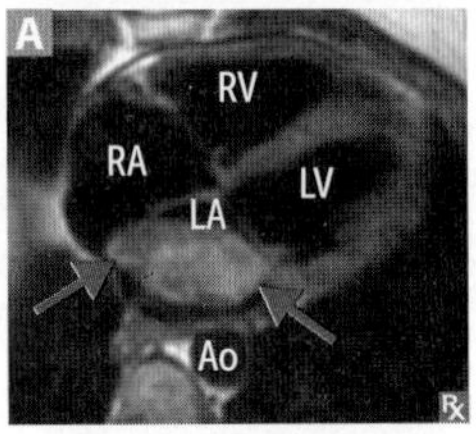	Most common 1° cardiac tumor in **adults** (arrows in A). 90% occur in the atria (mostly left atrium). Myxomas are usually described as a "ball valve" obstruction in the left atrium (associated with multiple syncopal episodes). IL-6 production by tumor → constitutional symptoms (eg, fever, weight loss). May auscultate early diastolic "tumor plop" sound. Histology: gelatinous material, myxoma cells immersed in glycosaminoglycans. **Adults** make **6 myxed** drinks.
Rhabdomyomas	Most frequent 1° cardiac tumor in children (associated with tuberous sclerosis). Histology: hamartomatous growths. More common in the ventricles.

Kussmaul sign	Paradoxical ↑ in JVP on inspiration (normally, inspiration → negative intrathoracic pressure → ↑ venous return → ↓ JVP). Impaired RV filling → blood backs up into vena cava → ↓ venous return as negative intrathoracic pressure is insufficient to bring blood to right heart → Kussmaul sign. May be seen with constrictive pericarditis, restrictive cardiomyopathy, right heart failure, massive pulmonary embolism, right atrial or ventricular tumors.

Hereditary hemorrhagic telangiectasia	Also called Osler-Weber-Rendu syndrome. Autosomal dominant disorder of blood vessels. Findings: blanching lesions (telangiectasias) on skin and mucous membranes, recurrent epistaxis, skin discolorations, arteriovenous malformations (AVMs), GI bleeding, hematuria.

▸ CARDIOVASCULAR—PHARMACOLOGY

Hypertension treatment

Primary (essential) hypertension	Thiazide diuretics, ACE inhibitors, angiotensin II receptor blockers (ARBs), dihydropyridine Ca^{2+} channel blockers.	
Hypertension with heart failure	Diuretics, ACE inhibitors/ARBs, β-blockers (compensated HF), aldosterone antagonists.	β-blockers must be used cautiously in decompensated HF and are contraindicated in cardiogenic shock. In HF, ARBs may be combined with the neprilysin inhibitor sacubitril.
Hypertension with diabetes mellitus	ACE inhibitors/ARBs, Ca^{2+} channel blockers, thiazide diuretics, β-blockers.	ACE inhibitors/ARBs are protective against diabetic nephropathy. β-blockers can mask hypoglycemia symptoms.
Hypertension in asthma	ARBs, Ca^{2+} channel blockers, thiazide diuretics, cardioselective β-blockers.	Avoid nonselective β-blockers to prevent β_2-receptor–induced bronchoconstriction. Avoid ACE inhibitors to prevent confusion between drug or asthma-related cough.
Hypertension in pregnancy	Nifedipine, methyldopa, labetalol, hydralazine.	New moms love hugs.

Cardiovascular agents and molecular targets

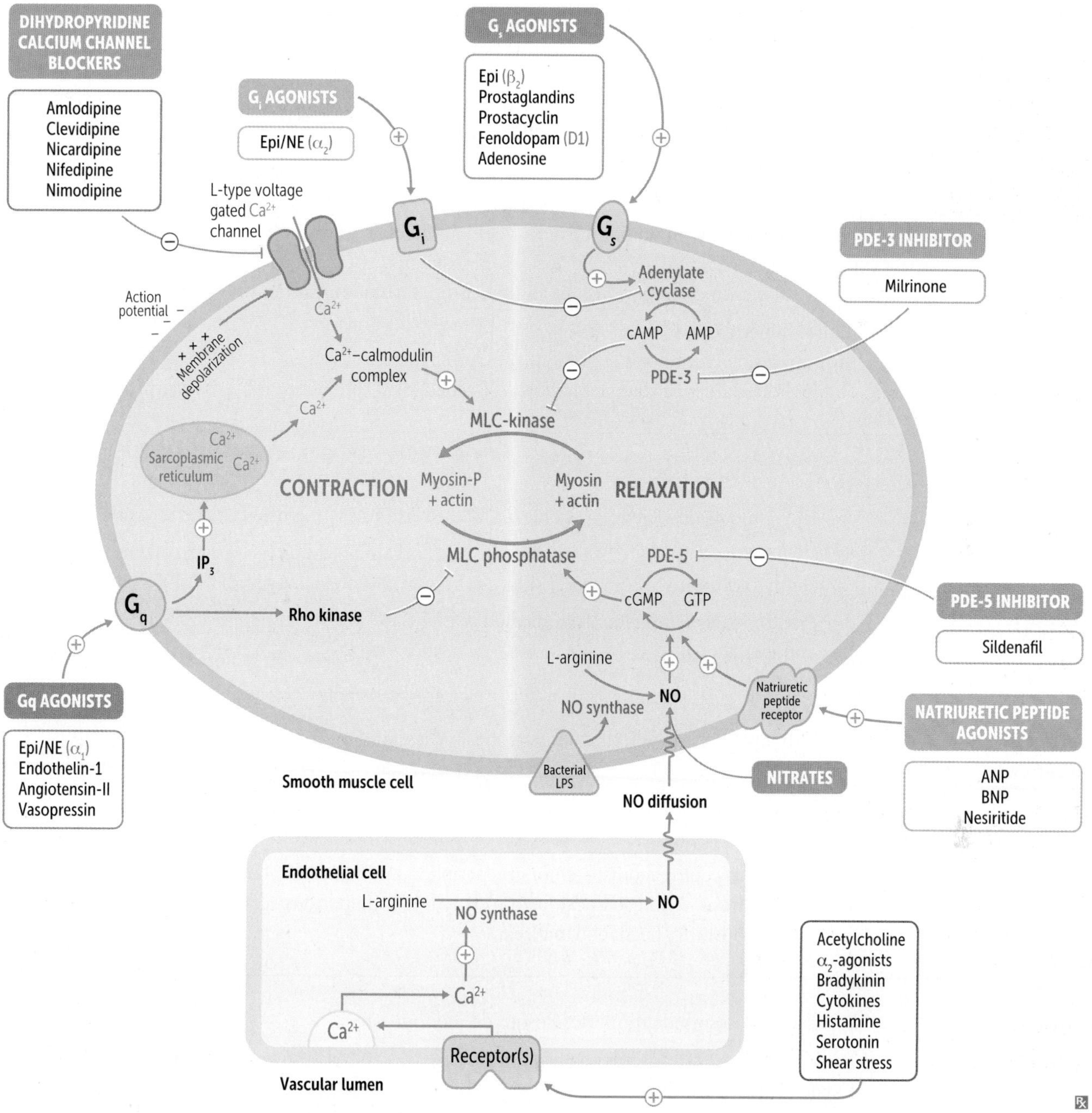

Calcium channel blockers	Amlodipine, clevidipine, nicardipine, nifedipine, nimodipine (dihydropyridines, act on vascular smooth muscle); diltiazem, verapamil (nondihydropyridines, act on heart).
MECHANISM	Block voltage-dependent L-type calcium channels of cardiac and smooth muscle → ↓ muscle contractility. Vascular smooth muscle—amlodipine = nifedipine > diltiazem > verapamil. Heart—verapamil > diltiazem > amlodipine = nifedipine.
CLINICAL USE	Dihydropyridines (except nimodipine): hypertension, angina (including vasospastic type), Raynaud phenomenon. Nimodipine: subarachnoid hemorrhage (prevents cerebral vasospasm). Nicardipine, clevidipine: hypertensive urgency or emergency. Nondihydropyridines: hypertension, angina, atrial fibrillation/flutter.
ADVERSE EFFECTS	Gingival hyperplasia. Dihydropyridine: peripheral edema, flushing, dizziness. Nondihydropyridine: cardiac depression, AV block, hyperprolactinemia (verapamil), constipation.

Hydralazine	
MECHANISM	↑ cGMP → smooth muscle relaxation. Vasodilates arterioles > veins; afterload reduction.
CLINICAL USE	Severe hypertension (particularly acute), HF (with organic nitrate). Safe to use during pregnancy. Frequently coadministered with a β-blocker to prevent reflex tachycardia.
ADVERSE EFFECTS	Compensatory tachycardia (contraindicated in angina/CAD), fluid retention, headache, angina, drug-induced lupus.

Hypertensive emergency	Treat with labetalol, clevidipine, fenoldopam, nicardipine, nitroprusside.
Nitroprusside	Short acting vasodilator (arteries = veins); ↑ cGMP via direct release of NO. Can cause cyanide toxicity (releases cyanide).
Fenoldopam	Dopamine D_1 receptor agonist—coronary, peripheral, renal, and splanchnic vasodilation. ↓ BP, ↑ natriuresis. Also used postoperatively as an antihypertensive. Can cause hypotension, tachycardia, flushing, headache, nausea.

Nitrates	Nitroglycerin, isosorbide dinitrate, isosorbide mononitrate.
MECHANISM	Vasodilate by ↑ NO in vascular smooth muscle → ↑ in cGMP and smooth muscle relaxation. Dilate veins >> arteries. ↓ preload.
CLINICAL USE	Angina, acute coronary syndrome, pulmonary edema.
ADVERSE EFFECTS	Reflex tachycardia (treat with β-blockers), hypotension, flushing, headache, "Monday disease" in industrial nitrate exposure: development of tolerance for the vasodilating action during the work week and loss of tolerance over the weekend → tachycardia, dizziness, headache upon reexposure. Contraindicated in right ventricular infarction, hypertrophic cardiomyopathy, and with concurrent PDE-5 inhibitor use.

Antianginal therapy Goal is reduction of myocardial O_2 consumption (MVO_2) by ↓ 1 or more of the determinants of MVO_2: end-diastolic volume, BP, HR, contractility.

COMPONENT	NITRATES	β-BLOCKERS	NITRATES + β-BLOCKERS
End-diastolic volume	↓	No effect or ↑	No effect or ↓
Blood pressure	↓	↓	↓
Contractility	↑ (reflex response)	↓	Little/no effect
Heart rate	↑ (reflex response)	↓	No effect or ↓
Ejection time	↓	↑	Little/no effect
MVO_2	↓	↓	↓↓

Verapamil is similar to β-blockers in effect.
Pindolol and acebutolol are partial β-agonists that should be used with caution in angina.

Ranolazine

MECHANISM	Inhibits the late phase of inward sodium current thereby reducing diastolic wall tension and oxygen consumption. Does not affect heart rate or blood pressure.
CLINICAL USE	Refractory angina.
ADVERSE EFFECTS	Constipation, dizziness, headache, nausea.

Sacubitril

MECHANISM	A neprilysin inhibitor; prevents degradation of bradykinin, natriuretic peptides, angiotensin II, and substance P → ↑ vasodilation, ↓ ECF volume.
CLINICAL USE	Used in combination with valsartan (an ARB) to treat HFrEF.
ADVERSE EFFECTS	Hypotension, hyperkalemia, cough, dizziness; contraindicated with ACE inhibitors due to angioedema (both drugs ↑ bradykinin).

Lipid-lowering agents

DRUG	LDL	HDL	TRIGLYCERIDES	MECHANISMS OF ACTION	ADVERSE EFFECTS/PROBLEMS
HMG-CoA reductase inhibitors Atorvastatin, simvastatin	↓↓↓	↑	↓	Inhibit conversion of HMG-CoA to mevalonate, a cholesterol precursor; → ↓ intrahepatic cholesterol → ↑ LDL receptor recycling → ↑ LDL catabolism ↓ in mortality in patients with CAD	Hepatotoxicity (↑ LFTs), myopathy (esp when used with fibrates or niacin)
Bile acid resins Cholestyramine, colestipol, colesevelam	↓↓	↑ slightly	↑ slightly	Prevent intestinal reabsorption of bile acids; liver must use cholesterol to make more	GI upset, ↓ absorption of other drugs and fat-soluble vitamins
Ezetimibe	↓↓	↑/—	↓/—	Prevents cholesterol absorption at small intestine brush border	Rare ↑ LFTs, diarrhea
Fibrates Gemfibrozil, bezafibrate, fenofibrate	↓	↑	↓↓↓	Activate PPAR-α → upregulate LPL → ↑ TG clearance Activate PPAR-α → induce HDL synthesis	Myopathy (↑ risk with statins), cholesterol gallstones (via inhibition of cholesterol 7α-hydroxylase)
Niacin	↓↓	↑↑	↓	Inhibits lipolysis (hormone-sensitive lipase) in adipose tissue; reduces hepatic VLDL synthesis	Flushed face (prostaglandin mediated; ↓ by NSAIDs or long-term use) Hyperglycemia Hyperuricemia
PCSK9 inhibitors Alirocumab, evolocumab	↓↓↓	↑	↓	Inactivation of LDL-receptor degradation → ↑ removal of LDL from bloodstream	Myalgias, delirium, dementia, other neurocognitive effects
Fish oil and marine omega-3 fatty acids	↑ slightly	↑ slightly	↓ at high doses	Believed to decrease FFA delivery to liver and decrease activity of TG-synthesizing enzymes	Nausea, fish-like taste

Lipid-lowering agents *(continued)*

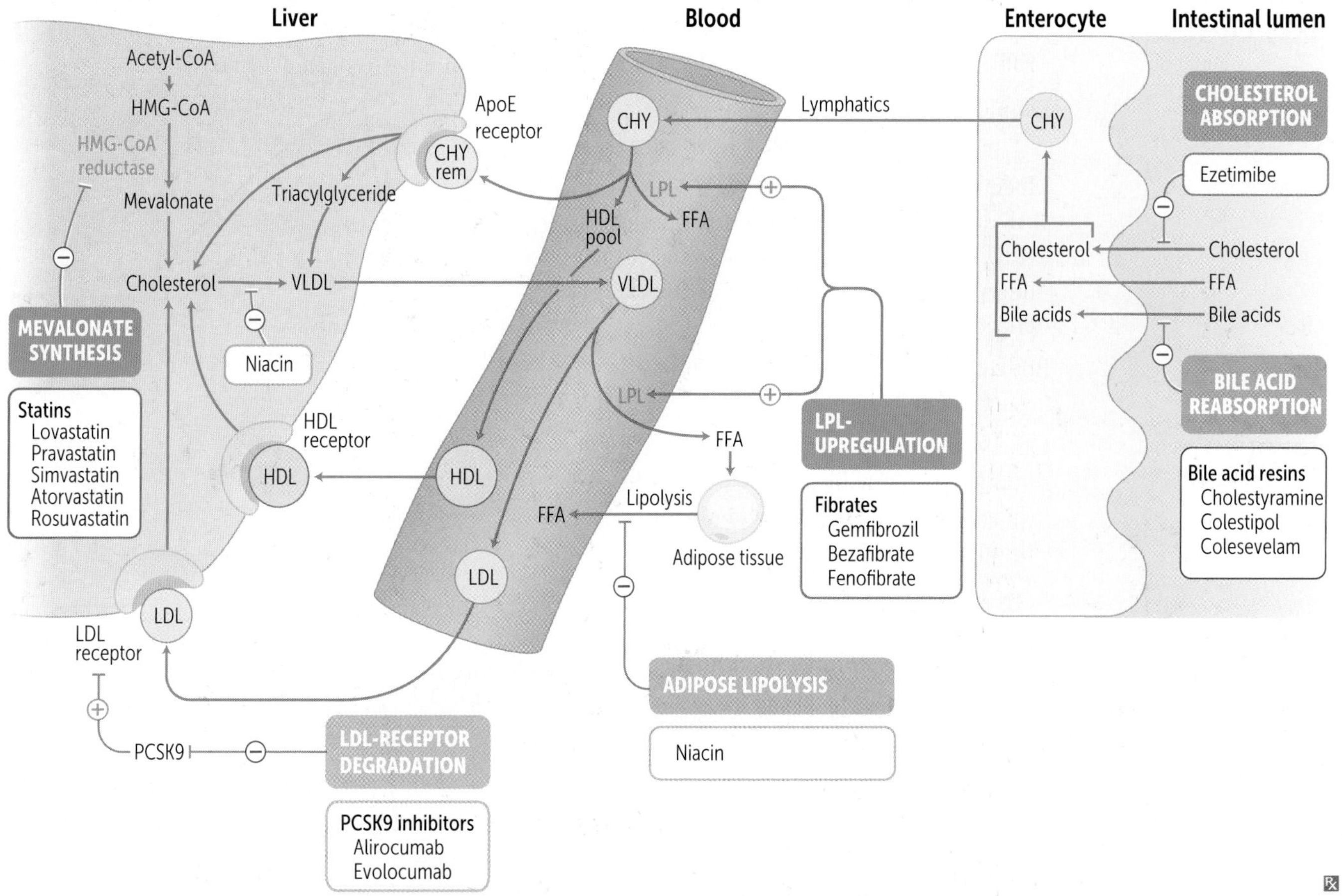

Cardiac glycosides	Digoxin.
MECHANISM	Direct inhibition of Na^+/K^+ ATPase → indirect inhibition of Na^+/Ca^{2+} exchanger. ↑ $[Ca^{2+}]_i$ → positive inotropy. Stimulates vagus nerve → ↓ HR. 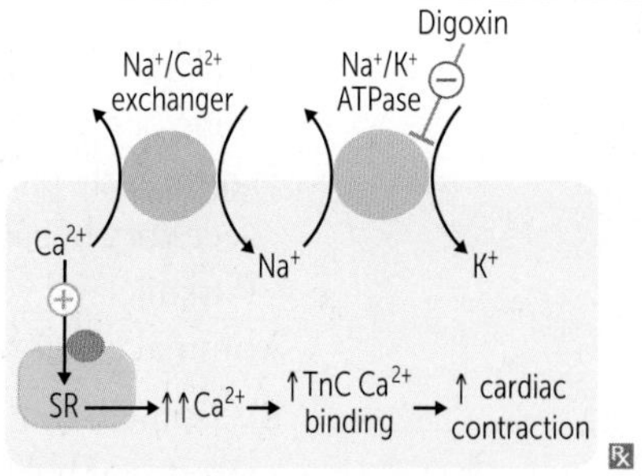
CLINICAL USE	HF (↑ contractility); atrial fibrillation (↓ conduction at AV node and depression of SA node).
ADVERSE EFFECTS	Cholinergic effects (nausea, vomiting, diarrhea), blurry **yellow** vision (think van **Glow**), arrhythmias, AV block. Can lead to hyperkalemia, which indicates poor prognosis. Factors predisposing to toxicity: renal failure (↓ excretion), hypokalemia (permissive for digoxin binding at K^+-binding site on Na^+/K^+ ATPase), drugs that displace digoxin from tissue-binding sites, and ↓ clearance (eg, verapamil, amiodarone, quinidine).
ANTIDOTE	Slowly normalize K^+, cardiac pacer, anti-digoxin Fab fragments, Mg^{2+}.

Antiarrhythmics—sodium channel blockers (class I)

Slow or block conduction (especially in depolarized cells). ↓ slope of phase 0 depolarization. ↑ action at faster HR. State dependent ↑ HR → shorter diastole, Na^+ channels spend less time in resting state (drugs dissociate during this state) → less time for drug to dissociate from receptor. Effect most pronounced in IC>IA>IB due to relative binding strength. **Fast** taxi **CAB**.

Class IA

Quinidine, **procainamide**, **disopyramide**. "The **queen proclaims Diso's pyramid**."

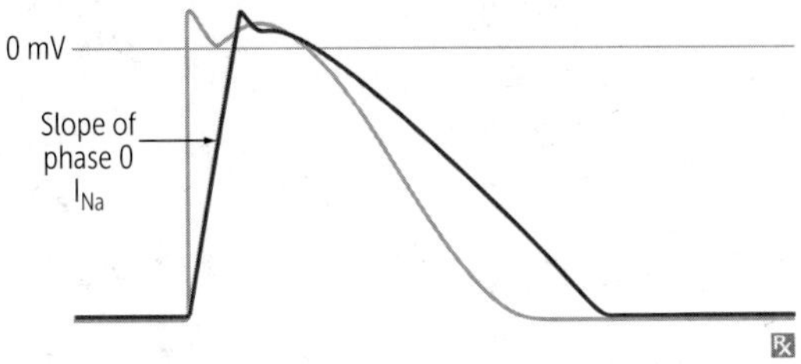

MECHANISM

Moderate Na^+ channel blockade.
↑ AP duration, ↑ effective refractory period (ERP) in ventricular action potential, ↑ QT interval, some potassium channel blocking effects.

CLINICAL USE

Both atrial and ventricular arrhythmias, especially re-entrant and ectopic SVT and VT.

ADVERSE EFFECTS

Cinchonism (headache, tinnitus with quinidine), reversible SLE-like syndrome (procainamide), HF (disopyramide), thrombocytopenia, torsades de pointes due to ↑ QT interval.

Class IB

Lidocaine, **phenytoin**, **mexiletine**. "I'd **B**uy **Lid**dy's **ph**ine **Mex**ican tacos."

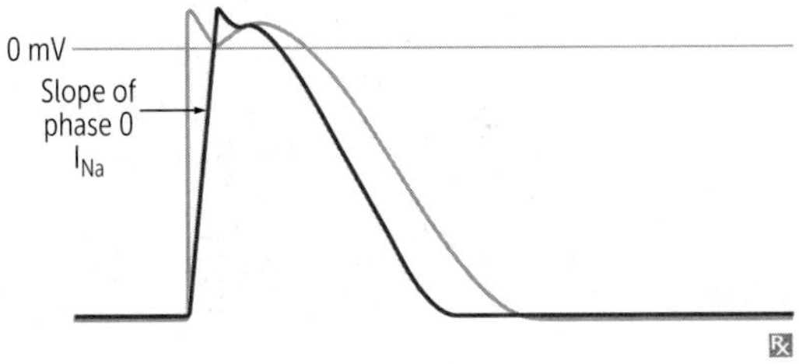

MECHANISM

Weak Na^+ channel blockade.
↓ AP duration. Preferentially affect ischemic or depolarized Purkinje and ventricular tissue.

CLINICAL USE

Acute ventricular arrhythmias (especially post-MI), digitalis-induced arrhythmias.
IB is **B**est post-MI.

ADVERSE EFFECTS

CNS stimulation/depression, cardiovascular depression.

Class IC

Flecainide, propafenone. "Can I have fries, please?"

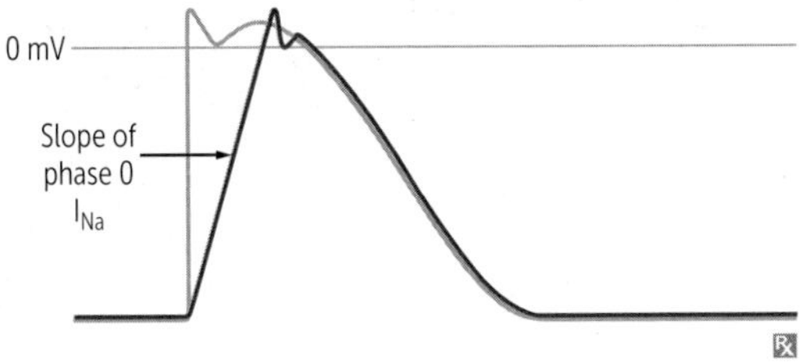

MECHANISM

Strong Na^+ channel blockade.
Significantly prolongs ERP in AV node and accessory bypass tracts. No effect on ERP in Purkinje and ventricular tissue.
Minimal effect on AP duration.

CLINICAL USE

SVTs, including atrial fibrillation. Only as a last resort in refractory VT.

ADVERSE EFFECTS

Proarrhythmic, especially post-MI (contraindicated). IC is **C**ontraindicated in structural and ischemic heart disease.

Antiarrhythmics—β-blockers (class II)

Metoprolol, propranolol, esmolol, atenolol, timolol, carvedilol.

MECHANISM	Decrease SA and AV nodal activity by ↓ cAMP, ↓ Ca^{2+} currents. Suppress abnormal pacemakers by ↓ slope of phase 4. AV node particularly sensitive—↑ PR interval. Esmolol very short acting.
CLINICAL USE	SVT, ventricular rate control for atrial fibrillation and atrial flutter.
ADVERSE EFFECTS	Impotence, exacerbation of COPD and asthma, cardiovascular effects (bradycardia, AV block, HF), CNS effects (sedation, sleep alterations). May mask the signs of hypoglycemia. Metoprolol can cause dyslipidemia. Propranolol can exacerbate vasospasm in vasospastic angina. β-blockers (except the nonselective α- and β-antagonists carvedilol and labetalol) cause unopposed α_1-agonism if given alone for pheochromocytoma or for cocaine toxicity (unsubstantiated). Treat β-blocker overdose with saline, atropine, glucagon.

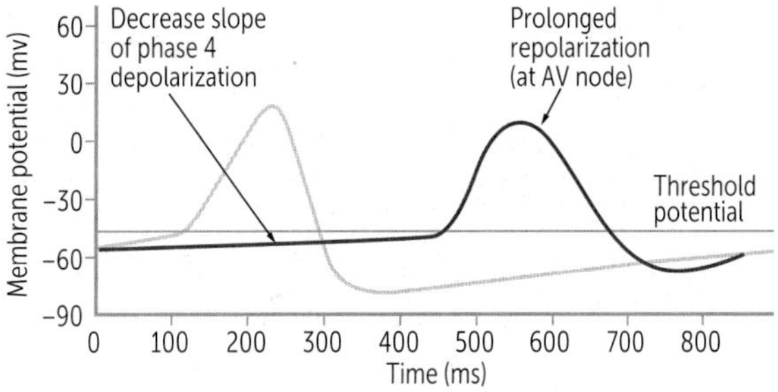

Pacemaker cell action potential

Antiarrhythmics—potassium channel blockers (class III)

Amiodarone, Ibutilide, Dofetilide, Sotalol. AIDS.

MECHANISM	↑ AP duration, ↑ ERP, ↑ QT interval.	
CLINICAL USE	Atrial fibrillation, atrial flutter; ventricular tachycardia (amiodarone, sotalol).	
ADVERSE EFFECTS	Sotalol—torsades de pointes, excessive β blockade. Ibutilide—torsades de pointes. Amiodarone—pulmonary fibrosis, hepatotoxicity, hypothyroidism or hyperthyroidism (amiodarone is 40% iodine by weight), acts as hapten (corneal deposits, blue/gray skin deposits resulting in photodermatitis), neurologic effects, constipation, cardiovascular effects (bradycardia, heart block, HF).	Remember to check PFTs, LFTs, and TFTs when using amiodarone. Amiodarone is lipophilic and has class I, II, III, and IV effects.

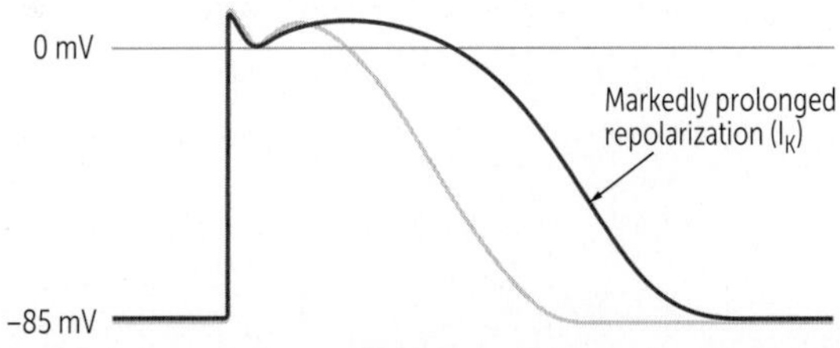

Cell action potential

Antiarrhythmics—calcium channel blockers (class IV)	Diltiazem, verapamil.
MECHANISM	Decrease conduction velocity, ↑ ERP, ↑ PR interval.
CLINICAL USE	Prevention of nodal arrhythmias (eg, SVT), rate control in atrial fibrillation.
ADVERSE EFFECTS	Constipation, flushing, edema, cardiovascular effects (HF, AV block, sinus node depression).

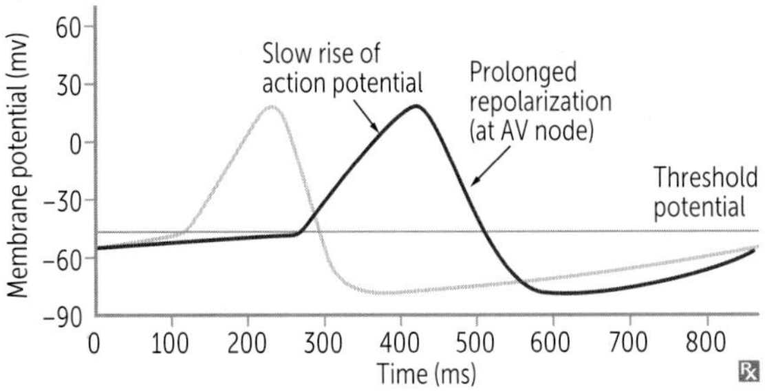

Other antiarrhythmics	
Adenosine	↑ K^+ out of cells → hyperpolarizing the cell and ↓ I_{Ca}, decreasing AV node conduction. Drug of choice in diagnosing/terminating certain forms of SVT. Very short acting (~ 15 sec). Effects blunted by theophylline and caffeine (both are adenosine receptor antagonists). Adverse effects include flushing, hypotension, chest pain, sense of impending doom, bronchospasm.
Magnesium	Effective in torsades de pointes and digoxin toxicity.

Ivabradine	
MECHANISM	**IV**abradine prolongs slow depolarization (phase "**IV**") by selectively inhibiting "funny" sodium channels (I_f).
CLINICAL USE	Chronic stable angina in patients who cannot take β-blockers. Chronic HFrEF.
ADVERSE EFFECTS	Luminous phenomena/visual brightness, hypertension, bradycardia.

Endocrine

"If you skew the endocrine system, you lose the pathways to self."

—Hilary Mantel

"Sometimes you need a little crisis to get your adrenaline flowing and help you realize your potential."

—Jeannette Walls, *The Glass Castle*

"Chocolate causes certain endocrine glands to secrete hormones that affect your feelings and behavior by making you happy."

—Elaine Sherman, *Book of Divine Indulgences*

The endocrine system comprises widely distributed organs that work in a highly integrated manner to orchestrate a state of hormonal equilibrium within the body. Generally speaking, endocrine diseases can be classified either as diseases of underproduction or overproduction, or as conditions involving the development of mass lesions—which themselves may be associated with underproduction or overproduction of hormones. Therefore, study the endocrine system first by learning the glands, their hormones, and their regulation, and then by integrating disease manifestations with diagnosis and management. Take time to learn the multisystem connections.

▶ ENDOCRINE—EMBRYOLOGY

Thyroid development

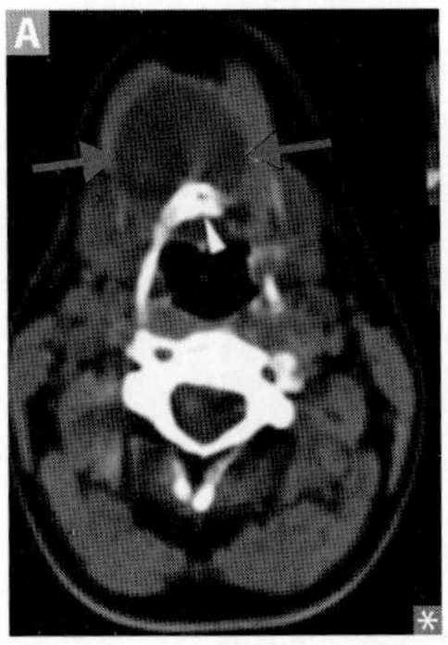

Thyroid diverticulum arises from floor of primitive pharynx and descends into neck. Connected to tongue by thyroglossal duct, which normally disappears but may persist as cysts or the pyramidal lobe of thyroid. Foramen cecum is normal remnant of thyroglossal duct.

Most common ectopic thyroid tissue site is the tongue (lingual thyroid). Removal may result in hypothyroidism if it is the only thyroid tissue present.

Thyroglossal duct cyst A presents as an anterior midline neck mass that moves with swallowing or protrusion of the tongue (vs persistent cervical sinus leading to pharyngeal cleft cyst in lateral neck).

Thyroid follicular cells derived from endoderm.

Parafollicular cells arise from 4th pharyngeal pouch.

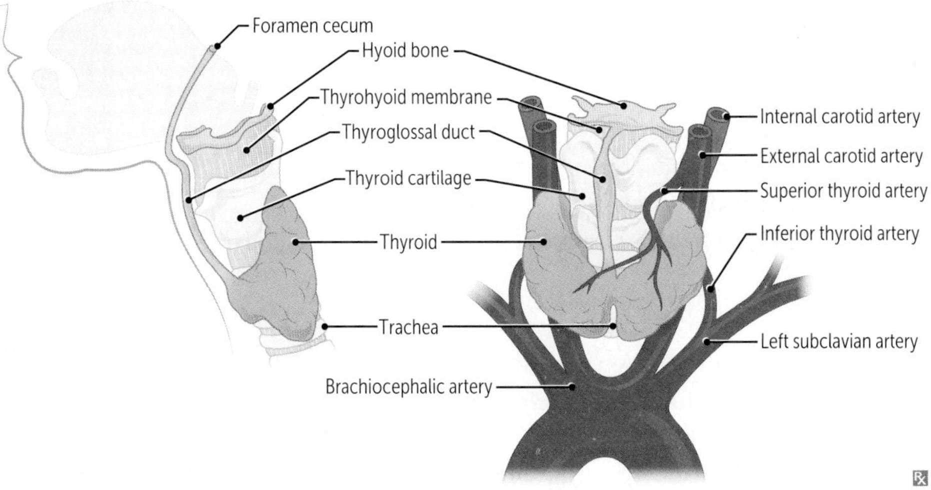

▸ ENDOCRINE—ANATOMY

Pituitary gland

Anterior pituitary (adenohypophysis)	Secretes FSH, LH, ACTH, TSH, prolactin, GH, and β-endorphin. Melanotropin (MSH) secreted from intermediate lobe of pituitary. Derived from oral ectoderm (Rathke pouch). ▪ α subunit—hormone subunit common to TSH, LH, FSH, and hCG. ▪ β subunit—determines hormone specificity.	Proopiomelanocortin derivatives—β-endorphin, ACTH, and MSH. Go pro with a BAM! FLAT PiG: FSH, LH, ACTH, TSH, PRL, GH. B-FLAT: Basophils—FSH, LH, ACTH, TSH. Acid PiG: Acidophils — PRL, GH.
Posterior pituitary (neurohypophysis)	Stores and releases vasopressin (antidiuretic hormone, or ADH) and oxytocin, both made in the hypothalamus (supraoptic and paraventricular nuclei) and transported to posterior pituitary via neurophysins (carrier proteins). Derived from neuroectoderm.	

Adrenal cortex and medulla

Adrenal cortex (derived from mesoderm) and medulla (derived from neural crest).

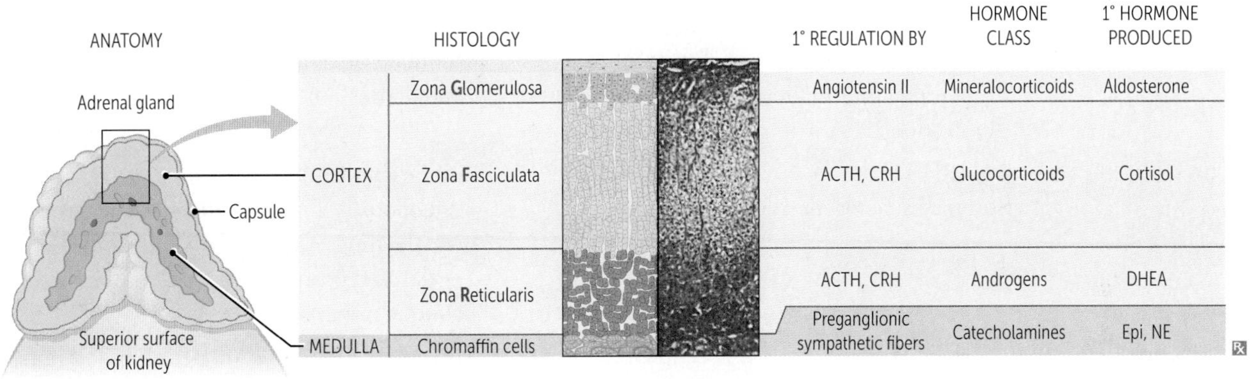
ANATOMY
Adrenal gland
Capsule
Superior surface of kidney
HISTOLOGY
CORTEX
MEDULLA
Zona Glomerulosa
Zona Fasciculata
Zona Reticularis
Chromaffin cells
1° REGULATION BY
HORMONE CLASS
1° HORMONE PRODUCED
Angiotensin II
Mineralocorticoids
Aldosterone
ACTH, CRH
Glucocorticoids
Cortisol
ACTH, CRH
Androgens
DHEA
Preganglionic sympathetic fibers
Catecholamines
Epi, NE

GFR corresponds with salt (mineralocorticoids), sugar (glucocorticoids), and sex (androgens). "The deeper you go, the sweeter it gets."

Endocrine pancreas cell types

Islets of Langerhans are collections of α, β, and δ endocrine cells. Islets arise from pancreatic buds.
α = glucagon (peripheral)
β = insulin (central)
δ = somatostatin (interspersed)

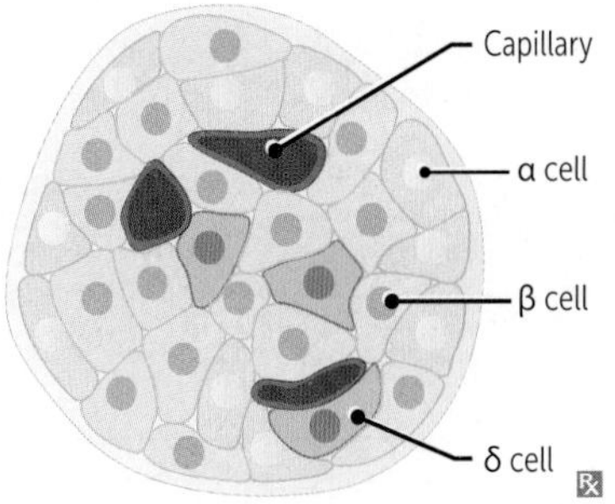
Capillary
α cell
β cell
δ cell

▸ ENDOCRINE—PHYSIOLOGY

Hypothalamic-pituitary hormones

HORMONE	FUNCTION	CLINICAL NOTES
ADH	↑ water permeability of distal convoluted tubule and collecting duct cells in kidney to ↑ water reabsorption	Stimulus for secretion is ↑ plasma osmolality, except in SIADH, in which ADH is elevated despite ↓ plasma osmolality
CRH	↑ ACTH, MSH, β-endorphin	↓ in chronic exogenous steroid use
Dopamine	↓ prolactin, TSH	Also called prolactin-inhibiting factor Dopamine antagonists (eg, antipsychotics) can cause galactorrhea due to hyperprolactinemia
GHRH	↑ GH	Analog (tesamorelin) used to treat HIV-associated lipodystrophy
GnRH	↑ FSH, LH	Suppressed by hyperprolactinemia Tonic GnRH analog (eg, leuprolide) suppresses hypothalamic–pituitary–gonadal axis. Pulsatile GnRH leads to puberty, fertility
MSH	↑ melanogenesis by melanocytes	Causes hyperpigmentation in Cushing disease, as MSH and ACTH share the same precursor molecule, proopiomelanocortin
Oxytocin	Causes uterine contractions during labor. Responsible for milk letdown reflex in response to suckling.	Modulates fear, anxiety, social bonding, mood, and depression
Prolactin	↓ GnRH Stimulates lactogenesis.	Pituitary prolactinoma → amenorrhea, osteoporosis, hypogonadism, galactorrhea Breastfeeding → ↑ prolactin → ↓ GnRH → delayed postpartum ovulation (natural contraception)
Somatostatin	↓ GH, TSH	Also called growth hormone inhibiting hormone (GHIH) Analogs used to treat acromegaly
TRH	↑ TSH, prolactin	↑ TRH (eg, in 1°/2° hypothyroidism) may increase prolactin secretion → galactorrhea

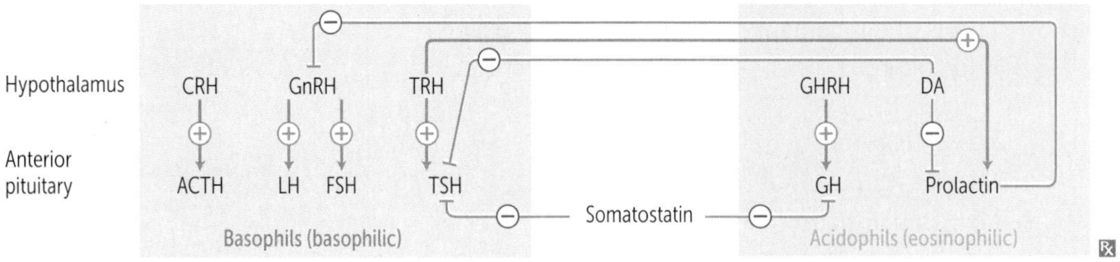

Growth hormone

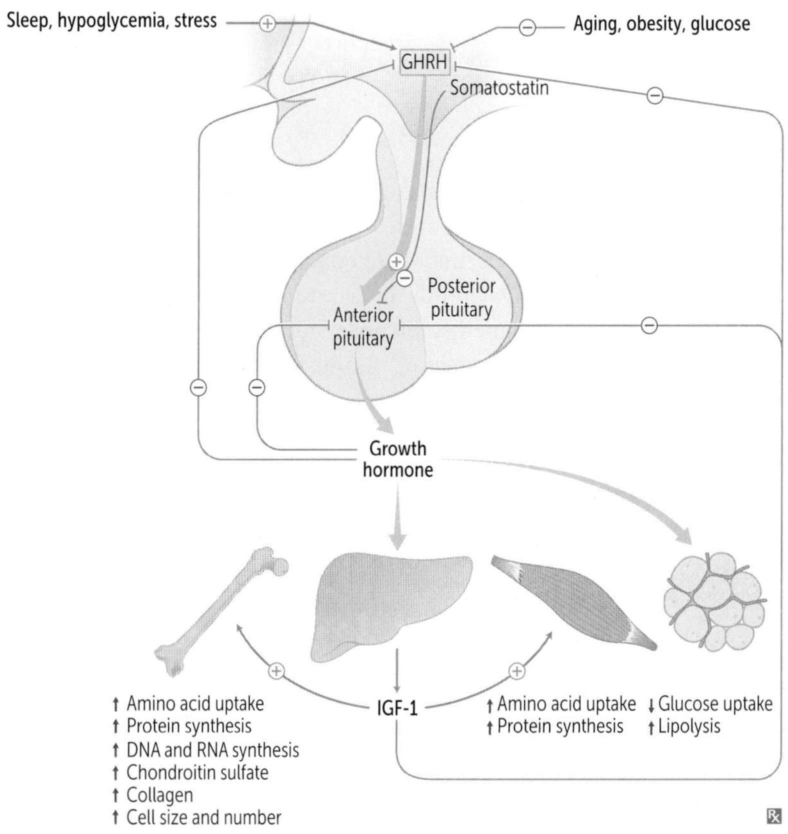
Sleep, hypoglycemia, stress
Aging, obesity, glucose
GHRH
Somatostatin
Posterior pituitary
Anterior pituitary
Growth hormone
IGF-1
↑ Amino acid uptake
↑ Protein synthesis
↑ DNA and RNA synthesis
↑ Chondroitin sulfate
↑ Collagen
↑ Cell size and number
↑ Amino acid uptake
↑ Protein synthesis
↓ Glucose uptake
↑ Lipolysis

Also called somatotropin. Secreted by anterior pituitary.

Stimulates linear growth and muscle mass through IGF-1 (somatomedin C) secretion by liver. ↑ insulin resistance (diabetogenic).

Released in pulses in response to growth hormone–releasing hormone (GHRH).

Secretion ↑ during exercise, deep sleep, puberty, hypoglycemia.

Secretion ↓ by glucose, somatostatin, somatomedin (regulatory molecule secreted by liver in response to GH acting on target tissues).

Excess secretion of GH (eg, pituitary adenoma) may cause acromegaly (adults) or gigantism (children). Treatment: somatostatin analogs (eg, octreotide) or surgery.

Antidiuretic hormone	Also called vasopressin.	
SOURCE	Synthesized in hypothalamus (supraoptic and paraventricular nuclei), stored and secreted by posterior pituitary.	
FUNCTION	Regulates blood pressure (V_1-receptors) and serum osmolality (V_2-receptors). Primary function is serum osmolality regulation (ADH ↓ serum osmolality, ↑ urine osmolality) via regulation of aquaporin channel insertion in principal cells of renal collecting duct.	ADH level is ↓ in central diabetes insipidus (DI), normal or ↑ in nephrogenic DI. Nephrogenic DI can be caused by mutation in V_2-receptor. Desmopressin (ADH analog) is a treatment for central DI and nocturnal enuresis.
REGULATION	Plasma osmolality (1°); hypovolemia.	

Prolactin

SOURCE	Secreted mainly by anterior pituitary.	Structurally homologous to growth hormone.
FUNCTION	Stimulates milk production in breast; inhibits ovulation in females and spermatogenesis in males by inhibiting GnRH synthesis and release.	Excessive amounts of prolactin associated with ↓ libido.
REGULATION	Prolactin secretion from anterior pituitary is tonically inhibited by dopamine from tuberoinfundibular pathway of hypothalamus. Prolactin in turn inhibits its own secretion by ↑ dopamine synthesis and secretion from hypothalamus. TRH ↑ prolactin secretion (eg, in 1° or 2° hypothyroidism).	Dopamine agonists (eg, bromocriptine) inhibit prolactin secretion and can be used in treatment of prolactinoma. Dopamine antagonists (eg, most antipsychotics, metoclopramide) and estrogens (eg, OCPs, pregnancy) stimulate prolactin secretion.

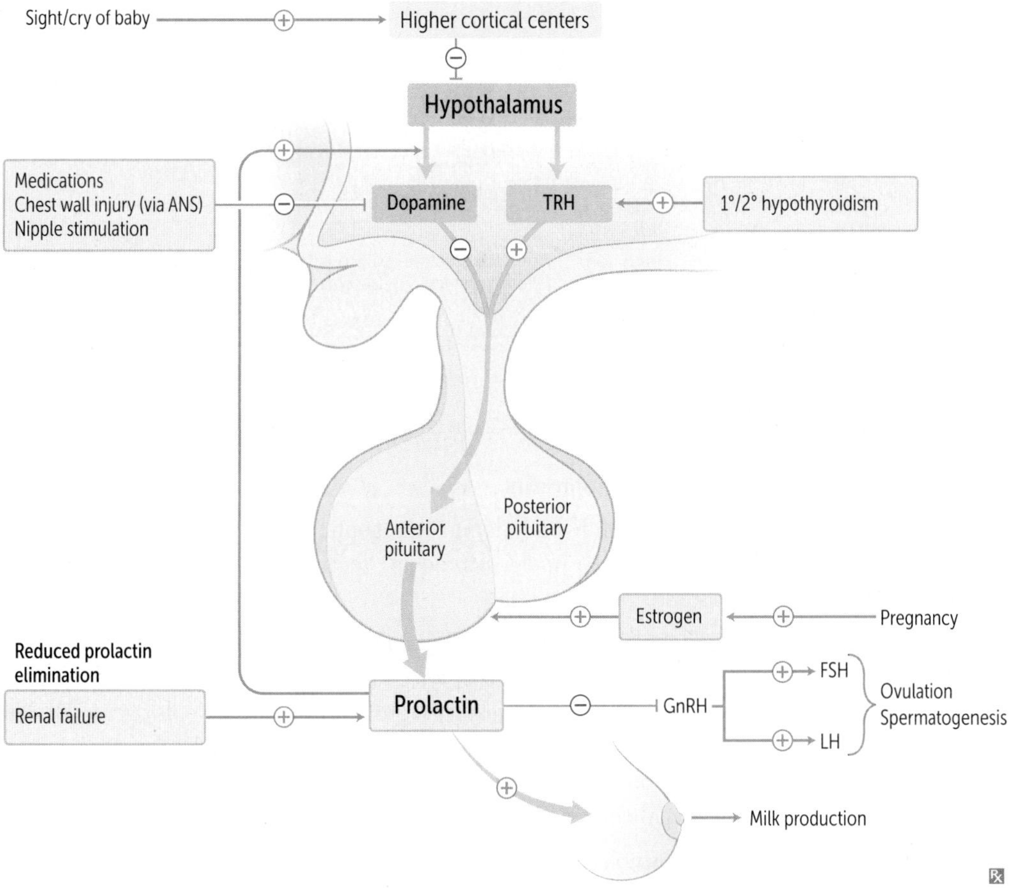

Thyroid hormones

Thyroid produces triiodothyronine (T_3) and thyroxine (T_4), iodine-containing hormones that control the body's metabolic rate.

SOURCE

Follicles of thyroid. 5′-deiodinase converts T_4 (the major thyroid product) to T_3 in peripheral tissue (5, 4, 3). Peripheral conversion is inhibited by glucocorticoids, β-blockers, and propylthiouracil (PTU). Reverse T_3 (rT_3) is a metabolically inactive byproduct of the peripheral conversion of T_4 and its production is increased by growth hormone and glucocorticoids. Functions of thyroid peroxidase include oxidation, organification of iodine, and coupling of monoiodotyrosine (MIT) and diiodotyrosine (DIT). Inhibited by PTU and methimazole. DIT + DIT = T_4. DIT + MIT = T_3. Wolff-Chaikoff effect—protective autoregulation; sudden exposure to excess iodine temporarily turns **off** thyroid peroxidase → ↓ T_3/T_4 production.

FUNCTION

Only free hormone is active. T_3 binds nuclear receptor with greater affinity than T_4. T_3 functions —7 B's:

- **B**rain maturation
- **B**one growth (synergism with GH)
- **β**-adrenergic effects. ↑ β_1 receptors in heart → ↑ CO, HR, SV, contractility; β-blockers alleviate adrenergic symptoms in thyrotoxicosis
- **B**asal metabolic rate ↑ (via ↑ Na^+/K^+-ATPase → ↑ O_2 consumption, RR, body temperature)
- **B**lood sugar (↑ glycogenolysis, gluconeogenesis)
- **B**reak down lipids (↑ lipolysis)
- Stimulates surfactant synthesis in **B**abies

REGULATION

TRH → ⊕ TSH release → ⊕ follicular cells. Thyroid-stimulating immunoglobulin (TSI) may ⊕ follicular cells in Graves disease.

Negative feedback primarily by free T_3/T_4:

- Anterior pituitary → ↓ sensitivity to TRH
- Hypothalamus → ↓ TRH secretion

Thyroxine-binding globulin (TBG) binds most T_3/T_4 in blood. Bound T_3/T_4 = inactive.

- ↑ TBG in pregnancy, OCP use (estrogen → ↑ TBG) → ↑ total T_3/T_4
- ↓ TBG in steroid use, nephrotic syndrome

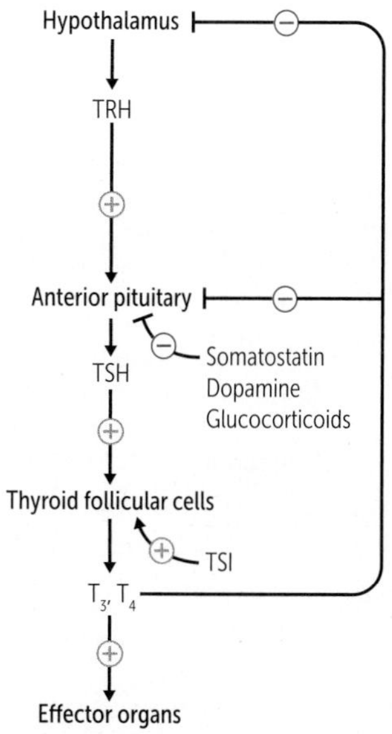

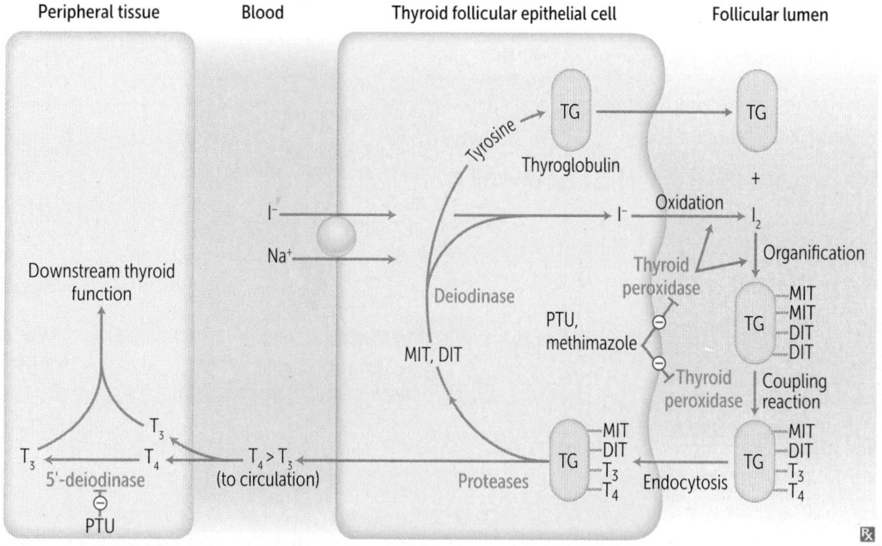

Parathyroid hormone

SOURCE	Chief cells of parathyroid	
FUNCTION	↑ free Ca^{2+} in the blood (1° function) ↑ Ca^{2+} and PO_4^{3-} absorption in GI system ↑ Ca^{2+} and PO_4^{3-} from bone resorption ↑ Ca^{2+} reabsorption from DCT ↓ PO_4^{3-} reabsorption in PCT ↑ 1,25-$(OH)_2D_3$ (calci**tri**ol) production by activating 1α-hydroxylase in **PCT** (**tri** to make D_3 in the **PCT**)	PTH ↑ serum Ca^{2+}, ↓ serum PO_4^{3-}, ↑ urine PO_4^{3-}, ↑ urine cAMP ↑ RANK-L (receptor activator of NF-κB ligand) secreted by osteoblasts and osteocytes; binds RANK (receptor) on osteoclasts and their precursors to stimulate osteoclasts and ↑ Ca^{2+} → bone resorption (intermittent PTH release can also stimulate bone formation) **PTH** = **P**hosphate-**T**rashing **H**ormone PTH-related peptide (PTHrP) functions like PTH and is commonly increased in malignancies (eg, squamous cell carcinoma of the lung, renal cell carcinoma)
REGULATION	↓ serum Ca^{2+} → ↑ PTH secretion ↑ serum PO_4^{3-} → ↑ PTH secretion ↓ serum Mg^{2+} → ↑ PTH secretion ↓↓ serum Mg^{2+} → ↓ PTH secretion Common causes of ↓ Mg^{2+} include diarrhea, aminoglycosides, diuretics, alcohol use disorder	

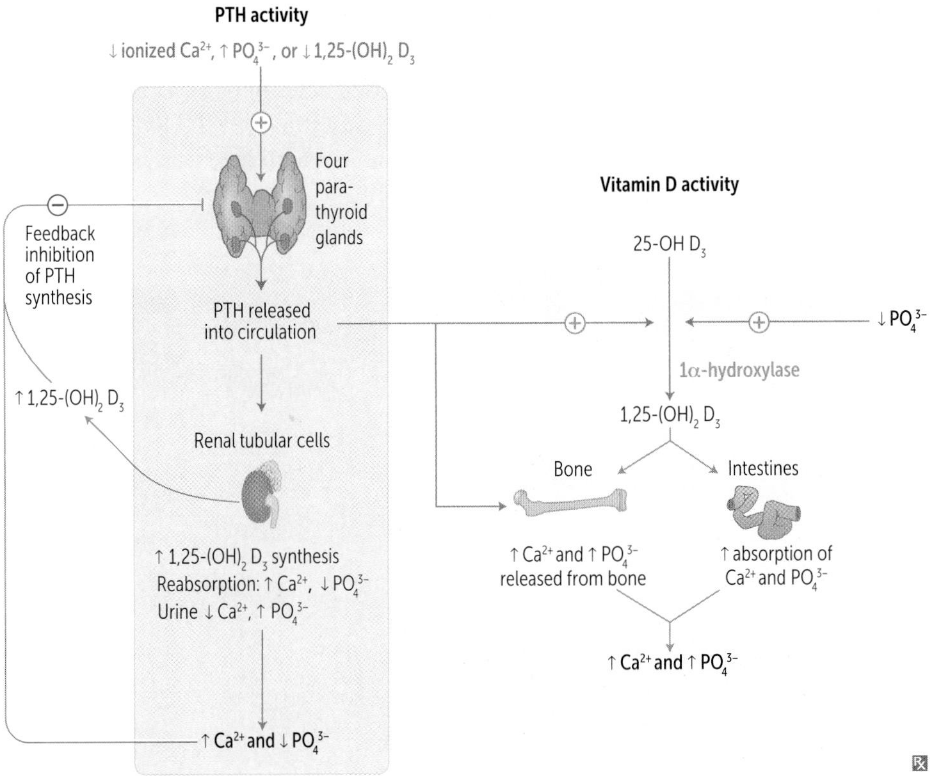

Calcium homeostasis	Plasma Ca^{2+} exists in three forms: ▪ Ionized/free (~ 45%, active form) ▪ Bound to albumin (~ 40%) ▪ Bound to anions (~ 15%)	↑ pH (less H^+) → albumin binds more Ca^{2+} → ↓ ionized Ca^{2+} (eg, cramps, pain, paresthesias, carpopedal spasm) → ↑ PTH ↓ pH (more H^+) → albumin binds less Ca^{2+} → ↑ ionized Ca^{2+} → ↓ PTH Ionized/free Ca^{2+} is 1° regulator of PTH; changes in pH alter PTH secretion, whereas changes in albumin concentration do not

Calcitonin

SOURCE	Parafollicular cells (C cells) of thyroid.	Calcitonin opposes actions of PTH. Not important in normal Ca^{2+} homeostasis Calcitonin tones down serum Ca^{2+} levels and keeps it in bones
FUNCTION	↓ bone resorption.	
REGULATION	↑ serum Ca^{2+} → ↑ calcitonin secretion.	

Glucagon

SOURCE	Made by α cells of pancreas.
FUNCTION	Promotes glycogenolysis, gluconeogenesis, lipolysis, ketogenesis. Elevates blood sugar levels to maintain homeostasis when bloodstream glucose levels fall too low (ie, fasting state).
REGULATION	Secreted in response to hypoglycemia. Inhibited by insulin, amylin, somatostatin, hyperglycemia.

Insulin

SYNTHESIS

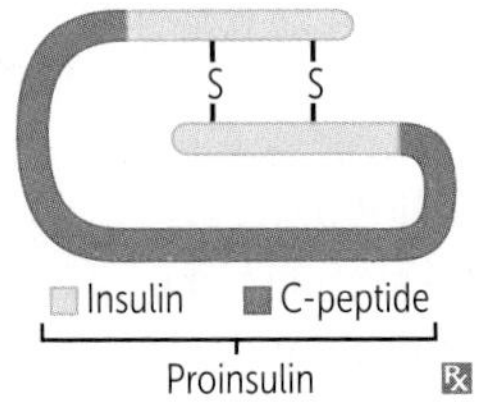

Preproinsulin (synthesized in RER of pancreatic β cells) → cleavage of "presignal" → proinsulin (stored in secretory granules) → cleavage of proinsulin → exocytosis of insulin and C-peptide equally. Insulin and C-peptide are ↑ in insulinoma and sulfonylurea use, whereas exogenous insulin lacks C-peptide.

FUNCTION

Binds **insulin** receptors (tyrosine kinase activity ❶), inducing glucose uptake (carrier-mediated transport) **into** insulin-dependent tissue ❷ and gene transcription.

Anabolic effects of insulin:
- ↑ glucose transport in skeletal muscle and adipose tissue
- ↑ glycogen synthesis and storage
- ↑ triglyceride synthesis
- ↑ Na^+ retention (kidneys)
- ↑ protein synthesis (muscles)
- ↑ cellular uptake of K^+ and amino acids
- ↓ glucagon release
- ↓ lipolysis in adipose tissue

Unlike glucose, insulin does not cross placenta.

Insulin-dependent glucose transporters:
- GLUT4: adipose tissue, striated muscle (exercise can also ↑ GLUT4 expression)

Insulin-independent transporters:
- GLUT1: RBCs, brain, cornea, placenta
- GLUT2 (**bi**directional): β islet cells, liver, kidney, GI tract (think 2-way street)
- GLUT3: brain, placenta
- GLUT5 (fructose): spermatocytes, GI tract
- SGLT1/SGLT2 (Na^+-glucose cotransporters): kidney, small intestine

Brain prefers glucose, but may use ketone bodies during starvation. RBCs utilize glucose, as they lack mitochondria for aerobic metabolism.

BRICK LIPS (insulin-independent glucose uptake): **B**rain, **R**BCs, **I**ntestine, **C**ornea, **K**idney, **L**iver, **I**slet (β) cells, **P**lacenta, **S**permatocytes.

REGULATION

Glucose is the major regulator of insulin release. ↑ insulin response with oral vs IV glucose due to incretins (eg, glucagon-like peptide 1 [GLP-1], glucose-dependent insulinotropic polypeptide [GIP]), which are released after meals and ↑ β cell sensitivity to glucose. Release ↓ by α_2, ↑ by β_2 stimulation (2 = regulates **insulin**).

Glucose enters β cells ❸ → ↑ ATP generated from glucose metabolism ❹ closes K^+ channels (target of sulfonylureas) ❺ and depolarizes β cell membrane ❻. Voltage-gated Ca^{2+} channels open → Ca^{2+} influx ❼ and stimulation of insulin exocytosis ❽.

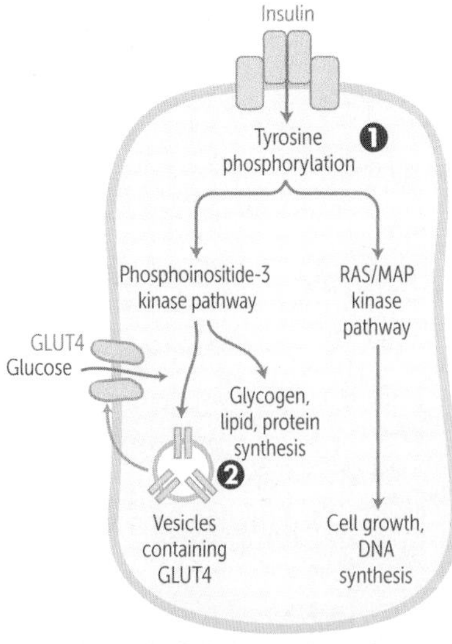

Insulin-dependent glucose uptake

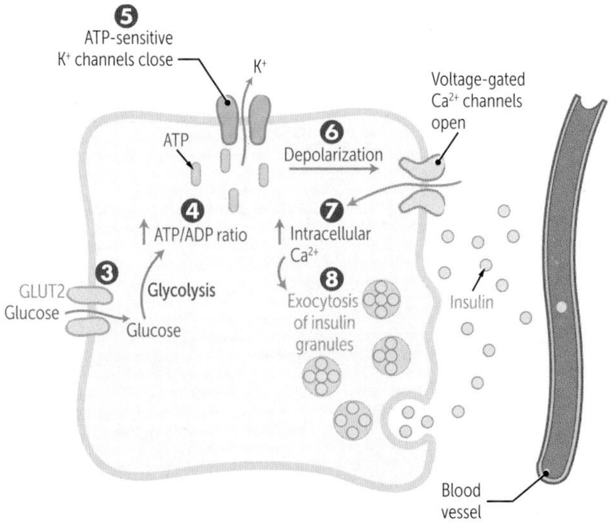

Insulin secretion by pancreatic β cells

Adrenal steroids and congenital adrenal hyperplasias

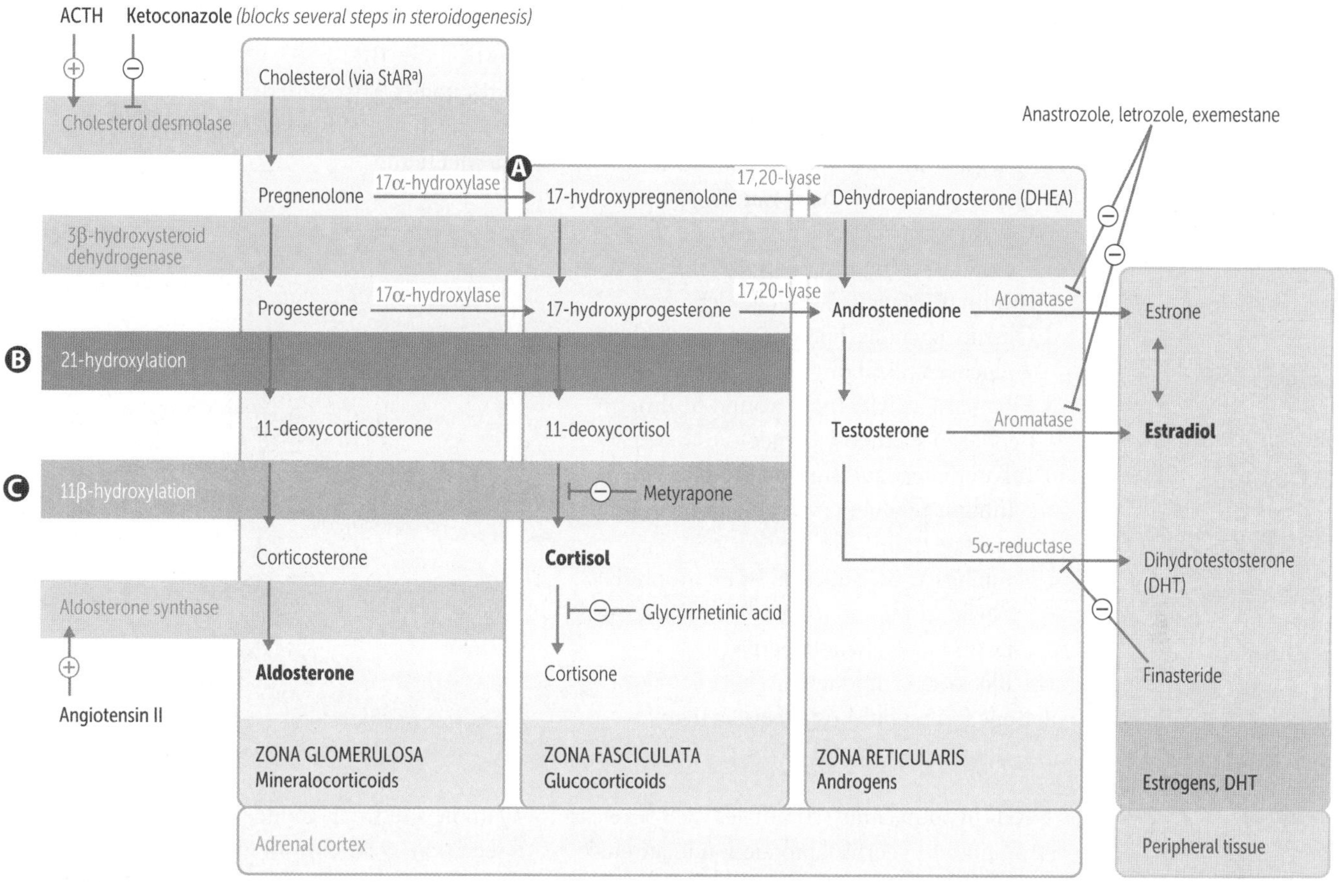

[a]Rate-limiting step.

ENZYME DEFICIENCY	MINERALOCORTICOIDS	[K⁺]	BP	CORTISOL	SEX HORMONES	LABS	PRESENTATION
A 17α-hydroxylase[a]	↑	↓	↑	↓	↓	↓ androstenedione	XY: ambiguous genitalia, undescended testes XX: lacks 2° sexual development
B 21-hydroxylase[a]	↓	↑	↓	↓	↑	↑ renin activity ↑ 17-hydroxy-progesterone	Most common Presents in infancy (salt wasting) or childhood (precocious puberty) XX: virilization
C 11β-hydroxylase[a]	↓ aldosterone ↑ 11-deoxycorti-costerone (results in ↑ BP)	↓	↑	↓	↑	↓ renin activity	Presents in infancy (severe hypertension) or childhood (precocious puberty) XX: virilization

[a]All congenital adrenal enzyme deficiencies are autosomal recessive disorders and most are characterized by skin hyperpigmentation (due to ↑ MSH production, which is coproduced and secreted with ACTH) and bilateral adrenal gland enlargement (due to ↑ ACTH stimulation).

If deficient enzyme starts with 1, it causes hypertension; if deficient enzyme ends with 1, it causes virilization in females.

Cortisol

SOURCE	Adrenal zona fasciculata.	Bound to corticosteroid-binding globulin.
FUNCTION	↑ Appetite ↑ Blood pressure: ▪ Upregulates α_1-receptors on arterioles → ↑ sensitivity to norepinephrine and epinephrine (permissive action) ▪ At high concentrations, can bind to mineralocorticoid (aldosterone) receptors ↑ Insulin resistance (diabetogenic) ↑ Gluconeogenesis, lipolysis, and proteolysis (↓ glucose utilization) ↓ Fibroblast activity (poor wound healing, ↓ collagen synthesis, ↑ striae) ↓ Inflammatory and Immune responses: ▪ Inhibits production of leukotrienes and prostaglandins ▪ Inhibits WBC adhesion → neutrophilia ▪ Blocks histamine release from mast cells ▪ Eosinopenia, lymphopenia ▪ Blocks IL-2 production ↓ Bone formation (↓ osteoblast activity)	Cortisol is **A BIG FIB**. Exogenous corticosteroids can cause reactivation of TB and candidiasis (blocks IL-2 production). 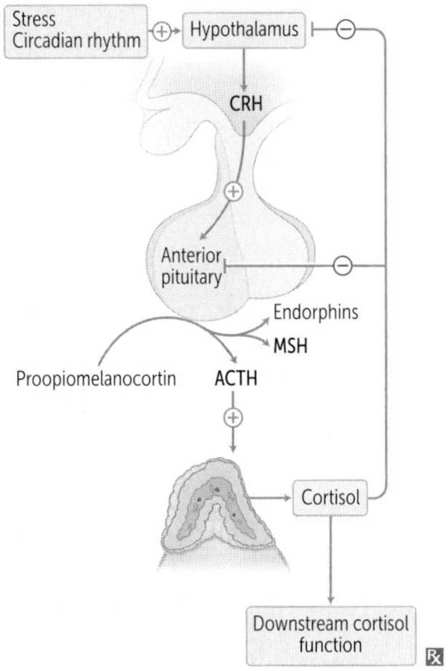
REGULATION	CRH (hypothalamus) stimulates ACTH release (pituitary) → cortisol production in adrenal zona fasciculata. Excess cortisol ↓ CRH, ACTH, and cortisol secretion.	Chronic stress may induce prolonged cortisol secretion, cortisol resistance, impaired immunocompetency, and dysregulation of HPA axis.

Appetite regulation

Ghrelin	Stimulates hunger (orexigenic effect) and GH release (via GH secretagog receptor). Produced by stomach. Sleep deprivation, fasting, or Prader-Willi syndrome → ↑ ghrelin production. **Ghrelin** makes you **ghrow hunghry**. Acts on lateral area of hypothalamus (hunger center) to ↑ appetite.
Leptin	Satiety hormone. Produced by adipose tissue. Mutation of leptin gene → severe obesity. Obese people have ↑ leptin due to ↑ adipose tissue but are tolerant or resistant to leptin's anorexigenic effect. Sleep deprivation or starvation → ↓ leptin production. **Leptin** keeps you **thin**. Acts on ventromedial area of hypothalamus (satiety center) to ↓ appetite.
Endocannabinoids	Act at cannabinoid receptors in hypothalamus and nucleus accumbens, two key brain areas for the homeostatic and hedonic control of food intake → ↑ appetite. Exogenous cannabinoids cause "the munchies."

Signaling pathways of endocrine hormones

cAMP	FSH, LH, ACTH, TSH, CRH, hCG, ADH (V_2-receptor), MSH, PTH, Calcitonin, Histamine (H_2-receptor), Glucagon, GHRH	FLAT ChAMPs CHuGG
cGMP	BNP, ANP, EDRF (NO)	BAD GraMPa Think vasodilation and diuresis
IP_3	GnRH, Oxytocin, ADH (V_1-receptor), TRH, Histamine (H_1-receptor), Angiotensin II, Gastrin	GOAT HAG
Intracellular receptor	Progesterone, Estrogen, Testosterone, Cortisol, Aldosterone, T_3/T_4, Vitamin D	PET CAT in TV
Receptor tyrosine kinase	IGF-1, FGF, PDGF, EGF, Insulin	MAP kinase pathway Get Found In the MAP
Serine/threonine kinase receptor	TGF-β	
Nonreceptor tyrosine kinase	G-CSF, Erythropoietin, Thrombopoietin Prolactin, Immunomodulators (eg, cytokines IL-2, IL-6, IFN), GH	JAK/STAT pathway Think acidophils and cytokines GET a JAKed PIG

Signaling pathways of steroid hormones

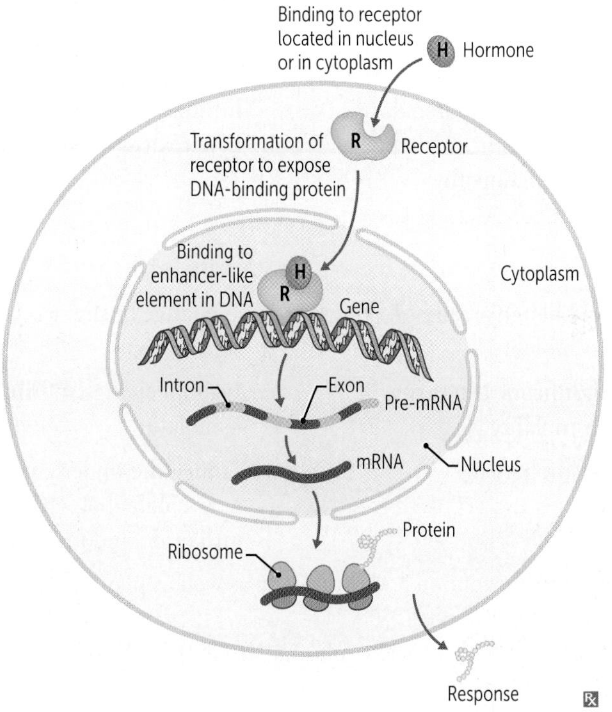
Binding to receptor located in nucleus or in cytoplasm
H
Hormone
Transformation of receptor to expose DNA-binding protein
R
Receptor
Binding to enhancer-like element in DNA
H
R
Gene
Cytoplasm
Intron
Exon
Pre-mRNA
mRNA
Nucleus
Protein
Ribosome
Response

Steroid hormones are lipophilic and therefore must circulate bound to specific binding globulins, which ↑ their solubility.

In males, ↑ sex hormone–binding globulin (SHBG) lowers free testosterone → gynecomastia.

In females, ↓ SHBG raises free testosterone → hirsutism.

↑ estrogen (eg, OCPs, pregnancy) → ↑ SHBG.

▶ ENDOCRINE—PATHOLOGY

Syndrome of inappropriate antidiuretic hormone secretion

Characterized by:
- Excessive free water retention
- Euvolemic hyponatremia with continued urinary Na^+ excretion
- Urine osmolality > serum osmolality

Body responds to water retention with ↓ aldosterone and ↑ ANP and BNP → ↑ urinary Na^+ secretion → normalization of extracellular fluid volume → euvolemic hyponatremia. Very low serum Na^+ levels can lead to cerebral edema, seizures. Correct slowly to prevent osmotic demyelination syndrome (formerly called central pontine myelinolysis).

SIADH causes include (**HELD**-up water):
- **H**ead trauma/CNS disorders
- **E**ctopic ADH (eg, small cell lung cancer)
- **L**ung disease
- **D**rugs (eg, SSRIs, carbamazepine, cyclophosphamide)

Treatment: fluid restriction (first line), salt tablets, IV hypertonic saline, diuretics, ADH antagonists (eg, conivaptan, tolvaptan, demeclocycline).

Primary polydipsia and diabetes insipidus

Characterized by the production of large amounts of dilute urine +/– thirst. Urine specific gravity <1.006. Urine osmolality usually <300 mOsm/kg. Diabetes insipidus (DI) is classified as central or nephrogenic depending on etiology.

	Primary polydipsia	Central DI	Nephrogenic DI
DEFINITION	Excessive water intake	↓ ADH release	ADH resistance
CAUSES	Psychiatric illnesses, hypothalamic lesions affecting thirst center	Idiopathic, tumors (eg, pituitary), infiltrative diseases (eg, sarcoidosis), trauma, surgery, hypoxic encephalopathy	Hereditary (ADH receptor mutation), drugs (eg, lithium, demeclocycline), hypercalcemia, hypokalemia
SERUM OSMOLALITY	↓	↑	↑
ADH LEVEL	↓ or normal	↓	Normal or ↑
WATER RESTRICTION[a]	Significant ↑ in urine osmolality (>700 mOsm/kg)	No change or slight ↑ in urine osmolality	No change or slight ↑ in urine osmolality
DESMOPRESSIN ADMINISTRATION[b]	—	Significant ↑ in urine osmolality (>50%)	Minimal change in urine osmolality
TREATMENT	Water restriction	Desmopressin	Manage the underlying cause. Low-solute diet, HCTZ, amiloride, indomethacin

[a]No water intake for 2-3 hours followed by hourly measurements of urine volume and osmolality as well as plasma Na^+ concentration and osmolality.

[b]Desmopressin (ADH analog) is administered if serum osmolality >295-300 mOsm/kg, plasma $Na^+ \geq 145$ mEq/L, or urine osmolality does not rise despite ↑ plasma osmolality.

Hypopituitarism

Undersecretion of pituitary hormones due to:

- Nonsecreting pituitary adenoma, craniopharyngioma
- Sheehan syndrome—ischemic infarct of pituitary following postpartum bleeding; pregnancy-induced pituitary growth → ↑ susceptibility to hypoperfusion. Usually presents with failure to lactate, absent menstruation, cold intolerance
- Empty sella syndrome—atrophy or compression of pituitary (which lies in the sella turcica), often idiopathic, common in obese females; associated with idiopathic intracranial hypertension
- Pituitary apoplexy—sudden hemorrhage of pituitary gland, often in the presence of an existing pituitary adenoma. Usually presents with sudden onset severe headache, visual impairment (eg, bitemporal hemianopia, diplopia due to CN III palsy), and features of hypopituitarism
- Brain injury
- Radiation

Treatment: hormone replacement therapy (corticosteroids, thyroxine, sex steroids, human growth hormone)

Acromegaly

Excess GH in adults. Typically caused by pituitary adenoma.

FINDINGS

Large tongue with deep furrows, deep voice, large hands and feet, coarsening of facial features with aging A, frontal bossing, diaphoresis (excessive sweating), impaired glucose tolerance (insulin resistance), hypertension. ↑ risk of colorectal polyps and cancer.

↑ GH in children → gigantism (↑ linear bone growth). HF most common cause of death.

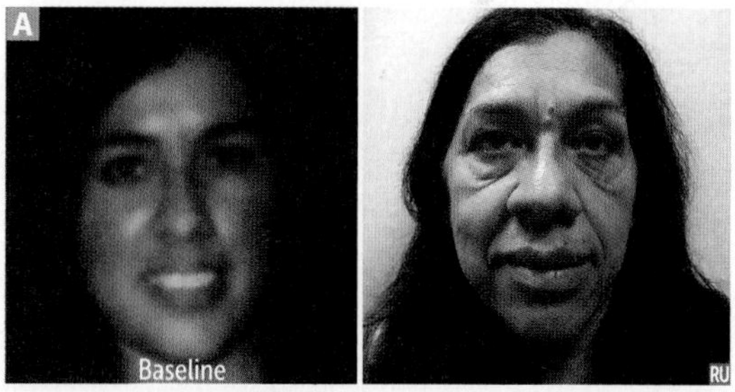

DIAGNOSIS

↑ serum IGF-1; failure to suppress serum GH following oral glucose tolerance test; pituitary mass seen on brain MRI.

TREATMENT

Pituitary adenoma resection. If not cured, treat with octreotide (somatostatin analog), pegvisomant (GH receptor antagonist), or dopamine agonists (eg, cabergoline).

Hypothyroidism vs hyperthyroidism

	Hypothyroidism	Hyperthyroidism
METABOLIC	Cold intolerance, ↓ sweating, weight gain (↓ basal metabolic rate → ↓ calorigenesis), hyponatremia (↓ free water clearance)	Heat intolerance, ↑ sweating, weight loss (↑ synthesis of Na^+-K^+ ATPase → ↑ basal metabolic rate → ↑ calorigenesis)
SKIN/HAIR	Dry, cool skin (due to ↓ blood flow); coarse, brittle hair; diffuse alopecia; brittle nails; puffy facies and generalized nonpitting edema (myxedema A) due to ↑ GAGs in interstitial spaces → ↑ osmotic pressure → water retention	Warm, moist skin (due to vasodilation); fine hair; onycholysis (B); pretibial myxedema in Graves disease
OCULAR	Periorbital edema C	Ophthalmopathy in Graves disease (including periorbital edema, exophthalmos), lid lag/retraction (↑ sympathetic stimulation of levator palpebrae superioris and superior tarsal muscle)
GASTROINTESTINAL	Constipation (↓ GI motility), ↓ appetite	Hyperdefecation/diarrhea (↑ GI motility), ↑ appetite
MUSCULOSKELETAL	Hypothyroid myopathy (proximal weakness, ↑ CK), carpal tunnel syndrome, myoedema (small lump rising on the surface of a muscle when struck with a hammer)	Thyrotoxic myopathy (proximal weakness, normal CK), osteoporosis/↑ fracture rate (T_3 directly stimulates bone resorption)
REPRODUCTIVE	Abnormal uterine bleeding, ↓ libido, infertility	Abnormal uterine bleeding, gynecomastia, ↓ libido, infertility
NEUROPSYCHIATRIC	Hypoactivity, lethargy, fatigue, weakness, depressed mood, ↓ reflexes (delayed/slow relaxing)	Hyperactivity, restlessness, anxiety, insomnia, fine tremors (due to ↑ β-adrenergic activity), ↑ reflexes (brisk)
CARDIOVASCULAR	Bradycardia, dyspnea on exertion (↓ cardiac output)	Tachycardia, palpitations, dyspnea, arrhythmias (eg, atrial fibrillation), chest pain and systolic HTN due to ↑ number and sensitivity of β-adrenergic receptors, ↑ expression of cardiac sarcolemmal ATPase and ↓ expression of phospholamban
LABS	↑ TSH (if 1°) ↓ free T_3 and T_4 Hypercholesterolemia (due to ↓ LDL receptor expression)	↓ TSH (if 1°) ↑ free T_3 and T_4 ↓ LDL, HDL, and total cholesterol

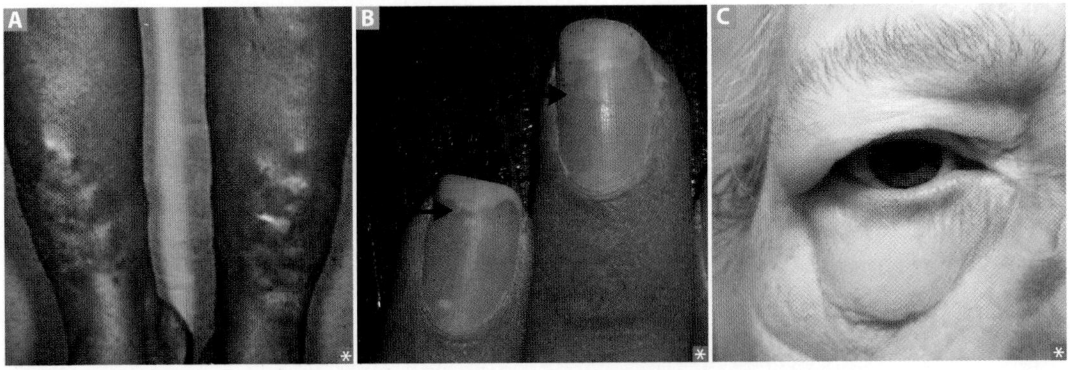

Hypothyroidism

Hashimoto thyroiditis	Also called chronic autoimmune thyroiditis. Most common cause of hypothyroidism in iodine-sufficient regions. Associated with HLA-DR3, ↑ risk of primary thyroid lymphoma (typically diffuse large B-cell lymphoma). Findings: moderately enlarged, **nontender** thyroid. May be preceded by transient hyperthyroid state ("Hashitoxicosis") due to follicular rupture and thyroid hormone release. Serology: ⊕ antithyroid peroxidase (antimicrosomal) and antithyroglobulin antibodies. Histology: Hürthle cells A, lymphoid aggregates with germinal centers B. Postpartum thyroiditis—mild, self-limited variant of Hashimoto thyroiditis arising < 1 year after delivery.
Subacute granulomatous thyroiditis	Also called de Quervain thyroiditis. Usually, a self-limited disease. Natural history: transient hyperthyroidism → euthyroid state → hypothyroidism. Often preceded by viral infection. Findings: ↑ ESR, jaw pain, very **tender** thyroid (de **Quervain** is associated with **pain**). Histology: granulomatous inflammation C.
Riedel thyroiditis	Also called invasive fibrous thyroiditis. May be part of IgG_4-related disease (eg, autoimmune pancreatitis, retroperitoneal fibrosis, noninfectious aortitis). Hypothyroidism occurs in ⅓ of patients. Fibrosis may extend to local structures (eg, trachea, esophagus), mimicking anaplastic carcinoma. Findings: slowly enlarging, hard (rock-like), fixed, **nontender** thyroid. Histology: thyroid replaced by fibrous tissue and inflammatory infiltrate D.
Congenital hypothyroidism	Formerly called cretinism. Most commonly caused by thyroid dysgenesis (abnormal thyroid gland development; eg, agenesis, hypoplasia, ectopy) or dyshormonogenesis (abnormal thyroid hormone synthesis; eg, mutations in thyroid peroxidase) in iodine-sufficient regions. Findings (6 P's): pot-bellied, pale, puffy-faced child E with protruding umbilicus, protuberant tongue F, and poor brain development.
Other causes	Iodine deficiency (most common cause worldwide; typically presents with goiter G), iodine excess (Wolff-Chaikoff effect), drugs (eg, amiodarone, lithium), nonthyroidal illness syndrome (also called euthyroid sick syndrome; ↓ T_3 with normal/↓ T_4 and TSH in critically ill patients).

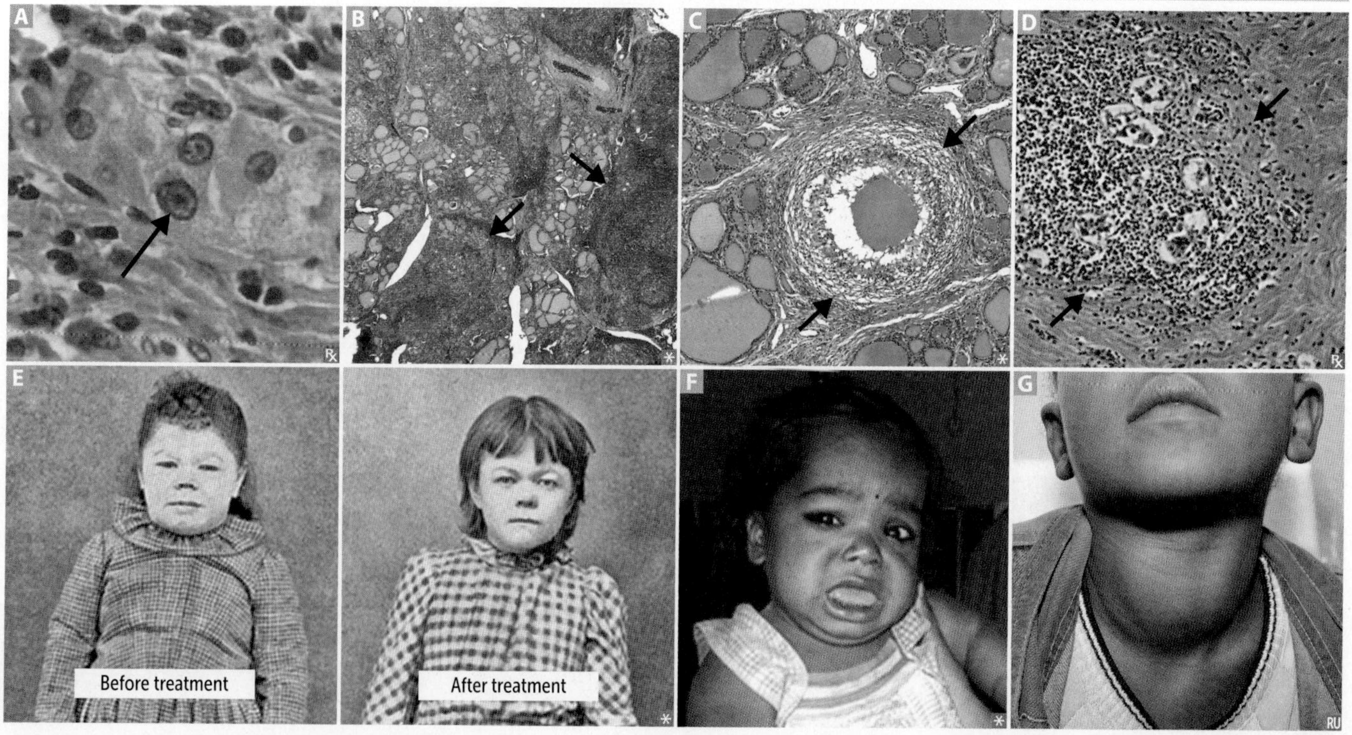
A
B
C
D
E
Before treatment
After treatment
F
G

Hyperthyroidism

Graves disease 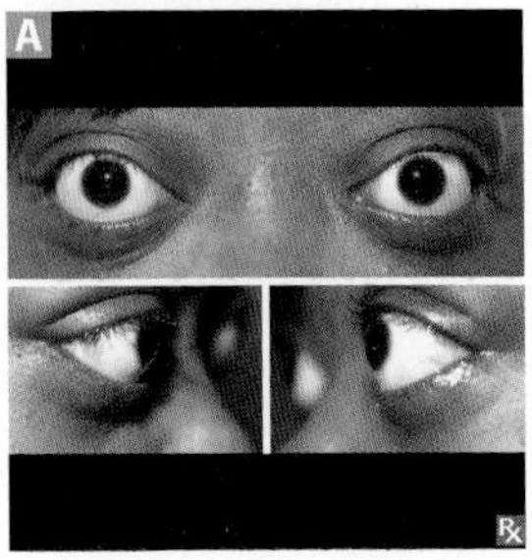	Most common cause of hyperthyroidism. Thyroid-stimulating immunoglobulin (IgG, can cause transient neonatal hyperthyroidism; type II hypersensitivity) stimulates TSH receptors on thyroid (hyperthyroidism, diffuse goiter), dermal fibroblasts (pretibial myxedema), and orbital fibroblasts (Graves orbitopathy). Activation of T-cells → lymphocytic infiltration of retroorbital space → ↑ cytokines (eg, TNF-α, IFN-γ) → ↑ fibroblast secretion of hydrophilic GAGs → ↑ osmotic muscle swelling, muscle inflammation, and adipocyte count → exophthalmos A. Often presents during stress (eg, pregnancy). Associated with HLA-DR3 and HLA-B8. Histology: tall, crowded follicular epithelial cells; scalloped colloid.
Toxic multinodular goiter	Focal patches of hyperfunctioning follicular cells distended with colloid working independently of TSH (due to TSH receptor mutations in 60% of cases). ↑ release of T_3 and T_4. Hot nodules are rarely malignant.
Thyroid storm	Uncommon but serious complication that occurs when hyperthyroidism is incompletely treated/untreated and then significantly worsens in the setting of acute stress such as infection, trauma, surgery. Presents with agitation, delirium, fever, diarrhea, coma, and tachyarrhythmia (cause of death). May see ↑ LFTs. Treat with the 4 P's: β-blockers (eg, propranolol), propylthiouracil, corticosteroids (eg, prednisolone), potassium iodide (Lugol iodine). Iodide load → ↓ T_4 synthesis → Wolff-Chaikoff effect.
Jod-Basedow phenomenon	Iodine-induced hyperthyroidism. Occurs when a patient with iodine deficiency and partially autonomous thyroid tissue (eg, autonomous nodule) is made iodine replete. Can happen after iodine IV contrast or amiodarone use. Opposite to Wolff-Chaikoff effect.
Causes of goiter	Smooth/diffuse: Graves disease, Hashimoto thyroiditis, iodine deficiency, TSH-secreting pituitary adenoma. Nodular: toxic multinodular goiter, thyroid adenoma, thyroid cancer, thyroid cyst.

Thyroid adenoma 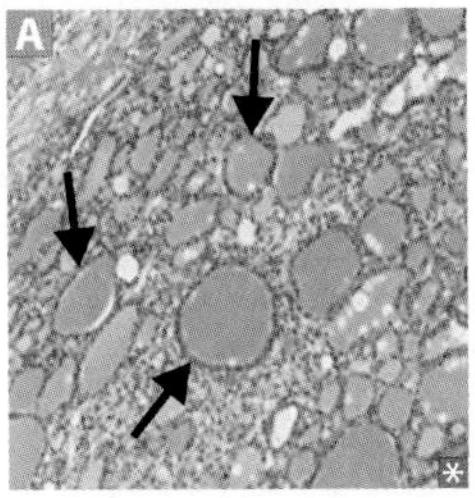	Benign solitary growth of the thyroid. Most are nonfunctional ("cold"), can rarely cause hyperthyroidism via autonomous thyroid hormone production ("hot" or "toxic"). Most common histology is follicular (arrows in A); absence of capsular or vascular invasion (unlike follicular carcinoma).

Thyroid cancer	Typically diagnosed with fine needle aspiration; treated with thyroidectomy. Complications of surgery include hypocalcemia (due to removal of parathyroid glands), transection of recurrent laryngeal nerve during ligation of inferior thyroid artery (leads to dysphagia and dysphonia [hoarseness]), and injury to the external branch of the superior laryngeal nerve during ligation of superior thyroid vascular pedicle (may lead to loss of tenor usually noticeable in professional voice users).
Papillary carcinoma 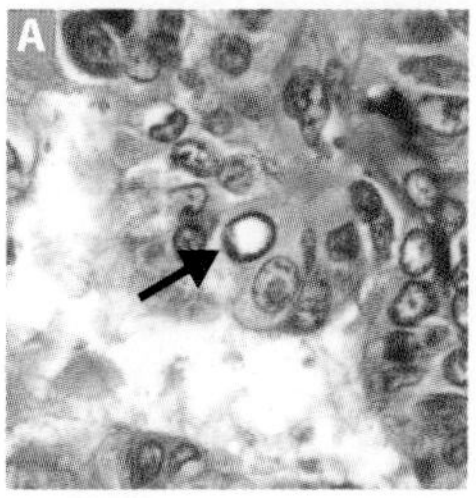	Most common. Empty-appearing nuclei with central clearing ("**Orphan Annie**" eyes) A, psam**Moma** bodies, nuclear grooves (**Papi** and **Moma** adopted **Orphan Annie**). ↑ risk with *RET/PTC* rearrangements and *BRAF* mutations, childhood irradiation. Papillary carcinoma: most prevalent, palpable lymph nodes. Good prognosis.
Follicular carcinoma	Good prognosis. Invades thyroid capsule and vasculature (unlike follicular adenoma), uniform follicles; hematogenous spread is common. Associated with *RAS* mutation and *PAX8-PPAR-γ* translocations. Fine needle aspiration cytology may not be able to distinguish between follicular adenoma and carcinoma.
Medullary carcinoma 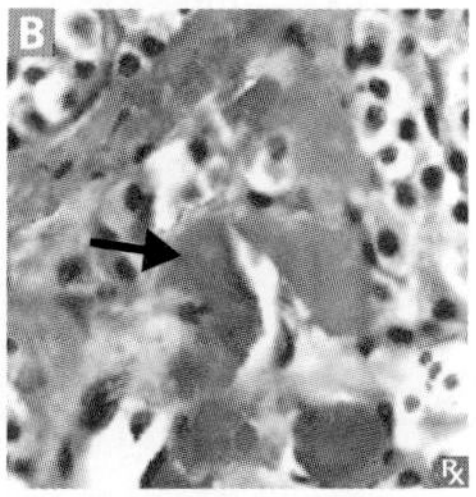	From parafollicular "**C** cells"; produces calcitonin, sheets of polygonal cells in an amyloid stroma B (stains with **C**ongo red). Associated with MEN 2A and 2B (*RET* mutations).
Undifferentiated/ anaplastic carcinoma	Older patients; presents with rapidly enlarging neck mass → compressive symptoms (eg, dyspnea, dysphagia, hoarseness); very poor prognosis. Associated with *TP53* mutation.

Diagnosing parathyroid disease

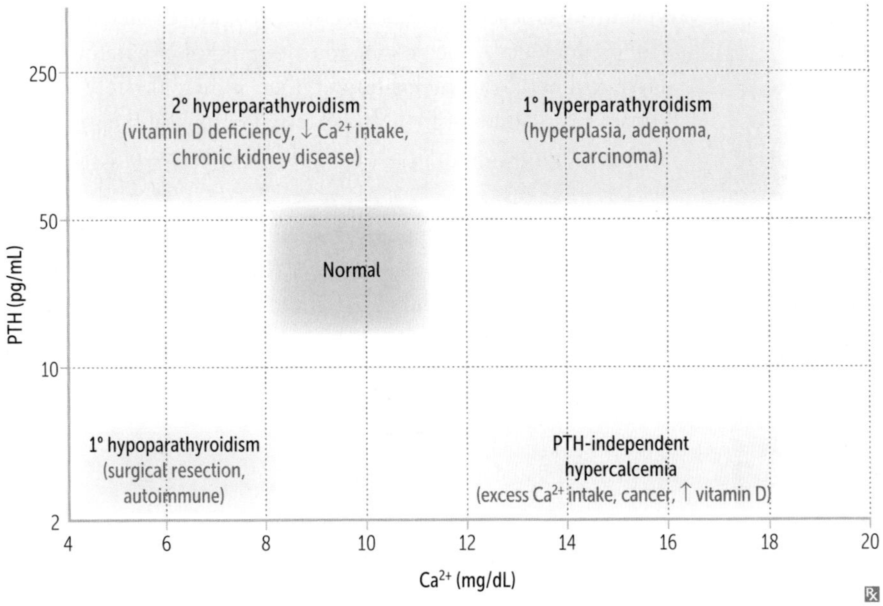

Hypoparathyroidism

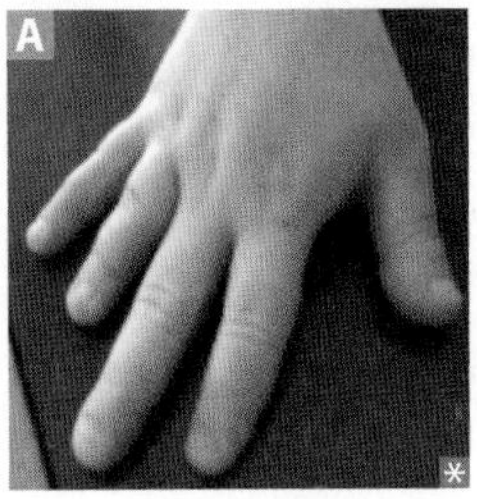

Due to injury to parathyroid glands or their blood supply (usually during surgery), autoimmune destruction, or DiGeorge syndrome. Findings: tetany, hypocalcemia, hyperphosphatemia.
Chvostek sign—tapping of facial nerve (tap the **C**heek) → contraction of facial muscles.
Trousseau sign—occlusion of brachial artery with BP cuff (cuff the **T**riceps) → carpal spasm.

Pseudohypoparathyroidism type 1A—autosomal dominant, maternally transmitted mutations (imprinted *GNAS* gene). GNAS1-inactivating mutation (coupled to PTH receptor) that encodes the G_s protein α subunit → inactivation of adenylate cyclase when PTH binds to its receptor → end-organ resistance (kidney and bone) to PTH.
Physical findings: Albright hereditary osteodystrophy (shortened 4th/5th digits A, short stature, round face, subcutaneous calcifications, developmental delay).
Labs: ↑ PTH, ↓ Ca^{2+}, ↑ PO_4^{3-}.

Pseudopseudohypoparathyroidism—autosomal dominant, paternally transmitted mutations (imprinted *GNAS* gene) but without end-organ resistance to PTH due to normal maternal allele maintaining renal responsiveness to PTH.
Physical findings: same as Albright hereditary osteodystrophy.
Labs: normal PTH, Ca^{2+}, PO_4^{3-}.

Lab values in hypocalcemia

DISORDER	Ca^{2+}	PO_4^{3-}	PTH
Vitamin D deficiency	↓	↓	↑
Hypoparathyroidism	↓	↑	↓
2° hyperparathyroidism (CKD)	↓	↑	↑
Pseudohypoparathyroidism	↓	↑	↑
Hyperphosphatemia	↓	↑	↑

Hyperparathyroidism

Primary hyperparathyroidism A 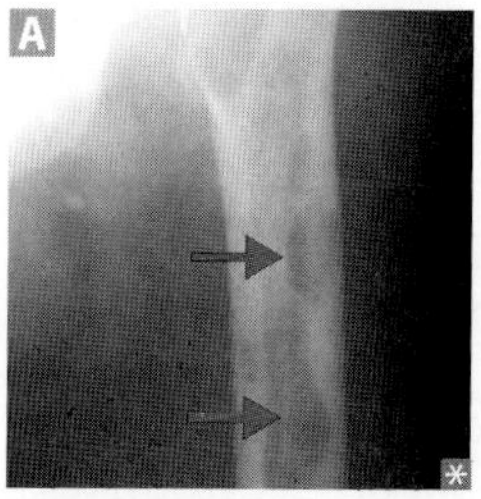	Usually due to parathyroid adenoma or hyperplasia. **Hypercalcemia**, hypercalciuria (renal **stones**), polyuria (**thrones**), hypophosphatemia, ↑ PTH, ↑ ALP, ↑ urinary cAMP. Most often asymptomatic. May present with **bone** pain, weakness, constipation ("**groans**"), abdominal/flank pain (kidney stones, acute pancreatitis), neuropsychiatric disturbances ("**psychiatric overtones**").	**Osteitis fibrosa cystica**—cystic **bone** spaces filled with brown fibrous tissue A ("brown tumor" consisting of osteoclasts and deposited hemosiderin from hemorrhages; causes bone pain). Due to ↑ PTH, classically associated with 1° (but also seen with 2°) hyperparathyroidism. "**Stones, thrones, bones, groans,** and **psychiatric overtones**."
Secondary hyperparathyroidism	2° hyperplasia due to ↓ Ca^{2+} absorption and/or ↑ PO_4^{3-}, most often in chronic kidney disease (causes hypovitaminosis D and hyperphosphatemia → ↓ Ca^{2+}). **Hypocalcemia**, hyperphosphatemia in chronic kidney disease (vs hypophosphatemia with most other causes), ↑ ALP, ↑ PTH.	**Renal osteodystrophy**—renal disease → 2° and 3° hyperparathyroidism → bone lesions.
Tertiary hyperparathyroidism	Refractory (autonomous) hyperparathyroidism resulting from chronic kidney disease. ↑↑ PTH, ↑ Ca^{2+}.	

Familial hypocalciuric hypercalcemia — Defective G-coupled Ca^{2+}-sensing receptors in multiple tissues (eg, parathyroids, kidneys). Higher than normal Ca^{2+} levels required to suppress PTH. Excessive renal Ca^{2+} reabsorption → mild hypercalcemia and hypocalciuria with normal to ↑ PTH levels.

Diabetes mellitus

ACUTE MANIFESTATIONS	Polydipsia, polyuria, polyphagia, weight loss, DKA (type 1), hyperosmolar hyperglycemic state (type 2). Rarely, can be caused by unopposed secretion of GH and epinephrine. Also seen in patients on glucocorticoid therapy (steroid diabetes).
CHRONIC COMPLICATIONS	Nonenzymatic glycation: ▪ Small vessel disease (diffuse thickening of basement membrane) → retinopathy (hemorrhage, exudates, microaneurysms, vessel proliferation), glaucoma, nephropathy. Nodular glomerulosclerosis → progressive proteinuria (initially microalbuminuria; ACE inhibitors and ARBs are renoprotective. Arteriolosclerosis (causing hypertension) → chronic kidney disease. ▪ Large vessel atherosclerosis, CAD, peripheral vascular occlusive disease, gangrene → limb loss, cerebrovascular disease. MI most common cause of death. Osmotic damage (sorbitol accumulation in organs with aldose reductase and ↓ or absent sorbitol dehydrogenase): ▪ Neuropathy: motor, sensory (glove and stocking distribution), autonomic degeneration (eg, GERD, gastroparesis, diabetic diarrhea). ▪ Cataracts.

DIAGNOSIS

TEST	DIAGNOSTIC CUTOFF	NOTES
HbA_{1c}	≥ 6.5%	Reflects average blood glucose over prior 3 months (influenced by RBC turnover)
Fasting plasma glucose	≥ 126 mg/dL	Fasting for > 8 hours
2-hour oral glucose tolerance test	≥ 200 mg/dL	2 hours after consumption of 75 g of glucose in water
Random plasma glucose	≥ 200 mg/dL	Presence of hyperglycemic symptoms is required

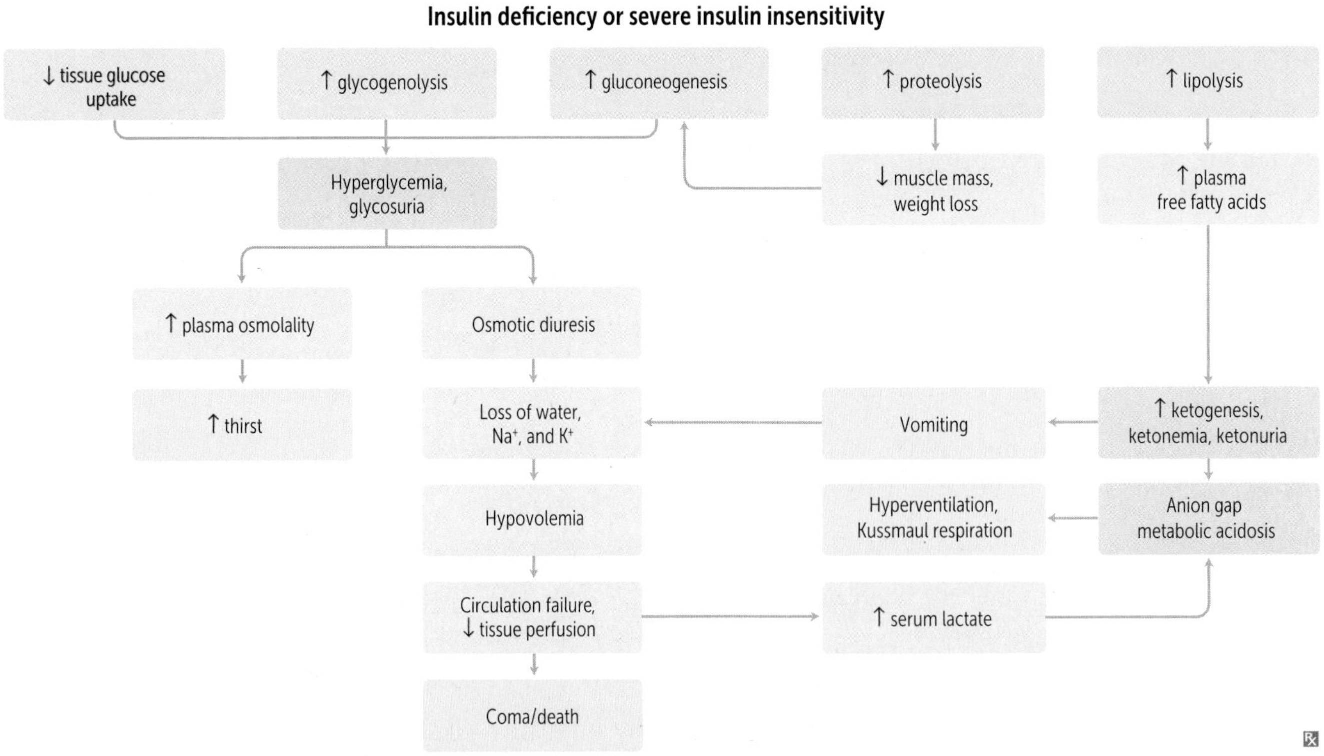

Type 1 vs type 2 diabetes mellitus

	Type 1	Type 2
1° DEFECT	Autoimmune T-cell–mediated destruction of β cells (eg, due to presence of glutamic acid decarboxylase antibodies)	↑ resistance to insulin, progressive pancreatic β-cell failure
INSULIN NECESSARY IN TREATMENT	Always	Sometimes
AGE (EXCEPTIONS COMMON)	< 30 yr	> 40 yr
ASSOCIATION WITH OBESITY	No	Yes
GENETIC PREDISPOSITION	Relatively weak (50% concordance in identical twins), polygenic	Relatively strong (90% concordance in identical twins), polygenic
ASSOCIATION WITH HLA SYSTEM	Yes, HLA-DR4 and -DR3 (4 – 3 = type 1)	No
GLUCOSE INTOLERANCE	Severe	Mild to moderate
INSULIN SENSITIVITY	High	Low
KETOACIDOSIS	Common	Rare
β-CELL NUMBERS IN THE ISLETS	↓	Variable (with amyloid deposits)
SERUM INSULIN LEVEL	↓	↑ initially, but ↓ in advanced disease
CLASSIC SYMPTOMS OF POLYURIA, POLYDIPSIA, POLYPHAGIA, WEIGHT LOSS	Common	Sometimes
HISTOLOGY	Islet leukocytic infiltrate	Islet amyloid polypeptide (IAPP) deposits

Hyperglycemic emergencies

	Diabetic ketoacidosis	Hyperosmolar hyperglycemic state
PATHOGENESIS	Insulin noncompliance or ↑ requirements due to ↑ stress (eg, infection) → excess lipolysis and ↑ ketogenesis from ↑ free fatty acids → ketone bodies (β-hydroxybutyrate > acetoacetate). **Insulin deficient, ketones present.**	Profound hyperglycemia → excessive osmotic diuresis → dehydration and ↑ serum osmolality → HHS. Classically seen in elderly patients with type 2 DM and limited ability to drink. **Insulin present, ketones absent.**
SIGNS/SYMPTOMS	**DKA** is **D**eadly: **D**elirium/psychosis, **K**ussmaul respirations (rapid, deep breathing), **A**bdominal pain/nausea/vomiting, **D**ehydration. Fruity breath odor due to exhaled acetone.	Thirst, polyuria, lethargy, focal neurologic deficits, seizures.
LABS	Hyperglycemia, ↑ H^+, ↓ HCO_3^- (↑ anion gap metabolic acidosis), ↑ urine and blood ketone levels, leukocytosis. Normal/↑ serum K^+, but depleted intracellular K^+ due to transcellular shift from ↓ insulin and acidosis. Osmotic diuresis → ↑ K^+ loss in urine → total body K^+ depletion.	Hyperglycemia (often > 600 mg/dL), ↑ serum osmolality (> 320 mOsm/kg), normal pH (no acidosis), no ketones. Normal/↑ serum K^+, ↓ intracellular K^+.
COMPLICATIONS	Life-threatening mucormycosis, cerebral edema, cardiac arrhythmias.	Can progress to coma and death if untreated.
TREATMENT	IV fluids, IV insulin, and K^+ (to replete intracellular stores). Glucose may be required to prevent hypoglycemia from insulin therapy.	

Hypoglycemia in diabetes mellitus

Usually occurs in patients treated with insulin or insulin secretagogues (eg, sulfonylureas, meglitinides) in the setting of high-dose treatment, inadequate food intake, and/or exercise.

- Neurogenic/autonomic symptoms: diaphoresis, tachycardia, tremor, anxiety, hunger. May allow perception of ↓ glucose (hypoglycemia awareness).
- Neuroglycopenic symptoms: altered mental status, seizures, death due to insufficient glucose in CNS.

Treatment: simple carbohydrates (eg, glucose tablets, fruit juice), IM glucagon, IV dextrose.

Cushing syndrome

ETIOLOGY

↑ cortisol due to a variety of causes:

- Exogenous corticosteroids → ↓ ACTH → bilateral adrenal atrophy. Most common cause.
- Primary adrenal adenoma, hyperplasia, or carcinoma → ↓ ACTH → atrophy of uninvolved adrenal gland.
- ACTH-secreting pituitary adenoma (Cushing disease); paraneoplastic ACTH secretion (eg, small cell lung cancer, bronchial carcinoids)→ bilateral adrenal hyperplasia. Cushing disease is responsible for the majority of endogenous cases of Cushing syndrome.

FINDINGS

CUSHING Syndrome: ↑ Cholesterol, ↑ Urinary free cortisol, Skin changes (thinning, striae A), Hypertension, Immunosuppression, Neoplasm (a cause, not a finding), Growth restriction (in children), ↑ Sugar (hyperglycemia, insulin resistance). Also, amenorrhea, moon facies B, buffalo hump, osteoporosis, ↑ weight (truncal obesity), hirsutism.

DIAGNOSIS

Screening tests include: ↑ free cortisol on 24-hr urinalysis, ↑ late night salivary cortisol, and no suppression with overnight low-dose dexamethasone test.

A

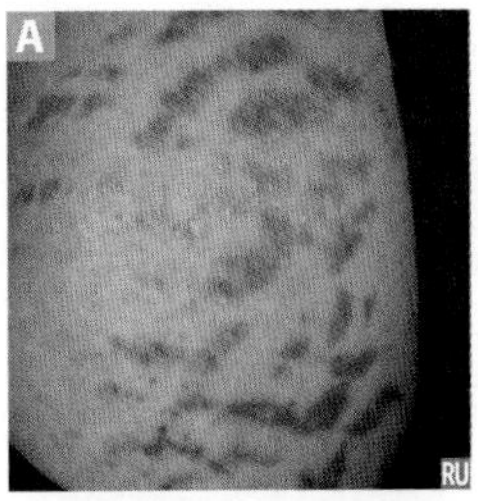

B

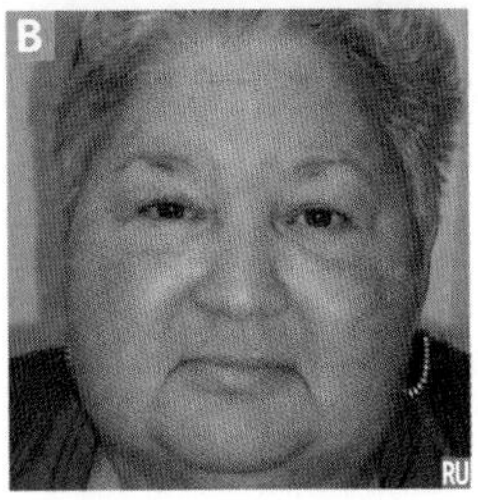

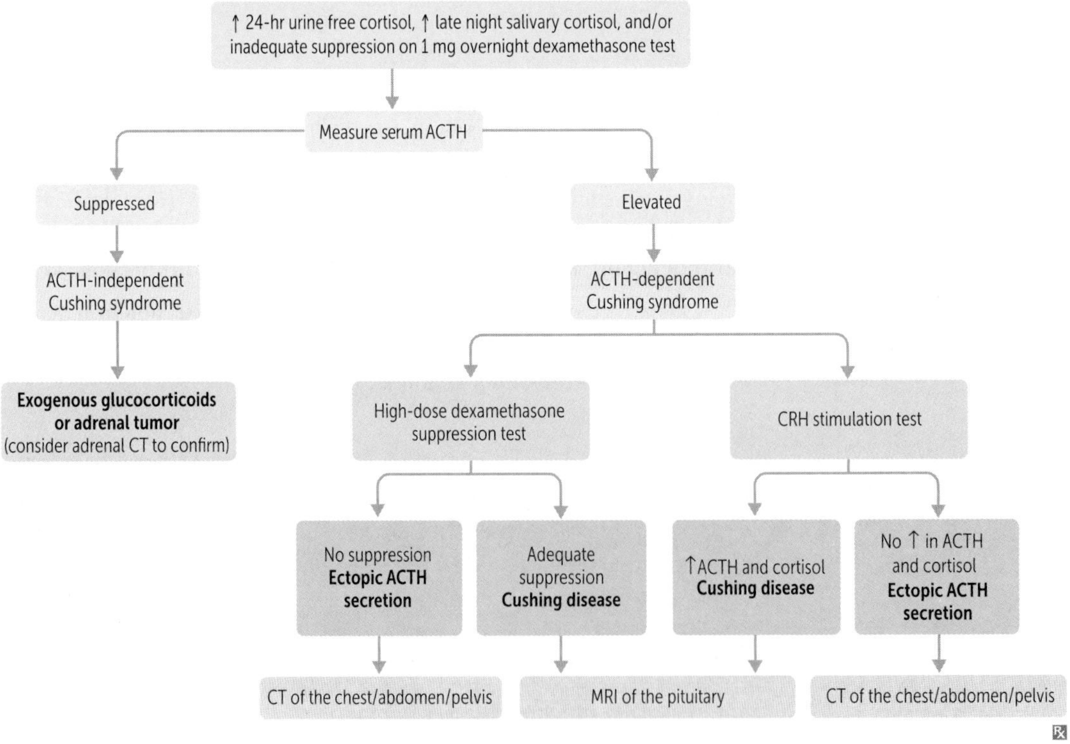

Nelson syndrome

Enlargement of pre-existing ACTH–secreting pituitary adenoma after bilateral adrenalectomy for refractory Cushing disease → ↑ ACTH (hyperpigmentation), mass effect (headaches, bitemporal hemianopia).
Treatment: transsphenoidal resection, postoperative pituitary irradiation for residual tumor.

Adrenal insufficiency

Inability of adrenal glands to generate enough glucocorticoids +/– mineralocorticoids for the body's needs. Can be acute or chronic. Symptoms include weakness, fatigue, orthostatic hypotension, muscle aches, weight loss, GI disturbances, sugar and/or salt cravings.
Treatment: glucocorticoid +/– mineralocorticoid replacement.

Primary adrenal insufficiency

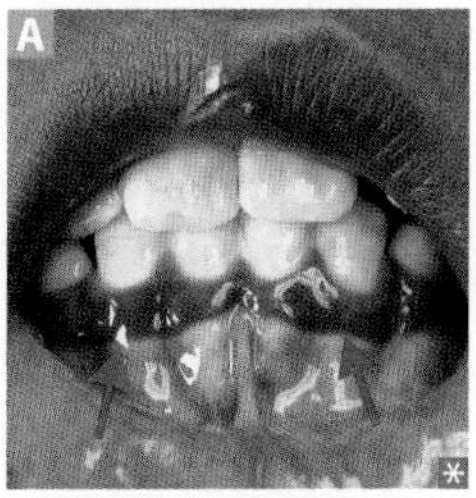

↓ gland function → ↓ cortisol, ↓ aldosterone → hypotension (hyponatremic volume contraction), hyperkalemia, metabolic acidosis, skin/mucosal hyperpigmentation A (↑ melanin synthesis due to ↑ MSH, a byproduct of POMC cleavage). Primary pigments the skin/mucosa.
Addison disease—chronic 1° adrenal insufficiency; caused by adrenal atrophy or destruction. Most commonly due to autoimmune adrenalitis (developed world) or TB (developing world).

Secondary and tertiary adrenal insufficiency

↓ pituitary ACTH secretion (secondary) or ↓ hypothalamic CRH secretion (tertiary). No hyperkalemia (aldosterone synthesis preserved due to functioning adrenal gland, intact RAAS), no hyperpigmentation.
2° adrenal insufficiency is due to pituitary pathologies, 3° adrenal insufficiency is most commonly due to abrupt cessation of chronic steroid therapy (HPA suppression). Tertiary from treatment.

Acute adrenal insufficiency

Also called adrenal (addisonian) crisis; often precipitated by acute stressors that ↑ steroid requirements (eg, infection) in patients with pre-existing adrenal insufficiency or on steroid therapy. May present with acute abdomen, nausea, vomiting, altered mental status, shock.
Waterhouse-Friderichsen syndrome—bilateral adrenal hemorrhage often due to meningococcemia. May present with acute adrenal insufficiency, fever, petechiae, sepsis.

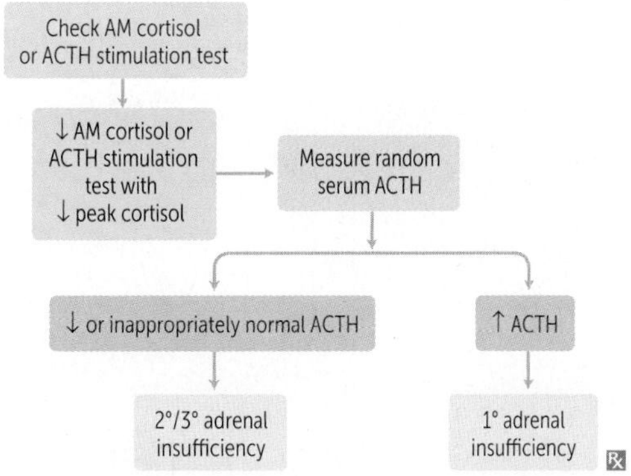

Hyperaldosteronism	Increased secretion of aldosterone from adrenal gland. Clinical features include hypertension, ↓ or normal K^+, metabolic alkalosis. 1° hyperaldosteronism does not directly cause edema due to aldosterone escape mechanism. However, certain 2° causes of hyperaldosteronism (eg, heart failure) impair the aldosterone escape mechanism, leading to worsening of edema.
Primary hyperaldosteronism	Seen in patients with bilateral adrenal hyperplasia or adrenal adenoma (Conn syndrome). ↑ aldosterone, ↓ renin. Leads to treatment-resistant hypertension.
Secondary hyperaldosteronism	Seen in patients with renovascular hypertension, juxtaglomerular cell tumors (renin-producing), and edema (eg, cirrhosis, heart failure, nephrotic syndrome).

Neuroendocrine tumors

Heterogeneous group of neoplasms originating from neuroendocrine cells (which have traits similar to nerve cells and hormone-producing cells).

Most neoplasms occur in the GI system (eg, carcinoid, gastrinoma), pancreas (eg, insulinoma, glucagonoma), and lungs (eg, small cell carcinoma). Also in thyroid (eg, medullary carcinoma) and adrenals (eg, pheochromocytoma).

Neuroendocrine cells (eg, pancreatic β cells, enterochromaffin cells) share a common biologic function through amine precursor uptake decarboxylase (APUD) despite differences in embryologic origin, anatomic site, and secretory products (eg, chromogranin A, neuron-specific enolase [NSE], synaptophysin, serotonin, histamine, calcitonin). Treatment: surgical resection, somatostatin analogs.

Neuroblastoma

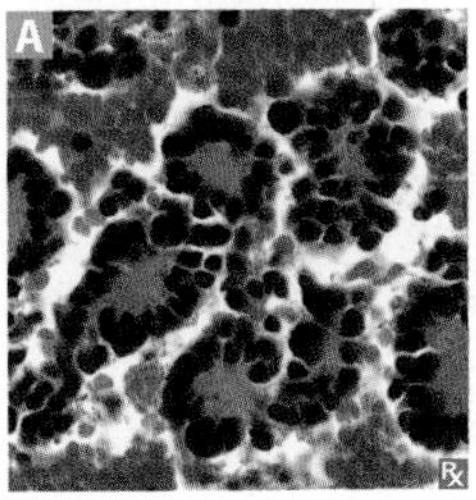

Most common tumor of the adrenal medulla in **children**, usually < 4 years old. Originates from neural crest cells. Occurs anywhere along the sympathetic chain.

Most common presentation is abdominal distension and a firm, irregular mass that can cross the midline (vs Wilms tumor, which is smooth and unilateral). Less likely to develop hypertension than with pheochromocytoma (neuroblastoma is normotensive). Can also present with opsoclonus-myoclonus syndrome ("dancing eyes-dancing feet").

↑ HVA and VMA (catecholamine metabolites) in urine. Homer-Wright rosettes (neuroblasts surrounding a central lumen A) characteristic of neuroblastoma and medulloblastoma. Bombesin and NSE ⊕. Associated with amplification of N-*myc* oncogene.

Pheochromocytoma

ETIOLOGY 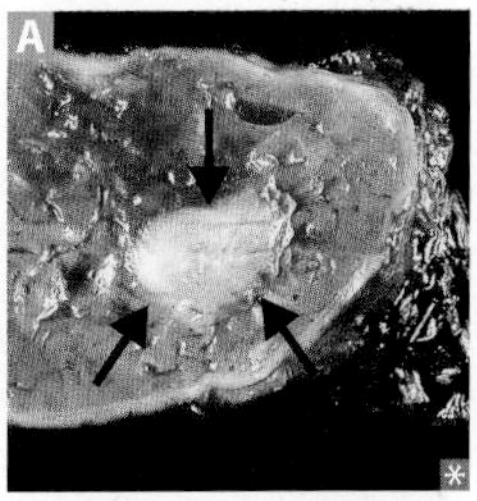	Most common tumor of the adrenal medulla in **adults** A. Derived from chromaffin cells (arise from neural crest). May be associated with germline mutations (eg, *NF-1*, *VHL*, *RET* [MEN 2A, 2B]).	Rule of 10's: 10% malignant 10% bilateral 10% extra-adrenal (eg, bladder wall, organ of Zuckerkandl) 10% calcify 10% kids
SYMPTOMS	Most tumors secrete epinephrine, norepinephrine, and dopamine, which can cause episodic hypertension. May also secrete EPO → polycythemia. Symptoms occur in "spells"—relapse and remit.	Episodic hyperadrenergic symptoms (5 P's): Pressure (↑ BP) Pain (headache) Perspiration Palpitations (tachycardia) Pallor
FINDINGS	↑ catecholamines and metanephrines (eg, homovanillic acid, vanillylmandelic acid) in urine and plasma.	Chromogranin, synaptophysin and NSE ⊕.
TREATMENT	Irreversible α-antagonists (eg, phenoxybenzamine) followed by β-blockers prior to tumor resection. α-blockade must be achieved before giving β-blockers to avoid a hypertensive crisis. A before B.	Phenoxybenzamine for pheochromocytoma.

Multiple endocrine neoplasias

All **MEN** syndromes have autosomal **dominant** inheritance.
The X-**MEN** are **dominant** over villains.

SUBTYPE	CHARACTERISTICS	COMMENTS
MEN 1	Pituitary tumors (prolactin or GH) Pancreatic endocrine tumors—Zollinger-Ellison syndrome, insulinomas, VIPomas, glucagonomas (rare) Parathyroid adenomas Associated with mutation of *MEN1* (menin, a tumor suppressor, chromosome 11), angiofibromas, collagenomas, meningiomas	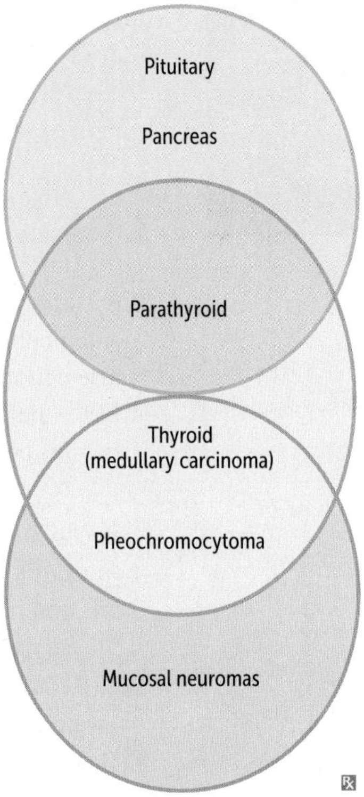 Pituitary Pancreas Parathyroid Thyroid (medullary carcinoma) Pheochromocytoma Mucosal neuromas
MEN 2A	Parathyroid hyperplasia Medullary thyroid carcinoma—neoplasm of parafollicular C cells; secretes calcitonin; prophylactic thyroidectomy required Pheochromocytoma (secretes catecholamines) Associated with mutation in *RET* (codes for receptor tyrosine kinase)	
MEN 2B 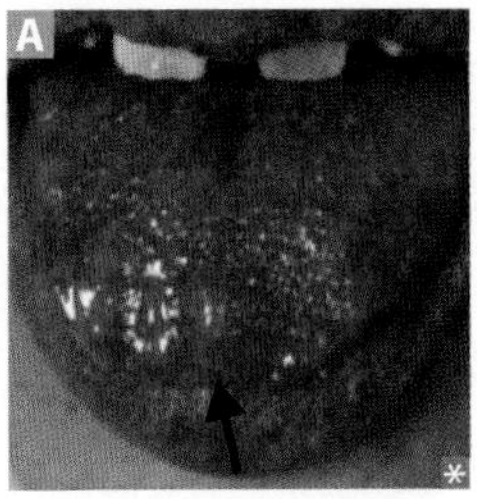 A	Medullary thyroid carcinoma Pheochromocytoma Mucosal neuromas A (oral/intestinal ganglioneuromatosis) Associated with marfanoid habitus; mutation in *RET* gene	MEN 1 = 3 P's: pituitary, parathyroid, and pancreas MEN 2A = 2 P's: parathyroid and pheochromocytoma MEN 2B = 1 P: pheochromocytoma

Pancreatic islet cell tumors

Insulinoma	Tumor of pancreatic β cells → overproduction of insulin → hypoglycemia. May see Whipple triad: low blood glucose, symptoms of hypoglycemia (eg, lethargy, syncope, diplopia), and resolution of symptoms after normalization of plasma glucose levels. Symptomatic patients have ↓ blood glucose and ↑ C-peptide levels (vs exogenous insulin use). ~ 10% of cases associated with MEN 1 syndrome. Treatment: surgical resection.
Glucagonoma	Tumor of pancreatic α cells → overproduction of glucagon. Presents with **6 D's**: **d**ermatitis (necrolytic migratory erythema), **d**iabetes (hyperglycemia), **DVT**, **d**eclining weight, **d**epression, **d**iarrhea. Treatment: octreotide, surgical resection.
Somatostatinoma	Tumor of pancreatic δ cells → overproduction of somatostatin → ↓ secretion of secretin, cholecystokinin, glucagon, insulin, gastrin, gastric inhibitory peptide (GIP). May present with diabetes/glucose intolerance, steatorrhea, gallstones, achlorhydria. Treatment: surgical resection; somatostatin analogs (eg, octreotide) for symptom control.

Carcinoid tumors

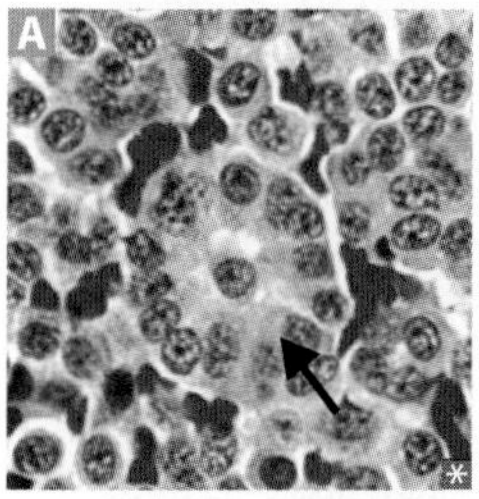

Carcinoid tumors arise from neuroendocrine cells, most commonly in the intestine or lung. Neuroendocrine cells secrete 5-HT, which undergoes hepatic first-pass metabolism and enzymatic breakdown by MAO in the lung. If 5-HT reaches the systemic circulation (eg, after liver metastasis), carcinoid tumor may present with **carcinoid syndrome**—episodic flushing, diarrhea, wheezing, right-sided valvular heart disease (eg, tricuspid regurgitation, pulmonic stenosis), niacin deficiency (pellagra).

Histology: prominent rosettes (arrow in A), chromogranin A ⊕, synaptophysin ⊕.

Treatment: surgical resection, somatostatin analog (eg, octreotide) or tryptophan hydroxylase inhibitor (eg, telotristat) for symptom control.

Rule of thirds:

- 1/3 metastasize
- 1/3 present with 2nd malignancy
- 1/3 are multiple

Zollinger-Ellison syndrome

Gastrin-secreting tumor (gastrinoma) of duodenum or pancreas. Acid hypersecretion causes recurrent ulcers in duodenum and jejunum. Presents with abdominal pain (peptic ulcer disease, distal ulcers), diarrhea (malabsorption). Positive secretin stimulation test: ↑ gastrin levels after administration of secretin, which normally inhibits gastrin release. May be associated with MEN 1.

▸ ENDOCRINE—PHARMACOLOGY

Diabetes mellitus therapy

All patients with diabetes mellitus should receive education on diet, exercise, blood glucose monitoring, and complication management. Treatment differs based on the type of diabetes and glycemic control:

- Type 1 DM—insulin replacement
- Type 2 DM—oral agents (metformin is first line), non-insulin injectables, insulin replacement; weight loss particularly helpful in lowering blood glucose
- Gestational DM—insulin replacement if nutrition therapy and exercise alone fail

Regular (short-acting) insulin is preferred for DKA (IV), hyperkalemia (+ glucose), stress hyperglycemia.

These drugs help To normalize pancreatic function (-glits, -glins, -glips, -glifs).

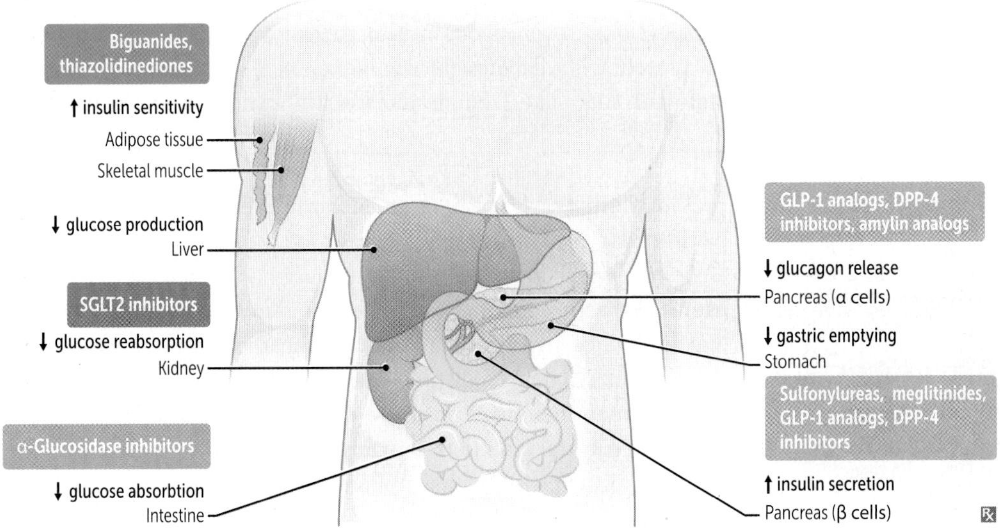

DRUG CLASS	MECHANISM	ADVERSE EFFECTS
Insulin preparations		
Rapid acting (1-hr peak): Lispro, Aspart, Glulisine (no **LAG**) Short acting (2–3 hr peak): regular Intermediate acting (4–10 hr peak): NPH Long acting (no real peak): detemir, glargine	Bind insulin receptor (tyrosine kinase activity) Liver: ↑ glucose storage as glycogen Muscle: ↑ glycogen, protein synthesis Fat: ↑ TG storage Cell membrane: ↑ K^+ uptake	Hypoglycemia, lipodystrophy, hypersensitivity reactions (rare), weight gain 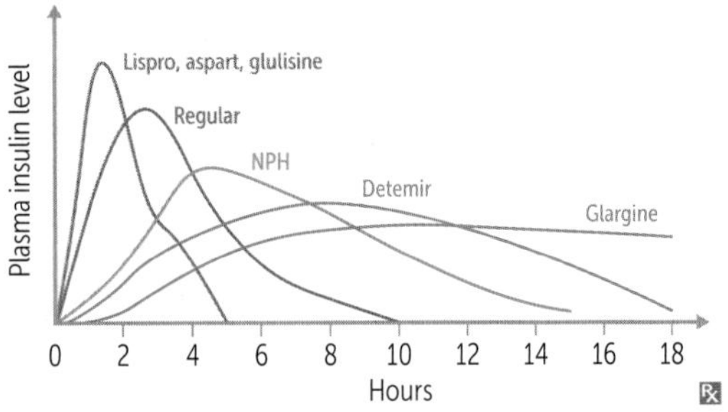

Diabetes mellitus therapy *(continued)*

DRUG CLASS	MECHANISM	ADVERSE EFFECTS
Increase insulin sensitivity		
Biguanides Metformin	Inhibit mGPD → inhibition of hepatic gluconeogenesis and the action of glucagon. ↑ glycolysis, peripheral glucose uptake (↑ insulin sensitivity).	GI upset, lactic acidosis (use with caution in renal insufficiency), vitamin B_{12} deficiency. Weight loss (often desired).
Thiazolidinediones "-glits" Pioglitazone, rosiglitazone	Activate PPAR-γ (a nuclear receptor) → ↑ insulin sensitivity and levels of adiponectin → regulation of glucose metabolism and fatty acid storage.	Weight gain, edema, HF, ↑ risk of fractures. Delayed onset of action (several weeks). Rosiglitazone: ↑ risk of MI, cardiovascular death.
Increase insulin secretion		
Sulfonylureas (1st gen) Chlorpropamide, tolbutamide		Disulfiram-like reaction with first-generation sulfonylureas only (rarely used).
Sulfonylureas (2nd gen) Glipizide, glyburide	Close K^+ channels in pancreatic B cell membrane → cell depolarizes → insulin release via ↑ Ca^{2+} influx.	Hypoglycemia (↑ risk in renal insufficiency), weight gain.
Meglitinides "-glins" Nateglinide, repaglinide		
Increase glucose-induced insulin secretion		
GLP-1 analogs Exenatide, liraglutide	↓ glucagon release, ↓ gastric emptying, ↑ glucose-dependent insulin release.	Nausea, vomiting, pancreatitis. Weight loss (often desired). ↑ satiety (often desired).
DPP-4 inhibitors "-glips" Linagliptin, saxagliptin, sitagliptin	Inhibit DPP-4 enzyme that deactivates GLP-1 → ↓ glucagon release, ↓ gastric emptying. ↑ glucose-dependent insulin release.	Respiratory and urinary infections, weight neutral. ↑ satiety (often desired).
Decrease glucose absorption		
Sodium-glucose co-transporter 2 inhibitors "-glifs" Canagliflozin, dapagliflozin, empagliflozin	Block reabsorption of glucose in proximal convoluted tubule.	Glucosuria (UTIs, vulvovaginal candidiasis), dehydration (orthostatic hypotension), weight loss. Use with caution in renal insufficiency (↓ efficacy with ↓ GFR).
α-glucosidase inhibitors Acarbose, miglitol	Inhibit intestinal brush-border α-glucosidases → delayed carbohydrate hydrolysis and glucose absorption → ↓ postprandial hyperglycemia.	GI upset, bloating. Not recommended in renal insufficiency.
Others		
Amylin analogs Pramlintide	↓ glucagon release, ↓ gastric emptying.	Hypoglycemia, nausea. ↑ satiety (often desired).

Thionamides	Propylthiouracil, methimazole.
MECHANISM	Block thyroid peroxidase, inhibiting the oxidation of iodide as well as the organification and coupling of iodine → inhibition of thyroid hormone synthesis. PTU also blocks 5′-deiodinase → ↓ Peripheral conversion of T_4 to T_3.
CLINICAL USE	Hyperthyroidism. PTU used in Primary (first) trimester of pregnancy (due to methimazole teratogenicity); methimazole used in second and third trimesters of pregnancy (due to risk of PTU-induced hepatotoxicity). Not used to treat Graves ophthalmopathy (treated with corticosteroids).
ADVERSE EFFECTS	Skin rash, agranulocytosis (rare), aplastic anemia, hepatotoxicity. PTU use has been associated with ANCA-positive vasculitis. Methimazole is a possible teratogen (can cause aplasia cutis).

Levothyroxine, liothyronine

MECHANISM	Hormone replacement for T_4 (levothyroxine) or T_3 (liothyronine).
CLINICAL USE	Hypothyroidism, myxedema. May be abused for weight loss. Distinguish exogenous hyperthyroidism from endogenous hyperthyroidism by using a combination of TSH receptor antibodies, radioactive iodine uptake, and/or measurement of thyroid blood flow on ultrasound.
ADVERSE EFFECTS	Tachycardia, heat intolerance, tremors, arrhythmias.

Hypothalamic/pituitary drugs

DRUG	CLINICAL USE
Conivaptan, tolvaptan	ADH antagonists SIADH (block action of ADH at V_2-receptor)
Demeclocycline	Interferes with ADH signaling, a tetracycline SIADH
Desmopressin	ADH analog Central DI, von Willebrand disease, sleep enuresis, hemophilia A
GH	GH deficiency, Turner syndrome
Oxytocin	Induction of labor (stimulates uterine contractions), control uterine hemorrhage
Somatostatin (octreotide)	Acromegaly, carcinoid syndrome, gastrinoma, glucagonoma, esophageal varices

Fludrocortisone

MECHANISM	Synthetic analog of aldosterone with glucocorticoid effects. **Fluid**rocortisone retains **fluid**.
CLINICAL USE	Mineralocorticoid replacement in 1° adrenal insufficiency.
ADVERSE EFFECTS	Similar to glucocorticoids; also edema, exacerbation of heart failure, hyperpigmentation.

Cinacalcet

MECHANISM	Sensitizes calcium-sensing receptor (CaSR) in parathyroid gland to circulating Ca^{2+} → ↓ PTH. Pronounce "Senacalcet."
CLINICAL USE	2° hyperparathyroidism in patients with CKD receiving hemodialysis, hypercalcemia in 1° hyperparathyroidism (if parathyroidectomy fails), or in parathyroid carcinoma.
ADVERSE EFFECTS	Hypocalcemia.

Sevelamer

MECHANISM	Nonabsorbable phosphate binder that prevents phosphate absorption from the GI tract.
CLINICAL USE	Hyperphosphatemia in CKD.
ADVERSE EFFECTS	Hypophosphatemia, GI upset.

Cation exchange resins

Patiromer, sodium polystyrene sulfonate, zirconium cyclosilicate.

MECHANISM	Bind K^+ in colon in exchange for other cations (eg, Na^+, Ca^{2+}) → K^+ excreted in feces.
CLINICAL USE	Hyperkalemia.
ADVERSE EFFECTS	Hypokalemia, GI upset.

▶ NOTES

Gastrointestinal

"A good set of bowels is worth more to a man than any quantity of brains."
—Josh Billings

"Man should strive to have his intestines relaxed all the days of his life."
—Moses Maimonides

"All right, let's not panic. I'll make the money by selling one of my livers. I can get by with one."
—Homer Simpson, *The Simpsons*

"The truth does not change according to our ability to stomach it emotionally."
—Flannery O'Connor

When studying the gastrointestinal system, be sure to understand the normal embryology, anatomy, and physiology and how the system is affected by various pathologies. Study not only disease pathophysiology, but also its specific findings, so that you can differentiate between two similar diseases. For example, what specifically makes ulcerative colitis different from Crohn disease? Also, be comfortable with basic interpretation of abdominal x-rays, CT scans, and endoscopic images.

▶ GASTROINTESTINAL—EMBRYOLOGY

Normal gastrointestinal embryology

Foregut—esophagus to duodenum at level of pancreatic duct and common bile duct insertion (ampulla of Vater).
Midgut—lower duodenum to proximal 2/3 of transverse colon.
Hindgut—distal 1/3 of transverse colon to anal canal above pectinate line.
Midgut:
- 6th week of development—physiologic herniation of midgut through umbilical ring
- 10th week of development—returns to abdominal cavity + rotates around superior mesenteric artery (SMA), total 270° counterclockwise

Ventral wall defects

Developmental defects due to failure of rostral fold closure (eg, sternal defects [ectopia cordis]), lateral fold closure (eg, omphalocele, gastroschisis), or caudal fold closure (eg, bladder exstrophy).

	Gastroschisis	Omphalocele
ETIOLOGY	Extrusion of abdominal contents through abdominal folds (typically right of umbilicus)	Failure of lateral walls to migrate at umbilical ring → persistent midline herniation of abdominal contents into umbilical cord
COVERAGE	Not covered by peritoneum or amnion A; "the guts come out of the gap (**schis**m) in the letter **G**"	Covered by peritoneum and amnion B (light gray shiny sac); "abdominal contents are **seal**ed in the letter **O**"
ASSOCIATIONS	Not associated with chromosome abnormalities; favorable prognosis	Associated with congenital anomalies (eg, trisomies 13 and 18, Beckwith-Wiedemann syndrome) and other structural abnormalities (eg, cardiac, GU, neural tube)

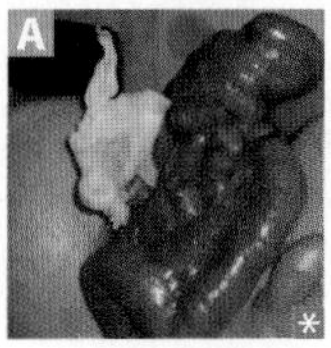
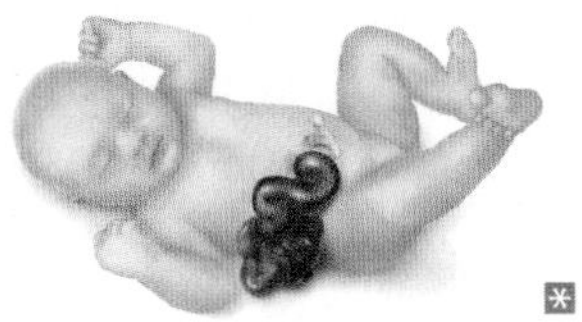
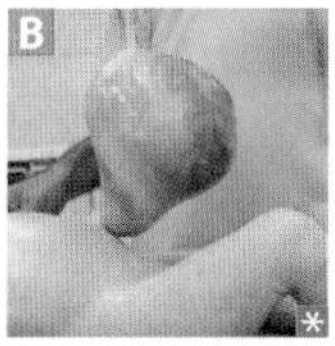
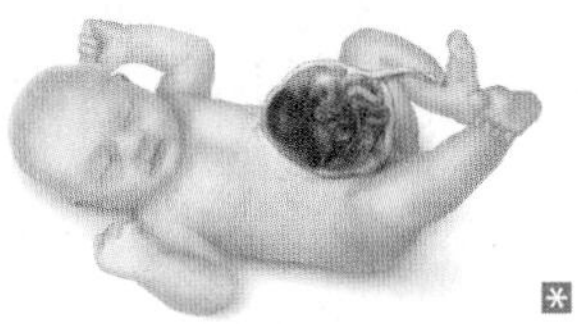

Congenital umbilical hernia

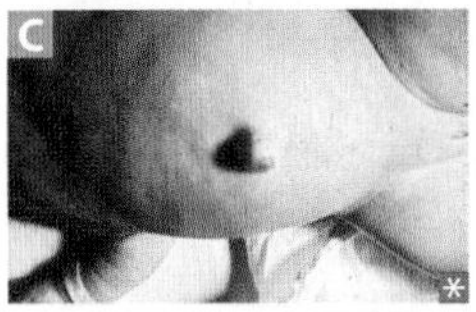

Failure of umbilical ring to close after physiologic herniation of midgut. Covered by skin C. Protrudes with ↑ intra-abdominal pressure (eg, crying). May be associated with congenital disorders (eg, Down syndrome, congenital hypothyroidism). Small defects usually close spontaneously.

Tracheoesophageal anomalies

Esophageal atresia (EA) with distal tracheoesophageal fistula (TEF) is the most common (85%) and often presents as polyhydramnios in utero (due to inability of fetus to swallow amniotic fluid). Neonates drool, choke, and vomit with first feeding. TEFs allow air to enter stomach (visible on CXR). Cyanosis is 2° to laryngospasm (to avoid reflux-related aspiration). Clinical test: failure to pass nasogastric tube into stomach.

In **H**-type, the fistula resembles the letter **H**. In pure EA, CXR shows gasless abdomen.

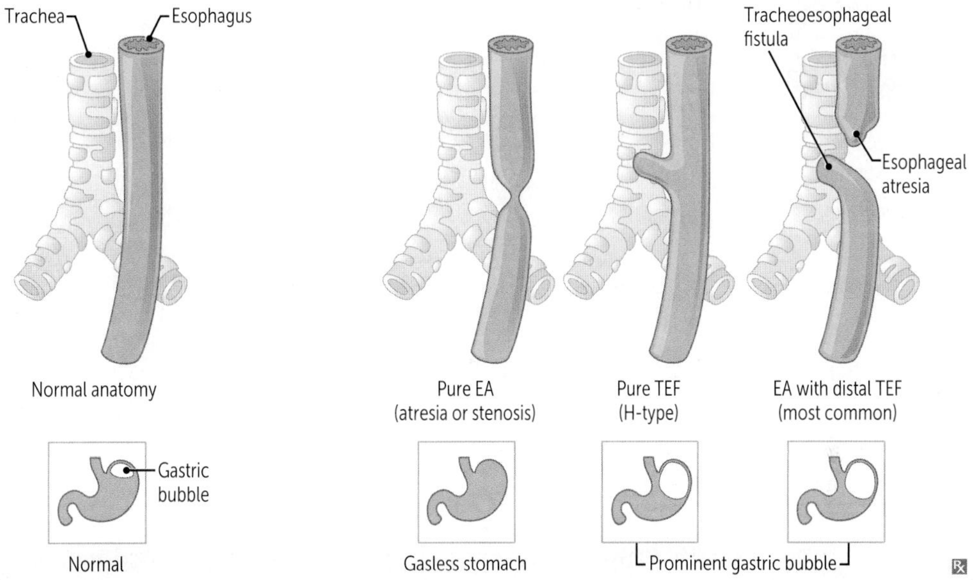

Intestinal atresia

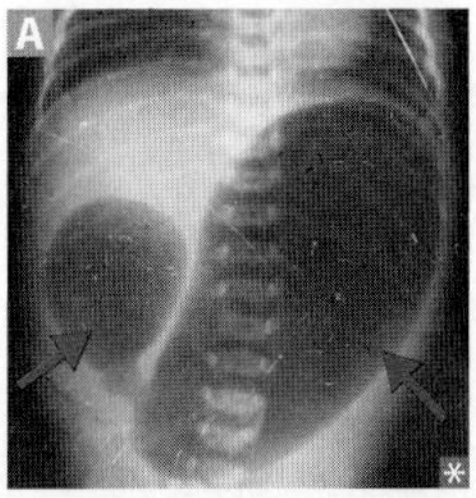

Presents with bilious vomiting and abdominal distension within first 1–2 days of life.

Duodenal atresia—failure to recanalize. X-ray A shows "double bubble" (dilated stomach, proximal duodenum). Associated with Down syndrome.

Jejunal and ileal atresia—disruption of mesenteric vessels (typically SMA) → ischemic necrosis of fetal intestine → segmental resorption: bowel becomes discontinuous. X-ray may show "triple bubble" (dilated stomach, duodenum, proximal jejunum) and gasless colon.

Hypertrophic pyloric stenosis

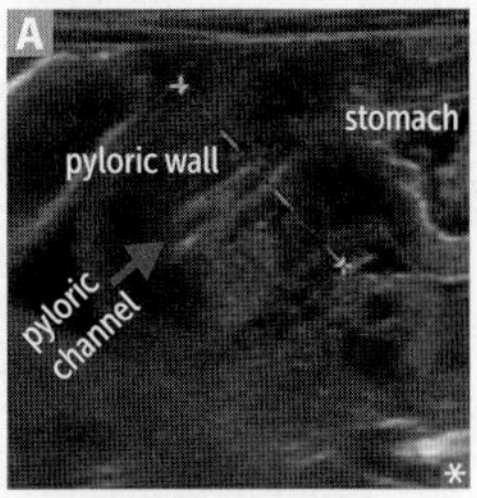

Most common cause of gastric outlet obstruction in infants (1:600). Palpable olive-shaped mass in epigastric region, visible peristaltic waves, and nonbilious projectile vomiting at ~ 2–6 weeks old. More common in firstborn males; associated with exposure to macrolides.

Results in hypokalemic hypochloremic metabolic alkalosis (2° to vomiting of gastric acid and subsequent volume contraction).

Ultrasound shows thickened and lengthened pylorus A.

Treatment: surgical incision of pyloric muscles (pyloromyotomy).

Pancreas and spleen embryology

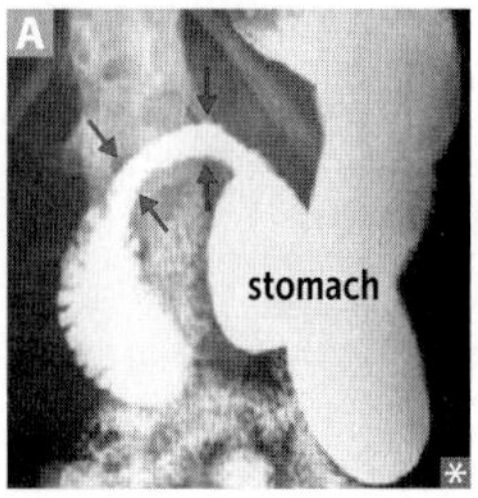
A
stomach

Pancreas—derived from foregut. Ventral pancreatic bud contributes to uncinate process and main pancreatic duct. The dorsal pancreatic bud alone becomes the body, tail, isthmus, and accessory pancreatic duct. Both the ventral and dorsal buds contribute to pancreatic head.

Annular pancreas—abnormal rotation of ventral pancreatic bud forms a ring of pancreatic tissue → encircles 2nd part of duodenum; may cause duodenal narrowing (arrows in A) and vomiting.

Pancreas divisum—ventral and dorsal parts fail to fuse at 7 weeks of development. Common anomaly; mostly asymptomatic, but may cause chronic abdominal pain and/or pancreatitis.

Spleen—arises in mesentery of stomach (hence is mesodermal) but has foregut supply (celiac trunk → splenic artery).

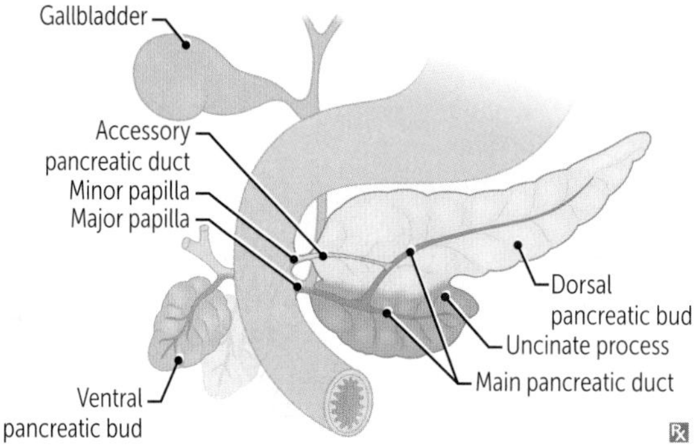
Gallbladder
Accessory pancreatic duct
Minor papilla
Major papilla
Dorsal pancreatic bud
Uncinate process
Main pancreatic duct
Ventral pancreatic bud

▶ GASTROINTESTINAL—ANATOMY

Retroperitoneal structures

Retroperitoneal structures A are posterior to (and outside of) the peritoneal cavity. Injuries to retroperitoneal structures can cause blood or gas accumulation in retroperitoneal space.

SAD PUCKER:
- Suprarenal (adrenal) glands [not shown]
- Aorta and IVC
- Duodenum (2nd through 4th parts)
- Pancreas (except tail)
- Ureters [not shown]
- Colon (descending and ascending)
- Kidneys
- Esophagus (thoracic portion) [not shown]
- Rectum (partially) [not shown]

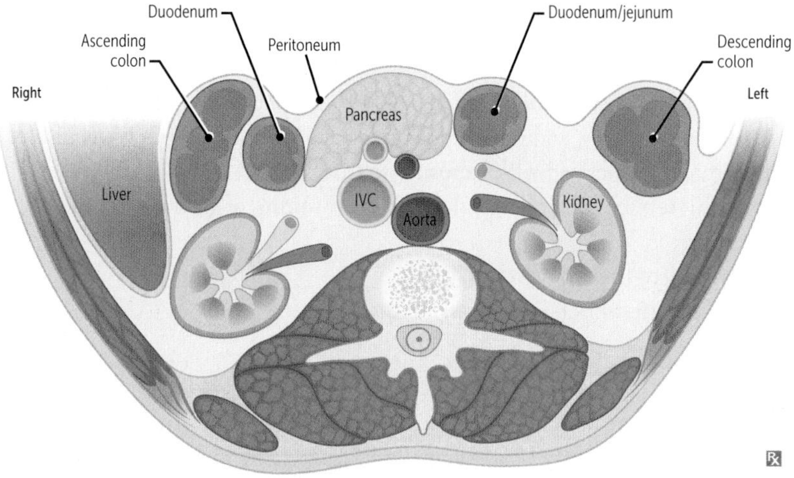
Duodenum
Ascending colon
Peritoneum
Duodenum/jejunum
Descending colon
Right
Left
Pancreas
Liver
IVC
Aorta
Kidney

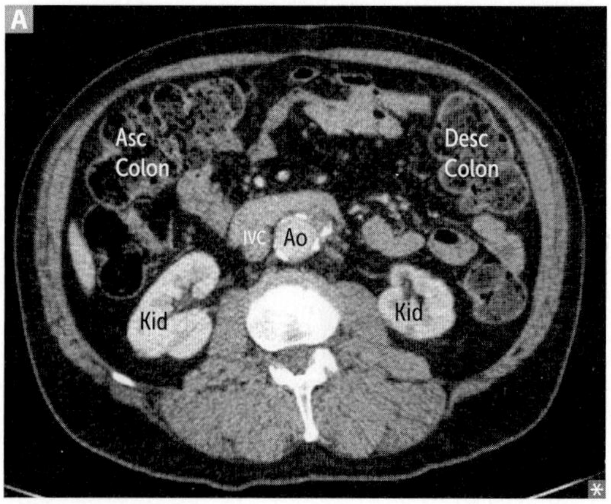
A
Asc Colon
Desc Colon
IVC
Ao
Kid
Kid

Important gastrointestinal ligaments

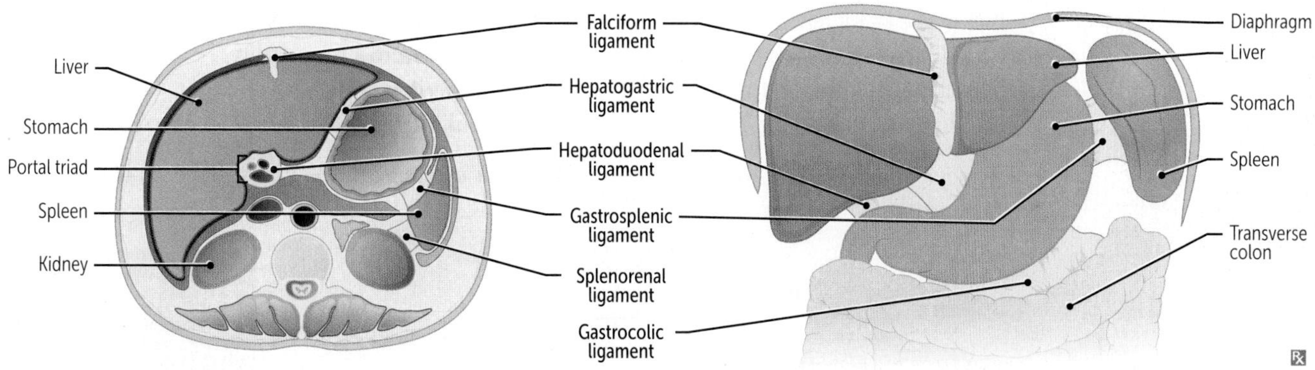

LIGAMENT	CONNECTS	STRUCTURES CONTAINED	NOTES
Falciform ligament	Liver to anterior abdominal wall	Ligamentum teres hepatis (derivative of fetal umbilical vein), patent paraumbilical veins	Derivative of ventral mesentery
Hepatoduodenal ligament	Liver to duodenum	Portal triad: proper hepatic artery, portal vein, common bile duct	Derivative of ventral mesentery Pringle maneuver—ligament is compressed manually or with a vascular clamp in omental foramen to control bleeding from hepatic inflow source Borders the omental foramen, which connects the greater and lesser sacs Part of lesser omentum
Hepatogastric ligament	Liver to lesser curvature of stomach	Gastric vessels	Derivative of ventral mesentery Separates greater and lesser sacs on the right May be cut during surgery to access lesser sac Part of lesser omentum
Gastrocolic ligament	Greater curvature and transverse colon	Gastroepiploic arteries	Derivative of dorsal mesentery Part of greater omentum
Gastrosplenic ligament	Greater curvature and spleen	Short gastrics, left gastroepiploic vessels	Derivative of dorsal mesentery Separates greater and lesser sacs on the left Part of greater omentum
Splenorenal ligament	Spleen to left pararenal space	Splenic artery and vein, tail of pancreas	Derivative of dorsal mesentery

Digestive tract anatomy

Layers of gut wall A (inside to outside—MSMS):

- Mucosa—epithelium, lamina propria, muscularis mucosa
- Submucosa—includes submucosal nerve plexus (Meissner), secretes fluid
- Muscularis externa—includes myenteric nerve plexus (Auerbach), motility
- Serosa (when intraperitoneal), adventitia (when retroperitoneal)

Ulcers can extend into submucosa, inner or outer muscular layer. Erosions are in mucosa only.

Frequency of basal electric rhythm (slow waves), which originate in the interstitial cells of Cajal: duodenum > ileum > stomach.

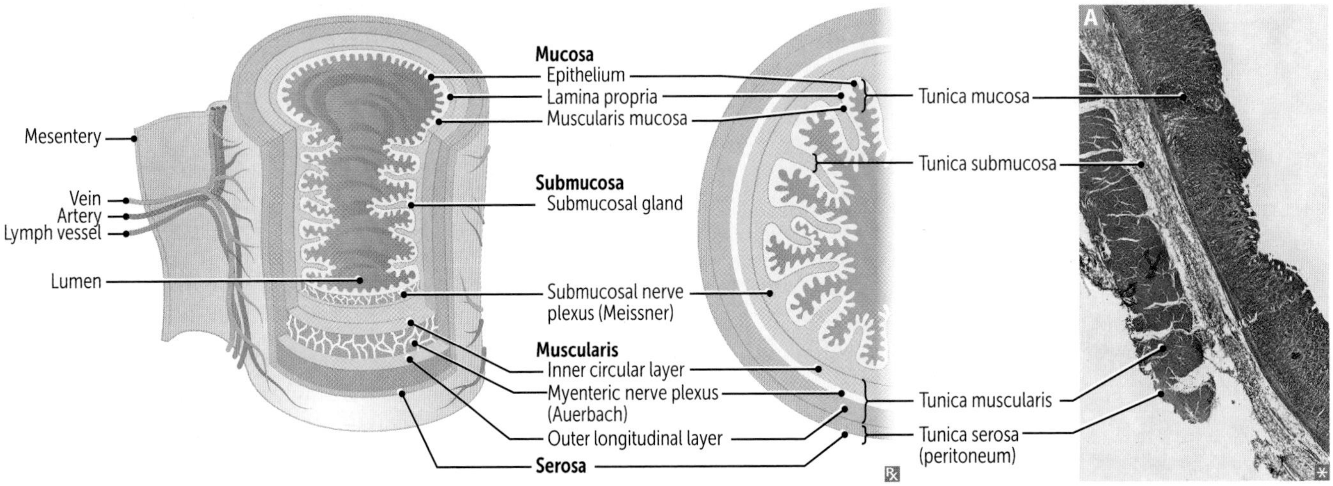

Digestive tract histology

Esophagus	Nonkeratinized stratified squamous epithelium. Upper 1/3, striated muscle; middle and lower 2/3 smooth muscle, with some overlap at the transition.
Stomach	Gastric glands A. Parietal cells are eosinophilic (pink, red arrow in B), chief cells are basophilic (black arrow in B).
Duodenum	Villi and microvilli ↑ absorptive surface. Brunner glands (bicarbonate-secreting cells of submucosa) and crypts of Lieberkühn (contain stem cells that replace enterocytes/goblet cells and Paneth cells that secrete defensins, lysozyme, and TNF).
Jejunum	Villi C, crypts of Lieberkühn, and plicae circulares (also present in distal duodenum).
Ileum	Villi, Peyer patches (arrow in D; lymphoid aggregates in lamina propria, submucosa), plicae circulares (proximal ileum), and crypts of Lieberkühn. Largest number of goblet cells in the small intestine.
Colon	Crypts of Lieberkühn with abundant goblet cells, but no villi E.

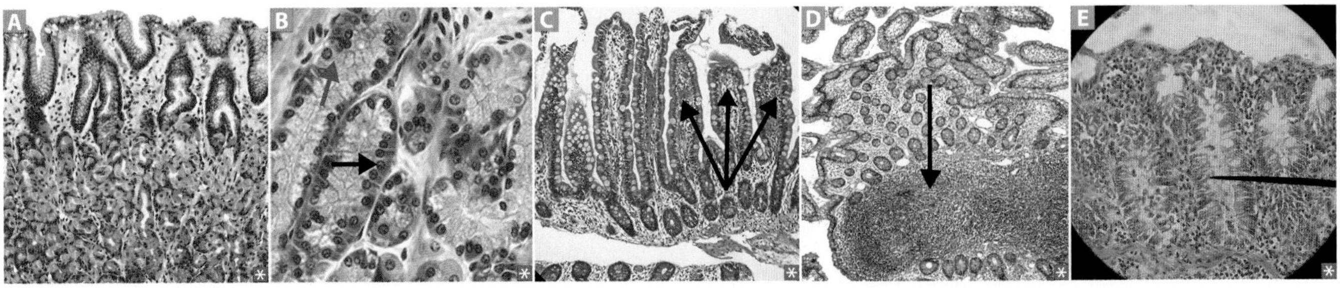

Abdominal aorta and branches

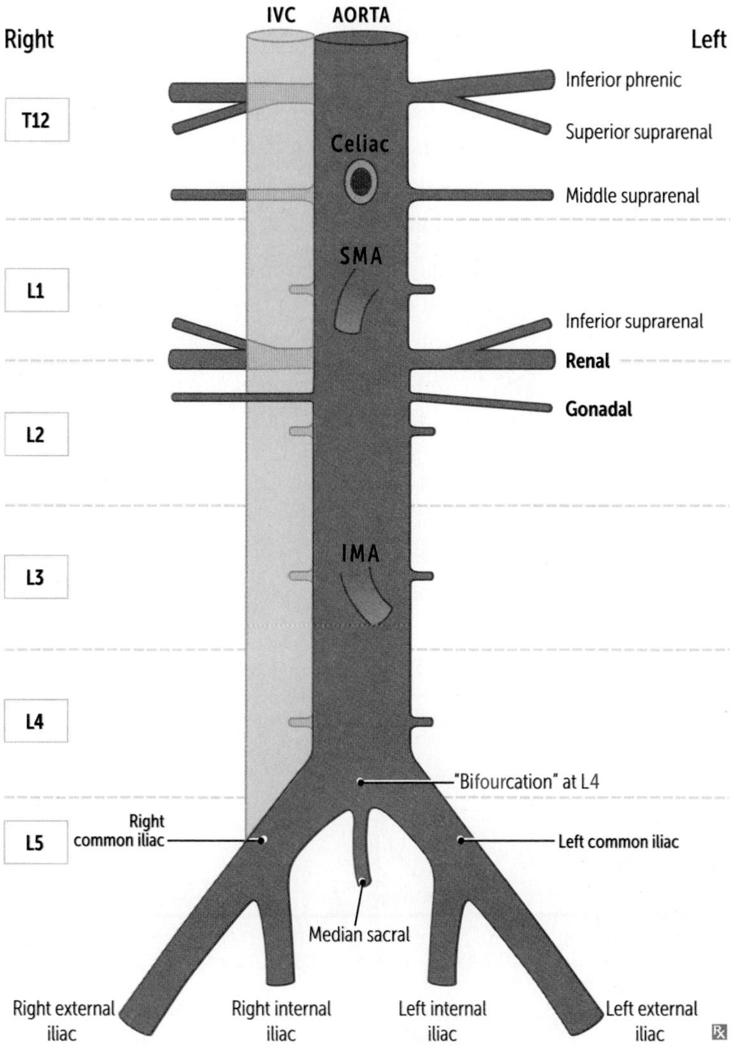
IVC
AORTA
Right
Left
T12
L1
L2
L3
L4
L5
Celiac
SMA
IMA
Inferior phrenic
Superior suprarenal
Middle suprarenal
Inferior suprarenal
Renal
Gonadal
"Bifourcation" at L4
Right common iliac
Left common iliac
Median sacral
Right external iliac
Right internal iliac
Left internal iliac
Left external iliac

Arteries supplying GI structures are single and branch anteriorly.

Arteries supplying non-GI structures are paired and branch laterally and posteriorly.

Two areas of the colon have dual blood supply from distal arterial branches ("watershed regions") → susceptible in colonic ischemia:

- Splenic flexure—SMA and IMA
- Rectosigmoid junction—the last sigmoid arterial branch from the IMA and superior rectal artery

Nutcracker syndrome—compression of left renal vein between superior mesenteric artery and aorta. May cause abdominal (flank) pain, gross hematuria (from rupture of thin-walled renal varicosities), left-sided varicocele.

Superior mesenteric artery syndrome—characterized by intermittent intestinal obstruction symptoms (primarily postprandial pain) when SMA and aorta compress transverse (third) portion of duodenum. Typically occurs in conditions associated with diminished mesenteric fat (eg, low body weight/malnutrition).

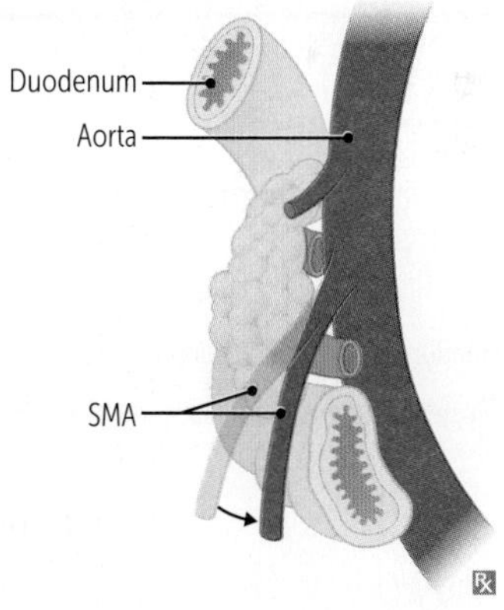
Duodenum
Aorta
SMA

Gastrointestinal blood supply and innervation

EMBRYONIC GUT REGION	ARTERY	PARASYMPATHETIC INNERVATION	VERTEBRAL LEVEL	STRUCTURES SUPPLIED
Foregut	Celiac	Vagus	T12/L1	Pharynx (vagus nerve only) and lower esophagus (celiac artery only) to proximal duodenum; liver, gallbladder, pancreas, spleen (mesoderm)
Midgut	SMA	Vagus	L1	Distal duodenum to proximal 2/3 of transverse colon
Hindgut	IMA	Pelvic	L3	Distal 1/3 of transverse colon to upper portion of anal canal

Celiac trunk

Branches of celiac trunk: common hepatic, splenic, and left gastric. These constitute the main blood supply of the foregut.

Strong anastomoses exist between:

- Left and right gastroepiploics
- Left and right gastrics

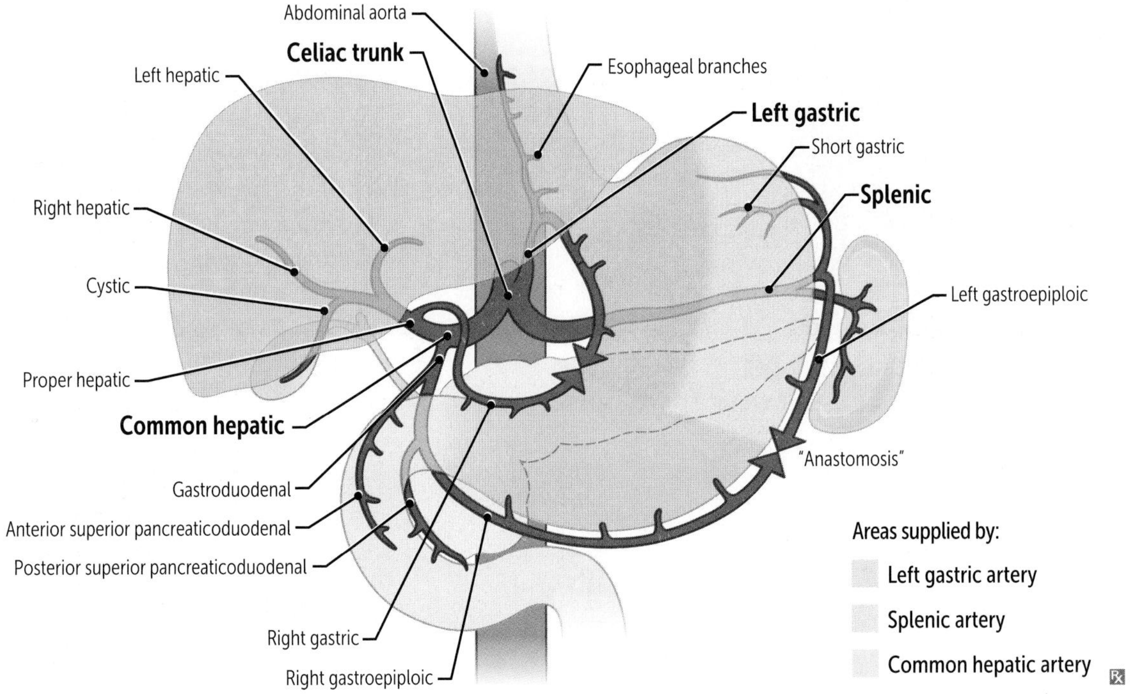

Portosystemic anastomoses

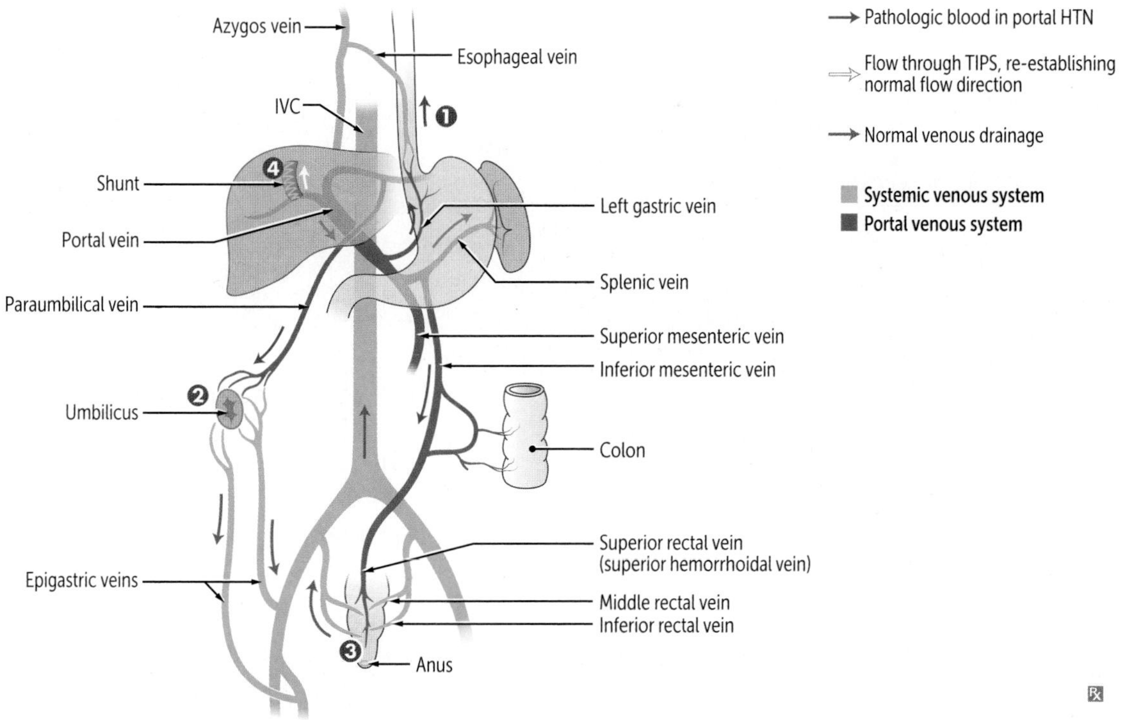

SITE OF ANASTOMOSIS	CLINICAL SIGN	PORTAL ↔ SYSTEMIC
❶ Esophagus	Esophageal varices	Left gastric ↔ esophageal (drains into azygos)
❷ Umbilicus	**Caput** medusae	Paraumbilical ↔ small epigastric veins of the anterior abdominal wall.
❸ Rectum	Anorectal varices	Superior rectal ↔ middle and inferior rectal

Varices of **gut, butt,** and **caput** (medusae) are commonly seen with portal hypertension.

❹ Treatment with a **T**ransjugular **I**ntrahepatic **P**ortosystemic **S**hunt (**TIPS**) between the portal vein and hepatic vein relieves portal hypertension by shunting blood to the systemic circulation, bypassing the liver. TIPS can precipitate hepatic encephalopathy due to ↓ clearance of ammonia from shunting.

Pectinate line

Also called dentate line. Formed where endoderm (hindgut) meets ectoderm.

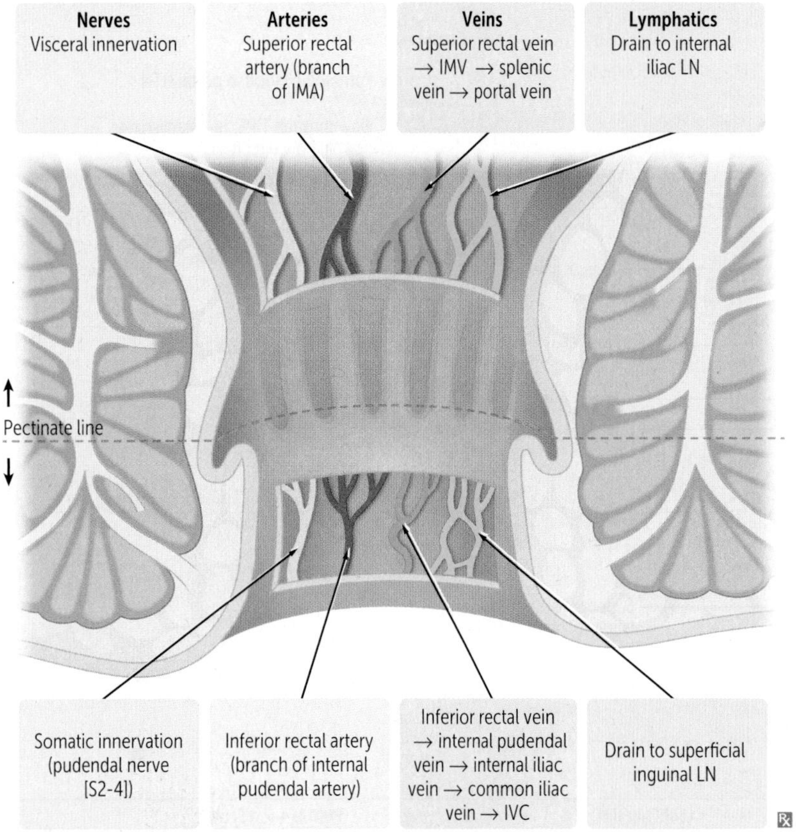

Nerves
Visceral innervation
Arteries
Superior rectal artery (branch of IMA)
Veins
Superior rectal vein → IMV → splenic vein → portal vein
Lymphatics
Drain to internal iliac LN
Pectinate line
Somatic innervation (pudendal nerve [S2-4])
Inferior rectal artery (branch of internal pudendal artery)
Inferior rectal vein → internal pudendal vein → internal iliac vein → common iliac vein → IVC
Drain to superficial inguinal LN

Above pectinate line: internal hemorrhoids, adenocarcinoma.

Internal hemorrhoids receive visceral innervation and are therefore **not painful**.

Below pectinate line: external hemorrhoids, anal fissures, squamous cell carcinoma.

External hemorrhoids receive somatic innervation (inferior rectal branch of pudendal nerve) and are therefore **painful** if thrombosed.

Anal fissure—tear in anoderm below pectinate line. Pain while pooping; blood on toilet paper. Located in the posterior midline because this area is poorly perfused. Associated with low-fiber diets and constipation.

Liver tissue architecture

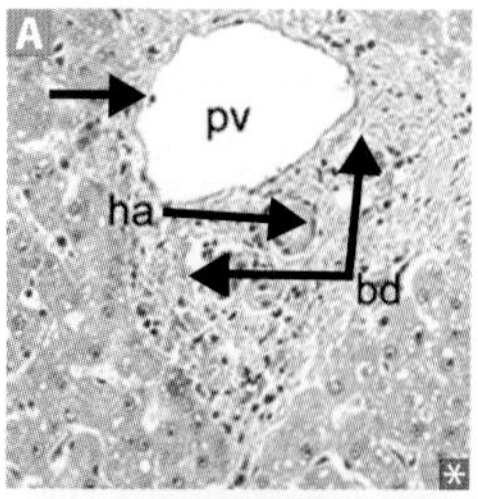
A
pv
ha
bd

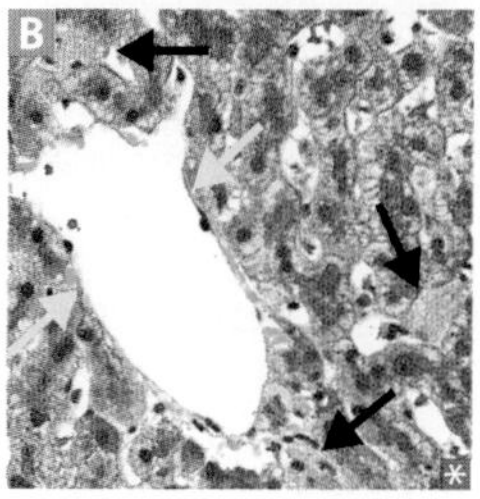
B

The functional unit of the liver is made up of hexagonally arranged lobules surrounding the central vein with portal triads on the edges (consisting of a portal vein, hepatic artery, bile ducts, as well as lymphatics) A.

Apical surface of hepatocytes faces bile canaliculi. Basolateral surface faces sinusoids.

Kupffer cells (specialized macrophages) located in sinusoids (black arrows in B; yellow arrows show central vein) clear bacteria and damaged or senescent RBCs.

Hepatic stellate (Ito) cells in space of Disse store vitamin A (when quiescent) and produce extracellular matrix (when activated). Responsible for hepatic fibrosis.

Zone I—periportal zone:

- Affected 1st by viral hepatitis
- Best oxygenated, most resistant to circulatory compromise
- Ingested toxins (eg, cocaine)

Zone II—intermediate zone:

- Yellow fever

Zone III—pericentral (centrilobular) zone:

- Affected 1st by ischemia (least oxygenated)
- High concentration of cytochrome P-450
- Most sensitive to metabolic toxins (eg, ethanol, CCl_4, halothane, rifampin, acetaminophen)
- Site of alcoholic hepatitis

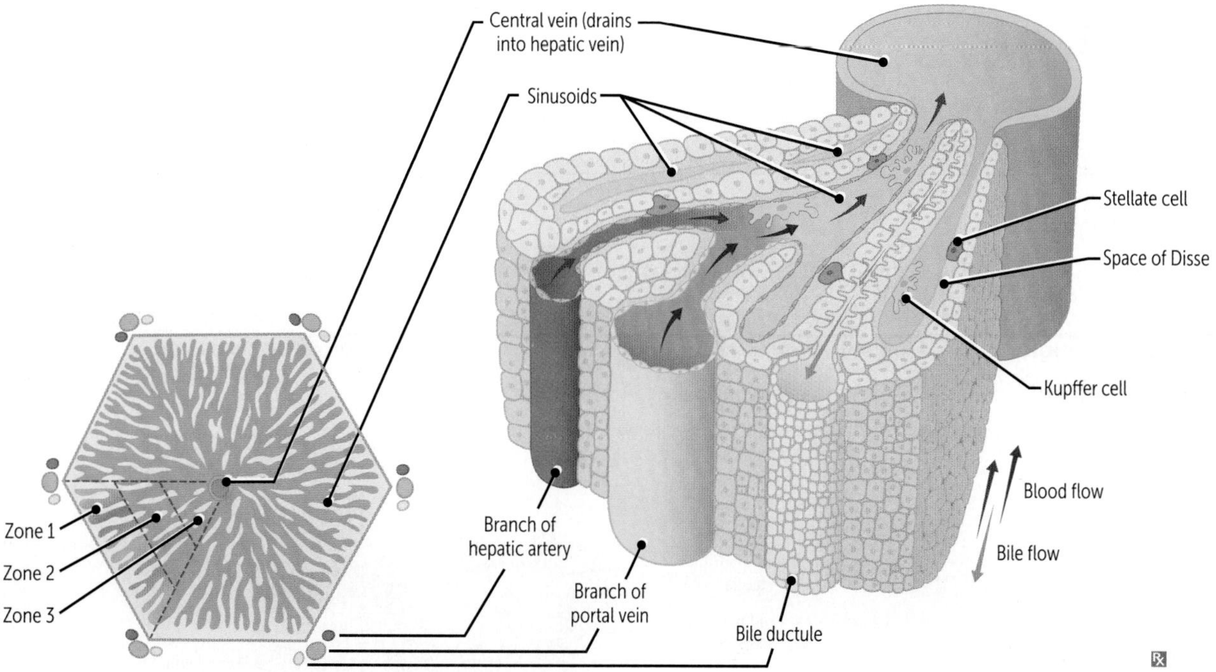
Central vein (drains into hepatic vein)
Sinusoids
Stellate cell
Space of Disse
Kupffer cell
Zone 1
Zone 2
Zone 3
Branch of hepatic artery
Branch of portal vein
Bile ductule
Blood flow
Bile flow

Biliary structures

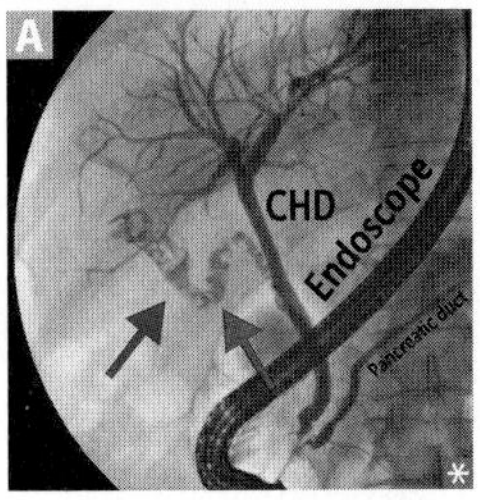

Cholangiography shows filling defects in gallbladder (blue arrow in A) and cystic duct (red arrow in A).

Gallstones that reach the confluence of the common bile and pancreatic ducts at the ampulla of Vater can block both the common bile and pancreatic ducts (double duct sign), causing both cholangitis and pancreatitis, respectively.

Tumors that arise in head of pancreas (usually ductal adenocarcinoma) can cause obstruction of common bile duct → enlarged gallbladder with painless jaundice (Courvoisier sign).

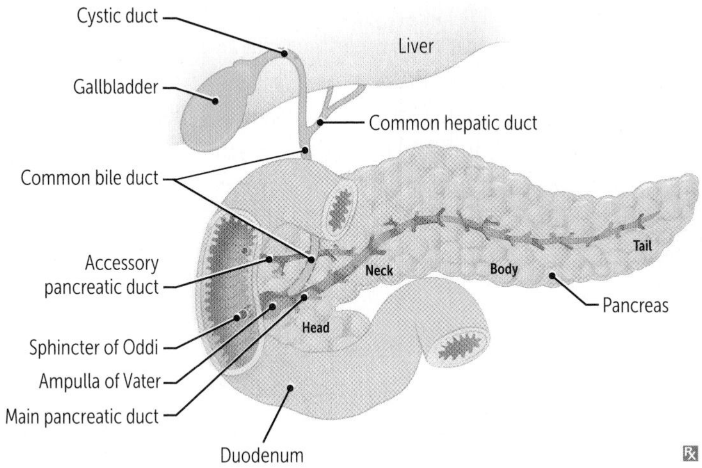

Femoral region

ORGANIZATION	**Lateral to medial**: nerve-artery-vein-lymphatics.	You go from **lateral to medial** to find your **navel**.
Femoral triangle	Contains femoral nerve, artery, vein.	**Venous** near the **penis**.
Femoral sheath	Fascial tube 3–4 cm below inguinal ligament. Contains femoral vein, artery, and canal (deep inguinal lymph nodes) but not femoral nerve.	

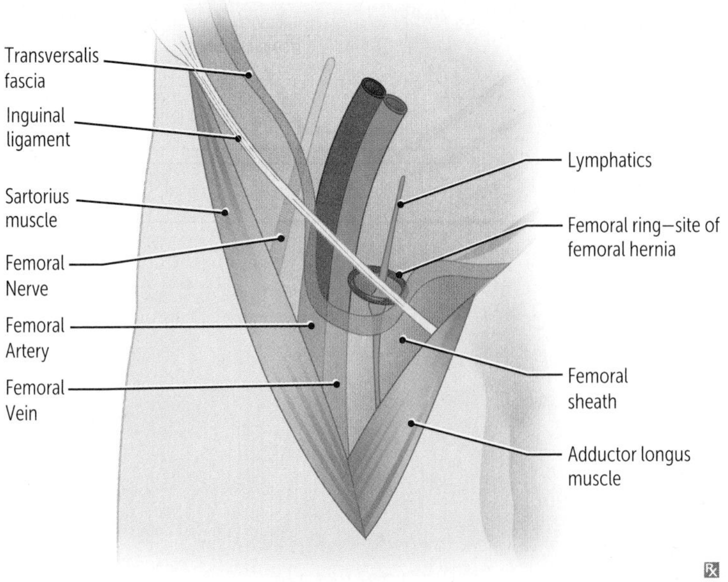

Inguinal canal

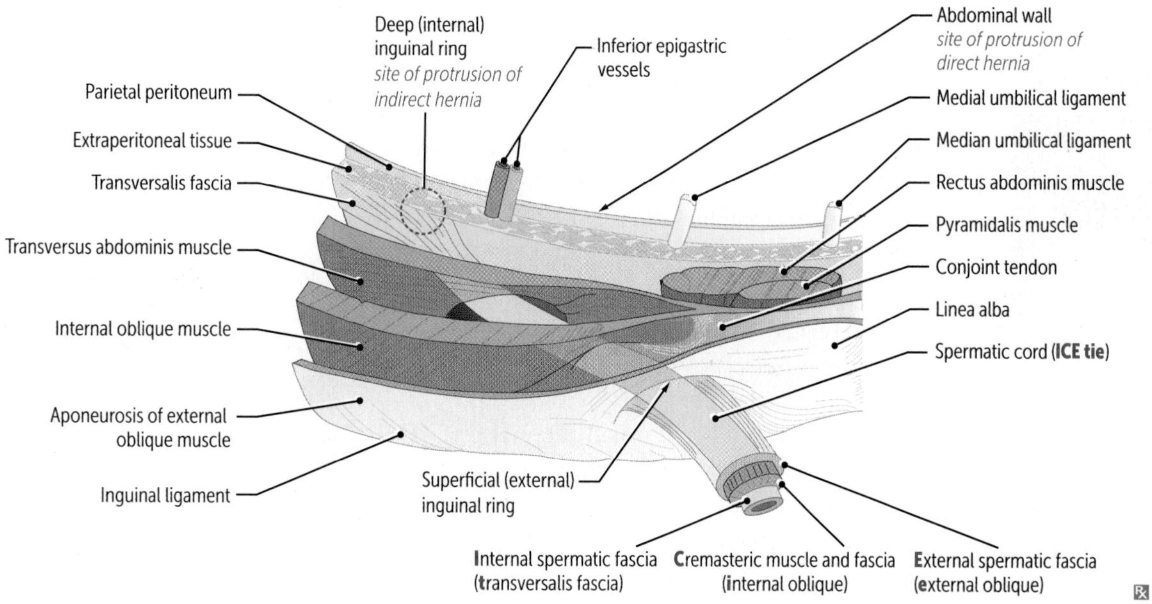
Deep (internal) inguinal ring
site of protrusion of indirect hernia
Inferior epigastric vessels
Abdominal wall
site of protrusion of direct hernia
Parietal peritoneum
Medial umbilical ligament
Extraperitoneal tissue
Median umbilical ligament
Transversalis fascia
Rectus abdominis muscle
Pyramidalis muscle
Transversus abdominis muscle
Conjoint tendon
Linea alba
Internal oblique muscle
Spermatic cord (ICE tie)
Aponeurosis of external oblique muscle
Inguinal ligament
Superficial (external) inguinal ring
Internal spermatic fascia (transversalis fascia)
Cremasteric muscle and fascia (internal oblique)
External spermatic fascia (external oblique)

Abdominal wall

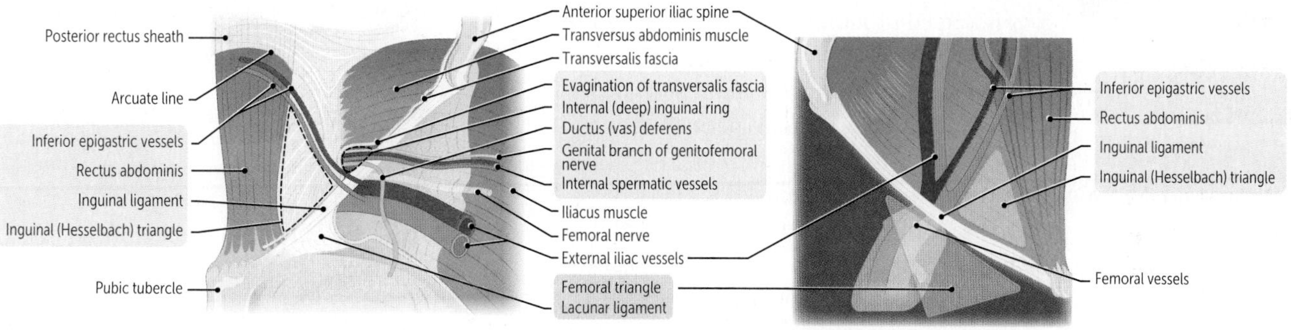
Posterior rectus sheath
Arcuate line
Inferior epigastric vessels
Rectus abdominis
Inguinal ligament
Inguinal (Hesselbach) triangle
Pubic tubercle
Anterior superior iliac spine
Transversus abdominis muscle
Transversalis fascia
Evagination of transversalis fascia
Internal (deep) inguinal ring
Ductus (vas) deferens
Genital branch of genitofemoral nerve
Internal spermatic vessels
Iliacus muscle
Femoral nerve
External iliac vessels
Femoral triangle
Lacunar ligament
Inferior epigastric vessels
Rectus abdominis
Inguinal ligament
Inguinal (Hesselbach) triangle
Femoral vessels

Anterior abdominal wall
(viewed from inside)

Anterior abdominal wall
(viewed from outside)

Hernias

Protrusion of peritoneum through an opening, usually at a site of weakness. Contents may be at risk for incarceration (not reducible back into abdomen/pelvis) and strangulation (ischemia and necrosis). Complicated hernias can present with tenderness, erythema, fever.

Diaphragmatic hernia

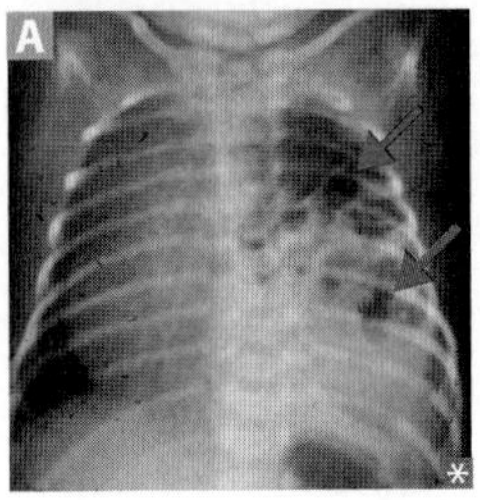

Abdominal structures enter the thorax. Most common causes:

- Infants—congenital defect of pleuroperitoneal membrane → left-sided herniation (right hemidiaphragm is relatively protected by liver) A.
- Adults—laxity/defect of phrenoesophageal membrane → **hiatal hernia** (herniation of stomach through esophageal hiatus).

Sliding hiatal hernia—gastroesophageal junction is displaced upward as gastric cardia slides into hiatus; "hourglass stomach." Most common type. Associated with GERD.

Paraesophageal hiatal hernia—gastroesophageal junction is usually normal but gastric fundus protrudes into the thorax.

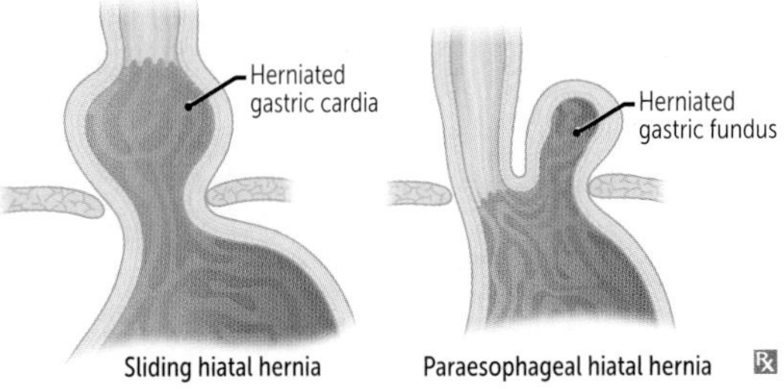

Indirect inguinal hernia

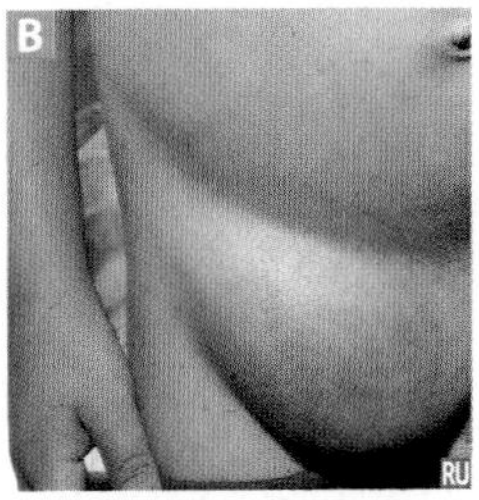

Goes through the internal (deep) inguinal ring, external (superficial) inguinal ring, and into the groin. Enters internal inguinal ring lateral to inferior epigastric vessels. Caused by failure of processus vaginalis to close (can form hydrocele). May be noticed in **in**fants or discovered in adulthood. Much more common in males B.

Follows the pathway of testicular descent. Covered by all 3 layers of spermatic fascia.

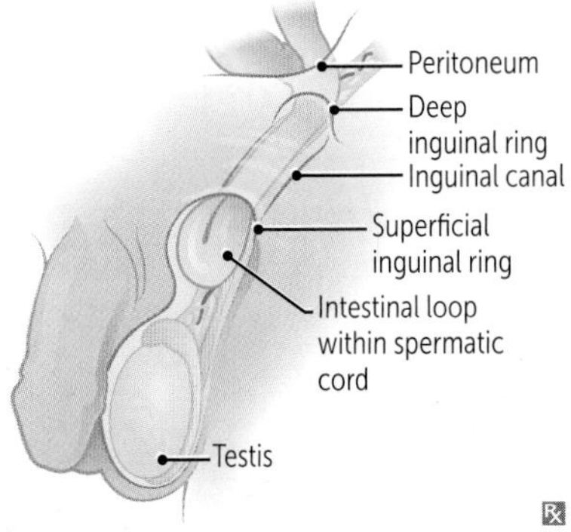

Direct inguinal hernia

Protrudes through inguinal (Hesselbach) triangle. Bulges directly through parietal peritoneum medial to the inferior epigastric vessels but lateral to the rectus abdominis. Goes through external (superficial) inguinal ring only. Covered by external spermatic fascia. Usually occurs in older males due to acquired weakness of transversalis fascia.

MDs don't **lie**:

- **M**edial to inferior epigastric vessels = **D**irect hernia.
- **L**ateral to inferior epigastric vessels = **i**ndirect hernia.

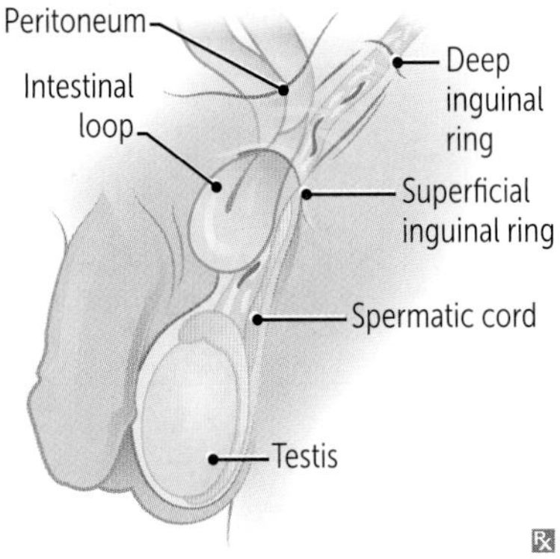

Femoral hernia

Protrudes below inguinal ligament through femoral canal below and lateral to pubic tubercle. More common in **fem**ales, but overall inguinal hernias are the most common.

More likely to present with incarceration or strangulation (vs inguinal hernia).

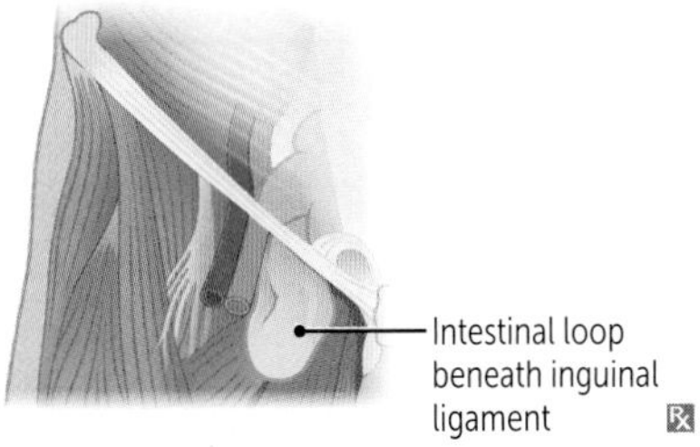

▶ GASTROINTESTINAL—PHYSIOLOGY

Gastrointestinal regulatory substances

REGULATORY SUBSTANCE	SOURCE	ACTION	REGULATION	NOTES
Gastrin	G cells (antrum of stomach, duodenum)	↑ gastric H^+ secretion ↑ growth of gastric mucosa ↑ gastric motility	↑ by stomach distention/alkalinization, amino acids, peptides, vagal stimulation via gastrin-releasing peptide (GRP) ↓ by pH < 1.5	↑ by chronic PPI use ↑ in chronic atrophic gastritis (eg, *H pylori*) ↑↑ in Zollinger-Ellison syndrome (gastrinoma)
Somatostatin	D cells (pancreatic islets, GI mucosa)	↓ gastric acid and pepsinogen secretion ↓ pancreatic and small intestine fluid secretion ↓ gallbladder contraction ↓ insulin and glucagon release	↑ by acid ↓ by vagal stimulation	Inhibits secretion of various hormones (encourages **somato-stasis**) Octreotide is an analog used to treat acromegaly, carcinoid syndrome, VIPoma, and variceal bleeding
Cholecystokinin	I cells (duodenum, jejunum)	↑ pancreatic secretion ↑ gallbladder contraction ↓ gastric emptying ↑ sphincter of Oddi relaxation	↑ by fatty acids, amino acids	Acts on neural muscarinic pathways to cause pancreatic secretion
Secretin	S cells (duodenum)	↑ pancreatic HCO_3^- secretion ↓ gastric acid secretion ↑ bile secretion	↑ by acid, fatty acids in lumen of duodenum	↑ HCO_3^- neutralizes gastric acid in duodenum, allowing pancreatic enzymes to function
Glucose-dependent insulinotropic peptide	K cells (duodenum, jejunum)	Exocrine: ↓ gastric H^+ secretion Endocrine: ↑ insulin release	↑ by fatty acids, amino acids, oral glucose	Also called gastric inhibitory peptide (GIP) Oral glucose load ↑ insulin compared to IV equivalent due to GIP secretion
Motilin	Small intestine	Produces migrating motor complexes (MMCs)	↑ in fasting state	Motilin receptor agonists (eg, erythromycin) are used to stimulate intestinal peristalsis.
Vasoactive intestinal polypeptide	Parasympathetic ganglia in sphincters, gallbladder, small intestine	↑ intestinal water and electrolyte secretion ↑ relaxation of intestinal smooth muscle and sphincters	↑ by distention and vagal stimulation ↓ by adrenergic input	VIPoma—non-α, non-β islet cell pancreatic tumor that secretes VIP; associated with **W**atery **D**iarrhea, **H**ypokalemia, **A**chlorhydria (**WDHA** syndrome)
Nitric oxide		↑ smooth muscle relaxation, including lower esophageal sphincter (LES)		Loss of NO secretion is implicated in ↑ LES tone of achalasia
Ghrelin	Stomach	↑ appetite ("ghrowlin' stomach")	↑ in fasting state ↓ by food	↑ in Prader-Willi syndrome ↓ after gastric bypass surgery

Gastrointestinal secretory products

PRODUCT	SOURCE	ACTION	REGULATION	NOTES
Intrinsic factor	Parietal cells (stomach A)	Vitamin B_{12}–binding protein (required for B_{12} uptake in terminal ileum)		Autoimmune destruction of parietal cells → chronic gastritis and pernicious anemia
Gastric acid	Parietal cells (stomach)	↓ stomach pH	↑ by histamine, vagal stimulation (ACh), gastrin ↓ by somatostatin, GIP, prostaglandin, secretin	
Pepsin	Chief cells (stomach)	Protein digestion	↑ by vagal stimulation (ACh), local acid	Pepsinogen (inactive) is converted to pepsin (active) in the presence of H^+
Bicarbonate	Mucosal cells (stomach, duodenum, salivary glands, pancreas) and Brunner glands (duodenum)	Neutralizes acid	↑ by pancreatic and biliary secretion with secretin	Trapped in mucus that covers the gastric epithelium

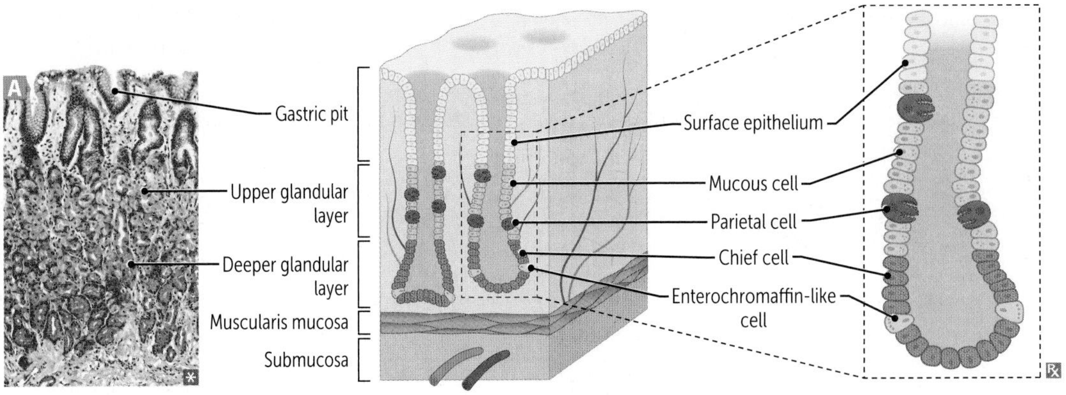
A
Gastric pit
Upper glandular layer
Deeper glandular layer
Muscularis mucosa
Submucosa
Surface epithelium
Mucous cell
Parietal cell
Chief cell
Enterochromaffin-like cell

Locations of gastrointestinal secretory cells

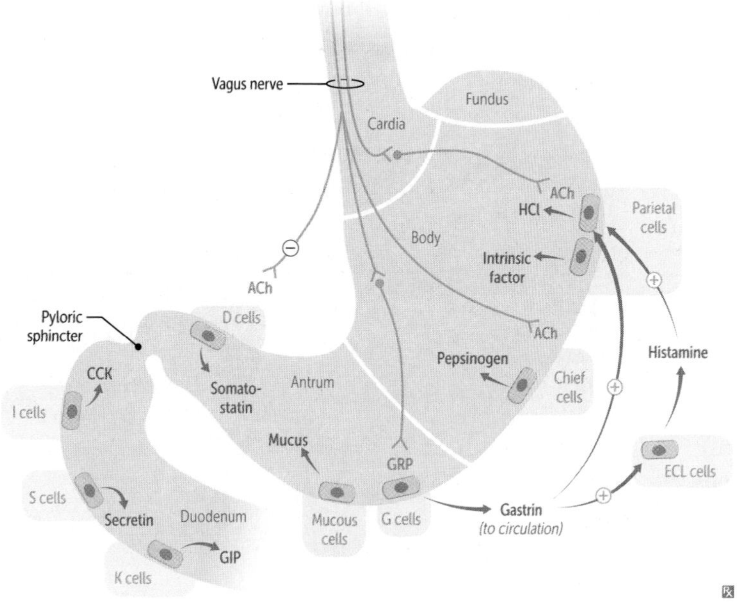

Gastrin ↑ acid secretion primarily through its effects on enterochromaffin-like (ECL) cells (leading to histamine release) rather than through its direct effect on parietal cells.

Pancreatic secretions Isotonic fluid; low flow → high Cl^-, high flow → high HCO_3^-.

ENZYME	ROLE	NOTES
α-amylase	Starch digestion	Secreted in active form
Lipases	Fat digestion	
Proteases	Protein digestion	Includes trypsin, chymotrypsin, elastase, carboxypeptidases Secreted as proenzymes also called zymogens
Trypsinogen	Converted to active enzyme trypsin → activation of other proenzymes and cleaving of additional trypsinogen molecules into active trypsin (positive feedback loop)	Converted to trypsin by enterokinase/enteropeptidase, a brush-border enzyme on duodenal and jejunal mucosa

Carbohydrate absorption

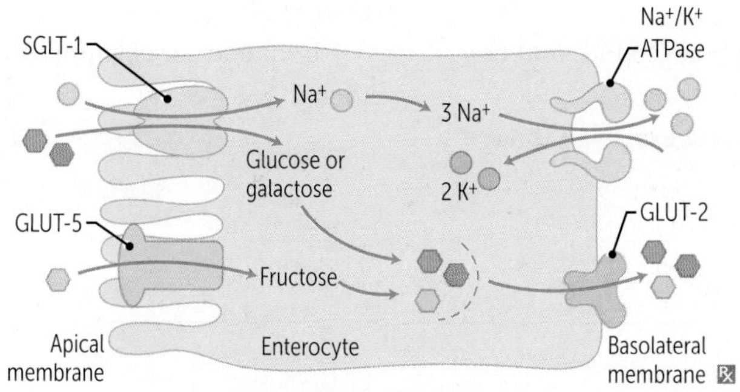

Only monosaccharides (glucose, galactose, fructose) are absorbed by enterocytes. Glucose and galactose are taken up by SGLT1 (Na^+ dependent). Fructose is taken up via facilitated diffusion by GLUT5. All are transported to blood by GLUT2.

D-xylose test: simple sugar that is passively absorbed in proximal small intestine; blood and urine levels ↓ with mucosal damage, normal in pancreatic insufficiency.

Vitamin and mineral absorption

Iron absorbed as Fe^{2+} in duodenum.
Folate absorbed in small bowel.
Vitamin **B_{12}** absorbed in terminal ileum along with bile salts, requires intrinsic factor.

Iron fist, **Bro**
Vitamin and mineral deficiencies may develop in patients with small bowel disease or after resection (eg, vitamin B_{12} deficiency after terminal ileum resection).

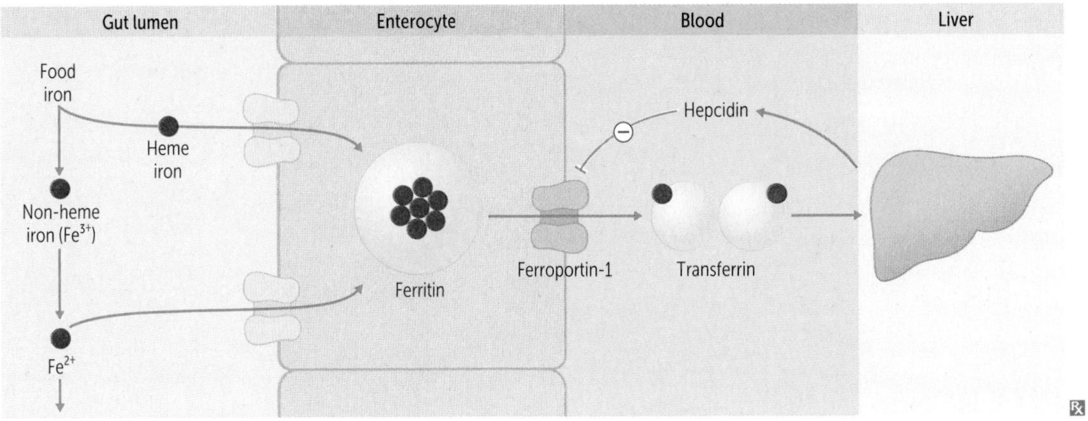

Peyer patches

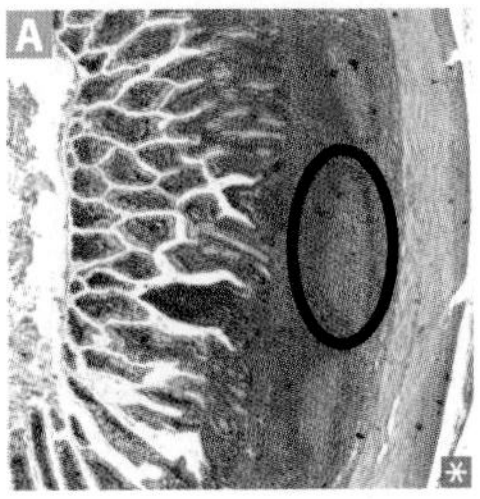

Unencapsulated lymphoid tissue A found in lamina propria and submucosa of ileum. Contain specialized **M** cells that sample and present antigens to i**M**mune cells.
B cells stimulated in germinal centers of Peyer patches differentiate into IgA-secreting plasma cells, which ultimately reside in lamina propria. IgA receives protective secretory component and is then transported across the epithelium to the gut to deal with intraluminal antigen.

Think of **IgA**, the **I**ntra-gut **A**ntibody

Bile

Composed of bile salts (bile acids conjugated to glycine or taurine, making them water soluble), phospholipids, cholesterol, bilirubin, water, and ions. Cholesterol 7α-hydroxylase catalyzes rate-limiting step of bile acid synthesis.
Functions:
- Digestion and absorption of lipids and fat-soluble vitamins
- Bilirubin and cholesterol excretion (body's 1° means of elimination)
- Antimicrobial activity (via membrane disruption)

↓ absorption of enteric bile salts at distal ileum (as in short bowel syndrome, Crohn disease) prevents normal fat absorption and may cause bile acid diarrhea.
Calcium, which normally binds oxalate, binds fat instead, so free oxalate is absorbed by gut → ↑ frequency of calcium oxalate kidney stones.

Bilirubin

Heme is metabolized by heme oxygenase to biliverdin, which is subsequently reduced to bilirubin. Unconjugated bilirubin is removed from blood by liver, conjugated with glucuronate, and excreted in bile.

Direct bilirubin: conjugated with glucuronic acid; water soluble (**di**ssolves in water).

Indirect bilirubin: unconjugated; water **in**soluble.

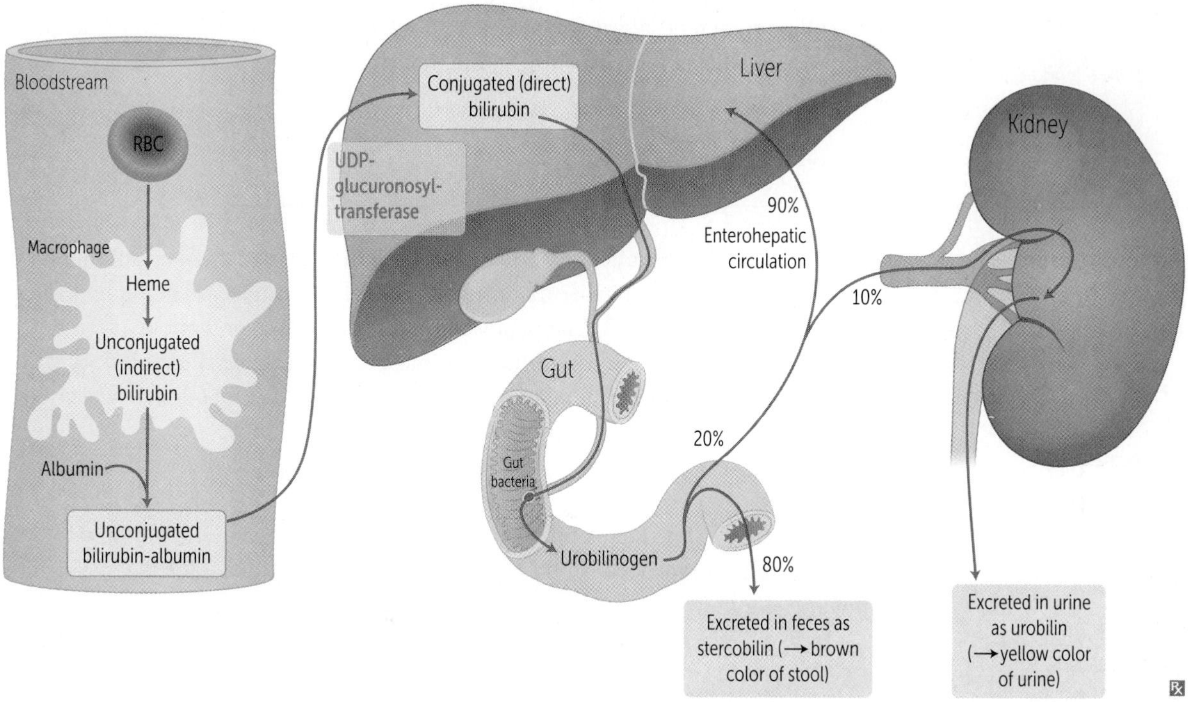

▶ GASTROINTESTINAL—PATHOLOGY

Sialolithiasis

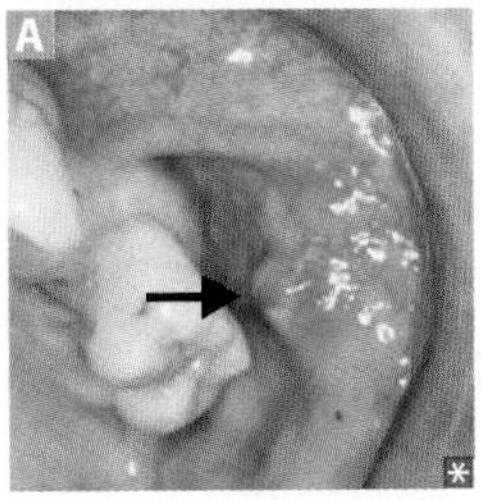

Stone(s) in salivary gland duct A. Can occur in 3 major salivary glands (parotid, submandibular, sublingual). Single stone more common in submandibular gland (Wharton duct).

Associated with salivary stasis (eg, dehydration) and trauma.

Presents as recurrent pre-/periprandial pain and swelling in affected gland.

Sialadenitis—inflammation of salivary gland due to obstruction, infection (eg, *S aureus*, mumps virus), or immune-mediated mechanisms (eg, Sjögren syndrome).

Salivary gland tumors

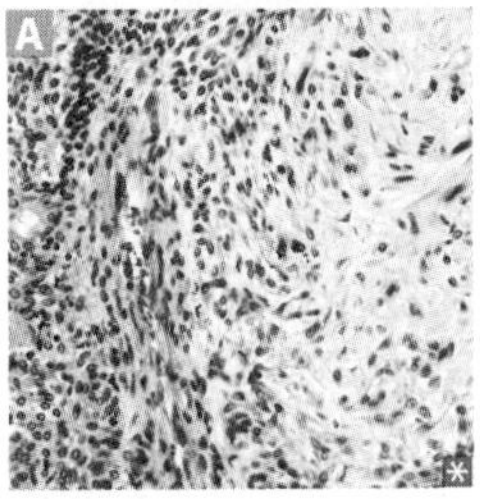

Most are benign and commonly affect parotid gland (80-85%). Nearly half of all submandibular gland neoplasms and most sublingual and minor salivary gland tumors are malignant. Typically present as painless mass/swelling. Facial paralysis or pain suggests malignant involvement.

- Pleomorphic adenoma (benign mixed tumor)—most common salivary gland tumor A. Composed of chondromyxoid stroma and epithelium and recurs if incompletely excised or ruptured intraoperatively. May undergo malignant transformation.
- Mucoepidermoid carcinoma—most common malignant tumor, has mucinous and squamous components.
- **War**thin tumor (papillary cystadenoma lymphomatosum)—benign cystic tumor with **germ**inal centers. Associated with tobacco **smoking**. Bilateral in 10%; multifocal in 10%. "**War**riors from **Germ**any love **smoking**."

Achalasia

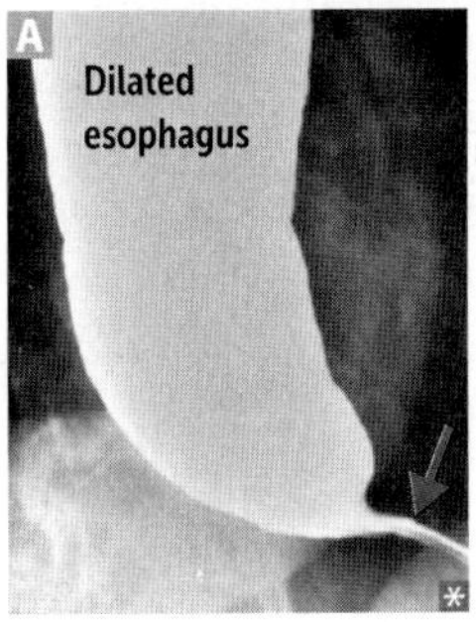

Failure of LES to relax due to degeneration of inhibitory neurons (containing NO and VIP) in the myenteric (Auerbach) plexus of esophageal wall.

1° achalasia is idiopathic. 2° achalasia may arise from Chagas disease (*T cruzi* infection) or extraesophageal malignancies (mass effect or paraneoplastic). **Chagas** disease can cause **achalasia**.

Presents with progressive dysphagia to solids and liquids (vs obstruction—primarily solids).

Associated with ↑ risk of esophageal cancer.

Manometry findings include uncoordinated or absent peristalsis with ↑ LES resting pressure.

Barium swallow shows dilated esophagus with area of distal stenosis ("bird's beak" A).

Treatment: surgery, endoscopic procedures (eg, botulinum toxin injection).

Esophageal pathologies

Gastroesophageal reflux disease	Commonly presents as heartburn, regurgitation, dysphagia. May also present as chronic cough, hoarseness (laryngopharyngeal reflux). Associated with asthma. Transient decreases in LES tone.
Eosinophilic esophagitis	Infiltration of eosinophils in the esophagus often in atopic patients. Etiology is multifactorial. Food allergens → dysphagia, food impaction. Esophageal rings and linear furrows often seen on endoscopy.
Esophagitis	Associated with reflux, infection in immunocompromised (*Candida:* white pseudomembrane A; HSV-1: punched-out ulcers; CMV: linear ulcers), caustic ingestion, or pill-induced esophagitis (eg, bisphosphonates, tetracycline, NSAIDs, iron, and potassium chloride).
Esophageal strictures	Associated with caustic ingestion, acid reflux, and esophagitis.
Plummer-Vinson syndrome	Triad of dysphagia, iron deficiency anemia, esophageal webs. ↑ risk of esophageal squamous cell carcinoma ("**Plumber dies**"). May be associated with glossitis.
Mallory-Weiss syndrome	Partial thickness, longitudinal lacerations of gastroesophageal junction, confined to mucosa/submucosa, due to severe vomiting. Often presents with hematemesis +/– abdominal/back pain. Usually found in patients with alcohol use disorder, bulimia nervosa.
Esophageal varices	Dilated submucosal veins (red arrows in B C) in lower 1/3 of esophagus 2° to portal hypertension. Common in patients with cirrhosis, may be source of life-threatening hematemesis.
Distal esophageal spasm	Formerly called diffuse esophageal spasm. Spontaneous, nonperistaltic (uncoordinated) contractions of the esophagus with normal LES pressure. Presents with dysphagia and angina-like chest pain. Barium swallow reveals "corkscrew" esophagus. Manometry is diagnostic. Treatment includes nitrates and CCBs.
Scleroderma esophageal involvement	Esophageal smooth muscle atrophy → ↓ LES pressure and distal esophageal dysmotility → acid reflux and dysphagia → stricture, Barrett esophagus, and aspiration. Part of CREST syndrome.
Esophageal perforation	Most commonly iatrogenic following esophageal instrumentation. Noniatrogenic causes include spontaneous rupture, foreign body ingestion, trauma, malignancy. May present with pneumomediastinum (arrows in D). Subcutaneous emphysema may be due to dissecting air (signs include crepitus in the neck region or chest wall). Boerhaave syndrome—transmural, usually distal esophageal rupture due to violent retching.

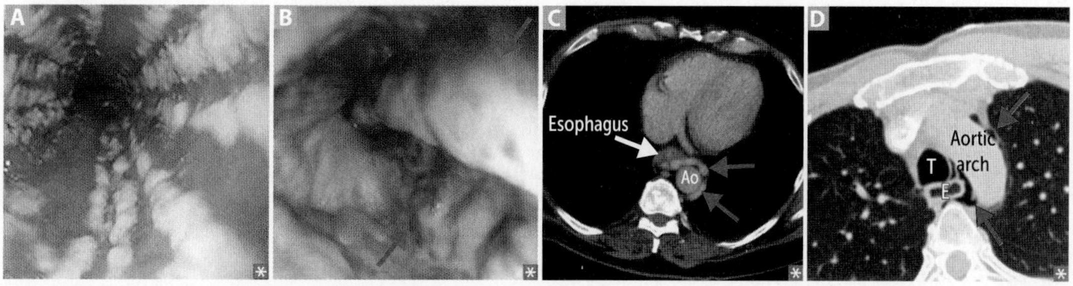

Barrett esophagus

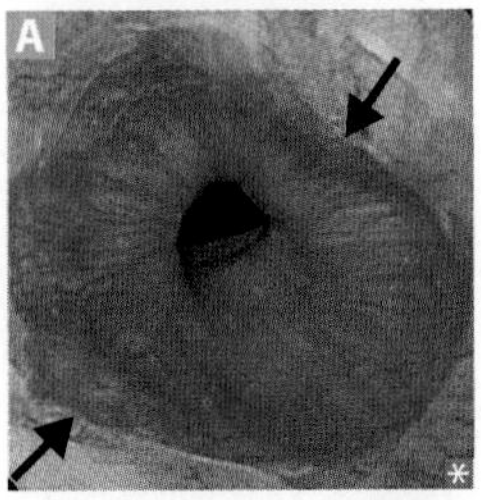

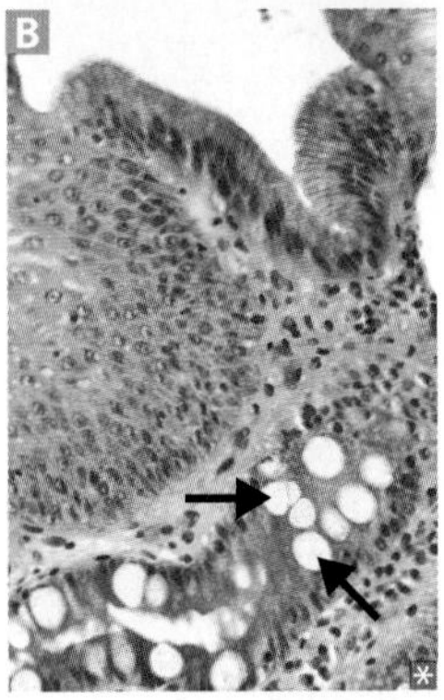

Specialized intestinal metaplasia (arrows in A)—replacement of nonkeratinized stratified squamous epithelium with intestinal epithelium (nonciliated columnar with goblet cells [arrows in B]) in distal esophagus. Due to chronic gastroesophageal reflux disease (GERD). Associated with ↑ risk of esophageal adenocarcinoma.

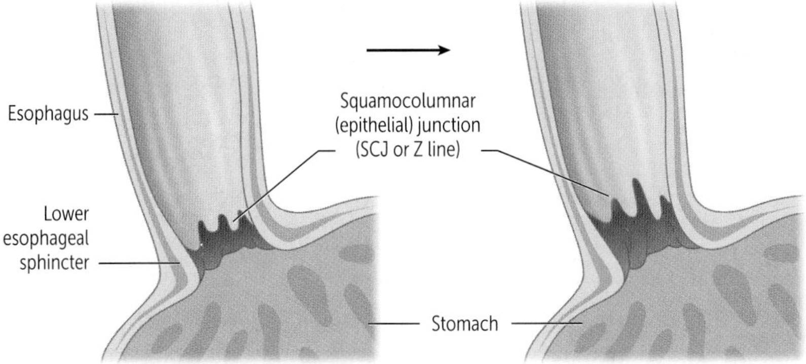

Esophageal cancer

Typically presents with progressive dysphagia (first solids, then liquids) and weight loss. Aggressive course due to lack of serosa in esophageal wall, allowing rapid extension. Poor prognosis due to advanced disease at presentation.

CANCER	PART OF ESOPHAGUS AFFECTED	RISK FACTORS	PREVALENCE
Squamous cell carcinoma	Upper 2/3	Alcohol, hot liquids, caustic strictures, smoking, achalasia	More common worldwide
Adenocarcinoma	Lower 1/3	Chronic GERD, Barrett esophagus, obesity, tobacco smoking	More common in America

Gastritis

Acute gastritis	Erosions can be caused by: ▪ NSAIDs—↓ PGE_2 → ↓ gastric mucosa protection ▪ **Burns** (**Curling** ulcer)—hypovolemia → mucosal ischemia ▪ **Brain** injury (**Cushing** ulcer)—↑ vagal stimulation → ↑ ACh → ↑ H^+ production	Especially common among patients with alcohol use disorder and those taking daily NSAIDs (eg, for rheumatoid arthritis) **Burned** by the **Curling** iron Always **Cush**ion the **brain**
Chronic gastritis	Mucosal inflammation, often leading to atrophy (hypochlorhydria → hypergastrinemia) and intestinal metaplasia (↑ risk of gastric cancers)	
H pylori	Most common. ↑ risk of peptic ulcer disease, MALT lymphoma	Affects antrum first and spreads to body of stomach
Autoimmune	Autoantibodies to the H^+/K^+ ATPase on parietal cells and to intrinsic factor. ↑ risk of pernicious anemia	Affects body/fundus of stomach

Ménétrier disease

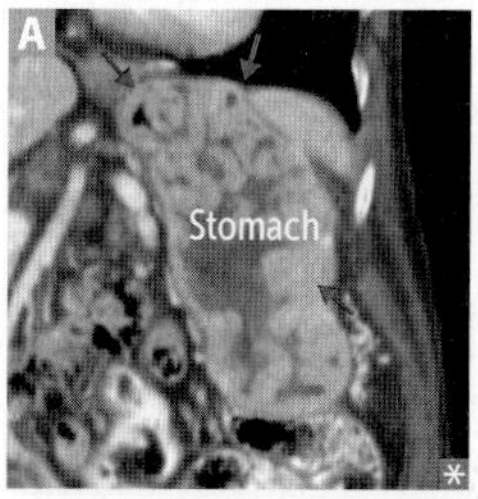

Hyperplasia of gastric mucosa → hypertrophied rugae ("**wavy**" like brain gyri A). Causes excess mucus production with resultant protein loss and parietal cell atrophy with ↓ acid production. Precancerous.

Presents with **W**eight loss, **A**norexia, **V**omiting, **E**pigastric pain, **E**dema (due to protein loss; pronounce "**WAVEE**").

Gastric cancer

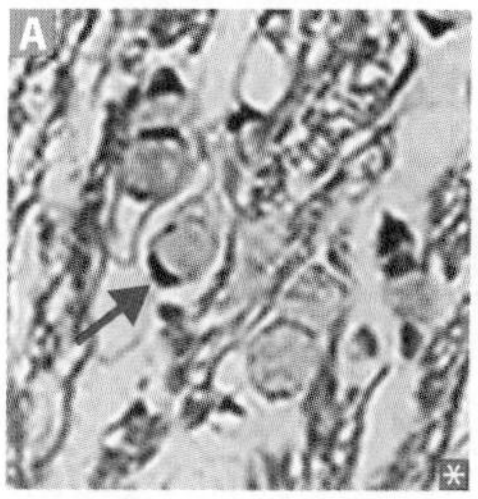

Most commonly gastric adenocarcinoma; lymphoma, GI stromal tumor, carcinoid (rare). Early aggressive local spread with node/liver metastases. Often presents late, with weight loss, abdominal pain, early satiety, and in some cases acanthosis nigricans or Leser-Trélat sign.

- Intestinal—associated with *H pylori*, dietary nitrosamines (smoked foods), tobacco smoking, achlorhydria, chronic gastritis. Commonly on lesser curvature; looks like ulcer with raised margins.
- Diffuse—not associated with *H pylori*; most cases due to E-cadherin mutation; signet ring cells (mucin-filled cells with peripheral nuclei) A; stomach wall grossly thickened and leathery (linitis plastica).

Virchow node—involvement of left supraclavicular node by metastasis from stomach.

Krukenberg tumor—metastasis to ovaries (typically bilateral). Abundant mucin-secreting, signet ring cells.

Sister Mary Joseph nodule—subcutaneous periumbilical metastasis.

Blumer shelf—palpable mass on digital rectal exam suggesting metastasis to rectouterine pouch (pouch of Douglas).

Peptic ulcer disease

	Gastric ulcer	Duodenal ulcer
PAIN	Can be greater with meals—weight loss	Decreases with meals—weight gain
H PYLORI INFECTION	~ 70%	~ 90%
MECHANISM	↓ mucosal protection against gastric acid	↓ mucosal protection or ↑ gastric acid secretion
OTHER CAUSES	NSAIDs	Zollinger-Ellison syndrome
RISK OF CARCINOMA	↑	Generally benign
OTHER	Biopsy margins to rule out malignancy	Benign-appearing ulcers are not routinely biopsied

Ulcer complications

Hemorrhage

Gastric, duodenal (posterior > anterior). Most common complication.
Ruptured gastric ulcer on the lesser curvature of stomach → bleeding from left gastric artery.
An ulcer on the posterior wall of duodenum → bleeding from gastroduodenal artery.

Obstruction

Pyloric channel, duodenal.

Perforation

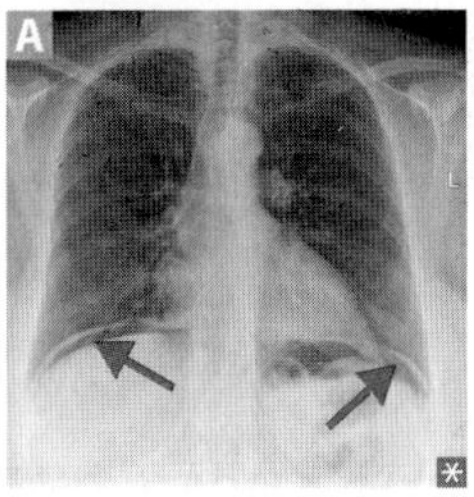

Duodenal (anterior > posterior).
Anterior duodenal ulcers can perforate into the anterior abdominal cavity, potentially leading to pneumoperitoneum.
May see free air under diaphragm (pneumoperitoneum) A with referred pain to the shoulder via irritation of phrenic nerve.

Acute gastrointestinal bleeding

Upper GI bleeding—originates **proximal** to ligament of Treitz (suspensory ligament of duodenum). Usually presents with hematemesis and/or melena. Associated with peptic ulcer disease, variceal hemorrhage.

Lower GI bleeding—originates **distal** to ligament of Treitz. Usually presents with hematochezia. Associated with IBD, diverticulosis, angiodysplasia, hemorrhoids, cancer.

Malabsorption syndromes

Can cause diarrhea, steatorrhea, weight loss, weakness, vitamin and mineral deficiencies. Screen for fecal fat (eg, Sudan stain).

Celiac disease

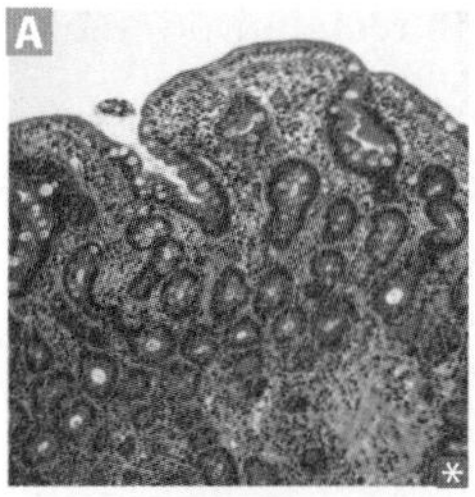

Also called gluten-sensitive enteropathy, celiac sprue. Autoimmune-mediated intolerance of gliadin (gluten protein found in wheat, barley, rye). Associated with HLA-DQ2, HLA-DQ8, northern European descent.

Primarily affects distal duodenum and/or proximal jejunum → malabsorption and steatorrhea.

Treatment: gluten-free diet.

Associated with dermatitis herpetiformis, ↓ bone density, moderately ↑ risk of malignancy (eg, T-cell lymphoma).

D-xylose test: abnormal.

Serology: ⊕ IgA anti-tissue transglutaminase (IgA tTG), anti-endomysial, and anti-deamidated gliadin peptide antibodies.

Histology: villous atrophy, crypt hyperplasia A, intraepithelial lymphocytosis.

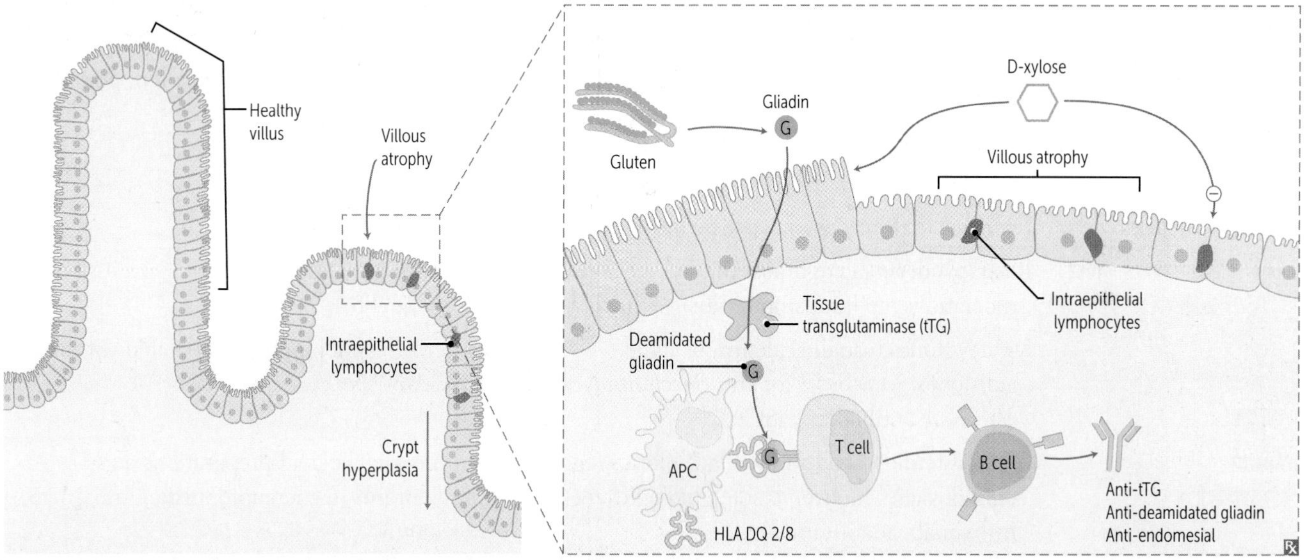

Lactose intolerance

Lactase deficiency. Normal-appearing villi, except when 2° to injury at tips of villi (eg, viral enteritis). Osmotic diarrhea with ↓ stool pH (colonic bacteria ferment lactose).

Lactose hydrogen breath test: ⊕ for lactose malabsorption if post-lactose breath hydrogen value rises > 20 ppm compared with baseline.

Pancreatic insufficiency

Due to chronic pancreatitis, cystic fibrosis, obstructing cancer. Causes malabsorption of fat and fat-soluble vitamins (A, D, E, K) as well as vitamin B_{12}.

↓ duodenal bicarbonate (and pH) and fecal elastase.

D-xylose test: normal.

Tropical sprue

Similar findings as celiac sprue (affects small bowel), but responds to antibiotics. Cause is unknown, but seen in residents of or recent visitors to tropics.

↓ mucosal absorption affecting duodenum and jejunum but can involve ileum with time. Associated with megaloblastic anemia due to folate deficiency and, later, B_{12} deficiency.

Whipple disease

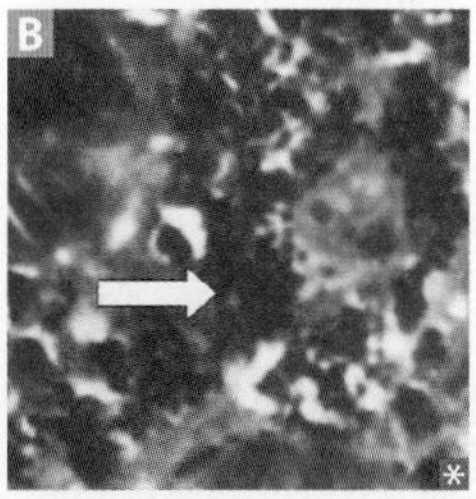

Infection with *Tropheryma whipplei* (intracellular gram ⊕); **PAS** ⊕ **foamy** macrophages in intestinal lamina propria B, mesenteric nodes. **C**ardiac symptoms, **A**rthralgias, and **N**eurologic symptoms are common. Diarrhea/steatorrhea occur later in disease course. Most common in older males.

PASs the foamy Whipped cream in a CAN.

Inflammatory bowel diseases

	Crohn disease	Ulcerative colitis
LOCATION	Any portion of the GI tract, usually the terminal ileum and colon. Skip lesions, rectal sparing.	Colitis = colon inflammation. Continuous colonic lesions, always with rectal involvement.
GROSS MORPHOLOGY	Transmural inflammation → fistulas. Cobblestone mucosa, creeping fat, bowel wall thickening ("string sign" on small bowel follow-through A), linear ulcers, fissures.	Mucosal and submucosal inflammation only. Friable mucosa with superficial and/or deep ulcerations (compare normal B with diseased C). Loss of haustra → "lead pipe" appearance on imaging.
MICROSCOPIC MORPHOLOGY	Noncaseating granulomas and lymphoid aggregates. Th1 mediated.	Crypt abscesses and ulcers, bleeding, no granulomas. Th2 mediated.
COMPLICATIONS	Malabsorption/malnutrition, colorectal cancer (↑ risk with pancolitis).	
	Fistulas (eg, enterovesical fistulae, which can cause recurrent UTI and pneumaturia), phlegmon/abscess, strictures (causing obstruction), perianal disease.	Fulminant colitis, toxic megacolon, perforation.
INTESTINAL MANIFESTATION	Diarrhea that may or may not be bloody.	Bloody diarrhea.
EXTRAINTESTINAL MANIFESTATIONS	Rash (pyoderma gangrenosum, erythema nodosum), eye inflammation (episcleritis, uveitis), oral ulcerations (aphthous stomatitis), arthritis (peripheral, spondylitis).	
	Kidney stones (usually calcium oxalate), gallstones. May be ⊕ for anti-*Saccharomyces cerevisiae* antibodies (ASCA).	1° sclerosing cholangitis. Associated with MPO-ANCA/p-ANCA.
TREATMENT	Corticosteroids, azathioprine, antibiotics (eg, ciprofloxacin, metronidazole), biologics (eg, infliximab, adalimumab).	5-aminosalicylic acid preparations (eg, mesalamine), 6-mercaptopurine, infliximab, colectomy.

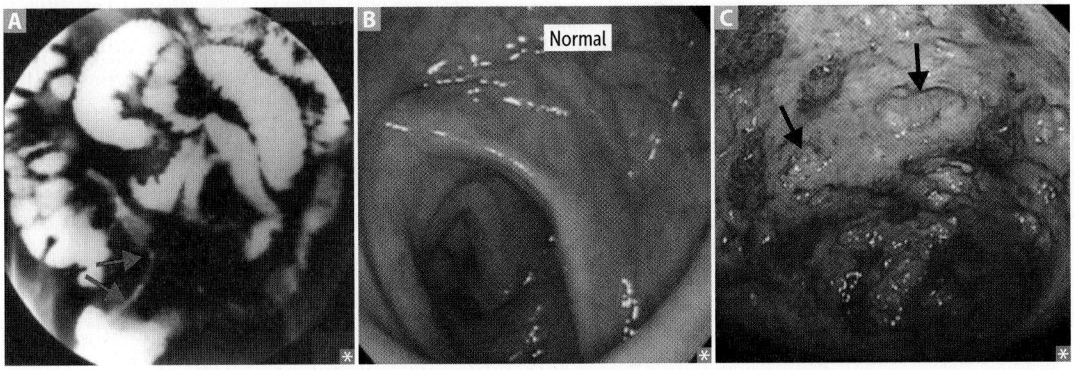

Microscopic colitis Inflammatory disease of colon that causes chronic watery diarrhea. Most common in older females. Colonic mucosa appears normal on endoscopy. Histology shows inflammatory infiltrate in lamina propria with thickened subepithelial collagen band or intraepithelial lymphocytes.

Irritable bowel syndrome

Recurrent abdominal pain associated with ≥ 2 of the following:
- Related to defecation
- Change in stool frequency
- Change in form (consistency) of stool

No structural abnormalities. Most common in middle-aged females. Chronic symptoms may be diarrhea-predominant, constipation-predominant, or mixed. Pathophysiology is multifaceted.
First-line treatment is lifestyle modification and dietary changes.

Appendicitis

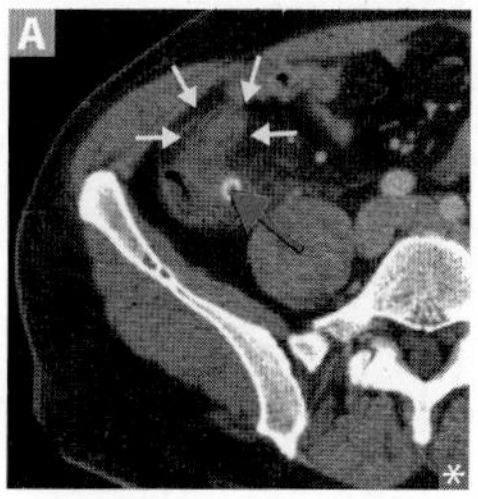

Acute inflammation of the appendix (yellow arrows in A), can be due to obstruction by fecalith (red arrow in A) (in adults) or lymphoid hyperplasia (in children).
Proximal obstruction of appendiceal lumen produces closed-loop obstruction → ↑ intraluminal pressure → stimulation of visceral afferent nerve fibers at T8-T10 → initial diffuse periumbilical pain → inflammation extends to serosa and irritates parietal peritoneum. Pain localized to RLQ/McBurney point (1/3 the distance from right anterior superior iliac spine to umbilicus). Nausea, fever; may perforate → peritonitis; may elicit psoas, obturator, and Rovsing signs, guarding and rebound tenderness on exam.
Treatment: appendectomy.

Diverticula of the GI tract

Diverticulum	Blind pouch A protruding from the alimentary tract that communicates with the lumen of the gut. Most diverticula (esophagus, stomach, duodenum, colon) are acquired and are termed "false diverticula."	"True" diverticulum—all gut wall layers outpouch (eg, Meckel). "False" diverticulum or pseudodiverticulum—only mucosa and submucosa outpouch. Occur especially where vasa recta perforate muscularis externa.
Diverticulosis	Many false diverticula of the colon B, commonly sigmoid. Common (in ~ 50% of people > 60 years). Caused by ↑ intraluminal pressure and focal weakness in colonic wall. Associated with obesity and diets low in fiber, high in total fat/red meat.	Often asymptomatic or associated with vague discomfort. Complications include diverticular bleeding (painless hematochezia), diverticulitis.
Diverticulitis	Inflammation of diverticula with wall thickening (red arrows in C) classically causing LLQ pain, fever, leukocytosis. Treat with antibiotics.	Complications: abscess, fistula (colovesical fistula → pneumaturia), obstruction (inflammatory stenosis), perforation (white arrows in C) (→ peritonitis). Hematochezia is rare.

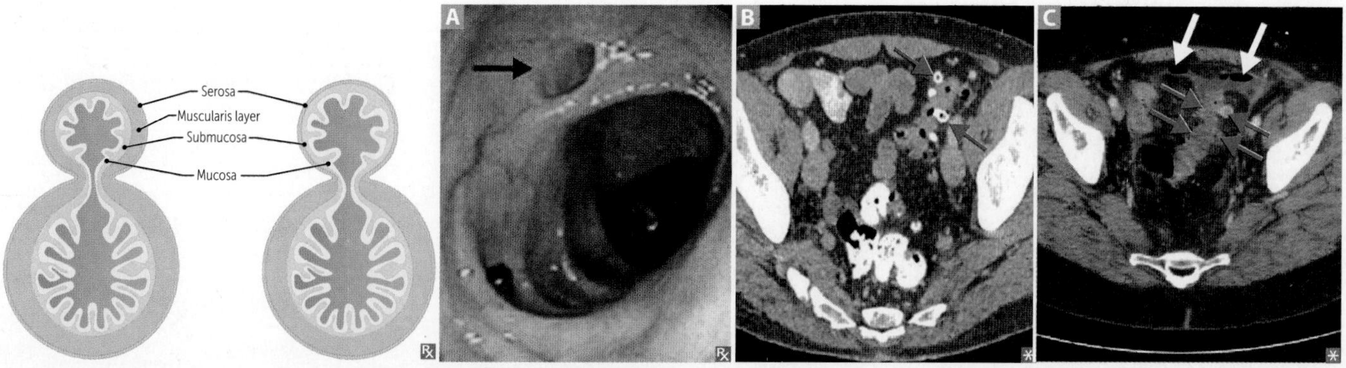

Zenker diverticulum

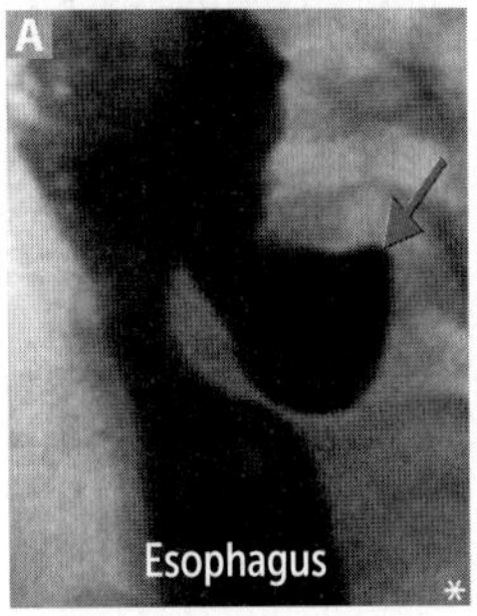
A
Esophagus

Pharyngoesophageal **false** diverticulum A. Esophageal dysmotility causes herniation of mucosal tissue at Killian triangle between the thyropharyngeal and cricopharyngeal parts of the inferior pharyngeal constrictor. Presenting symptoms: dysphagia, obstruction, gurgling, aspiration, foul breath, neck mass. Most common in elderly males.

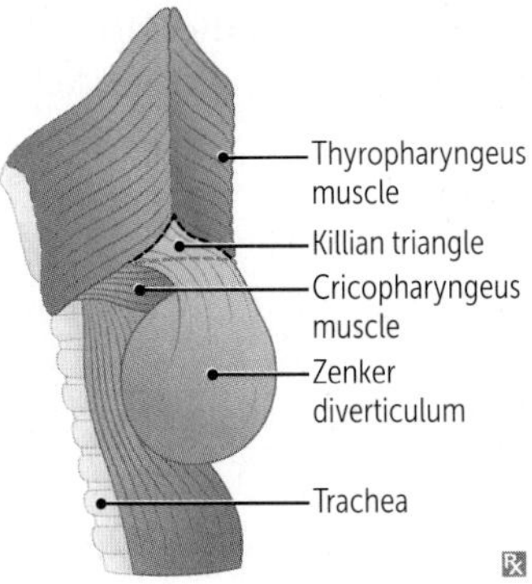
Thyropharyngeus muscle
Killian triangle
Cricopharyngeus muscle
Zenker diverticulum
Trachea

Meckel diverticulum

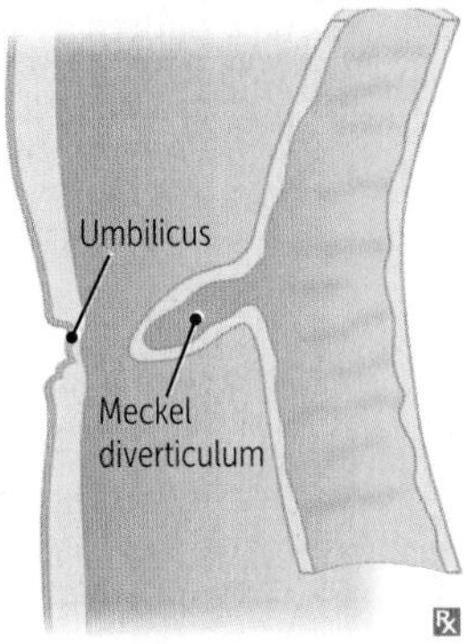
Umbilicus
Meckel diverticulum

True diverticulum. Persistence of the vitelline (omphalomesenteric) duct. May contain ectopic acid–secreting gastric mucosa and/or pancreatic tissue. Most common congenital anomaly of GI tract. Can cause hematochezia/melena (less common), RLQ pain, intussusception, volvulus, or obstruction near terminal ileum.

Diagnosis: ^{99m}Tc-pertechnetate scan (aka Meckel scan) for uptake by heterotopic gastric mucosa.

The rule of 2's:
- 2 times as likely in males.
- 2 inches long.
- 2 feet from the ileocecal valve.
- 2% of population.
- Commonly presents in first 2 years of life.
- May have 2 types of epithelia (gastric/pancreatic).

Hirschsprung disease

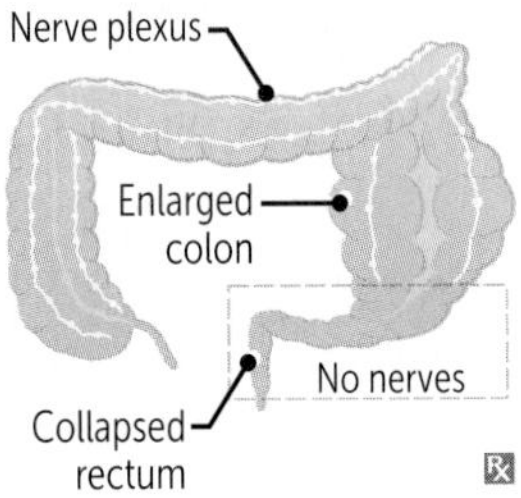
Nerve plexus
Enlarged colon
No nerves
Collapsed rectum

Congenital megacolon characterized by lack of ganglion cells/enteric nervous plexuses (Auerbach and Meissner plexuses) in distal segment of colon. Due to failure of neural crest cell migration. Associated with loss of function mutations in *RET*.

Presents with bilious emesis, abdominal distention, and failure to pass meconium within 48 hours → chronic constipation. Normal portion of the colon proximal to the aganglionic segment is dilated, resulting in a "transition zone."

Risk ↑ with Down syndrome.

Explosive expulsion of feces (squirt sign) → empty rectum on digital exam.

Diagnosed by absence of ganglion cells on rectal suction biopsy.

Treatment: resection.

RET mutation in the **RE**c**T**um.

Malrotation

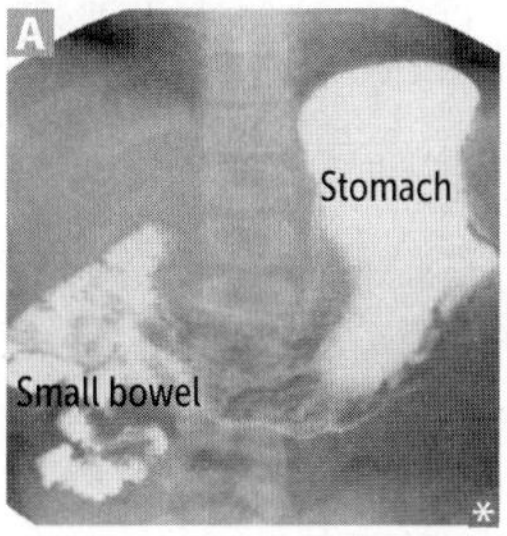

Anomaly of midgut rotation during fetal development → improper positioning of bowel (small bowel clumped on the right side) A, formation of fibrous bands (Ladd bands).

Can lead to volvulus, duodenal obstruction.

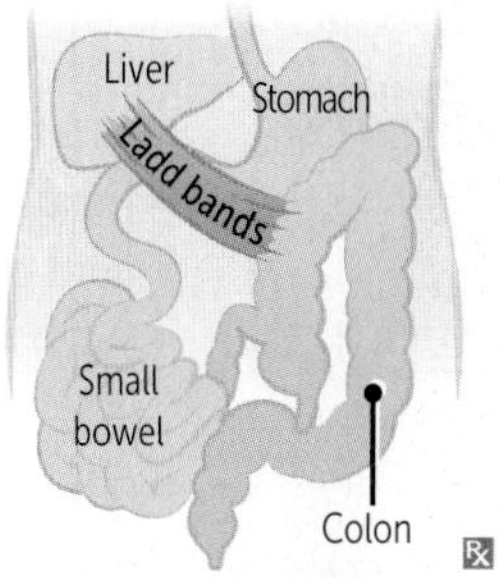

Intussusception

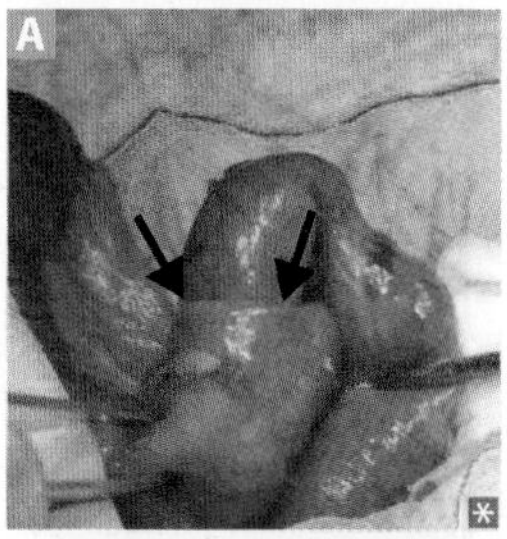

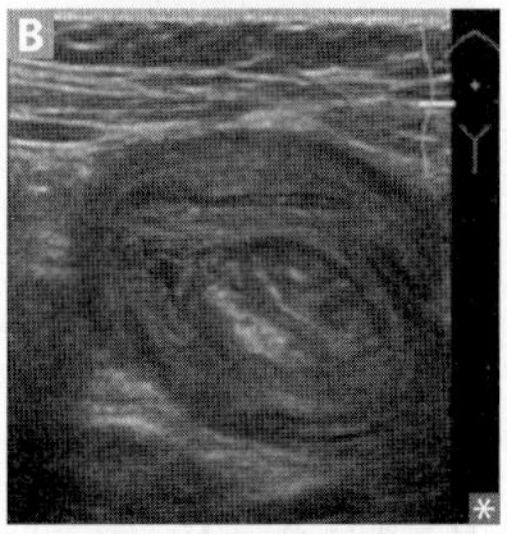

Telescoping A of proximal bowel segment into a distal segment, commonly at the ileocecal junction. Most commonly idiopathic, but may be due to lead point.

Compromised blood supply → intermittent, severe, abdominal pain often with "currant jelly" dark red stools.

Majority of cases in infants, unusual in adults.

Most common pathologic lead point:

- Children—Meckel diverticulum
- Adults—intraluminal mass/tumor

Physical exam—sausage-shaped mass in right abdomen, patient may draw legs to chest to ease pain.

Imaging—Ultrasound/CT may show "target sign" B.

May be associated with IgA vasculitis (HSP), recent viral infection (eg, adenovirus; Peyer patch hypertrophy creates lead point).

Volvulus

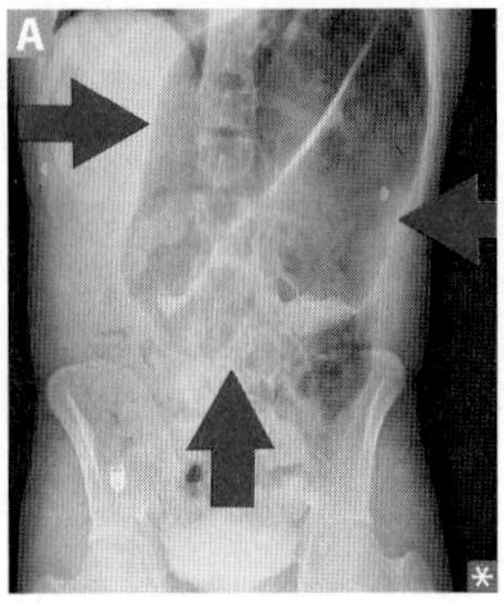

Twisting of portion of bowel around its mesentery; can lead to obstruction and infarction. Can occur throughout the GI tract.

- Midgut volvulus more common in infants and children (minors)
- Sigmoid volvulus (coffee bean sign on x-ray A) more common in seniors (elderly)

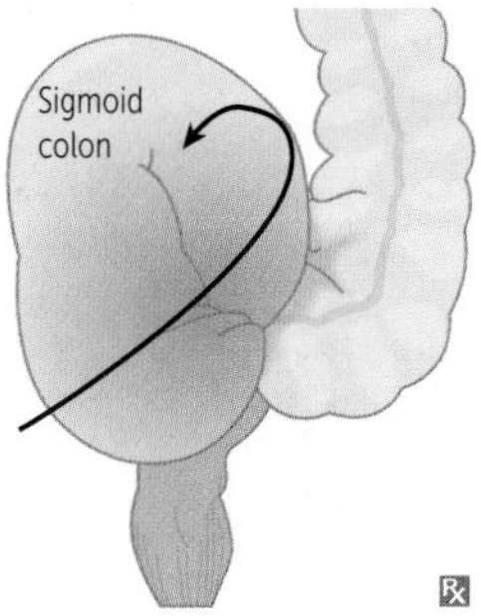

Other intestinal disorders

Acute mesenteric ischemia	Critical blockage of intestinal blood flow (often embolic occlusion of SMA) → small bowel necrosis A → abdominal pain out of proportion to physical findings. May see red "currant jelly" stools.
Adhesion	Fibrous band of scar tissue; commonly forms after surgery. Most common cause of small bowel obstruction, demonstrated by multiple dilated small bowel loops on x-ray (arrows in B).
Angiodysplasia	Tortuous dilation of vessels C → hematochezia. Most often found in the right-sided colon. More common in older patients. Confirmed by angiography. Associated with end-stage renal disease, von Willebrand disease, aortic stenosis.
Chronic mesenteric ischemia	"Intestinal angina": atherosclerosis of celiac artery, SMA, or IMA → intestinal hypoperfusion → postprandial epigastric pain → food aversion and weight loss.
Colonic ischemia	Crampy abdominal pain followed by hematochezia. Commonly occurs at watershed areas (splenic flexure, rectosigmoid junction). Typically affects elderly. Thumbprint sign on imaging due to mucosal edema/hemorrhage.
Ileus	Intestinal hypomotility without obstruction → constipation and ↓ flatus; distended/tympanic abdomen with ↓ bowel sounds. Associated with abdominal surgeries, opiates, hypokalemia, sepsis. No transition zone on imaging. Treatment: bowel rest, electrolyte correction, cholinergic drugs (stimulate intestinal motility).
Meconium ileus	Meconium plug obstructs intestine, prevents stool passage at birth. Associated with cystic fibrosis.
Necrotizing enterocolitis	Seen in premature, formula-fed infants with immature immune system. Necrosis of intestinal mucosa (most commonly terminal ileum and proximal colon), which can lead to pneumatosis intestinalis (arrows in D), pneumoperitoneum, portal venous gas.

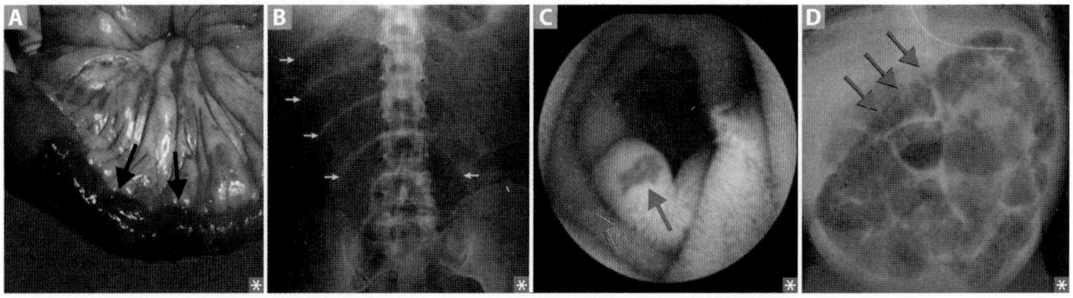

Colonic polyps Growths of tissue within the colon A. Grossly characterized as flat, sessile, or pedunculated on the basis of protrusion into colonic lumen. Generally classified by histologic type.

HISTOLOGIC TYPE	CHARACTERISTICS
Generally nonneoplastic	
Hamartomatous polyps	Solitary lesions do not have significant risk of transformation. Growths of normal colonic tissue with distorted architecture. Associated with Peutz-Jeghers syndrome and juvenile polyposis.
Hyperplastic polyps	Most common; generally smaller and predominantly located in rectosigmoid region. Occasionally evolves into serrated polyps and more advanced lesions.
Inflammatory pseudopolyps	Due to mucosal erosion in inflammatory bowel disease.
Mucosal polyps	Small, usually < 5 mm. Look similar to normal mucosa. Clinically insignificant.
Submucosal polyps	May include lipomas, leiomyomas, fibromas, and other lesions.
Potentially malignant	
Adenomatous polyps	Neoplastic, via chromosomal instability pathway with mutations in *APC* and *KRAS*. Tubular B histology has less malignant potential than villous C ("**villous** histology is **villainous**"); tubulovillous has intermediate malignant potential. Usually asymptomatic; may present with occult bleeding.
Serrated polyps	Neoplastic. Characterized by CpG island methylator phenotype (CIMP; cytosine base followed by guanine, linked by a phosphodiester bond). Defect may silence *MMR* gene (DNA mismatch repair) expression. Mutations lead to microsatellite instability and mutations in *BRAF*. "Saw-tooth" pattern of crypts on biopsy. Up to 20% of cases of sporadic CRC.

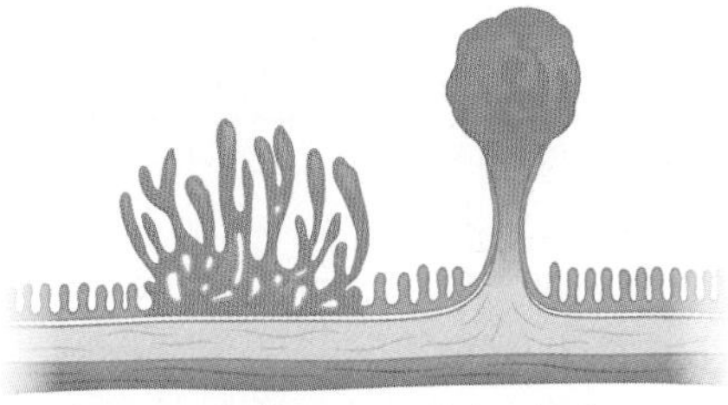

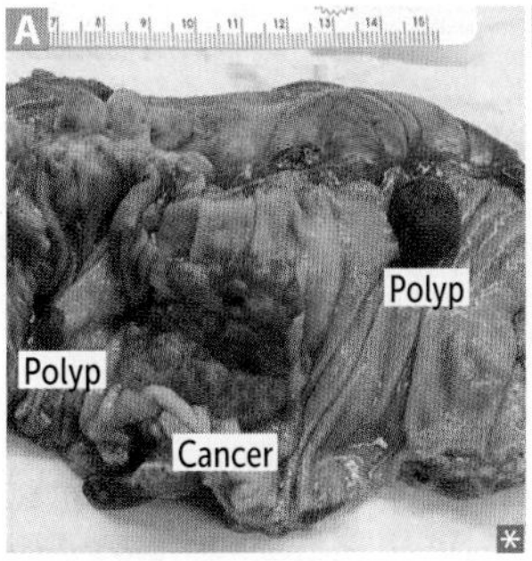

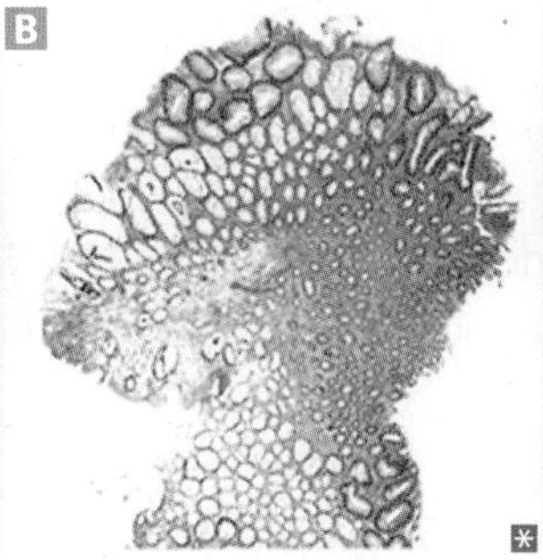

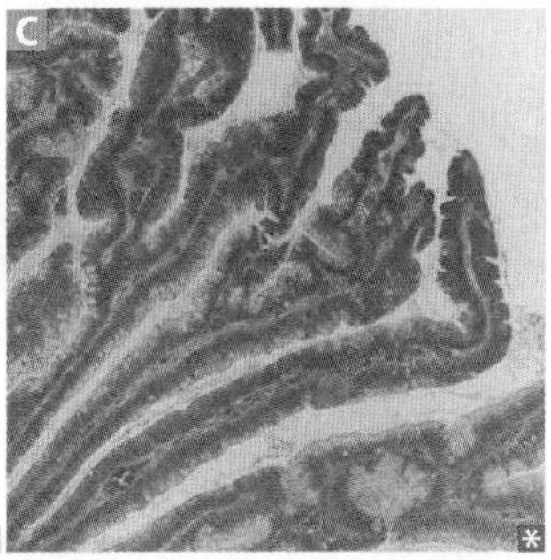

Polyposis syndromes

Familial adenomatous polyposis	Autosomal dominant mutation of *APC* tumor suppressor gene on chromosome 5q21-q22. 2-hit hypothesis. Thousands of polyps arise starting after puberty; pancolonic; always involves rectum. Prophylactic colectomy or else 100% progress to CRC.
Gardner syndrome	FAP + osseous and soft tissue tumors (eg, osteomas of skull or mandible), congenital hypertrophy of retinal pigment epithelium, impacted/supernumerary teeth.
Turcot syndrome	FAP or Lynch syndrome + malignant CNS tumor (eg, medulloblastoma, glioma). **Turcot** = **Turban**.
Peutz-Jeghers syndrome	Autosomal dominant syndrome featuring numerous hamartomas throughout GI tract, along with hyperpigmented macules on mouth, lips, hands, genitalia. Associated with ↑ risk of breast and GI cancers (eg, colorectal, stomach, small bowel, pancreatic).
Juvenile polyposis syndrome	Autosomal dominant syndrome in children (typically < 5 years old) featuring numerous hamartomatous polyps in the colon, stomach, small bowel. Associated with ↑ risk of CRC.

Lynch syndrome Previously called hereditary nonpolyposis colorectal cancer (HNPCC). Autosomal dominant mutation of mismatch repair genes (eg, *MLH1*, *MSH2*) with subsequent microsatellite instability. ~ 80% progress to CRC. Proximal colon is always involved. Associated with endometrial, ovarian, and skin cancers.

Colorectal cancer

DIAGNOSIS

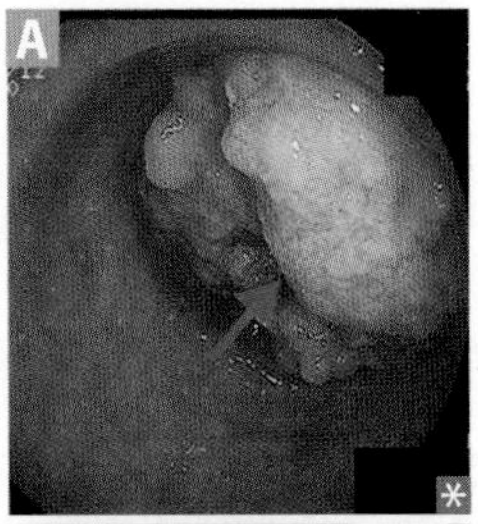

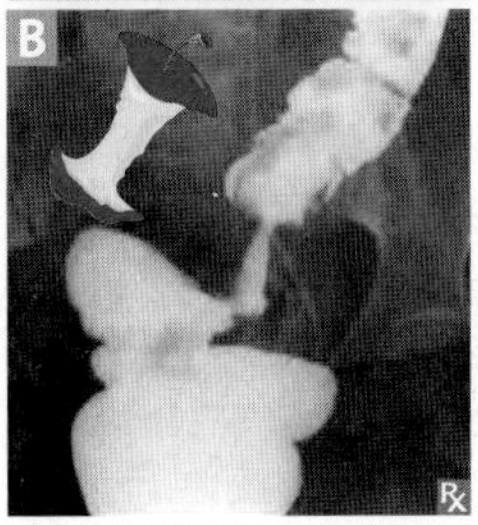

Iron deficiency anemia in males (especially > 50 years old) and postmenopausal females raises suspicion.

Screening:

- Average risk: screen at age 50 with colonoscopy (polyp seen in A); alternatives include flexible sigmoidoscopy, fecal occult blood testing (FOBT), fecal immunochemical testing (FIT), FIT-fecal DNA, CT colonography.
- Patients with a first-degree relative who has colon cancer: screen at age 40 with colonoscopy, or 10 years prior to the relative's presentation.
- Patients with IBD are screened more regularly.

"Apple core" lesion seen on barium enema x-ray B.

CEA tumor marker: good for monitoring recurrence, should not be used for screening.

EPIDEMIOLOGY

Most patients are > 50 years old. ~ 25% have a family history.

PRESENTATION

Rectosigmoid > ascending > descending.

Most are asymptomatic. Right side (cecal, ascending) associated with occult bleeding; left side (rectosigmoid) associated with hematochezia and obstruction (narrower lumen → ↓ stool caliber).

Ascending—exophytic mass, iron deficiency anemia, weight loss.

Descending—infiltrating mass, partial obstruction, colicky pain, hematochezia.

Can present with *S bovis* (*gallolyticus*) bacteremia/endocarditis or as an episode of diverticulitis.

RISK FACTORS

Adenomatous and serrated polyps, familial cancer syndromes, IBD, tobacco use, diet of processed meat with low fiber.

Molecular pathogenesis of colorectal cancer

Chromosomal instability pathway: mutations in *APC* cause FAP and most sporadic cases of CRC via adenoma-carcinoma sequence.

Microsatellite instability pathway: mutations or methylation of mismatch repair genes (eg, *MLH1*) cause Lynch syndrome and some sporadic CRC via serrated polyp pathway. Usually leads to right-sided CRC.

Overexpression of COX-2 has been linked to colorectal cancer, NSAIDs may be chemopreventive.

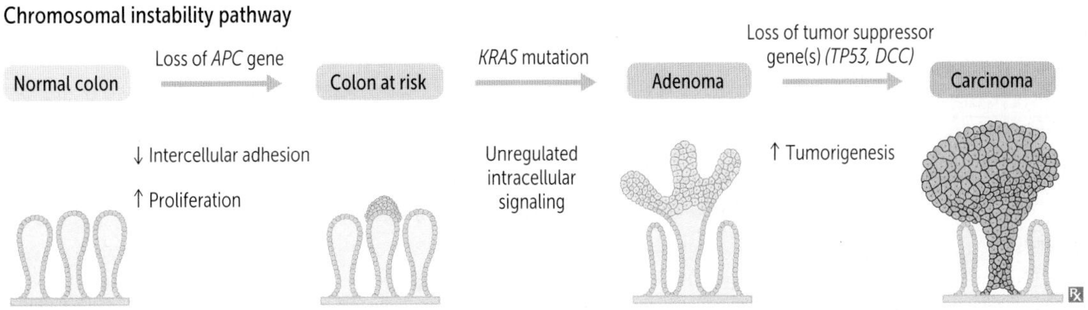
Chromosomal instability pathway
Normal colon
Loss of APC gene
Colon at risk
KRAS mutation
Adenoma
Loss of tumor suppressor gene(s) (TP53, DCC)
Carcinoma
↓ Intercellular adhesion
↑ Proliferation
Unregulated intracellular signaling
↑ Tumorigenesis

Cirrhosis and portal hypertension

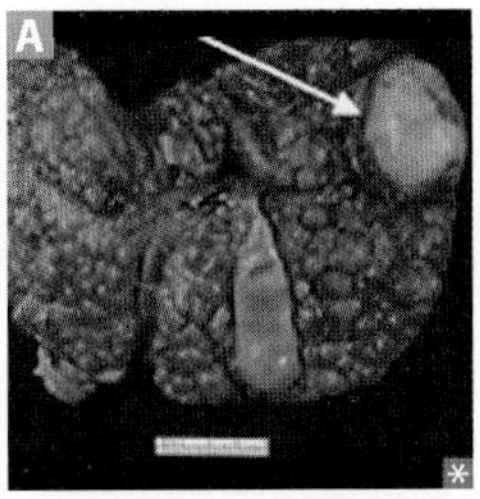

Cirrhosis—diffuse bridging fibrosis (via stellate cells) and regenerative nodules (arrows show splenomegaly) disrupt normal architecture of liver; ↑ risk for hepatocellular carcinoma (white arrow in A). Etiologies include alcohol, nonalcoholic steatohepatitis, chronic viral hepatitis, autoimmune hepatitis, biliary disease, genetic/metabolic disorders.

Portal hypertension—↑ pressure in portal venous system. Etiologies include cirrhosis (most common cause in developed countries), vascular obstruction (eg, portal vein thrombosis, Budd-Chiari syndrome), schistosomiasis.

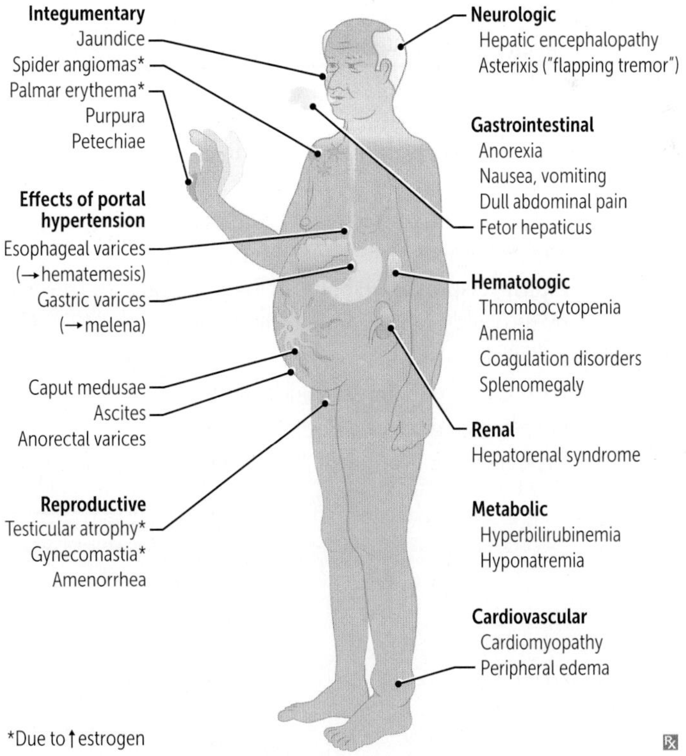
Integumentary
Jaundice
Spider angiomas*
Palmar erythema*
Purpura
Petechiae
Effects of portal hypertension
Esophageal varices (→hematemesis)
Gastric varices (→melena)
Caput medusae
Ascites
Anorectal varices
Reproductive
Testicular atrophy*
Gynecomastia*
Amenorrhea
*Due to ↑ estrogen
Neurologic
Hepatic encephalopathy
Asterixis ("flapping tremor")
Gastrointestinal
Anorexia
Nausea, vomiting
Dull abdominal pain
Fetor hepaticus
Hematologic
Thrombocytopenia
Anemia
Coagulation disorders
Splenomegaly
Renal
Hepatorenal syndrome
Metabolic
Hyperbilirubinemia
Hyponatremia
Cardiovascular
Cardiomyopathy
Peripheral edema

Spontaneous bacterial peritonitis

Also called 1° bacterial peritonitis. Common and potentially fatal bacterial infection in patients with cirrhosis and ascites. Often asymptomatic, but can cause fevers, chills, abdominal pain, ileus, or worsening encephalopathy. Commonly caused by gram ⊖ organisms (eg, *E coli*, *Klebsiella*) or less commonly gram ⊕ *Streptococcus*.

Diagnosis: paracentesis with ascitic fluid absolute neutrophil count (ANC) > 250 cells/mm^3. Empiric first-line treatment is 3rd generation cephalosporin (eg, cefotaxime).

Serum markers of liver pathology

ENZYMES RELEASED IN LIVER DAMAGE	
Aspartate aminotransferase and alanine aminotransferase	↑ in most liver disease: ALT > AST ↑ in **alcoholic** liver disease: **AST** > ALT (ratio usually > 2:1, AST does not typically exceed 500 U/L in alcoholic hepatitis). Make a to**AST** with **alcohol** AST > ALT in nonalcoholic liver disease suggests progression to advanced fibrosis or cirrhosis ↑↑↑ aminotransferases (>1000 U/L): differential includes drug-induced liver injury (eg, acetaminophen toxicity), ischemic hepatitis, acute viral hepatitis, autoimmune hepatitis
Alkaline phosphatase	↑ in cholestasis (eg, biliary obstruction), infiltrative disorders, bone disease
γ-glutamyl transpeptidase	↑ in various liver and biliary diseases (just as ALP can), but not in bone disease; associated with alcohol use
FUNCTIONAL LIVER MARKERS	
Bilirubin	↑ in various liver diseases (eg, biliary obstruction, alcoholic or viral hepatitis, cirrhosis), hemolysis
Albumin	↓ in advanced liver disease (marker of liver's biosynthetic function)
Prothrombin time	↑ in advanced liver disease (↓ production of clotting factors, thereby measuring the liver's biosynthetic function)
Platelets	↓ in advanced liver disease (↓ thrombopoietin, liver sequestration) and portal hypertension (splenomegaly/splenic sequestration)

Reye syndrome

Rare, often fatal childhood hepatic encephalopathy.

Associated with viral infection (especially VZV and influenza) that has been treated with aspirin. Aspirin metabolites ↓ β-oxidation by reversible inhibition of mitochondrial enzymes.

Findings: mitochondrial abnormalities, fatty liver (microvesicular fatty changes), hypoglycemia, vomiting, hepatomegaly, coma.

Avoid aspirin (**ASA**) in children, except in Kaw**ASA**ki disease.

Salicylates aren't a ray (**Reye**) of sun**SHINE** for kids:
- **S**teatosis of liver/hepatocytes
- **H**ypoglycemia/**H**epatomegaly
- **I**nfection (VZV, influenza)
- **N**ot awake (coma)
- **E**ncephalopathy

Alcoholic liver disease

Hepatic steatosis	Macrovesicular fatty change A that may be reversible with alcohol cessation.
Alcoholic hepatitis	Requires sustained, long-term consumption. Swollen and necrotic hepatocytes with neutrophilic infiltration. Mallory bodies B (intracytoplasmic eosinophilic inclusions of damaged keratin filaments).
Alcoholic cirrhosis	Final and usually irreversible form. Sclerosis around central vein (arrows in C) may be seen in early disease. Regenerative nodules surrounded by fibrous bands in response to chronic liver injury → portal hypertension and end-stage liver disease.

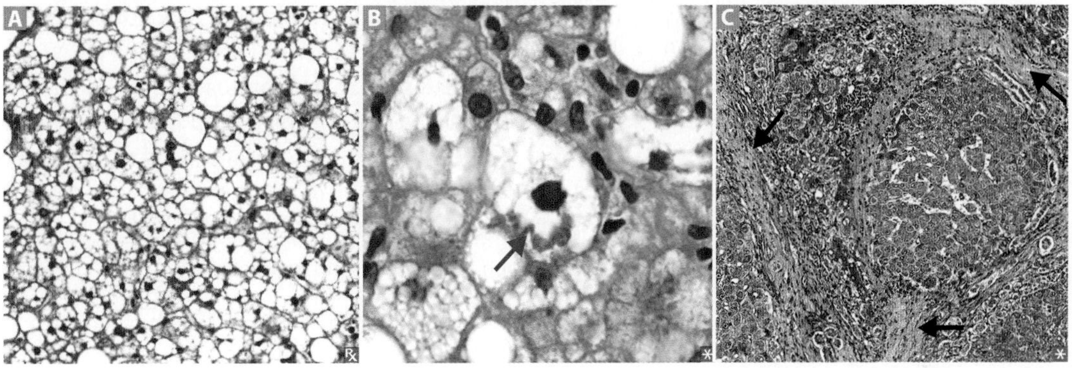

Nonalcoholic fatty liver disease

Metabolic syndrome (insulin resistance); obesity → fatty infiltration of hepatocytes A → cellular "ballooning" and eventual necrosis. May cause cirrhosis and HCC. Independent of alcohol use.

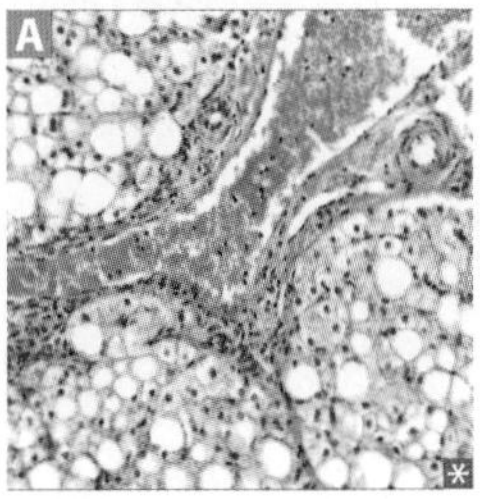

Autoimmune hepatitis

Chronic inflammatory liver disease. More common in females. May be asymptomatic or present with fatigue, nausea, pruritus. May be associated with ⊕ antinuclear, anti-smooth muscle and anti-liver/kidney microsomal-1 antibodies. Labs: ↑ ALT and AST. Histology: portal and periportal lymphoplasmacytic infiltrate.

Hepatic encephalopathy

Cirrhosis → portosystemic shunts → ↓ NH_3 metabolism → neuropsychiatric dysfunction. Reversible neuropsychiatric dysfunction ranging from disorientation/asterixis (mild) to difficult arousal or coma (severe).

Triggers:

- ↑ NH_3 production and absorption (due to GI bleed, constipation, infection).
- ↓ NH_3 removal (due to renal failure, diuretics, bypassed hepatic blood flow post-TIPS).

Treatment: lactulose (↑ NH_4^+ generation) and rifaximin (↓ NH_3-producing gut bacteria).

Liver tumors

Hepatic hemangioma	Also known as cavernous hemangioma. Most common benign liver tumor (venous malformation) A; typically occurs at age 30–50 years. Biopsy contraindicated because of risk of hemorrhage.
Focal nodular hyperplasia	Second most common benign liver tumor; occurs predominantly in females aged 35–50 years. Hyperplastic reaction of hepatocytes to an aberrant dystrophic artery. Marked by central stellate scar. Usually asymptomatic and detected incidentally.
Hepatic adenoma	Rare, benign tumor, often related to oral contraceptive or anabolic steroid use; may regress spontaneously or rupture (abdominal pain and shock).
Hepatocellular carcinoma	Also known as hepatoma. Most common 1° malignant liver tumor in adults B. Associated with HBV (+/– cirrhosis) and all other causes of cirrhosis (including HCV, alcoholic and nonalcoholic fatty liver disease, autoimmune disease, hemochromatosis, Wilson disease, α_1-antitrypsin deficiency) and specific carcinogens (eg, aflatoxin from *Aspergillus*). Findings: anorexia, jaundice, tender hepatomegaly. May lead to decompensation of previously stable cirrhosis (eg, ascites) and Budd-Chiari syndrome. Spreads hematogenously. Diagnosis: ↑ α-fetoprotein; ultrasound or contrast CT/MRI C; biopsy if diagnosis is uncertain
Hepatic angiosarcoma	Rare, malignant tumor of endothelial origin; associated with exposure to arsenic, vinyl chloride.
Metastases	Most common malignant liver tumors overall; 1° sources include GI, breast, lung cancers. Metastases are rarely solitary.

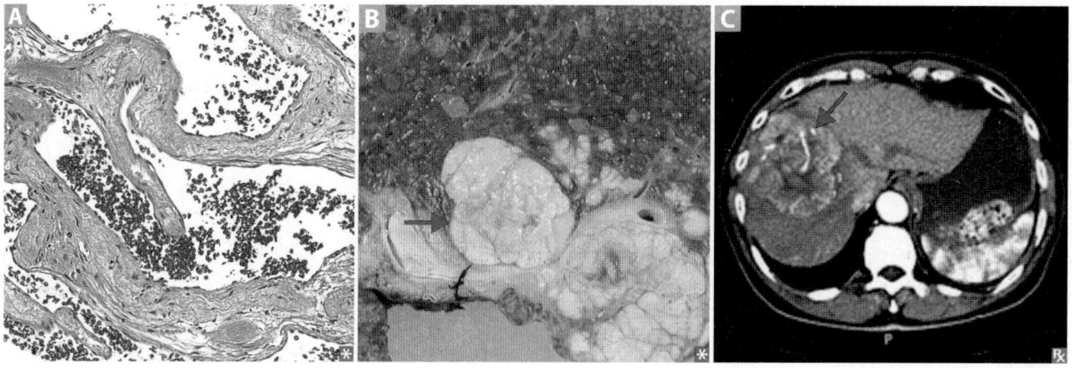

Budd-Chiari syndrome

Hepatic venous outflow tract obstruction (eg, due to thrombosis, compression) with centrilobular congestion and necrosis → congestive liver disease (hepatomegaly, ascites, varices, abdominal pain, liver failure). Absence of JVD. Associated with hypercoagulable states, polycythemia vera, postpartum state, HCC. May cause nutmeg liver (mottled appearance).

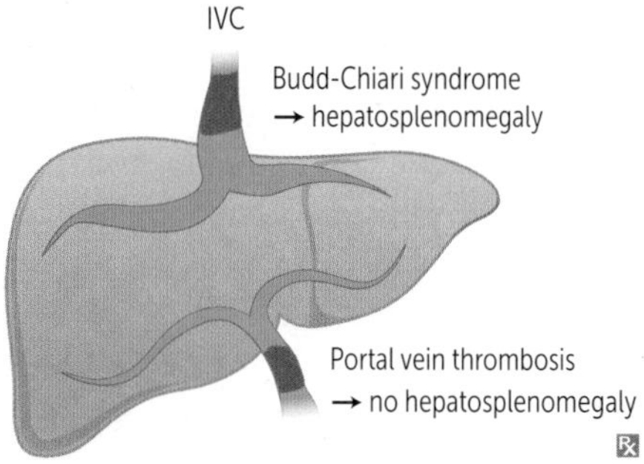

α_1-antitrypsin deficiency

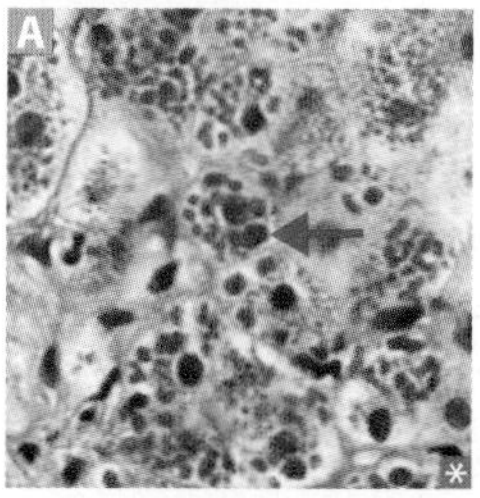

Misfolded gene product protein aggregates in hepatocellular ER → cirrhosis with PAS ⊕ globules A in liver. Codominant trait.
Often presents in young patients with liver damage and dyspnea without a history of tobacco smoking.

In lungs, ↓ α_1-antitrypsin → uninhibited elastase in alveoli → ↓ elastic tissue → panacinar emphysema.

Jaundice

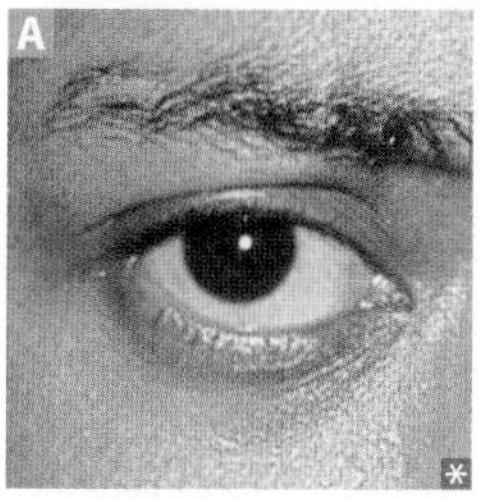

Abnormal yellowing of the skin and/or sclera A due to bilirubin deposition. Hyperbilirubinemia 2° to ↑ production or ↓ clearance (impaired hepatic uptake, conjugation, excretion).

HOT Liver—common causes of ↑ bilirubin level:
Hemolysis
Obstruction
Tumor
Liver disease

Conjugated (direct) hyperbilirubinemia	Biliary tract obstruction: gallstones, cholangiocarcinoma, pancreatic or liver cancer, liver fluke. Biliary tract disease: ▪ 1° sclerosing cholangitis ▪ 1° biliary cholangitis Excretion defect: Dubin-Johnson syndrome, Rotor syndrome.
Unconjugated (indirect) hyperbilirubinemia	Hemolytic, physiologic (newborns), Crigler-Najjar, Gilbert syndrome.
Mixed (direct and indirect) hyperbilirubinemia	Hepatitis, cirrhosis.

Physiologic neonatal jaundice

At birth, lower activity of UDP-glucuronosyltransferase → unconjugated hyperbilirubinemia → jaundice/kernicterus (deposition of unconjugated, lipid-soluble bilirubin in the brain, particularly basal ganglia).
Occurs after first 24 hours of life and usually resolves without treatment in 1–2 weeks.
Treatment: phototherapy (non-UV) isomerizes unconjugated bilirubin to water-soluble form.

Biliary atresia

Most common reason for pediatric liver transplantation.
Fibro-obliterative destruction of bile ducts → cholestasis.
Often presents as a newborn with persistent jaundice after 2 weeks of life, darkening urine, acholic stools, hepatomegaly.
Labs: ↑ direct bilirubin and GGT.

Hereditary hyperbilirubinemias	All autosomal recessive.
❶ **Gilbert syndrome**	Mildly ↓ UDP-glucuronosyltransferase conjugation. Asymptomatic or mild jaundice usually with stress, illness, or fasting. ↑ unconjugated bilirubin without overt hemolysis. Relatively common, benign condition.
❷ **Crigler-Najjar syndrome, type I**	Absent UDP-glucuronosyltransferase. Presents early in life, but some patients may not have neurologic signs until later in life. Findings: jaundice, kernicterus (bilirubin deposition in brain), ↑ unconjugated bilirubin. Treatment: plasmapheresis and phototherapy (does not conjugate UCB; but does ↑ polarity and ↑ water solubility to allow excretion). Liver transplant is curative. Type II is less severe and responds to phenobarbital, which ↑ liver enzyme synthesis.
❸ **Dubin-Johnson syndrome**	Conjugated hyperbilirubinemia due to defective liver excretion. Grossly black (**D**ark) liver due to impaired excretion of epinephrine metabolites. Benign.
❹ **Rotor syndrome**	Phenotypically similar to Dubin-Johnson, but milder in presentation without black (**R**egular) liver. Due to impaired hepatic storage of conjugated bilirubin.

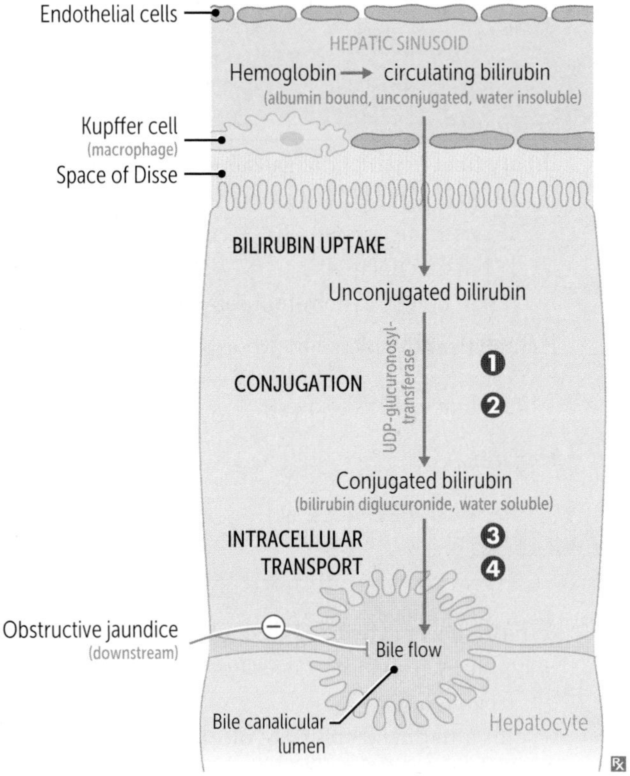

Wilson disease

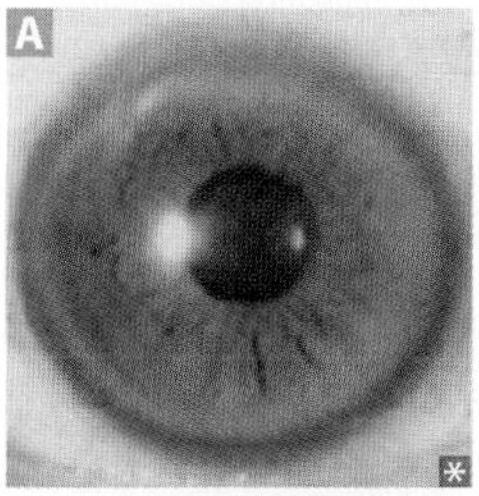

Also called hepatolenticular degeneration. Autosomal recessive mutations in hepatocyte copper-transporting ATPase (*ATP7B* gene; chromosome 13) → ↓ copper incorporation into apoceruloplasmin and excretion into bile → ↓ serum ceruloplasmin. Copper accumulates, especially in liver, brain (eg, basal ganglia), cornea, kidneys; ↑ urine copper.

Presents before age 40 with liver disease (eg, hepatitis, acute liver failure, cirrhosis), neurologic disease (eg, dysarthria, dystonia, tremor, parkinsonism), psychiatric disease, Kayser-Fleischer rings (deposits in Descemet membrane of cornea) A, hemolytic anemia, renal disease (eg, Fanconi syndrome).

Treatment: chelation with penicillamine or trientine, oral zinc. Liver transplant in acute liver failure related to Wilson disease.

Hemochromatosis

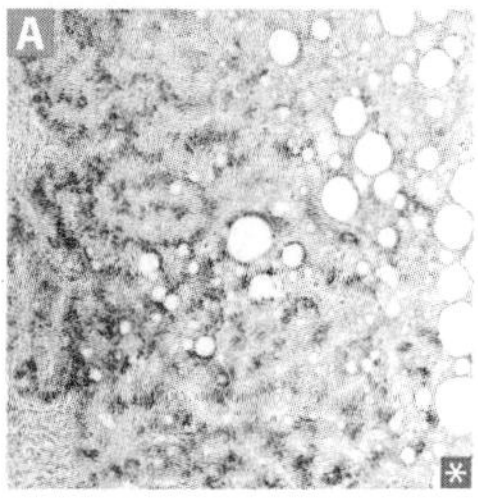

Autosomal recessive. Mutation in *HFE* gene, located on chromosome 6. Leads to abnormal **iron** sensing and ↑ intestinal absorption (↑ ferritin, ↑ iron, ↓ TIBC → ↑ transferrin saturation). Iron overload can also be 2° to chronic transfusion therapy (eg, β-thalassemia major). Iron accumulates, especially in liver, pancreas, skin, heart, pituitary, joints. Hemosiderin (iron) can be identified on liver MRI or biopsy with Prussian blue stain A.

Presents after age 40 when total body iron > 20 g; iron loss through menstruation slows progression in females. Classic triad of cirrhosis, diabetes mellitus, skin pigmentation ("bronze diabetes"). Also causes restrictive cardiomyopathy (classic) or dilated cardiomyopathy (reversible), hypogonadism, arthropathy (calcium pyrophosphate deposition; especially metacarpophalangeal joints). HCC is common cause of death.

Treatment: repeated phlebotomy, iron (**Fe**) chelation with de**fe**rasirox, de**fe**roxamine, de**fe**riprone.

Biliary tract disease

May present with pruritus, jaundice, dark urine, light-colored stool, hepatosplenomegaly. Typically with cholestatic pattern of LFTs (↑ conjugated bilirubin, ↑ cholesterol, ↑ ALP, ↑ GGT).

	PATHOLOGY	EPIDEMIOLOGY	ADDITIONAL FEATURES
Primary sclerosing cholangitis	Unknown cause of concentric "onion skin" bile duct fibrosis → alternating strictures and dilation with "beading" of intra- and extrahepatic bile ducts on ERCP, magnetic resonance cholangiopancreatography (MRCP).	Classically in middle-aged males with ulcerative colitis.	Associated with ulcerative colitis. MPO-ANCA/p-ANCA ⊕. ↑ IgM. Can lead to 2° biliary cirrhosis. ↑ risk of cholangiocarcinoma and gallbladder cancer.
Primary biliary cholangitis	Autoimmune reaction → lymphocytic infiltrate +/− granulomas → destruction of lobular bile ducts.	Classically in middle-aged females.	Anti-mitochondrial antibody ⊕, ↑ IgM. Associated with other autoimmune conditions (eg, Hashimoto thyroiditis, rheumatoid arthritis, celiac disease). Treatment: ursodiol.
Secondary biliary cirrhosis	Extrahepatic biliary obstruction → ↑ pressure in intrahepatic ducts → injury/ fibrosis and bile stasis.	Patients with known obstructive lesions (gallstones, biliary strictures, pancreatic carcinoma).	May be complicated by acute cholangitis.

Cholelithiasis and related pathologies

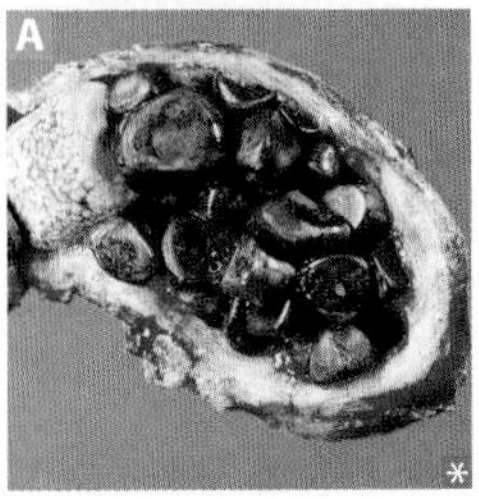

↑ cholesterol and/or bilirubin, ↓ bile salts, and gallbladder stasis all cause stones.

2 types of stones:

- Cholesterol stones (radiolucent with 10–20% opaque due to calcifications)—80% of stones. Associated with obesity, Crohn disease, advanced age, estrogen therapy, multiparity, rapid weight loss, medications (eg, fibrates).
- Pigment stones A (black = radiopaque, Ca^{2+} bilirubinate, hemolysis; brown = radiolucent, infection). Associated with Crohn disease, chronic hemolysis, alcoholic cirrhosis, advanced age, biliary infections, total parenteral nutrition (TPN).

Risk factors (4 F's):

1. Female
2. Fat (obesity)
3. Fertile (multiparity)
4. Forty

Most common complication is cholecystitis; can also cause acute pancreatitis, acute cholangitis.

Diagnose with ultrasound. Treat with elective cholecystectomy if symptomatic.

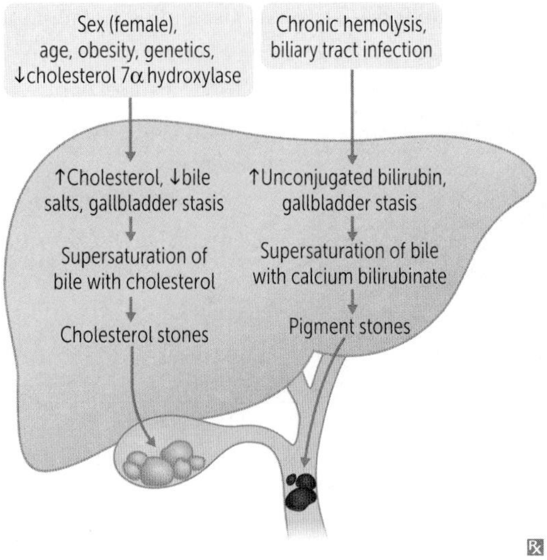
Sex (female), age, obesity, genetics, ↓cholesterol 7α hydroxylase
Chronic hemolysis, biliary tract infection
↑Cholesterol, ↓bile salts, gallbladder stasis
↑Unconjugated bilirubin, gallbladder stasis
Supersaturation of bile with cholesterol
Supersaturation of bile with calcium bilirubinate
Cholesterol stones
Pigment stones

RELATED PATHOLOGIES	CHARACTERISTICS
Biliary colic	Associated with nausea/vomiting and dull RUQ pain. Neurohormonal activation (eg, by CCK after a fatty meal) triggers contraction of gallbladder, forcing stone into cystic duct. Labs are normal, ultrasound shows cholelithiasis.
Choledocholithiasis	Presence of gallstone(s) in common bile duct, often leading to elevated ALP, GGT, direct bilirubin, and/or AST/ALT.
Cholecystitis 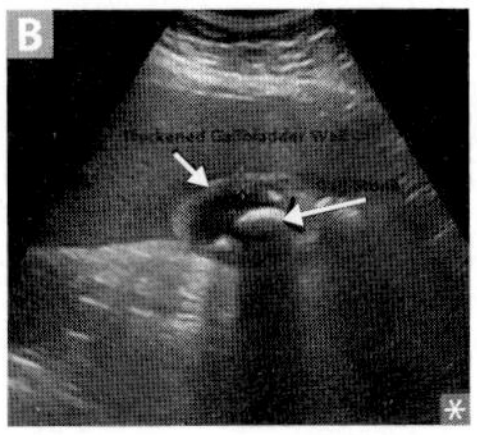	Acute or chronic inflammation of gallbladder. Calculous cholecystitis—most common type; due to gallstone impaction in the cystic duct resulting in inflammation and gallbladder wall thickening (arrows in B); can produce 2° infection. Acalculous cholecystitis—due to gallbladder stasis, hypoperfusion, or infection (CMV); seen in critically ill patients. Murphy sign: inspiratory arrest on RUQ palpation due to pain. Pain may radiate to right shoulder (due to irritation of phrenic nerve). ↑ ALP if bile duct becomes involved (eg, acute cholangitis). Diagnose with ultrasound or cholescintigraphy (HIDA scan). Failure to visualize gallbladder on HIDA scan suggests obstruction. Gallstone ileus—fistula between gallbladder and GI tract → stone enters GI lumen → obstructs at ileocecal valve (narrowest point); can see air in biliary tree (pneumobilia). Rigler triad: radiographic findings of pneumobilia, small bowel obstruction, gallstone (usually in iliac fossa).

Cholelithiasis and related pathologies *(continued)*

RELATED PATHOLOGIES	CHARACTERISTICS
Porcelain gallbladder 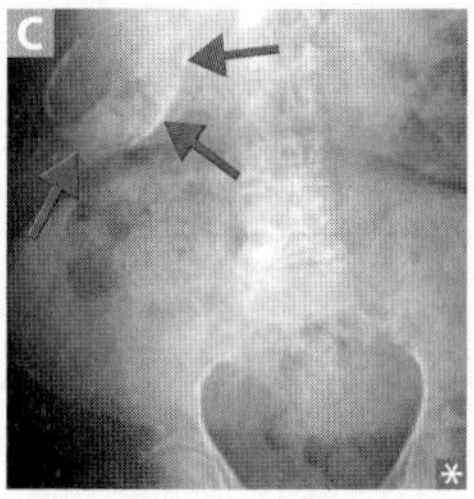	Calcified gallbladder due to chronic cholecystitis; usually found incidentally on imaging C. Treatment: prophylactic cholecystectomy generally recommended due to ↑ risk of gallbladder cancer (mostly adenocarcinoma).
Acute cholangitis	Also called ascending cholangitis. Infection of biliary tree usually due to obstruction that leads to stasis/bacterial overgrowth. Charcot triad of cholangitis includes jaundice, fever, RUQ pain. Reynolds pentad is Charcot triad plus altered mental status and shock (hypotension).

Cholangiocarcinoma	Malignant tumor of bile duct epithelium. Risk factors include 1° sclerosing cholangitis, liver fluke infections. Usually presents late with fatigue, weight loss, abdominal pain, jaundice. Imaging may show biliary tract obstruction. Histology: infiltrating neoplastic glands associated with desmoplastic stroma.
Acute pancreatitis 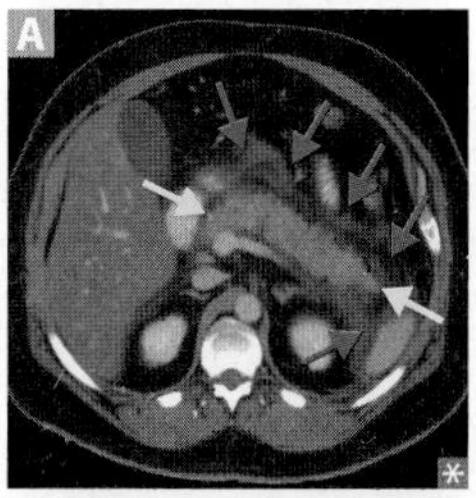 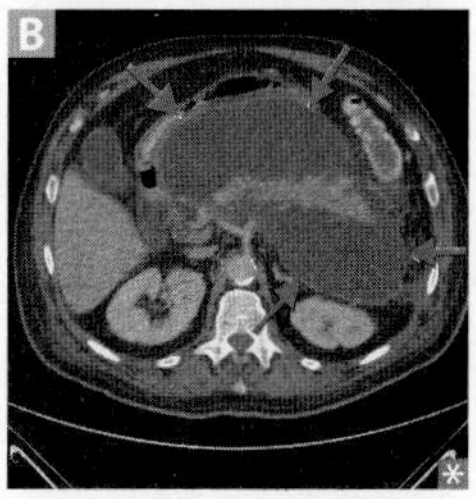	Autodigestion of pancreas by pancreatic enzymes (A shows pancreas [yellow arrows] surrounded by edema [red arrows]). Causes: **I**diopathic, **G**allstones, **E**thanol, **T**rauma, **S**teroids, **M**umps, **A**utoimmune disease, **S**corpion sting, **H**ypercalcemia/**H**ypertriglyceridemia (> 1000 mg/dL), **E**RCP, **D**rugs (eg, sulfa drugs, NRTIs, protease inhibitors). **I GET SMASHED**. Diagnosis by 2 of 3 criteria: acute epigastric pain often radiating to the back, ↑ serum amylase or lipase (more specific) to 3× upper limit of normal, or characteristic imaging findings. Complications: pseudocyst B (lined by granulation tissue, not epithelium), abscess, necrosis, hemorrhage, infection, organ failure (ALI/ARDS, shock, renal failure), hypocalcemia (precipitation of Ca^{2+} soaps).
Chronic pancreatitis 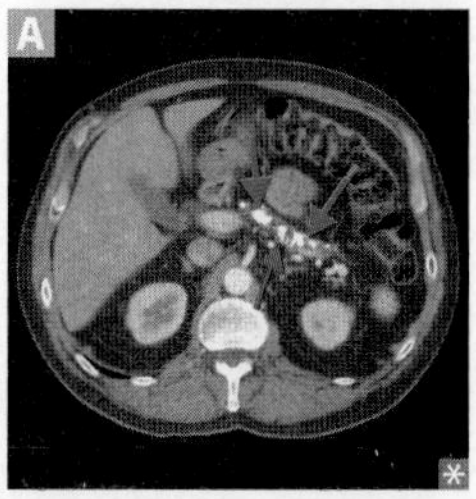	Chronic inflammation, atrophy, calcification of the pancreas A. Major risk factors include alcohol use disorder and genetic predisposition (eg, cystic fibrosis); can be idiopathic. Complications include pancreatic insufficiency and pseudocysts. Pancreatic insufficiency (typically when <10% pancreatic function) may manifest with steatorrhea, fat-soluble vitamin deficiency, diabetes mellitus. Amylase and lipase may or may not be elevated (almost always elevated in acute pancreatitis).

Pancreatic adenocarcinoma

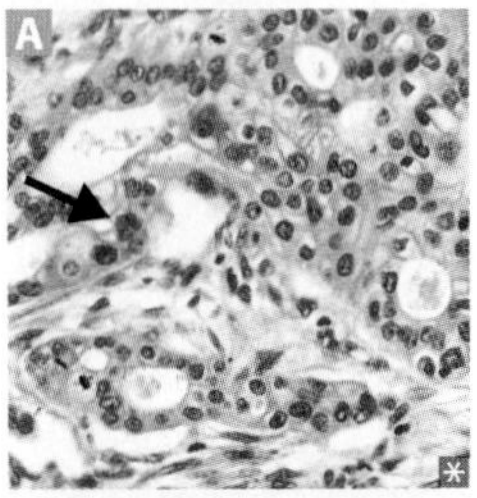

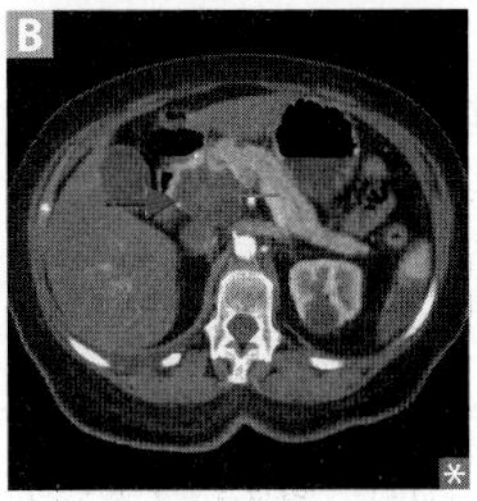

Very aggressive tumor arising from pancreatic ducts (disorganized glandular structure with cellular infiltration A); often metastatic at presentation, with average survival ~ 1 year after diagnosis. Tumors more common in pancreatic head B (lead to obstructive jaundice). Associated with CA 19-9 tumor marker (also CEA, less specific).

Risk factors:

- Tobacco smoking
- Chronic pancreatitis (especially > 20 years)
- Diabetes
- Age > 50 years

Often presents with:

- Abdominal pain radiating to back
- Weight loss (due to malabsorption and anorexia)
- Migratory thrombophlebitis—redness and tenderness on palpation of extremities (Trousseau syndrome)
- Obstructive jaundice with palpable, nontender gallbladder (Courvoisier sign)

▸ GASTROINTESTINAL—PHARMACOLOGY

Acid suppression therapy

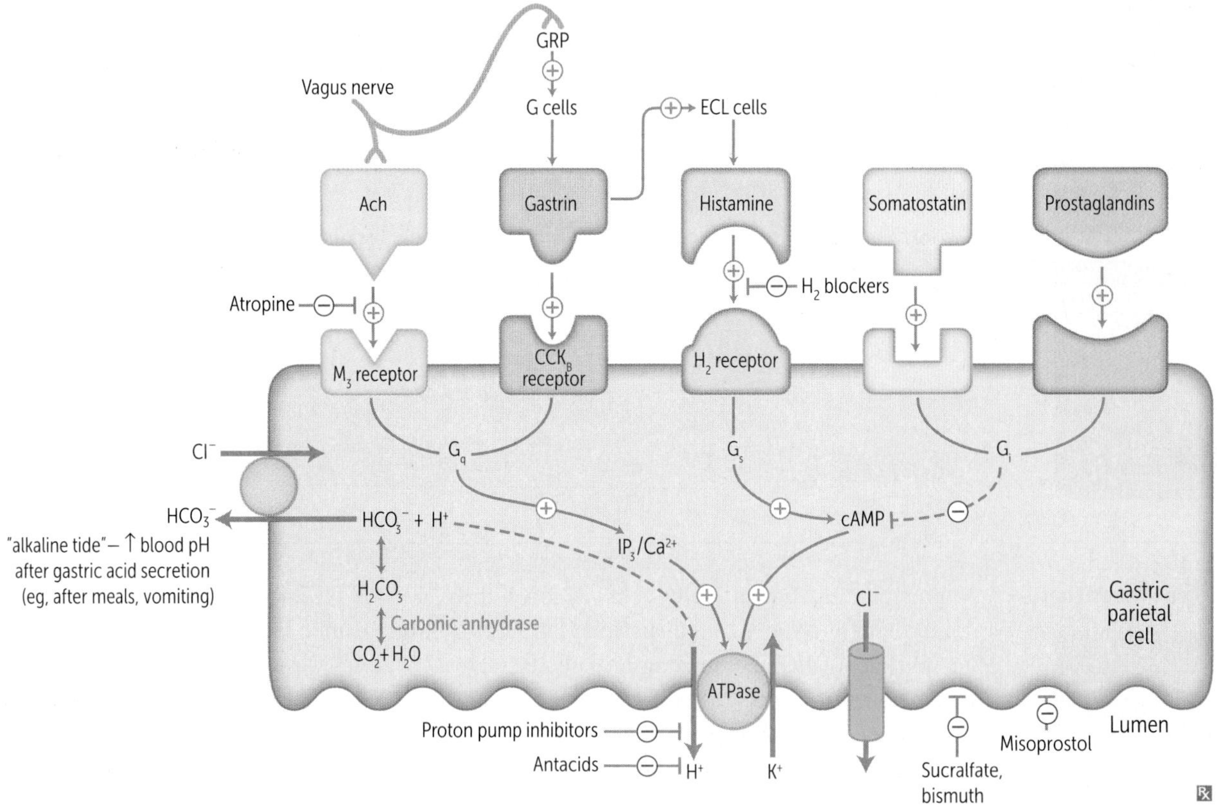

H_2-blockers	Cimetidine, famotidine, nizatidine.	Take H_2 blockers before you **dine**. Think "**table for 2**" to remember H_2.
MECHANISM	Reversible block of histamine H_2-receptors → ↓ H^+ secretion by parietal cells.	
CLINICAL USE	Peptic ulcer, gastritis, mild esophageal reflux.	
ADVERSE EFFECTS	Cimetidine is a potent inhibitor of cytochrome P-450 (multiple drug interactions); it also has antiandrogenic effects (prolactin release, gynecomastia, impotence, ↓ libido in males); can cross blood-brain barrier (confusion, dizziness, headaches) and placenta. Cimetidine ↓ renal excretion of creatinine. Other H_2 blockers are relatively free of these effects.	

Proton pump inhibitors	Omeprazole, lansoprazole, esomeprazole, pantoprazole, dexlansoprazole.
MECHANISM	Irreversibly inhibit H^+/K^+ ATPase in stomach parietal cells.
CLINICAL USE	Peptic ulcer, gastritis, esophageal reflux, Zollinger-Ellison syndrome, component of therapy for *H pylori*, stress ulcer prophylaxis.
ADVERSE EFFECTS	↑ risk of *C difficile* infection, pneumonia, acute interstitial nephritis. Vitamin B_{12} malabsorption; ↓ serum Mg^{2+} and ↓ Ca^{2+} absorption (potentially leading to increased fracture risk in elderly).

Antacids	Can affect absorption, bioavailability, or urinary excretion of other drugs by altering gastric and urinary pH or by delaying gastric emptying. All can cause hypokalemia. Overuse can also cause the following problems:	
Aluminum hydroxide	Constipation, Hypophosphatemia, Osteodystrophy, Proximal muscle weakness, Seizures	**Aluminimum** amount of feces **CHOPS**
Calcium carbonate	Hypercalcemia (milk-alkali syndrome), rebound acid ↑	Can chelate and ↓ effectiveness of other drugs (eg, tetracycline)
Magnesium hydroxide	Diarrhea, hyporeflexia, hypotension, cardiac arrest	**Mg^{2+} = Must go 2 the bathroom**

Bismuth, sucralfate	
MECHANISM	Bind to ulcer base, providing physical protection and allowing HCO_3^- secretion to reestablish pH gradient in the mucous layer. Sucralfate requires acidic environment, not given with PPIs/H_2 blockers.
CLINICAL USE	↑ ulcer healing, travelers' diarrhea (bismuth). Bismuth also used in quadruple therapy for *H pylori* gastritis.

Misoprostol	
MECHANISM	PGE_1 analog. ↑ production and secretion of gastric mucous barrier, ↓ acid production.
CLINICAL USE	Prevention of NSAID-induced peptic ulcers (NSAIDs block PGE_1 production). Also used off-label for induction of labor (ripens cervix).
ADVERSE EFFECTS	Diarrhea. Contraindicated in patients of childbearing potential (abortifacient).

Octreotide

MECHANISM	Long-acting somatostatin analog; inhibits secretion of various splanchnic vasodilatory hormones.
CLINICAL USE	Acute variceal bleeds, acromegaly, VIPoma, carcinoid tumors.
ADVERSE EFFECTS	Nausea, cramps, steatorrhea. ↑ risk of cholelithiasis due to CCK inhibition.

Sulfasalazine

MECHANISM	A combination of sulfapyridine (antibacterial) and 5-aminosalicylic acid (anti-inflammatory). Activated by colonic bacteria.
CLINICAL USE	Ulcerative colitis, Crohn disease (colitis component).
ADVERSE EFFECTS	Malaise, nausea, sulfonamide toxicity, reversible oligospermia.

Loperamide

MECHANISM	Agonist at μ-opioid receptors; slows gut motility. Poor CNS penetration (low addictive potential).
CLINICAL USE	Diarrhea.
ADVERSE EFFECTS	Constipation, nausea.

Ondansetron

MECHANISM	$5\text{-}HT_3$ antagonist. Acts peripherally (↓ vagal stimulation) and centrally. Potent antiemetic.
CLINICAL USE	Control vomiting postoperatively and in patients undergoing cancer chemotherapy.
ADVERSE EFFECTS	Headache, constipation, QT interval prolongation, serotonin syndrome.

Aprepitant

MECHANISM	Substance P antagonist. Blocks NK_1 (neurokinin-1) receptors in brain.
CLINICAL USE	Antiemetic for chemotherapy-induced nausea and vomiting.

Metoclopramide

MECHANISM	D_2 receptor antagonist. ↑ resting tone, contractility, LES tone, motility, promotes gastric emptying. Does not influence colon transport time.
CLINICAL USE	Diabetic and postoperative gastroparesis, antiemetic, persistent GERD.
ADVERSE EFFECTS	↑ parkinsonian effects, tardive dyskinesia. Restlessness, drowsiness, fatigue, depression, diarrhea. Drug interaction with digoxin and diabetic agents. Contraindicated in patients with small bowel obstruction, Parkinson disease (due to D_2-receptor blockade), ↓ seizure threshold.

Orlistat

MECHANISM	Inhibits gastric and pancreatic lipase → ↓ breakdown and absorption of dietary fats. Taken with fat-containing meals.
CLINICAL USE	Weight loss.
ADVERSE EFFECTS	Abdominal pain, flatulence, bowel urgency/frequent bowel movements, steatorrhea; ↓ absorption of fat-soluble vitamins.

Laxatives

Indicated for constipation or patients on opiates requiring a bowel regimen.

	EXAMPLES	MECHANISM	ADVERSE EFFECTS
Bulk-forming laxatives	Psyllium, methylcellulose	Soluble fibers draw water into gut lumen, forming a viscous liquid that promotes peristalsis	Bloating
Osmotic laxatives	Magnesium hydroxide, magnesium citrate, polyethylene glycol, lactulose	Provides osmotic load to draw water into GI lumen Lactulose also treats hepatic encephalopathy: gut flora degrade lactulose into metabolites (lactic acid, acetic acid) that promote nitrogen excretion as NH_4^+	Diarrhea, dehydration; may be misused by patients with bulimia nervosa; overuse may cause metabolic alkalosis
Stimulants	Senna, bisacodyl	Enteric nerve stimulation → colonic contraction	Diarrhea, melanosis coli; overuse may cause metabolic alkalosis
Emollients	Docusate	Promotes incorporation of water and fat into stool	Diarrhea; overuse may cause metabolic alkalosis

▶ NOTES

HIGH-YIELD SYSTEMS

Hematology and Oncology

"You're always somebody's type! (blood type, that is)"

—BloodLink

"The best blood will at some time get into a fool or a mosquito."

—Austin O'Malley

"A life touched by cancer is not a life destroyed by cancer."

—Drew Boswell, *Climbing the Cancer Mountain*

"Without hair, a queen is still a queen."

—Prajakta Mhadnak

"Blood can circulate forever if you keep donating it."

—Anonymous

When studying hematology, pay close attention to the many cross connections to immunology. Make sure you master the different types of anemias. Be comfortable interpreting blood smears. When reviewing oncologic drugs, focus on mechanisms and adverse effects rather than details of clinical uses, which may be lower yield.

Please note that solid tumors are covered in their respective organ system chapters.

▶ HEMATOLOGY AND ONCOLOGY—EMBRYOLOGY

Fetal erythropoiesis

Fetal erythropoiesis occurs in:
- Yolk sac (3–8 weeks)
- Liver (6 weeks–birth)
- Spleen (10–28 weeks)
- Bone marrow (18 weeks to adult)

Young liver synthesizes blood.

Hemoglobin development

Embryonic globins: ζ and ε.
Fetal hemoglobin (HbF) = $\alpha_2\gamma_2$.
Adult hemoglobin (HbA_1) = $\alpha_2\beta_2$.
HbF has higher affinity for O_2 due to less avid binding of 2,3-BPG, allowing HbF to extract O_2 from maternal hemoglobin (HbA_1 and HbA_2) across the placenta. HbA_2 ($\alpha_2\delta_2$) is a form of adult hemoglobin present in small amounts.

From fetal to adult hemoglobin:
Alpha always; gamma goes, becomes beta.

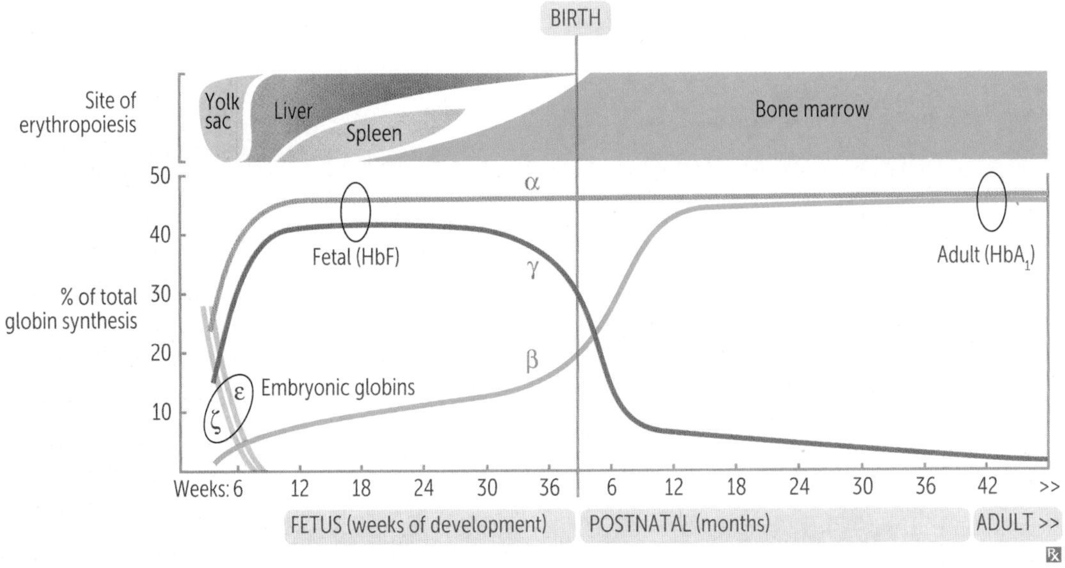

Blood groups

	ABO classification				Rh classification	
	A	B	AB	O	Rh⊕	Rh⊖
RBC type	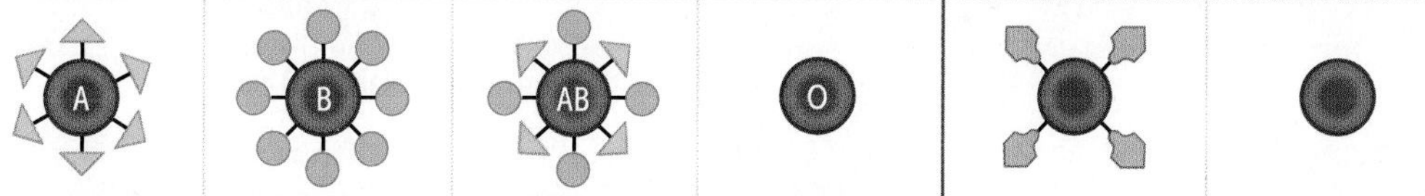					
Group antigens on RBC surface	A	B	A & B	None	Rh (D)	None
Antibodies in plasma	Anti-B IgM	Anti-A IgM	None	Anti-A Anti-B IgG (predominantly), IgM	None	Anti-D IgG
Clinical relevance Compatible RBC types to receive	A, O	B, O	AB, A, B, O	O	Rh⊕, Rh⊖	Rh⊖
Compatible RBC types to donate to	A, AB	B, AB	AB	A, B, AB, O	Rh⊕	Rh⊕, Rh⊖

Hemolytic disease of the fetus and newborn

Also known as erythroblastosis fetalis.

	Rh hemolytic disease	ABO hemolytic disease
INTERACTION	Rh ⊖ pregnant patient; Rh ⊕ fetus.	Type O pregnant patient; type A or B fetus.
MECHANISM	First pregnancy: patient exposed to fetal blood (often during delivery) → formation of maternal anti-D IgG. Subsequent pregnancies: anti-D IgG crosses placenta → attacks fetal and newborn RBCs → hemolysis.	Preexisting pregnant patient anti-A and/or anti-B IgG antibodies cross the placenta → attack fetal and newborn RBCs → hemolysis.
PRESENTATION	Hydrops fetalis, jaundice shortly after birth, kernicterus.	Mild jaundice in the neonate within 24 hours of birth. Unlike Rh hemolytic disease, can occur in firstborn babies and is usually less severe.
TREATMENT/PREVENTION	Prevent by administration of anti-D IgG to Rh ⊖ pregnant patients during third trimester and early postpartum period (if fetus Rh ⊕). Prevents maternal anti-D IgG production.	Treatment: phototherapy or exchange transfusion.

▸ HEMATOLOGY AND ONCOLOGY—ANATOMY

Hematopoiesis

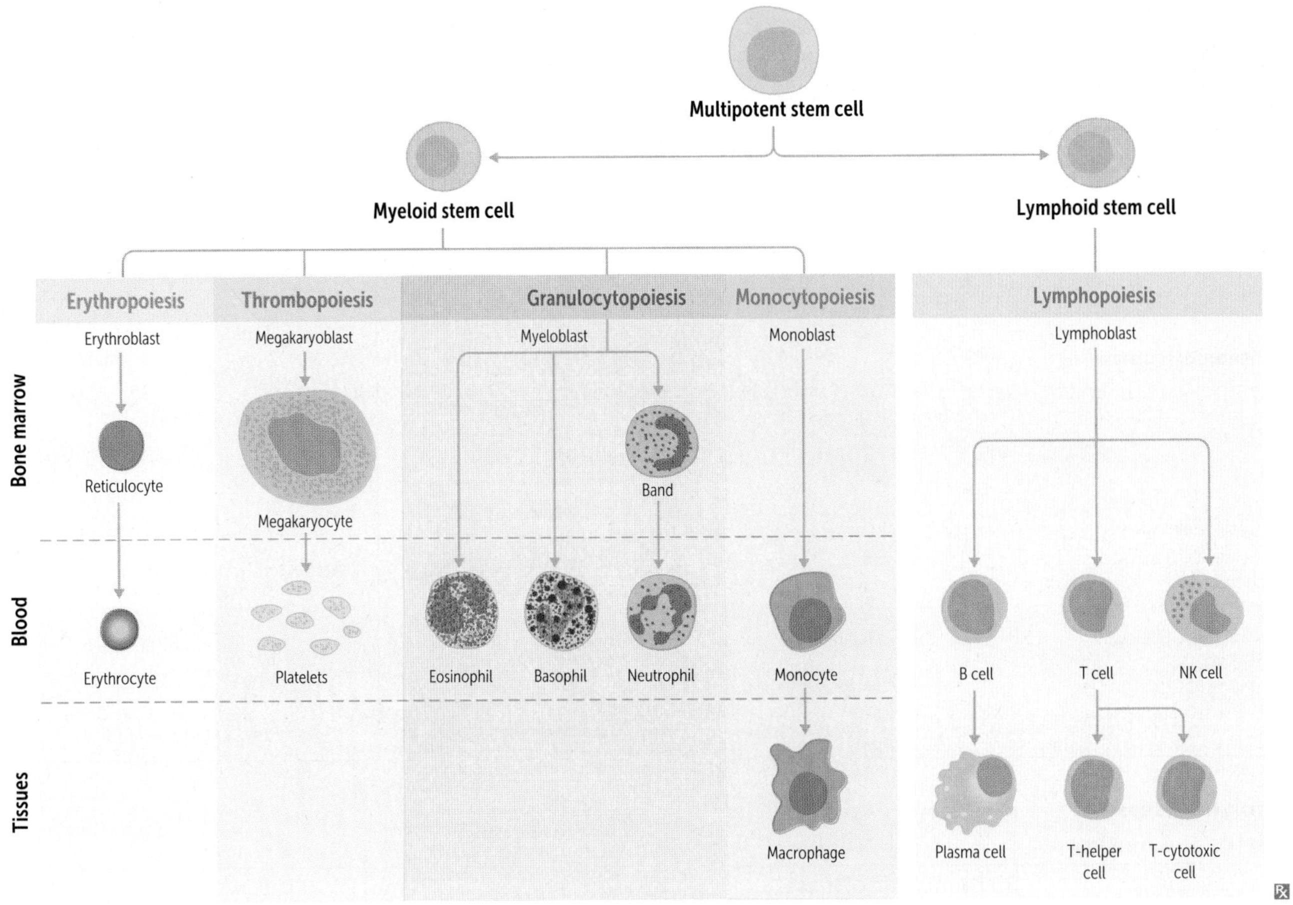

Neutrophils

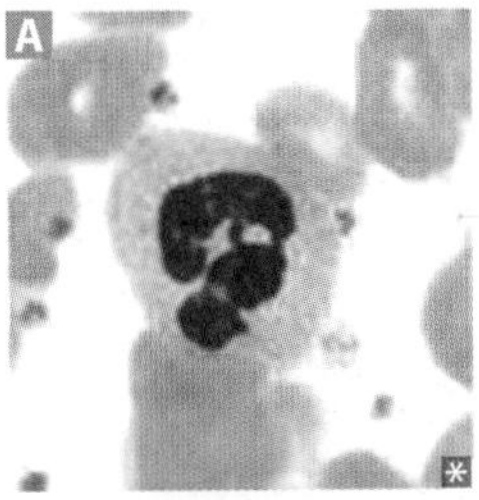

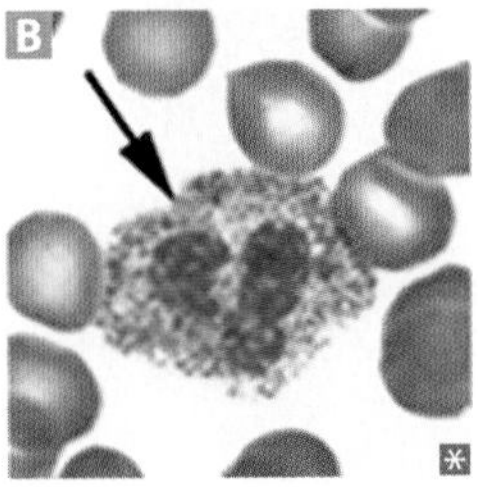

Acute inflammatory response cells. Phagocytic. Multilobed nucleus A. Specific granules contain leukocyte alkaline phosphatase (LAP), collagenase, lysozyme, and lactoferrin. Azurophilic granules (lysosomes) contain proteinases, acid phosphatase, myeloperoxidase, and β-glucuronidase.

Inflammatory states (eg, bacterial infection) cause neutrophilia and changes in neutrophil morphology, such as left shift, toxic granulation (dark blue, coarse granules), Döhle bodies (light blue, peripheral inclusions, arrow in B), and cytoplasmic vacuoles.

Neutrophil chemotactic agents: C5a, IL-8, LTB_4, 5-HETE (leukotriene precursor), kallikrein, platelet-activating factor, N-formylmethionine (bacterial proteins).

Hypersegmented neutrophils (nucleus has 6+ lobes) are seen in vitamin B_{12}/folate deficiency.

Left shift—↑ neutrophil precursors (eg, band cells, metamyelocytes) in peripheral blood. Reflects states of ↑ myeloid proliferation (eg, inflammation, CML).

Leukoerythroblastic reaction—left shift accompanied by immature RBCs. Suggests bone marrow infiltration (eg, myelofibrosis, metastasis).

Erythrocytes

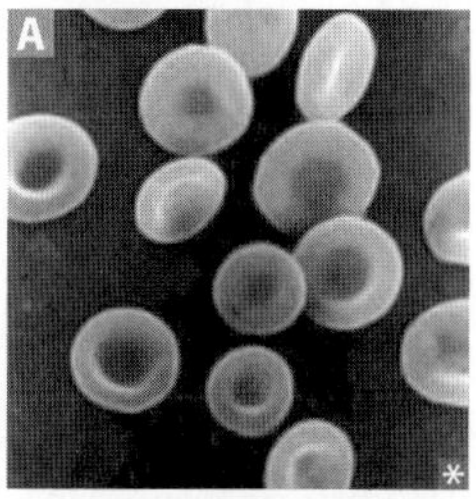

Carry O_2 to tissues and CO_2 to lungs. Anucleate and lack organelles; biconcave A, with large surface area-to-volume ratio for rapid gas exchange. Life span of ~120 days in healthy adults; 60-90 days in neonates. Source of energy is glucose (90% used in glycolysis, 10% used in HMP shunt). Membranes contain Cl^-/HCO_3^- antiporter, which allow RBCs to export HCO_3^- and transport CO_2 from the periphery to the lungs for elimination.

Erythro = red; *cyte* = cell.

Erythrocytosis = polycythemia = ↑ Hct.
Anisocytosis = varying sizes.
Poikilocytosis = varying shapes.

Reticulocyte = immature RBC; reflects erythroid proliferation.
Bluish color (polychromasia) on Wright-Giemsa stain of reticulocytes represents residual ribosomal RNA.

Thrombocytes (platelets)

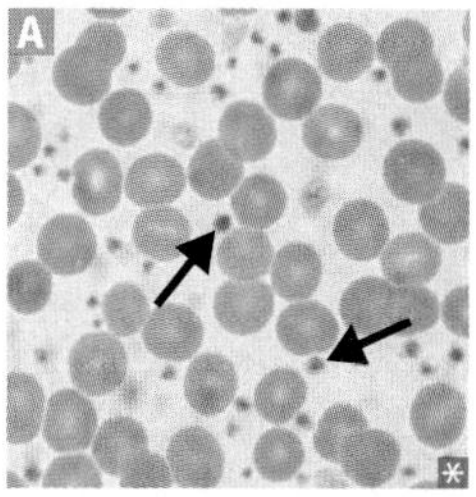

Involved in 1° hemostasis. Anucleate, small cytoplasmic fragments A derived from megakaryocytes. Life span of 8–10 days (pl8lets). When activated by endothelial injury, aggregate with other platelets and interact with fibrinogen to form platelet plug. Contain dense granules (Ca^{2+}, ADP, Serotonin, Histamine; **CASH**) and α granules (vWF, fibrinogen, fibronectin, platelet factor 4). Approximately ⅓ of platelet pool is stored in the spleen.

Thrombocytopenia or ↓ platelet function results in petechiae.
vWF receptor: GpIb.
Fibrinogen receptor: GpIIb/IIIa.
Thrombopoietin stimulates megakaryocyte proliferation.
Alfa granules contain vWF, fibrinogen, fibronectin, platelet factor four.

Monocytes

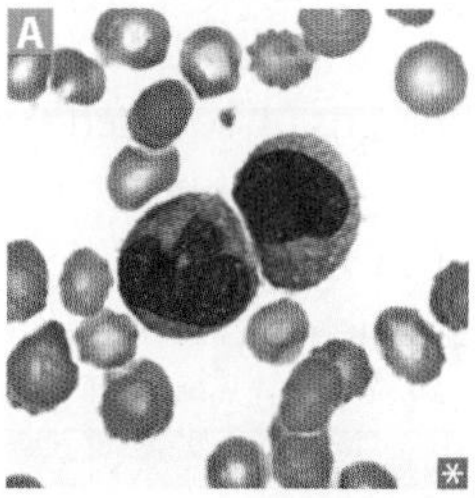

Found in blood, differentiate into macrophages in tissues.
Large, kidney-shaped nucleus A. Extensive "frosted glass" cytoplasm.

Mono = one (nucleus); *cyte* = cell.

Macrophages

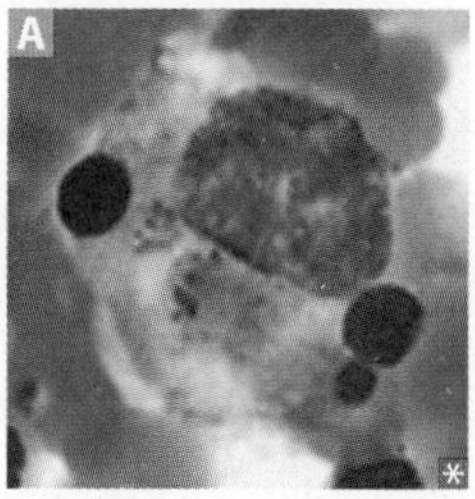

Phagocytose bacteria, cellular debris, and senescent RBCs. Long life in tissues. Differentiate from circulating blood monocytes A. Activated by γ-interferon. Can function as antigen-presenting cell via MHC II. Important cellular component of granulomas (eg, TB, sarcoidosis), where they may fuse to form giant cells.

Macro = large; *phage* = eater.
Macrophage naming varies by specific tissue type (eg, Kupffer cells in liver, histiocytes in connective tissue, Langerhans cells in skin, osteoclasts in bone, microglial cells in brain).
Lipid A from bacterial LPS binds CD14 on macrophages to initiate septic shock.

Eosinophils

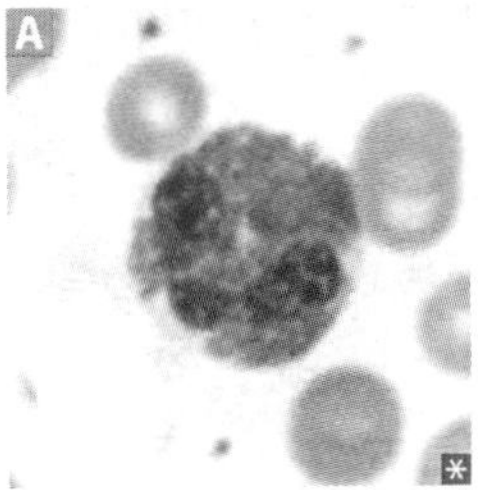

Defend against helminthic infections (major basic protein). Bilobate nucleus. Packed with large eosinophilic granules of uniform size A. Highly phagocytic for antigen-antibody complexes.

Produce histaminase, major basic protein (MBP, a helminthotoxin), eosinophil peroxidase, eosinophil cationic protein, and eosinophil-derived neurotoxin.

Eosin = pink dye; *philic* = loving.

Causes of eosinophilia (**PACMAN E**ats):
- **P**arasites
- **A**sthma
- **C**hronic adrenal insufficiency
- **M**yeloproliferative disorders
- **A**llergic processes
- **N**eoplasia (eg, Hodgkin lymphoma)
- **E**osinophilic granulomatosis with polyangiitis

Basophils

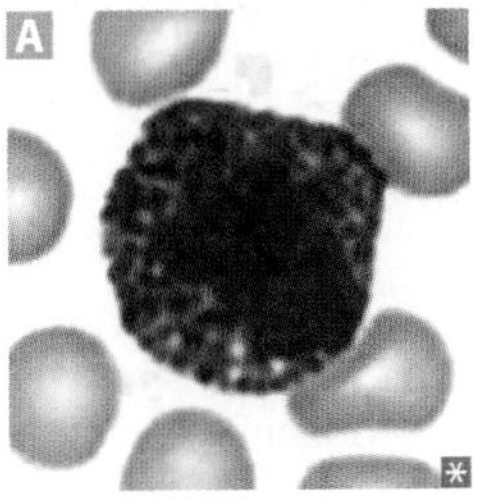

Mediate allergic reaction. Densely basophilic granules A contain heparin (anticoagulant) and histamine (vasodilator). Leukotrienes synthesized and released on demand.

Basophilic—stains readily with **basic** stains.

Basophilia is uncommon, but can be a sign of myeloproliferative disorders, particularly CML.

Mast cells

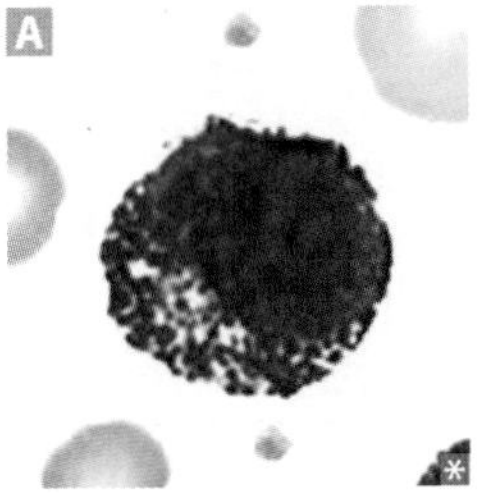

Mediate local tissue allergic reactions. Contain basophilic granules A. Originate from same precursor as basophils but are not the same cell type. Can bind the Fc portion of IgE to membrane. Activated by tissue trauma, C3a and C5a, surface IgE cross-linking by antigen (IgE receptor aggregation) → degranulation → release of histamine, heparin, tryptase, and eosinophil chemotactic factors.

Involved in type I hypersensitivity reactions.

Cromolyn sodium prevents mast cell degranulation (used for asthma prophylaxis).

Vancomycin, opioids, and radiocontrast dye can elicit IgE-independent mast cell degranulation.

Mastocytosis—rare; proliferation of mast cells in skin and/or extracutaneous organs. Associated with c-*KIT* mutations and ↑ serum tryptase. ↑ histamine → flushing, pruritus, hypotension, abdominal pain, diarrhea, peptic ulcer disease.

Dendritic cells

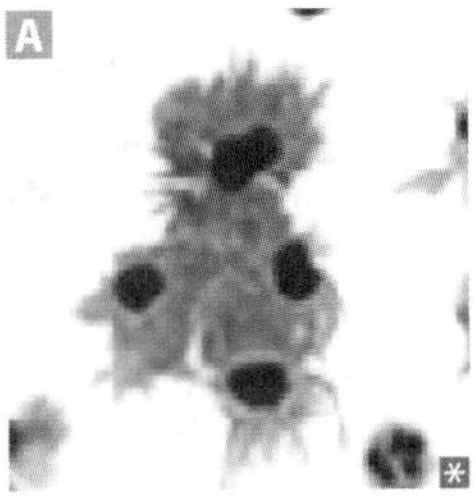

Highly phagocytic antigen-presenting cells (APCs) A. Function as link between innate and adaptive immune systems. Express MHC class II and Fc receptors on surface. Can present exogenous antigens on MHC class I (cross-presentation).

Lymphocytes

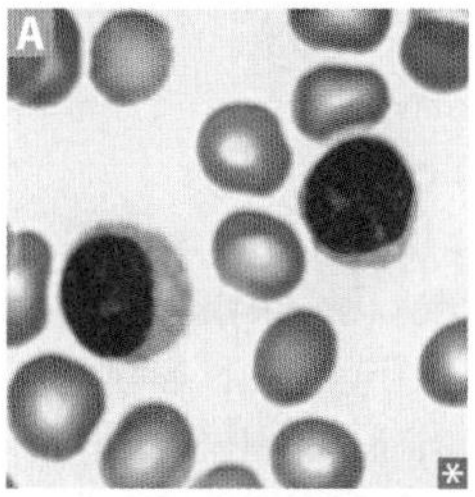

Refer to B cells, T cells, and NK cells. B cells and T cells mediate adaptive immunity. NK cells are part of the innate immune response. Round, densely staining nucleus with small amount of pale cytoplasm A.

Natural killer cells

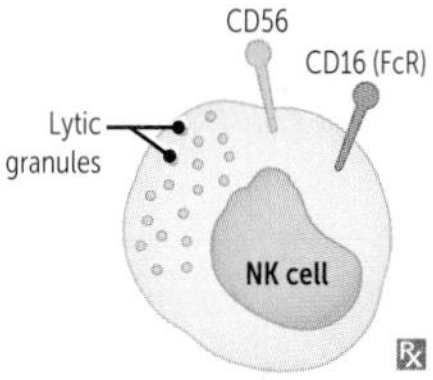

Important in innate immunity, especially against intracellular pathogens. Larger than B and T cells, with distinctive cytoplasmic lytic granules (containing perforin and granzymes) that, when released, act on target cells to induce apoptosis. Distinguish between healthy and infected cells by identifying cell surface proteins (induced by stress, malignant transformation, or microbial infections).

B cells

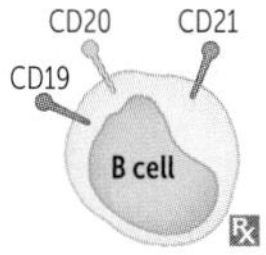

Mediate humoral immune response. Originate from stem cells in bone marrow and matures in marrow. Migrate to peripheral lymphoid tissue (follicles of lymph nodes, white pulp of spleen, unencapsulated lymphoid tissue). When antigen is encountered, B cells differentiate into plasma cells (which produce antibodies) and memory cells. Can function as an APC.

B = bone marrow.

T cells

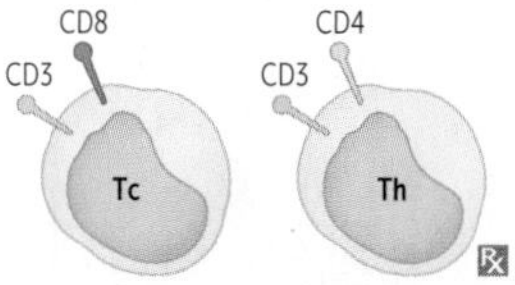

Mediate cellular immune response. Originate from stem cells in the bone marrow, but mature in the thymus. Differentiate into cytotoxic T cells (express CD8, recognize MHC I), helper T cells (express CD4, recognize MHC II), and regulatory T cells. CD28 (costimulatory signal) necessary for T-cell activation. Most circulating lymphocytes are T cells (80%).

T = thymus.

CD4+ helper T cells are the primary target of HIV.

Rule of 8: MHC II × CD4 = 8; MHC I × CD8 = 8.

Plasma cells

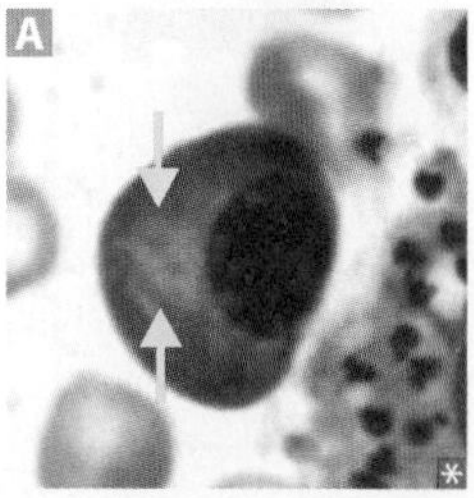

Produce large amounts of antibody specific to a particular antigen. "Clock-face" chromatin distribution and eccentric nucleus, abundant RER, and well-developed Golgi apparatus (arrows in A). Found in bone marrow and normally do not circulate in peripheral blood.

Multiple myeloma is a plasma cell dyscrasia.

▶ HEMATOLOGY AND ONCOLOGY—PHYSIOLOGY

Hemoglobin electrophoresis

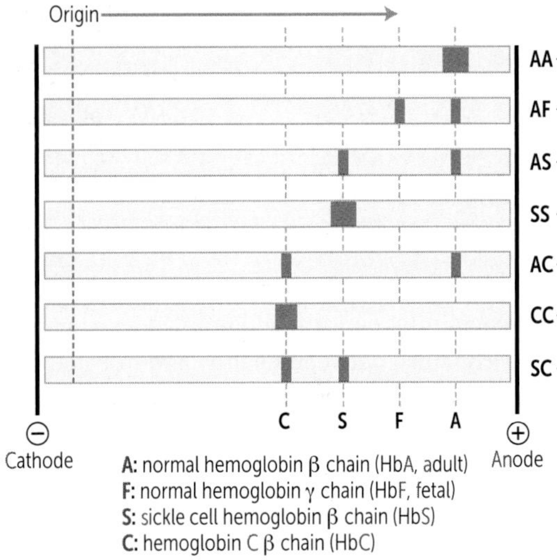
Origin
AA → Normal adult
AF → Normal newborn
AS → Sickle cell trait
SS → Sickle cell disease
AC → Hb C trait
CC → Hb C disease
SC → Hb SC disease
C S F A
⊖ Cathode
⊕ Anode
A: normal hemoglobin β chain (HbA, adult)
F: normal hemoglobin γ chain (HbF, fetal)
S: sickle cell hemoglobin β chain (HbS)
C: hemoglobin C β chain (HbC)

On a gel, hemoglobin migrates from the negatively charged cathode to the positively charged anode. HbA migrates the farthest, followed by HbF, HbS, and HbC. This is because the missense mutations in HbS and HbC replace glutamic acid ⊖ with valine (neutral) and lysine ⊕, respectively, making HbC and HbS more positively charged than HbA.

A Fat **S**anta **C**laus **can**'t (**ca**thode → **an**ode) go far.

Coombs test

Also called antiglobulin test. Detects the presence of antibodies against circulating RBCs.

Direct Coombs test—anti-Ig antibody (Coombs reagent) added to patient's RBCs. RBCs agglutinate if RBCs are coated with Ig. Used for AIHA diagnosis.

Indirect Coombs test—normal RBCs added to patient's serum. If serum has anti-RBC surface Ig, RBCs agglutinate when Coombs reagent is added. Used for pretransfusion testing.

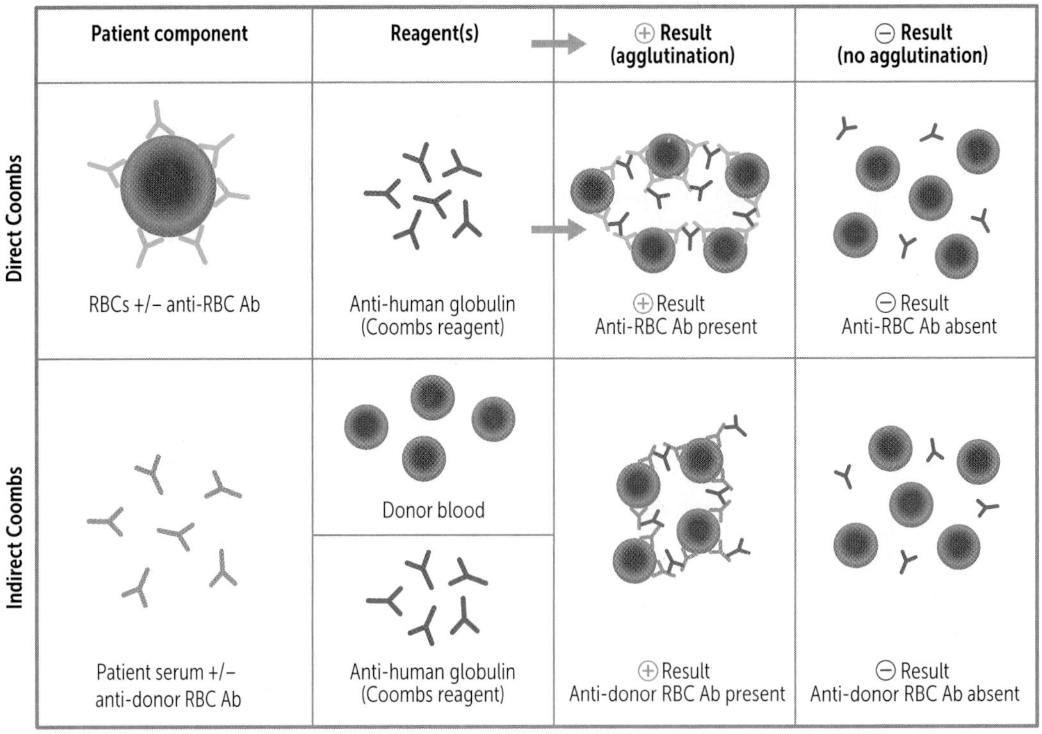
Patient component
Reagent(s)
⊕ Result (agglutination)
⊖ Result (no agglutination)
Direct Coombs
RBCs +/– anti-RBC Ab
Anti-human globulin (Coombs reagent)
⊕ Result Anti-RBC Ab present
⊖ Result Anti-RBC Ab absent
Indirect Coombs
Patient serum +/– anti-donor RBC Ab
Donor blood
Anti-human globulin (Coombs reagent)
⊕ Result Anti-donor RBC Ab present
⊖ Result Anti-donor RBC Ab absent

Platelet plug formation (primary hemostasis)

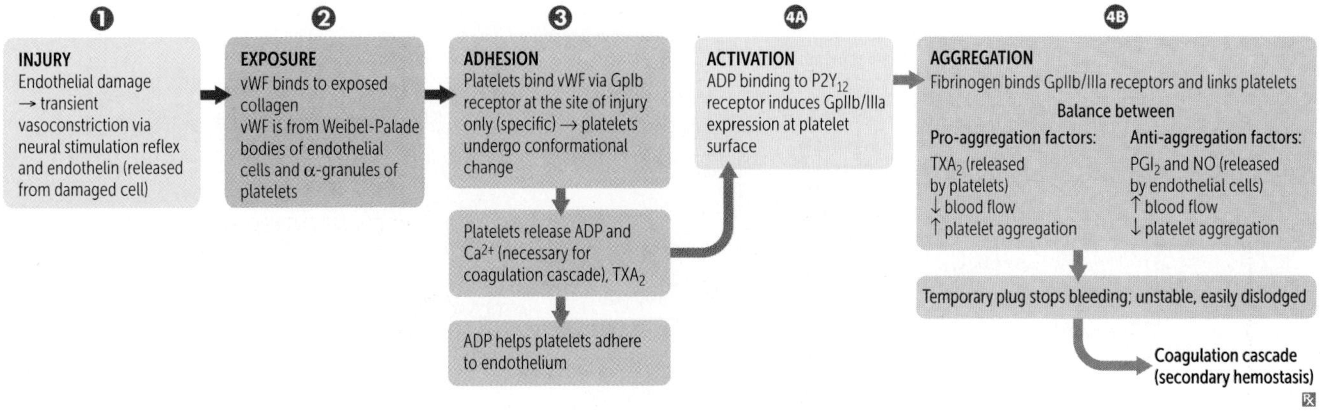
1
INJURY
Endothelial damage → transient vasoconstriction via neural stimulation reflex and endothelin (released from damaged cell)
2
EXPOSURE
vWF binds to exposed collagen
vWF is from Weibel-Palade bodies of endothelial cells and α-granules of platelets
3
ADHESION
Platelets bind vWF via GpIb receptor at the site of injury only (specific) → platelets undergo conformational change
Platelets release ADP and Ca2+ (necessary for coagulation cascade), TXA2
ADP helps platelets adhere to endothelium
4A
ACTIVATION
ADP binding to P2Y12 receptor induces GpIIb/IIIa expression at platelet surface
4B
AGGREGATION
Fibrinogen binds GpIIb/IIIa receptors and links platelets
Balance between
Pro-aggregation factors:
TXA2 (released by platelets)
↓ blood flow
↑ platelet aggregation
Anti-aggregation factors:
PGI2 and NO (released by endothelial cells)
↑ blood flow
↓ platelet aggregation
Temporary plug stops bleeding; unstable, easily dislodged
Coagulation cascade (secondary hemostasis)

Thrombogenesis

Formation of insoluble fibrin mesh.

Aspirin irreversibly inhibits cyclooxygenase, thereby inhibiting TXA_2 synthesis.

Clopidogrel, prasugrel, ticagrelor, and ticlopidine inhibit ADP-induced expression of GpIIb/IIIa by blocking $P2Y_{12}$ receptor.

Abciximab, eptifibatide, and tirofiban inhibit GpIIb/IIIa directly.

Ristocetin activates vWF to bind GpIb. Failure of aggregation with ristocetin assay occurs in von Willebrand disease and Bernard-Soulier syndrome. Desmopressin promotes the release of vWF and factor VIII from endothelial cells.

vWF carries/protects factor **VIII**; volks**W**agen **F**actories make gr**8** cars.

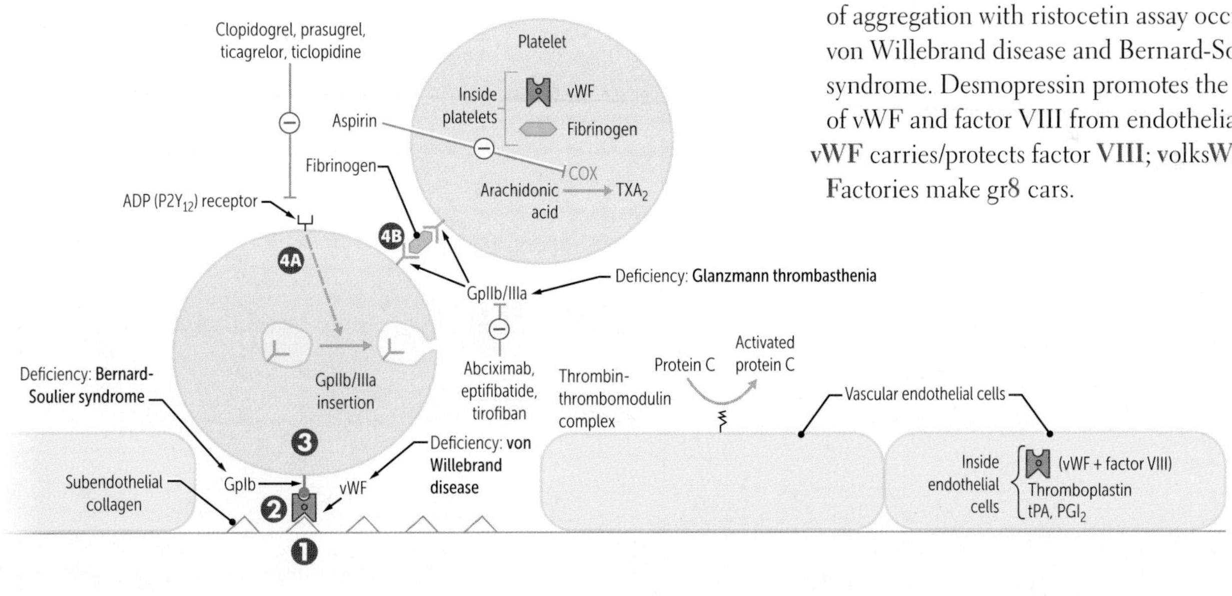
Clopidogrel, prasugrel, ticagrelor, ticlopidine
Aspirin
Platelet
Inside platelets
vWF
Fibrinogen
COX
Arachidonic acid
TXA2
Fibrinogen
ADP (P2Y12) receptor
4A
4B
GpIIb/IIIa
Deficiency: Glanzmann thrombasthenia
GpIIb/IIIa insertion
Abciximab, eptifibatide, tirofiban
Deficiency: Bernard-Soulier syndrome
3
Deficiency: von Willebrand disease
Subendothelial collagen
GpIb
vWF
2
1
Thrombin-thrombomodulin complex
Protein C
Activated protein C
Vascular endothelial cells
Inside endothelial cells
(vWF + factor VIII)
Thromboplastin
tPA, PGI2

Coagulation and kinin pathways

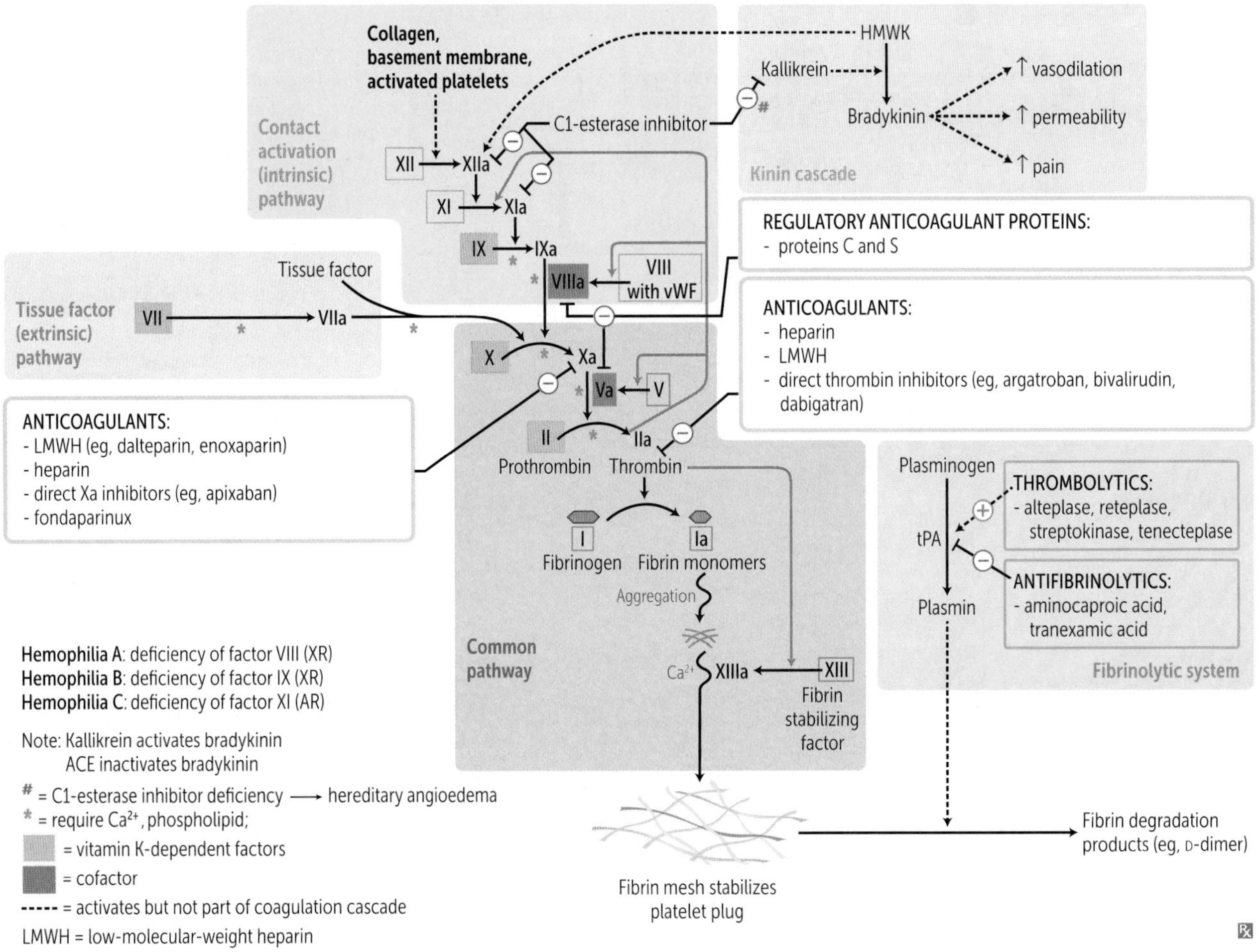

Vitamin K–dependent coagulation

Procoagulation

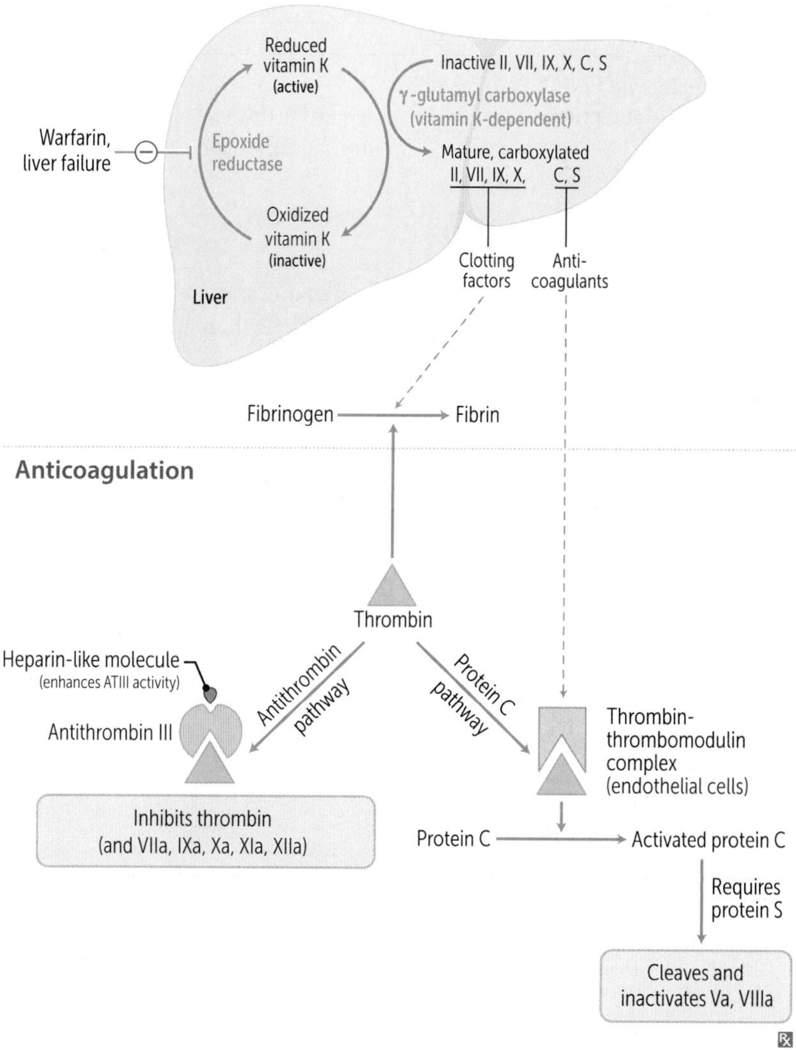

Vitamin K deficiency—↓ synthesis of factors II, VII, IX, X, protein C, protein S.

Warfarin inhibits vitamin K epoxide reductase. Vitamin K administration can potentially reverse inhibitory effect of warfarin on clotting factor synthesis (delayed). FFP or PCC administration reverses action of warfarin immediately and can be given with vitamin K in cases of severe bleeding.

Neonates lack enteric bacteria, which produce vitamin K. Early administration of vitamin K overcomes neonatal deficiency/coagulopathy.

Factor VII (**s**even)—shortest half-life.

Factor II (**two**)—longest (**too** long) half-life.

Anticoagulation

Antithrombin inhibits thrombin (factor IIa) and factors VIIa, IXa, Xa, XIa, XIIa.

Heparin enhances the activity of antithrombin.

Principal targets of antithrombin: thrombin and factor Xa.

Factor V Leiden mutation produces a factor V resistant to inhibition by activated protein C.

tPA is used clinically as a thrombolytic.

▶ HEMATOLOGY AND ONCOLOGY—PATHOLOGY

RBC morphology

TYPE	EXAMPLE	ASSOCIATED PATHOLOGY	NOTES
Acanthocytes ("spur cells")	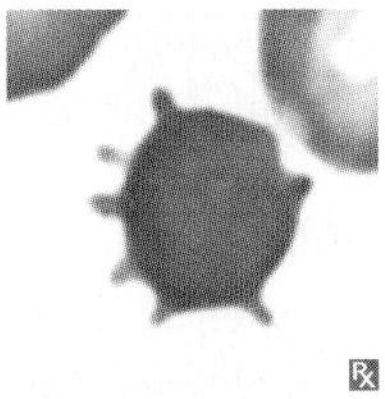	Liver disease, abetalipoproteinemia, vitamin E deficiency	Projections of varying size at irregular intervals (**acanth**ocytes are **asym**metric).
Echinocytes ("burr cells")	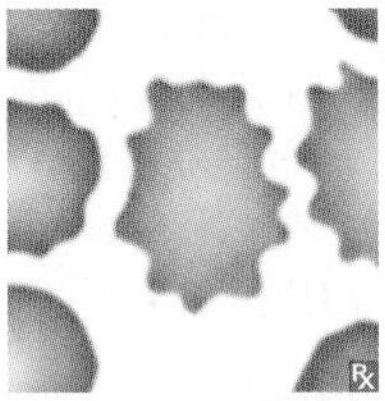	Liver disease, ESRD, pyruvate kinase deficiency	Smaller and more uniform projections than acanthocytes (**echin**ocytes are **even**).
Dacrocytes ("teardrop cells")	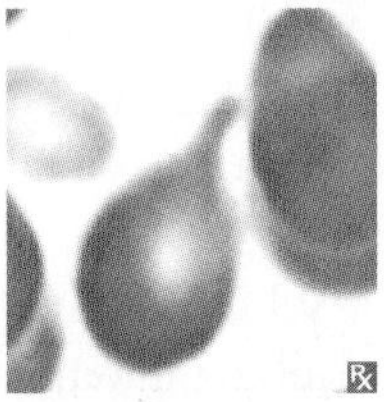	Bone marrow infiltration (eg, myelofibrosis)	RBC "sheds a **tear**" because it's mechanically squeezed out of its home in the bone marrow
Schistocytes (eg, "helmet" cells)	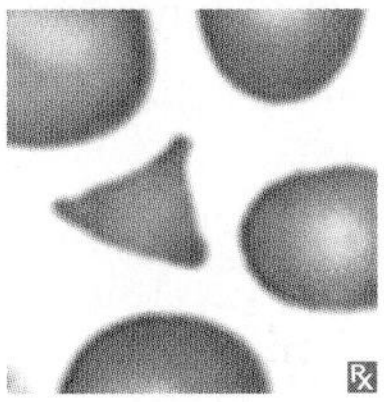	MAHAs (eg, DIC, TTP/HUS, HELLP syndrome), mechanical hemolysis (eg, heart valve prosthesis)	Fragmented RBCs
Degmacytes ("bite cells")	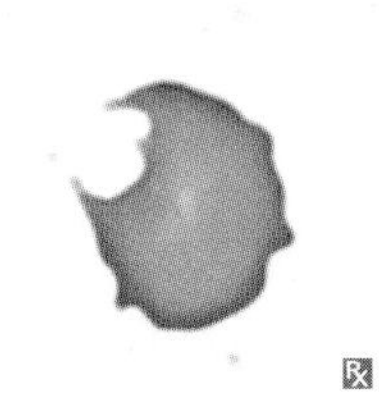	G6PD deficiency	Due to removal of Heinz bodies by splenic macrophages (they "**deg**" them out of/**bite** them off of RBCs)
Elliptocytes	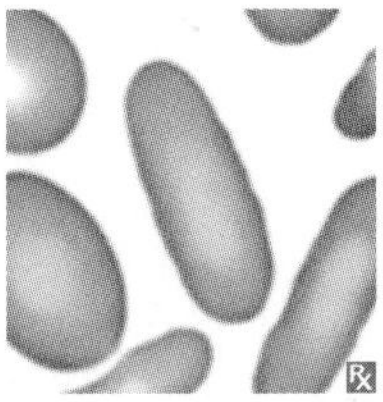	Hereditary elliptocytosis	Caused by mutation in genes encoding RBC membrane proteins (eg, spectrin)

RBC morphology *(continued)*

TYPE	EXAMPLE	ASSOCIATED PATHOLOGY	NOTES
Spherocytes	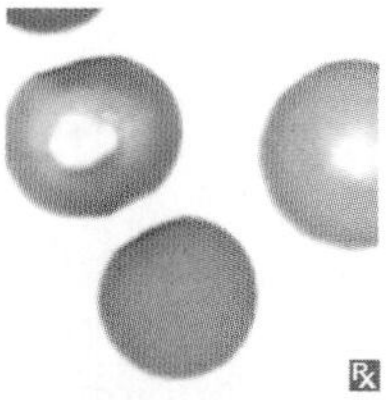	Hereditary spherocytosis, autoimmune hemolytic anemia	Small, spherical cells without central pallor ↓ surface area-to-volume ratio
Macro-ovalocytes	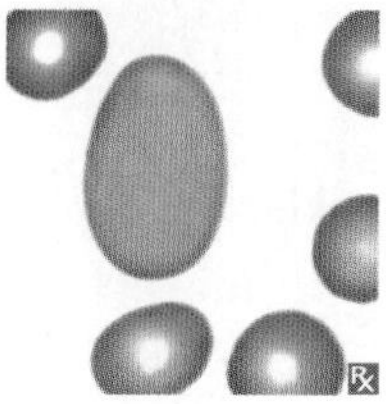	Megaloblastic anemia (also hypersegmented PMNs)	
Target cells	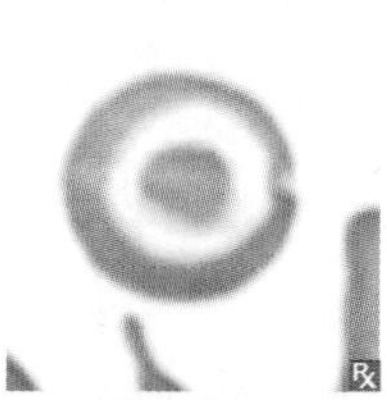	**H**bC disease, **A**splenia, **L**iver disease, **T**halassemia	"**HALT**," said the hunter to his **target** ↑ surface area-to-volume ratio
Sickle cells	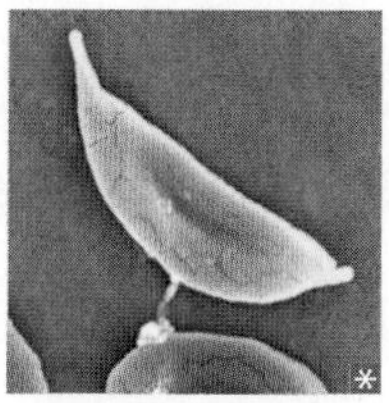	Sickle cell anemia	Sickling occurs with low O_2 conditions (eg, high altitude, acidosis)

RBC inclusions

TYPE	EXAMPLE	ASSOCIATED PATHOLOGY	NOTES
Bone marrow			
Iron granules	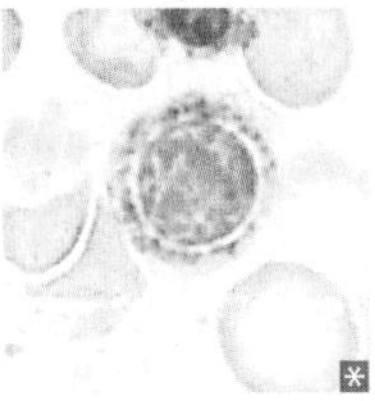	Sideroblastic anemias (eg, lead poisoning, myelodysplastic syndromes, chronic alcohol overuse)	Perinuclear mitochondria with excess iron (forming ring in ringed sideroblasts) Require Prussian blue stain to be visualized
Peripheral smear			
Howell-Jolly bodies	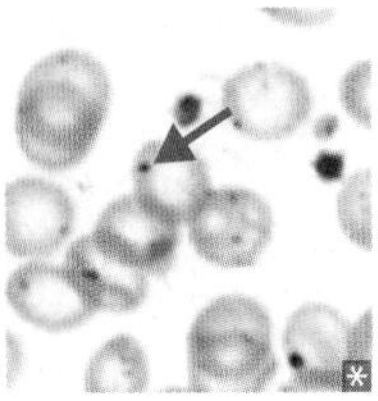	Functional hyposplenia (eg, sickle cell disease), asplenia	Basophilic nuclear remnants (do not contain iron) Usually removed by splenic macrophages
Basophilic stippling	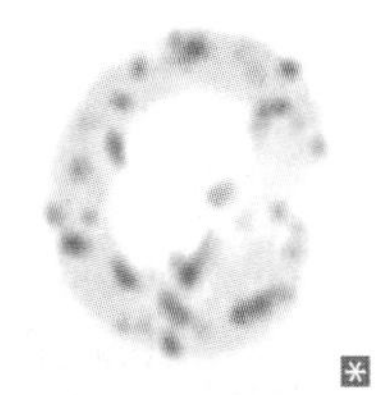	Sideroblastic anemias, thalassemias	Basophilic ribosomal precipitates (do not contain iron)
Pappenheimer bodies	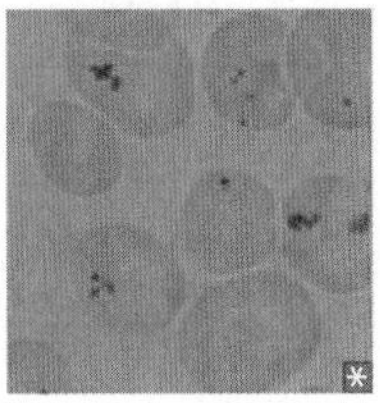	Sideroblastic anemia	Basophilic granules (contain iron)
Heinz bodies	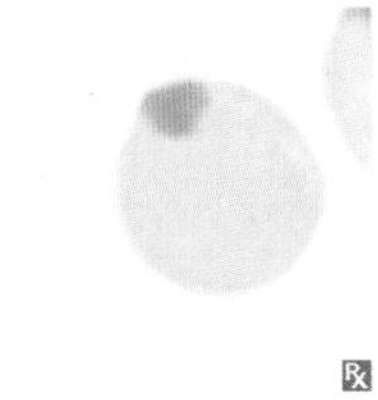	G6PD deficiency	Denatured and precipitated hemoglobin (contain iron) Phagocytic removal of Heinz bodies → bite cells Requires supravital stain (eg, crystal violet) to be visualized

Anemias

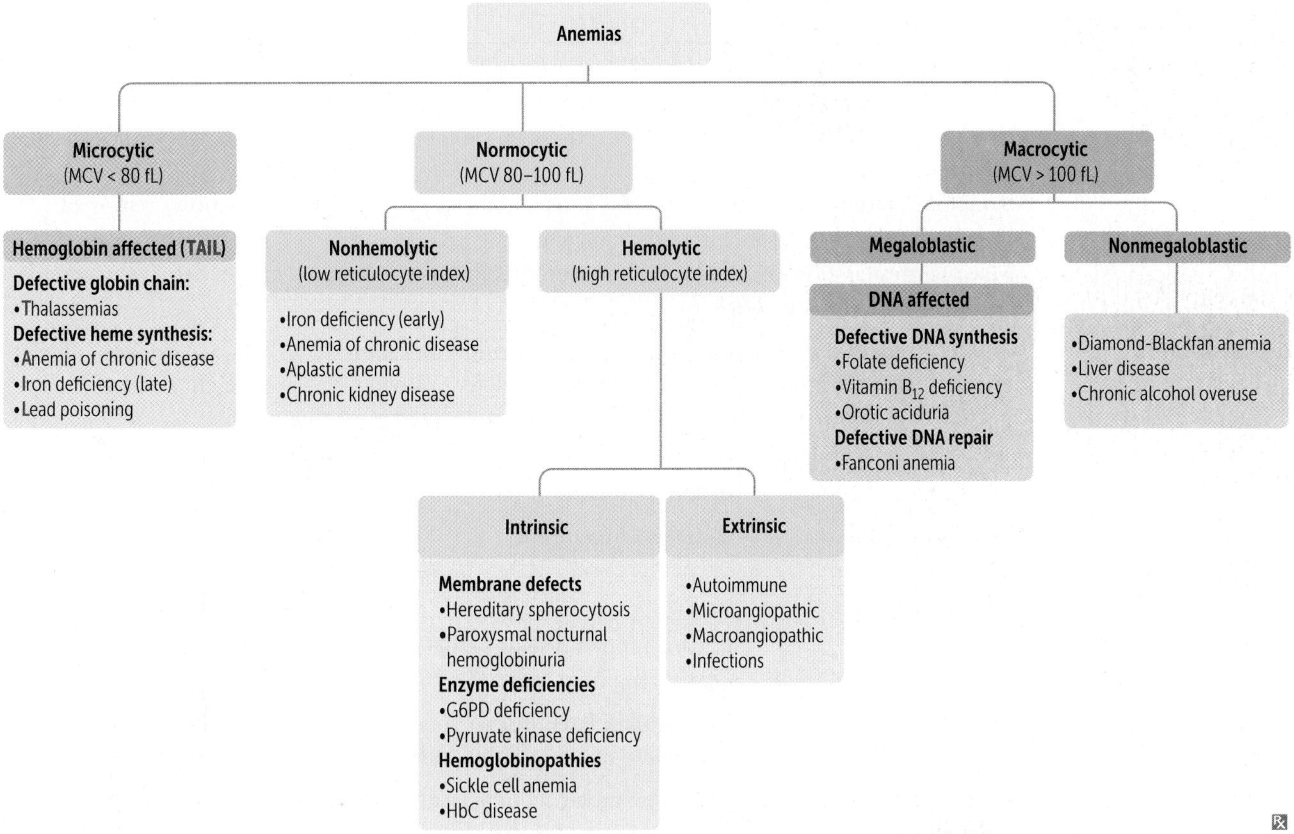
Anemias
Microcytic (MCV < 80 fL)
Normocytic (MCV 80–100 fL)
Macrocytic (MCV > 100 fL)
Hemoglobin affected (TAIL)
Defective globin chain:
•Thalassemias
Defective heme synthesis:
•Anemia of chronic disease
•Iron deficiency (late)
•Lead poisoning
Nonhemolytic (low reticulocyte index)
•Iron deficiency (early)
•Anemia of chronic disease
•Aplastic anemia
•Chronic kidney disease
Hemolytic (high reticulocyte index)
Intrinsic
Membrane defects
•Hereditary spherocytosis
•Paroxysmal nocturnal hemoglobinuria
Enzyme deficiencies
•G6PD deficiency
•Pyruvate kinase deficiency
Hemoglobinopathies
•Sickle cell anemia
•HbC disease
Extrinsic
•Autoimmune
•Microangiopathic
•Macroangiopathic
•Infections
Megaloblastic
DNA affected
Defective DNA synthesis
•Folate deficiency
•Vitamin B12 deficiency
•Orotic aciduria
Defective DNA repair
•Fanconi anemia
Nonmegaloblastic
•Diamond-Blackfan anemia
•Liver disease
•Chronic alcohol overuse

Reticulocyte production index

Also called corrected reticulocyte count. Used to correct falsely elevated reticulocyte count in anemia. Measures appropriate bone marrow response to anemic conditions (effective erythropoiesis). High RPI (>3) indicates compensatory RBC production; low RPI (<2) indicates inadequate response to correct anemia. Calculated as:

$$\text{RPI} = \frac{\text{reticulocyte \%} \times \text{actual Hct}}{\text{normal Hct } (\approx 45\%)}$$

Microcytic, hypochromic anemias

MCV < 80 fL.

Iron deficiency

↓ iron due to chronic bleeding (eg, GI loss, menorrhagia), malnutrition, absorption disorders, GI surgery (eg, gastrectomy), or ↑ demand (eg, pregnancy) → ↓ final step in heme synthesis.

Labs: ↓ iron, ↑ TIBC, ↓ ferritin, ↑ free erythrocyte protoporphyrin, ↑ RDW, ↓ RI. Microcytosis and hypochromasia (↑ central pallor) A.

Symptoms: fatigue, conjunctival pallor B, pica (persistent craving and compulsive eating of nonfood substances), spoon nails (koilonychia).

May manifest as glossitis, cheilosis, **Plummer-Vinson syndrome** (triad of iron deficiency anemia, esophageal webs, and dysphagia).

α-thalassemia

α-globin gene deletions on chromosome 16 → ↓ α-globin synthesis. May have *cis* deletion (deletions occur on same chromosome) or *trans* deletion (deletions occur on separate chromosomes). Normal is αα/αα. Often ↑ RBC count, in contrast to iron deficiency anemia.

NUMBER OF α-GLOBIN GENES DELETED	DISEASE	CLINICAL OUTCOME
1 (α α/α –)	α-thalassemia minima	No anemia (silent carrier)
2 (α –/α –; *trans*) or (α α/– –; *cis*)	α-thalassemia minor	Mild microcytic, hypochromic anemia; *cis* deletion may worsen outcome for the carrier's offspring
3 (– –/– α)	Hemoglobin H disease (HbH); excess β-globin forms β_4	Moderate to severe microcytic hypochromic anemia
4 (– –/– –)	Hemoglobin Barts disease; no α-globin, excess γ-globin forms γ_4	Hydrops fetalis; incompatible with life

β-thalassemia

Point mutations in splice sites and promoter sequences on chromosome 11 → ↓ β-globin synthesis. ↑ prevalence in people of Mediterranean descent.

β-thalassemia minor (heterozygote): β chain is underproduced. Usually asymptomatic. Diagnosis confirmed by ↑ HbA_2 (> 3.5%) on electrophoresis.

β-thalassemia major (homozygote): β chain is absent → severe microcytic, hypochromic anemia with target cells and increased anisopoikilocytosis C requiring blood transfusion (2° hemochromatosis). Marrow expansion ("crew cut" on skull x-ray) → skeletal deformities (eg, "chipmunk" facies). Extramedullary hematopoiesis → hepatosplenomegaly. ↑ risk of parvovirus B19–induced aplastic crisis. ↑ HbF ($\alpha_2\gamma_2$), HbA_2 ($\alpha_2\delta_2$). HbF is protective in the infant and disease becomes symptomatic only after 6 months, when fetal hemoglobin declines.

HbS/β-thalassemia heterozygote: mild to moderate sickle cell disease depending on amount of β-globin production.

Microcytic, hypochromic anemias *(continued)*

Lead poisoning

Lead inhibits ferrochelatase and ALA dehydratase → ↓ heme synthesis and ↑ RBC protoporphyrin. Also inhibits rRNA degradation → RBCs retain aggregates of rRNA (basophilic stippling).

Symptoms of LEAD poisoning:

- Lead Lines on gingivae (Burton lines) and on metaphyses of long bones D on x-ray.
- Encephalopathy and Erythrocyte basophilic stippling.
- Abdominal colic and sideroblastic Anemia.
- Drops—wrist and foot drop.

Treatment: chelation with succimer, EDTA, dimercaprol.

Exposure risk ↑ in old houses with chipped paint (children) and workplace (adults).

Sideroblastic anemia

Causes: genetic (eg, X-linked defect in ALA synthase gene), acquired (myelodysplastic syndromes), and reversible (alcohol is most common; also lead poisoning, vitamin B_6 deficiency, copper deficiency, drugs [eg, isoniazid, linezolid]).

Lab findings: ↑ iron, normal/↓ TIBC, ↑ ferritin. Ringed sideroblasts (with iron-laden, Prussian blue–stained mitochondria) seen in bone marrow E. Peripheral blood smear: basophilic stippling of RBCs. Some acquired variants may be normocytic or macrocytic.

Treatment: pyridoxine (B_6, cofactor for ALA synthase).

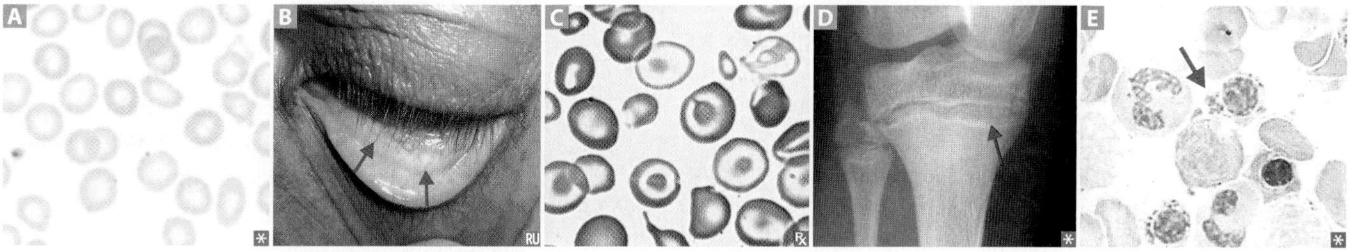

Interpretation of iron studies

	Iron deficiency	Chronic disease	Hemochromatosis	Pregnancy/ OCP use
Serum iron	↓	↓	↑	—
Transferrin or TIBC	↑	↓[a]	↓	↑
Ferritin	↓	↑	↑	—
% transferrin saturation (serum iron/TIBC)	↓↓	—/↓	↑↑	↓

↑↓ = 1° disturbance.

Transferrin—transports iron in blood.

TIBC—indirectly measures transferrin.

Ferritin—1° iron storage protein of body.

[a]Evolutionary reasoning—pathogens use circulating iron to thrive. The body has adapted a system in which iron is stored within the cells of the body and prevents pathogens from acquiring circulating iron.

Macrocytic anemias MCV > 100 fL.

	DESCRIPTION	FINDINGS
Megaloblastic anemia 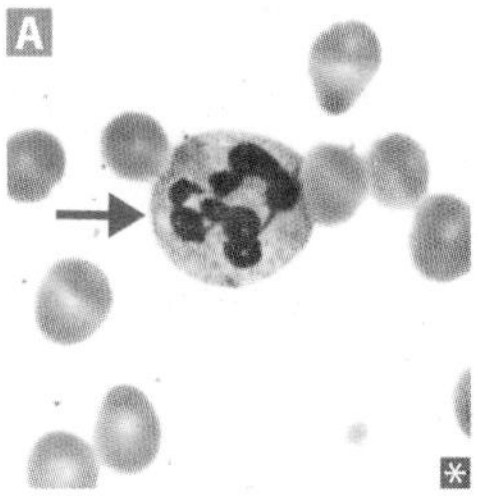	Impaired DNA synthesis → maturation of nucleus of precursor cells in bone marrow delayed relative to maturation of cytoplasm. Causes: vitamin B_{12} deficiency, folate deficiency, medications (eg, hydroxyurea, phenytoin, methotrexate, sulfa drugs).	RBC macrocytosis, hypersegmented neutrophils (arrow in A), glossitis.
Folate deficiency	Causes: malnutrition (eg, chronic alcohol overuse), malabsorption, drugs (eg, methotrexate, trimethoprim, phenytoin), ↑ requirement (eg, hemolytic anemia, pregnancy).	↑ homocysteine, normal methylmalonic acid. **No neurologic symptoms** (vs B_{12} deficiency).
Vitamin B_{12} (cobalamin) deficiency	Causes: pernicious anemia, malabsorption (eg, Crohn disease), pancreatic insufficiency, gastrectomy, insufficient intake (eg, veganism), *Diphyllobothrium latum* (fish tapeworm).	↑ homocysteine, ↑ methylmalonic acid. **Neurologic symptoms:** reversible dementia, subacute combined degeneration (due to involvement of B_{12} in fatty acid pathways and myelin synthesis): spinocerebellar tract, lateral corticospinal tract, dorsal column dysfunction. Folate supplementation in vitamin B_{12} deficiency can correct the anemia, but worsens neurologic symptoms. Historically diagnosed with the Schilling test, a test that determines if the cause is dietary insufficiency vs malabsorption. Anemia 2° to insufficient intake may take several years to develop due to liver's ability to store B_{12} (vs folate deficiency, which takes weeks to months).
Orotic aciduria	Inability to convert orotic acid to UMP (de novo pyrimidine synthesis pathway) because of defect in UMP synthase. Autosomal recessive. Presents in children as failure to thrive, developmental delay, and megaloblastic anemia refractory to folate and B_{12}. No hyperammonemia (vs ornithine transcarbamylase deficiency—↑ orotic acid with hyperammonemia).	Orotic acid in urine. Treatment: uridine monophosphate or uridine triacetate to bypass mutated enzyme.
Nonmegaloblastic anemia	Macrocytic anemia in which DNA synthesis is normal. Causes: chronic alcohol overuse, liver disease.	RBC macrocytosis without hypersegmented neutrophils.
Diamond-Blackfan anemia	A congenital form of pure red cell aplasia (vs Fanconi anemia, which causes pancytopenia). Rapid-onset anemia within 1st year of life due to intrinsic defect in erythroid progenitor cells.	↑ % HbF (but ↓ total Hb). Short stature, craniofacial abnormalities, and upper extremity malformations (triphalangeal thumbs) in up to 50% of cases.

Normocytic, normochromic anemias	Normocytic, normochromic anemias are classified as nonhemolytic or hemolytic. The hemolytic anemias are further classified according to the cause of the hemolysis (intrinsic vs extrinsic to the RBC) and by the location of the hemolysis (intravascular vs extravascular). Hemolysis can lead to increases in LDH, reticulocytes, unconjugated bilirubin, pigmented gallstones, and urobilinogen in urine.
Intravascular hemolysis	Findings: ↓ haptoglobin, ↑ schistocytes on blood smear. Characteristic hemoglobinuria, hemosiderinuria, and urobilinogen in urine. Notable causes are mechanical hemolysis (eg, prosthetic valve), paroxysmal nocturnal hemoglobinuria, microangiopathic hemolytic anemias.
Extravascular hemolysis	Mechanism: macrophages in spleen clear RBCs. Findings: spherocytes in peripheral smear (most commonly due to hereditary spherocytosis and autoimmune hemolytic anemia), no hemoglobinuria/hemosiderinuria. Can present with urobilinogen in urine.

Nonhemolytic, normocytic anemias

	DESCRIPTION	FINDINGS
Anemia of chronic disease	Inflammation (eg, ↑ IL-6) → ↑ hepcidin (released by liver, binds ferroportin on intestinal mucosal cells and macrophages, thus inhibiting iron transport) → ↓ release of iron from macrophages and ↓ iron absorption from gut. Associated with conditions such as chronic infections, neoplastic disorders, chronic kidney disease, and autoimmune diseases (eg, SLE, rheumatoid arthritis).	↓ iron, ↓ TIBC, ↑ ferritin. Normocytic, but can become microcytic. Treatment: address underlying cause of inflammation, judicious use of blood transfusion, consider erythropoiesis-stimulating agents such as EPO (eg, in chronic kidney disease).
Aplastic anemia 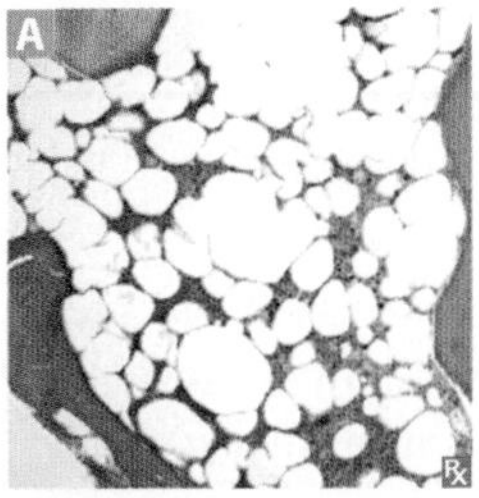	Failure or destruction of hematopoietic stem cells. Causes (reducing volume from inside diaphysis): ▪ Radiation ▪ Viral agents (eg, EBV, HIV, hepatitis viruses) ▪ Fanconi anemia (autosomal recessive DNA repair defect → bone marrow failure); normocytosis or macrocytosis on CBC ▪ Idiopathic (immune mediated, 1° stem cell defect); may follow acute hepatitis ▪ Drugs (eg, benzene, chloramphenicol, alkylating agents, antimetabolites)	↓ reticulocyte count, ↑ EPO. Pancytopenia characterized by anemia, leukopenia, and thrombocytopenia (not to be confused with aplastic crisis, which causes anemia only). Normal cell morphology, but hypocellular bone marrow with fatty infiltration A (dry bone marrow tap). Symptoms: fatigue, malaise, pallor, purpura, mucosal bleeding, petechiae, infection. Treatment: withdrawal of offending agent, immunosuppressive regimens (eg, antithymocyte globulin, cyclosporine), bone marrow allograft, RBC/platelet transfusion, bone marrow stimulation (eg, GM-CSF).

Intrinsic hemolytic anemias

	DESCRIPTION	FINDINGS
Hereditary spherocytosis	Primarily autosomal dominant. Due to defect in proteins interacting with RBC membrane skeleton and plasma membrane (eg, ankyrin, band 3, protein 4.2, spectrin). Small, round RBCs with less surface area and no central pallor (↑ MCHC) → premature removal by spleen (extravascular hemolysis).	Splenomegaly, pigmented gallstones, aplastic crisis (parvovirus B19 infection). Labs: ↓ mean fluorescence of RBCs in eosin 5-maleimide (EMA) binding test, ↑ fragility in osmotic fragility test. Normal to ↓ MCV with abundance of RBCs. Treatment: splenectomy.
G6PD deficiency	X-linked recessive. G6PD defect → ↓ NADPH → ↓ reduced glutathione → ↑ RBC susceptibility to oxidative stress (eg, sulfa drugs, antimalarials, **fava beans**) → hemolysis. Causes extravascular and intravascular hemolysis.	Back pain, hemoglobinuria a few days after oxidant **stress**. Labs: blood smear shows RBCs with **Heinz** bodies and **bite** cells. "**Stress** makes me eat **bites** of **fava beans** with **Heinz** ketchup."
Pyruvate kinase deficiency	Autosomal recessive. Pyruvate kinase defect → ↓ ATP → rigid RBCs → extravascular hemolysis. Increases levels of 2,3-BPG → ↓ hemoglobin affinity for O_2.	Hemolytic anemia in a newborn. Labs: blood smear shows burr cells.
Paroxysmal nocturnal hemoglobinuria	Hematopoietic stem cell mutation → ↑ complement-mediated intravascular hemolysis, especially at night. Acquired *PIGA* mutation → impaired GPI anchor synthesis for decay-accelerating factor (DAF/CD55) and membrane inhibitor of reactive lysis (MIRL/CD59), which protect RBC membrane from complement.	Triad: Coombs ⊖ hemolytic anemia, pancytopenia, venous thrombosis (eg, Budd-Chiari syndrome). Pink/red urine in morning. Associated with aplastic anemia, acute leukemias. Labs: CD55/59 ⊖ RBCs on flow cytometry. Treatment: eculizumab (targets terminal complement protein C5).
Sickle cell anemia 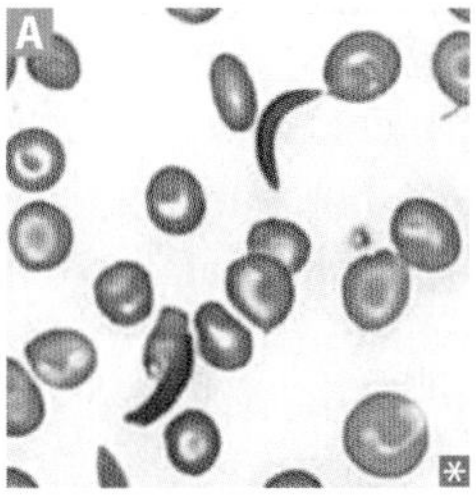	Point mutation in β-globin gene → single amino acid substitution (glutamic acid → valine). Mutant HbA is termed HbS. Causes extravascular and intravascular hemolysis. Pathogenesis: low O_2, high altitude, or acidosis precipitates sickling (deoxygenated HbS polymerizes) → anemia, vaso-occlusive disease. Newborns are initially asymptomatic because of ↑ HbF and ↓ HbS. Heterozygotes (sickle cell trait) have resistance to malaria. Most common autosomal recessive disease in Black population. Sickle cells are crescent-shaped RBCs A. "Crew cut" on skull x-ray due to marrow expansion from ↑ erythropoiesis (also seen in thalassemias).	Complications in sickle cell disease: ▪ Aplastic crisis (transient arrest of erythropoiesis due to parvovirus B19). ▪ Autosplenectomy (Howell-Jolly bodies) → ↑ risk of infection by encapsulated organisms (eg, *S pneumoniae*). ▪ Splenic infarct/sequestration crisis. ▪ *Salmonella* osteomyelitis. ▪ Painful vaso-occlusive crises: dactylitis (painful swelling of hands/feet), priapism, acute chest syndrome (respiratory distress, new pulmonary infiltrates on CXR, common cause of death), avascular necrosis, stroke. ▪ Sickling in renal medulla (↓ Po_2) → renal papillary necrosis → hematuria. Hb electrophoresis: ↓↓ HbA, ↑ HbF, ↑↑ HbS. Treatment: hydroxyurea (↑ HbF), hydration.
HbC disease	Glutamic acid–to-lycine (lysine) mutation in β-globin. Causes extravascular hemolysis.	Patients with HbSC (1 of each mutant gene) have milder disease than HbSS patients. Blood smear in homozygotes: hemoglobin crystals inside RBCs, target cells.

Extrinsic hemolytic anemias

	DESCRIPTION	FINDINGS
Autoimmune hemolytic anemia 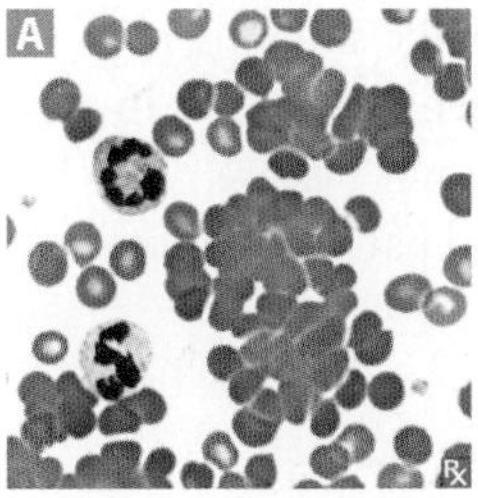	A normocytic anemia that is usually idiopathic and Coombs ⊕. Two types: ▪ Warm AIHA–chronic anemia in which primarily IgG causes extravascular hemolysis. Seen in SLE and CLL and with certain drugs (eg, β-lactams, α-methyldopa). "Warm weather is Good." ▪ Cold AIHA–acute anemia in which primarily IgM + complement cause RBC agglutination and extravascular hemolysis upon exposure to cold → painful, blue fingers and toes. Seen in CLL, *Mycoplasma pneumoniae* infections, infectious mononucleosis.	Spherocytes and agglutinated RBCs A on peripheral blood smear. Warm AIHA treatment: steroids, rituximab, splenectomy (if refractory). Cold AIHA treatment: cold avoidance, rituximab.
Microangiopathic hemolytic anemia	RBCs are damaged when passing through obstructed or narrowed vessels. Causes intravascular hemolysis. Seen in DIC, TTP/HUS, SLE, HELLP syndrome, hypertensive emergency.	Schistocytes (eg, "helmet cells") are seen on peripheral blood smear due to mechanical destruction (*schisto* = to split) of RBCs.
Macroangiopathic hemolytic anemia	Prosthetic heart valves and aortic stenosis may also cause hemolytic anemia 2° to mechanical destruction of RBCs.	Schistocytes on peripheral blood smear.
Hemolytic anemia due to infection	↑ destruction of RBCs (eg, malaria, *Babesia*).	

Leukopenias

CELL TYPE	CELL COUNT	CAUSES
Neutropenia	Absolute neutrophil count < 1500 cells/mm^3 Severe infections typical when < 500 cells/mm^3	Sepsis/postinfection, drugs (including chemotherapy), aplastic anemia, SLE, radiation
Lymphopenia	Absolute lymphocyte count < 1500 cells/mm^3 (< 3000 cells/mm^3 in children)	HIV, DiGeorge syndrome, SCID, SLE, corticosteroids[a], radiation, sepsis, postoperative
Eosinopenia	Absolute eosinophil count < 30 cells/mm^3	Cushing syndrome, corticosteroids[a]

[a]Corticosteroids cause neutrophilia, despite causing eosinopenia and lymphopenia. Corticosteroids ↓ activation of neutrophil adhesion molecules, impairing migration out of the vasculature to sites of inflammation. In contrast, corticosteroids sequester eosinophils in lymph nodes and cause apoptosis of lymphocytes.

Heme synthesis, porphyrias, and lead poisoning

The porphyrias are hereditary or acquired conditions of defective heme synthesis that lead to the accumulation of heme precursors. Lead inhibits specific enzymes needed in heme synthesis, leading to a similar condition.

CONDITION	AFFECTED ENZYME	ACCUMULATED SUBSTRATE	PRESENTING SYMPTOMS
Lead poisoning 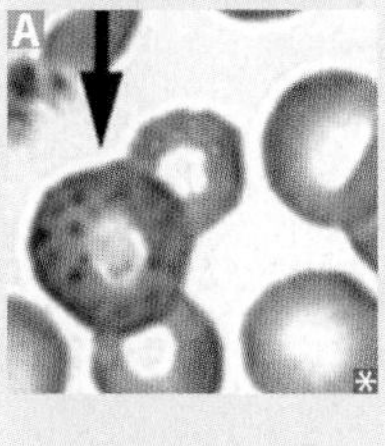	Ferrochelatase and ALA dehydratase	Protoporphyrin, ALA (blood)	Microcytic anemia (basophilic stippling in peripheral smear A, ringed sideroblasts in bone marrow), GI and kidney disease. Children—exposure to lead paint → mental deterioration. Adults—environmental exposure (eg, batteries, ammunition) → headache, memory loss, demyelination (peripheral neuropathy).
Acute intermittent porphyria	Porphobilinogen deaminase, previously called uroporphyrinogen I synthase (autosomal dominant mutation)	Porphobilinogen, ALA	Symptoms (5 P's): ▪ Painful abdomen ▪ Port wine–colored Pee ▪ Polyneuropathy ▪ Psychological disturbances ▪ Precipitated by factors that ↑ ALA synthase (eg, drugs [CYP450 inducers], alcohol, starvation) Treatment: hemin and glucose.
Porphyria cutanea tarda 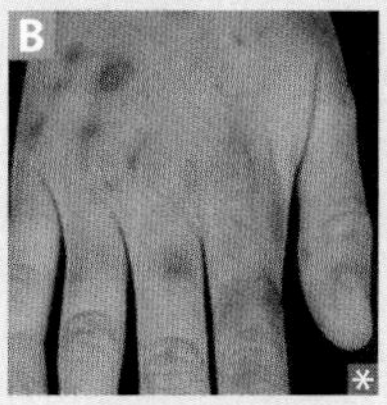	Uroporphyrinogen decarboxylase	Uroporphyrin (tea-colored urine)	Blistering cutaneous photosensitivity and hyperpigmentation B. Most common porphyria. Exacerbated with alcohol consumption. Causes: familial, hepatitis C. Treatment: phlebotomy, sun avoidance, antimalarials (eg, hydroxychloroquine).

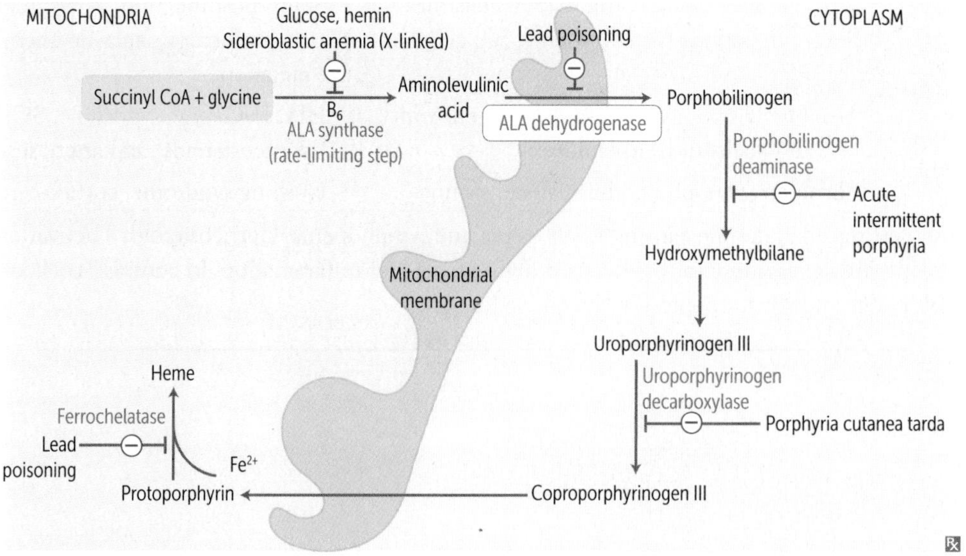
MITOCHONDRIA
Glucose, hemin
Sideroblastic anemia (X-linked)
Lead poisoning
CYTOPLASM
Succinyl CoA + glycine
B6
ALA synthase
(rate-limiting step)
Aminolevulinic acid
ALA dehydrogenase
Porphobilinogen
Porphobilinogen deaminase
Acute intermittent porphyria
Hydroxymethylbilane
Mitochondrial membrane
Uroporphyrinogen III
Uroporphyrinogen decarboxylase
Porphyria cutanea tarda
Heme
Ferrochelatase
Lead poisoning
Fe2+
Protoporphyrin
Coproporphyrinogen III

Iron poisoning

	Acute	Chronic
FINDINGS	High mortality rate associated with accidental ingestion by children (adult iron tablets may look like candy).	Seen in patients with 1° (hereditary) or 2° (eg, chronic blood transfusions for thalassemia or sickle cell disease) hemochromatosis.
MECHANISM	Cell death due to formation of free radicals and peroxidation of membrane lipids.	
SYMPTOMS/SIGNS	Abdominal pain, vomiting, GI bleeding. Radiopaque pill seen on x-ray. May progress to anion gap metabolic acidosis and multiorgan failure. Leads to scarring with GI obstruction.	Arthropathy, cirrhosis, cardiomyopathy, diabetes mellitus and skin pigmentation ("bronze diabetes"), hypogonadism.
TREATMENT	Chelation (eg, deferoxamine, deferasirox), gastric lavage.	Phlebotomy (patients without anemia) or chelation.

Coagulation disorders

PT—tests function of common and extrinsic pathway (factors I, II, V, VII, and X). Defect → ↑ **PT** (**P**lay **T**ennis **outside** [**extrinsic** pathway]).

INR (international normalized ratio) = patient PT/control PT. 1 = normal, > 1 = prolonged. Most common test used to follow patients on warfarin, which prolongs INR.

PTT—tests function of common and **intrinsic** pathway (all factors except VII and XIII). Defect → ↑ **PTT** (**P**lay **T**able **T**ennis **inside**).

Coagulation disorders can be due to clotting factor deficiencies or acquired factor inhibitors (most commonly against factor VIII). Diagnosed with a mixing study, in which normal plasma is added to patient's plasma. Clotting factor deficiencies should correct (the PT or PTT returns to within the appropriate normal range), whereas factor inhibitors will not correct.

DISORDER	PT	PTT	MECHANISM AND COMMENTS
Hemophilia A, B, or C 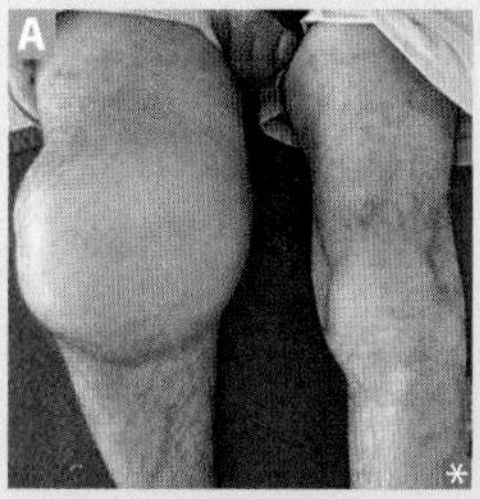	—	↑	Intrinsic pathway coagulation defect (↑ PTT). ▪ A: deficiency of factor **VIII**; X-linked recessive. Pronounce "hemophilia **eight**." ▪ B: deficiency of factor IX; X-linked recessive. ▪ C: deficiency of factor XI; autosomal recessive. Hemorrhage in hemophilia—hemarthroses (bleeding into joints, eg, knee A), easy bruising, bleeding after trauma or surgery (eg, dental procedures). Treatment: desmopressin, factor VIII concentrate, emicizumab (A); factor IX concentrate (B); factor XI concentrate (C).
Vitamin K deficiency	↑	↑	General coagulation defect. Bleeding time normal. ↓ activity of factors II, VII, IX, X, protein C, protein S.

Platelet disorders

All platelet disorders have ↑ bleeding time (BT), mucous membrane bleeding, and microhemorrhages (eg, petechiae, epistaxis). Platelet count (PC) is usually low, but may be normal in qualitative disorders.

DISORDER	PC	BT	NOTES
Bernard-Soulier syndrome	–/↓	↑	Autosomal recessive defect in adhesion. ↓ GpIb → ↓ platelet-to-vWF adhesion. Labs: abnormal ristocetin test, large platelets.
Glanzmann thrombasthenia	–	↑	Autosomal recessive defect in aggregation. ↓ GpIIb/IIIa (↓ integrin $\alpha_{IIb}\beta_3$) → ↓ platelet-to-platelet aggregation and defective platelet plug formation. Labs: blood smear shows no platelet clumping.
Immune thrombocytopenia	↓	↑	Destruction of platelets in spleen. Anti-GpIIb/IIIa antibodies → splenic macrophages phagocytose platelets. May be idiopathic or 2° to autoimmune disorders (eg, SLE), viral illness (eg, HIV, HCV), malignancy (eg, CLL), or drug reactions. Labs: ↑ megakaryocytes on bone marrow biopsy, ↓ platelet count. Treatment: steroids, IVIG, rituximab, TPO receptor agonists (eg, eltrombopag, romiplostim), or splenectomy for refractory ITP.

Thrombotic microangiopathies

Disorders overlap significantly in symptomatology.

	Thrombotic thrombocytopenic purpura	Hemolytic-uremic syndrome
EPIDEMIOLOGY	Typically females	Typically children
PATHOPHYSIOLOGY	Inhibition or deficiency of ADAMTS13 (a vWF metalloprotease) → ↓ degradation of vWF multimers → ↑ large vWF multimers → ↑ platelet adhesion and aggregation (microthrombi formation)	Commonly caused by Shiga toxin-producing *Escherichia coli* (STEC) infection (serotype O157:H7)
PRESENTATION	Triad of thrombocytopenia (↓ platelets), microangiopathic hemolytic anemia (↓ Hb, schistocytes, ↑ LDH), acute kidney injury (↑ Cr)	
DIFFERENTIATING SYMPTOMS	Triad + fever + neurologic symptoms	Triad + bloody diarrhea
LABS	Normal PT and PTT helps distinguish TTP and HUS (coagulation pathway is not activated) from DIC (coagulation pathway is activated)	
TREATMENT	Plasma exchange, steroids, rituximab	Supportive care

Mixed platelet and coagulation disorders

DISORDER	PC	BT	PT	PTT	NOTES
von Willebrand disease	—	↑	—	—/↑	Intrinsic pathway coagulation defect: ↓ vWF → ↑ PTT (vWF carries/protects factor VIII). Defect in platelet plug formation: ↓ vWF → defect in platelet-to-vWF adhesion. Most are autosomal dominant. Mild but most common inherited bleeding disorder. No platelet aggregation with ristocetin cofactor assay. Treatment: desmopressin, which releases vWF stored in endothelium.
Disseminated intravascular coagulation	↓	↑	↑	↑	Widespread clotting factor activation → deficiency in clotting factors → bleeding state (eg, blood oozing from puncture sites). Causes: **S**nake bites, **S**epsis (gram ⊖), **T**rauma, **O**bstetric complications, acute **P**ancreatitis, malignancy, nephrotic syndrome, transfusion (**SSTOP** making new thrombi). Labs: schistocytes, ↑ fibrin degradation products (D-dimers), ↓ fibrinogen, ↓ factors V and VIII.

Hereditary thrombophilias

All autosomal dominant. Lead to hypercoagulable state.

DISEASE	DESCRIPTION
Antithrombin deficiency	Has no direct effect on the PT, PTT, or thrombin time but diminishes the increase in PTT following standard heparin dosing. Can also be acquired: renal failure/nephrotic syndrome → antithrombin loss in urine → ↓ inhibition of factors IIa and Xa.
Factor V Leiden	Production of mutant factor V (guanine → adenine DNA point mutation → Arg506Gln mutation near the cleavage site) that is resistant to degradation by activated protein C. Complications include DVT, cerebral vein thrombosis, recurrent pregnancy loss.
Protein C or S deficiency	↓ ability to inactivate factors Va and VIIIa. ↑ risk of warfarin-induced skin necrosis. Together, protein **C** **C**ancels, and protein **S** **S**tops, coagulation.
Prothrombin *G20210A* mutation	Point mutation in 3′ untranslated region → ↑ production of prothrombin → ↑ plasma levels and venous clots.

Blood transfusion therapy

COMPONENT	DOSAGE EFFECT	CLINICAL USE
Packed RBCs	↑ Hb and O_2 carrying capacity	Acute blood loss, severe anemia
Platelets	↑ platelet count (↑ ~ 5000/mm³/unit)	Stop significant bleeding (thrombocytopenia, qualitative platelet defects)
Fresh frozen plasma/ prothrombin complex concentrate	↑ coagulation factor levels; FFP contains all coagulation factors and plasma proteins; PCC generally contains factors II, VII, IX, and X, as well as protein C and S	Cirrhosis, immediate anticoagulation reversal
Cryoprecipitate	Contains fibrinogen, factor VIII, factor XIII, vWF, and fibronectin	Coagulation factor deficiencies involving fibrinogen and factor VIII

Blood transfusion risks include infection transmission (low), transfusion reactions, iron overload (may lead to 2° hemochromatosis), hypocalcemia (citrate is a Ca^{2+} chelator), and hyperkalemia (RBCs may lyse in old blood units).

Leukemia vs lymphoma

Leukemia	Lymphoid or myeloid neoplasm with widespread involvement of bone marrow. Tumor cells are usually found in peripheral blood.
Lymphoma	Discrete tumor mass arising from lymph nodes. Variable clinical presentation (eg, arising in atypical sites, leukemic presentation).

Hodgkin vs non-Hodgkin lymphoma

Hodgkin	Non-Hodgkin
Both may present with constitutional ("B") signs/symptoms: low-grade fever, night sweats, weight loss.	
Localized, single group of nodes with contiguous spread (stage is strongest predictor of prognosis). Better prognosis.	Multiple lymph nodes involved; extranodal involvement common; noncontiguous spread. Worse prognosis.
Characterized by Reed-Sternberg cells.	Majority involve B cells; a few are of T-cell lineage.
Bimodal distribution: young adulthood and > 55 years; more common in males except for nodular sclerosing type.	Can occur in children and adults.
Associated with EBV.	May be associated with autoimmune diseases and viral infections (eg, HIV, EBV, HTLV).

Hodgkin lymphoma

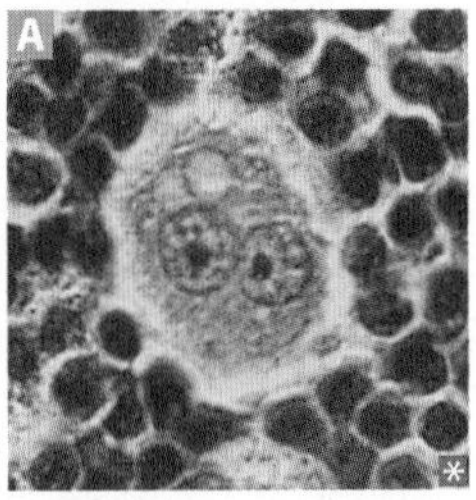

Contains Reed-Sternberg cells: distinctive tumor giant cells; binucleate or bilobed with the 2 halves as mirror images ("owl eyes" A). RS cells are CD15+ and CD30+ B-cell origin. 2 owl eyes × 15 = 30.

SUBTYPE	NOTES
Nodular sclerosis	Most common
Lymphocyte **rich**	**Best** prognosis (the **rich** have **better** bank accounts)
Mixed cellularity	Eosinophilia; seen in immunocompromised patients
Lymphocyte **depleted**	**Worst** prognosis (the **poor** have **worse** bank accounts); seen in immunocompromised patients

Non-Hodgkin lymphoma

TYPE	OCCURS IN	GENETICS	COMMENTS
Neoplasms of mature B cells			
Burkitt lymphoma	Adolescents or young adults	t(8;14)—translocation of c-*myc* (8) and heavy-chain Ig (14)	"Starry sky" appearance, sheets of lymphocytes with interspersed "tingible body" macrophages (arrows in A). Associated with EBV. Jaw lesion B in endemic form in Africa; pelvis or abdomen in sporadic form.
Diffuse large B-cell lymphoma	Usually older adults, but 20% in children	Mutations in *BCL-2*, *BCL-6*	Most common type of non-Hodgkin lymphoma in adults.
Follicular lymphoma	Adults	t(14;18)—translocation of heavy-chain Ig (14) and *BCL-2* (18)	Indolent course with painless "waxing and waning" lymphadenopathy. Bcl-2 normally inhibits apoptosis.
Mantle cell lymphoma	Adult males >> adult females	t(11;14)—translocation of cyclin D1 (11) and heavy-chain Ig (14), CD5+	Very aggressive, patients typically present with late-stage disease.
Marginal zone lymphoma	Adults	t(11;18)	Associated with chronic inflammation (eg, Sjögren syndrome, chronic gastritis [MALT lymphoma; may regress with *H pylori* eradication]).
Primary central nervous system lymphoma	Adults	EBV related; associated with HIV/AIDS	Considered an AIDS-defining illness. Variable presentation: confusion, memory loss, seizures. CNS mass (often single, ring-enhancing lesion on MRI) in immunocompromised patients C, needs to be distinguished from toxoplasmosis via CSF analysis or other lab tests.
Neoplasms of mature T cells			
Adult T-cell lymphoma	Adults	Caused by HTLV (associated with IV drug use)	Adults present with cutaneous lesions; common in Japan (T-cell in Tokyo), West Africa, and the Caribbean. Lytic bone lesions, hypercalcemia.
Mycosis fungoides/ Sézary syndrome	Adults		Mycosis fungoides: skin patches and plaques D (cutaneous T-cell lymphoma), characterized by atypical CD4+ cells with "cerebriform" nuclei and intraepidermal neoplastic cell aggregates (Pautrier microabscess). May progress to Sézary syndrome (T-cell leukemia).

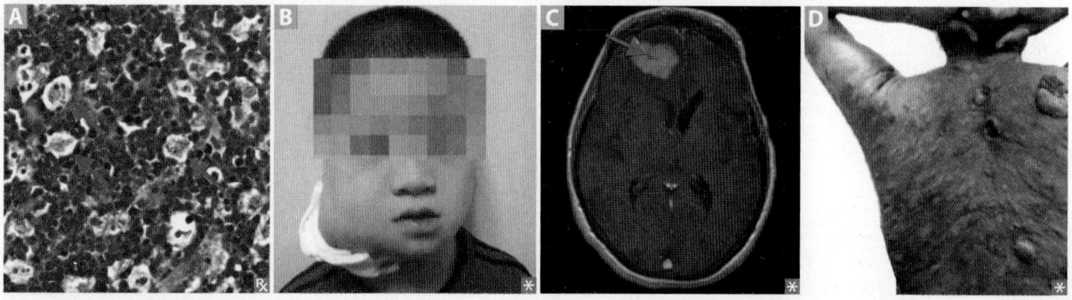

Plasma cell dyscrasias 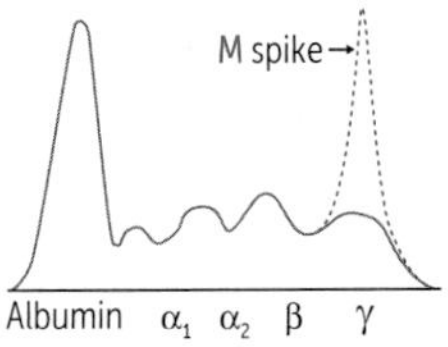	Characterized by monoclonal immunoglobulin (paraprotein) overproduction due to plasma cell disorder. Labs: serum protein electrophoresis (SPEP) or free light chain (FLC) assay for initial tests (M spike on SPEP represents overproduction of a monoclonal Ig fragment). For urinalysis, use 24-hr urine protein electrophoresis (UPEP) to detect light chain, as routine urine dipstick detects only albumin. Confirm with bone marrow biopsy.
Multiple myeloma	Overproduction of IgG (55% of cases) > IgA. Clinical features: **CRAB** ▪ Hyper**C**alcemia ▪ **R**enal involvement ▪ **A**nemia ▪ **B**one lytic lesions ("punched out" on X-ray A) → back pain. Peripheral blood smear shows rouleaux formation B (RBCs stacked like poker chips). Urinalysis shows Ig light chains (Bence Jones proteinuria) with ⊖ urine dipstick. Bone marrow analysis shows > 10% monoclonal plasma cells with clock-face chromatin C and intracytoplasmic inclusions containing IgG. Complications: ↑ infection risk, 1° amyloidosis (AL).

Waldenstrom macroglobulinemia	Overproduction of IgM (**macro**globulinemia because IgM is the **largest** Ig).
	Clinical features:
	▪ Peripheral neuropathy
	▪ No CRAB findings
	▪ Hyperviscosity syndrome:
	  ▪ Headache
	  ▪ Blurry vision
	  ▪ Raynaud phenomenon
	  ▪ Retinal hemorrhages
	Bone marrow analysis shows >10% small lymphocytes with intranuclear pseudoinclusions containing IgM (lymphoplasmacytic lymphoma).
	Complication: thrombosis.

Monoclonal gammopathy of undetermined significance	Overproduction of any Ig type. Usually asymptomatic. No CRAB findings. Bone marrow analysis shows < 10% monoclonal plasma cells. Complication: 1-2% risk per year of transitioning to multiple myeloma.

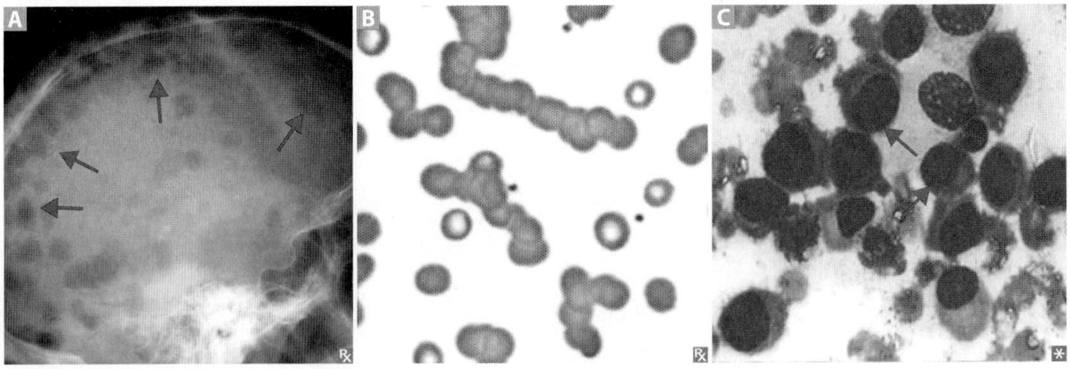

Myelodysplastic syndromes

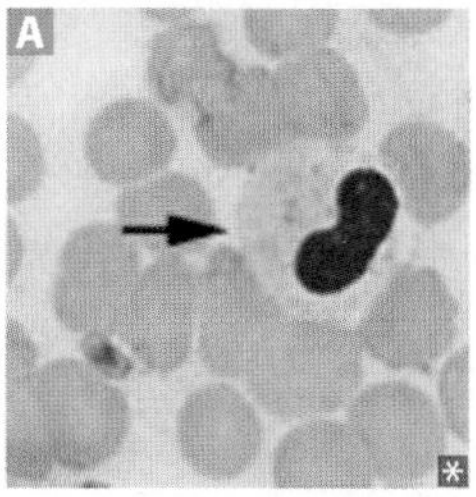

Stem cell disorders involving ineffective hematopoiesis → defects in cell maturation of nonlymphoid lineages. Bone marrow blasts <20% (vs >20% in AML). Caused by de novo mutations or environmental exposure (eg, radiation, benzene, chemotherapy). Risk of transformation to AML.

Pseudo-Pelger-Huët anomaly—neutrophils with bilobed ("**duet**") nuclei A. Associated with myelodysplastic syndromes or drugs (eg, immunosuppressants).

Leukemias Unregulated growth and differentiation of WBCs in bone marrow → marrow failure → anemia (↓ RBCs), infections (↓ mature WBCs), and hemorrhage (↓ platelets). Usually presents with ↑ circulating WBCs (malignant leukocytes in blood), although some cases present with normal/↓ WBCs.

Leukemic cell infiltration of liver, spleen, lymph nodes, and skin (leukemia cutis) possible.

TYPE	NOTES
Lymphoid neoplasms	
Acute lymphoblastic leukemia/lymphoma	Most frequently occurs in children; less common in adults (worse prognosis). T-cell ALL can present as mediastinal mass (presenting as SVC-like syndrome). Associated with Down syndrome. Peripheral blood and bone marrow have ↑↑↑ lymphoblasts A. TdT+ (marker of pre-T and pre-B cells), CD10+ (marker of pre-B cells). Most responsive to therapy. May spread to CNS and testes. t(12;21) → better prognosis; t(9;22) (Philadelphia chromosome) → worse prognosis.
Chronic lymphocytic leukemia/small lymphocytic lymphoma	Age > 60 years. Most common adult leukemia. CD20+, CD23+, CD5+ B-cell neoplasm. Often asymptomatic, progresses slowly; smudge cells B in peripheral blood smear; autoimmune hemolytic anemia. **CLL** = **C**rushed **L**ittle **L**ymphocytes (smudge cells). Richter transformation—CLL/SLL transformation into an aggressive lymphoma, most commonly diffuse large B-cell lymphoma (DLBCL).
Hairy cell leukemia	Adult males. Mature B-cell tumor. Cells have filamentous, hair-like projections (fuzzy appearing on LM C). Peripheral lymphadenopathy is uncommon. Causes marrow fibrosis → dry tap on aspiration. Patients usually present with massive splenomegaly and pancytopenia. Stains **TRAP** (**T**artrate-**R**esistant **A**cid **P**hosphatase) ⊕ (**TRAP**ped in a **hairy** situation). TRAP stain largely replaced with flow cytometry. Associated with *BRAF* mutations. Treatment: purine analogs (cladribine, pentostatin).
Myeloid neoplasms	
Acute myelogenous leukemia	Median onset 65 years. Auer rods D; myeloperoxidase ⊕ cytoplasmic inclusions seen mostly in APL (formerly M3 AML); ↑↑↑ circulating myeloblasts on peripheral smear. Risk factors: prior exposure to alkylating chemotherapy, radiation, myeloproliferative disorders, Down syndrome (typically acute megakaryoblastic leukemia [formerly M7 AML]). APL: t(15;17), responds to all-*trans* retinoic acid (vitamin A) and arsenic trioxide, which induce differentiation of promyelocytes; DIC is a common presentation.
Chronic myelogenous leukemia	Peak incidence: 45—85 years; median age: 64 years. Defined by the Philadelphia chromosome (t[9;22], *BCR-ABL*) and myeloid stem cell proliferation. Presents with dysregulated production of mature and maturing granulocytes (eg, neutrophils, metamyelocytes, myelocytes, basophils E) and splenomegaly. May accelerate and transform to AML or ALL ("blast crisis"). Responds to BCR-ABL tyrosine kinase inhibitors (eg, imatinib).

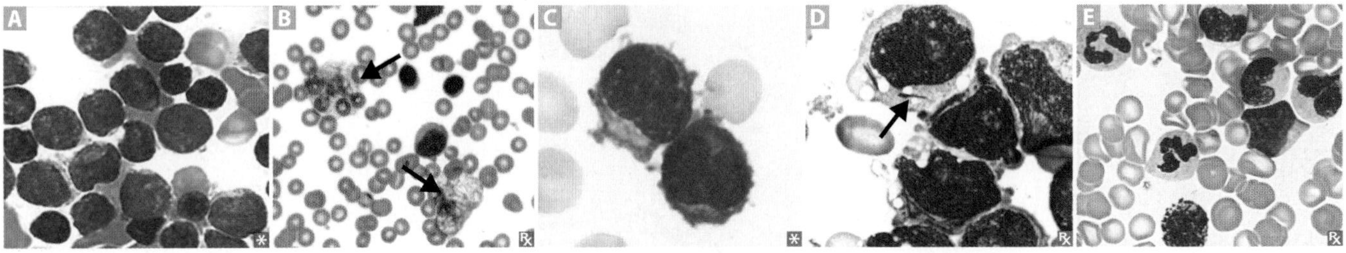

Myeloproliferative neoplasms

Malignant hematopoietic neoplasms with varying impacts on WBCs and myeloid cell lines.

Polycythemia vera

Primary polycythemia. Disorder of ↑ RBCs, usually due to acquired *JAK2* mutation. May present as intense itching after shower (aquagenic pruritus). Rare but classic symptom is erythromelalgia (severe, burning pain and red-blue coloration) due to episodic blood clots in vessels of the extremities A.

↓ EPO (vs 2° polycythemia, which presents with endogenous or artificially ↑ EPO).

Treatment: phlebotomy, hydroxyurea, ruxolitinib (JAK1/2 inhibitor).

Essential thrombocythemia

Characterized by massive proliferation of megakaryocytes and platelets. Symptoms include bleeding and thrombosis. Blood smear shows markedly increased number of platelets, which may be large or otherwise abnormally formed B. Erythromelalgia may occur.

Myelofibrosis

Atypical megakaryocyte hyperplasia → ↑ TGF-β secretion → ↑ fibroblast activity → obliteration of bone marrow with fibrosis C. Associated with massive splenomegaly and "**teardrop**" RBCs D. "Bone marrow **cries** because it's fibrosed and is a dry tap."

	RBCs	WBCs	PLATELETS	PHILADELPHIA CHROMOSOME	*JAK2* MUTATIONS
Polycythemia vera	↑	↑	↑	⊖	⊕
Essential thrombocythemia	–	–	↑	⊖	⊕ (30–50%)
Myelofibrosis	↓	Variable	Variable	⊖	⊕ (30–50%)
CML	↓	↑	↑	⊕	⊖

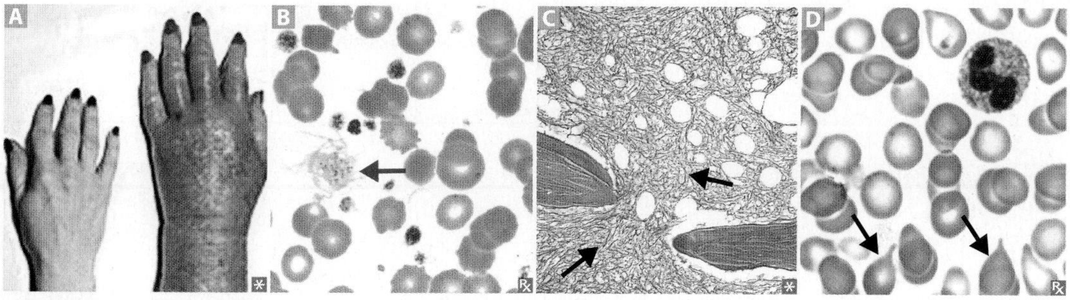

Leukemoid reaction vs chronic myelogenous leukemia

	Leukemoid reaction	Chronic myelogenous leukemia
DEFINITION	Reactive neutrophilia >50,000 cells/mm^3	Myeloproliferative neoplasm ⊕ for *BCR-ABL*
NEUTROPHIL MORPHOLOGY	Toxic granulation, Döhle bodies, cytoplasmic vacuoles	Pseudo-Pelger-Huët anomaly
LAP SCORE	↑	↓ (LAP enzyme ↓ in malignant neutrophils)
EOSINOPHILS AND BASOPHILS	Normal	↑

Polycythemia

	PLASMA VOLUME	RBC MASS	O_2 SATURATION	EPO LEVELS	ASSOCIATIONS
Relative	↓	–	–	–	Dehydration, burns.
Appropriate absolute	–	↑	↓	↑	Lung disease, congenital heart disease, high altitude.
Inappropriate absolute	–	↑	–	↑	Exogenous EPO: athlete abuse ("blood doping"). Inappropriate EPO secretion: malignancy (eg, RCC, HCC).
Polycythemia vera	↑	↑↑	–	↓	EPO ↓ in PCV due to negative feedback suppressing renal EPO production.

↑↓ = 1° disturbance

Chromosomal translocations

TRANSLOCATION	ASSOCIATED DISORDER	NOTES
t(8;14)	Burkitt (Burk-8) lymphoma (c-*myc* activation)	The Ig heavy chain genes on chromosome 14 are constitutively expressed. When other genes (eg, *c-myc* and *BCL-2*) are translocated next to this heavy chain gene region, they are overexpressed.
t(11;14)	Mantle cell lymphoma (cyclin D1 activation)	
t(11;18)	Marginal zone lymphoma	
t(14;18)	Follicular lymphoma (*BCL-2* activation)	
t(15;17)	APL (formerly M3 type of AML)	
t(9;22) (**Philadelphia** chromosome)	**CML** (*BCR-ABL* hybrid), ALL (less common); **Philadelphia CreaML** cheese	

Langerhans cell histiocytosis

Collective group of proliferative disorders of Langerhans cells. Presents in a child as lytic bone lesions A and skin rash or as recurrent otitis media with a mass involving the mastoid bone. Cells are functionally immature and do not effectively stimulate primary T cells via antigen presentation. Cells express S-100 (mesodermal origin) and CD1a. Birbeck granules ("tennis rackets" or rod shaped on EM) are characteristic B.

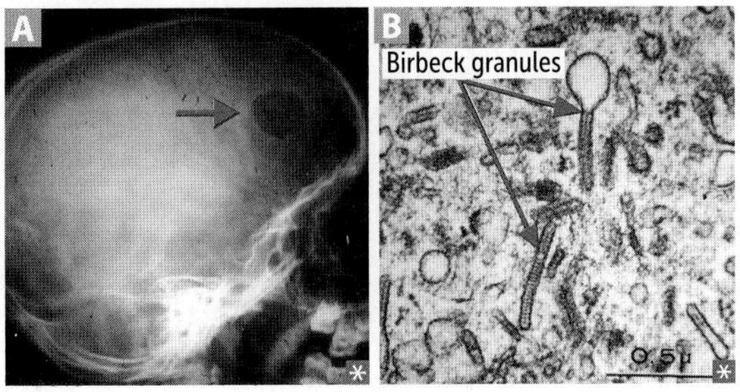

Tumor lysis syndrome

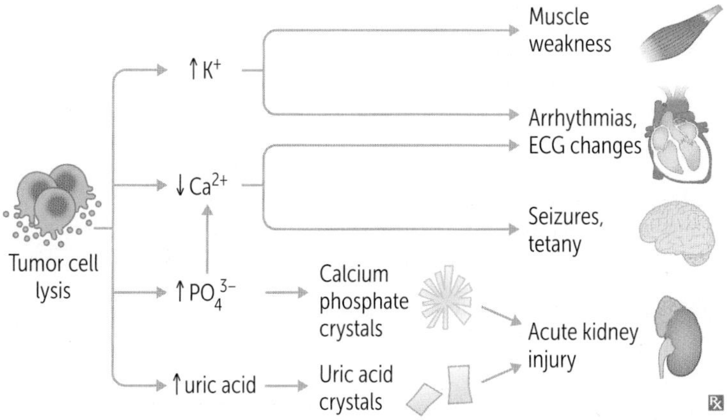
Tumor cell lysis
↑K+
↓Ca2+
↑PO43–
↑uric acid
Muscle weakness
Arrhythmias, ECG changes
Seizures, tetany
Calcium phosphate crystals
Uric acid crystals
Acute kidney injury

Oncologic emergency triggered by massive tumor cell lysis, seen most often with lymphomas/leukemias. Usually caused by treatment initiation, but can occur spontaneously with fast-growing cancers. Release of K^+ → hyperkalemia, release of PO_4^{3-} → hyperphosphatemia, hypocalcemia due to Ca^{2+} sequestration by PO_4^{3-}. ↑ nucleic acid breakdown → hyperuricemia → acute kidney injury. Prevention and treatment include aggressive hydration, allopurinol, rasburicase.

Hemophagocytic lymphohistiocytosis

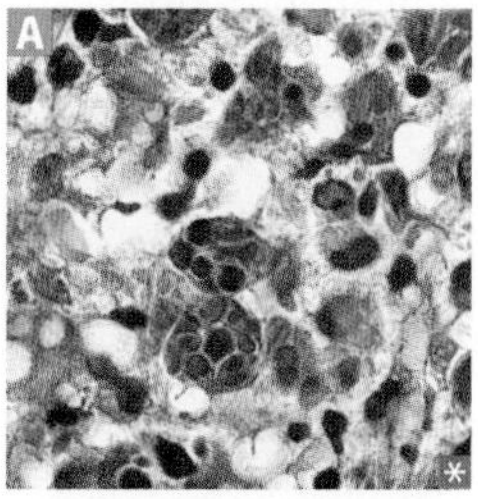
A

Systemic overactivation of macrophages and cytotoxic T cells → fever, pancytopenia, hepatosplenomegaly, ↑↑ serum ferritin levels. Can be inherited or 2° to strong immunologic activation (eg, after EBV infection, malignancy). Bone marrow biopsy shows macrophages phagocytosing marrow elements A.

▸ HEMATOLOGY AND ONCOLOGY—PHARMACOLOGY

Heparin

MECHANISM	Activates antithrombin, which ↓ action primarily of factors IIa (thrombin) and Xa. Short half-life.
CLINICAL USE	Immediate anticoagulation for pulmonary embolism (PE), acute coronary syndrome, MI, deep venous thrombosis (DVT). Used during pregnancy (does not cross placenta). Monitor PTT.
ADVERSE EFFECTS	Bleeding (reverse with protamine sulfate), heparin-induced thrombocytopenia (HIT), osteoporosis (with long-term use), drug-drug interactions. ▪ HIT type 1—mild (platelets >100,000/mm³), transient, nonimmunologic drop in platelet count that typically occurs within the first 2 days of heparin administration. Not clinically significant. ▪ HIT type 2—development of IgG antibodies against heparin-bound platelet factor 4 (PF4) that typically occurs 5–10 days after heparin administration. Antibody-heparin-PF4 complex binds and activates platelets → removal by splenic macrophages and thrombosis →↓↓ platelet count. Highest risk with unfractionated heparin.
NOTES	Low-molecular-weight heparins (eg, enoxaparin, dalteparin) act mainly on factor Xa. Fondaparinux acts only on factor Xa. Have better bioavailability and 2–4× longer half life than unfractionated heparin; can be administered subcutaneously and without lab monitoring. LMWHs undergo renal clearance (vs hepatic clearance of unfractionated heparin) and must be used with caution in patients with renal insufficiency. Not easily reversible.

Warfarin

MECHANISM	Inhibits vitamin K epoxide reductase by competing with vitamin K → inhibition of vitamin K–dependent γ-carboxylation of clotting factors II, VII, IX, and X and proteins C and S. Metabolism affected by polymorphisms in the gene for vitamin K epoxide reductase complex (*VKORC1*). In laboratory assay, has effect on extrinsic pathway and ↑ PT. Long half-life. "The ex-PresidenT went to war(farin)."
CLINICAL USE	Chronic anticoagulation (eg, venous thromboembolism prophylaxis and prevention of stroke in atrial fibrillation). Not used in pregnant patients (because warfarin, unlike heparin, crosses placenta). Monitor PT/INR.
ADVERSE EFFECTS 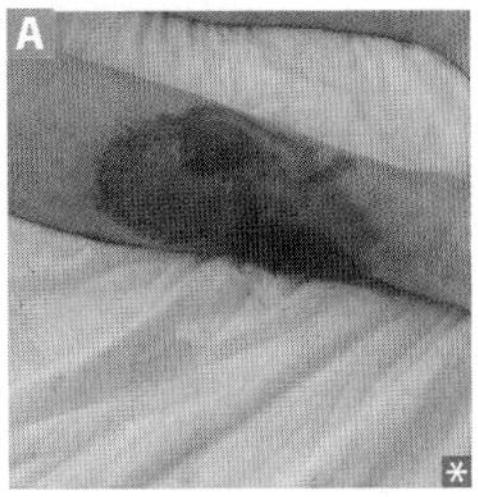	Bleeding, teratogenic effects, skin/tissue necrosis A, drug-drug interactions (metabolized by cytochrome P-450 [CYP2C9]). Initial risk of hypercoagulation: protein C has shorter half-life than factors II and X. Existing protein C depletes before existing factors II and X deplete, and before warfarin can reduce factors II and X production → hypercoagulation. Skin/tissue necrosis within first few days of large doses believed to be due to small vessel microthrombosis. Heparin "bridging": heparin frequently used when starting warfarin. Heparin's activation of antithrombin enables anticoagulation during initial, transient hypercoagulable state caused by warfarin. Initial heparin therapy reduces risk of recurrent venous thromboembolism and skin/tissue necrosis. For reversal of warfarin, give vitamin K. For rapid reversal, give FFP or PCC.

Heparin vs warfarin

	Heparin	Warfarin
ROUTE OF ADMINISTRATION	Parenteral (IV, SC)	Oral
SITE OF ACTION	Blood	Liver
ONSET OF ACTION	Rapid (seconds)	Slow, limited by half-lives of normal clotting factors
DURATION OF ACTION	Hours	Days
MONITORING	PTT (intrinsic pathway)	PT/INR (extrinsic pathway)
CROSSES PLACENTA	No	Yes (teratogenic)

Direct coagulation factor inhibitors

DRUG	MECHANISM	CLINICAL USE	ADVERSE EFFECTS
Bivalirudin, argatroban, dabigatran	Directly inhibit thrombin (factor IIa)	Venous thromboembolism, atrial fibrillation. Can be used in HIT, when heparin is BAD for the patient	Bleeding (reverse dabigatran with idarucizumab) Dabigatran is the only oral agent in class Do not require lab monitoring
Apixaban, edoxaban, rivaroxaban	Directly inhibit factor Xa	Treatment and prophylaxis for DVT and PE; stroke prophylaxis in patients with atrial fibrillation	Bleeding (reverse with andexanet alfa) Oral agents that do not usually require lab monitoring

Anticoagulation reversal

ANTICOAGULANT	REVERSAL AGENT	NOTES
Heparin	Protamine sulfate	⊕ charged peptide that binds ⊖ charged heparin
Warfarin	Vitamin K (slow) +/– FFP or PCC (rapid)	
Dabigatran	Idarucizumab	Monoclonal antibody Fab fragments
Direct factor Xa inhibitors	Andexanet alfa	Recombinant modified factor Xa (inactive)

Antiplatelets

All work by ↓ platelet aggregation.

DRUG	MECHANISM	CLINICAL USE	ADVERSE EFFECTS
Aspirin	Irreversibly blocks COX → ↓ TXA_2 release	Acute coronary syndrome; coronary stenting. ↓ incidence or recurrence of thrombotic stroke	Gastric ulcers, tinnitus, allergic reactions, renal injury
Clopidogrel, prasugrel, ticagrelor, ticlopidine	Block ADP ($P2Y_{12}$) receptor → ↓ ADP-induced expression of GpIIb/IIIa	Same as aspirin; dual antiplatelet therapy	Neutropenia (ticlopidine); TTP may be seen
Abciximab, eptifibatide, tirofiban	Block GpIIb/IIIa (fibrinogen receptor) on activated platelets. Abciximab is made from monoclonal antibody Fab fragments	Unstable angina, percutaneous coronary intervention	Bleeding, thrombocytopenia
Cilostazol, dipyridamole	Block phosphodiesterase → ↓ cAMP in platelets	Intermittent claudication, stroke prevention, cardiac stress testing, prevention of coronary stent restenosis	Nausea, headache, facial flushing, hypotension, abdominal pain

Thrombolytics

Alteplase (tPA), reteplase (rPA), streptokinase, tenecteplase (TNK-tPA).

MECHANISM	Directly or indirectly aid conversion of plasminogen to plasmin, which cleaves thrombin and fibrin clots. ↑ PT, ↑ PTT, no change in platelet count.
CLINICAL USE	Early MI, early ischemic stroke, direct thrombolysis of severe PE.
ADVERSE EFFECTS	Bleeding. Contraindicated in patients with active bleeding, history of intracranial bleeding, recent surgery, known bleeding diatheses, or severe hypertension. Nonspecific reversal with antifibrinolytics (eg, aminocaproic acid, tranexamic acid), platelet transfusions, and factor corrections (eg, cryoprecipitate, FFP, PCC).

Cancer therapy—cell cycle

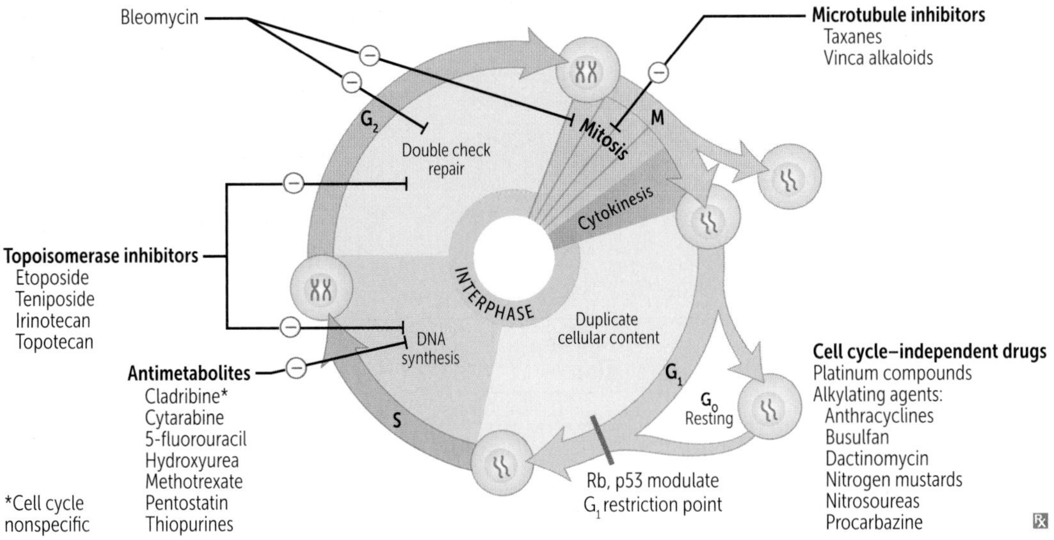
Bleomycin
Microtubule inhibitors
Taxanes
Vinca alkaloids
G2
M
Mitosis
Double check repair
Cytokinesis
Topoisomerase inhibitors
Etoposide
Teniposide
Irinotecan
Topotecan
INTERPHASE
Duplicate cellular content
DNA synthesis
Antimetabolites
Cladribine*
Cytarabine
5-fluorouracil
Hydroxyurea
Methotrexate
Pentostatin
Thiopurines
*Cell cycle nonspecific
S
G1
G0 Resting
Rb, p53 modulate G1 restriction point
Cell cycle–independent drugs
Platinum compounds
Alkylating agents:
Anthracyclines
Busulfan
Dactinomycin
Nitrogen mustards
Nitrosoureas
Procarbazine

Cancer therapy—targets

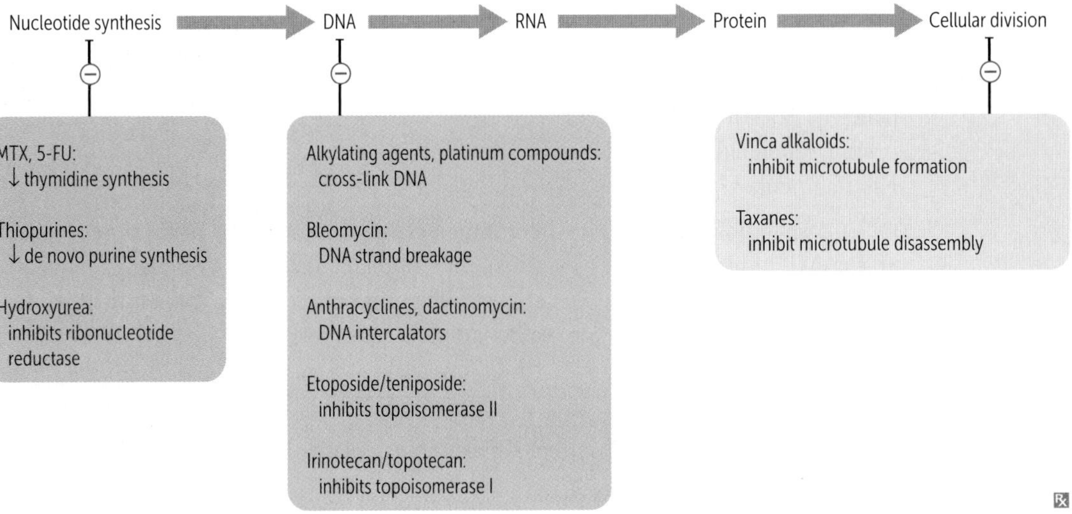
Nucleotide synthesis
DNA
RNA
Protein
Cellular division
MTX, 5-FU:
↓ thymidine synthesis
Thiopurines:
↓ de novo purine synthesis
Hydroxyurea:
inhibits ribonucleotide reductase
Alkylating agents, platinum compounds:
cross-link DNA
Bleomycin:
DNA strand breakage
Anthracyclines, dactinomycin:
DNA intercalators
Etoposide/teniposide:
inhibits topoisomerase II
Irinotecan/topotecan:
inhibits topoisomerase I
Vinca alkaloids:
inhibit microtubule formation
Taxanes:
inhibit microtubule disassembly

Antibody-drug conjugates

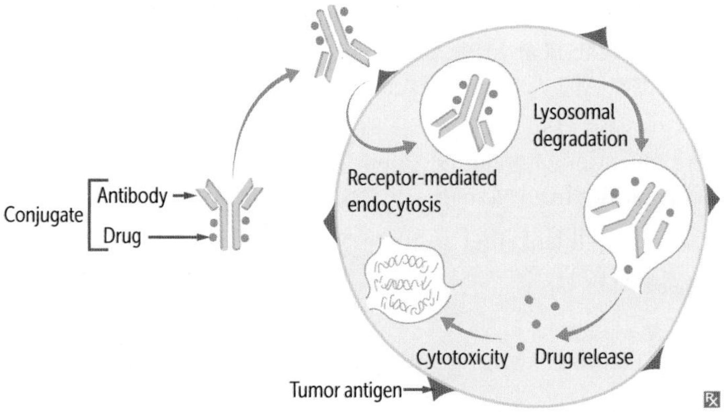
Lysosomal degradation
Receptor-mediated endocytosis
Conjugate
Antibody
Drug
Cytotoxicity
Drug release
Tumor antigen

Formed by linking monoclonal antibodies with cytotoxic chemotherapeutic drugs. Antibody selectivity against tumor antigens allows targeted drug delivery to tumor cells while sparing healthy cells → ↑ efficacy and ↓ toxicity.

Example: ado-trastuzumab emtansine (T-DM1) for HER2 ⊕ breast cancer.

Antitumor antibiotics All are cell cycle nonspecific, except bleomycin which is G_2/M phase specific.

DRUG	MECHANISM	CLINICAL USE	ADVERSE EFFECTS
Bleomycin	Induces free radical formation → breaks in DNA strands	Testicular cancer, Hodgkin lymphoma	Pulmonary fibrosis, skin hyperpigmentation
Dactinomycin (actinomycin D)	Intercalates into DNA, preventing RNA synthesis	Wilms tumor, Ewing sarcoma, rhabdomyosarcoma	Myelosuppression
Anthracyclines Doxorubicin, daunorubicin	Generate free radicals Intercalate in DNA → breaks in DNA → ↓ replication Inhibit topoisomerase II	Solid tumors, leukemias, lymphomas	Dilated cardiomyopathy (often irreversible; prevent with dexrazoxane), myelosuppression, alopecia

Antimetabolites All are S-phase specific except cladribine, which is cell cycle nonspecific.

DRUG	MECHANISM	CLINICAL USE	ADVERSE EFFECTS
Thiopurines Azathioprine, 6-mercaptopurine	Purine (thiol) analogs → ↓ de novo purine synthesis AZA is converted to 6-MP, which is then activated by HGPRT	Rheumatoid arthritis, IBD, SLE, ALL; steroid-refractory disease Prevention of organ rejection Weaning from steroids	Myelosuppression; GI, liver toxicity 6-MP is inactivated by xanthine oxidase (↑ toxicity with allopurinol or febuxostat)
Cladribine, pentostatin	Purine analogs → multiple mechanisms (eg, inhibition of ADA, DNA strand breaks)	Hairy cell leukemia	Myelosuppression
Cytarabine (arabinofuranosyl cytidine)	Pyrimidine analog → DNA chain termination Inhibits DNA polymerase	Leukemias (AML), lymphomas	Myelosuppression
5-Fluorouracil	Pyrimidine analog bioactivated to 5-FdUMP → thymidylate synthase inhibition → ↓ dTMP → ↓ DNA synthesis Capecitabine is a prodrug	Colon cancer, pancreatic cancer, actinic keratosis, basal cell carcinoma (topical) Effects enhanced with the addition of leucovorin	Myelosuppression, palmar-plantar erythrodysesthesia (hand-foot syndrome)
Hydroxyurea	Inhibits ribonucleotide reductase → ↓ DNA synthesis	Myeloproliferative disorders (eg, CML, polycythemia vera), sickle cell disease (↑ HbF)	Severe myelosuppression, megaloblastic anemia
Methotrexate	Folic acid analog that competitively inhibits dihydrofolate reductase → ↓ dTMP → ↓ DNA synthesis	Cancers: leukemias (ALL), lymphomas, choriocarcinoma, sarcomas Nonneoplastic: ectopic pregnancy, medical abortion (with misoprostol), rheumatoid arthritis, psoriasis, IBD, vasculitis	Myelosuppression (reversible with leucovorin "rescue"), hepatotoxicity, mucositis (eg, mouth ulcers), pulmonary fibrosis, folate deficiency (teratogenic), nephrotoxicity

Alkylating agents All are cell cycle nonspecific.

DRUG	MECHANISM	CLINICAL USE	ADVERSE EFFECTS
Busulfan	Cross-links DNA	Used to ablate patient's bone marrow before bone marrow transplantation	Severe myelosuppression (in almost all cases), pulmonary fibrosis, hyperpigmentation
Nitrogen mustards Cyclophosphamide, ifosfamide	Cross-link DNA Require bioactivation by liver	Solid tumors, leukemia, lymphomas, rheumatic disease (eg, SLE, granulomatosis with polyangiitis)	Myelosuppression, SIADH, Fanconi syndrome (ifosfamide), hemorrhagic cystitis and bladder cancer (prevent with mesna)
Nitrosoureas Carmustine, lomustine	Cross-link DNA Require bioactivation Cross blood-brain barrier → CNS entry	Brain tumors (including **glio**blastoma multiforme) Put **nitro** in your **Mus**tang and travel the **globe**	CNS toxicity (convulsions, dizziness, ataxia)
Procarbazine	Mechanism unknown Weak MAO inhibitor	Hodgkin lymphoma, brain tumors	Bone marrow suppression, pulmonary toxicity, leukemia, disulfiram-like reaction

Platinum compounds Cisplatin, carboplatin, oxaliplatin.

MECHANISM	Cross-link DNA. Cell cycle nonspecific.
CLINICAL USE	Solid tumors (eg, testicular, bladder, ovarian, GI, lung), lymphomas.
ADVERSE EFFECTS	Nephrotoxicity (eg, Fanconi syndrome; prevent with amifostine), peripheral neuropathy, ototoxicity.

Microtubule inhibitors All are M-phase specific.

DRUG	MECHANISM	CLINICAL USE	ADVERSE EFFECTS
Taxanes Docetaxel, paclitaxel	Hyper**stabilize** polymerized microtubules → prevent mitotic spindle breakdown	Various tumors (eg, ovarian and breast carcinomas)	Myelosuppression, neuropathy, hypersensitivity **Tax**es **stabilize** society
Vinca alkaloids Vincristine, vinblastine	Bind β-tubulin and inhibit its polymerization into microtubules → prevent mitotic spindle formation	Solid tumors, leukemias, Hodgkin and non-Hodgkin lymphomas	Vin**cris**tine (**cris**ps the nerves): neurotoxicity (axonal neuropathy), constipation (including ileus) Vin**blast**ine (**blast**s the marrow): myelosuppression

Topoisomerase inhibitors All cause ↑ DNA degradation resulting in cell cycle arrest in S and G_2 phases.

DRUG	MECHANISM	CLINICAL USE	ADVERSE EFFECTS
Irinotecan, topotecan	Inhibit topoisomerase **I** "-**tecone**"	Colon, ovarian, small cell lung cancer	Severe myelosuppression, diarrhea
Etoposide, teniposide	Inhibit topoisomerase **II** "-**bothside**"	Testicular, small cell lung cancer, leukemia, lymphoma	Myelosuppression, alopecia

Tamoxifen

MECHANISM	Selective estrogen receptor modulator with complex mode of action: antagonist in breast tissue, partial agonist in endometrium and bone. Blocks the binding of estrogen to ER in ER ⊕ cells.
CLINICAL USE	Prevention and treatment of breast cancer, prevention of gynecomastia in patients undergoing prostate cancer therapy.
ADVERSE EFFECTS	Hot flashes, ↑ risk of thromboembolic events (eg, DVT, PE) and endometrial cancer.

Anticancer monoclonal antibodies Work against extracellular targets to neutralize them or to promote immune system recognition (eg, ADCC by NK cells).

AGENT	TARGET	CLINICAL USE	ADVERSE EFFECTS
Alemtuzumab	CD52	Chronic **lym**phocytic leukemia (CLL), multiple sclerosis.	↑ risk of infections and autoimmunity (eg, ITP)
Bevacizumab	VEGF (inhibits blood vessel formation)	Colorectal cancer (CRC), renal cell carcinoma (RCC), non–small cell lung cancer (NSCLC), angioproliferative retinopathy	Hemorrhage, blood clots, impaired wound healing
Cetuximab, panitumumab	EGFR	Metastatic CRC (wild-type RAS), head and neck cancer	Rash, elevated LFTs, diarrhea
Rituximab	CD20	Non-Hodgkin lymphoma, CLL, rheumatoid arthritis, ITP, TTP, AIHA, multiple sclerosis	↑ risk of PML in patients with JC virus
Trastuzumab	HER2 ("**trust HER**")	Breast cancer, gastric cancer	Dilated **cardiomyopathy** (often reversible). "**Heart**ceptin"
Pembrolizumab, nivolumab, cemiplimab	PD-1	Various tumors (eg, NSCLC, RCC, melanoma, urothelial carcinoma)	↑ risk of autoimmunity (eg, dermatitis, enterocolitis, hepatitis, pneumonitis, endocrinopathies)
Atezolizumab, durvalumab, avelumab	PD-L1		
Ipilimumab	CTLA-4		

Anticancer small molecule inhibitors

AGENT	TARGET	CLINICAL USE	ADVERSE EFFECTS
Alectinib	ALK	Non–small cell lung cancer	Edema, rash, diarrhea
Erlotinib, gefitinib, afatinib	EGFR	Non–small cell lung cancer	Rash, diarrhea
Imatinib, dasatinib, nilotinib	BCR-ABL (also other tyrosine kinases [eg, c-KIT])	CML, ALL, GISTs	Myelosuppression, ↑ LFTs, edema, myalgias
Ruxolitinib	JAK1/2	Polycythemia vera	Bruises, ↑ LFTs
Bortezomib, ixazomib, carfilzomib	Proteasome (induce arrest at G2-M phase → apoptosis)	Multiple myeloma, mantle cell lymphoma	Peripheral neuropathy, herpes zoster reactivation
Vemurafenib, encorafenib, dabrafenib	BRAF	Melanoma Often co-administered with MEK inhibitors (eg, trametinib)	Rash, fatigue, nausea, diarrhea
Palbociclib	Cyclin-dependent kinase 4/6 (induces arrest at G1-S phase → apoptosis)	Breast cancer	Myelosuppression, pneumonitis
Olaparib	Poly(ADP-ribose) polymerase (↓ DNA repair)	Breast, ovarian, pancreatic, and prostate cancers	Myelosuppression, edema, diarrhea

Amelioration of adverse effects of chemotherapy

DRUG	MECHANISM	CLINICAL USE
Amifostine	Free radical scavenger	Nephrotoxicity from platinum compounds
Dexrazoxane	Iron chelator	Cardiotoxicity from anthracyclines
Leucovorin (folinic acid)	Tetrahydrofolate precursor	Myelosuppression from methotrexate (leucovorin "rescue"); also enhances the effects of 5-FU
Mesna	Sulfhydryl compound that binds acrolein (toxic metabolite of cyclophosphamide/ifosfamide)	Hemorrhagic cystitis from cyclophosphamide/ifosfamide
Rasburicase	Recombinant uricase that catalyzes metabolism of uric acid to allantoin	Tumor lysis syndrome
Ondansetron, granisetron	5-HT_3 receptor antagonists	Acute nausea and vomiting (usually within 1-2 hr after chemotherapy)
Prochlorperazine, metoclopramide	D_2 receptor antagonists	
Aprepitant, fosaprepitant	NK_1 receptor antagonists	Delayed nausea and vomiting (>24 hr after chemotherapy)
Filgrastim, sargramostim	Recombinant G(M)-CSF	Neutropenia
Epoetin alfa	Recombinant erythropoietin	Anemia

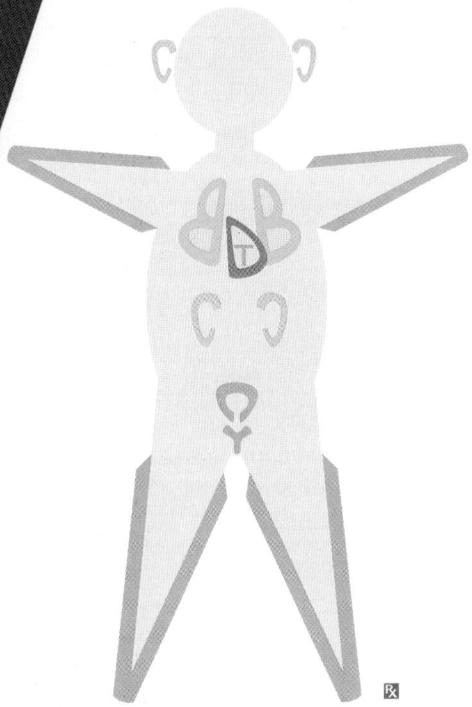

Cisplatin, Carboplatin → ototoxicity

Vincristine → peripheral neuropathy
Bleomycin, Busulfan → pulmonary fibrosis
Doxorubicin, Daunorubicin → cardiotoxicity
Trastuzumab → cardiotoxicity
Cisplatin, Carboplatin → nephrotoxicity

CYclophosphamide → hemorrhagic cystitis

Nonspecific common toxicities of nearly all cytotoxic chemotherapies include myelosuppression (neutropenia, anemia, thrombocytopenia), GI toxicity (nausea, vomiting, mucositis), alopecia.

HIGH-YIELD SYSTEMS

Musculoskeletal, Skin, and Connective Tissue

"Rigid, the skeleton of habit alone upholds the human frame."

—Virginia Woolf, *Mrs. Dalloway*

"Beauty may be skin deep, but ugly goes clear to the bone."

—Redd Foxx

"The finest clothing made is a person's own skin, but, of course, society demands something more than this."

—Mark Twain

"To thrive in life you need three bones. A wishbone. A backbone. And a funny bone."

—Reba McEntire

This chapter provides information you will need to understand certain anatomical dysfunctions, rheumatic diseases, and dermatologic conditions. Be able to interpret 3D anatomy in the context of radiologic imaging. For the rheumatic diseases, create instructional cases or personas that include the most likely presentation and symptoms: risk factors, gender, important markers (eg, autoantibodies), and other epidemiologic factors. Doing so will allow you to answer the higher order questions that are likely to be asked on the exam.

▶ MUSCULOSKELETAL, SKIN, AND CONNECTIVE TISSUE—ANATOMY AND PHYSIOLOGY

Rotator cuff muscles

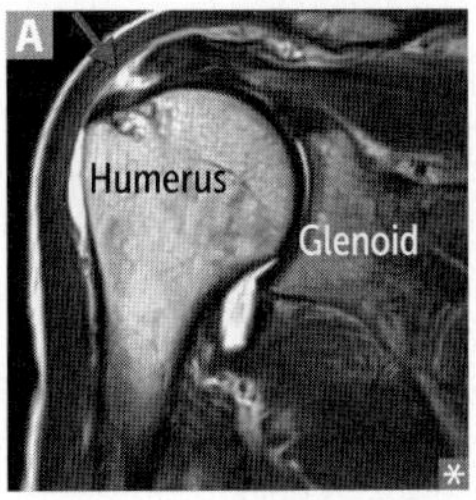

Shoulder muscles that form the rotator cuff:

- Supraspinatus (suprascapular nerve)—abducts arm initially (before the action of the deltoid); most common rotator cuff injury (trauma or degeneration and impingement → tendinopathy or tear [arrow in A]), assessed by "empty/full can" test
- Infraspinatus (suprascapular nerve)—externally rotates arm; pitching injury
- teres minor (axillary nerve)—adducts and externally rotates arm
- Subscapularis (upper and lower subscapular nerves)—internally rotates and adducts arm

Innervated primarily by C5-C6.

SItS (small t is for teres minor).

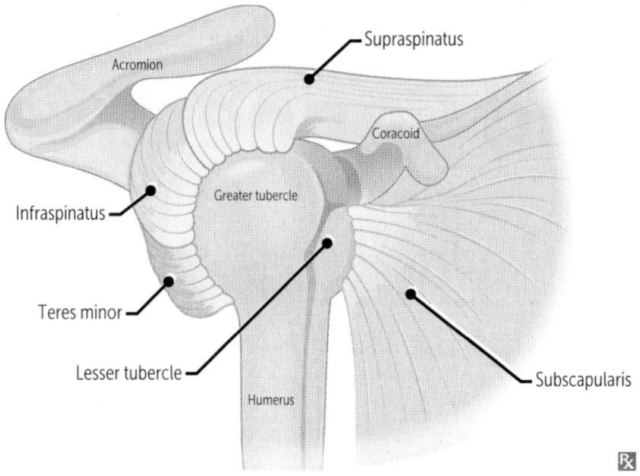

Arm abduction

DEGREE	MUSCLE	NERVE
0°–15°	Supraspinatus	Suprascapular
15°–90°	Deltoid	Axillary
> 90°	Trapezius	Accessory
> 90°	Serratus Anterior	Long Thoracic (SALT)

Upper extremity nerves

NERVE	CAUSES OF INJURY	PRESENTATION
Axillary (C5-C6)	Fractured surgical neck of humerus Anterior dislocation of humerus	Flattened deltoid Loss of arm abduction at shoulder (> 15°) Loss of sensation over deltoid and lateral arm
Musculocutaneous (C5-C7)	Upper trunk compression	↓ biceps (C5-6) reflex Loss of forearm flexion and supination Loss of sensation over radial and dorsal forearm
Radial (C5-T1)	Compression of axilla, eg, due to crutches or sleeping with arm over chair ("Saturday night palsy") Midshaft fracture of humerus Repetitive pronation/supination of forearm, eg, due to screwdriver use ("finger drop")	Injuries above the elbow cause loss of sensation over posterior arm/forearm and dorsal hand, wrist drop (loss of elbow, wrist, and finger extension) with ↓ grip strength (wrist extension necessary for maximal action of flexors) Injuries below the elbow cause distal paresthesias without wrist drop Tricep function and posterior arm sensation spared in midshaft fracture

Upper extremity nerves *(continued)*

NERVE	CAUSES OF INJURY	PRESENTATION
Median (C5-T1)	Supracondylar fracture of humerus → proximal lesion of the nerve Carpal tunnel syndrome and wrist laceration → distal lesion of the nerve	"Ape hand" and "Hand of benediction" Loss of wrist flexion and function of the lateral two **L**umbricals, **O**pponens pollicis, **A**bductor pollicis brevis, **F**lexor pollicis brevis (**LOAF**) Loss of sensation over thenar eminence and dorsal and palmar aspects of lateral 3½ fingers with proximal lesion
Ulnar (C8-T1)	Fracture of medial epicondyle of humerus "funny bone" (proximal lesion) Fractured hook of hamate (distal lesion) from fall on outstretched hand	"Ulnar claw" on digit extension Radial deviation of wrist upon flexion (proximal lesion) ↓ flexion of ulnar fingers, abduction and adduction of fingers (interossei), thumb adduction, actions of ulnar 2 lumbrical muscles Loss of sensation over ulnar 1½ fingers including hypothenar eminence
Recurrent branch of median nerve (C5-T1)	Superficial laceration of palm	"Ape hand" Loss of thenar muscle group: opposition, abduction, and flexion of thumb No loss of sensation

Humerus fractures, proximally to distally, follow the **ARM** (**A**xillary → **R**adial → **M**edian)

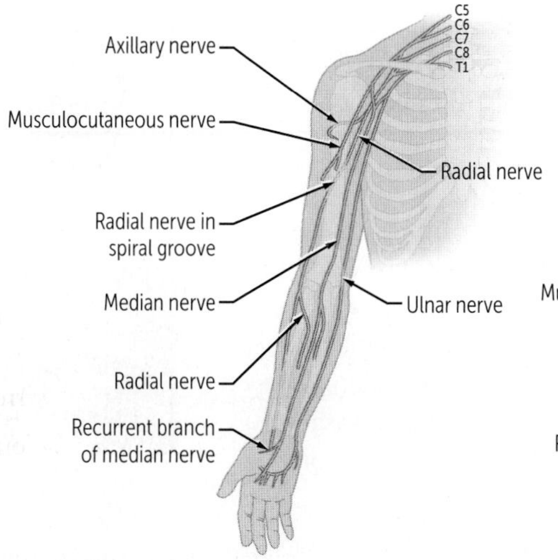

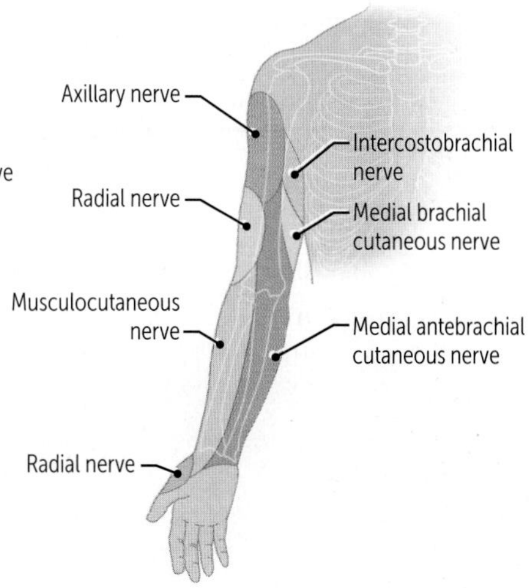

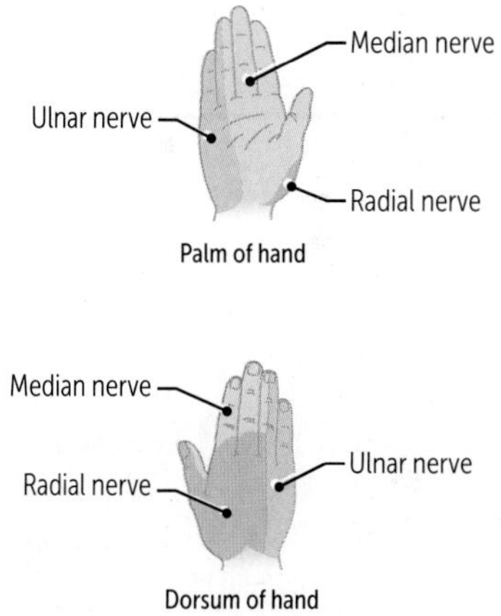

Brachial plexus lesions

1. Erb palsy ("waiter's tip")
2. Klumpke palsy (claw hand)
3. Wrist drop
4. Winged scapula
5. Deltoid paralysis
6. "Saturday night palsy" (wrist drop)
7. Difficulty flexing elbow, variable sensory loss
8. Decreased thumb function, "hand of benediction"
9. Intrinsic muscles of hand, claw hand

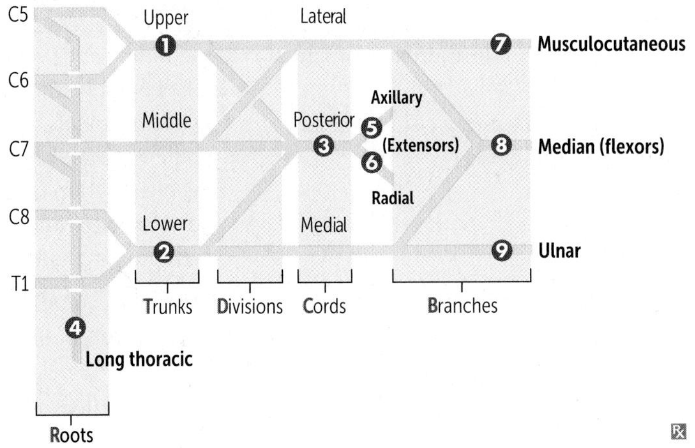

Divisions of brachial plexus:
Randy
Travis
Drinks
Cold
Beer

CONDITION	INJURY	CAUSES	MUSCLE DEFICIT	FUNCTIONAL DEFICIT	PRESENTATION
Erb palsy ("waiter's tip")	Traction or tear of **upper** trunk: C5-C6 roots	Infants—lateral traction on neck during delivery Adults—trauma	Deltoid, supraspinatus	Abduction (arm hangs by side)	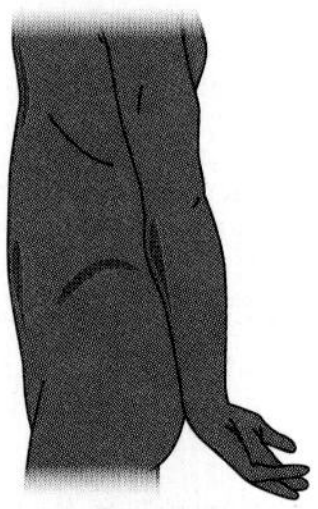
			Infraspinatus, supraspinatus	Lateral rotation (arm medially rotated)	
			Biceps brachii Herb gets **DIB**s on **tips**	Flexion, supination (arm extended and pronated)	
Klumpke palsy	Traction or tear of **lower** trunk: C8-T1 roots	Infants—upward force on arm during delivery Adults—trauma (eg, grabbing a tree branch to break a fall)	Intrinsic hand muscles: lumbricals, interossei, thenar, hypothenar	Claw hand: lumbricals normally flex MCP joints and extend DIP and PIP joints	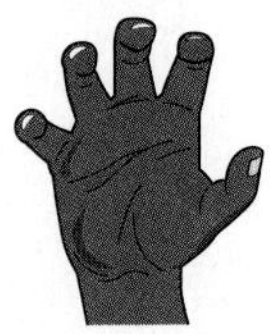
Thoracic outlet syndrome	Compression of **lower** trunk and subclavian vessels, most commonly within the scalene triangle	Cervical rib (arrows in A), Pancoast tumor	Same as Klumpke palsy	Atrophy of intrinsic hand muscles; ischemia, pain, and edema due to vascular compression	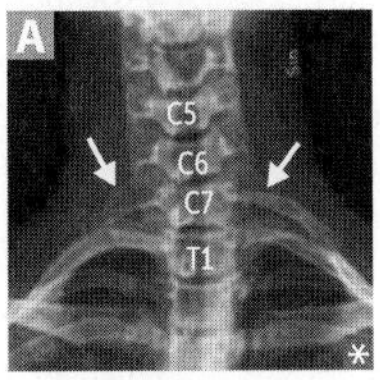
Winged scapula	Lesion of long thoracic nerve, roots C5-C7 ("**wings** of **heaven**")	Axillary node dissection after mastectomy, stab wounds	Serratus anterior	Inability to anchor scapula to thoracic cage → cannot abduct arm above horizontal position B	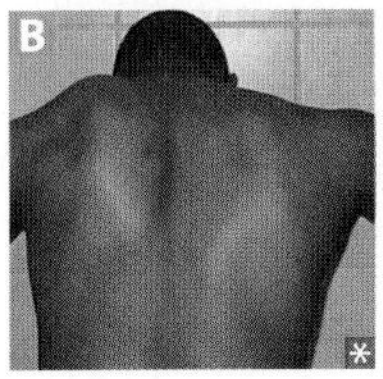

Wrist region

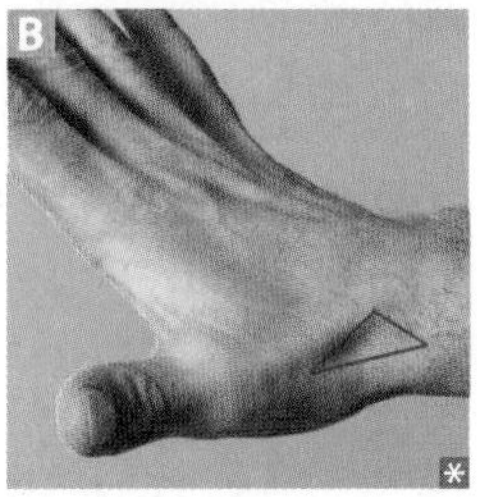

Scaphoid, lunate, triquetrum, pisiform, hamate, capitate, trapezoid, trapezium A. (So long to pinky, here comes the thumb)

Scaphoid (palpable in anatomic snuff box B) is the most commonly fractured carpal bone, typically due to a fall on an outstretched hand. Complications of proximal scaphoid fractures include avascular necrosis and nonunion due to retrograde blood supply from a branch of the radial artery. Occult fracture not always seen on initial x-ray.

Dislocation of lunate may impinge median nerve and cause carpal tunnel syndrome.

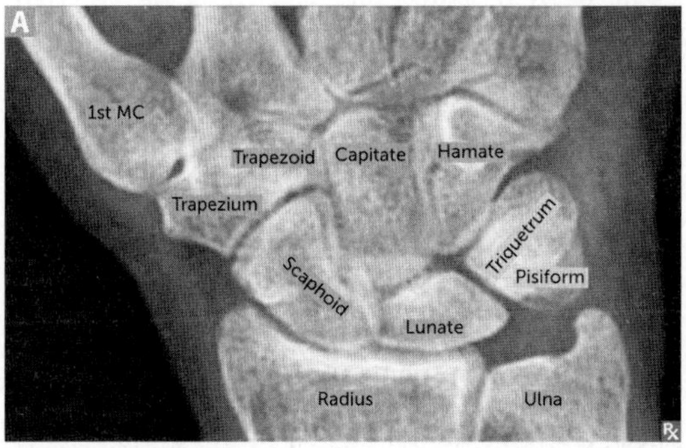

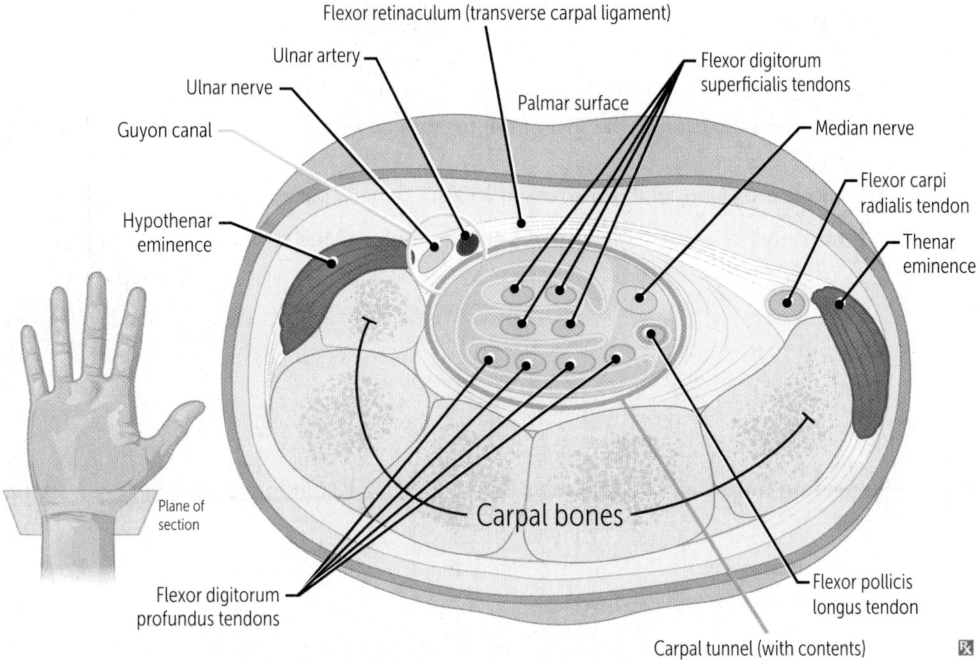

Hand muscles

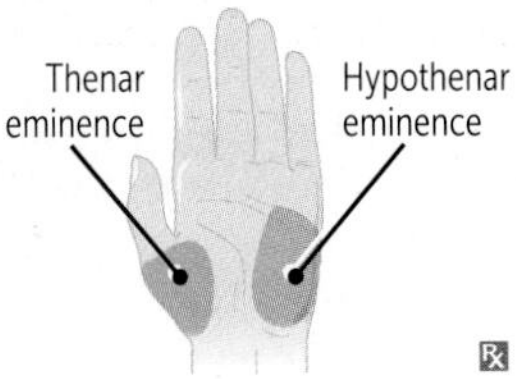

Thenar (median)—Opponens pollicis, Abductor pollicis brevis, Flexor pollicis brevis, superficial head (deep head by ulnar nerve).
Hypothenar (ulnar)—Opponens digiti minimi, Abductor digiti minimi, Flexor digiti minimi brevis.

Both groups perform the same functions: Oppose, Abduct, and Flex (OAF).

Dorsal interossei (ulnar)—abduct the fingers.
Palmar interossei (ulnar)—adduct the fingers.

DAB = Dorsals ABduct.
PAD = Palmars ADduct.

Lumbricals (1st/2nd, median; 3rd/4th, ulnar)—flex at the MCP joint, extend PIP and DIP joints.

Distortions of the hand

At rest, a balance exists between the extrinsic flexors and extensors of the hand, as well as the intrinsic muscles of the hand—particularly the lumbrical muscles (flexion of MCP, extension of DIP and PIP joints).
"Clawing"—seen best with **distal** lesions of median or ulnar nerves. Remaining extrinsic flexors of the digits exaggerate the loss of the lumbricals → fingers extend at MCP, flex at DIP and PIP joints.
Deficits less pronounced in **proximal** lesions; deficits present during voluntary flexion of the digits.

SIGN	"Ulnar claw"	"Hand of benediction"	"Median claw"	"OK gesture"
PRESENTATION	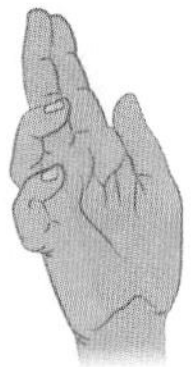	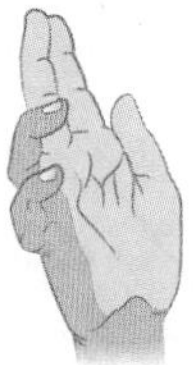	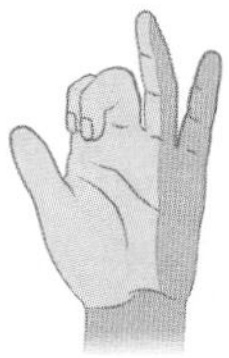	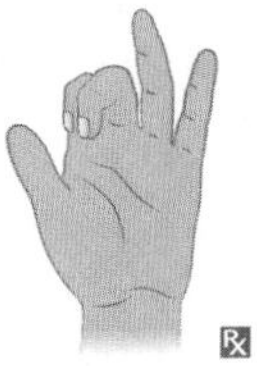
CONTEXT	Extending fingers/at rest	Making a fist	Extending fingers/at rest	Making a fist
LOCATION OF LESION	Distal ulnar nerve	Proximal median nerve	Distal median nerve	Proximal ulnar nerve

Note: Atrophy of the thenar eminence can be seen in median nerve lesions, while atrophy of the hypothenar eminence can be seen in ulnar nerve lesions.

Actions of hip muscles

ACTION	MUSCLES
Abductors	Gluteus medius, gluteus minimus
Adductors	Adductor magnus, adductor longus, adductor brevis
Extensors	Gluteus maximus, semitendinosus, semimembranosus
Flexors	Iliopsoas, rectus femoris, tensor fascia lata, pectineus, sartorius
Internal rotation	Gluteus medius, gluteus minimus, tensor fascia latae
External rotation	Iliopsoas, gluteus maximus, piriformis, obturator

Lower extremity nerves

NERVE	INNERVATION	CAUSE OF INJURY	PRESENTATION/COMMENTS
Iliohypogastric (T12-L1)	Sensory—suprapubic region Motor—transversus abdominis and internal oblique	Abdominal surgery	Burning or tingling pain in surgical incision site radiating to inguinal and suprapubic region
Genitofemoral nerve (L1-L2)	Sensory—scrotum/labia majora, medial thigh Motor—cremaster	Laparoscopic surgery	↓ upper medial thigh and anterior thigh sensation beneath the inguinal ligament (lateral part of the femoral triangle); absent cremasteric reflex
Lateral femoral cutaneous (L2-L3)	Sensory—anterior and lateral thigh	Tight clothing, obesity, pregnancy, pelvic procedures	↓ thigh sensation (anterior and lateral)
Obturator (L2-L4) 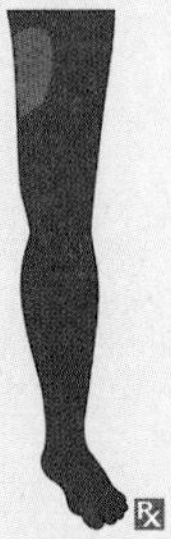	Sensory—medial thigh Motor—obturator externus, adductor longus, adductor brevis, gracilis, pectineus, adductor magnus	Pelvic surgery	↓ thigh sensation (medial) and adduction
Femoral (L2-L4) 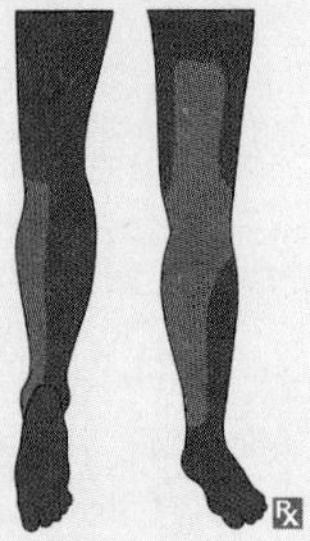	Sensory—anterior thigh, medial leg Motor—quadriceps, iliacus, pectineus, sartorius	Pelvic fracture	↓ leg extension (↓ patellar reflex)
Sciatic (L4-S3)	Motor—semitendinosus, semimembranosus, biceps femoris, adductor magnus	Herniated disc, posterior hip dislocation	Splits into common peroneal and tibial nerves
Common (fibular) peroneal (L4-S2) 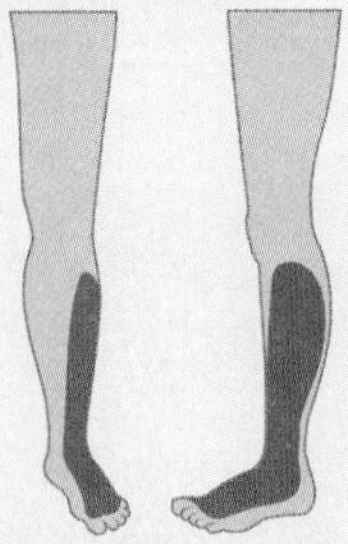	Superficial peroneal nerve: ▪ Sensory—dorsum of foot (except webspace between hallux and 2nd digit) ▪ Motor—peroneus longus and brevis Deep peroneal nerve: ▪ Sensory—webspace between hallux and 2nd digit ▪ Motor—tibialis anterior	Trauma or compression of lateral aspect of leg, fibular neck fracture	PED = Peroneal Everts and Dorsiflexes; if injured, foot dropPED Loss of sensation on dorsum of foot Foot drop—inverted and plantarflexed at rest, loss of eversion and dorsiflexion; "steppage gait"

Lower extremity nerves *(continued)*

NERVE	INNERVATION	CAUSE OF INJURY	PRESENTATION/COMMENTS
Tibial (L4-S3) 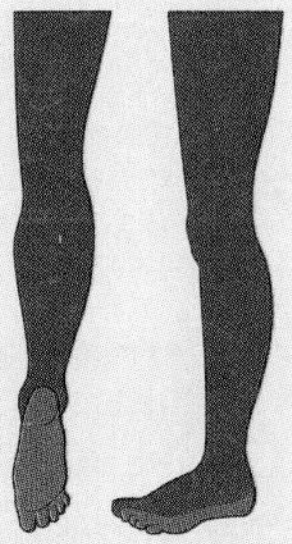	Sensory—sole of foot Motor—biceps femoris (long head), triceps surae, plantaris, popliteus, flexor muscles of foot	Knee trauma, Baker cyst (proximal lesion); tarsal tunnel syndrome (distal lesion)	TIP = Tibial Inverts and Plantarflexes; if injured, can't stand on TIPtoes Inability to curl toes and loss of sensation on sole; in proximal lesions, foot everted at rest with weakened inversion and plantar flexion
Superior gluteal (L4-S1) 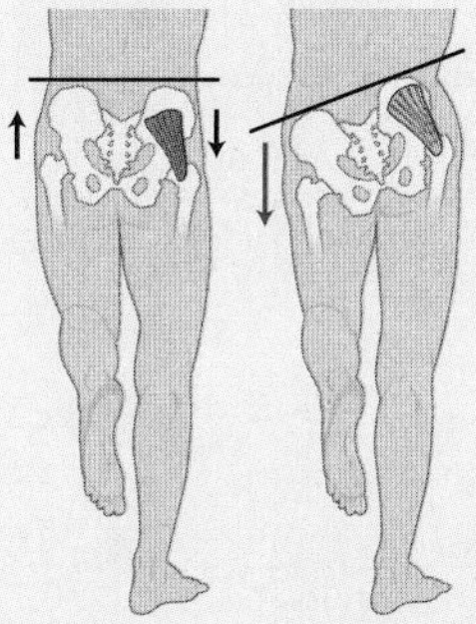 	Motor—gluteus medius, gluteus minimus, tensor fascia latae	Iatrogenic injury during intramuscular injection to superomedial gluteal region (prevent by choosing superolateral quadrant, preferably anterolateral region)	Trendelenburg sign/gait—pelvis tilts because weight-bearing leg cannot maintain alignment of pelvis through hip abduction Lesion is contralateral to the side of the hip that drops, ipsilateral to extremity on which the patient stands
Inferior gluteal (L5-S2)	Motor—gluteus maximus	Posterior hip dislocation	Difficulty climbing stairs, rising from seated position; loss of hip extension
Pudendal (S2-S4)	Sensory—perineum Motor—external urethral and anal sphincters	Stretch injury during childbirth, prolonged cycling, horseback riding	↓ sensation in perineum and genital area; can cause fecal and/or urinary incontinence Can be blocked with local anesthetic during childbirth using ischial spine as a landmark for injection

Knee exam

Lateral femoral condyle to anterior tibia: ACL.
Medial femoral condyle to posterior tibia: PCL.
LAMP.

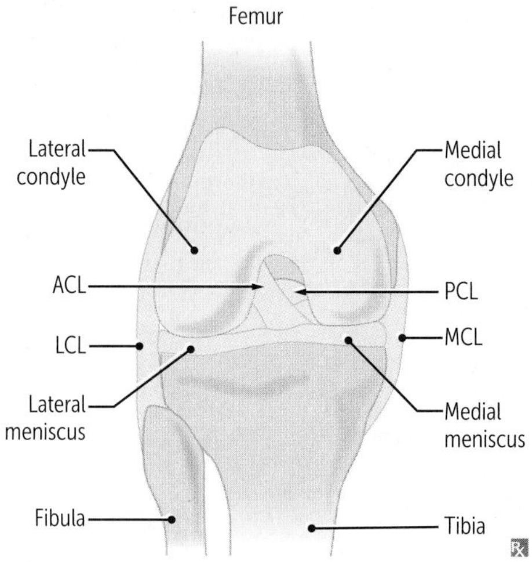

TEST	PROCEDURE	
Anterior drawer sign	Bending knee at 90° angle, ↑ anterior gliding of tibia (relative to femur) due to ACL injury Lachman test also tests ACL, but is more sensitive (↑ anterior gliding of tibia [relative to femur] with knee bent at 30° angle)	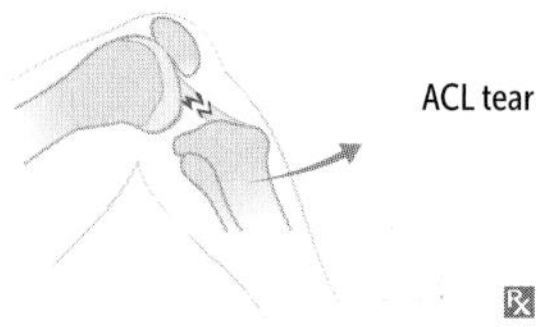
Posterior drawer sign	Bending knee at 90° angle, ↑ posterior gliding of tibia due to PCL injury	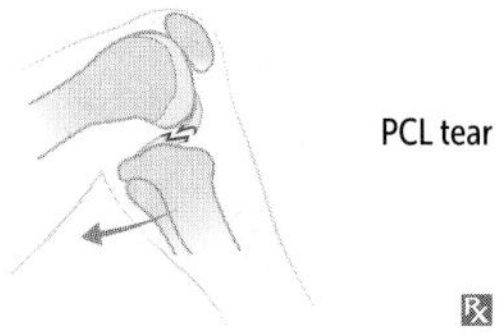
Abnormal passive abduction	Also called valgus stress test. Knee either extended or at ~ 30° angle, lateral (valgus) force → medial space widening of tibia → MCL injury	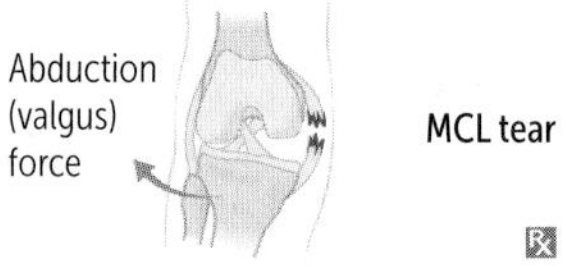
Abnormal passive adduction	Also called varus stress test. Knee either extended or at ~ 30° angle, medial (varus) force → lateral space widening of tibia → LCL injury	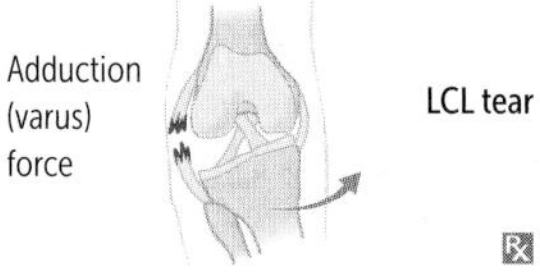
McMurray test	During flexion and extension of knee with rotation of tibia/foot (**LIME**): ▪ Pain, "popping" on internal rotation and varus force → Lateral meniscal tear (**I**nternal rotation stresses lateral meniscus) ▪ Pain, "popping" on external rotation and valgus force → **M**edial meniscal tear (**E**xternal rotation stresses medial meniscus)	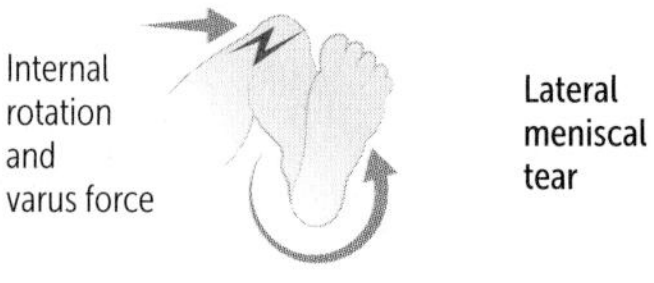 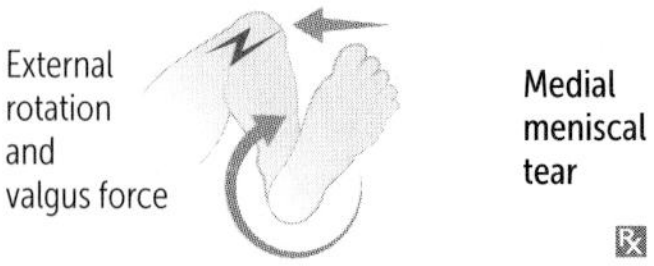

Ankle sprains

Anterior talofibular ligament—most common ankle sprain overall, classified as a low ankle sprain. Due to overinversion/supination of foot. Always tears first.

Anterior inferior tibiofibular ligament—most common high ankle sprain.

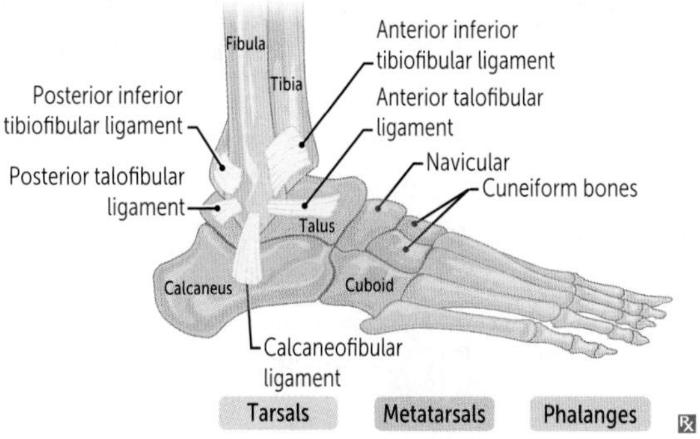

Signs of lumbosacral radiculopathy

Paresthesia and weakness related to specific lumbosacral spinal nerves. Intervertebral disc (nucleus pulposus) herniates posterolaterally through annulus fibrosus (outer ring) into central canal due to thin posterior longitudinal ligament and thicker anterior longitudinal ligament along midline of vertebral bodies. Nerve affected is usually below the level of herniation.

Disc level herniation	L3-L4	L4-L5	L5-S1
Nerve root affected	L4	L5	S1
Dermatome affected	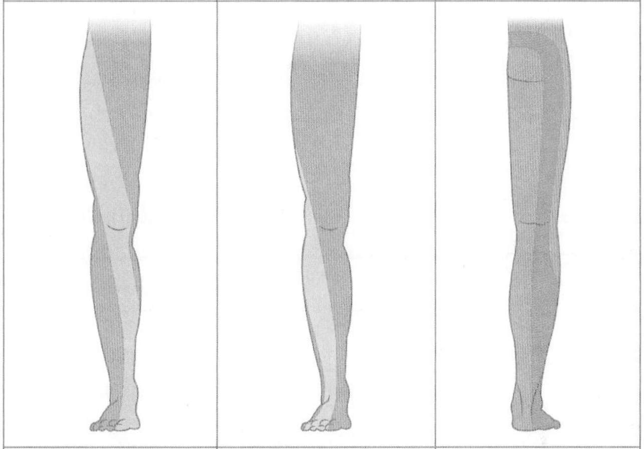		
Clinical findings	Weakness of knee extension ↓patellar reflex	Weakness of dorsiflexion Difficulty in heel walking	Weakness of plantar flexion Difficulty in toe walking ↓Achilles reflex

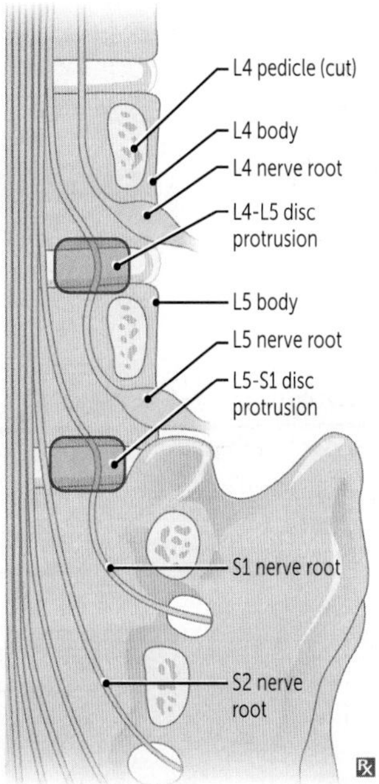

Neurovascular pairing

Nerves and arteries are frequently named together by the bones/regions with which they are associated. The following are exceptions to this naming convention.

LOCATION	NERVE	ARTERY
Axilla/lateral thorax	Long thoracic	Lateral thoracic
Surgical neck of humerus	Axillary	Posterior circumflex
Midshaft of humerus	Radial	Deep brachial
Distal humerus/cubital fossa	Median	Brachial
Popliteal fossa	Tibial	Popliteal
Posterior to medial malleolus	Tibial	Posterior tibial

Motoneuron action potential to muscle contraction

T-tubules are extensions of plasma membrane in contact with the sarcoplasmic reticulum, allowing for coordinated contraction of striated muscles.

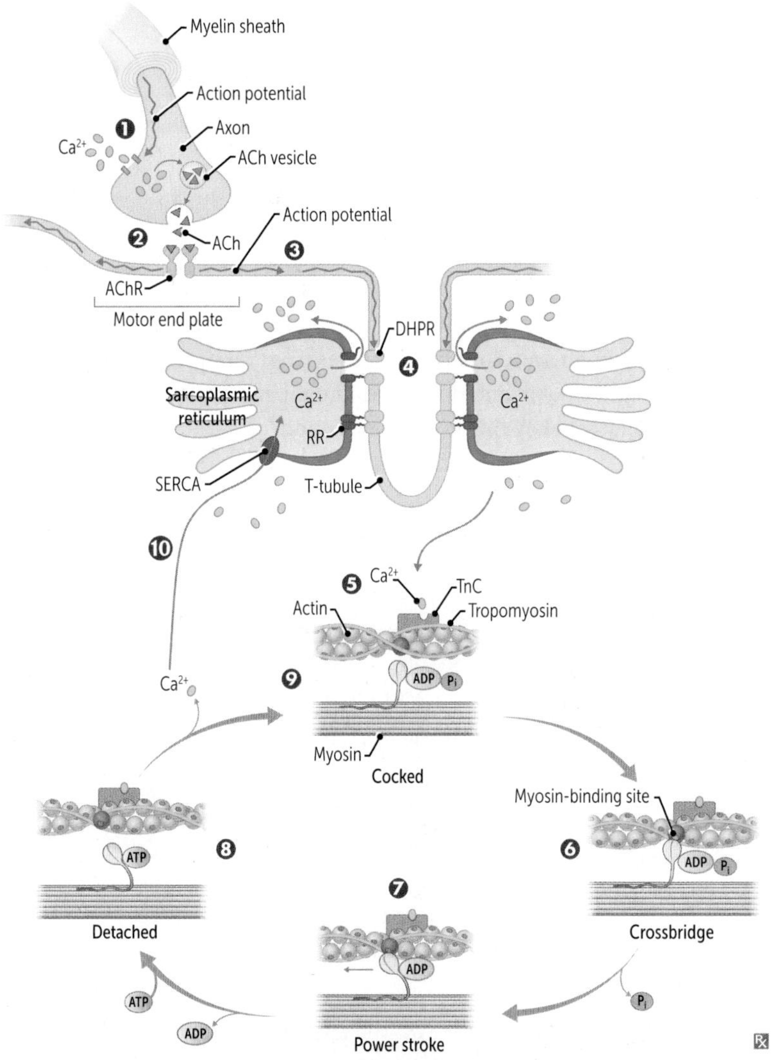

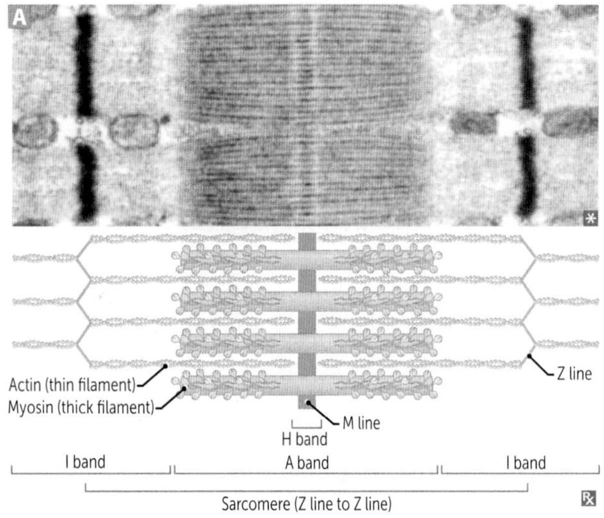

❶ Action potential opens presynaptic voltage-gated Ca^{2+} channels, inducing acetylcholine (ACh) release.

❷ Postsynaptic ACh binding leads to muscle cell depolarization at the motor end plate.

❸ Depolarization travels over the entire muscle cell and deep into the muscle via the T-tubules.

❹ Membrane depolarization induces conformational changes in the voltage-sensitive dihydropyridine receptor (DHPR) and its mechanically coupled ryanodine receptor (RR) → Ca^{2+} release from the sarcoplasmic reticulum into the cytoplasm.

❺ Tropomyosin is blocking myosin-binding sites on the actin filament. Released Ca^{2+} binds to troponin C (TnC), shifting tropomyosin to expose the myosin-binding sites.

❻ The myosin head binds strongly to actin, forming a crossbridge. P_i is then released, initiating the power stroke.

❼ During the power stroke, force is produced as myosin pulls on the thin filament A. Muscle shortening occurs, with shortening of **H** and **I** bands and between **Z** lines (**HIZ** shrinkage). The A band remains the same length (**A** band is **A**lways the same length). ADP is released at the end of the power stroke.

❽ Binding of new ATP molecule causes detachment of myosin head from actin filament. Ca^{2+} is resequestered.

❾ ATP hydrolysis into ADP and P_i results in myosin head returning to high-energy position (cocked). The myosin head can bind to a new site on actin to form a crossbridge if Ca^{2+} remains available.

❿ Reuptake of calcium by sarco(endo)plasmic reticulum Ca^{2+} ATPase (SERCA) → muscle relaxation.

Types of skeletal muscle fibers

	Type I	Type II
CONTRACTION VELOCITY	Slow	Fast
FIBER COLOR	Red	White
PREDOMINANT METABOLISM	Oxidative phosphorylation → sustained contraction	Anaerobic glycolysis
MITOCHONDRIA, MYOGLOBIN	↑	↓
TYPE OF TRAINING	Endurance training	Weight/resistance training, sprinting
NOTES	Think "1 slow red ox"	Think "2 fast white antelopes"

Skeletal muscle adaptations

	Atrophy	Hypertrophy
MYOFIBRILS	↓ (removal via ubiquitin-proteasome system)	↑ (addition of sarcomeres in parallel)
MYONUCLEI	↓ (selective apoptosis)	↑ (fusion of satellite cells)

Vascular smooth muscle contraction and relaxation

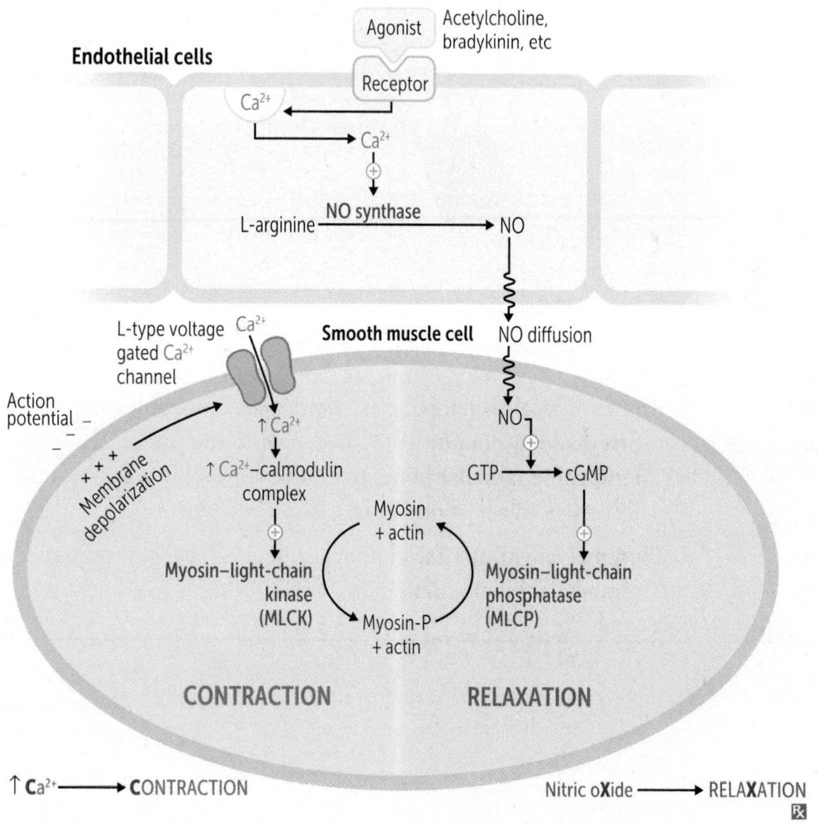

Muscle proprioceptors

Specialized sensory receptors that relay information about muscle dynamics.

	Muscle stretch receptors	Golgi tendon organ
PATHWAY	❶ ↑ length and speed of stretch → ❷ via dorsal root ganglion (DRG) → ❸ activation of inhibitory interneuron and α motor neuron → ❹ simultaneous inhibition of antagonist muscle (prevents overstretching) and activation of agonist muscle (contraction).	❶ ↑ tension → ❷ via DRG → ❸ activation of inhibitory interneuron → ❹ inhibition of agonist muscle (reduced tension within muscle and tendon)
LOCATION/INNERVATION	Body of muscle/type Ia and II sensory axons	Tendons/type Ib sensory axons
ACTIVATION BY	↑ muscle stretch. Responsible for deep tendon reflexes	↑ muscle tension

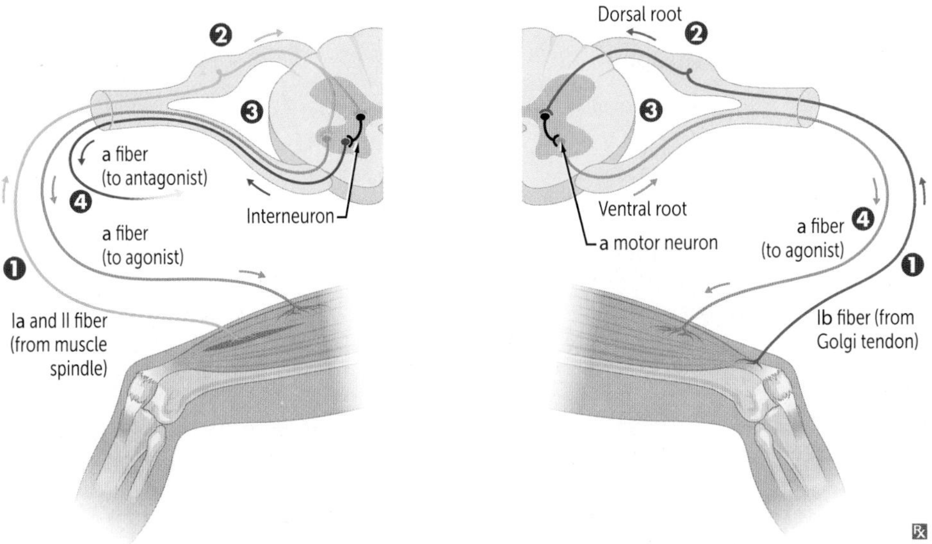

Bone formation

Endochondral ossification	Bones of axial skeleton, appendicular skeleton, and base of skull. Cartilaginous model of bone is first made by chondrocytes. Osteoclasts and osteoblasts later replace with woven bone and then remodel to lamellar bone. In adults, woven bone occurs after fractures and in Paget disease. Defective in achondroplasia.
Membranous ossification	Bones of calvarium, facial bones, and clavicle. Woven bone formed directly without cartilage. Later remodeled to lamellar bone.

Cell biology of bone

Osteoblast	Builds bone by secreting collagen and catalyzing mineralization in alkaline environment via ALP. Differentiates from mesenchymal stem cells in periosteum. Osteoblastic activity measured by bone ALP, osteocalcin, propeptides of type I procollagen.
Osteoclast	Dissolves ("crushes") bone by secreting H^+ and collagenases. Differentiates from a fusion of monocyte/macrophage lineage precursors. RANK receptors on osteoclasts are stimulated by RANKL (RANK ligand, expressed on osteoblasts). OPG (osteoprotegerin, a RANKL decoy receptor) binds RANKL to prevent RANK-RANKL interaction → ↓ osteoclast activity.
Parathyroid hormone	At low, intermittent levels, exerts anabolic effects (building bone) on osteoblasts and osteoclasts (indirect). Chronically ↑ PTH levels (1° hyperparathyroidism) cause catabolic effects (osteitis fibrosa cystica).
Estrogen	Inhibits apoptosis in bone-forming osteoblasts and induces apoptosis in bone-resorbing osteoclasts. Causes closure of epiphyseal plate during puberty. Estrogen deficiency (surgical or postmenopausal) → ↑ cycles of remodeling and bone resorption → ↑ risk of osteoporosis.

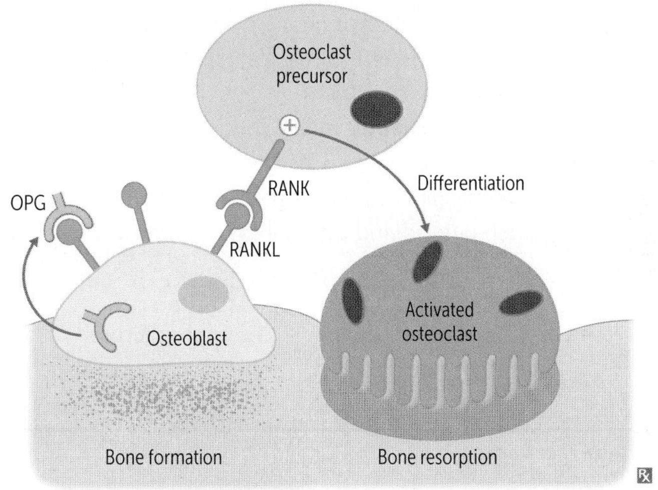

▶ MUSCULOSKELETAL, SKIN, AND CONNECTIVE TISSUE—PATHOLOGY

Overuse injuries of the elbow

Medial epicondylitis (golfer's elbow)	Repetitive flexion or idiopathic → pain near medial epicondyle.
Lateral epicondylitis (tennis elbow)	Repetitive extension (backhand shots) or idiopathic → pain near lateral epicondyle.

Clavicle fractures

Common in children and as birth trauma. Usually caused by a fall on outstretched hand or by direct trauma to shoulder. Weakest point at the junction of middle and lateral thirds; fractures at the middle third segment are most common A. Presents as shoulder drop, shortened clavicle (lateral fragment is depressed due to arm weight and medially rotated by arm adductors [eg, pectoralis major]).

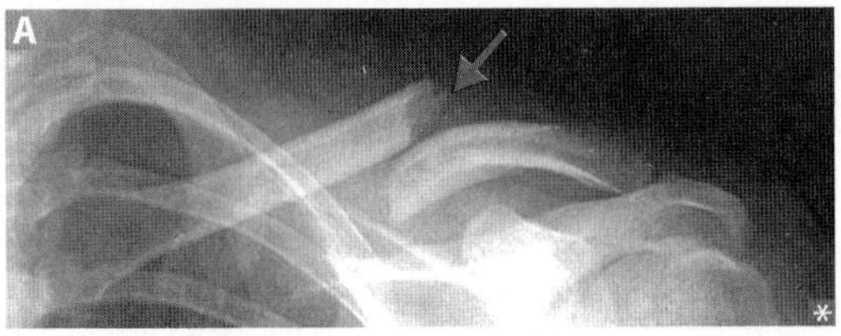

Wrist and hand injuries

Guyon canal syndrome

Compression of ulnar nerve at wrist. Classically seen in cyclists due to pressure from handlebars.

Carpal tunnel syndrome

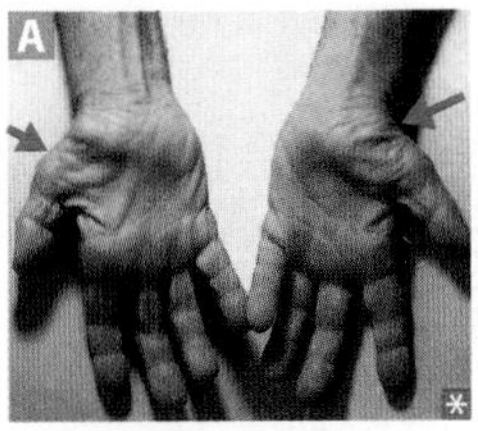

Entrapment of median nerve in carpal tunnel (between transverse carpal ligament and carpal bones) → nerve compression → paresthesia, pain, and numbness in distribution of median nerve. Thenar eminence atrophies A but sensation spared, because palmar cutaneous branch enters hand external to carpal tunnel.

Suggested by ⊕ Tinel sign (percussion of wrist causes tingling) and Phalen maneuver (90° flexion of wrist causes tingling).
Associated with pregnancy (due to edema), rheumatoid arthritis, hypothyroidism, diabetes, acromegaly, dialysis-related amyloidosis; may be associated with repetitive use.

Metacarpal neck fracture

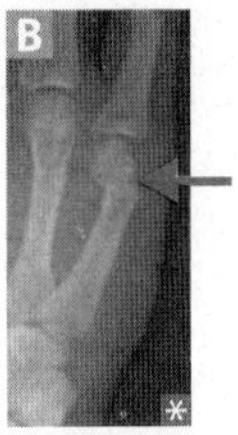

Also called boxer's fracture. Common fracture caused by direct blow with a closed fist (eg, from punching a wall). Most commonly seen in the 5th metacarpal B.

Common knee conditions

"Unhappy triad"	Common injury in contact sports due to laterally directed force to a planted foot. Consists of damage to the ACL A, MCL, and medial meniscus (attached to MCL). However, lateral meniscus involvement is more common than medial meniscus involvement in conjunction with ACL and MCL injury. Presents with acute pain and signs of joint instability.
Prepatellar bursitis	Inflammation of the prepatellar bursa in front of the kneecap (red arrow in B). Can be caused by repeated trauma or pressure from excessive kneeling (also called "housemaid's knee").
Popliteal cyst	Also called Baker cyst. Popliteal fluid collection (red arrow in C) in gastrocnemius-semimembranosus bursa commonly communicating with synovial space and related to chronic joint disease (eg, osteoarthritis, rheumatoid arthritis).

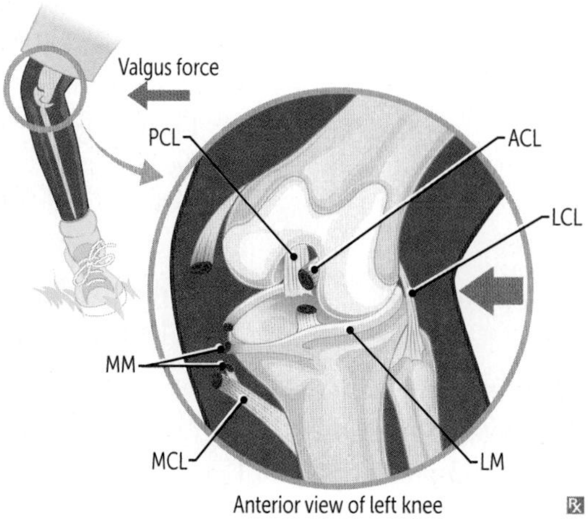

Anterior view of left knee

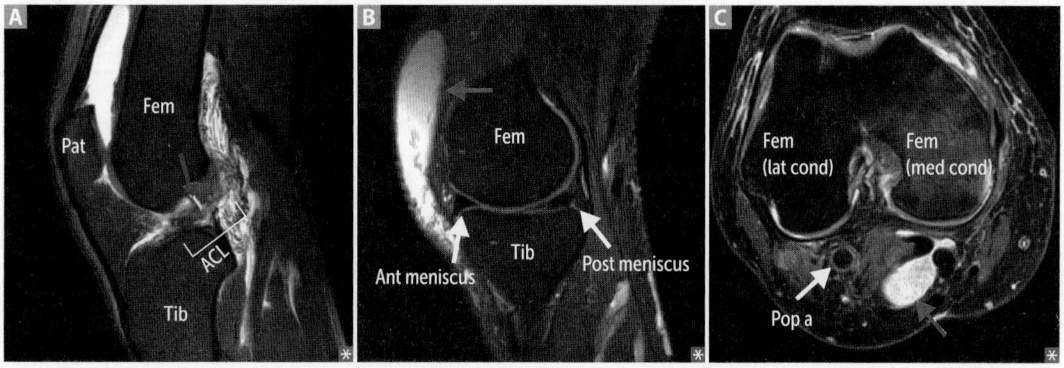

Common musculoskeletal conditions

De Quervain tenosynovitis	Noninflammatory thickening of abductor pollicis longus and extensor pollicis brevis tendons → pain or tenderness at radial styloid. ⊕ Finkelstein test (pain at radial styloid with active or passive stretch of thumb tendons). ↑ risk in new parent (lifting baby), golfers, racquet sport players, "thumb" texters. 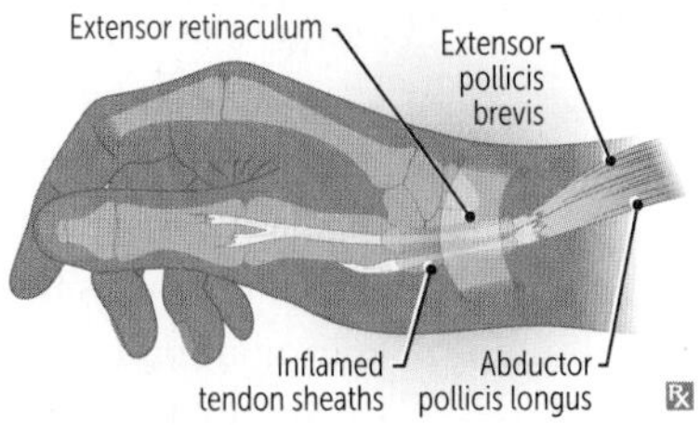
Ganglion cyst	Fluid-filled swelling overlying joint or tendon sheath, most commonly at dorsal side of wrist. Arises from herniation of dense connective tissue. Usually resolves spontaneously.
Iliotibial band syndrome	Overuse injury of lateral knee that occurs primarily in runners. Pain develops 2° to friction of iliotibial band against lateral femoral epicondyle.
Limb compartment syndrome	↑ pressure within fascial compartment of a limb → venous outflow obstruction and arteriolar collapse → anoxia and necrosis. Causes include significant long bone fractures, reperfusion injury, animal venoms. Presents with severe pain and tense, swollen compartments with passive stretch of muscles in the affected compartment. Increased serum creatine kinase and motor deficits are late signs of irreversible muscle and nerve damage. 5 Ps: pain, palor, paresthesia, pulselessness, paralysis.
Medial tibial stress syndrome	Also called shin splints. Common cause of shin pain and diffuse tenderness in runners and military recruits. Caused by bone resorption that outpaces bone formation in tibial cortex.
Plantar fasciitis	Inflammation of plantar aponeurosis characterized by heel pain (worse with first steps in the morning or after period of inactivity) and tenderness.
Temporomandibular disorders	Group of disorders that involve the temporomandibular joint (TMJ) and muscles of mastication. Multifactorial etiology; associated with TMJ trauma, poor head and neck posture, abnormal trigeminal nerve pain processing, psychological factors. Present with dull, constant unilateral facial pain that worsens with jaw movement, otalgia, headache, TMJ dysfunction (eg, limited range of motion).

Childhood musculoskeletal conditions

Radial head subluxation

Also called nursemaid's elbow. Common elbow injury in children < 5 years. Caused by a sudden pull on the arm → immature annular ligament slips over head of radius. Injured arm held in slightly flexed and pronated position.

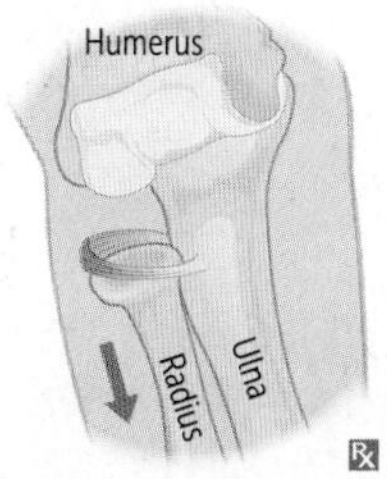

Osgood-Schlatter disease

Also called traction apophysitis. Overuse injury caused by repetitive strain and chronic avulsion of the secondary ossification center of proximal tibial tubercle. Occurs in adolescents after growth spurt. Common in running and jumping athletes. Presents with progressive anterior knee pain.

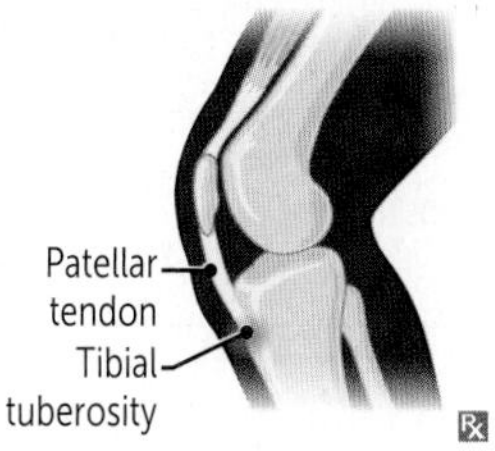

Patellofemoral syndrome

Overuse injury that commonly presents in young, female athletes as anterior knee pain. Exacerbated by prolonged sitting or weight-bearing on a flexed knee.

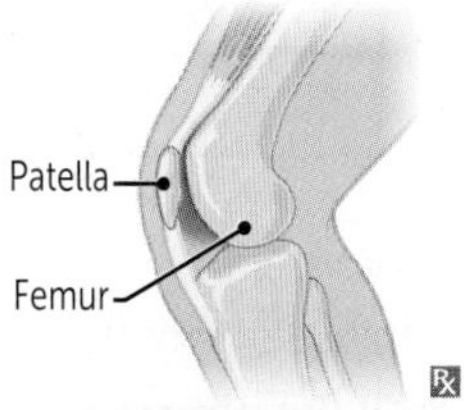

Developmental dysplasia of the hip

Abnormal acetabulum development in newborns. Risk factor is breech presentation. Results in hip instability/dislocation. Commonly tested with Ortolani and Barlow maneuvers (manipulation of newborn hip reveals a "clunk"). Confirmed via ultrasound (x-ray not used until ~4–6 months because cartilage is not ossified).

Legg-Calvé-Perthes disease

Idiopathic avascular necrosis of femoral head. Commonly presents between 5–7 years with insidious onset of hip pain that may cause child to limp. More common in males (4:1 ratio). Initial x-ray often normal.

Slipped capital femoral epiphysis

Classically presents in an obese young adolescent with hip/knee pain and altered gait. Increased axial force on femoral head → epiphysis displaces relative to femoral neck (like a scoop of ice cream slipping off a cone). Diagnosed via x-ray.

Common pediatric fractures

Greenstick fracture

Incomplete fracture extending partway through width of bone A following bending stress; bone fails on tension side; compression side intact (compare to torus fracture). Bone is bent like a green twig.

Torus (buckle) fracture

Axial force applied to immature bone → cortex buckles on compression (concave) side and fractures B. Tension (convex) side remains solid (intact).

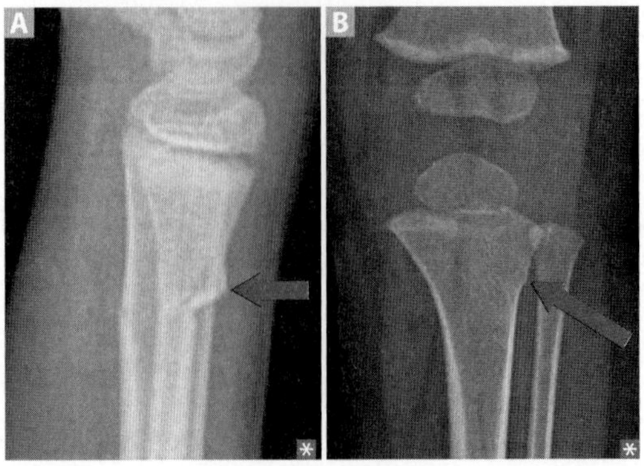
A
B

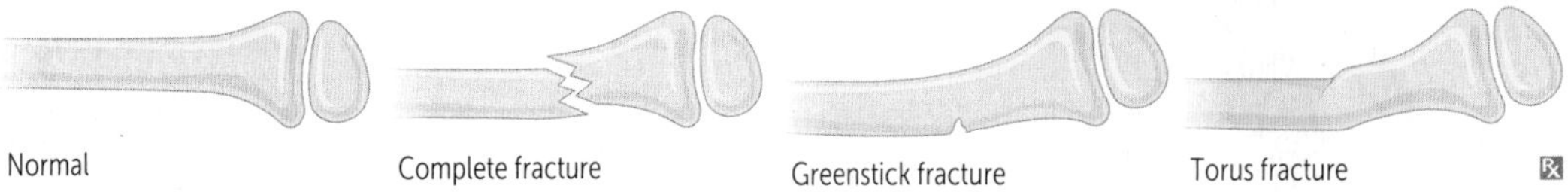
Normal
Complete fracture
Greenstick fracture
Torus fracture

Achondroplasia

Failure of longitudinal bone growth (endochondral ossification) → short limbs. Membranous ossification is not affected → large head relative to limbs. Constitutive activation of fibroblast growth factor receptor (FGFR3) actually inhibits chondrocyte proliferation. > 85% of mutations occur sporadically; autosomal dominant with full penetrance (homozygosity is lethal). Associated with ↑ paternal age. Most common cause of short-limbed dwarfism.

Osteoporosis

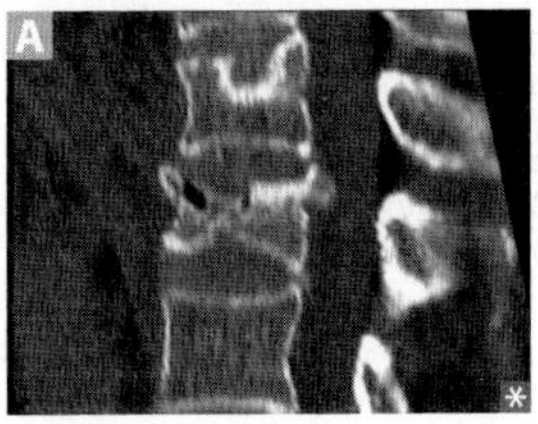
A

Trabecular (spongy) and cortical bone lose mass despite normal bone mineralization and lab values (serum Ca^{2+} and PO_4^{3-}).

Most commonly due to ↑ bone resorption related to ↓ estrogen levels and old age. Can be 2° to drugs (eg, steroids, alcohol, anticonvulsants, anticoagulants, thyroid replacement therapy) or other conditions (eg, hyperparathyroidism, hyperthyroidism, multiple myeloma, malabsorption syndromes, anorexia).

Diagnosed by bone mineral density measurement by DEXA (dual-energy X-ray absorptiometry) at the lumbar spine, total hip, and femoral neck, with a T-score of ≤ −2.5 or by a fragility fracture (eg, fall from standing height, minimal trauma) at hip or vertebra. One-time screening recommended in females ≥ 65 years old.

Prophylaxis: regular weight-bearing exercise and adequate Ca^{2+} and vitamin D intake throughout adulthood.

Treatment: bisphosphonates, teriparatide, SERMs, rarely calcitonin; denosumab (monoclonal antibody against RANKL).

Can lead to vertebral compression fractures A—acute back pain, loss of height, kyphosis. Also can present with fractures of femoral neck, distal radius (Colles fracture).

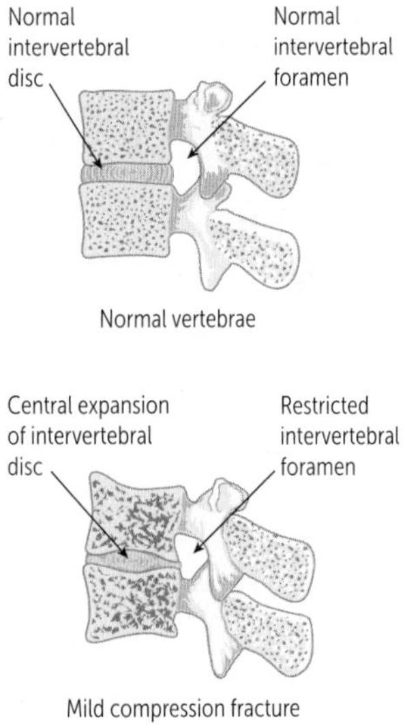
Normal intervertebral disc
Normal intervertebral foramen
Normal vertebrae
Central expansion of intervertebral disc
Restricted intervertebral foramen
Mild compression fracture

Osteopetrosis

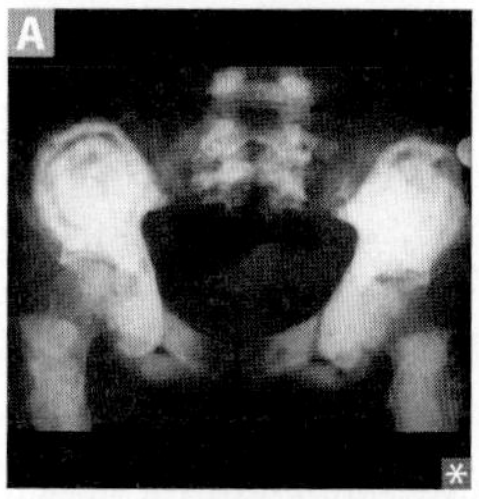
A

Failure of normal bone resorption due to defective osteoclasts → thickened, dense bones that are prone to fracture. Mutations (eg, carbonic anhydrase II) impair ability of osteoclast to generate acidic environment necessary for bone resorption. Overgrowth of cortical bone fills marrow space → pancytopenia, extramedullary hematopoiesis. Can result in cranial nerve impingement and palsies due to narrowed foramina.

X-rays show diffuse symmetric sclerosis (bone-in-bone, "stone bone" A). Bone marrow transplant is potentially curative as osteoclasts are derived from monocytes.

Osteomalacia/rickets

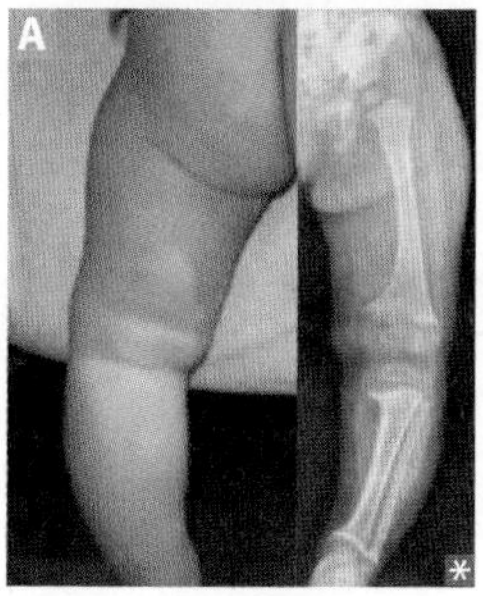
A

Defective mineralization of osteoid (osteomalacia) or cartilaginous growth plates (rickets, only in children). Most commonly due to vitamin D deficiency.

X-rays show osteopenia and pseudofractures in osteomalacia, epiphyseal widening and metaphyseal cupping/fraying in rickets. Children with rickets have pathologic bow legs (genu varum A), bead-like costochondral junctions (rachitic rosary B), craniotabes (soft skull).

↓ vitamin D → ↓ serum Ca^{2+} → ↑ PTH secretion → ↓ serum PO_4^{3-}.

Hyperactivity of osteoblasts → ↑ ALP.

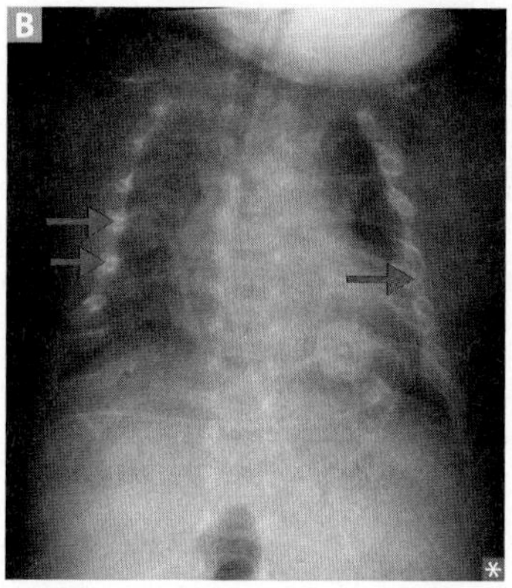
B

Osteitis deformans

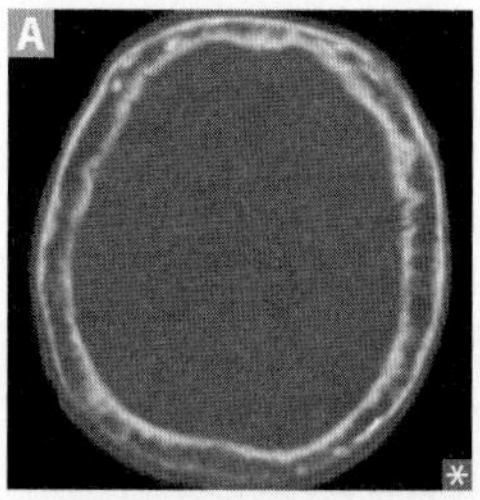
A

Also called Paget disease of bone. Common, localized disorder of bone remodeling caused by ↑ osteoclastic activity followed by ↑ osteoblastic activity that forms poor-quality bone. Serum Ca^{2+}, phosphorus, and PTH levels are normal. ↑ ALP. Mosaic pattern of woven and lamellar bone (osteocytes within lacunae in chaotic juxtapositions); long bone chalk-stick fractures. ↑ blood flow from ↑ arteriovenous shunts may cause high-output heart failure. ↑ risk of osteosarcoma.

Hat size can be increased due to skull thickening A; hearing loss is common due to skull deformity.

Stages of Paget disease:

- Lytic—osteoclasts
- Mixed—osteoclasts + osteoblasts
- Sclerotic—osteoblasts
- Quiescent—minimal osteoclast/osteoblast activity

Treatment: bisphosphonates.

Avascular necrosis of bone

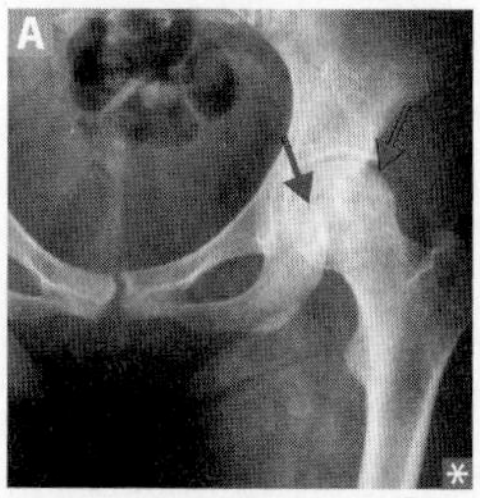
A

Infarction of bone and marrow, usually very painful. Most common site is femoral head (watershed zone) A (due to insufficiency of medial circumflex femoral artery). Causes include Corticosteroids, chronic Alcohol overuse, Sickle cell disease, Trauma, SLE, "the Bends" (caisson/decompression disease), LEgg-Calvé-Perthes disease (idiopathic), Gaucher disease, Slipped capital femoral epiphysis—CASTS Bend LEGS.

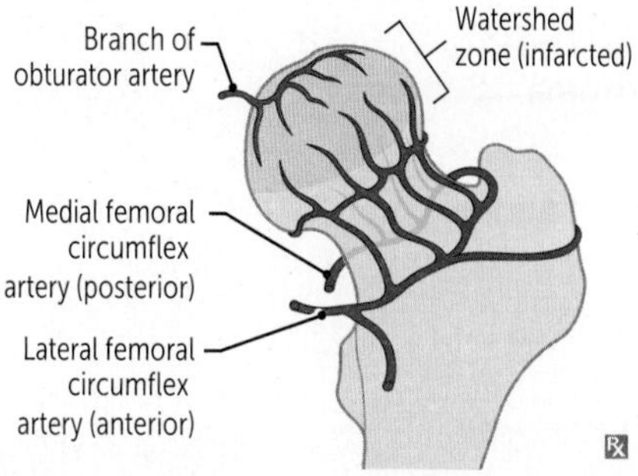
Branch of obturator artery
Watershed zone (infarcted)
Medial femoral circumflex artery (posterior)
Lateral femoral circumflex artery (anterior)

Lab values in bone disorders

DISORDER	SERUM Ca^{2+}	PO_4^{3-}	ALP	PTH	COMMENTS
Osteoporosis	—	—	—	—	↓ bone mass
Osteopetrosis	—/↓	—	—	—	Dense, brittle bones. Ca^{2+} ↓ in severe, malignant disease
Paget disease of bone	—	—	↑	—	Abnormal "mosaic" bone architecture
Osteitis fibrosa cystica Primary hyperparathyroidism	↑	↓	↑	↑	"Brown tumors" due to fibrous replacement of bone, subperiosteal thinning Idiopathic or parathyroid hyperplasia, adenoma, carcinoma
Secondary hyperparathyroidism	↓	↑	↑	↑	Often as compensation for CKD (↓ PO_4^{3-} excretion and production of activated vitamin D)
Osteomalacia/rickets	↓	↓	↑	↑	Soft bones; vitamin D deficiency also causes 2° hyperparathyroidism
Hypervitaminosis D	↑	↑	—	↓	Caused by oversupplementation or granulomatous disease (eg, sarcoidosis)

↑ ↓ = 1° change.

Primary bone tumors Metastatic disease is more common than 1° bone tumors. Benign bone tumors that start with **o** are more common in boys.

TUMOR TYPE	EPIDEMIOLOGY	LOCATION	CHARACTERISTICS
Benign tumors			
Osteochondroma	Most common benign bone tumor Males < 25 years old	Metaphysis of long bones	Lateral bony projection of growth plate (continuous with marrow space) covered by cartilaginous cap A Rarely transforms to chondrosarcoma
Osteoma	Middle age	Surface of facial bones	Associated with Gardner syndrome
Osteoid osteoma	Adults < 25 years old Males > females	Cortex of long bones	Presents as bone pain (worse at night) that is relieved by NSAIDs Bony mass (< 2 cm) with radiolucent osteoid core B
Osteoblastoma	Males > females	Vertebrae	Similar histology to osteoid osteoma Larger size (> 2 cm), pain unresponsive to NSAIDs
Chondroma		Medulla of small bones of hand and feet	Benign tumor of cartilage
Giant cell tumor	20–40 years old	Epiphysis of long bones (often in knee region)	Locally aggressive benign tumor Neoplastic mononuclear cells that express RANKL and reactive multinucleated giant (osteoclast-like) cells. "Osteoclastoma" "Soap bubble" appearance on x-ray C

Primary bone tumors *(continued)*

TUMOR TYPE	EPIDEMIOLOGY	LOCATION	CHARACTERISTICS
Malignant tumors			
Osteosarcoma (osteogenic sarcoma)	Accounts for 20% of 1° bone cancers. Peak incidence of 1° tumor in males < 20 years. Less common in elderly; usually 2° to predisposing factors, such as Paget disease of bone, bone infarcts, radiation, familial retinoblastoma, Li-Fraumeni syndrome.	Metaphysis of long bones (often in knee region).	Pleomorphic osteoid-producing cells (malignant osteoblasts). Presents as painful enlarging mass or pathologic fractures. **Cod**man triangle D (from elevation of periosteum) or **sun**burst pattern on x-ray E (think of an **osteocod** [bone fish] swimming in the **sun**). Aggressive. 1° usually responsive to treatment (surgery, chemotherapy), poor prognosis for 2°.
Chondrosarcoma		Medulla of pelvis, proximal femur and humerus.	Tumor of malignant chondrocytes.
Ewing sarcoma	Most common in White patients. Generally males < 15 years old.	Diaphysis of long bones (especially femur), pelvic flat bones.	Anaplastic small blue cells of neuroectodermal origin (resemble lymphocytes) F. Differentiate from conditions with similar morphology (eg, lymphoma, chronic osteomyelitis) by testing for t(**11**;**22**) (fusion protein EWS-FLI1). "Onion skin" periosteal reaction in bone. Aggressive with early metastases, but responsive to chemotherapy. 11 + 22 = 33 (Patrick **Ewing**'s jersey number).

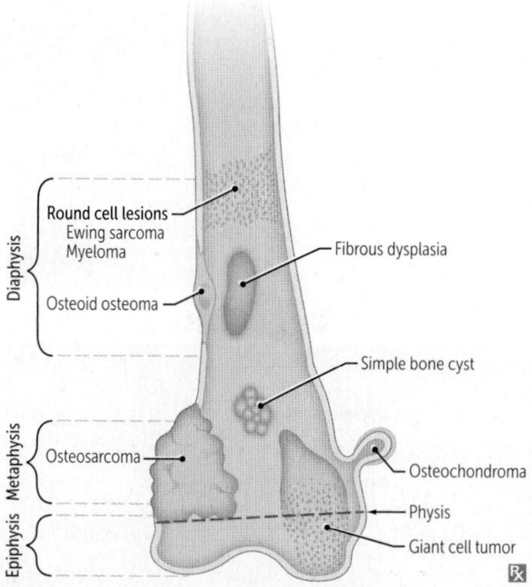

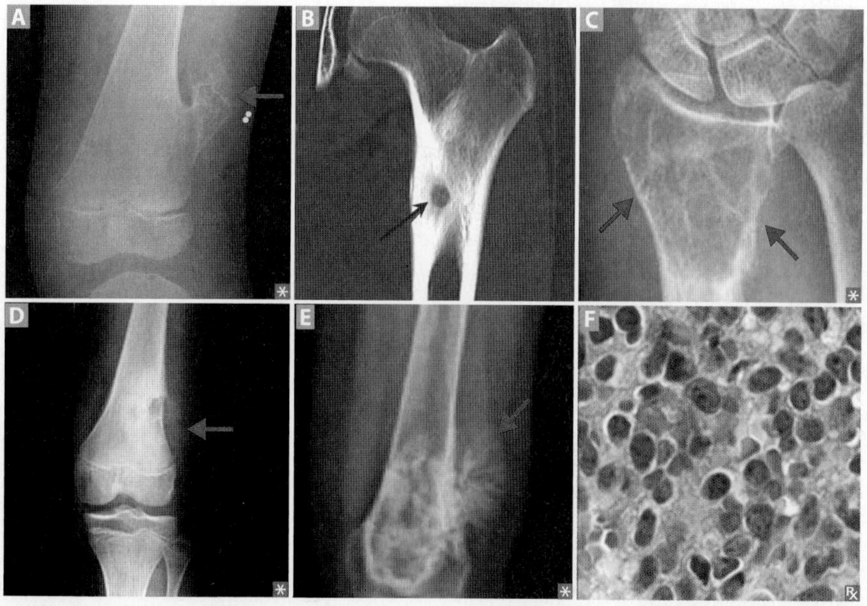

Osteoarthritis vs rheumatoid arthritis

	Osteoarthritis A	Rheumatoid arthritis B
PATHOGENESIS	Mechanical—wear and tear destroys articular cartilage (degenerative joint disorder) → inflammation with inadequate repair. Chondrocytes mediate degradation and inadequate repair.	Autoimmune—inflammation C induces formation of pannus (proliferative granulation tissue), which erodes articular cartilage and bone.
PREDISPOSING FACTORS	Age, female, obesity, joint trauma.	Female, HLA-DR4 (4-walled "**rheum**"), tobacco smoking. ⊕ rheumatoid factor (IgM antibody that targets IgG Fc region; in 80%), anti-cyclic citrullinated peptide antibody (more specific).
PRESENTATION	Pain in weight-bearing joints after use (eg, at the end of the day), improving with rest. Asymmetric joint involvement. Knee cartilage loss begins medially ("bowlegged"). No systemic symptoms.	Pain, swelling, and morning stiffness lasting > 1 hour, improving with use. Symmetric joint involvement. Systemic symptoms (fever, fatigue, weight loss). Extraarticular manifestations common.*
JOINT FINDINGS	Osteophytes (bone spurs), joint space narrowing, subchondral sclerosis and cysts. Synovial fluid noninflammatory (WBC < 2000/mm^3). Development of Heberden nodes D (at DIP) and Bouchard nodes E (at PIP), and 1st CMC; not MCP.	Erosions, juxta-articular osteopenia, soft tissue swelling, subchondral cysts, joint space narrowing. Deformities: cervical subluxation, ulnar finger deviation, swan neck F, boutonniere G. Involves MCP, PIP, wrist; not DIP or 1st CMC.
TREATMENT	Activity modification, acetaminophen, NSAIDs, intra-articular glucocorticoids.	NSAIDs, glucocorticoids, disease-modifying agents (eg, methotrexate, sulfasalazine), biologic agents (eg, TNF-α inhibitors).

*Extraarticular manifestations include rheumatoid nodules (fibrinoid necrosis with palisading histiocytes) in subcutaneous tissue and lung (+ pneumoconiosis → Caplan syndrome), interstitial lung disease, pleuritis, pericarditis, anemia of chronic disease, neutropenia + splenomegaly (Felty syndrome), AA amyloidosis, Sjögren syndrome, scleritis, carpal tunnel syndrome.

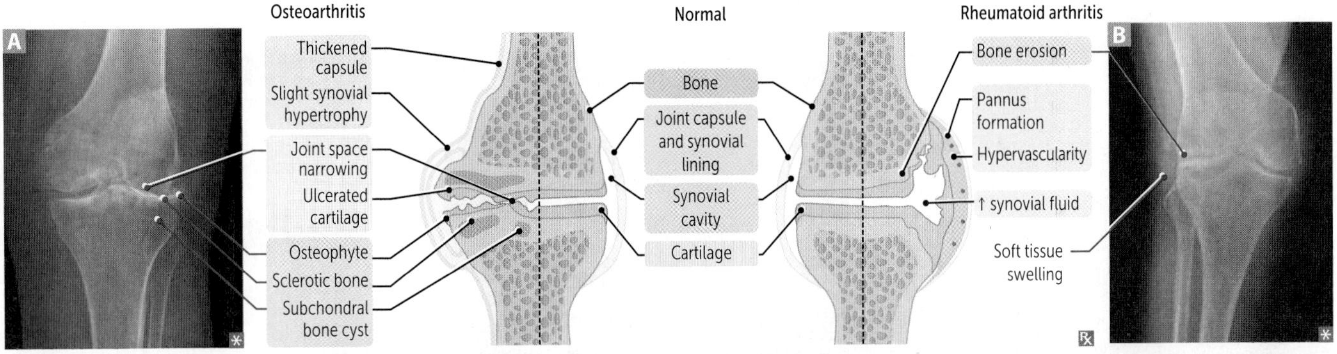

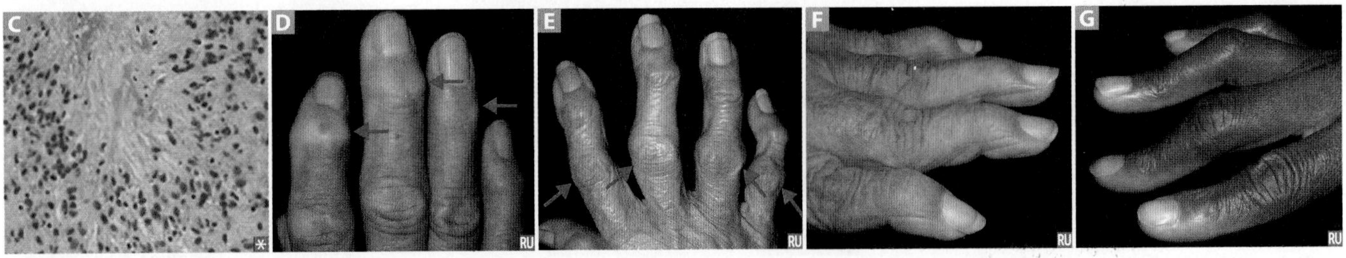

Gout

FINDINGS	Acute inflammatory monoarthritis caused by precipitation of monosodium urate crystals in joints A. Risk factors: male sex, hypertension, obesity, diabetes, dyslipidemia, alcohol use. Strongest risk factor is hyperuricemia, which can be caused by: ▪ Underexcretion of uric acid (90% of patients)—largely idiopathic, potentiated by renal failure; can be exacerbated by certain medications (eg, thiazide diuretics). ▪ Overproduction of uric acid (10% of patients)—Lesch-Nyhan syndrome, PRPP excess, ↑ cell turnover (eg, tumor lysis syndrome), von Gierke disease. Crystals are needle shaped and ⊖ birefringent under polarized light (yellow under parallel light, blue under perpendicular light B). Serum uric acid levels may be normal during an acute attack.
SYMPTOMS	Asymmetric joint distribution. Joint is swollen, red, and painful. Classic manifestation is painful MTP joint of big toe (podagra). Tophus formation C (often on external ear, olecranon bursa, or Achilles tendon). Acute attack tends to occur after a large meal with foods rich in purines (eg, red meat, seafood), trauma, surgery, dehydration, diuresis, or alcohol consumption (alcohol metabolites compete for same excretion sites in kidney as uric acid → ↓ uric acid secretion and subsequent buildup in blood).
TREATMENT	Acute: NSAIDs (eg, indomethacin), glucocorticoids, colchicine. Chronic (preventive): xanthine oxidase inhibitors (eg, allopurinol, febuxostat).

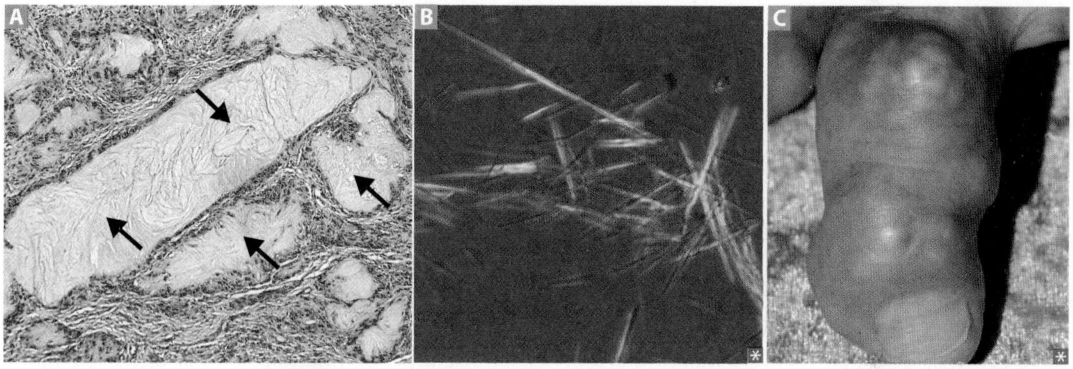

Calcium pyrophosphate deposition disease

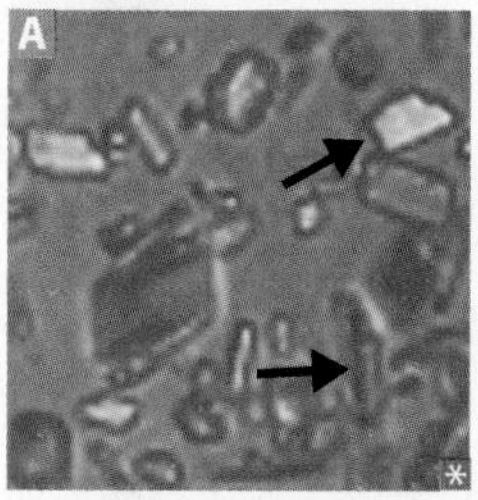

Previously called pseudogout. Deposition of calcium pyrophosphate crystals within the joint space. Occurs in patients > 50 years old; both sexes affected equally. Usually idiopathic, sometimes associated with hemochromatosis, hyperparathyroidism, joint trauma.

Pain and swelling with acute inflammation (pseudogout) and/or chronic degeneration (pseudo-osteoarthritis). Most commonly affected joint is the knee.

Chondrocalcinosis (cartilage calcification) on x-ray.

Crystals are rhomboid and weakly ⊕ birefringent under polarized light (blue when parallel to light) A.

Acute treatment: NSAIDs, colchicine, glucocorticoids.

Prophylaxis: colchicine.

The **blue P's—blue** (when **p**arallel), **p**ositive birefringence, calcium **p**yrophosphate, **p**seudogout

Systemic juvenile idiopathic arthritis

Systemic arthritis seen in < 16 year olds. Usually presents with daily spiking fevers, salmon-pink macular rash, arthritis (commonly 2+ joints). Associated with anterior uveitis. Frequently presents with leukocytosis, thrombocytosis, anemia, ↑ ESR, ↑ CRP. Treatment: NSAIDs, steroids, methotrexate, TNF inhibitors.

Sjögren syndrome

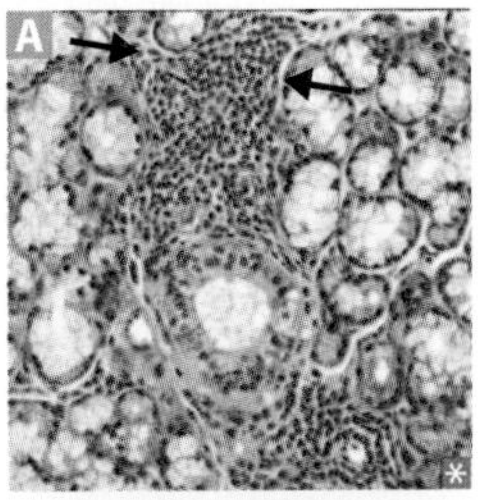

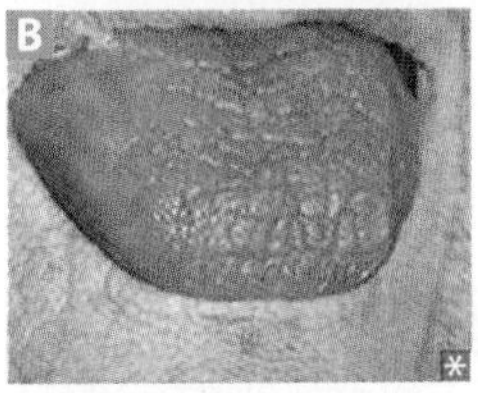

Autoimmune disorder characterized by destruction of exocrine glands (especially lacrimal and salivary) by lymphocytic infiltrates A. Predominantly affects females 40–60 years old.

Findings:

- Inflammatory joint pain
- Keratoconjunctivitis sicca (↓ tear production and subsequent corneal damage)
- Xerostomia (↓ saliva production) → mucosal atrophy, fissuring of the tongue B
- Presence of antinuclear antibodies, rheumatoid factor (can be positive in the absence of rheumatoid arthritis), antiribonucleoprotein antibodies: SS-A (anti-Ro) and/or SS-B (anti-La)
- Bilateral parotid enlargement

Anti-SSA and anti-SSB may also be seen in SLE.

A common 1° disorder or a 2° syndrome associated with other autoimmune disorders (eg, rheumatoid arthritis, SLE, systemic sclerosis).

Complications: dental caries; mucosa-associated lymphoid tissue (MALT) lymphoma (may present as parotid enlargement); ↑ risk of giving birth to baby with neonatal lupus.

Focal lymphocytic sialadenitis on labial salivary gland biopsy can confirm diagnosis.

Septic arthritis

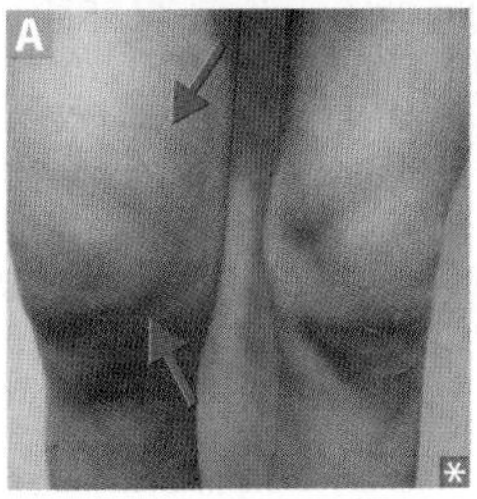

S aureus, *Streptococcus*, and *Neisseria gonorrhoeae* are common causes. Affected joint is swollen A, red, and painful. Synovial fluid purulent (WBC > 50,000/mm^3).

Disseminated gonococcal infection—STI that presents as either purulent arthritis (eg, knee) or triad of polyarthralgia, tenosynovitis (eg, hand), dermatitis (eg, pustules).

Seronegative spondyloarthritis	Arthritis without rheumatoid factor (no anti-IgG antibody). Strong association with HLA-B27 (MHC class I serotype). Subtypes (**PAIR**) share variable occurrence of inflammatory back pain (associated with morning stiffness, improves with exercise), peripheral arthritis, enthesitis (inflamed insertion sites of tendons, eg, Achilles), dactylitis ("sausage fingers"), uveitis.	
Psoriatic arthritis	Associated with skin psoriasis and nail lesions. Asymmetric and patchy involvement A. Dactylitis and "pencil-in-cup" deformity of DIP on x-ray B.	Seen in fewer than $1/3$ of patients with psoriasis.
Ankylosing spondylitis	Symmetric involvement of spine and sacroiliac joints → ankylosis (joint fusion), uveitis, aortic regurgitation.	Bamboo spine (vertebral fusion) C. Costovertebral and costosternal ankylosis may cause restrictive lung disease. Monitor degree of reduced chest wall expansion to assess disease severity. More common in males.
Inflammatory bowel disease	Crohn disease and ulcerative colitis are often associated with spondyloarthritis.	
Reactive arthritis	Classic triad: ▪ Conjunctivitis ▪ Urethritis ▪ Arthritis	"Can't see, can't pee, can't bend my knee." Associated with infections by *Shigella*, *Campylobacter*, *E coli*, *Salmonella*, *Chlamydia*, *Yersinia*. "She Caught Every Student Cheating Yesterday and overreacted."

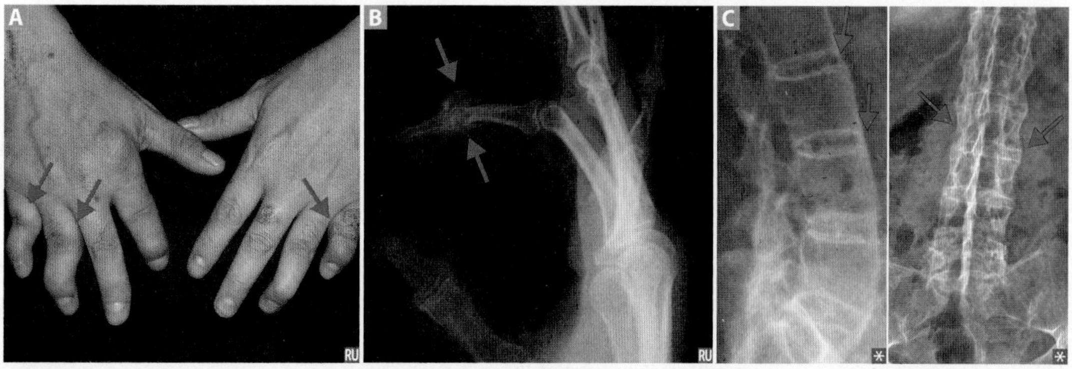

Systemic lupus erythematosus

Systemic, remitting, and relapsing autoimmune disease. Organ damage primarily due to a type III hypersensitivity reaction and, to a lesser degree, a type II hypersensitivity reaction. Associated with deficiency of early complement proteins (eg, C1q, C4, C2) → ↓ clearance of immune complexes. Classic presentation: rash, joint pain, and fever in a female of reproductive age. ↑ prevalence in Black, Caribbean, Asian, and Hispanic populations.

A

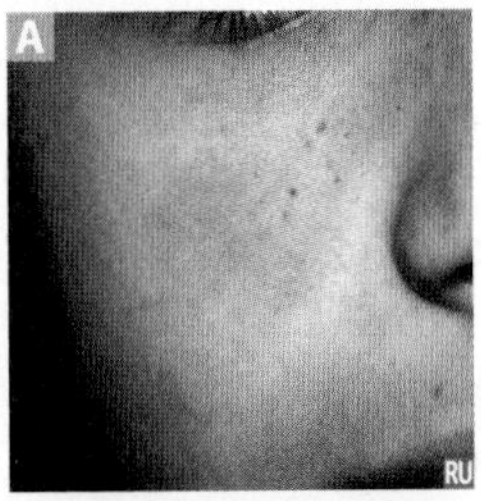

B

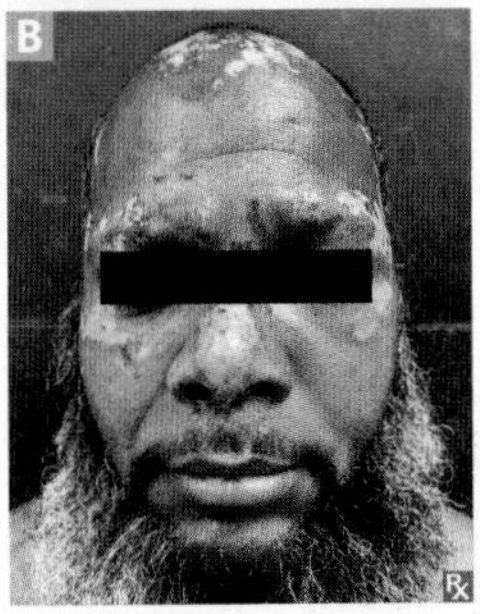

Libman-Sacks Endocarditis—nonbacterial, verrucous thrombi usually on mitral or aortic valve and can be present on either surface of the valve (but usually on undersurface). LSE in SLE.

Lupus nephritis (glomerular deposition of DNA-anti-DNA immune complexes) can be nephritic or nephrotic (causing hematuria or proteinuria). Most common and severe type is diffuse proliferative.

Common causes of death in SLE: infections, cardiovascular disease (accelerated CAD), kidney disease (most common). Immune complexes kill.

In an anti-SSA ⊕ pregnant patient, ↑ risk of newborn developing **neonatal lupus** → congenital heart block, periorbital/diffuse rash, transaminitis, and cytopenias at birth.

RASH OR PAIN:
- Rash (malar A or discoid B)
- Arthritis (nonerosive)
- Serositis (eg, pleuritis, pericarditis)
- Hematologic disorders (eg, cytopenias)
- Oral/nasopharyngeal ulcers (usually painless)
- Renal disease
- Photosensitivity
- Antinuclear antibodies
- Immunologic disorder (anti-dsDNA, anti-Sm, antiphospholipid)
- Neurologic disorders (eg, seizures, psychosis)

Mixed connective tissue disease

Features of SLE, systemic sclerosis, and/or polymyositis. Associated with anti-U1 RNP antibodies (speckled ANA).

Antiphospholipid syndrome

1° or 2° autoimmune disorder (most commonly in SLE).

Diagnosed based on clinical criteria including history of thrombosis (arterial or venous) or spontaneous abortion along with laboratory findings of lupus anticoagulant, anticardiolipin, anti-β_2 glycoprotein I antibodies.

Treatment: systemic anticoagulation.

Anticardiolipin antibodies can cause false-positive VDRL/RPR.

Lupus anticoagulant can cause prolonged PTT that is not corrected by the addition of normal platelet-free plasma.

Polymyalgia rheumatica

SYMPTOMS	Pain and stiffness in proximal muscles (eg, shoulders, hips), often with fever, malaise, weight loss. Does not cause muscular weakness. More common in females > 50 years old; associated with giant cell (temporal) arteritis.
FINDINGS	↑ ESR, ↑ CRP, normal CK.
TREATMENT	Rapid response to low-dose corticosteroids.

Fibromyalgia

Most common in females 20–50 years old. Chronic, widespread musculoskeletal pain associated with "tender points," stiffness, paresthesias, poor sleep, fatigue, cognitive disturbance ("fibro fog"). Treatment: regular exercise, antidepressants (TCAs, SNRIs), neuropathic pain agents (eg, gabapentin).

Polymyositis/dermatomyositis

Nonspecific: ⊕ ANA, ↑ CK. Specific: ⊕ anti-Jo-1 (histidyl-tRNA synthetase), ⊕ anti-SRP (signal recognition particle), ⊕ anti-Mi-2 (helicase).

Polymyositis

Progressive symmetric proximal muscle weakness, characterized by endomysial inflammation with CD8+ T cells. Most often involves shoulders.

Dermatomyositis

Clinically similar to polymyositis, but also involves Gottron papules A, photodistributed facial erythema (eg, heliotrope [violaceous] edema of the eyelids B), "shawl and face" rash C, darkening and thickening of fingertips and sides resulting in irregular, "dirty"-appearing marks. ↑ risk of occult malignancy. Perimysial inflammation and atrophy with CD4+ T cells.

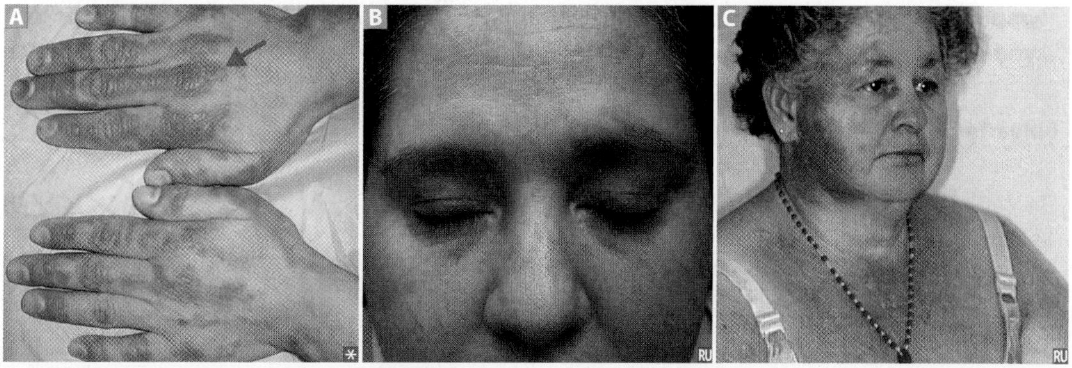

Myositis ossificans

Heterotopic ossification involving skeletal muscle (eg, quadriceps). Associated with blunt muscle trauma. Presents as painful soft tissue mass. Imaging shows eggshell calcification. Histology shows metaplastic bone surrounding area of fibroblastic proliferation. Benign, but may be mistaken for sarcoma.

Vasculitides

	EPIDEMIOLOGY/PRESENTATION	NOTES
Large-vessel vasculitis		
Giant cell (temporal) arteritis	Females > 50 years old. Unilateral headache, possible temporal artery tenderness, jaw claudication. May lead to irreversible blindness due to anterior ischemic optic neuropathy. Associated with polymyalgia rheumatica.	Most commonly affects branches of carotid artery. Focal granulomatous inflammation A. ↑ ESR. Treat with high-dose corticosteroids prior to temporal artery biopsy to prevent blindness.
Takayasu arteritis	Usually Asian females < 40 years old. "Pulseless disease" (weak upper extremity pulses), fever, night sweats, arthritis, myalgias, skin nodules, ocular disturbances.	Granulomatous thickening and narrowing of aortic arch and proximal great vessels B. ↑ ESR. Treatment: corticosteroids.
Medium-vessel vasculitis		
Buerger disease (thromboangiitis obliterans)	Heavy tobacco smoking history, males < 40 years old. Intermittent claudication. May lead to gangrene C, autoamputation of digits, superficial nodular phlebitis. Raynaud phenomenon is often present.	Segmental thrombosing vasculitis with vein and nerve involvement. Treatment: smoking cessation.
Kawasaki disease (mucocutaneous lymph node syndrome)	Usually Asian children < 4 years old. Conjunctival injection, **R**ash (polymorphous → desquamating), **A**denopathy (cervical), **S**trawberry tongue (oral mucositis) D, **H**and-foot changes (edema, erythema), fever.	**CRASH** and **burn** on a **Kawasaki**. May develop coronary artery aneurysms E; thrombosis or rupture can cause death. Treatment: IV immunoglobulin and aspirin.
Polyarteritis nodosa	Usually middle-aged males. Hepatitis B seropositivity in 30% of patients. Fever, weight loss, malaise, headache. GI: abdominal pain, melena. Hypertension, neurologic dysfunction, cutaneous eruptions, renal damage.	Typically involves renal and visceral vessels, not pulmonary arteries. Different stages of transmural inflammation with fibrinoid necrosis. Innumerable renal microaneurysms F and spasms on arteriogram (string of pearls appearance). Treatment: corticosteroids, cyclophosphamide.
Small-vessel vasculitis		
Behçet syndrome	↑ incidence in people of Turkish and eastern Mediterranean descent. Recurrent aphthous ulcers, genital ulcerations, uveitis, erythema nodosum. Can be precipitated by HSV or parvovirus. Flares last 1–4 weeks.	Immune complex vasculitis. Associated with HLA-B51.
Cutaneous small-vessel vasculitis	Occurs 7-10 days after certain medications (penicillin, cephalosporins, phenytoin, allopurinol) or infections (eg, HCV, HIV). Palpable purpura, no visceral involvement.	Immune complex–mediated leukocytoclastic vasculitis; late involvement indicates systemic vasculitis.

Vasculitides *(continued)*

	EPIDEMIOLOGY/PRESENTATION	NOTES
Small-vessel vasculitis *(continued)*		
Eosinophilic granulomatosis with polyangiitis	Asthma, sinusitis, skin nodules or purpura, peripheral neuropathy (eg, wrist/foot drop). Can also involve heart, GI, kidneys (pauci-immune glomerulonephritis).	Formerly called Churg-Strauss syndrome. Granulomatous, necrotizing vasculitis with eosinophilia G. MPO-ANCA/p-ANCA, ↑ IgE level.
Granulomatosis with polyangiitis	Upper respiratory tract: perforation of nasal septum, chronic sinusitis, otitis media, mastoiditis. Lower respiratory tract: hemoptysis, cough, dyspnea. Renal: hematuria, red cell casts.	Triad: ▪ Focal necrotizing vasculitis ▪ Necrotizing granulomas in lung and upper airway ▪ Necrotizing glomerulonephritis PR3-ANCA/c-ANCA H (anti-proteinase 3). CXR: large nodular densities. Treatment: corticosteroids in combination with rituximab or cyclophosphamide.
Immunoglobulin A vasculitis	Most common childhood systemic vasculitis. Often follows URI. Classic triad of Henoch-Schönlein purpura ▪ Hinge pain (arthralgias) ▪ Stomach pain (abdominal pain associated with intussusception) ▪ Palpable purpura on buttocks/legs I	Formerly called Henoch-Schönlein purpura. Vasculitis 2° to IgA immune complex deposition. Associated with IgA nephropathy (Berger disease). Treatment: supportive care, possibly corticosteroids.
Microscopic polyangiitis	Necrotizing vasculitis commonly involving lung, kidneys, and skin with pauci-immune glomerulonephritis and palpable purpura. Presentation similar to granulomatosis with polyangiitis but without nasopharyngeal involvement.	No granulomas. MPO-ANCA/p-ANCA J (anti-myeloperoxidase). Treatment: cyclophosphamide, corticosteroids.
Mixed cryoglobulinemia	Often due to viral infections, especially HCV. Triad of palpable purpura, weakness, arthralgias. May also have peripheral neuropathy and renal disease (eg, glomerulonephritis).	Cryoglobulins are immunoglobulins that precipitate in the Cold. Vasculitis due to mixed IgG and IgM immune complex deposition.

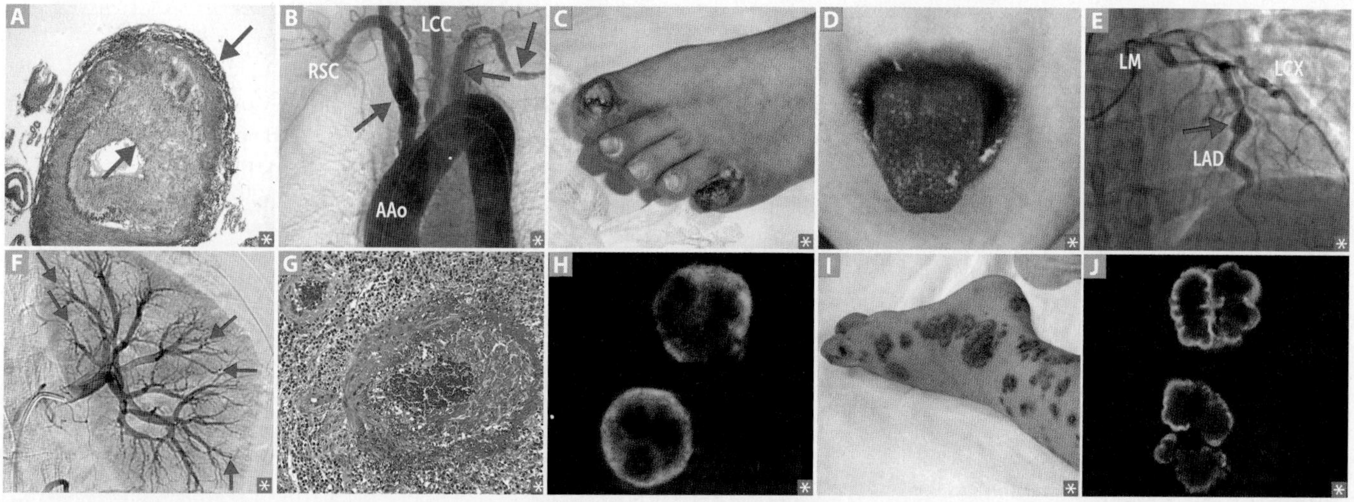

Neuromuscular junction diseases

	Myasthenia gravis	Lambert-Eaton myasthenic syndrome
FREQUENCY	Most common NMJ disorder	Uncommon
PATHOPHYSIOLOGY	Autoantibodies to postsynaptic ACh receptor	Autoantibodies to presynaptic Ca^{2+} channel → ↓ ACh release
CLINICAL	Fatigable muscle weakness—ptosis; diplopia; proximal weakness; respiratory muscle involvement → dyspnea; bulbar muscle involvement → dysphagia, difficulty chewing Spared reflexes Worsens with muscle use	Proximal muscle weakness, autonomic symptoms (dry mouth, constipation, impotence) Hyporeflexia Improves with muscle use
ASSOCIATED WITH	Thymoma, thymic hyperplasia	Small cell lung cancer
AChE INHIBITOR ADMINISTRATION	Reverses symptoms (pyridostigmine for treatment)	Minimal effect

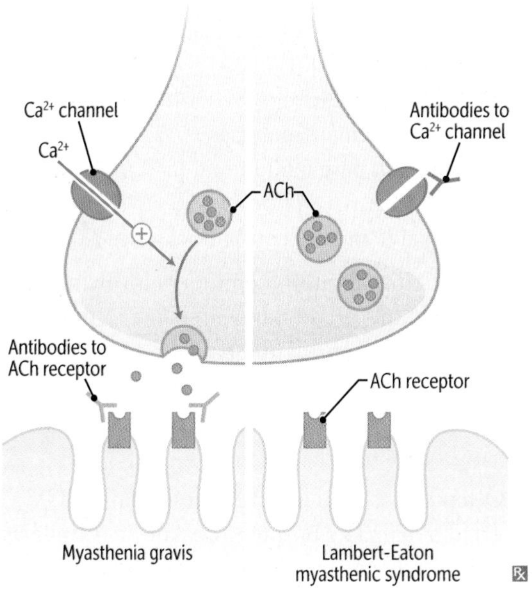

Raynaud phenomenon

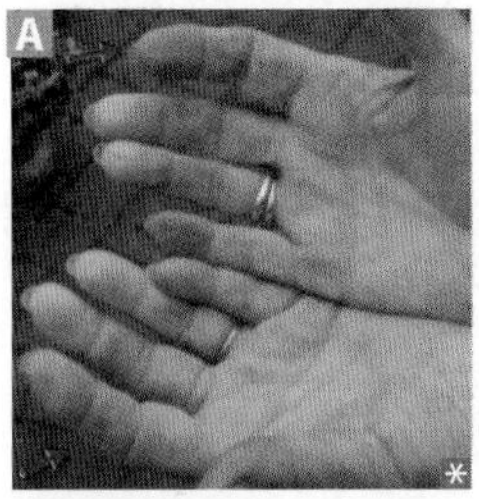

↓ blood flow to skin due to arteriolar (small vessel) vasospasm in response to cold or stress: color change from white (ischemia) to blue (hypoxia) to red (reperfusion). Most often in the fingers A and toes. Called **Raynaud disease** when 1° (idiopathic), **Raynaud syndrome** when 2° to a disease process such as mixed connective tissue disease, SLE, or CREST syndrome (limited form of systemic sclerosis). Digital ulceration (critical ischemia) seen in 2° Raynaud syndrome. Treat with calcium channel blockers.

Scleroderma

Systemic sclerosis. Triad of autoimmunity, noninflammatory vasculopathy, and collagen deposition with fibrosis. Commonly sclerosis of skin, manifesting as puffy, taut skin A without wrinkles, fingertip pitting B. Can involve other systems, eg, renal (scleroderma renal crisis; treat with ACE inhibitors), pulmonary (interstitial fibrosis, pulmonary HTN), GI (esophageal dysmotility and reflux), cardiovascular. 75% female. 2 major types:

- **Diffuse scleroderma**—widespread skin involvement, rapid progression, early visceral involvement. Associated with anti-Scl-70 antibody (anti-DNA topoisomerase-I antibody) and anti-RNA polymerase III.
- **Limited scleroderma**—limited skin involvement confined to fingers and face. Also with CREST syndrome: Calcinosis cutis C, anti-Centromere antibody, Raynaud phenomenon, Esophageal dysmotility, Sclerodactyly, and Telangiectasia. More benign clinical course.

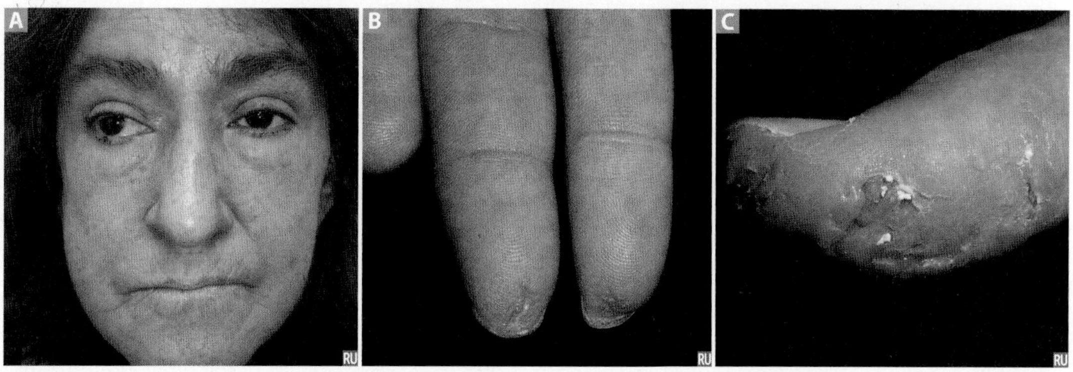
A
B
C
RU
RU
RU

▶ MUSCULOSKELETAL, SKIN, AND CONNECTIVE TISSUE—DERMATOLOGY

Skin layers

Skin has 3 layers: epidermis, dermis, subcutaneous fat (hypodermis, subcutis).
Epidermal layers: come, let's get sunburned.

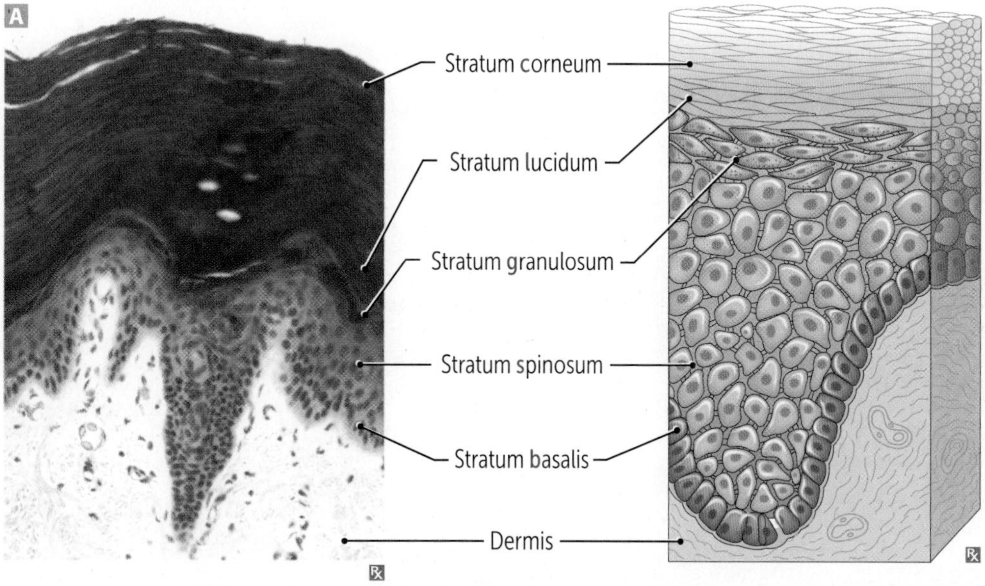
A
Stratum corneum
Stratum lucidum
Stratum granulosum
Stratum spinosum
Stratum basalis
Dermis

Epithelial cell junctions

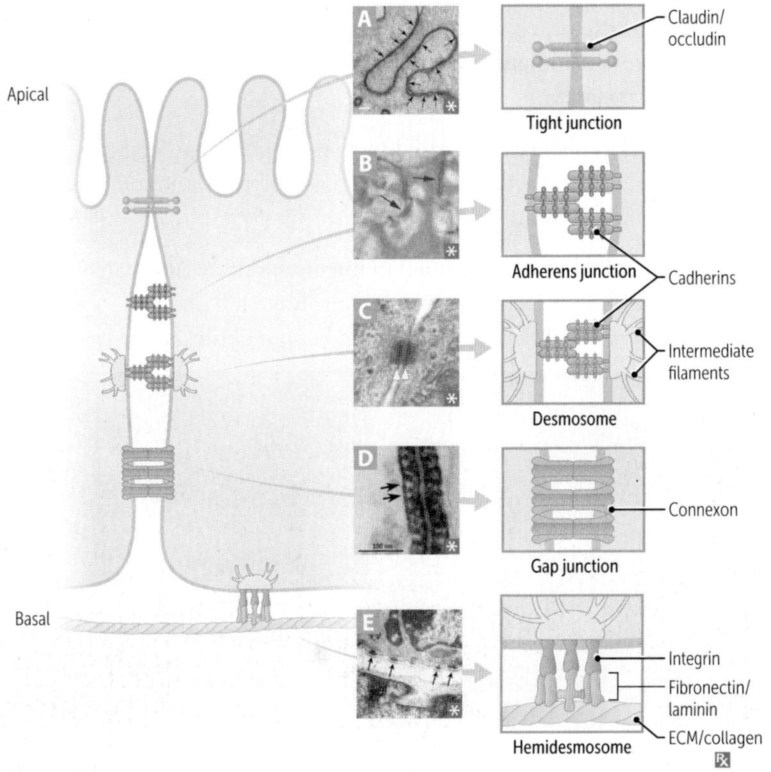

Tight junctions (zonula occludens) A–prevents paracellular movement of solutes; composed of claudins and occludins.

Adherens junction (belt desmosome, zonula adherens) B–forms "belt" connecting actin cytoskeletons of adjacent cells with **cad**herins (**Ca**$^{2+}$-dependent **ad**hesion proteins). Loss of E-cadherin promotes metastasis.

Desmosome (spot desmosome, macula adherens) C–structural support via intermediate filament interactions. Autoantibodies to desmoglein 1 and/or 3 → pemphigus vulgaris.

Gap junction D–channel proteins called connexons permit electrical and chemical communication between cells.

Hemidesmosome E–connects keratin in basal cells to underlying basement membrane. Autoantibodies → **bullo**us pemphigoid. (Hemidesmosomes are down "**bullow**.")

Integrins–membrane proteins that maintain **integr**ity of basolateral membrane by binding to collagen, laminin, and fibronectin in basement membrane.

Dermatologic macroscopic terms

LESION	CHARACTERISTICS	EXAMPLES
Macule	Flat lesion with well-circumscribed change in skin color < 1 cm	Freckle (ephelide), labial macule A
Patch	Macule > 1 cm	Large birthmark (congenital nevus) B
Papule	Elevated solid skin lesion < 1 cm	Mole (nevus) C, acne
Plaque	Papule > 1 cm	Psoriasis D
Vesicle	Small fluid-containing blister < 1 cm	Chickenpox (varicella), shingles (zoster) E
Bulla	Large fluid-containing blister > 1 cm	Bullous pemphigoid F
Pustule	Vesicle containing pus	Pustular psoriasis G
Wheal	Transient smooth papule or plaque	Hives (urticaria) H
Scale	Flaking off of stratum corneum	Eczema, psoriasis, SCC I
Crust	Dry exudate	Impetigo J

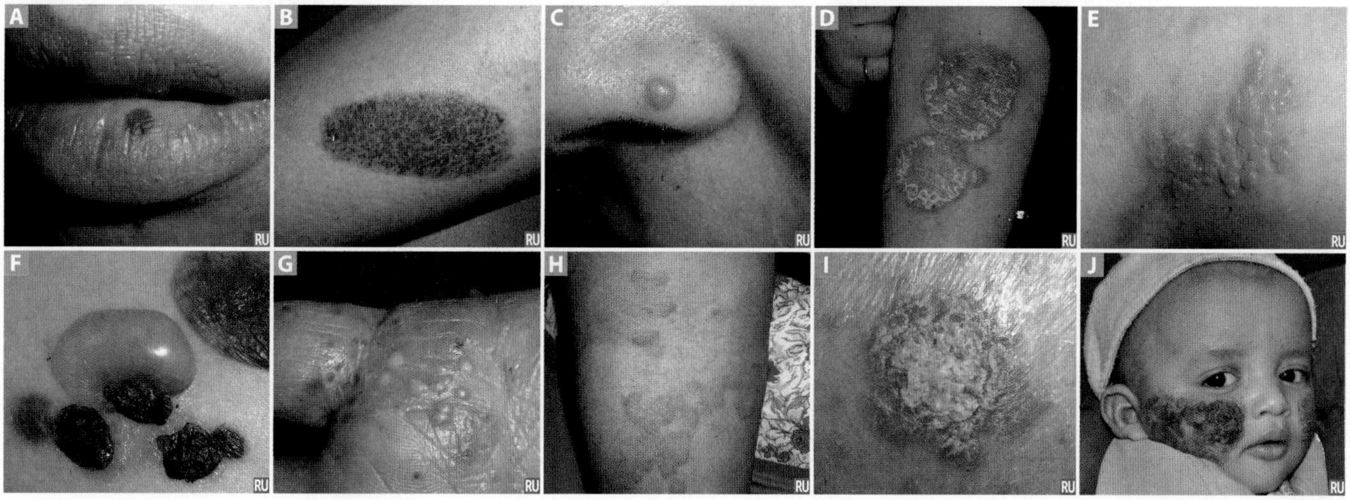

Dermatologic microscopic terms

LESION	CHARACTERISTICS	EXAMPLES
Dyskeratosis	Abnormal premature keratinization	Squamous cell carcinoma
Hyperkeratosis	↑ thickness of stratum corneum	Psoriasis, calluses
Parakeratosis	Retention of nuclei in stratum corneum	Psoriasis, actinic keratosis
Hypergranulosis	↑ thickness of stratum granulosum	Lichen planus
Spongiosis	Epidermal accumulation of edematous fluid in intercellular spaces	Eczematous dermatitis
Acantholysis	Separation of epidermal cells	Pemphigus vulgaris
Acanthosis	Epidermal hyperplasia (↑ spinosum)	Acanthosis nigricans, psoriasis

Pigmented skin disorders

Albinism	Normal melanocyte number with ↓ melanin production A due to ↓ tyrosinase activity or defective tyrosine transport. ↑ risk of skin cancer.
Melasma (chloasma)	Acquired hyperpigmentation associated with pregnancy ("mask of pregnancy" B) or OCP use. More common in pregnant patients with darker skin tones.
Vitiligo	Irregular patches of complete depigmentation C. Caused by destruction of melanocytes (believed to be autoimmune). Associated with other autoimmune disorders.

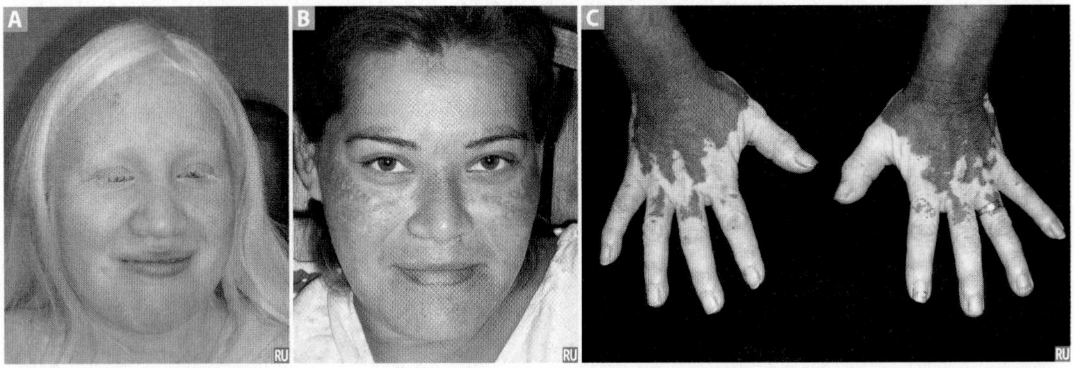

Seborrheic dermatitis

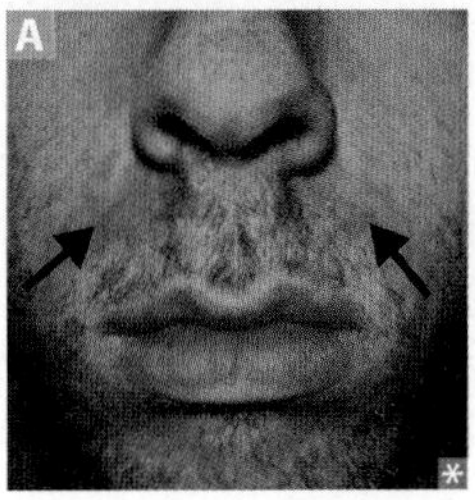

Erythematous, well-demarcated plaques A with greasy yellow scales in areas rich in sebaceous glands, such as scalp, face, and periocular region. Common in both infants (cradle cap) and adults, associated with Parkinson disease. Sebaceous glands are not inflamed, but play a role in disease development. Possibly associated with *Malassezia* spp. Treatment: topical antifungals and corticosteroids.

Common skin disorders

Acne	Multifactorial etiology—↑ sebum/androgen production, abnormal keratinocyte desquamation, *Cutibacterium acnes* colonization of the pilosebaceous unit (comedones), and inflammation (papules/pustules A, nodules, cysts). Treatment: retinoids, benzoyl peroxide, and antibiotics.
Atopic dermatitis (eczema)	Type I hypersensitivity reaction. Pruritic eruption, commonly on skin flexures. Associated with other atopic diseases (asthma, allergic rhinitis, food allergies); ↑ serum IgE. Mutations in filaggrin gene predispose (via skin barrier dysfunction). Often appears on face in infancy B and then in antecubital fossa C in children and adults.
Allergic contact dermatitis	Type IV hypersensitivity reaction secondary to contact allergen (eg, nickel D, poison ivy, neomycin E).
Melanocytic nevus	Common mole. Benign, but melanoma can arise in congenital or atypical moles. Intradermal nevi are papular F. Junctional nevi are flat macules G.
Pseudofolliculitis barbae	Foreign body inflammatory facial skin disorder characterized by firm, hyperpigmented papules and pustules that are painful and pruritic. Located on cheeks, jawline, and neck. Commonly occurs as a result of shaving ("razor bumps"), primarily affects Black males.
Psoriasis	Papules and plaques with silvery scaling H, especially on knees and elbows. Acanthosis with parakeratotic scaling (nuclei still in stratum corneum), Munro microabscesses. ↑ stratum spinosum, ↓ stratum granulosum. Auspitz sign (I)—pinpoint bleeding spots from exposure of dermal papillae when scales are scraped off. Associated with nail pitting and psoriatic arthritis.
Rosacea	Inflammatory facial skin disorder characterized by erythematous papules and pustules J, but no comedones. May be associated with facial flushing in response to external stimuli (eg, alcohol, heat). Complications include ocular involvement, rhinophyma (bulbous deformation of nose).
Seborrheic keratosis	Flat, greasy, pigmented squamous epithelial proliferation of immature keratinocytes with keratin-filled cysts (horn cysts) K. Looks "stuck on." Lesions occur on head, trunk, and extremities. Common benign neoplasm of older persons. Leser-Trélat sign L—rapid onset of multiple seborrheic keratoses, indicates possible malignancy (eg, GI adenocarcinoma).
Verrucae	Warts; caused by low-risk HPV strains. Soft, tan-colored, cauliflower-like papules M. Epidermal hyperplasia, hyperkeratosis, koilocytosis. Condyloma acuminatum on anus or genitals N.
Urticaria	Hives. Pruritic wheals that form after mast cell degranulation O. Characterized by superficial dermal edema and lymphatic channel dilation.

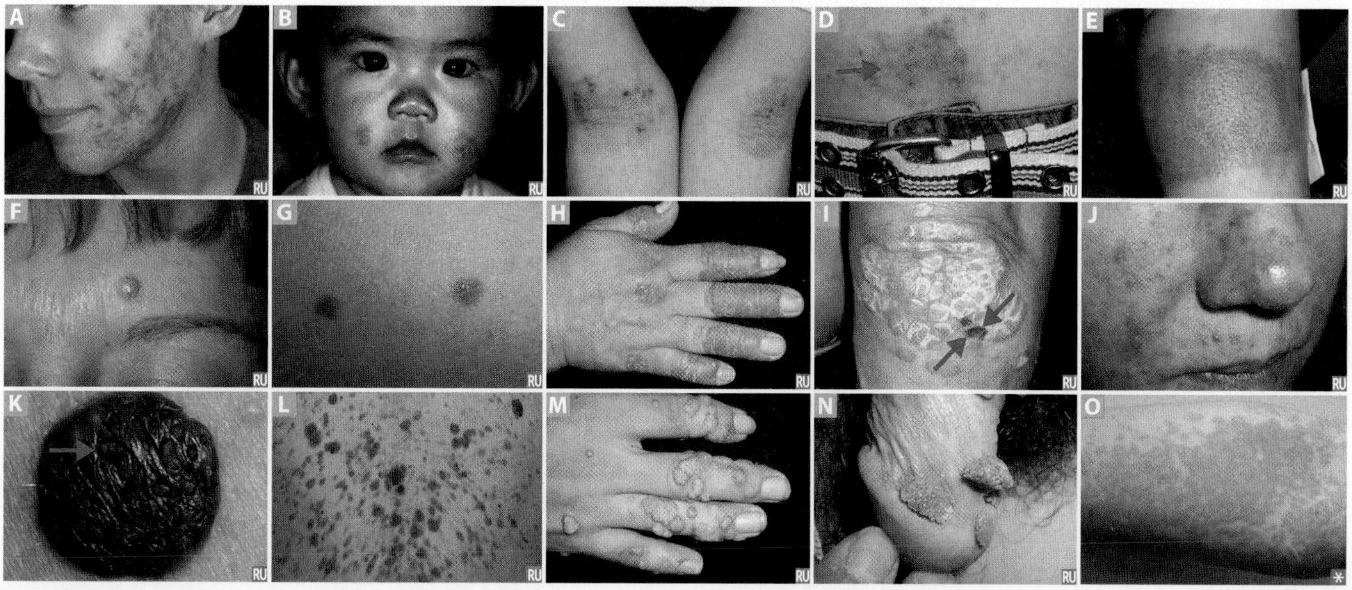

Vascular tumors of skin

Angiosarcoma	Rare blood vessel malignancy typically occurring in the head, neck, and breast areas. Usually in elderly, on sun-exposed areas. Associated with radiation therapy and chronic postmastectomy lymphedema. Hepatic angiosarcoma associated with vinyl chloride and arsenic exposures. Very aggressive and difficult to resect due to delay in diagnosis.
Bacillary angiomatosis	Benign capillary skin papules A found in patients with AIDS. Caused by *Bartonella* infections. Frequently mistaken for Kaposi sarcoma, but has neutrophilic infiltrate.
Cherry hemangioma	Benign capillary hemangioma B commonly appearing in middle-aged adults. Does not regress. Frequency ↑ with age.
Glomus tumor	Benign, painful, red-blue tumor, commonly under fingernails C. Arises from modified smooth muscle cells of the thermoregulatory glomus body.
Kaposi sarcoma	Endothelial malignancy most commonly affecting the skin, mouth, GI tract, respiratory tract. Classically seen in older Eastern European males, patients with AIDS, and organ transplant patients. Associated with HHV-8 and HIV. Lymphocytic infiltrate, unlike bacillary angiomatosis.
Pyogenic granuloma	Polypoid lobulated capillary hemangioma D that can ulcerate and bleed. Associated with trauma and pregnancy.
Strawberry hemangioma	Benign capillary hemangioma of infancy E. Appears in first few weeks of life (1/200 births); grows rapidly and regresses spontaneously by 5–8 years old.

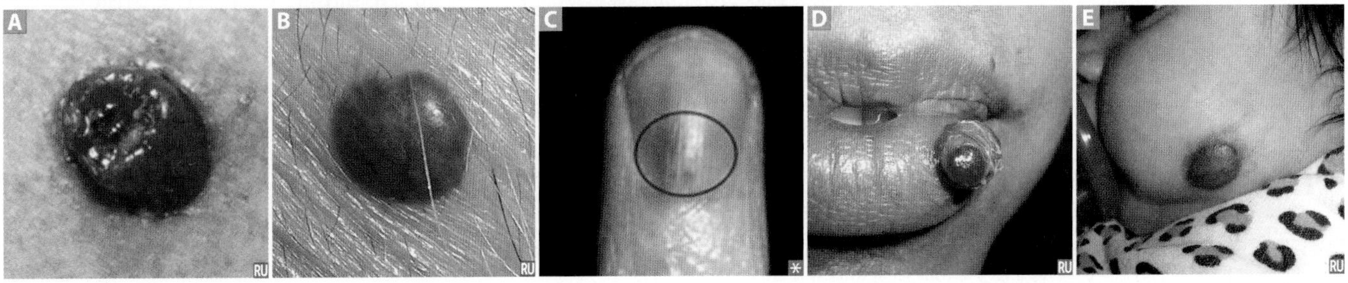

Skin infections

Bacterial infections	
Impetigo	Skin infection involving superficial epidermis. Usually from *S aureus* or *S pyogenes*. Highly contagious. Honey-colored crusting A. Bullous impetigo B has bullae and is usually caused by *S aureus*.
Erysipelas	Infection involving upper dermis and superficial lymphatics, usually from *S pyogenes*. Presents with well-defined, raised demarcation between infected and normal skin C.
Cellulitis	Acute, painful, spreading infection of deeper dermis and subcutaneous tissues. Usually from *S pyogenes* or *S aureus*. Often starts with a break in skin from trauma or another infection D.
Abscess	Collection of pus from a walled-off infection within deeper layers of skin E. Offending organism is almost always *S aureus*.
Necrotizing fasciitis	Deeper tissue injury, usually from anaerobic bacteria or *S pyogenes*. Pain may be out of proportion to exam findings. Results in crepitus from methane and CO_2 production. "Flesh-eating bacteria." Causes bullae and skin necrosis → violaceous color of bullae, surrounding skin F. Surgical emergency.
Staphylococcal scalded skin syndrome	Exotoxin destroys keratinocyte attachments in stratum granulosum only (vs toxic epidermal necrolysis, which destroys epidermal-dermal junction). Characterized by fever and generalized erythematous rash with sloughing of the upper layers of the epidermis G that heals completely. ⊕ Nikolsky sign (separation of epidermis upon manual stroking of skin). Commonly seen in newborns and children/adults with renal insufficiency.
Viral infections	
Herpes	Herpes virus infections (HSV1 and HSV2) of skin can occur anywhere from mucosal surfaces to normal skin. These include herpes labialis, herpes genitalis, herpetic whitlow H (finger).
Molluscum contagiosum	Umbilicated papules I caused by a poxvirus. While frequently seen in children, it may be sexually transmitted in adults.
Varicella zoster virus	Causes varicella (chickenpox) and zoster (shingles). Varicella presents with multiple crops of lesions in various stages from vesicles to crusts. Zoster is a reactivation of the virus in dermatomal distribution (unless it is disseminated).
Hairy leukoplakia	Irregular, white, painless plaques on lateral tongue that cannot be scraped off J. EBV mediated. Occurs in patients living with HIV, organ transplant recipients. Contrast with thrush (scrapable) and leukoplakia (precancerous).

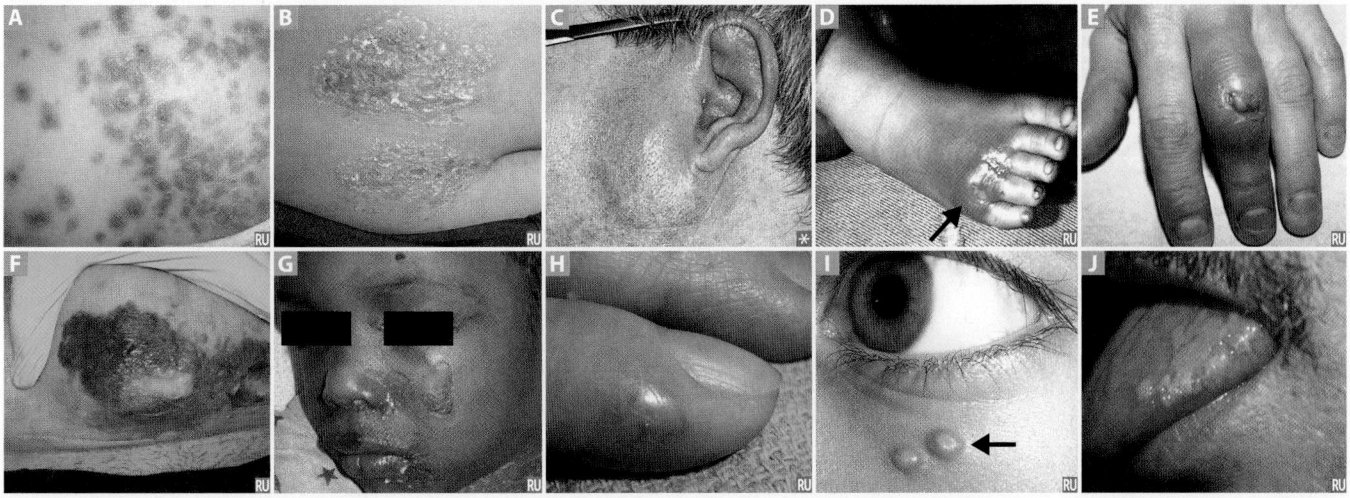

Autoimmune blistering skin disorders

	Pemphigus vulgaris	Bullous pemphigoid
PATHOPHYSIOLOGY	Potentially fatal. Most commonly seen in older adults. Type II hypersensitivity reaction. IgG antibodies against desmoglein-1 and/or desmoglein-3 (component of desmosomes, which connect keratinocytes in the stratum spinosum).	Less severe than pemphigus vulgaris. Most commonly seen in older adults. Type II hypersensitivity reaction. IgG antibodies against hemidesmosomes (epidermal basement membrane; antibodies are "bullow" the epidermis).
GROSS MORPHOLOGY	Flaccid intraepidermal bullae A caused by acantholysis (separation of keratinocytes, "row of tombstones" on H&E stain); oral mucosa is involved. Nikolsky sign ⊕.	Tense blisters C containing eosinophils; oral mucosa spared. Nikolsky sign ⊖.
IMMUNOFLUORESCENCE	Reticular pattern around epidermal cells B.	Linear pattern at epidermal-dermal junction D.

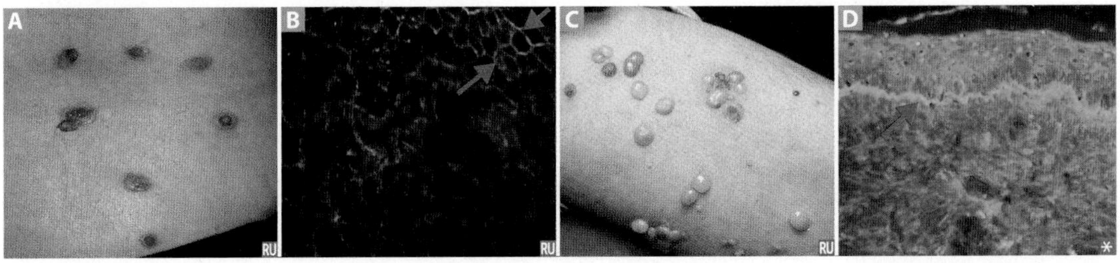

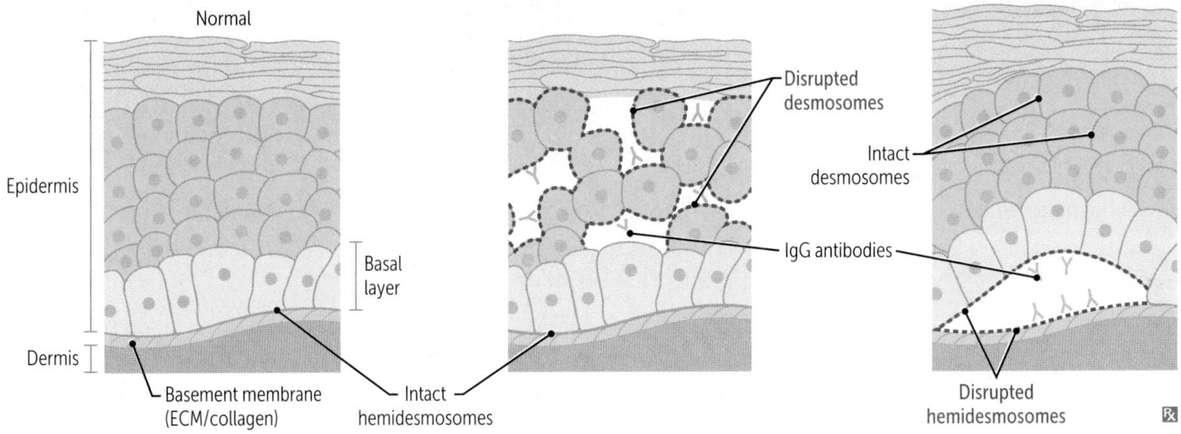

Other blistering skin disorders

Dermatitis herpetiformis	Pruritic papules, vesicles, and bullae (often found on elbows, knees, buttocks) A. Deposits of IgA at tips of dermal papillae. Associated with celiac disease. Treatment: dapsone, gluten-free diet.
Erythema multiforme	Associated with infections (eg, *Mycoplasma pneumoniae*, HSV), drugs (eg, sulfa drugs, β-lactams, phenytoin). Presents with multiple types of lesions—macules, papules, vesicles, target lesions (look like targets with multiple rings and dusky center showing epithelial disruption) B.
Stevens-Johnson syndrome	Characterized by fever, bullae formation and necrosis, sloughing of skin at dermal-epidermal junction (⊕ Nikolsky), high mortality rate. Typically mucous membranes are involved C D. Targetoid skin lesions may appear, as seen in erythema multiforme. Usually associated with adverse drug reaction. Toxic epidermal necrolysis (TEN) E F is more severe form of SJS involving > 30% body surface area. 10–30% involvement denotes SJS-TEN.

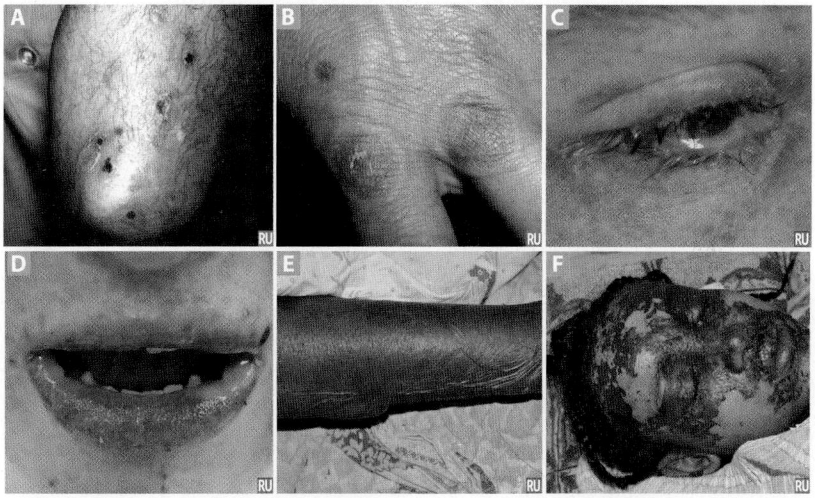

Lower extremity ulcers

	Venous ulcer	Arterial ulcer	Neuropathic ulcer
ETIOLOGY	Chronic venous insufficiency; most common ulcer type	Peripheral artery disease (eg, atherosclerotic stenosis)	Peripheral neuropathy (eg, diabetic foot)
LOCATION	Gaiter area (ankle to midcalf), typically over malleoli	Distal toes, anterior shin, pressure points	Bony prominences (eg, metatarsal heads, heel)
APPEARANCE	Irregular border, shallow, exudative A	Symmetric with well-defined punched out appearance B	Hyperkeratotic edge with undermined borders C
PAIN	Mild to moderate	Severe	Absent
ASSOCIATED SIGNS	Telangiectasias, varicose veins, edema, stasis dermatitis (erythematous eczematous patches)	Signs of arterial insufficiency including cold, pale, atrophic skin with hair loss and nail dystrophy, absent pulses	Claw toes, Charcot joints, absent reflexes

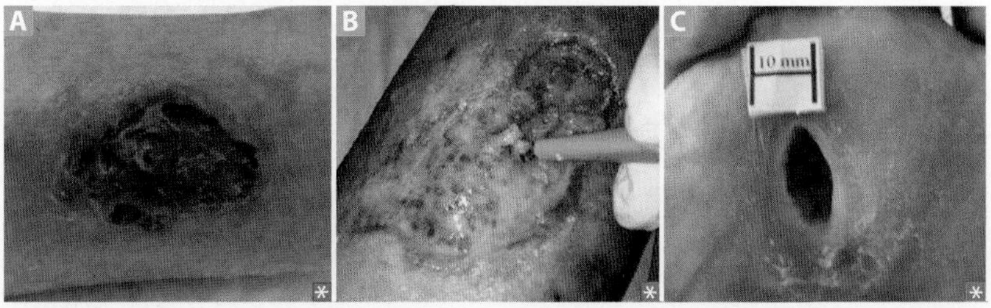

Miscellaneous skin disorders

Acanthosis nigricans	Epidermal hyperplasia causing symmetric, hyperpigmented thickening of skin, especially in axilla or on neck A B. Associated with insulin resistance (eg, diabetes, obesity, Cushing syndrome, PCOS), visceral malignancy (eg, gastric adenocarcinoma).
Actinic keratosis	Premalignant lesions caused by sun exposure. Small, rough, erythematous or brownish papules or plaques C D. Risk of squamous cell carcinoma is proportional to degree of epithelial dysplasia.
Erythema nodosum	Painful, raised inflammatory lesions of subcutaneous fat (panniculitis), usually on anterior shins. Often idiopathic, but can be associated with sarcoidosis, coccidioidomycosis, histoplasmosis, TB, streptococcal infections E, leprosy F, inflammatory bowel disease.
Lichen Planus	Pruritic, purple, polygonal planar papules and plaques are the 6 P's of lichen Planus G H. Mucosal involvement manifests as Wickham striae (reticular white lines) and hypergranulosis. Sawtooth infiltrate of lymphocytes at dermal-epidermal junction. Associated with hepatitis C.
Pityriasis rosea	"Herald patch" I followed days later by other scaly erythematous plaques, often in a "Christmas tree" distribution on trunk J. Multiple pink plaques with collarette scale. Self-resolving in 6–8 weeks.
Sunburn	Acute cutaneous inflammatory reaction due to excessive UV irradiation. Causes DNA mutations, inducing apoptosis of keratinocytes. UVB is dominant in sunBurn, UVA in tAnning and photoAging. Exposure to UVA and UVB ↑ risk of skin cancer.

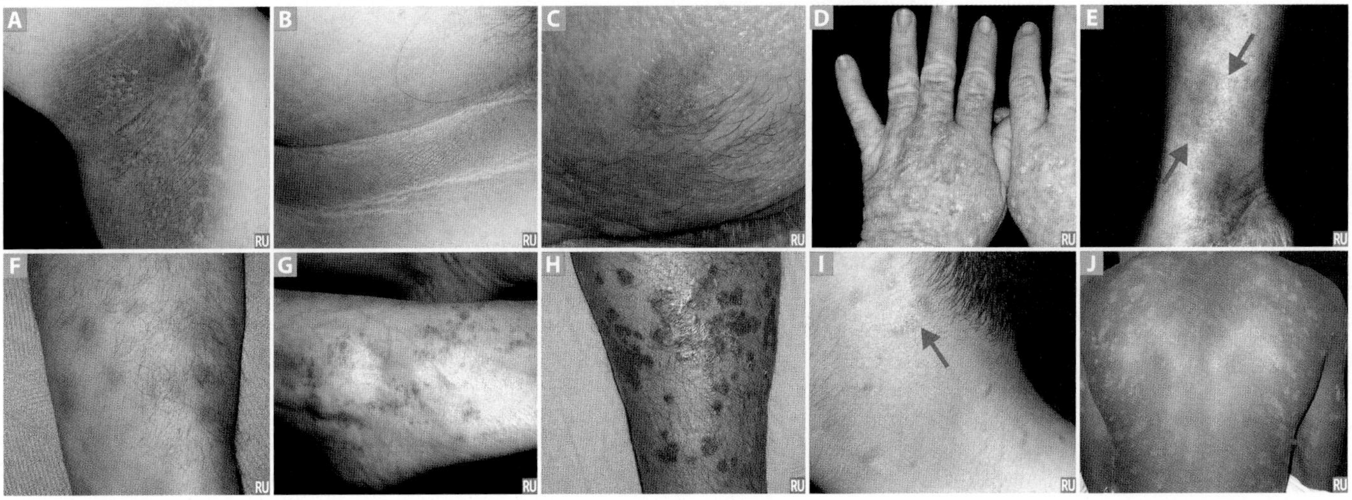

Rule of 9's

The extent of a burn injury can be estimated as a percentage of the body surface area.

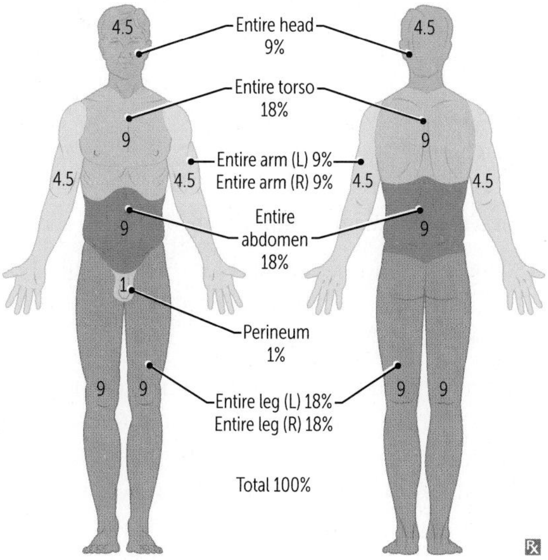

4.5
Entire head
9%
4.5
Entire torso
18%
9
9
4.5
4.5
Entire arm (L) 9%
Entire arm (R) 9%
4.5
4.5
Entire abdomen
18%
9
9
1
Perineum
1%
9
9
Entire leg (L) 18%
Entire leg (R) 18%
9
9
Total 100%

Burn classification

DEPTH	INVOLVEMENT	APPEARANCE	SENSATION
Superficial burn	Epidermis only	Similar to sunburn; localized, dry, blanching redness with no blisters	Painful
Superficial partial-thickness burn	Epidermis and papillary dermis	Blisters, blanches with pressure, swollen, warm	Painful to temperature and air
Deep partial-thickness burn	Epidermis and reticular dermis	Blisters (easily unroofed), does not blanch with pressure	Painless; perception of pressure only
Full-thickness burn	Epidermis and full-thickness dermis	White, waxy, dry, inelastic, leathery, does not blanch with pressure	Painless; perception of deep pressure only
Deeper injury burn	Epidermis, dermis, and involvement of underlying tissue (eg, fascia, muscle)	White, dry, inelastic, does not blanch with pressure	Painless; some perception of deep pressure

Skin cancer

Basal cell carcinoma more common above **upper lip**

Squamous cell carcinoma more common below **lower lip**

Sun exposure strongly predisposes to skin cancer.

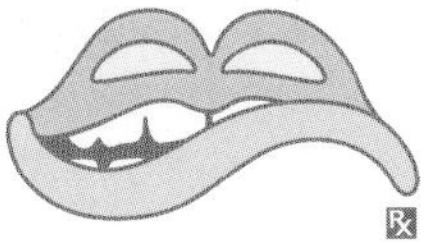

Basal cell carcinoma

Most common skin cancer. Found in sun-exposed areas of body (eg, face). Locally invasive, but rarely metastasizes. Waxy, pink, pearly nodules, commonly with telangiectasias, rolled borders A, central crusting or ulceration. BCCs also appear as nonhealing ulcers with infiltrating growth B or as a scaling plaque (superficial BCC) C. Basal cell tumors have "palisading" (aligned) nuclei D.

Keratoacanthoma

Seen in middle-aged and elderly individuals. Rapidly growing, resembles squamous cell carcinoma. Presents as dome-shaped nodule with keratin-filled center. Grows rapidly (4-6 weeks) and may spontaneously regress E.

Melanoma

Common tumor with significant risk of metastasis. S-100 tumor marker. Associated with dysplastic nevi; people with lighter skin tones are at ↑ risk. Depth of tumor (Breslow thickness) correlates with risk of metastasis. Look for the ABCDEs: Asymmetry, Border irregularity, Color variation, Diameter > 6 mm, and Evolution over time. At least 4 different types of melanoma, including superficial spreading F, nodular G, lentigo maligna H, and acral lentiginous (highest prevalence in people with darker skin tones) I. Often driven by activating mutation in BRAF kinase. Primary treatment is excision with appropriately wide margins. Advanced melanoma also treated with immunotherapy (eg, ipilimumab) and/or BRAF inhibitors (eg, vemurafenib).

Squamous cell carcinoma

Second most common skin cancer. Associated with immunosuppression, chronic nonhealing wounds, and occasionally arsenic exposure. Commonly appears on face J, lower lip K, ears, hands. Locally invasive, may spread to lymph nodes, and will rarely metastasize. Ulcerative red lesions. Histopathology: keratin "pearls" L.

Actinic keratosis, a scaly plaque, is a precursor to squamous cell carcinoma.

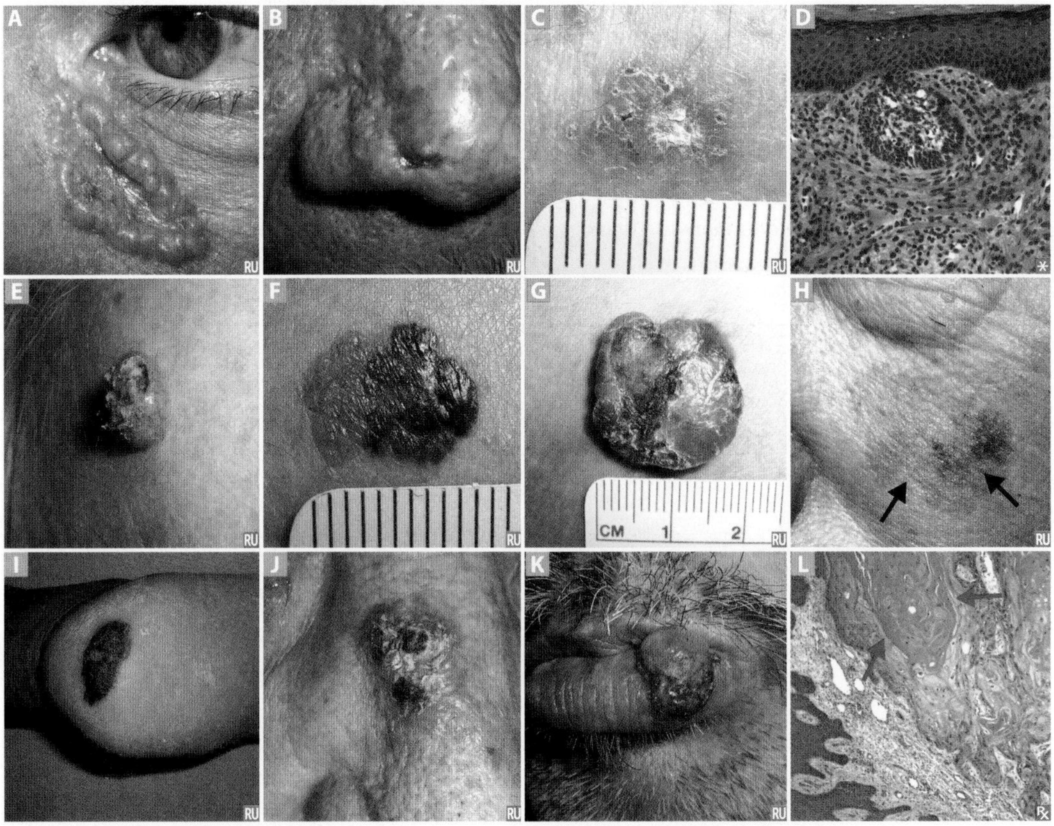

▶ MUSCULOSKELETAL, SKIN, AND CONNECTIVE TISSUE—PHARMACOLOGY

Arachidonic acid pathways

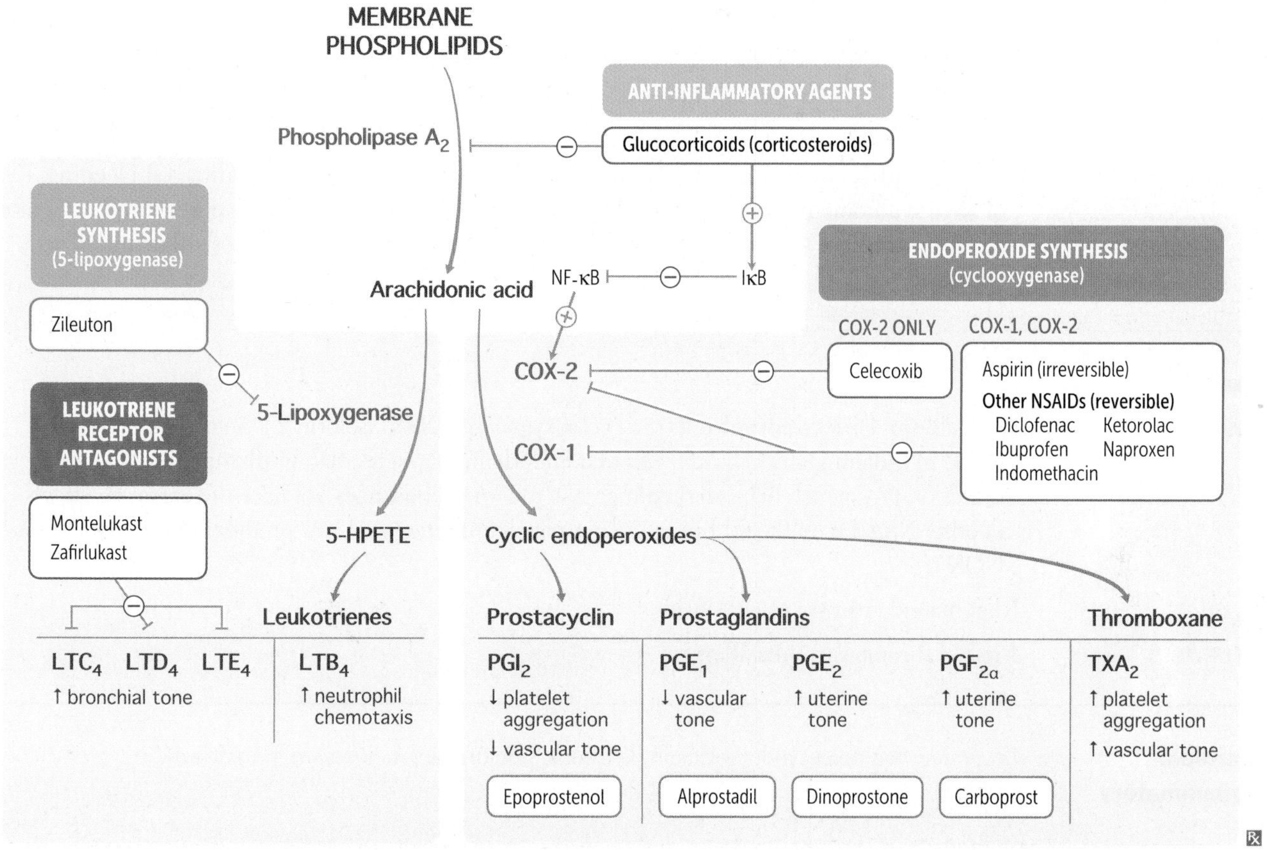

LTB_4 is a **neutrophil** chemotactic agent. **Neutrophils** arrive "**B4**" others.

PGI_2 inhibits platelet aggregation and promotes vasodilation. **P**latelet-**G**athering **I**nhibitor.

Acetaminophen

MECHANISM	Reversibly inhibits cyclooxygenase, mostly in CNS. Inactivated peripherally.
CLINICAL USE	Antipyretic, analgesic, but not anti-inflammatory. Used instead of aspirin to avoid Reye syndrome in children with viral infection.
ADVERSE EFFECTS	Overdose produces hepatic necrosis; acetaminophen metabolite (NAPQI) depletes glutathione and forms toxic tissue byproducts in liver. N-acetylcysteine is antidote—regenerates glutathione.

Aspirin

MECHANISM	NSAID that irreversibly inhibits cyclooxygenase (both COX-1 and COX-2) by covalent acetylation → ↓ synthesis of TXA_2 and prostaglandins. ↑ bleeding time. No effect on PT, PTT. Effect lasts until new platelets are produced.
CLINICAL USE	Low dose (< 300 mg/day): ↓ platelet aggregation. Intermediate dose (300–2400 mg/day): antipyretic and analgesic. High dose (2400–4000 mg/day): anti-inflammatory.
ADVERSE EFFECTS	Gastric ulceration, tinnitus (CN VIII), allergic reactions (especially in patients with asthma or nasal polyps). Chronic use can lead to acute kidney injury, interstitial nephritis, GI bleeding. Risk of Reye syndrome in children treated with aspirin for viral infection. Toxic doses cause respiratory alkalosis early, but transitions to mixed metabolic acidosis-respiratory alkalosis. Treatment of overdose: $NaHCO_3$.

Celecoxib

MECHANISM	Reversibly and **selectively** inhibits the cyclooxygenase (**COX**) isoform 2 ("**Selecoxib**"), which is found in inflammatory cells and vascular endothelium and mediates inflammation and pain; spares COX-1, which helps maintain gastric mucosa. Thus, does not have the corrosive effects of other NSAIDs on the GI lining. Spares platelet function as TXA_2 production is dependent on COX-1.
CLINICAL USE	Rheumatoid arthritis, osteoarthritis.
ADVERSE EFFECTS	↑ risk of thrombosis, sulfa allergy.

Nonsteroidal anti-inflammatory drugs

Ibuprofen, naproxen, indomethacin, ketorolac, diclofenac, meloxicam, piroxicam.

MECHANISM	Reversibly inhibit cyclooxygenase (both COX-1 and COX-2). Block prostaglandin synthesis.
CLINICAL USE	Antipyretic, analgesic, anti-inflammatory. Indomethacin is used to close a PDA.
ADVERSE EFFECTS	Interstitial nephritis, gastric ulcer (prostaglandins protect gastric mucosa), renal ischemia (prostaglandins vasodilate afferent arteriole), aplastic anemia.

Leflunomide

MECHANISM	Reversibly inhibits dihydroorotate dehydrogenase, preventing pyrimidine synthesis. Suppresses T-cell proliferation.
CLINICAL USE	Rheumatoid arthritis, psoriatic arthritis.
ADVERSE EFFECTS	Diarrhea, hypertension, hepatotoxicity, teratogenicity.

Bisphosphonates

Alendronate, ibandronate, risedronate, zoledronate.

MECHANISM	Pyrophosphate analogs; bind hydroxyapatite in bone, inhibiting osteoclast activity.
CLINICAL USE	Osteoporosis, hypercalcemia, Paget disease of bone, metastatic bone disease, osteogenesis imperfecta.
ADVERSE EFFECTS	Esophagitis (if taken orally, patients are advised to take with water and remain upright for 30 minutes), osteonecrosis of jaw, atypical femoral stress fractures.

Teriparatide

MECHANISM	Recombinant PTH analog. ↑ osteoblastic activity when administered in pulsatile fashion.
CLINICAL USE	Osteoporosis. Causes ↑ bone growth compared to antiresorptive therapies (eg, bisphosphonates).
ADVERSE EFFECTS	↑ risk of osteosarcoma (avoid use in patients with Paget disease of the bone or unexplained elevation of alkaline phosphatase). Avoid in patients who have had prior cancers or radiation therapy. Transient hypercalcemia.

Gout drugs

Chronic gout drugs (preventive)	
Allopurinol	Competitive inhibitor of xanthine oxidase → ↓ conversion of hypoxanthine and xanthine to urate. Also used in lymphoma and leukemia to prevent tumor lysis–associated urate nephropathy. ↑ concentrations of xanthine oxidase active metabolites, azathioprine, and 6-MP.
Pegloticase	Recombinant uricase catalyzing uric acid to allantoin (a more water-soluble product).
Febuxostat	Inhibits xanthine oxidase. Think, "febu-**xo**-**stat** makes **X**anthine **O**xidase **stat**ic."
Probenecid	Inhibits reabsorption of uric acid in proximal convoluted tubule (also inhibits secretion of penicillin). Can precipitate uric acid calculi.
Acute gout drugs	
NSAIDs	Any NSAID. Use salicylates with caution (may decrease uric acid excretion, particularly at low doses).
Glucocorticoids	Oral, intra-articular, or parenteral.
Colchicine	Binds and stabilizes tubulin to inhibit microtubule polymerization, impairing neutrophil chemotaxis and degranulation. Acute and prophylactic value. GI, neuromyopathic side effects. Can also cause myelosupression, nephrotoxicity.

All painful flares are preventable.

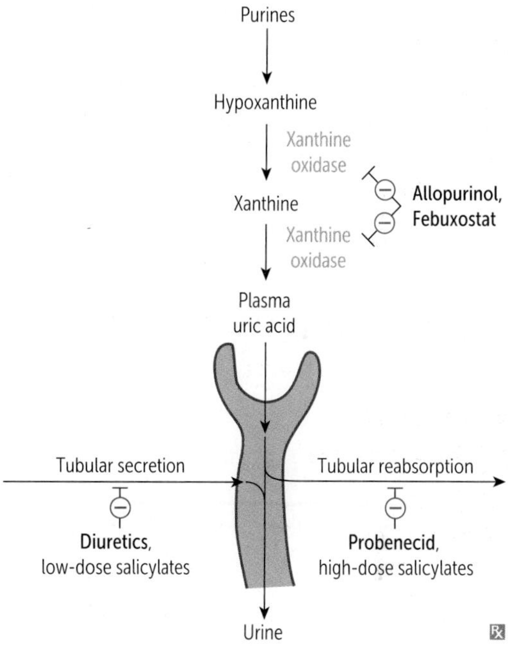
Purines
Hypoxanthine
Xanthine oxidase
Xanthine
Xanthine oxidase
Allopurinol, Febuxostat
Plasma uric acid
Tubular secretion
Tubular reabsorption
Diuretics, low-dose salicylates
Probenecid, high-dose salicylates
Urine

TNF-α inhibitors

DRUG	MECHANISM	CLINICAL USE	ADVERSE EFFECTS
Etanercept	Fusion protein (decoy receptor for TNF-α + IgG_1 Fc), produced by recombinant DNA. Etanercept intercepts TNF.	Rheumatoid arthritis, psoriasis, ankylosing spondylitis	Predisposition to infection, including reactivation of latent TB, since TNF is important in granuloma formation and stabilization. Can also lead to drug-induced lupus.
Infliximab, adalimumab, certolizumab, golimumab	Anti-TNF-α monoclonal antibody.	Inflammatory bowel disease, rheumatoid arthritis, ankylosing spondylitis, psoriasis	

HIGH-YIELD SYSTEMS

Neurology and Special Senses

"We are all now connected by the Internet, like neurons in a giant brain."
—Stephen Hawking

"Anything's possible if you've got enough nerve."
—J.K. Rowling, *Harry Potter and the Order of the Phoenix*

"I like nonsense; it wakes up the brain cells."
—Dr. Seuss

"I believe in an open mind, but not so open that your brains fall out."
—Arthur Hays Sulzberger

"The chief function of the body is to carry the brain around."
—Thomas Edison

"Exactly how [the brain] operates remains one of the biggest unsolved mysteries, and it seems the more we probe its secrets, the more surprises we find."
—Neil deGrasse Tyson

Understand the difference between the findings and underlying anatomy of upper motor neuron and lower motor neuron lesions. Know the major motor, sensory, cerebellar and visual pathways and their respective locations in the CNS. Connect key neurological associations with certain pathologies (eg, cerebellar lesions, stroke manifestations, Brown-Séquard syndrome). Recognize common findings on MRI/CT (eg, ischemic and hemorrhagic stroke) and on neuropathology (eg, neurofibrillary tangles and Lewy bodies). High-yield medications include those used to treat epilepsy, Parkinson disease, migraine, and pain (eg, opioids).

▶ NEUROLOGY—EMBRYOLOGY

Neural development

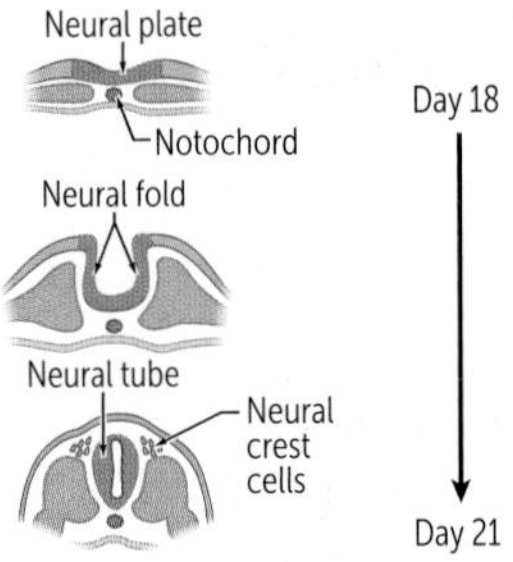

Notochord induces overlying ectoderm to differentiate into neuroectoderm and form neural plate.
Neural plate gives rise to neural tube and neural crest cells.
Notochord becomes nucleus pulposus of intervertebral disc in adults.

Alar plate (dorsal): sensory; regulated by TGF-β (including bone morphogenetic protein [*BMP*])
Basal plate (ventral): motor; regulated by sonic hedgehog gene (*SHH*)
— Same orientation as spinal cord

Regional specification of developing brain

Telencephalon is the 1st part. **Diencephalon** is the **2nd** part. The rest are arranged alphabetically: **mesencephalon, metencephalon, myelencephalon.**

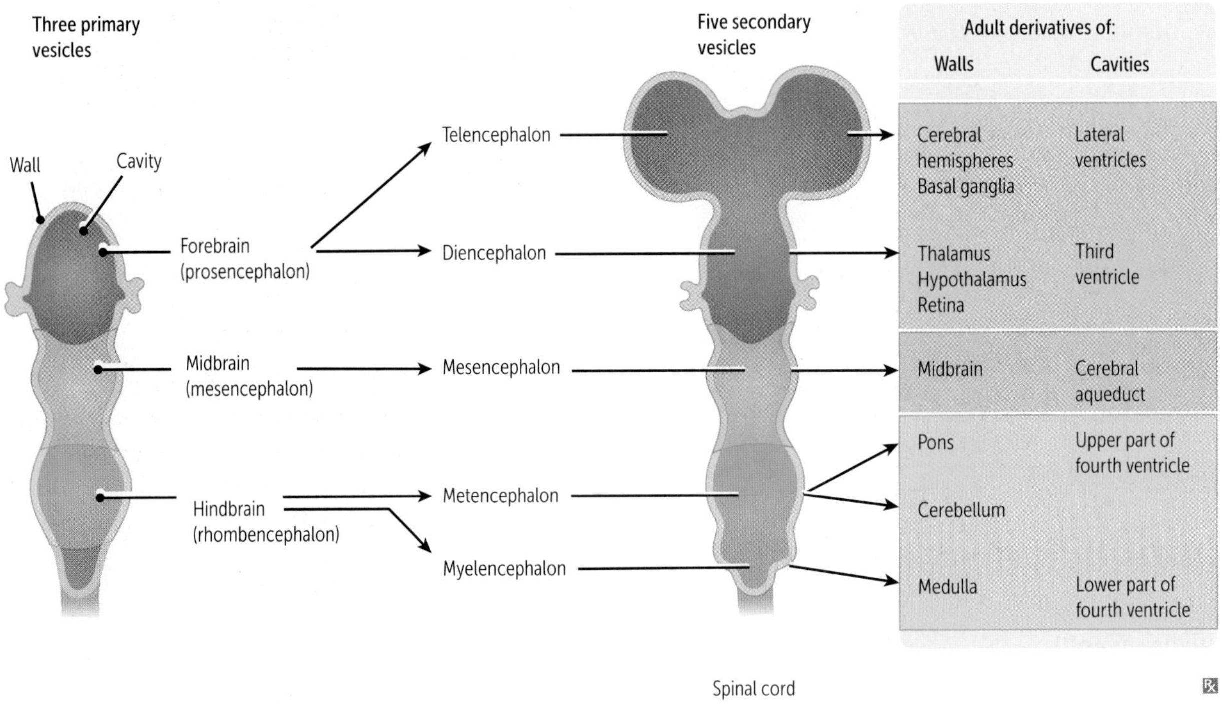

Central and peripheral nervous systems origins

Neuroepithelia in neural tube—CNS neurons, CNS glial cells (astrocytes, oligodendrocytes, ependymal cells).
Neural crest—PNS neurons (dorsal root ganglia, autonomic ganglia [sympathetic, parasympathetic, enteric]), PNS glial cells (Schwann cells, satellite cells), adrenal medulla, melanocytes, face/branchial arch mesenchyme.
Mesoderm—microglia (like macrophages).

Neural tube defects	Neuropores fail to fuse by the 4th week of development → persistent connection between amniotic cavity and spinal canal. Associated with diabetes and folate deficiency during pregnancy. ↑ α-fetoprotein (AFP) in amniotic fluid and serum (except spina bifida occulta = normal AFP). ↑ acetylcholinesterase (AChE) in amniotic fluid is a helpful confirmatory test.
Spina bifida occulta	Failure of caudal neuropore to close, but no herniation. Usually seen at lower vertebral levels. Dura is intact. Associated with tuft of hair or skin dimple at level of bony defect.
Meningocele	Meninges (but no neural tissue) herniate through bony defect.
Myelomeningocele	Meninges and neural tissue (eg, cauda equina) herniate through bony defect.
Myeloschisis	Also called rachischisis. Exposed, unfused neural tissue without skin/meningeal covering.
Anencephaly	Failure of rostral neuropore to close → no forebrain, open calvarium. Clinical findings: polyhydramnios (no swallowing center in brain).

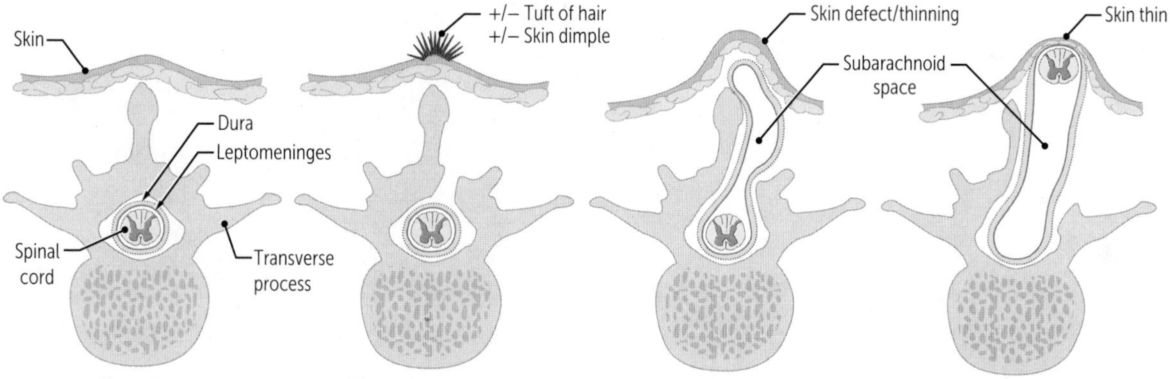

Holoprosencephaly

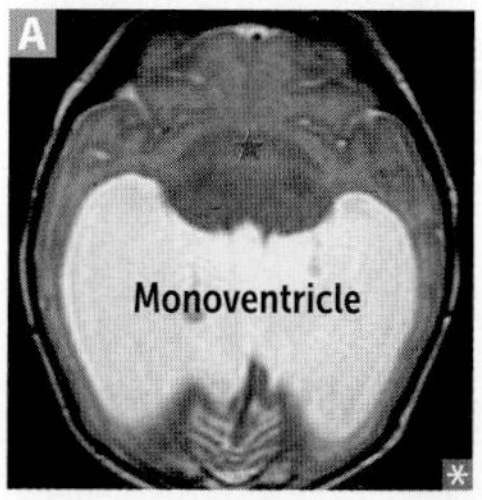

Developmental field defect characterized by failure of embryonic forebrain (prosencephalon) to separate into 2 cerebral hemispheres; usually occurs during weeks 3–4 of development. May be related to mutations in sonic hedgehog signaling pathway. Associated with other midline defects including cleft lip/palate (moderate form) and cyclopia (severe form). ↑ risk for pituitary dysfunction (eg, diabetes insipidus). May be seen with Patau syndrome (trisomy 13) and maternal alcohol use.

MRI reveals monoventricle A and fusion of basal ganglia (star in A).

Lissencephaly

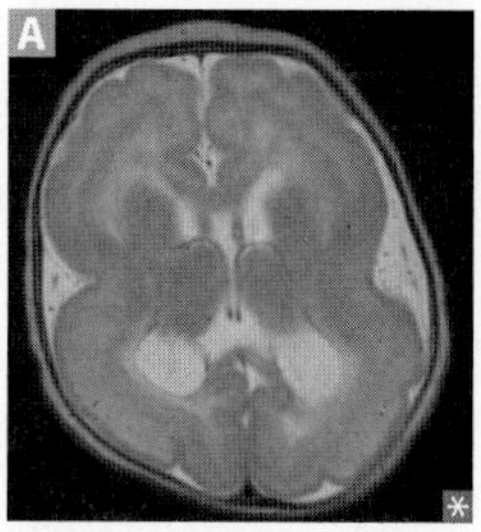

Failure of neuronal migration resulting in a "smooth brain" that lacks sulci and gyri A. May be associated with microcephaly, ventriculomegaly, hydrocephalus.

Posterior fossa malformations

Chiari I malformation	Ectopia of cerebellar **tonsils** inferior to foramen magnum (1 structure) A. Congenital, usually asymptomatic in childhood, manifests in adulthood with headaches and cerebellar symptoms. Associated with spinal cavitations (eg, syringomyelia).
Chiari II malformation	Herniation of **cerebellum** (vermis and tonsils) and **medulla** (2 structures) through foramen magnum → noncommunicating hydrocephalus. Usually associated with aqueductal stenosis, lumbosacral myelomeningocele (may present as paralysis/sensory loss at and below the level of the lesion). More severe than Chiari I, usually presents early in life.
Dandy-Walker malformation	Agenesis of cerebellar vermis → cystic enlargement of 4th ventricle (arrow in B) that fills the enlarged posterior fossa. Associated with noncommunicating hydrocephalus, spina bifida.

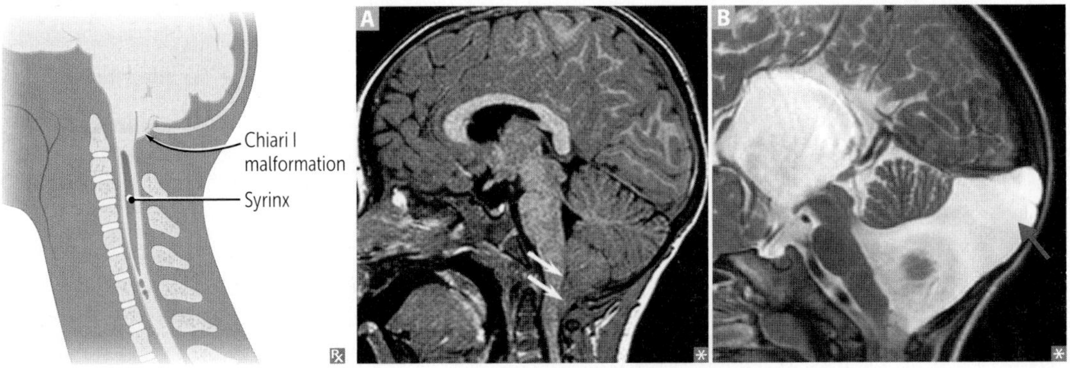
Chiari I malformation
Syrinx
A
B

Syringomyelia

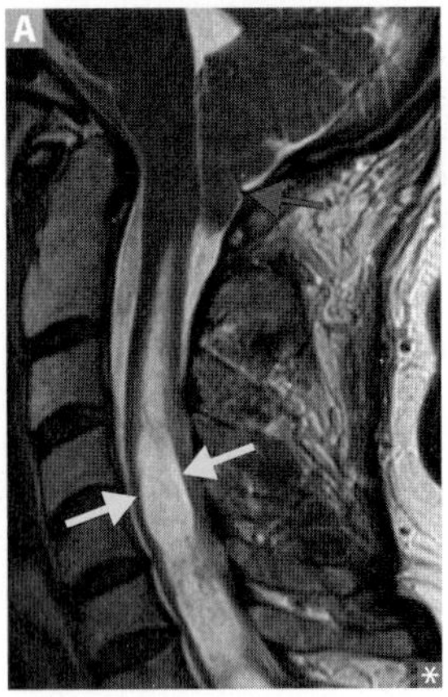
A

Cystic cavity (syrinx) within central canal of spinal cord (yellow arrows in A). Fibers crossing in anterior white commissure (spinothalamic tract) are typically damaged first. Results in a "cape-like," bilateral, symmetrical loss of pain and temperature sensation in upper extremities (fine touch sensation is preserved).

Associated with Chiari I malformation (red arrow in A shows low-lying cerebellar tonsils), scoliosis and other congenital malformations; acquired causes include trauma and tumors. Most common location cervical > thoracic >> lumbar. **Syrinx** = tube, as in "**syringe**."

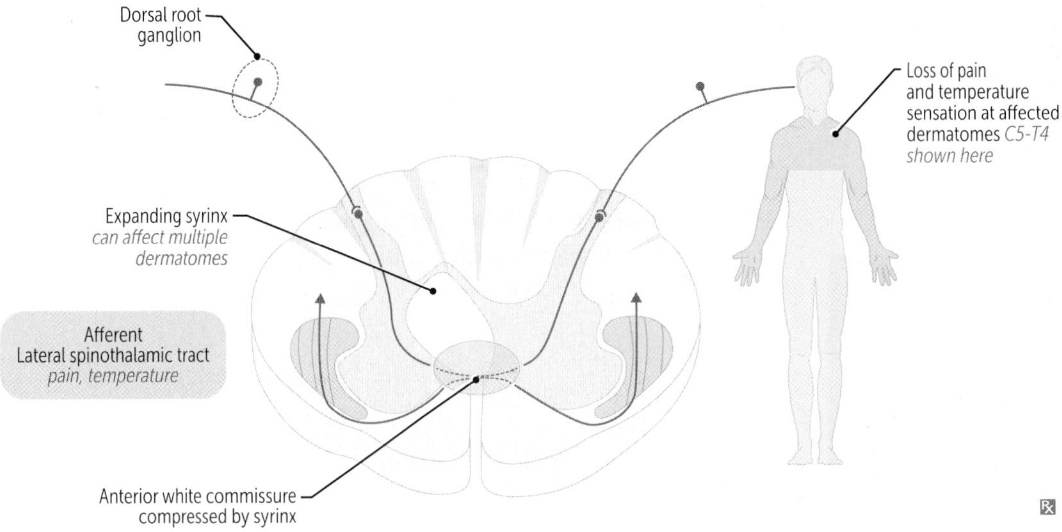
Dorsal root ganglion
Loss of pain and temperature sensation at affected dermatomes *C5-T4 shown here*
Expanding syrinx *can affect multiple dermatomes*
Afferent
Lateral spinothalamic tract
pain, temperature
Anterior white commissure compressed by syrinx

Tongue development

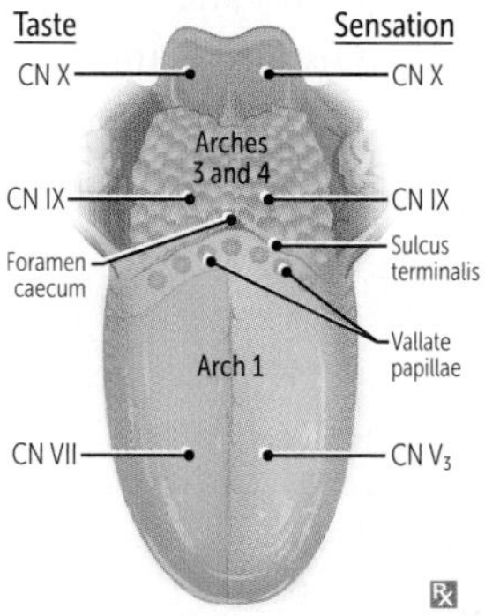
Taste
Sensation
CN X
CN X
Arches 3 and 4
CN IX
CN IX
Foramen caecum
Sulcus terminalis
Vallate papillae
Arch 1
CN VII
CN V_3

1st pharyngeal arch forms anterior 2/3 of tongue (sensation via CN V_3, taste via CN VII).
3rd and 4th pharyngeal arches form posterior 1/3 of tongue (sensation and taste mainly via CN IX, extreme posterior via CN X).
Motor innervation is via CN XII to hyoglossus (retracts and depresses tongue), genioglossus (protrudes tongue), and styloglossus (draws sides of tongue upward to create a trough for swallowing).
Motor innervation is via CN X to palatoglossus (elevates posterior tongue during swallowing).

Taste—CN VII, IX, X (solitary nucleus).
Pain—CN V_3, IX, X.
Motor—CN X, XII.

The **genie** comes **out** of the lamp in **style**.

CN **10** innervates palat**en**glossus.

▶ NEUROLOGY—ANATOMY AND PHYSIOLOGY

Neurons

Signal-transmitting cells of the nervous system. Permanent cells—do not divide in adulthood.
Signal-relaying cells with dendrites (receive input), cell bodies, and axons (send output). Cell bodies and dendrites can be seen on Nissl staining (stains RER). RER is not present in the axon. Neuron markers: neurofilament protein, synaptophysin.

Astrocytes

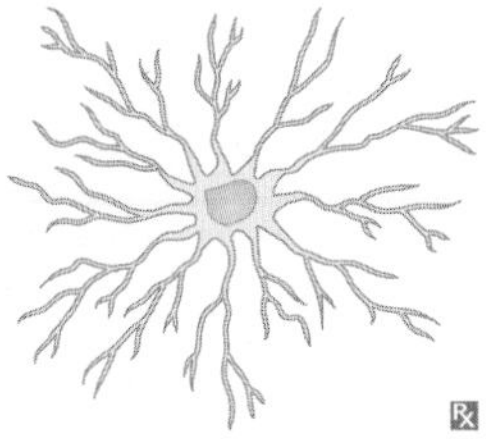

Most common glial cell type in CNS.
Physical support, repair, removal of excess neurotransmitter, component of blood-brain barrier, glycogen fuel reserve buffer. Reactive gliosis in response to neural injury.

Derived from neuroectoderm.
Astrocyte marker: GFAP.

Microglia

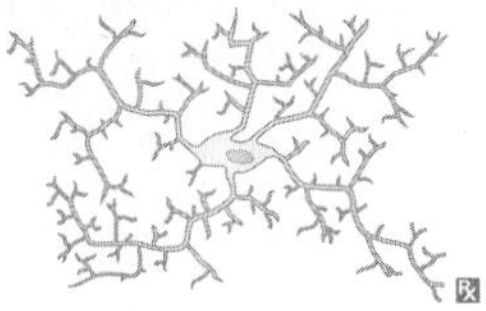

Phagocytic scavenger cells of CNS. Activation in response to tissue damage → release of inflammatory mediators (eg, nitric oxide, glutamate). Not readily discernible by Nissl stain.

Derived from mesoderm.
HIV-infected microglia fuse to form multinucleated giant cells in CNS seen in HIV-associated dementia.

Ependymal cells

Ciliated simple columnar glial cells lining ventricles and central canal of spinal cord. Apical surfaces are covered with cilia (which circulate CSF) and microvilli (which help with CSF absorption).

Derived from neuroectoderm.
Specialized ependymal cells (choroid plexus) produce CSF.

Myelin 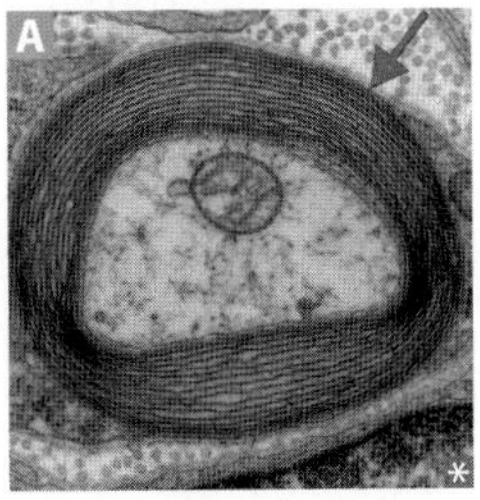	↑ conduction velocity of signals transmitted down axons → saltatory conduction of action potential at the nodes of Ranvier, where there are high concentrations of Na^+ channels. In CNS (including CN II), myelin is synthesized by oligodendrocytes; in PNS (including CN III-XII), myelin is synthesized by Schwann cells.	Myelin (arrow in A) wraps and insulates axons: ↓ membrane capacitance, ↑ membrane resistance, ↑ space (length) constant, ↓ time constant. CNS: Oligodendrocytes. PNS: Schwann cells. COPS
Schwann cells 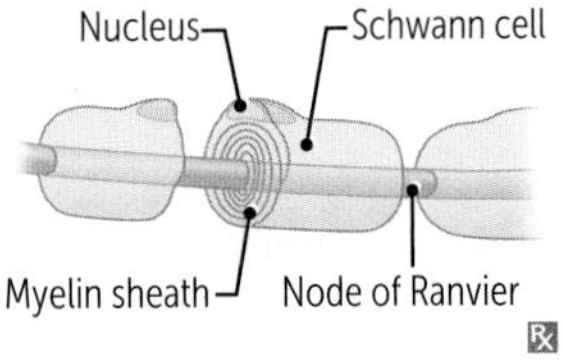	Promote axonal regeneration. Derived from neural crest.	Each "Schwone" cell myelinates only 1 PNS axon. Injured in Guillain-Barré syndrome. Schwann cell marker: S100.
Oligodendrocytes 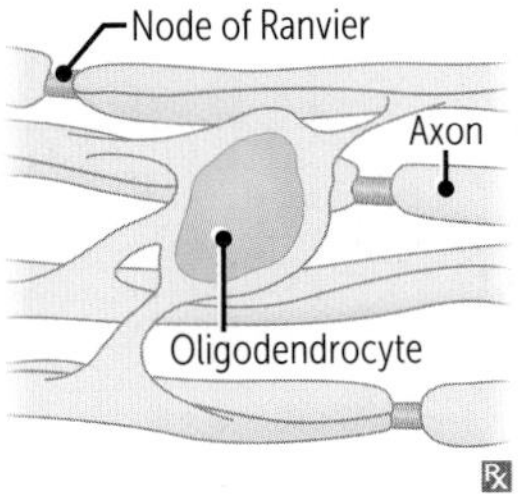	Myelinate axons of neurons in CNS. Each oligodendrocyte can myelinate many axons (~ 30). Predominant type of glial cell in white matter.	Derived from neuroectoderm. "Fried egg" appearance histologically. Injured in multiple sclerosis, progressive multifocal leukoencephalopathy (PML), leukodystrophies.

Neuron action potential

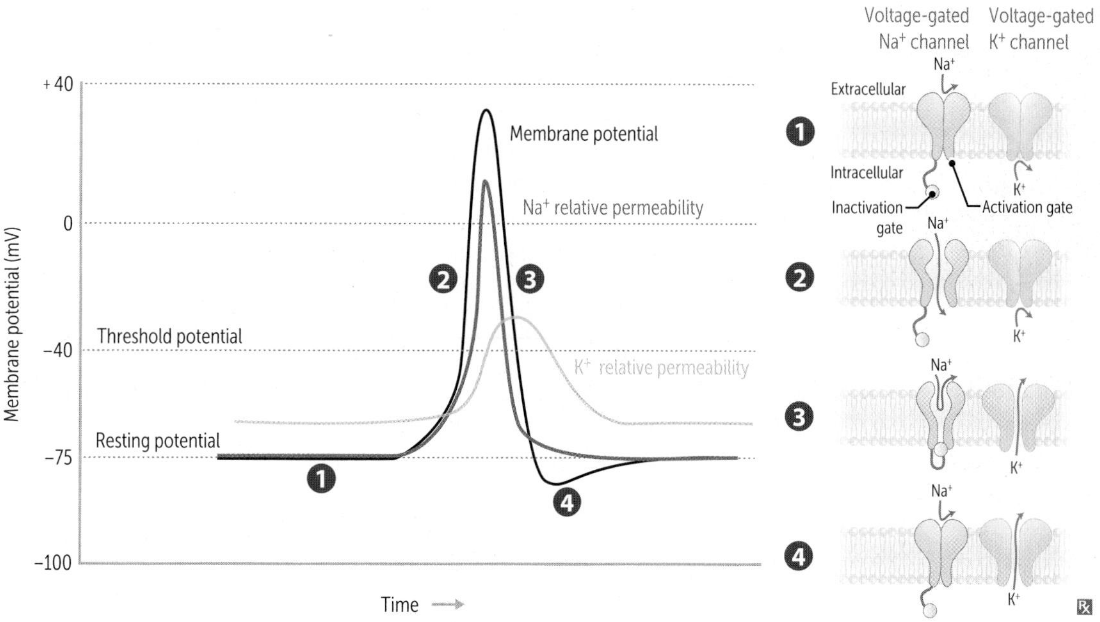

❶ Resting membrane potential: membrane is more permeable to K^+ than Na^+ at rest. Voltage-gated Na^+ and K^+ channels are closed.

❷ Membrane depolarization: Na^+ activation gate opens → Na^+ flows inward.

❸ Membrane repolarization: Na^+ inactivation gate closes at peak potential, thus stopping Na^+ inflow. K^+ activation gate gate opens → K^+ flows outward.

❹ Membrane hyperpolarization: K^+ activation gates are slow to close → excess K^+ efflux and brief period of hyperpolarization. Voltage-gated Na^+ channels switch back to resting state. Na^+/K^+ pump restores ions concentration.

Sensory receptors

RECEPTOR TYPE	SENSORY NEURON FIBER TYPE	LOCATION	SENSES
Free nerve endings	Aδ—fast, myelinated fibers C—slow, unmyelinated A Delta plane is fast, but a taxC is slow	All tissues except cartilage and eye lens; numerous in skin	Pain, temperature
Meissner corpuscles	Large, myelinated fibers; adapt quickly	Glabrous (hairless) skin	Dynamic, fine/light touch, position sense, low-frequency vibration, skin indentation
Pacinian corpuscles	Large, myelinated fibers; adapt quickly	Deep skin layers, ligaments, joints	High-frequency vibration, pressure
Merkel discs	Large, myelinated fibers; adapt slowly	Finger tips, superficial skin	Pressure, deep static touch (eg, shapes, edges)
Ruffini corpuscles	Large, myelinated fiber intertwined among collagen fiber bundles; adapt slowly	Finger tips, joints	Stretch, joint angle change

Peripheral nerve

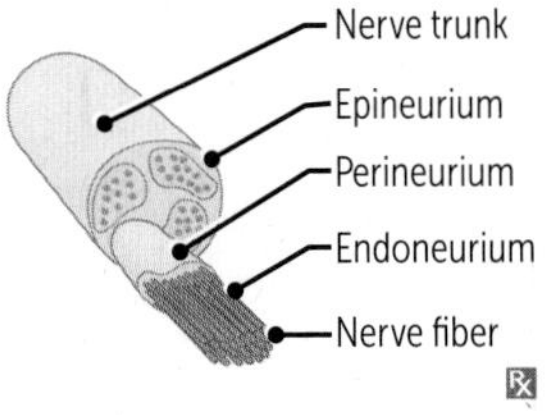

Endoneurium—thin, supportive connective tissue that ensheathes and supports individual myelinated nerve fibers. May be affected in Guillain-Barré syndrome.
Perineurium (blood-nerve permeability barrier)—surrounds a fascicle of nerve fibers.
Epineurium—dense connective tissue that surrounds entire nerve (fascicles and blood vessels).

Endo = inner
Peri = around
Epi = outer

Chromatolysis

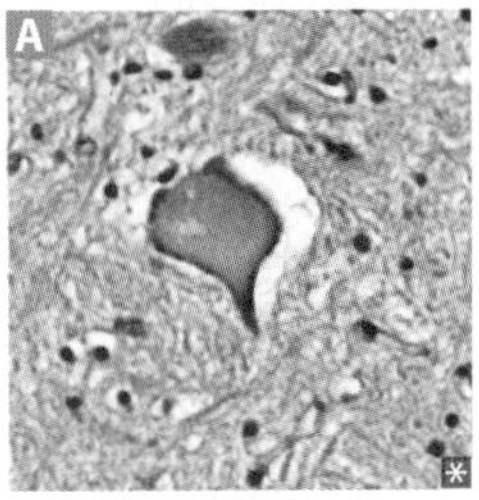

Reaction of neuronal cell body to axonal injury. Changes reflect ↑ protein synthesis in effort to repair the damaged axon. Characterized by:
- Round cellular swelling A
- Displacement of the nucleus to the periphery
- Dispersion of Nissl substance throughout cytoplasm

Wallerian degeneration—disintegration of the axon and myelin sheath distal to site of axonal injury with macrophages removing debris.
Proximal to the injury, the axon retracts, and the cell body sprouts new protrusions that grow toward other neurons for potential reinnervation. Serves as a preparation for axonal regeneration and functional recovery.

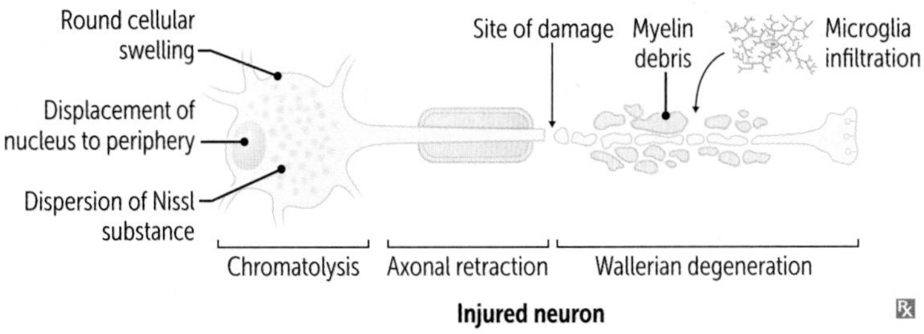

Neurotransmitter changes with disease

	LOCATION OF SYNTHESIS	ANXIETY	DEPRESSION	SCHIZOPHRENIA	ALZHEIMER DISEASE	HUNTINGTON DISEASE	PARKINSON DISEASE
Acetylcholine	Basal nucleus of Meynert (forebrain)				↓	↓	↑
Dopamine	Ventral tegmentum, SNc (midbrain)		↓	↑		↑	↓
GABA	Nucleus accumbens (basal ganglia)	↓				↓	
Norepinephrine	Locus ceruleus (pons)	↑	↓				
Serotonin	Raphe nuclei (brain stem)	↓	↓				↓

Meninges

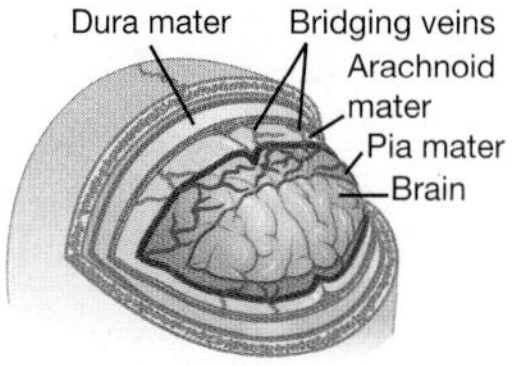

Three membranes that surround and protect the brain and spinal cord:

- Dura mater—thick outer layer closest to skull. Derived from mesoderm.
- Arachnoid mater—middle layer, contains web-like connections. Derived from neural crest.
- Pia mater—thin, fibrous inner layer that firmly adheres to brain and spinal cord. Derived from neural crest.

CSF flows in the subarachnoid space, located between arachnoid and pia mater.

Epidural space—potential space between dura mater and skull/vertebral column containing fat and blood vessels. Site of blood collection associated with middle meningeal artery injury.

Blood-brain barrier

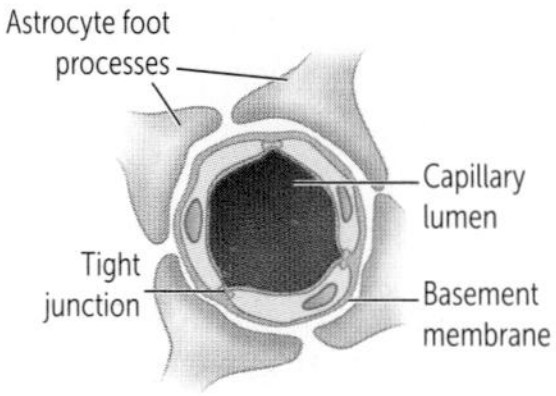

Prevents circulating blood substances (eg, bacteria, drugs) from reaching the CSF/CNS. Formed by 4 structures:

- Tight junctions between nonfenestrated capillary endothelial cells
- Basement membrane
- Astrocyte foot processes
- Pericytes

Glucose and amino acids cross slowly by carrier-mediated transport mechanisms.

Nonpolar/lipid-soluble substances cross rapidly via diffusion.

Circumventricular organs with fenestrated capillaries and no blood-brain barrier allow molecules in blood to affect brain function (eg, area postrema—vomiting after chemotherapy; OVLT [organum vasculosum lamina terminalis]—osmoreceptors) or neurosecretory products to enter circulation (eg, neurohypophysis—ADH release).

Infarction and/or neoplasm destroys endothelial cell tight junctions → vasogenic edema.

Hyperosmolar agents (eg, mannitol) can disrupt the BBB → ↑ permeability of medications.

Vomiting center

Coordinated by nucleus tractus solitarius (NTS) in the medulla, which receives information from the chemoreceptor trigger zone (CTZ, located within area postrema (pronounce "puke"-strema) in 4th ventricle), GI tract (via vagus nerve), vestibular system, and CNS.

CTZ and adjacent vomiting center nuclei receive input from 5 major receptors: muscarinic (M_1), dopamine (D_2), histamine (H_1), serotonin (5-HT_3), and neurokinin (NK-1) receptors.

- 5-HT_3, D_2, and NK-1 antagonists used to treat chemotherapy-induced vomiting.
- H_1 and M_1 antagonists treat motion sickness; H_1 antagonists treat hyperemesis gravidarum.

Sleep physiology

Sleep cycle is regulated by the circadian rhythm, which is driven by suprachiasmatic nucleus (SCN) of the hypothalamus. Circadian rhythm controls nocturnal release of ACTH, prolactin, melatonin, norepinephrine: SCN → norepinephrine release → pineal gland → ↑ melatonin. SCN is regulated by environment (eg, light).

Two stages: rapid-eye movement (REM) and non-REM.

Alcohol, benzodiazepines, and barbiturates are associated with ↓ REM sleep and N3 sleep; norepinephrine also ↓ REM sleep.

Benzodiazepines are useful for night terrors and sleepwalking by ↓ N3 and REM sleep.

SLEEP STAGE (% OF TOTAL SLEEP TIME IN YOUNG ADULTS)	DESCRIPTION	EEG WAVEFORM AND NOTES
Awake (eyes open)	Alert, active mental concentration.	**Beta** (highest frequency, lowest amplitude).
Awake (eyes closed)		**Alpha**.
Non-REM sleep		
Stage N1 (5%)	Light sleep.	**Theta**.
Stage N2 (45%)	Deeper sleep; when bruxism ("**twoth**" [tooth] grinding) occurs.	Sleep spindles and K complexes.
Stage N3 (25%)	Deepest non-REM sleep (slow-wave sleep); **sleepwalking**, night terrors, and **bedwetting** occur (**wee** and **flee** in N3).	**Delta** (lowest frequency, highest amplitude), deepest sleep stage.
REM sleep (25%)	Loss of motor tone, ↑ brain O_2 use, variable pulse/BP, ↑ ACh. REM is when dreaming, nightmares, and penile/clitoral tumescence occur; may serve memory processing function. Extraocular movements due to activity of PPRF (paramedian pontine reticular formation/conjugate gaze center). Occurs every 90 minutes, and duration ↑ through the night.	**Beta**. Changes in elderly: ↓ REM, ↓ N3, ↑ sleep latency, ↑ early awakenings. Changes in depression: ↑ REM sleep time, ↓ REM latency, ↓ N3, repeated nighttime awakenings, early morning awakening (terminal insomnia). Change in narcolepsy: ↓ REM latency. At night, **BATS Drink Blood**.

Hypothalamus	Maintains homeostasis by regulating Thirst and water balance, controlling Adenohypophysis (anterior pituitary) and Neurohypophysis (posterior pituitary) release of hormones produced in the hypothalamus, and regulating Hunger, Autonomic nervous system, Temperature, and Sexual urges (TAN HATS). Inputs (areas not protected by blood-brain barrier): OVLT (senses change in osmolarity), area postrema (found in dorsal medulla, responds to emetics).	
Lateral nucleus	Hunger. Destruction → anorexia, failure to thrive (infants). Stimulated by ghrelin, inhibited by leptin.	Lateral injury makes you lean.
Ventromedial nucleus	Satiety. Destruction (eg, craniopharyngioma) → hyperphagia. Stimulated by leptin.	Ventromedial injury makes you very massive.
Anterior nucleus	Cooling, parasympathetic.	A/C = Anterior Cooling.
Posterior nucleus	Heating, sympathetic.	Heating controlled by posterior nucleus ("hot pot").
Suprachiasmatic nucleus	Circadian rhythm.	SCN is a Sun-Censing Nucleus.
Supraoptic and paraventricular nuclei	Synthesize ADH and oxytocin.	SAD POX: Supraoptic = ADH, Paraventricular = OXytocin. ADH and oxytocin are carried by neurophysins down axons to posterior pituitary, where these hormones are stored and released.
Preoptic nucleus	Thermoregulation, sexual behavior. Releases GnRH.	Failure of GnRH-producing neurons to migrate from olfactory pit → Kallmann syndrome.

Thalamus Major relay for all ascending sensory information except olfaction.

NUCLEI	INPUT	SENSES	DESTINATION	MNEMONIC
Ventral posterolateral nucleus	Spinothalamic and dorsal columns/medial lemniscus	Vibration, pain, pressure, proprioception (conscious), light touch, temperature	1° somatosensory cortex (parietal lobe)	
Ventral posteromedial nucleus	Trigeminal and gustatory pathway	Face sensation, taste	1° somatosensory cortex (parietal lobe)	Very pretty makeup goes on the face
Lateral geniculate nucleus	CN II, optic chiasm, optic tract	Vision	1° visual cortex (occipital lobe)	Lateral = light
Medial geniculate nucleus	Superior olive and inferior colliculus of tectum	Hearing	1° auditory cortex (temporal lobe)	Medial = music
Ventral anterior and lateral nuclei	Basal ganglia, cerebellum	Motor	Motor cortices (frontal lobe)	Venus astronauts love to move

Limbic system

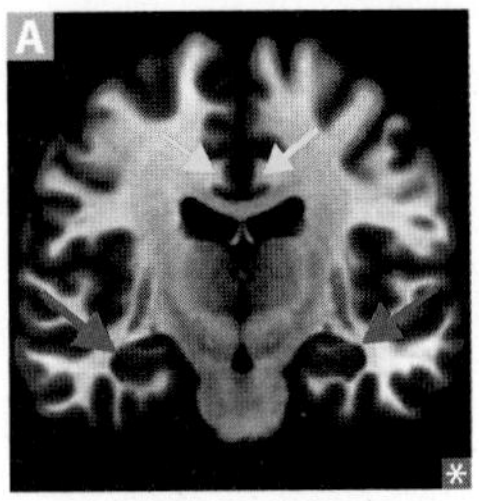

Collection of neural structures involved in emotion, long-term memory, olfaction, behavior modulation, ANS function.
Consists of hippocampus (red arrows in A), amygdalae, mammillary bodies, anterior thalamic nuclei, cingulate gyrus (yellow arrows in A), entorhinal cortex. Responsible for feeding, fleeing, fighting, feeling, and sex.

The famous 5 F's.

Dopaminergic pathways

Commonly altered by drugs (eg, antipsychotics) and movement disorders (eg, Parkinson disease).

PATHWAY	SYMPTOMS OF ALTERED ACTIVITY	NOTES
Mesocortical	↓ activity → "negative" symptoms (eg, anergia, apathy, lack of spontaneity)	Antipsychotic drugs have limited effect
Mesolimbic	↑ activity → "positive" symptoms (eg, delusions, hallucinations)	1° therapeutic target of antipsychotic drugs → ↓ positive symptoms (eg, in schizophrenia)
Nigrostriatal	↓ activity → extrapyramidal symptoms (eg, dystonia, akathisia, parkinsonism, tardive dyskinesia)	Major dopaminergic pathway in brain Significantly affected by movement disorders and antipsychotic drugs
Tuberoinfundibular	↓ activity → ↑ prolactin → ↓ libido, sexual dysfunction, galactorrhea, gynecomastia (in males)	

Cerebellum

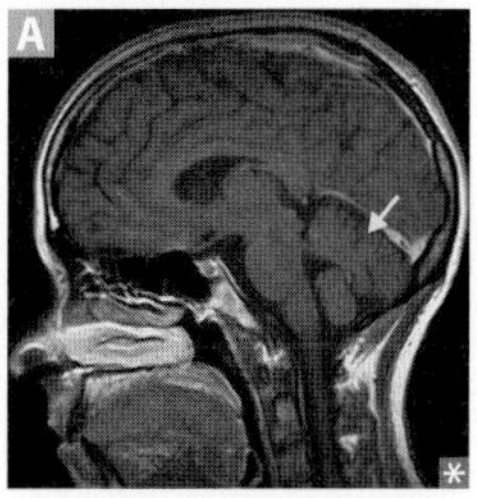
A

Modulates movement; aids in coordination and balance A.
- Ipsilateral (unconscious) proprioceptive information via inferior cerebellar peduncle from spinal cord
- Deep nuclei (lateral → medial)—dentate, emboliform, globose, fastigial

Lateral lesions—affect voluntary movement of extremities (**lateral** structures); when injured, propensity to fall toward injured (ipsilateral) side.

Medial lesions (eg, vermis, fastigial nuclei, flocculonodular lobe)—truncal ataxia (wide-based cerebellar gait), nystagmus, head tilting. Generally result in bilateral motor deficits affecting axial and proximal limb musculature (**medial structures**).

Tests: **finger-to-nose**, gait, heel-to-shin, dysdiadochokinesis.

Don't eat greasy foods.

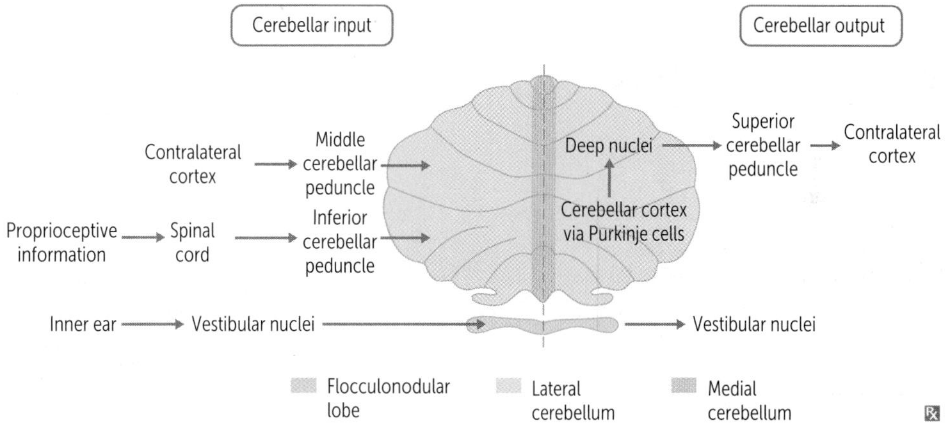
Cerebellar input
Cerebellar output
Contralateral cortex
Middle cerebellar peduncle
Proprioceptive information
Spinal cord
Inferior cerebellar peduncle
Deep nuclei
Cerebellar cortex via Purkinje cells
Superior cerebellar peduncle
Contralateral cortex
Inner ear
Vestibular nuclei
Vestibular nuclei
Flocculonodular lobe
Lateral cerebellum
Medial cerebellum

Basal ganglia

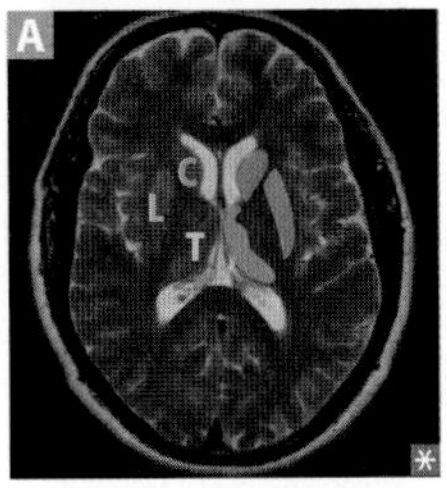

Important in voluntary movements and adjusting posture A.
Receives cortical input, provides negative feedback to cortex to modulate movement.
Striatum = putamen (motor) + Caudate (cognitive).
Lentiform = putamen + globus pallidus.

D_1 **R**eceptor = **D1Rect** pathway.
Indirect (D_2) = **I**nhibitory.

Direct (excitatory) pathway—SNc input to the striatum via the nigrostriatal dopaminergic pathway releases GABA, which inhibits GABA release from the GPi, disinhibiting the Thalamus via the GPi (↑ motion).
Indirect (inhibitory) pathway—SNc input to the striatum via the nigrostriatal dopaminergic pathway releases GABA that disinhibits STN via GPe inhibition, and STN stimulates GPi to inhibit the thalamus (↓ motion).

Dopamine binds to D_1, stimulating the excitatory pathway, and to D_2, inhibiting the inhibitory pathway → ↑ motion.

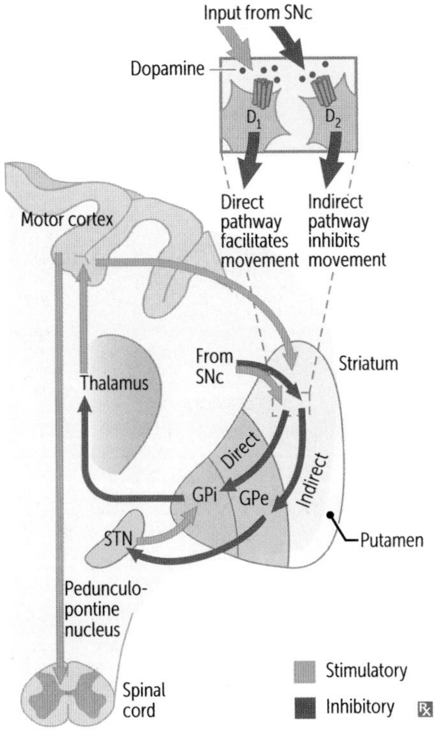

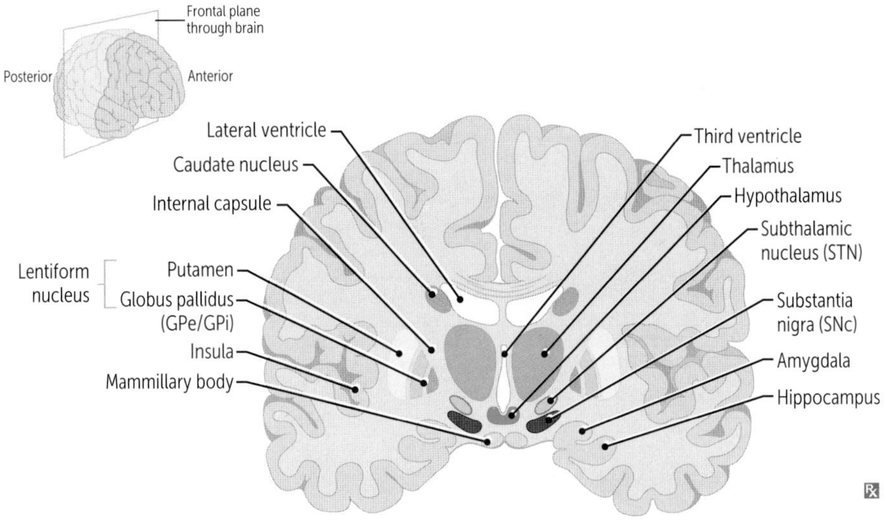

Cerebral cortex regions

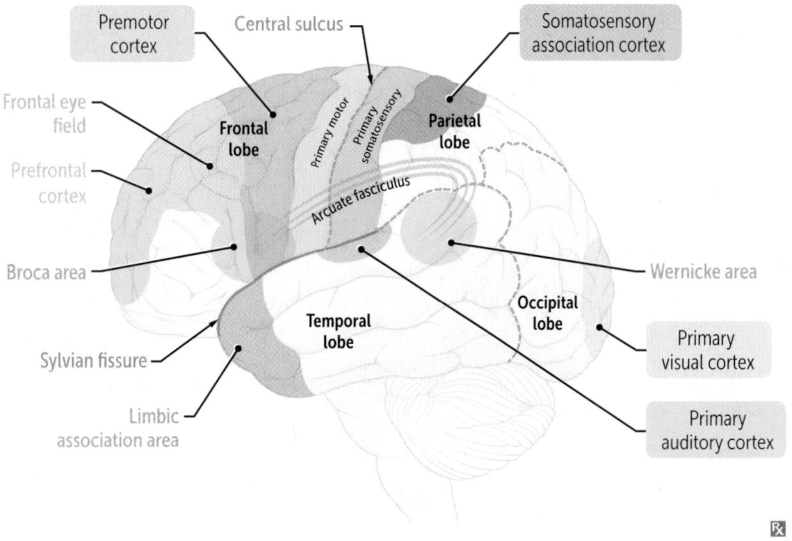

Cerebral perfusion

Relies on tight autoregulation. Primarily driven by P_{CO_2} (P_{O_2} also modulates perfusion in severe hypoxia).

Also relies on a pressure gradient between mean arterial pressure (MAP) and intracranial pressure (ICP). ↓ blood pressure or ↑ ICP → ↓ cerebral perfusion pressure (CPP).

Cushing reflex—triad of hypertension, bradycardia, and respiratory depression in response to ↑ ICP.

Therapeutic hyperventilation → ↓ P_{CO_2} → vasoconstriction → ↓ cerebral blood flow → ↓ ICP. May be used to treat acute cerebral edema (eg, 2° to stroke) unresponsive to other interventions.

CPP = MAP – ICP. If CPP = 0, there is no cerebral perfusion → brain death.

Hypoxemia increases CPP only if P_{O_2} < 50 mm Hg.

CPP is directly proportional to P_{CO_2} until P_{CO_2} > 90 mm Hg.

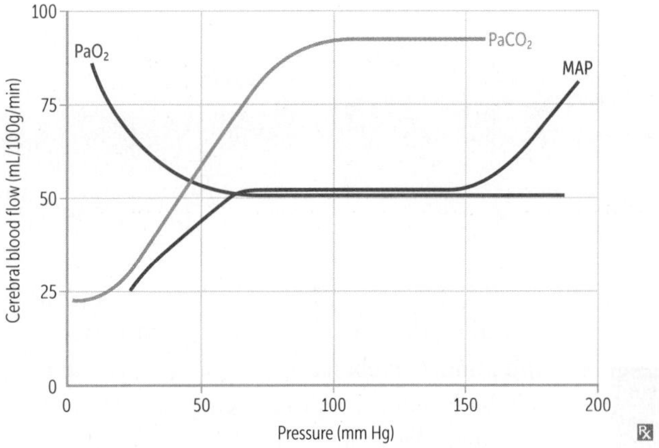

Homunculus

Topographic representation of motor and sensory areas in the cerebral cortex. Distorted appearance is due to certain body regions being more richly innervated and thus having ↑ cortical representation.

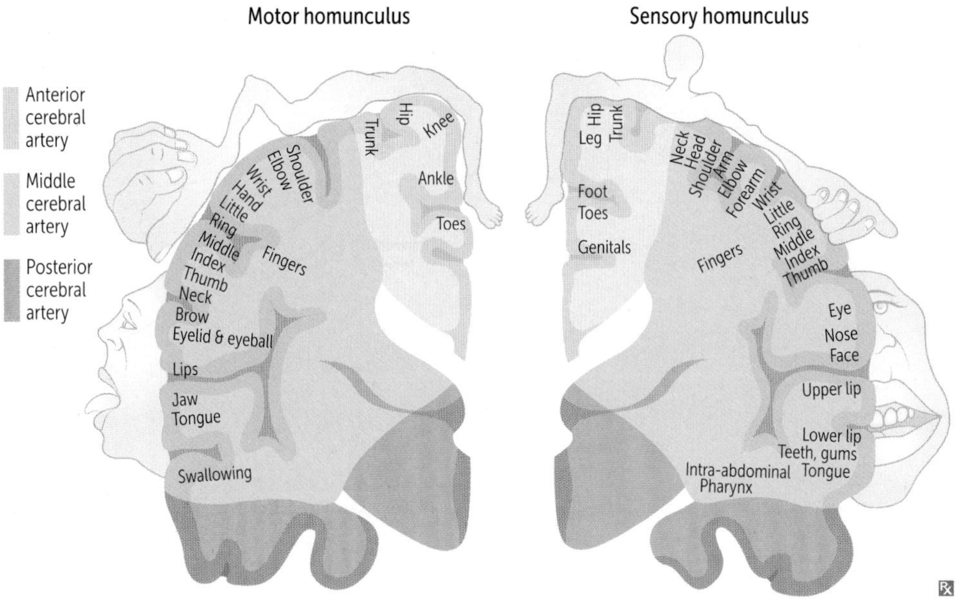

Cerebral arteries—cortical distribution

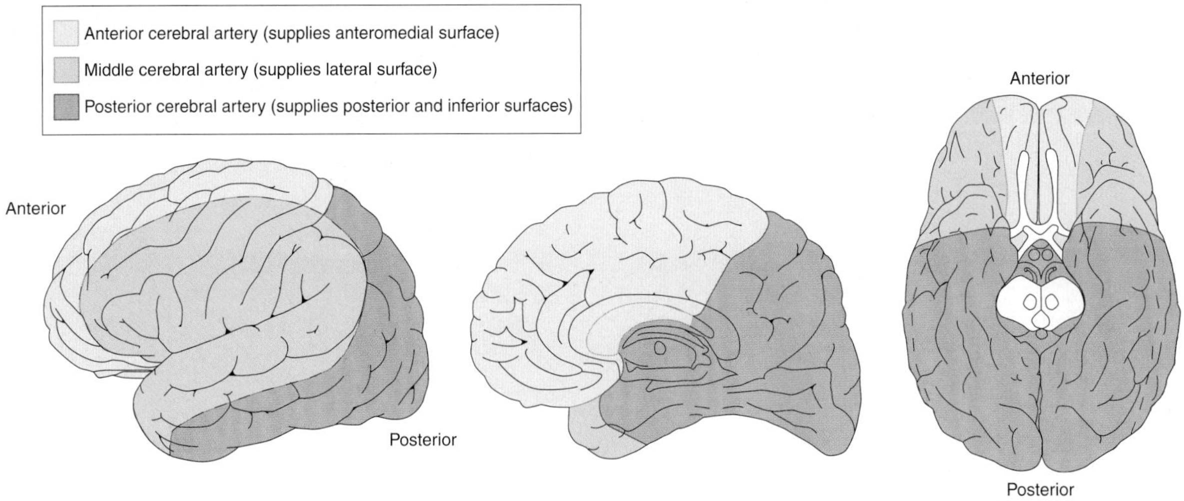

Watershed zones

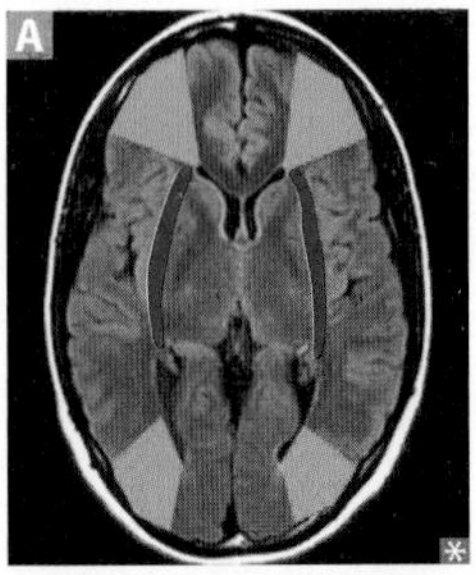

Cortical border zones occur between anterior and middle cerebral arteries and posterior and middle cerebral arteries (blue areas in A).

Internal border zones occur between the superficial and deep vascular territories of the middle cerebral artery (red areas in A).

Common locations for brain metastases.

Infarct due to severe hypoperfusion:

- ACA-MCA watershed infarct—proximal upper and lower extremity weakness ("man-in-a-barrel syndrome").
- PCA-MCA watershed infarct—higher-order visual dysfunction.

Circle of Willis

System of anastomoses between anterior and posterior blood supplies to brain.

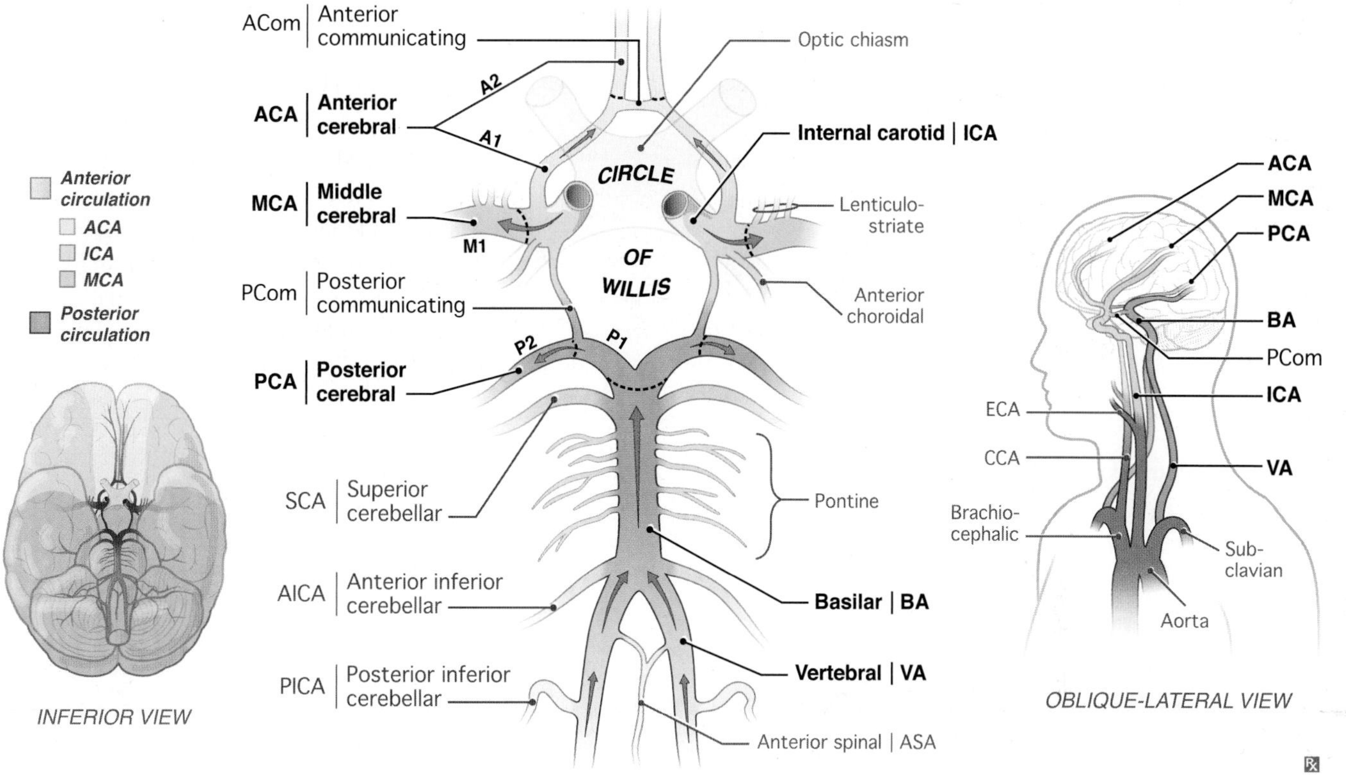

Dural venous sinuses

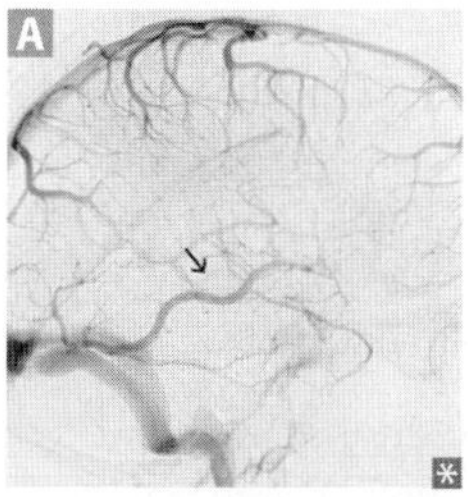

Large venous channels A that run through the periosteal and meningeal layers of the dura mater. Drain blood from cerebral veins (arrow) and receive CSF from arachnoid granulations. Empty into internal jugular vein.

Venous sinus thrombosis—presents with signs/symptoms of ↑ ICP (eg, headache, seizures, papilledema, focal neurologic deficits). May lead to venous hemorrhage. Associated with hypercoagulable states (eg, pregnancy, OCP use, factor V Leiden).

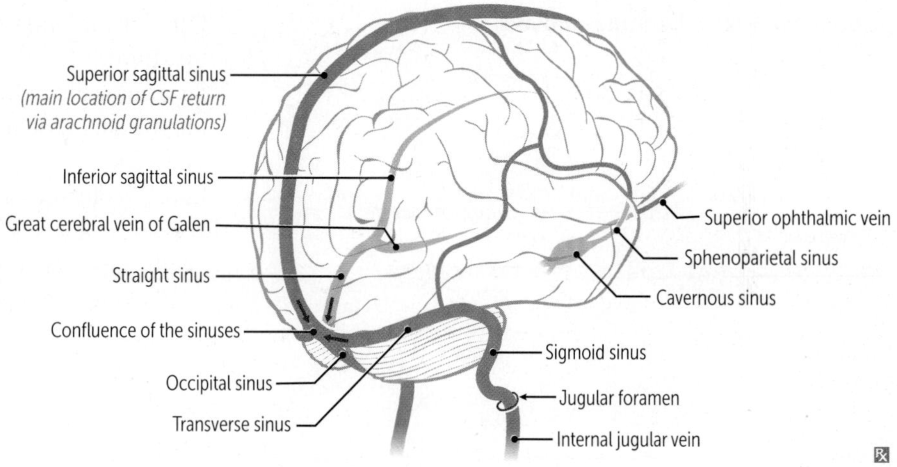

Ventricular system

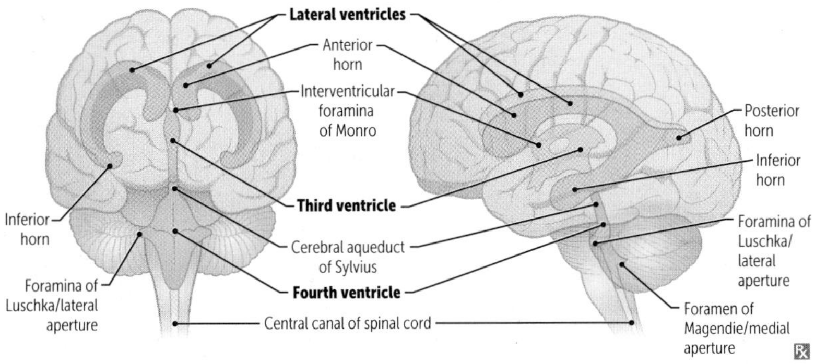

Lateral ventricles → 3rd ventricle via right and left interventricular foramina of Monro.

3rd ventricle → 4th ventricle via cerebral aqueduct of Sylvius.

4th ventricle → subarachnoid space via:
- Foramina of Luschka = lateral.
- Foramen of Magendie = medial.

CSF made by choroid plexuses located in the lateral and fourth ventricles. Travels to subarachnoid space via foramina of Luschka and Magendie, is reabsorbed by arachnoid granulations, and then drains into dural venous sinuses.

Brain stem—ventral view

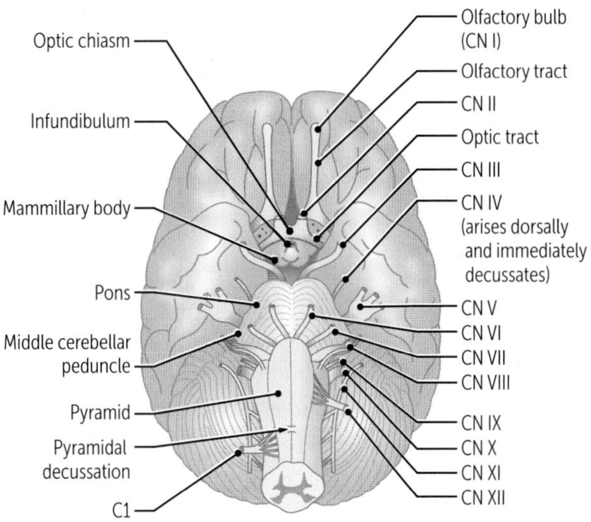

4 CN are above pons (I, II, III, IV).
4 CN exit the pons (V, VI, VII, VIII).
4 CN are in medulla (IX, X, XI, XII).
4 CN nuclei are medial (III, IV, VI, XII).
"Factors of 12, except 1 and 2."

Brain stem—dorsal view (cerebellum removed)

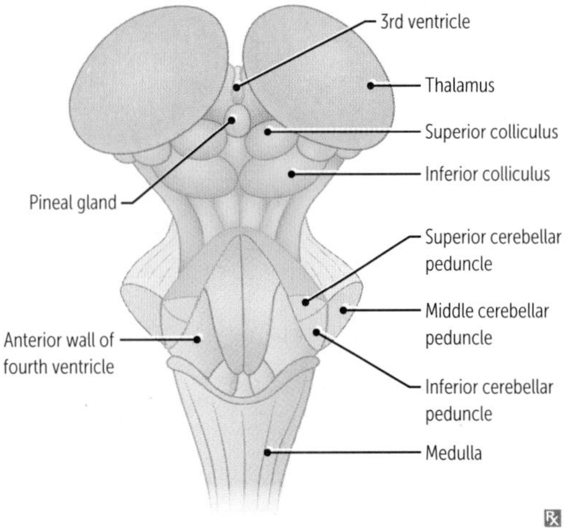

Pineal gland—melatonin secretion, circadian rhythms.

Superior colliculi—direct eye movements to stimuli (noise/movements) or objects of interest.

Inferior colliculi—auditory.

Your eyes are **above** your ears, and the superior colliculus (visual) is **above** the inferior colliculus (auditory).

Cranial nerve nuclei	Located in tegmentum portion of brain stem (between dorsal and ventral portions): ▪ Midbrain—nuclei of CN III, IV ▪ Pons—nuclei of CN V, VI, VII, VIII ▪ Medulla—nuclei of CN IX, X, XII ▪ Spinal cord—nucleus of CN XI	Lateral nuclei = sensory (alar plate). —Sulcus limitans— Medial nuclei = motor (basal plate).

Vagal nuclei

NUCLEUS	FUNCTION	CRANIAL NERVES
Nucleus tractus solitarius	Visceral sensory information (eg, taste, baroreceptors, gut distention) May play a role in vomiting	VII, IX, X
Nucleus ambiguus	Motor innervation of pharynx, larynx, upper esophagus (eg, swallowing, palate elevation)	IX, X, XI (cranial portion)
Dorsal motor nucleus	Sends autonomic (parasympathetic) fibers to heart, lungs, upper GI	X

Cranial nerves and vessel pathways

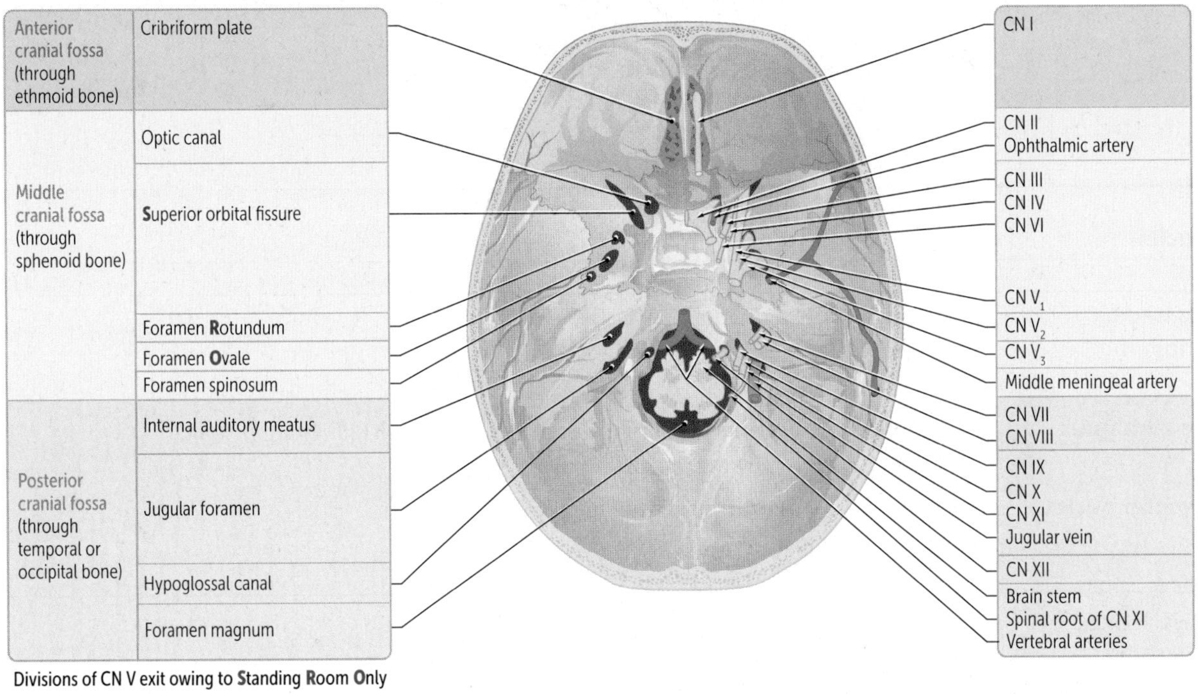

Anterior cranial fossa (through ethmoid bone)
Cribriform plate
Middle cranial fossa (through sphenoid bone)
Optic canal
Superior orbital fissure
Foramen Rotundum
Foramen Ovale
Foramen spinosum
Posterior cranial fossa (through temporal or occipital bone)
Internal auditory meatus
Jugular foramen
Hypoglossal canal
Foramen magnum
CN I
CN II
Ophthalmic artery
CN III
CN IV
CN VI
CN V1
CN V2
CN V3
Middle meningeal artery
CN VII
CN VIII
CN IX
CN X
CN XI
Jugular vein
CN XII
Brain stem
Spinal root of CN XI
Vertebral arteries

Divisions of CN V exit owing to **S**tanding **R**oom **O**nly

Cranial nerves and arteries

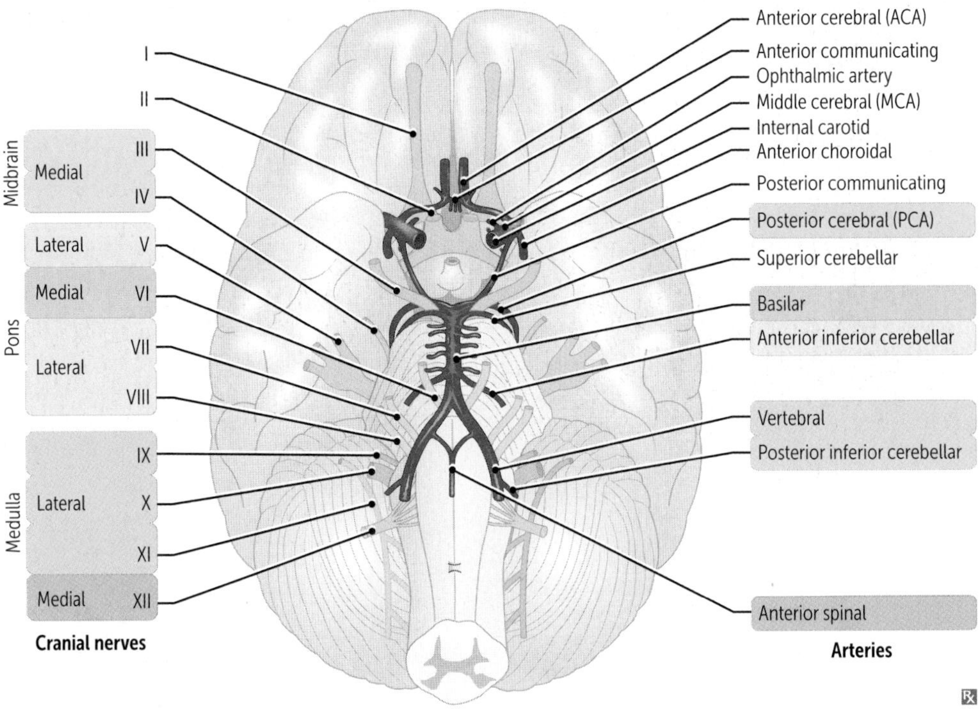

I
II
Midbrain
Medial
III
IV
Pons
Lateral
V
Medial
VI
Lateral
VII
VIII
Medulla
Lateral
IX
X
XI
Medial
XII
Cranial nerves
Anterior cerebral (ACA)
Anterior communicating
Ophthalmic artery
Middle cerebral (MCA)
Internal carotid
Anterior choroidal
Posterior communicating
Posterior cerebral (PCA)
Superior cerebellar
Basilar
Anterior inferior cerebellar
Vertebral
Posterior inferior cerebellar
Anterior spinal
Arteries

Cranial nerves

NERVE	CN	FUNCTION	TYPE	MNEMONIC
Olfactory	I	Smell (only CN without thalamic relay to cortex)	Sensory	Some
Optic	II	Sight	Sensory	Say
Oculomotor	III	Eye movement (SR, IR, MR, IO), pupillary constriction (sphincter pupillae: pretectal nucleus, Edinger-Westphal nuclei, muscarinic receptors), accommodation, eyelid opening (levator palpebrae)	Motor	Marry
Trochlear	IV	Eye movement (SO)	Motor	Money
Trigeminal	V	Mastication, facial sensation (ophthalmic, maxillary, mandibular divisions), somatosensation from anterior 2/3 of tongue, dampening of loud noises (tensor tympani)	Both	But
Abducens	VI	Eye movement (LR)	Motor	My
Facial	VII	Facial movement, taste from anterior 2/3 of tongue (chorda tympani), lacrimation, salivation (submandibular and sublingual glands are innervated by CN seven), eye closing (orbicularis oculi), auditory volume modulation (stapedius)	Both	Brother
Vestibulocochlear	VIII	Hearing, balance	Sensory	Says
Glossopharyngeal	IX	Taste and sensation from posterior 1/3 of tongue, swallowing, salivation (parotid gland), monitoring carotid body and sinus chemo- and baroreceptors, and elevation of pharynx/larynx (stylopharyngeus)	Both	Big
Vagus	X	Taste from supraglottic region, swallowing, soft palate elevation, midline uvula, talking, cough reflex, parasympathetics to thoracoabdominal viscera, monitoring aortic arch chemo- and baroreceptors	Both	Brains
Accessory	XI	Head turning, shoulder shrugging (SCM, trapezius)	Motor	Matter
Hypoglossal	XII	Tongue movement	Motor	Most

Cranial nerve reflexes

REFLEX	AFFERENT	EFFERENT
Corneal	V_1 ophthalmic (nasociliary branch)	Bilateral VII (temporal branch—orbicularis oculi)
Cough	X	X (also phrenic and spinal nerves)
Gag	IX	X
Jaw jerk	V_3 (sensory—muscle spindle from masseter)	V_3 (motor—masseter)
Lacrimation	V_1 (loss of reflex does not preclude emotional tears)	VII
Pupillary	II	III

Mastication muscles

3 muscles close jaw: masseter, temporalis, medial pterygoid. Lateral pterygoids protrude the jaw. All are innervated by trigeminal nerve (V_3).

M's munch.

Spinal nerves

There are 31 pairs of spinal nerves: 8 cervical, 12 thoracic, 5 lumbar, 5 sacral, 1 coccygeal.
Nerves C1–C7 exit above the corresponding vertebrae (eg, C3 exits above the 3rd cervical vertebra). C8 spinal nerve exits below C7 and above T1. All other nerves exit below (eg, L2 exits below the 2nd lumbar vertebra).

Spinal cord—lower extent

In adults, spinal cord ends at lower border of L1–L2 vertebrae. Subarachnoid space (which contains the CSF) extends to lower border of S2 vertebra. Lumbar puncture is usually performed between L3–L4 or L4–L5 (level of cauda equina).

Goal of lumbar puncture is to obtain sample of CSF without damaging spinal cord. To **keep** the cord **alive**, keep the spinal needle between L3 and L5.

Needle passes through:

❶ skin
❷ fascia and fat
❸ supraspinous ligament
❹ interspinous ligament
❺ ligamentum flavum
❻ epidural space
(epidural anesthesia needle stops here)
❼ dura mater
❽ arachnoid mater
❾ subarachnoid space
(CSF collection occurs here)

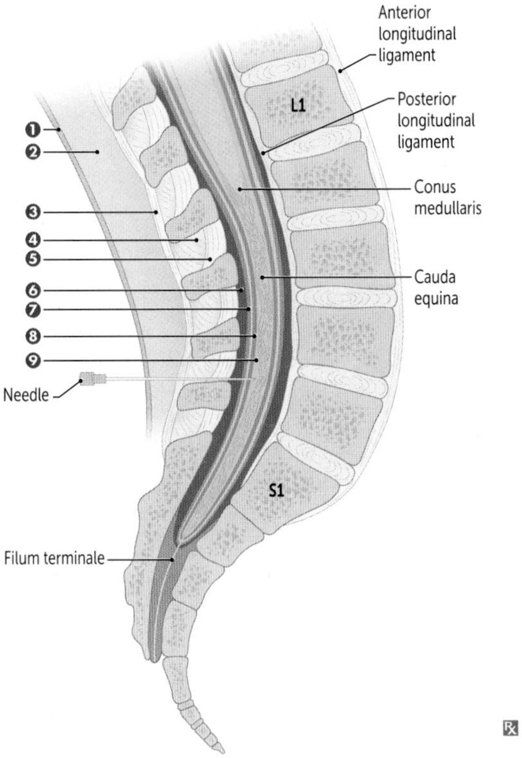

Spinal cord and associated tracts

Legs (lumbosacral) are lateral in lateral corticospinal, spinothalamic tracts. Thoracic spinal cord section in A.

Dorsal columns are organized as you are, with hands at sides. "Arms outside, legs inside."

A

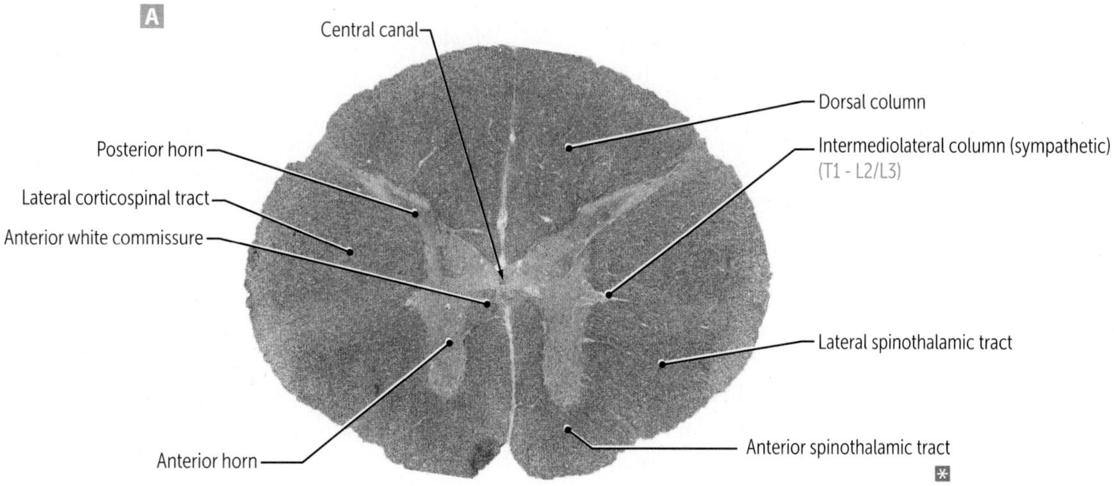
Central canal
Dorsal column
Posterior horn
Intermediolateral column (sympathetic)
(T1 - L2/L3)
Lateral corticospinal tract
Anterior white commissure
Lateral spinothalamic tract
Anterior horn
Anterior spinothalamic tract

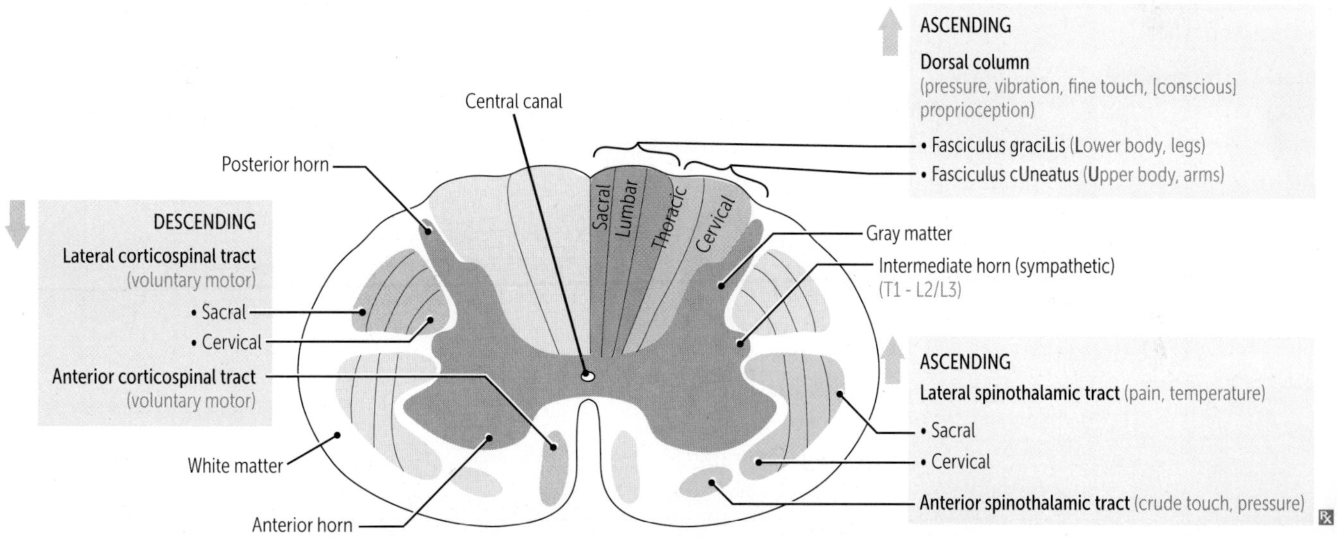
ASCENDING
Dorsal column
(pressure, vibration, fine touch, [conscious] proprioception)
• Fasciculus graciLis (Lower body, legs)
• Fasciculus cUneatus (Upper body, arms)
Central canal
Posterior horn
Sacral
Lumbar
Thoracic
Cervical
Gray matter
Intermediate horn (sympathetic)
(T1 - L2/L3)
DESCENDING
Lateral corticospinal tract
(voluntary motor)
• Sacral
• Cervical
Anterior corticospinal tract
(voluntary motor)
White matter
Anterior horn
ASCENDING
Lateral spinothalamic tract (pain, temperature)
• Sacral
• Cervical
Anterior spinothalamic tract (crude touch, pressure)

Spinal tract anatomy and functions

Ascending tracts synapse and then cross.

TRACT	FUNCTION	1ST-ORDER NEURON	SYNAPSE 1	2ND-ORDER NEURON	SYNAPSE 2 + PROJECTIONS
Ascending tracts					
Dorsal column	Pressure, vibration, fine touch, (conscious) proprioception	Sensory nerve ending → bypasses pseudounipolar cell body in dorsal root ganglion → enters spinal cord → ascends ipsilaterally in dorsal columns	Nucleus gracilis, nucleus cuneatus (ipsilateral medulla)	Decussates in medulla → ascends contralaterally as the medial lemniscus	VPL (thalamus) → sensory cortex
Spinothalamic tract	Lateral: pain, temperature Anterior: crude touch, pressure	Sensory nerve ending (Aδ and C fibers) → bypasses pseudounipolar cell body in dorsal root ganglion → enters spinal cord	Ipsilateral gray matter (spinal cord)	Decussates in spinal cord as the anterior white commissure → ascends contralaterally	VPL (thalamus) → sensory cortex
Descending tract					
Lateral corticospinal tract	Voluntary movement of contralateral limbs	UMN: cell body in 1° motor cortex → descends ipsilaterally (through posterior limb of internal capsule and cerebral peduncle), most fibers decussate at caudal medulla (pyramidal decussation) → descends contralaterally	Cell body of anterior horn (spinal cord)	LMN: leaves spinal cord	NMJ → muscle fibers

Clinical reflexes

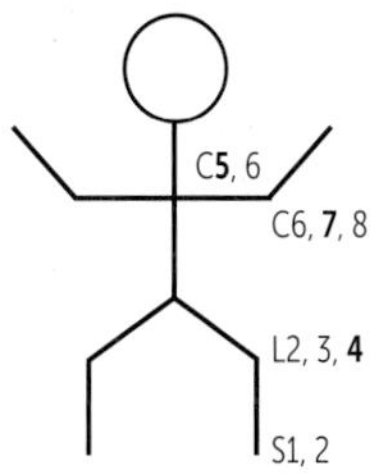

Reflexes count up in order (main nerve root in **bold**):
- **Achilles reflex** = **S1**, S2 ("buckle my shoe")
- **Patellar reflex** = L2-**L4** ("kick the door")
- **Biceps and brachioradialis reflexes** = **C5**, C6 ("pick up sticks")
- **Triceps reflex** = C6, **C7**, C8 ("lay them straight")

Additional reflexes:
- **Cremasteric reflex** = L1, L2 ("testicles move")
- **Anal wink reflex** = S3, S4 ("winks galore")

Reflex grading:
- 0: absent
- 1: hypoactive
- 2: normal
- 3: hyperactive
- 4: clonus

Primitive reflexes

CNS reflexes that are present in a healthy infant, but are absent in a neurologically intact adult. Normally disappear within 1st year of life. These primitive reflexes are inhibited by a mature/developing frontal lobe. They may reemerge in adults following frontal lobe lesions → loss of inhibition of these reflexes.

Moro reflex	"Hang on for life" reflex—abduct/extend arms when startled, and then draw together.
Rooting reflex	Movement of head toward one side if cheek or mouth is stroked (nipple seeking).
Sucking reflex	Sucking response when roof of mouth is touched.
Palmar reflex	Curling of fingers if palm is stroked.
Plantar reflex	Dorsiflexion of large toe and fanning of other toes with plantar stimulation. Babinski sign—presence of this reflex in an adult, which may signify a UMN lesion.
Galant reflex	Stroking along one side of the spine while newborn is in ventral suspension (face down) causes lateral flexion of lower body toward stimulated side.

Landmark dermatomes

DERMATOME	CHARACTERISTICS
C2	Posterior half of skull
C3	High turtleneck shirt Diaphragm and gallbladder pain referred to the right shoulder via phrenic nerve C3, 4, 5 keeps the diaphragm alive
C4	Low-collar shirt
C6	Includes thumbs Thumbs up sign on left hand looks like a 6
T4	At the nipple T4 at the teat pore
T7	At the xiphoid process 7 letters in xiphoid
T10	At the umbilicus (belly butten) Point of referred pain in early appendicitis
L1	At the Inguinal Ligament
L4	Includes the kneecaps Down on ALL 4's
S2, S3, S4	Sensation of penile and anal zones S2, 3, 4 keep the penis off the floor

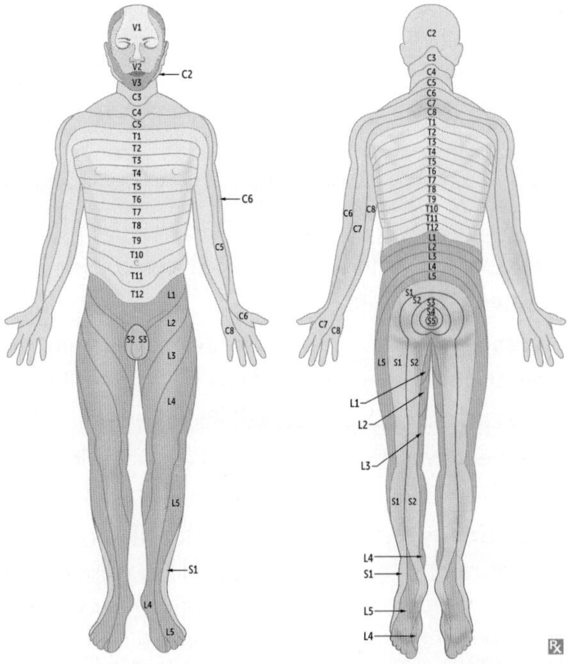

▶ NEUROLOGY—PATHOLOGY

Common brain lesions

AREA OF LESION	CONSEQUENCE	EXAMPLES/COMMENTS
Frontal lobe	Disinhibition and deficits in concentration, orientation, judgment; may have reemergence of primitive reflexes	
Frontal eye fields	Destructive lesions (eg, MCA stroke): eyes look toward brain lesion (ie, away from side of hemiplegia)	
Paramedian pontine reticular formation	Eyes look away from brain lesion (ie, toward side of hemiplegia)	
Medial longitudinal fasciculus	Internuclear ophthalmoplegia (impaired adduction of ipsilateral eye; nystagmus of contralateral eye with abduction)	Multiple sclerosis
Dominant parietal cortex	Agraphia, acalculia, finger agnosia, left-right disorientation	Gerstmann syndrome
Nondominant parietal cortex	Agnosia of the contralateral side of the world	Hemispatial neglect syndrome
Hippocampus (bilateral)	Anterograde amnesia—inability to make new memories	
Basal ganglia	May result in tremor at rest, chorea, athetosis	Parkinson disease, Huntington disease, Wilson disease
Subthalamic nucleus	Contralateral hemiballismus	
Mammillary bodies (bilateral)	Wernicke-Korsakoff syndrome—Confusion, Ataxia, Nystagmus, Ophthalmoplegia, memory loss (anterograde and retrograde amnesia), confabulation, personality changes	Wernicke problems come in a **CAN O'** beer and other conditions associated with thiamine deficiency
Amygdala (bilateral)	Klüver-Bucy syndrome—disinhibited behavior (eg, hyperphagia, hypersexuality, hyperorality)	HSV-1 encephalitis
Dorsal midbrain	Parinaud syndrome—vertical gaze palsy, pupillary light-near dissociation, lid retraction, convergence-retraction nystagmus	Stroke, hydrocephalus, pinealoma
Reticular activating system (midbrain)	Reduced levels of arousal and wakefulness	Coma
Cerebellar hemisphere	Intention tremor, limb ataxia, loss of balance; damage to cerebellum → ipsilateral deficits; fall toward side of lesion	Cerebellar hemispheres are **lateral**ly located—affect **lateral** limbs
Cerebellar vermis	Truncal ataxia (wide-based, "drunken sailor" gait), nystagmus	Vermis is **central**ly located—affects **central** body Degeneration associated with chronic alcohol use
Red nucleus (midbrain)	Decorticate (flexor) posturing—lesion above red nucleus, presents with flexion of upper extremities and extension of lower extremities Decerebrate (extensor) posturing—lesion at or below red nucleus, presents with extension of upper and lower extremities	Worse prognosis with decerebrate posturing In de**cor**ticate posturing, your hands are near the **cor** (heart)

Ischemic brain disease/stroke

Irreversible neuronal injury begins after 5 minutes of hypoxia. Most **vulnerable: hippocampus**, neocortex, cerebellum (**Purkinje** cells), **watershed** areas ("**vulnerable hippos need pure water**").

Stroke imaging: noncontrast CT to exclude hemorrhage (before tPA can be given). CT detects ischemic changes in 6–24 hr. Diffusion-weighted MRI can detect ischemia within 3–30 min.

TIME SINCE ISCHEMIC EVENT	12–24 HOURS	24–72 HOURS	3–5 DAYS	1–2 WEEKS	> 2 WEEKS
Histologic features	Eosinophilic cytoplasm + pyknotic nuclei (red neurons)	Necrosis + neutrophils	Macrophages (microglia)	Reactive gliosis (astrocytes) + vascular proliferation	Glial scar

Ischemic stroke

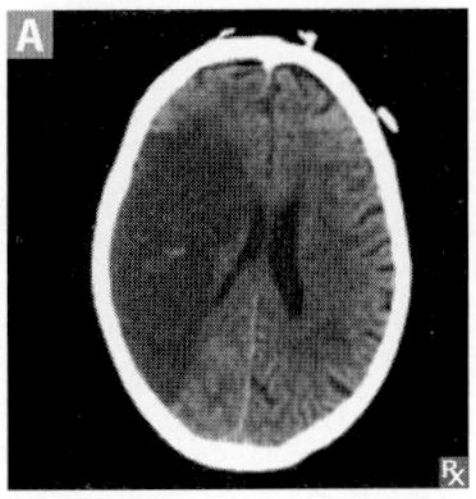

Acute blockage of vessels → disruption of blood flow and subsequent ischemia → infarction → liquefactive necrosis.

3 types:

- Thrombotic—due to a clot forming directly at site of infarction (commonly the MCA A), usually over a ruptured atherosclerotic plaque.
- Embolic—embolus from another part of the body obstructs vessel. Can affect multiple vascular territories. Examples: atrial fibrillation, carotid artery stenosis, DVT with patent foramen ovale (paradoxical embolism), infective endocarditis.
- Hypoxic—due to hypoperfusion or hypoxemia. Common during cardiovascular surgeries, tends to affect watershed areas.

Treatment: tPA (if within 3–4.5 hr of onset and no hemorrhage/risk of hemorrhage) and/or thrombectomy (if large artery occlusion). Reduce risk with medical therapy (eg, aspirin, clopidogrel); optimum control of blood pressure, blood sugars, lipids; smoking cessation; and treat conditions that ↑ risk (eg, atrial fibrillation, carotid artery stenosis).

Transient ischemic attack

Brief, reversible episode of focal neurologic dysfunction without acute infarction (⊖ MRI), with the majority resolving in < 15 minutes; ischemia (eg, embolus, small vessel stenosis). May present with amaurosis fugax (transient visual loss) due to retinal artery emboli from carotid artery disease.

Neonatal intraventricular hemorrhage

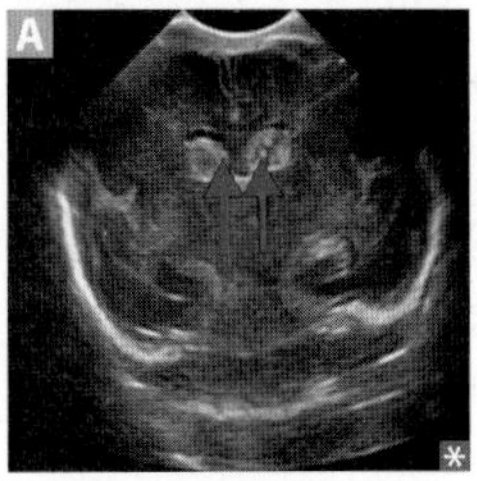

Bleeding into ventricles (arrows in A show blood in intraventricular spaces on ultrasound). Increased risk in premature and low-birth-weight infants. Originates in germinal matrix, a highly vascularized layer within the subventricular zone. Due to reduced glial fiber support and impaired autoregulation of BP in premature infants. Can present with altered level of consciousness, bulging fontanelle, hypotension, seizures, coma.

Intracranial hemorrhage

Epidural hematoma

Rupture of middle meningeal artery (branch of maxillary artery), often 2° to skull fracture (circle in A) involving the pterion (thinnest area of the lateral skull). Might present with transient loss of consciousness → recovery ("lucid interval") → rapid deterioration due to hematoma expansion.

Scalp hematoma (arrows in A) and rapid intracranial expansion (arrows in B) under systemic arterial pressure → transtentorial herniation, CN III palsy.

CT shows biconvex (lentiform), hyperdense blood collection B **not crossing suture lines**.

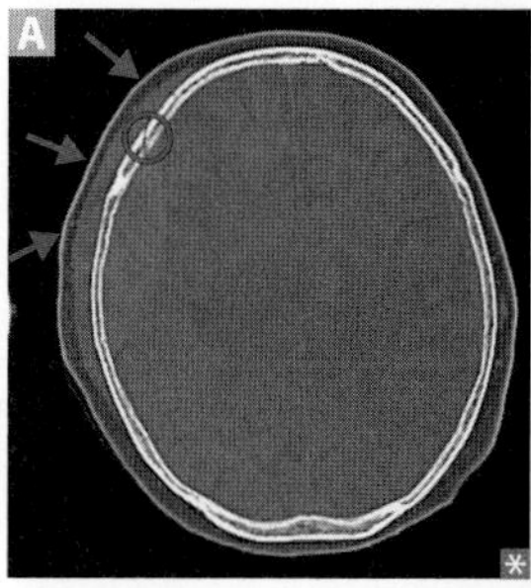
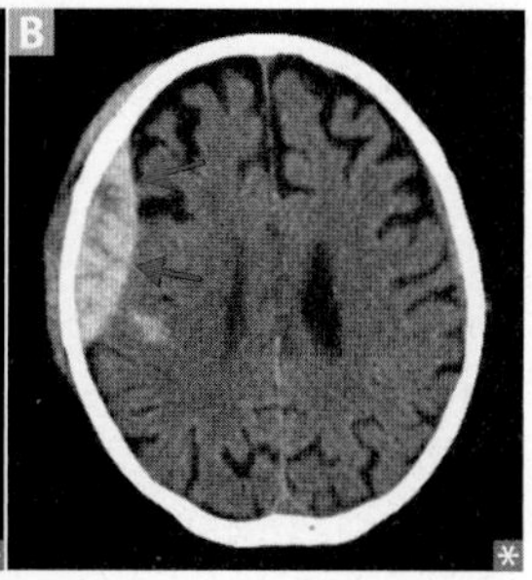

Subdural hematoma

Rupture of bridging veins. Can be acute (traumatic, high-energy impact → hyperdense on CT) or chronic (associated with mild trauma, cerebral atrophy, elderly, chronic alcohol overuse → hypodense on CT). Also seen in shaken babies. Predisposing factors: brain atrophy, trauma.

Crescent-shaped hemorrhage (red arrows in C and D) that **crosses suture lines**. Can cause midline shift (yellow arrow in C), findings of "acute on chronic" hemorrhage (blue arrows in D).

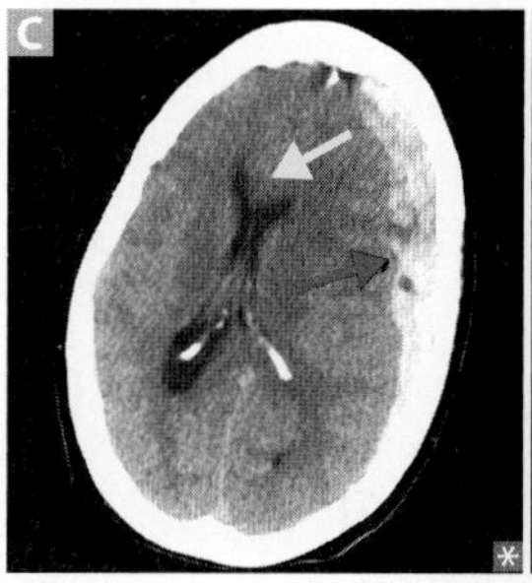
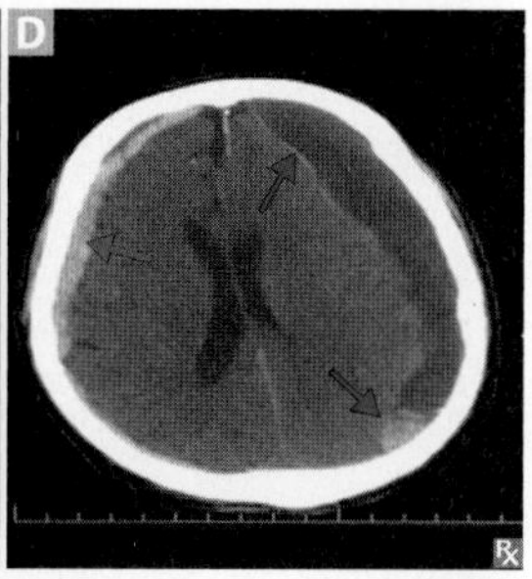

Subarachnoid hemorrhage

Bleeding E F due to trauma, or rupture of an aneurysm (such as a saccular aneurysm E) or arteriovenous malformation. Rapid time course. Patients complain of "worst headache of my life." Bloody or yellow (xanthochromic) lumbar puncture.

Vasospasm can occur due to blood breakdown or rebleed 3–10 days after hemorrhage → ischemic infarct; nimodipine used to prevent/reduce vasospasm. ↑ risk of developing communicating and/or obstructive hydrocephalus.

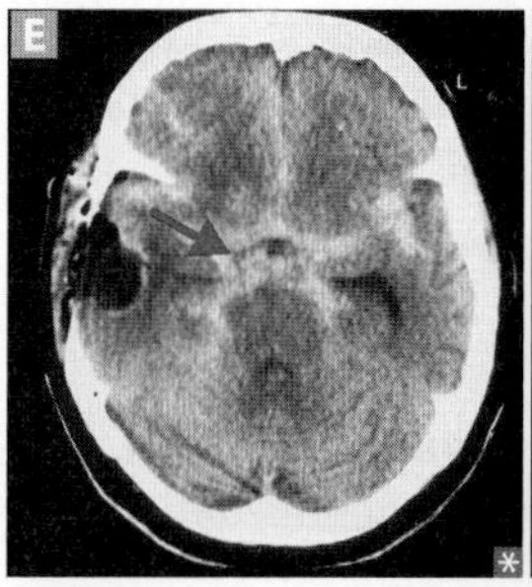
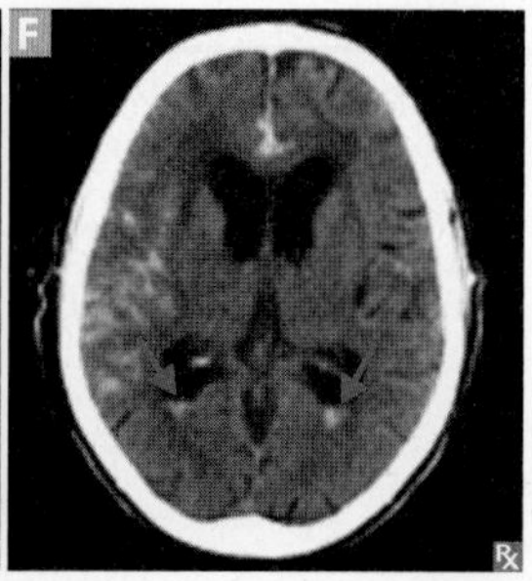

Intraparenchymal hemorrhage

Most commonly caused by systemic hypertension. Also seen with amyloid angiopathy (recurrent lobar hemorrhagic stroke in elderly), vascular malformations, vasculitis, neoplasm. May be 2° to reperfusion injury in ischemic stroke.

Hypertensive hemorrhages (Charcot-Bouchard microaneurysm) most often occur in putamen of basal ganglia (lenticulostriate vessels G), followed by thalamus, pons, and cerebellum H.

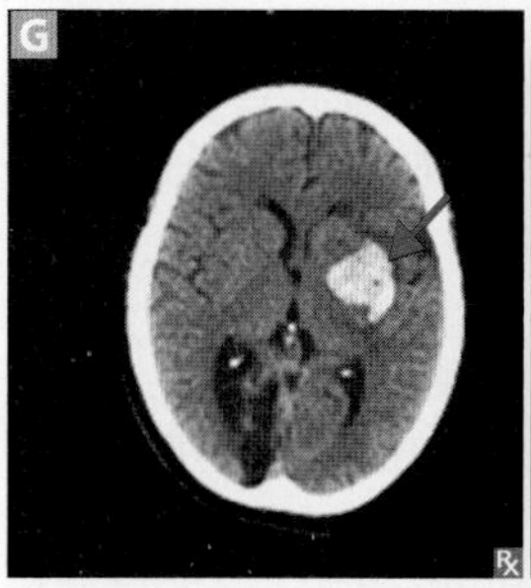
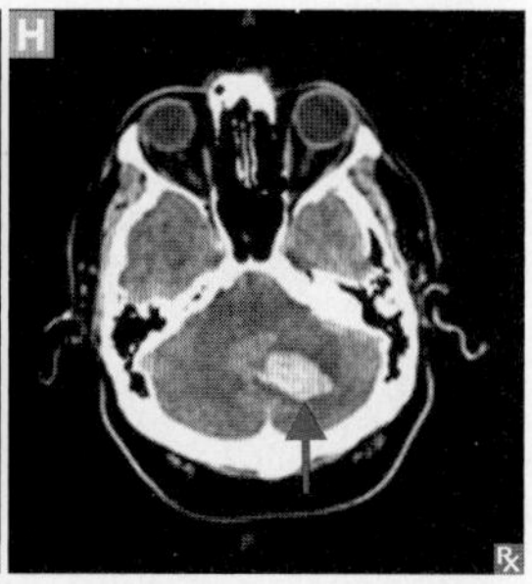

Effects of strokes

ARTERY	AREA OF LESION	SYMPTOMS	NOTES
Anterior circulation			
Anterior cerebral artery	Motor and sensory cortices—lower limb.	Contralateral paralysis and sensory loss—lower limb, urinary incontinence.	
Middle cerebral artery	Motor and sensory cortices **A**—upper limb and face. Temporal lobe (Wernicke area); frontal lobe (Broca area).	Contralateral paralysis and sensory loss—face and upper limb. Aphasia if in dominant (usually left) hemisphere. Hemineglect if lesion affects nondominant (usually right) hemisphere.	Wernicke aphasia is associated with right superior quadrant visual field defect due to temporal lobe involvement.
Lenticulo-striate artery	Striatum, internal capsule.	Contralateral paralysis. Absence of cortical signs (eg, neglect, aphasia, visual field loss).	Pure motor stroke (most common). Common location of lacunar infarcts **B**, due to microatheroma and hyaline arteriosclerosis (lipohyalinosis) 2° to unmanaged hypertension.
Posterior circulation			
Posterior cerebral artery	Occipital lobe **C**.	Contralateral hemianopia with macular sparing; alexia without agraphia (dominant hemisphere, extending to splenium of corpus callosum); prosopagnosia (nondominant hemisphere).	
Basilar artery	Pons, medulla, lower midbrain. Corticospinal and corticobulbar tracts. Ocular cranial nerve nuclei, paramedian pontine reticular formation.	If RAS spared, consciousness is preserved. Quadriplegia; loss of voluntary facial, mouth, and tongue movements. Loss of horizontal, but not vertical, eye movements.	**Locked**-in syndrome (**locked in the basement**).
Anterior inferior cerebellar artery	Facial nucleus. Vestibular nuclei. Spinothalamic tract, spinal trigeminal nucleus. Sympathetic fibers. Middle and inferior cerebellar peduncles. Labyrinthine artery.	Paralysis of face (LMN lesion vs UMN lesion in cortical stroke), ↓ lacrimation, ↓ salivation, ↓ taste from anterior 2/3 of tongue. Vomiting, vertigo, nystagmus ↓ pain and temperature sensation from contralateral body, ipsilateral face. Ipsilateral Horner syndrome. Ipsilateral ataxia, dysmetria. Ipsilateral sensorineural deafness, vertigo.	Lateral pontine syndrome. Facial nucleus effects are specific to AICA lesions.

Effects of strokes *(continued)*

ARTERY	AREA OF LESION	SYMPTOMS	NOTES
Posterior inferior cerebellar artery	Nucleus ambiguus (CN IX, X, XI).	**Dysphagia, hoarseness**, ↓ gag reflex, hiccups.	Lateral medullary (Wallenberg) syndrome.
	Vestibular nuclei.	Vomiting, vertigo, nystagmus	Nucleus ambiguus effects are specific to PICA lesions D.
	Lateral spinothalamic tract, spinal trigeminal nucleus.	↓ pain and temperature sensation from contralateral body, ipsilateral face.	"Don't **pick a** (**PICA**) **horse** (hoarseness) that **can't eat** (dysphagia)."
	Sympathetic fibers.	Ipsilateral Horner syndrome.	
	Inferior cerebellar peduncle.	Ipsilateral ataxia, dysmetria.	
Anterior spinal artery	Corticospinal tract.	Contralateral paralysis—upper and lower limbs.	Medial Medullary syndrome—caused by infarct of paramedian branches of ASA and/or vertebral arteries. **Ants** love **M&M's**.
	Medial lemniscus.	↓ contralateral proprioception.	
	Caudal medulla—hypoglossal nerve.	Ipsilateral hypoglossal dysfunction (tongue deviates ipsilaterally).	

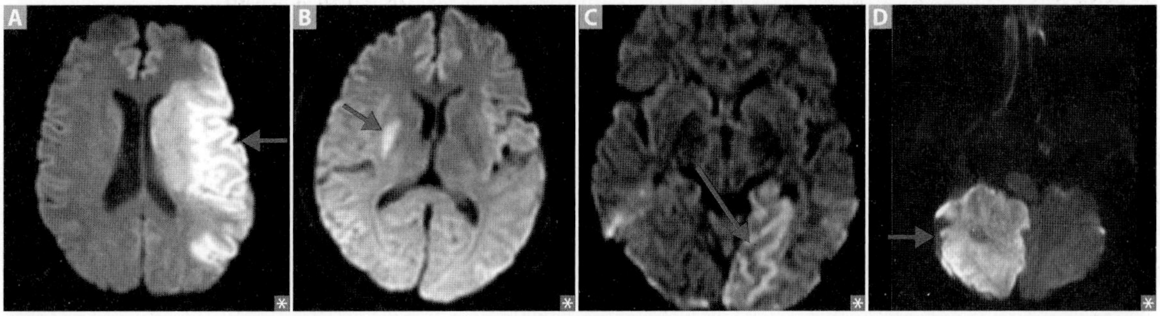

Central poststroke pain syndrome

Neuropathic pain due to thalamic lesions. Initial paresthesias followed in weeks to months by allodynia (ordinarily painless stimuli cause pain) and dysesthesia (altered sensation) on the contralateral side. Occurs in 10% of stroke patients.

Diffuse axonal injury

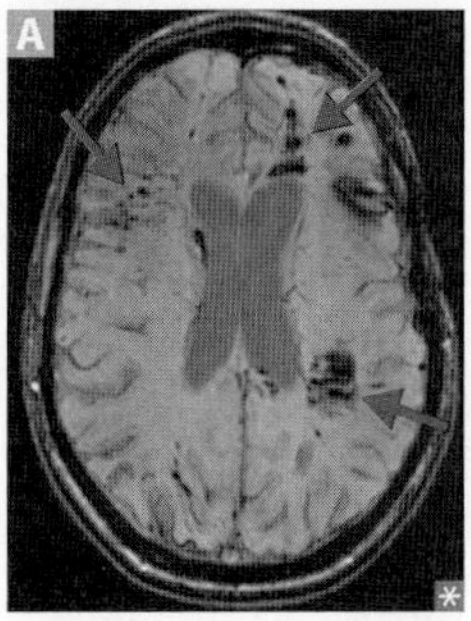

Traumatic shearing of white matter tracts during rapid acceleration and/or deceleration of the brain (eg, motor vehicle accident). Usually results in devastating neurologic injury, often causing coma or persistent vegetative state. MRI shows multiple lesions (punctate hemorrhages) involving white matter tracts A.

Aphasia

Aphasia—higher-order language deficit (inability to understand/produce/use language appropriately); caused by pathology in dominant cerebral hemisphere (usually left).
Dysarthria—motor inability to produce speech (movement deficit).

TYPE	COMMENTS
Broca (expressive)	Broca area in inferior frontal gyrus of frontal lobe. Associated with defective language production. Patients appear frustrated, insight intact. Broca = broken boca (*boca* = mouth in Spanish).
Wernicke (receptive)	Wernicke area in superior temporal gyrus of temporal lobe. Associated with impaired language comprehension. Patients do not have insight. Wernicke is a word salad and makes no sense.
Conduction	Can be caused by damage to arCuate fasciculus.
Global	Broca and Wernicke areas affected.

Aneurysms

Abnormal dilation of an artery due to weakening of vessel wall.

Saccular aneurysm

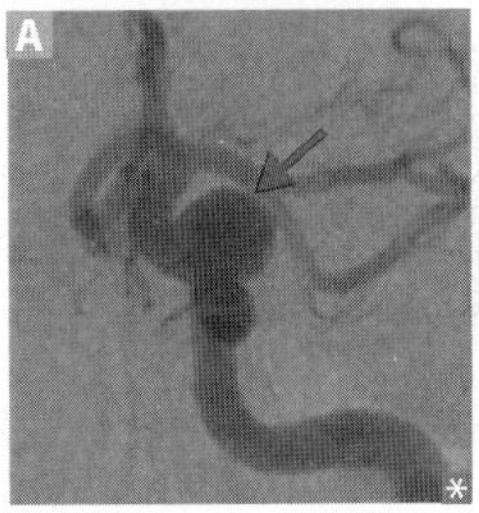

Also called berry aneurysm A. Occurs at bifurcations in the circle of Willis. Most common site is junction of ACom and ACA. Associated with ADPKD, Ehlers-Danlos syndrome. Other risk factors: advanced age, hypertension, tobacco smoking.

Usually clinically silent until rupture (most common complication) → subarachnoid hemorrhage ("worst headache of my life" or "thunderclap headache") → focal neurologic deficits. Can also cause symptoms via direct compression of surrounding structures by growing aneurysm.

- ACom—compression → bitemporal hemianopia (compression of optic chiasm); visual acuity deficits; rupture → ischemia in ACA distribution → contralateral lower extremity hemiparesis, sensory deficits.
- MCA—rupture → ischemia in MCA distribution → contralateral upper extremity and lower facial hemiparesis, sensory deficits.
- PCom—compression → ipsilateral CN III palsy → mydriasis ("blown pupil"); may also see ptosis, "down and out" eye.

Charcot-Bouchard microaneurysm

Common, associated with chronic hypertension; affects small vessels (eg, lenticulostriate arteries in basal ganglia, thalamus) and can cause hemorrhagic intraparenchymal strokes. Not visible on angiography.

Fever vs heat stroke

	Fever	Heat stroke
PATHOPHYSIOLOGY	Cytokine activation during inflammation (eg, infection)	Inability of body to dissipate heat (eg, exertion)
TEMPERATURE	Usually < 40°C (104°F)	Usually > 40°C (104°F)
COMPLICATIONS	Febrile seizure (benign, usually self-limiting)	CNS dysfunction (eg, confusion), end-organ damage, acute respiratory distress syndrome, rhabdomyolysis
MANAGEMENT	Acetaminophen or ibuprofen for comfort (does not prevent future febrile seizures), antibiotic therapy if indicated	Rapid external cooling, rehydration and electrolyte correction

Seizures	Characterized by synchronized, high-frequency neuronal firing. Variety of forms.	
Partial (focal) seizures	Affect single area of the brain. Most commonly originate in medial temporal lobe. Types: ▪ Simple partial (consciousness intact)—motor, sensory, autonomic, psychic ▪ Complex partial (impaired consciousness, automatisms)	Epilepsy—disorder of recurrent, unprovoked seizures (febrile seizures are not epilepsy). Status epilepticus—continuous (≥ 5 min) or recurring seizures that may result in brain injury. Causes of seizures by age: ▪ Children—genetic, infection (febrile), trauma, congenital, metabolic ▪ Adults—tumor, trauma, stroke, infection ▪ Elderly—stroke, tumor, trauma, metabolic, infection
Generalized seizures	Diffuse. Types: ▪ Absence (petit mal)—3 Hz spike-and-wave discharges, short (usually 10 seconds) and frequent episodes of blank stare, no postictal confusion. Can be triggered by hyperventilation ▪ Myoclonic—quick, repetitive jerks ▪ Tonic-clonic (grand mal)—alternating stiffening and movement, postictal confusion, urinary incontinence, tongue biting ▪ Tonic—stiffening ▪ Atonic—"drop" seizures (falls to floor); commonly mistaken for fainting	

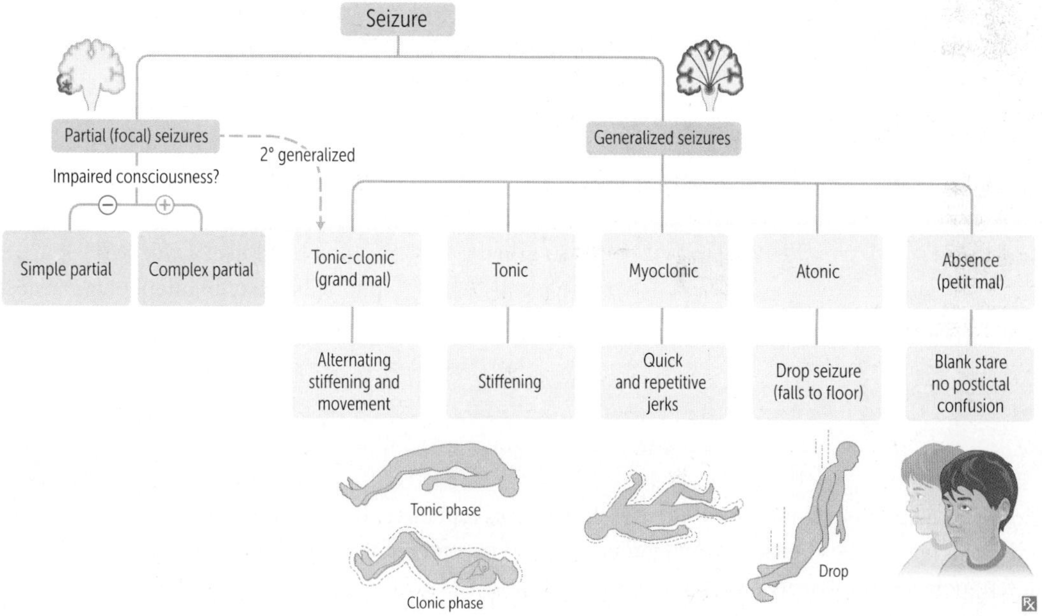

Headaches

Pain due to irritation of structures such as the dura, cranial nerves, or extracranial structures. Primary headaches include cluster, migraine, and tension; migraine and tension headaches are more common in females. Secondary headaches include subarachnoid hemorrhage, meningitis, hydrocephalus, neoplasia, giant cell (temporal) arteritis.

CLASSIFICATION	LOCALIZATION	DURATION	DESCRIPTION	TREATMENT
Cluster[a] 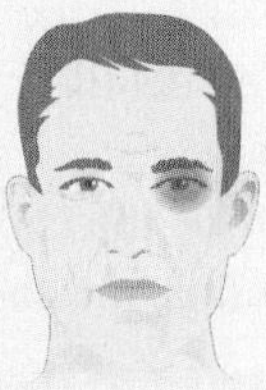	Unilateral	15 min–3 hr; repetitive	Excruciating periorbital pain ("suicide headache") with autonomic symptoms (eg, lacrimation, rhinorrhea, conjunctival injection). May present with Horner syndrome. More common in males.	Acute: sumatriptan, 100% O_2. Prophylaxis: verapamil.
Migraine 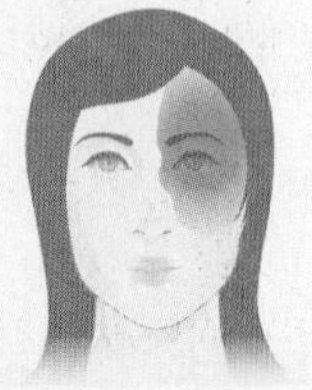	Unilateral	4–72 hr	Pulsating pain with nausea, photophobia, and/or phonophobia. May have "aura." Due to irritation of CN V, meninges, or blood vessels (release of vasoactive neuropeptides [eg, substance P, calcitonin gene-related peptide]).	Acute: NSAIDs, triptans, dihydroergotamine, antiemetics (eg, prochlorperazine, metoclopramide). Prophylaxis: lifestyle changes (eg, sleep, exercise, diet), β-blockers, amitriptyline, topiramate, valproate, botulinum toxin, anti-CGRP monoclonal antibodies. POUND–Pulsatile, One-day duration, Unilateral, Nausea, Disabling.
Tension 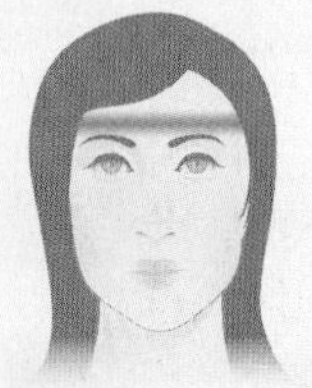	Bilateral	> 30 min (typically 4–6 hr); constant	Steady, "band-like" pain. No photophobia or phonophobia. No aura.	Acute: analgesics, NSAIDs, acetaminophen. Prophylaxis: TCAs (eg, amitriptyline), behavioral therapy.

[a]Compare with **trigeminal neuralgia**, which produces repetitive, unilateral, shooting/shock-like pain in the distribution of CN V. Triggered by chewing, talking, touching certain parts of the face. Lasts (typically) for seconds to minutes, but episodes often increase in intensity and frequency over time. First-line therapy: carbamazepine.

Movement disorders

DISORDER	PRESENTATION	CHARACTERISTIC LESION	NOTES
Akathisia	Restlessness and intense urge to move		Can be seen with neuroleptic use or as a side effect of Parkinson treatment
Asterixis	Extension of wrists causes "flapping" motion		Associated with hepatic encephalopathy, Wilson disease, and other metabolic derangements
Athetosis	Slow, snake-like, writhing movements; especially seen in the fingers	Basal ganglia	Seen in Huntington disease
Chorea	Sudden, jerky, purposeless movements	Basal ganglia	*Chorea* = dancing Seen in Huntington disease and in acute rheumatic fever (Sydenham chorea)
Dystonia	Sustained, involuntary muscle contractions		Writer's cramp, blepharospasm, torticollis Treatment: botulinum toxin injection
Essential tremor	High-frequency tremor with sustained posture (eg, outstretched arms), worsened with movement or when anxious		Often familial Patients often self-medicate with alcohol, which ↓ tremor amplitude Treatment: nonselective β-blockers (eg, propranolol), barbiturates (primidone)
Intention tremor	Slow, zigzag motion when pointing/extending toward a target	Cerebellar dysfunction	
Resting tremor	Uncontrolled movement of distal appendages (most noticeable in hands); tremor alleviated by intentional movement	Substantia nigra (**Park**inson disease)	Occurs at rest; "pill-rolling tremor" of Parkinson disease When you **park** your car, it is at **rest**
Hemiballismus	Sudden, wild flailing of one side of the body	Contralateral subthalamic nucleus (eg, lacunar stroke)	Pronounce "**Half-of-body** is going **ballistic**"
Myoclonus	Sudden, brief, uncontrolled muscle contraction		Jerks; hiccups; common in metabolic abnormalities (eg, renal and liver failure), Creutzfeldt-Jakob disease
Restless legs syndrome	Uncomfortable sensations in legs causing irresistible urge to move them; relieved by movement; worse at rest/nightime		Associated with iron deficiency, CKD Treatment: dopamine agonists (pramipexole, ropinirole)

Neurodegenerative disorders

↓ in cognitive ability, memory, or function with intact consciousness.
Must rule out depression as cause of dementia (called pseudodementia). Other reversible causes of dementia: hypothyroidism, vitamin B_{12} deficiency, neurosyphilis, normal pressure hydrocephalus.

DISEASE	DESCRIPTION	HISTOLOGIC/GROSS FINDINGS
Parkinson disease	Parkinson **TRAPSS** your body: **T**remor (pill-rolling tremor at rest) **R**igidity (cogwheel) **A**kinesia (or bradykinesia) **P**ostural instability **S**huffling gait **S**mall handwriting (micrographia) Dementia is usually a late finding. MPTP, a contaminant in illegal drugs, is metabolized to MPP+, which is toxic to substantia nigra.	Loss of dopaminergic neurons (ie, depigmentation) of substantia nigra pars compacta. Lewy bodies: composed of α-synuclein (intracellular eosinophilic inclusions A).
Huntington disease	Autosomal dominant trinucleotide $(CAG)_n$ repeat expansion in the **hunt**ingtin (*HTT*) gene on chromosome 4 (**4 letters**). Symptoms manifest between ages 20 and 50: chorea, athetosis, aggression, depression, dementia (sometimes initially mistaken for substance use). Anticipation results from expansion of CAG repeats. Caudate loses ACh and GABA.	Atrophy of caudate and putamen with ex vacuo ventriculomegaly. ↑ dopamine, ↓ GABA, ↓ ACh in brain. Neuronal death via NMDA-R binding and glutamate excitotoxicity.
Alzheimer disease	Most common cause of dementia in elderly. Down syndrome patients have ↑ risk of developing early-onset Alzheimer disease, as APP is located on chromosome 21. ↓ ACh. Associated with the following altered proteins: ▪ ApoE-2: ↓ risk of sporadic form ▪ ApoE-4: ↑ risk of sporadic form ▪ APP, presenilin-1, presenilin-2: familial forms (10%) with earlier onset	Widespread cortical atrophy (normal cortex B; cortex in Alzheimer disease C), especially hippocampus (arrows in B and C). Narrowing of gyri and widening of sulci. Senile plaques D in gray matter: extracellular β-amyloid core; may cause amyloid angiopathy → intracranial hemorrhage; Aβ (amyloid-β) synthesized by cleaving amyloid precursor protein (APP). Neurofibrillary tangles E: intracellular, hyperphosphorylated tau protein = insoluble cytoskeletal elements; number of tangles correlates with degree of dementia. Hirano bodies—intracellular eosinophilic proteinaceous rods in hippocampus.
Frontotemporal dementia	Formerly called Pick disease. Early changes in personality and behavior (behavioral variant), or aphasia (primary progressive aphasia). May have associated movement disorders.	Frontotemporal lobe degeneration F. Inclusions of hyperphosphorylated tau (round Pick bodies G) or ubiquitinated TDP-43.

Neurodegenerative disorders *(continued)*

DISEASE	DESCRIPTION	HISTOLOGIC/GROSS FINDINGS
Lewy body dementia	Visual hallucinations ("haLewycinations"), dementia with fluctuating cognition/alertness, REM sleep behavior disorder, and parkinsonism. Called Lewy body dementia if cognitive and motor symptom onset < 1 year apart, otherwise considered dementia 2° to Parkinson disease.	Intracellular Lewy bodies A primarily in cortex.
Vascular dementia	Result of multiple arterial infarcts and/or chronic ischemia. Step-wise decline in cognitive ability with late-onset memory impairment. 2nd most common cause of dementia in elderly.	MRI or CT shows multiple cortical and/or subcortical infarcts.
Creutzfeldt-Jakob disease	Rapidly progressive (weeks to months) dementia with myoclonus ("startle myoclonus") and ataxia. Associated with periodic sharp waves on EEG and ↑ 14-3-3 protein in CSF. May be transmitted by contaminated materials (eg, corneal transplant, neurosurgical equipment). Fatal.	Spongiform cortex (vacuolation without inflammation). Prions ($PrP^c \rightarrow PrP^{sc}$ sheet [β-pleated sheet resistant to proteases]) H.
HIV-associated dementia	Subcortical dysfunction associated with advanced HIV infection. Characterized by cognitive deficits, gait disturbance, irritability, depressed mood.	Diffuse gray matter and subcortical atrophy. Microglial nodules with multinucleated giant cells.

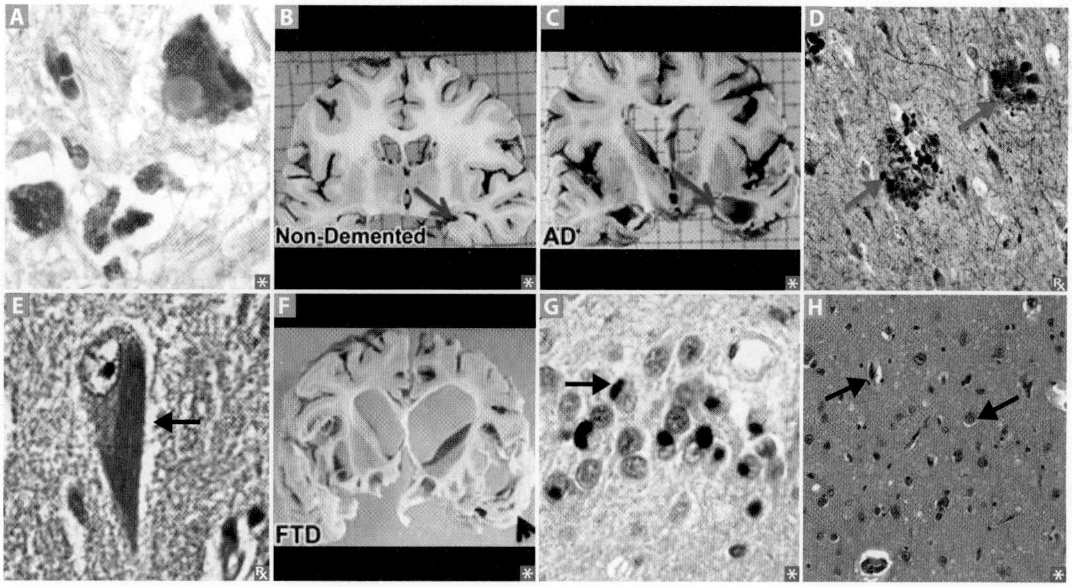

Idiopathic intracranial hypertension	Also called pseudotumor cerebri. ↑ ICP with no obvious findings on imaging. Risk factors include **female** sex, **T**etracyclines, **O**besity, vitamin **A** excess, **D**anazol (**female TOAD**). Associated with cerebral venous sinus stenosis. Findings: headache, tinnitus, diplopia (usually from CN VI palsy), no change in mental status. Impaired optic nerve axoplasmic flow → papilledema. Visual field testing shows enlarged blind spot and peripheral constriction. Lumbar puncture reveals ↑ opening pressure and provides temporary headache relief. Treatment: weight loss, acetazolamide, invasive procedures for refractory cases (eg, CSF shunt placement, optic nerve sheath fenestration surgery for visual loss).

Hydrocephalus	↑ CSF volume → ventricular dilation +/– ↑ ICP.
Communicating	
Communicating hydrocephalus	↓ CSF absorption by arachnoid granulations (eg, arachnoid scarring post-meningitis) → ↑ ICP, papilledema, herniation.
Normal pressure hydrocephalus	Affects the elderly; idiopathic; CSF pressure elevated only episodically; does not result in increased subarachnoid space volume. Expansion of ventricles A distorts the fibers of the corona radiata → triad of **urinary incontinence**, **gait apraxia** (magnetic gait), and **cognitive dysfunction**. "**Wet, wobbly**, and **wacky**." Symptoms potentially reversible with CSF drainage via lumbar puncture or shunt placement.
Noncommunicating (obstructive)	
Noncommunicating hydrocephalus	Caused by structural blockage of CSF circulation within ventricular system (eg, stenosis of aqueduct of Sylvius, colloid cyst blocking foramen of Monro, tumor B).
Hydrocephalus mimics	
Ex vacuo ventriculomegaly	Appearance of ↑ CSF on imaging C, but is actually due to ↓ brain tissue and neuronal atrophy (eg, Alzheimer disease, advanced HIV, frontotemporal dementia, Huntington disease). ICP is normal; NPH triad is not seen.

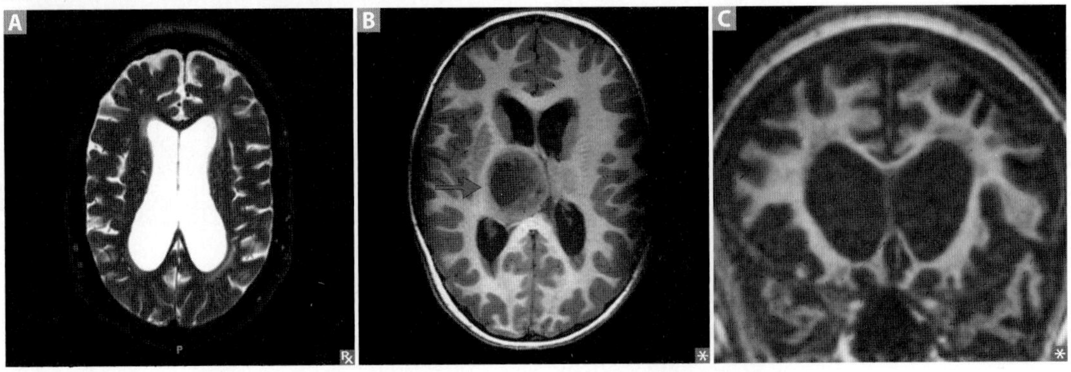

Multiple sclerosis

Autoimmune inflammation and demyelination of CNS (brain and spinal cord) with subsequent axonal damage. Can present with:

- Acute optic neuritis (painful unilateral visual loss associated with Marcus Gunn pupil)
- Brain stem/cerebellar syndromes (eg, diplopia, ataxia, scanning speech, intention tremor, nystagmus/INO [bilateral > unilateral])
- Pyramidal tract demyelination (eg, weakness, spasticity)
- Spinal cord syndromes (eg, electric shock-like sensation along cervical spine on neck flexion, neurogenic bladder, paraparesis, sensory manifestations affecting the trunk or one or more extremity)

Symptoms may exacerbate with increased body temperature (eg, hot bath, exercise). Relapsing and remitting is most common clinical course. Most often affects females in their 20s and 30s; more common in individuals who grew up farther from equator and with low serum vitamin D levels.

FINDINGS

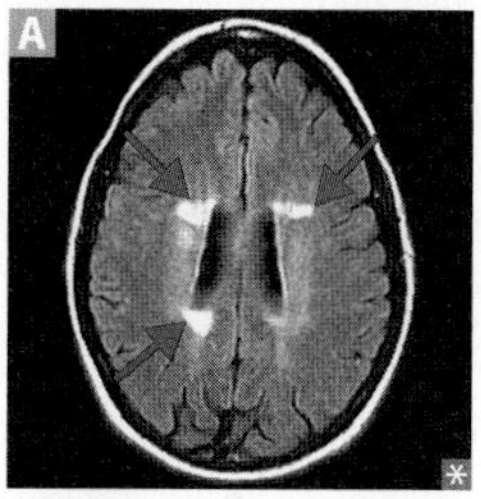

↑ IgG level and myelin basic protein in CSF. Oligoclonal bands are diagnostic. MRI is gold standard. Periventricular plaques A (areas of oligodendrocyte loss and reactive gliosis). Multiple white matter lesions disseminated in space and time.

TREATMENT

Stop relapses and halt/slow progression with disease-modifying therapies (eg, β-interferon, glatiramer, natalizumab). Treat acute flares with IV steroids. Symptomatic treatment for neurogenic bladder (catheterization, muscarinic antagonists), spasticity (baclofen, $GABA_B$ receptor agonists), pain (TCAs, anticonvulsants).

Other demyelinating and dysmyelinating disorders

Osmotic demyelination syndrome

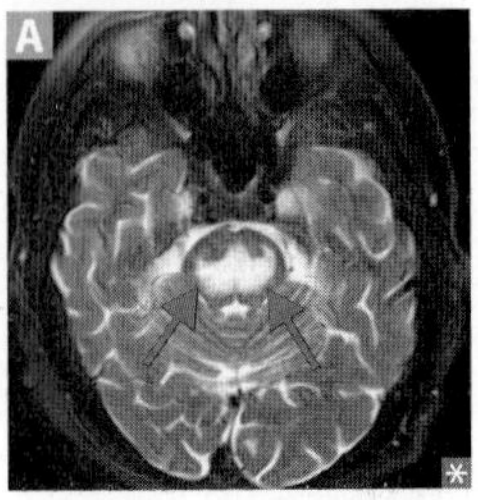

Also called central pontine myelinolysis. Massive axonal demyelination in pontine white matter A 2° to rapid osmotic changes, most commonly iatrogenic correction of hyponatremia but also rapid shifts of other osmolytes (eg, glucose). Acute paralysis, dysarthria, dysphagia, diplopia, loss of consciousness. Can cause "locked-in syndrome."

Correcting serum Na^+ too fast:

- "From low to high, your pons will die" (osmotic demyelination syndrome)
- "From high to low, your brains will blow" (cerebral edema/herniation)

Acute inflammatory demyelinating polyneuropathy

Most common subtype of **Guillain-Barré syndrome**.

Autoimmune condition that destroys Schwann cells via inflammation and demyelination of motor fibers, sensory fibers, peripheral nerves (including CN III-XII). Likely facilitated by molecular mimicry and triggered by inoculations or stress. Despite association with infections (eg, *Campylobacter jejuni*, viruses [eg, Zika]), no definitive causal link to any pathogen.

Results in symmetric ascending muscle weakness/paralysis and depressed/absent DTRs beginning in lower extremities. Facial paralysis (usually bilateral) and respiratory failure are common. May see autonomic dysregulation (eg, cardiac irregularities, hypertension, hypotension) or sensory abnormalities. Most patients survive with good functional recovery.

↑ CSF protein with normal cell count (albuminocytologic dissociation).

Respiratory support is critical until recovery. Disease-modifying treatment: plasma exchange or IV immunoglobulins. No role for steroids.

Acute disseminated (postinfectious) encephalomyelitis

Multifocal inflammation and demyelination after infection or vaccination. Presents with rapidly progressive multifocal neurologic symptoms, altered mental status.

Charcot-Marie-Tooth disease

Also called hereditary motor and sensory neuropathy. Group of progressive hereditary nerve disorders related to the defective production of proteins involved in the structure and function of peripheral nerves or the myelin sheath. Typically autosomal dominant and associated with foot deformities (eg, pes cavus, hammer toe), lower extremity weakness (eg, foot drop), and sensory deficits (Can't Move Toes). Most common type, CMT1A, is caused by *PMP22* gene duplication.

Progressive multifocal leukoencephalopathy

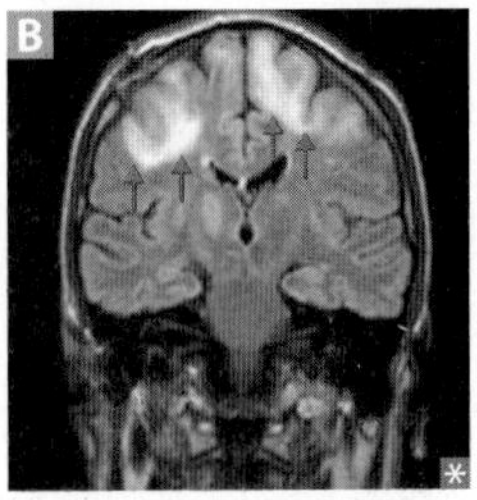

Demyelination of CNS B due to destruction of oligodendrocytes (2° to reactivation of latent JC virus infection). Associated with severe immunosuppression (eg, lymphomas and leukemias, AIDS, organ transplantation). Rapidly progressive, usually fatal. Predominantly involves parietal and occipital areas; visual symptoms are common. ↑ risk associated with natalizumab and rituximab.

Other disorders

Krabbe disease, metachromatic leukodystrophy, adrenoleukodystrophy.

Neurocutaneous disorders

DISORDER	GENETICS	PRESENTATION	NOTES
Sturge-Weber syndrome	Congenital nonhereditary anomaly of neural crest derivatives. Somatic mosaicism of an activating mutation in one copy of the *GNAQ* gene.	Capillary vascular malformation → port-wine stain A (nevus flammeus or non-neoplastic birthmark) in CN V_1/V_2 distribution; ipsilateral leptomeningeal angioma with calcifications B → seizures/epilepsy; intellectual disability; episcleral hemangioma → ↑ IOP → early-onset glaucoma.	Also called encephalotrigeminal angiomatosis.
Tuberous sclerosis	AD, variable expression. Mutation in tumor suppressor genes *TSC1* on chromosome 9 (hamartin), *TSC2* on chromosome 16 (tuberin; pronounce "twoberin").	Hamartomas in CNS and skin, angiofibromas C, mitral regurgitation, ash-leaf spots D, cardiac rhabdomyoma, intellectual disability, renal angiomyolipoma E, seizures, shagreen patches.	Autosomal dominant. ↑ incidence of subependymal giant cell astrocytomas and ungual fibromas.
Neurofibromatosis type I	AD, 100% penetrance. Mutation in *NF1* tumor suppressor gene on chromosome 17 (encodes neurofibromin, a negative RAS regulator).	Café-au-lait spots F, Intellectual disability, Cutaneous neurofibromas G, Lisch nodules (pigmented iris hamartomas H), Optic gliomas, Pheochromocytomas, Seizures/focal neurologic Signs (often from meningioma), bone lesions (eg, sphenoid dysplasia).	Also called von Recklinghausen disease. 17 letters in "von Recklinghausen." CICLOPSS.
Neurofibromatosis type II	AD. Mutation in *NF2* tumor suppressor gene (merlin) on chromosome 22.	Bilateral vestibular schwannomas, juvenile cataracts, meningiomas, ependymomas.	NF2 affects 2 ears, 2 eyes.
von Hippel-Lindau disease	AD. Deletion of *VHL* gene on chromosome 3p. pVHL ubiquitinates hypoxia-inducible factor 1a.	Hemangioblastomas (high vascularity with hyperchromatic nuclei I) in retina, brain stem, cerebellum, spine J; Angiomatosis; bilateral Renal cell carcinomas; Pheochromocytomas.	Numerous tumors, benign and malignant. HARP. VHL = 3 letters = chromosome 3; associated with RCC (also 3 letters).

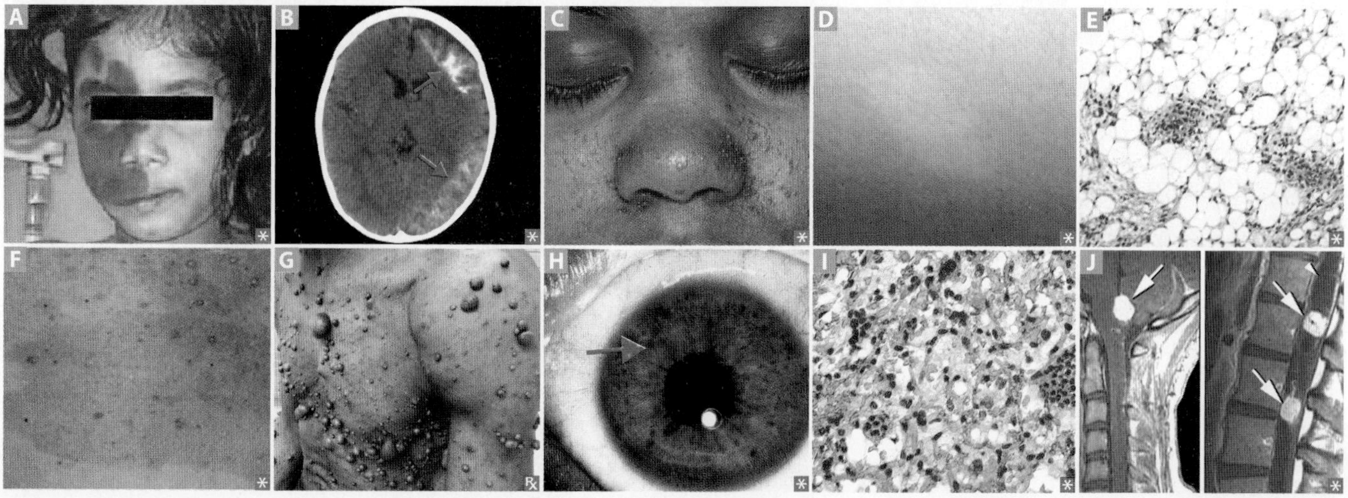

Adult primary brain tumors

TUMOR	DESCRIPTION	HISTOLOGY
Glioblastoma	Grade IV astrocytoma. Common, highly malignant 1° brain tumor with ~ 1-year median survival. Found in cerebral hemispheres. Can cross corpus callosum ("butterfly glioma" A). Associated with *EGFR* amplification.	Astrocyte origin, GFAP ⊕. "Pseudopalisading" pleomorphic tumor cells B border central areas of necrosis, hemorrhage, and/or microvascular proliferation.
Oligodendroglioma	Relatively rare, slow growing. Most often in frontal lobes C. Often calcified.	Oligodendrocyte origin. "Fried egg" cells—round nuclei with clear cytoplasm D. "Chicken-wire" capillary pattern.
Meningioma	Common, typically benign. Females > males. Most often occurs near surfaces of brain and in parasagittal region. Extra-axial (external to brain parenchyma) and may have a dural attachment ("tail" E). Often asymptomatic; may present with seizures or focal neurologic signs. Resection and/or radiosurgery.	Arachnoid cell origin. Spindle cells concentrically arranged in a whorled pattern F; psammoma bodies (laminated calcifications).
Hemangioblastoma	Most often cerebellar G. Associated with von Hippel-Lindau syndrome when found with retinal angiomas. Can produce erythropoietin → 2° polycythemia.	Blood vessel origin. Closely arranged, thin-walled capillaries with minimal intervening parenchyma H.

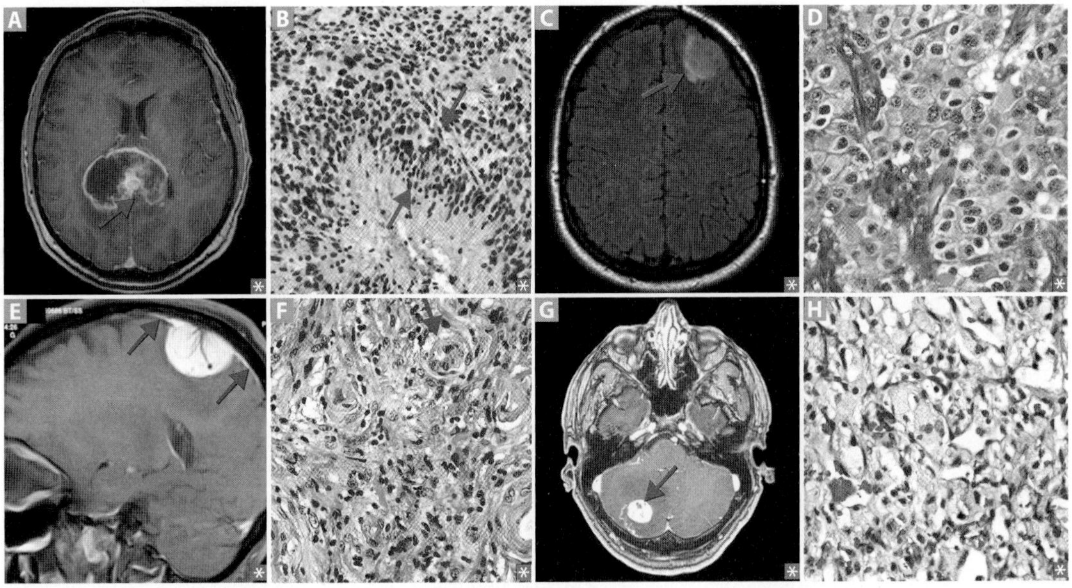

Adult primary brain tumors *(continued)*

TUMOR	DESCRIPTION	HISTOLOGY
Pituitary adenoma	May be nonfunctioning (silent) or hyperfunctioning (hormone-producing). Nonfunctional tumors present with mass effect (eg, bitemporal hemianopia [due to pressure on optic chiasm I]). Pituitary apoplexy → hyper- or hypopituitarism. Prolactinoma classically presents as galactorrhea, amenorrhea, ↓ bone density due to suppression of estrogen in females and as ↓ libido, infertility in males. Treatment: dopamine agonists (eg, bromocriptine, cabergoline), transsphenoidal resection.	Hyperplasia of only one type of endocrine cells found in pituitary. Most commonly from lactotrophs (prolactin) J → hyperprolactinemia. Less commonly, from somatotrophs (GH) → acromegaly, gigantism; corticotrophs (ACTH) → Cushing disease. Rarely, from thyrotrophs (TSH), gonadotrophs (FSH, LH).
Schwannoma	Classically at the cerebellopontine angle K, benign, involving CNs V, VII, and VIII, but can be along any peripheral nerve. Often localized to CN VIII in internal acoustic meatus → vestibular schwannoma (can present as hearing loss and tinnitus). Bilateral vestibular schwannomas found in NF-2. Resection or stereotactic radiosurgery.	Schwann cell origin, S-100 ⊕. Biphasic, dense, hypercellular areas containing spindle cells alternating with hypocellular, myxoid areas L.

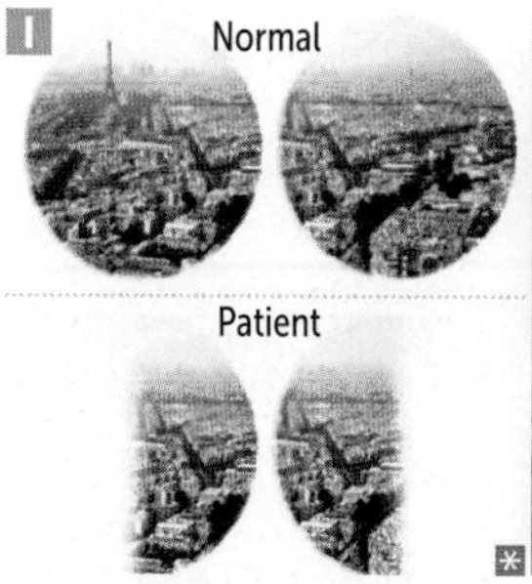
I
Normal
Patient

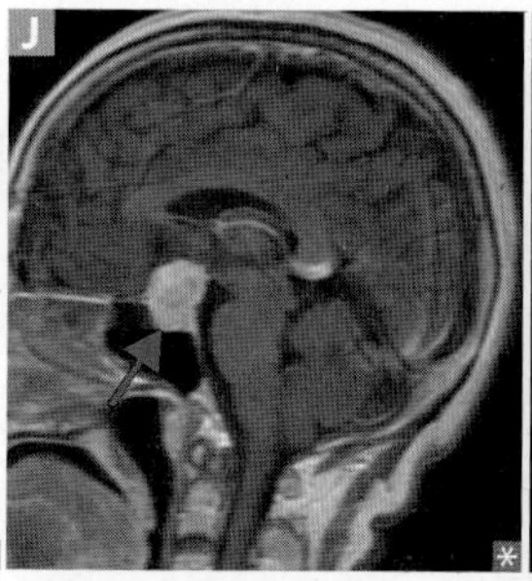
J

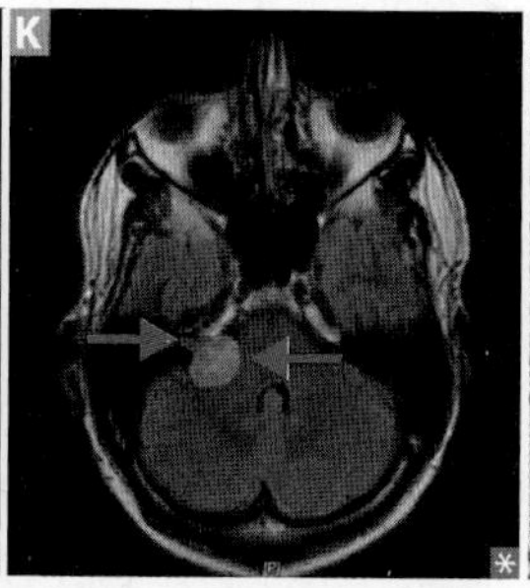
K

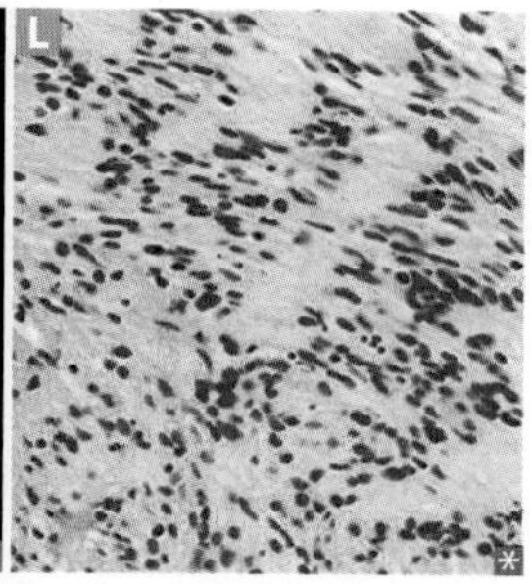
L

Childhood primary brain tumors

TUMOR	DESCRIPTION	HISTOLOGY
Pilocytic astrocytoma	Low-grade astrocytoma. Most common 1° brain tumor in childhood. Usually well circumscribed. In children, most often found in posterior fossa A (eg, cerebellum). May be supratentorial. Benign; good prognosis.	Astrocyte origin, GFAP ⊕. Bipolar neoplastic cells with hair-like projections. Associated with microcysts and Rosenthal fibers (eosinophilic, corkscrew fibers B). Cystic + solid (gross).
Medulloblastoma	Most common malignant brain tumor in childhood. Commonly involves cerebellum C. Can compress 4th ventricle, causing noncommunicating hydrocephalus → headaches, papilledema. Can involve the cerebellar vermis → truncal ataxia. Can send "drop metastases" to spinal cord.	Form of primitive neuroectodermal tumor (PNET). Homer-Wright rosettes, small blue cells D. Synaptophysin ⊕.
Ependymoma	Most commonly found in 4th ventricle E. Can cause hydrocephalus. Poor prognosis.	Ependymal cell origin. Characteristic perivascular pseudorosettes F. Rod-shaped blepharoplasts (basal ciliary bodies) found near the nucleus.
Craniopharyngioma	Most common childhood supratentorial tumor. May be confused with pituitary adenoma (both cause bitemporal hemianopia). Associated with a high recurrence rate.	Derived from remnants of Rathke pouch (ectoderm). Calcification is common G H. Cholesterol crystals found in "motor oil"-like fluid within tumor.
Pinealoma	Tumor of pineal gland. Can cause Parinaud syndrome (compression of tectum → vertical gaze palsy); obstructive hydrocephalus (compression of cerebral aqueduct); precocious puberty in males (hCG production).	Similar to germ cell tumors (eg, testicular seminoma).

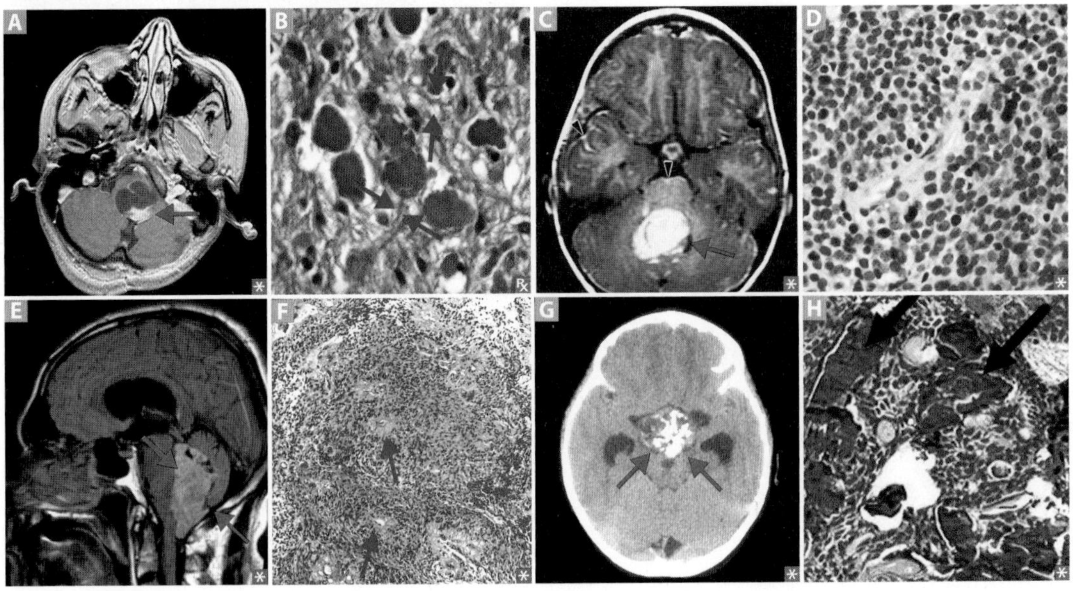

Herniation syndromes

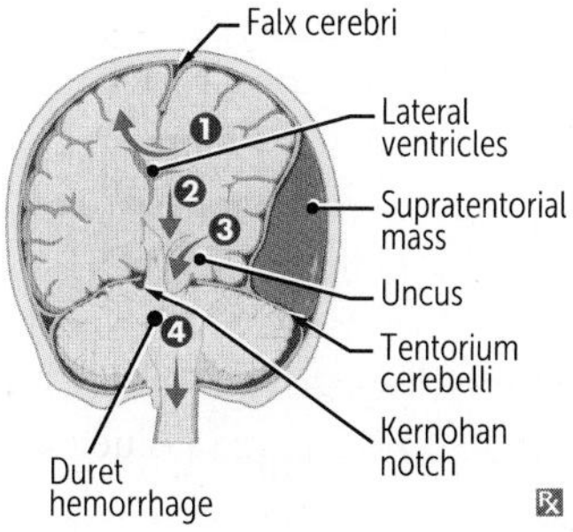
Falx cerebri
Lateral ventricles
Supratentorial mass
Uncus
Tentorium cerebelli
Kernohan notch
Duret hemorrhage

❶ Cingulate (subfalcine) herniation under falx cerebri	Can compress anterior cerebral artery.
❷ Central/downward transtentorial herniation	Caudal displacement of brain stem → rupture of paramedian basilar artery branches → Duret hemorrhages. Usually fatal.
❸ Uncal transtentorial herniation	Uncus = medial temporal lobe. Early herniation → ipsilateral blown pupil (unilateral CN III compression), contralateral hemiparesis. Late herniation → coma, Kernohan phenomenon (misleading contralateral blown pupil and ipsilateral hemiparesis due to contralateral compression against Kernohan notch).
❹ Cerebellar tonsillar herniation into the foramen magnum	Coma and death result when these herniations compress the brain stem.

Motor neuron signs

SIGN	UMN LESION	LMN LESION	COMMENTS
Weakness	+	+	**Lower** motor neuron (LMN) = everything **lowered** (less muscle mass, ↓ muscle tone, ↓ reflexes, downgoing toes)
Atrophy	–	+	
Fasciculations	–	+	
Reflexes	↑	↓	**Upper** motor neuron (UMN) = everything **up** (tone, DTRs, toes)
Tone	↑	↓	
Babinski	+	–	Fasciculations = muscle twitching Positive Babinski is normal in infants
Spastic paresis	+	–	
Flaccid paralysis	–	+	
Clasp knife spasticity	+	–	

Spinal lesions

AREA AFFECTED	DISEASE	CHARACTERISTICS
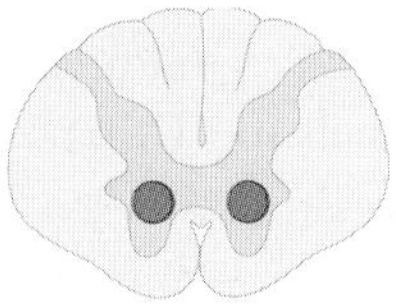	**Spinal muscular atrophy**	Congenital degeneration of anterior horns. LMN symptoms only, symmetric weakness. "Floppy baby" with marked hypotonia (flaccid paralysis) and tongue fasciculations. Autosomal recessive *SMN1* mutation → defective snRNP assembly. SMA type 1 is called Werdnig-Hoffmann disease.
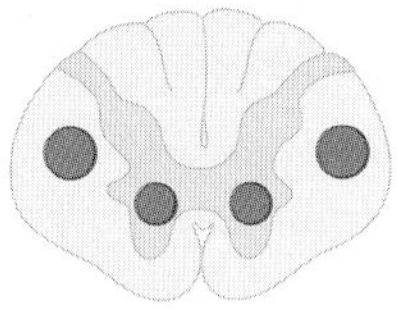	**Amyotrophic lateral sclerosis**	Also called **Lou** Gehrig disease. Combined UMN (corticobulbar/corticospinal) and LMN (medullary and spinal cord) degeneration. No sensory or bowel/bladder deficits. Can be caused by defect in superoxide dismutase 1. LMN deficits: flaccid limb weakness, fasciculations, atrophy, bulbar palsy (dysarthria, dysphagia, tongue atrophy). UMN deficits: spastic limb weakness, hyperreflexia, clonus, pseudobulbar palsy (dysarthria, dysphagia, emotional lability). Fatal (most often from respiratory failure). Treatment: "ri**Lou**zole".
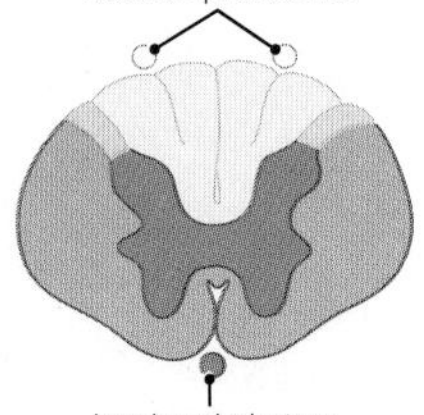	**Complete occlusion of anterior spinal artery**	Spares dorsal columns and Lissauer tract; mid-thoracic ASA territory is watershed area, as artery of Adamkiewicz supplies ASA below T8. Can be caused by aortic aneurysm repair. Presents with UMN deficit below the lesion (corticospinal tract), LMN deficit at the level of the lesion (anterior horn), and loss of pain and temperature sensation below the lesion (spinothalamic tract).
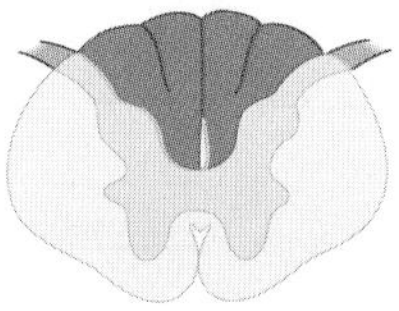	**Tabes dorsalis**	Caused by 3° syphilis. Results from degeneration/demyelination of dorsal columns and roots → progressive sensory ataxia (impaired proprioception → poor coordination). ⊕ Romberg sign and absent DTRs. Associated with Charcot joints, shooting pain, Argyll Robertson pupils.
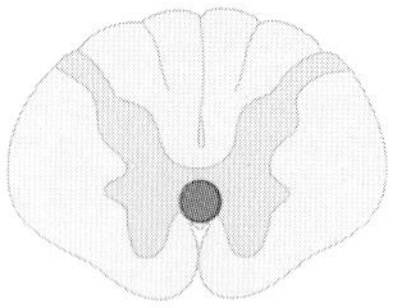	**Syringomyelia**	Syrinx expands and damages anterior white commissure of spinothalamic tract (2nd-order neurons) → bilateral symmetric loss of pain and temperature sensation in cape-like distribution. Seen with Chiari I malformation. Can affect other tracts.
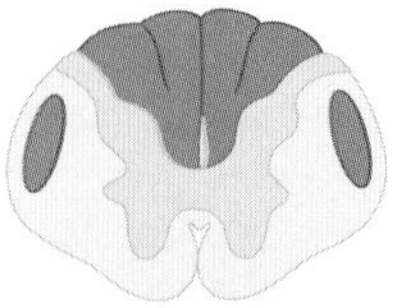	**Vitamin B_{12} deficiency**	Subacute combined degeneration (**SCD**)—demyelination of **S**pinocerebellar tracts, lateral **C**orticospinal tracts, and **D**orsal columns. Ataxic gait, paresthesia, impaired position/vibration sense (⊕ Romberg sign), UMN symptoms.
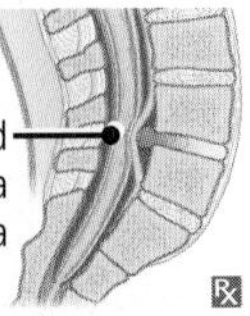	**Cauda equina syndrome**	Compression of spinal roots L2 and below, often due to intervertebral disc herniation or tumor. Radicular pain, absent knee and ankle reflexes, loss of bladder and anal sphincter control, saddle anesthesia.

Poliomyelitis

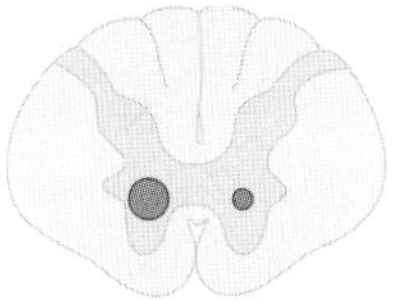

Caused by poliovirus (fecal-oral transmission). Replicates in lymphoid tissue of oropharynx and small intestine before spreading via bloodstream to CNS. Infection causes destruction of cells in anterior horn of spinal cord (LMN death).

Signs of LMN lesion: asymmetric weakness (vs symmetric weakness in spinal muscular atrophy), hypotonia, flaccid paralysis, fasciculations, hyporeflexia, muscle atrophy. Respiratory muscle involvement leads to respiratory failure. Signs of infection: malaise, headache, fever, nausea, etc.

CSF shows ↑ WBCs (lymphocytic pleocytosis) and slight ↑ of protein (with no change in CSF glucose). Virus recovered from stool or throat.

Brown-Séquard syndrome

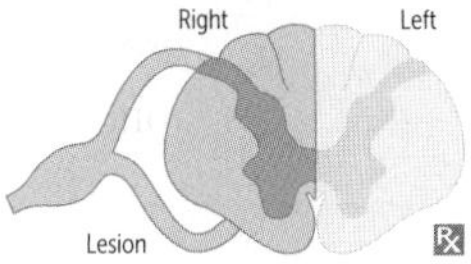

Hemisection of spinal cord. Findings:

❶ Ipsilateral loss of all sensation **at** level of lesion

❷ Ipsilateral LMN signs (eg, flaccid paralysis) **at** level of lesion

❸ Ipsilateral UMN signs **below** level of lesion (due to corticospinal tract damage)

❹ Ipsilateral loss of proprioception, vibration, and light (2-point discrimination) touch **below** level of lesion (due to dorsal column damage)

❺ Contralateral loss of pain, temperature, and crude (non-discriminative) touch **below** level of lesion (due to spinothalamic tract damage)

If lesion occurs above T1, patient may present with ipsilateral Horner syndrome due to damage of oculosympathetic pathway.

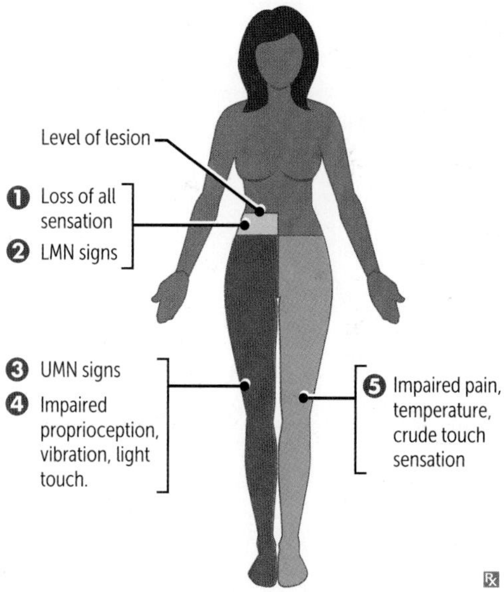

Friedreich ataxia

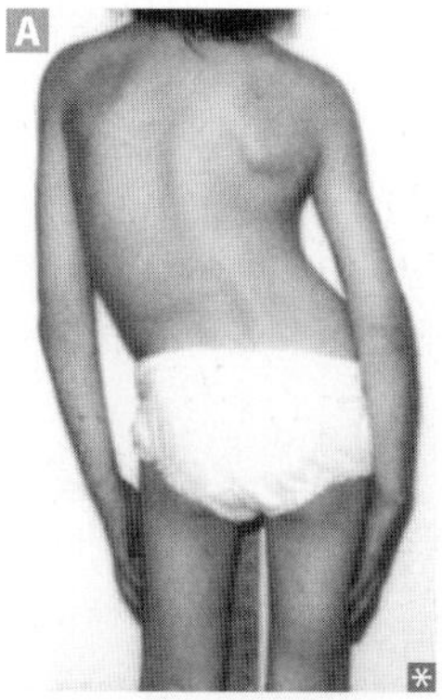

Autosomal recessive trinucleotide repeat disorder $(GAA)_n$ on chromosome 9 in gene that encodes frataxin (iron-binding protein). Leads to impairment in mitochondrial functioning. Degeneration of lateral corticospinal tract (spastic paralysis), spinocerebellar tract (ataxia), dorsal columns (↓ vibratory sense, proprioception), and dorsal root ganglia (loss of DTRs). **Staggering** gait, frequent **falling**, nystagmus, dysarthria, pes cavus, hammer toes, **diabetes** mellitus, **hypertrophic cardiomyopathy** (cause of death). Presents in childhood with kyphoscoliosis A.

Friedreich is fratastic (**frataxin**): he's your favorite **frat** brother, always **staggering** and **falling** but has a **sweet**, **big heart**. Ataxic GAAit.

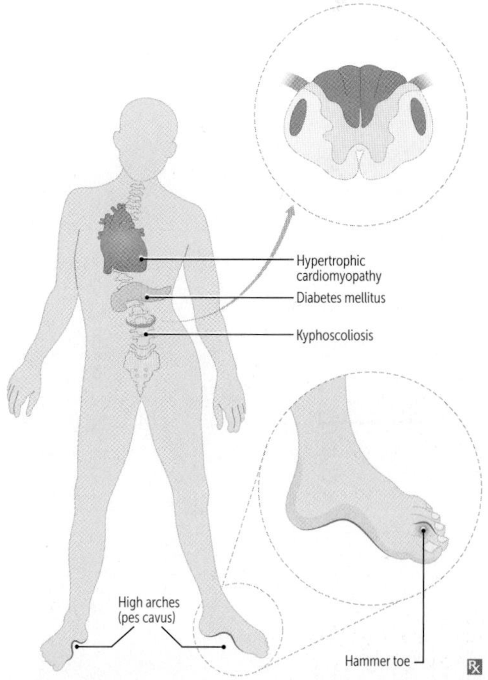

Common cranial nerve lesions

CN V motor lesion	Jaw deviates **toward** side of lesion due to unopposed force from the opposite pterygoid muscle.
CN X lesion	Uvula deviates **away** from side of lesion. Weak side collapses and uvula points away.
CN XI lesion	Weakness turning head to contralateral side of lesion (SCM). Shoulder droop on side of lesion (trapezius). The left SCM contracts to help turn the head to the right.
CN XII lesion	LMN lesion. Tongue deviates **toward** side of lesion ("lick your wounds") due to weakened tongue muscles on affected side.

Facial nerve lesions

A

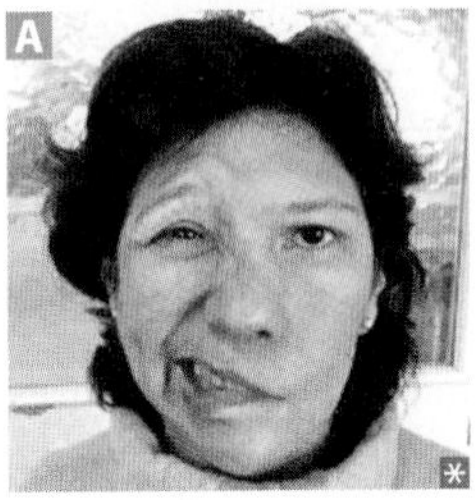

Bell palsy is the most common cause of peripheral facial palsy A. Usually develops after HSV reactivation. Treatment: corticosteroids +/– acyclovir. Most patients gradually recover function, but aberrant regeneration can occur. Other causes of peripheral facial palsy include Lyme disease, herpes zoster (Ramsay Hunt syndrome), sarcoidosis, tumors (eg, parotid gland), diabetes mellitus.

	Upper motor neuron lesion	Lower motor neuron lesion
LESION LOCATION	Motor cortex, connection from motor cortex to facial nucleus in pons	Facial nucleus, anywhere along CN VII
AFFECTED SIDE	Contralateral	Ipsilateral
MUSCLES INVOLVED	Lower muscles of facial expression	Upper and lower muscles of facial expression
FOREHEAD INVOLVED?	Spared, due to bilateral UMN innervation	Affected
OTHER SYMPTOMS	Variable; depends on size of lesion	Incomplete eye closure (dry eyes, corneal ulceration), hyperacusis, loss of taste sensation to anterior tongue

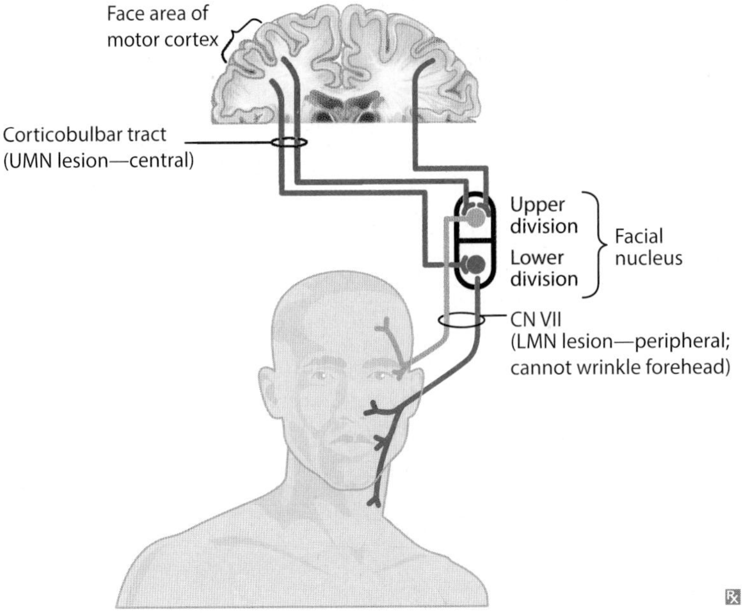

▸ NEUROLOGY—OTOLOGY

Auditory anatomy and physiology

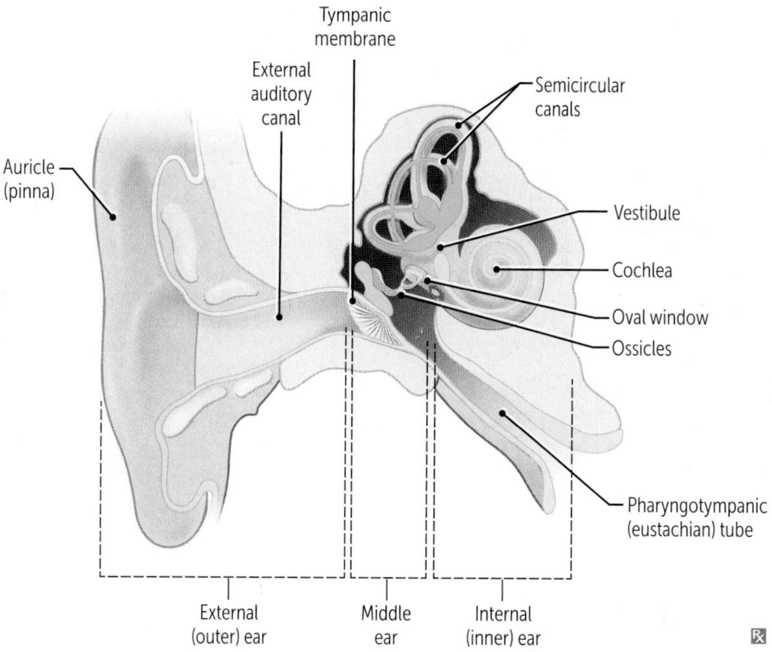

Outer ear	Visible portion of ear (pinna), includes auditory canal and tympanic membrane. Transfers sound waves via vibration of tympanic membrane.
Middle ear	Air-filled space with three bones called the ossicles (malleus, incus, stapes). Ossicles conduct and amplify sound from tympanic membrane to inner ear.
Inner ear	Snail-shaped, fluid-filled cochlea. Contains basilar membrane that vibrates 2° to sound waves. Vibration transduced via specialized hair cells → auditory nerve signaling → brain stem. Each frequency leads to vibration at specific location on basilar membrane (tonotopy): ▪ Low frequency heard at apex near helicotrema (wide and flexible). ▪ High frequency heard best at base of cochlea (thin and rigid).

Types of hearing loss

Noise-induced hearing loss	Damage to stereociliated cells in organ of Corti. Loss of high-frequency hearing first. Sudden extremely loud noises can produce hearing loss due to tympanic membrane rupture.
Presbycusis	Aging-related progressive bilateral/symmetric sensorineural hearing loss (often of higher frequencies) due to destruction of hair cells at the cochlear base (preserved low-frequency hearing at apex).

Diagnosing hearing loss

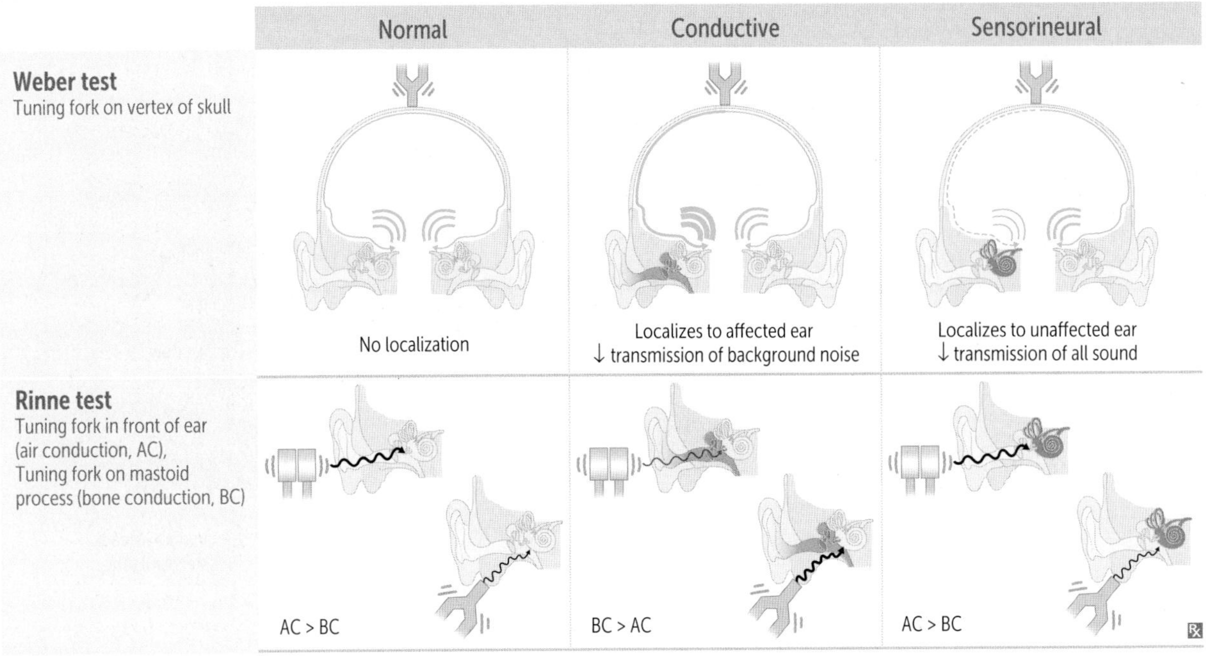
Normal
Conductive
Sensorineural
Weber test
Tuning fork on vertex of skull
No localization
Localizes to affected ear
↓ transmission of background noise
Localizes to unaffected ear
↓ transmission of all sound
Rinne test
Tuning fork in front of ear (air conduction, AC),
Tuning fork on mastoid process (bone conduction, BC)
AC > BC
BC > AC
AC > BC

Cholesteatoma

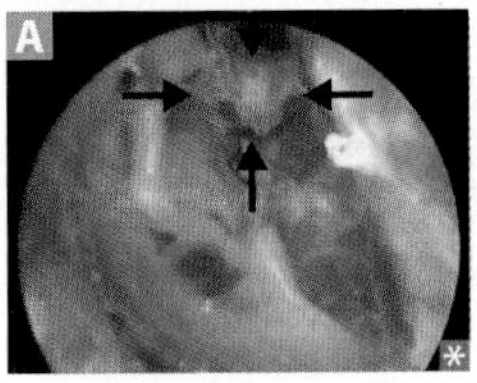
A

Overgrowth of desquamated keratin debris within the middle ear space (A, arrows). Can be congenital or acquired (eg, 2° to recurrent/chronic otitis media). May erode ossicles, mastoid air cells → conductive hearing loss. Often presents with painless otorrhea.

Vertigo

Sensation of spinning while actually stationary. Subtype of "dizziness," but distinct from "lightheadedness." Peripheral vertigo more common than central vertigo.

Peripheral vertigo

Due to inner ear pathologies such as semicircular canal debris (benign paroxysmal positional vertigo, BPPV), vestibular nerve infection, Ménière disease—triad of sensorineural hearing loss, vertigo, tinnitus; endolymphatic hydrops → ↑ endolymph within the inner ear.

Treatment: antihistamines, anticholinergics, antiemetics (symptomatic relief); low-salt diet +/– diuretics (Ménière disease); Epley maneuver (BPPV).

Central vertigo

Brain stem or cerebellar lesion (eg, stroke affecting vestibular nuclei, demyelinating disease, or posterior fossa tumor). Findings: directional or purely vertical nystagmus, skew deviation (vertical misalignment of the eyes), diplopia, dysmetria. Focal neurologic findings.

▸ NEUROLOGY—OPHTHALMOLOGY

Normal eye anatomy

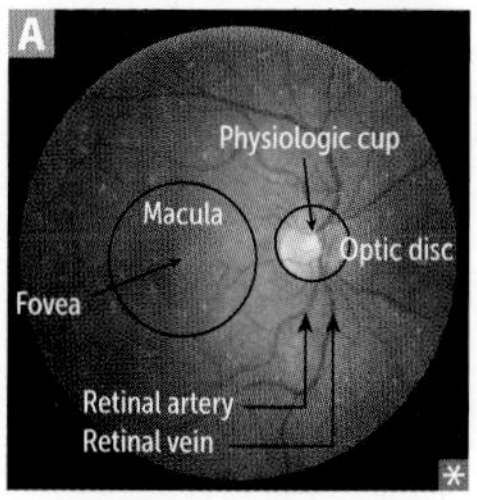

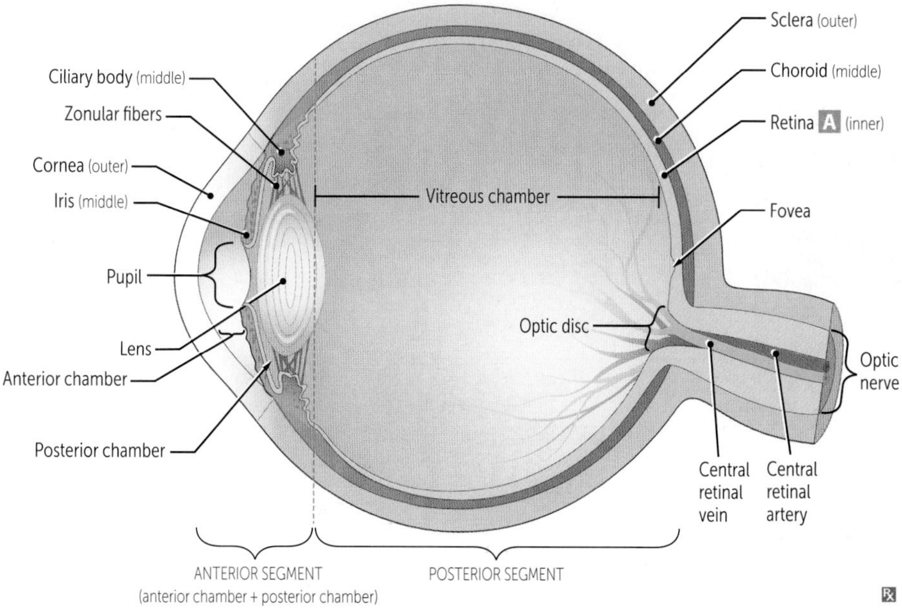

Conjunctivitis

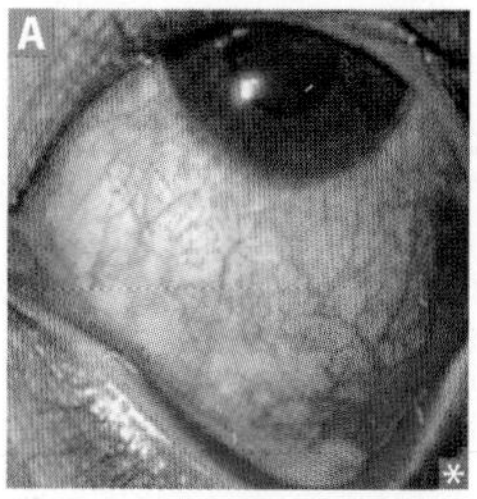

Inflammation of the conjunctiva → red eye A.
Allergic—itchy eyes, bilateral.
Bacterial—pus; treat with antibiotics.
Viral—most common, often adenovirus; sparse mucous discharge, swollen preauricular node, ↑ lacrimation; self-resolving.

Refractive errors	Common cause of impaired vision, correctable with glasses.
Hyperopia	Also called "farsightedness." Eye too short for refractive power of cornea and lens → light focused behind retina. Correct with convex (converging) lenses.
Myopia	Also called "nearsightedness." Eye too long for refractive power of cornea and lens → light focused in front of retina. Correct with concave (diverging) lens.
Astigmatism	Abnormal curvature of cornea → different refractive power at different axes. Correct with cylindrical lens.

Presbyopia

Aging-related impaired accommodation (focusing on near objects), primarily due to ↓ lens elasticity, changes in lens curvature, ↓ strength of the ciliary muscle. Patients often need "reading glasses" (magnifiers).

Cataract

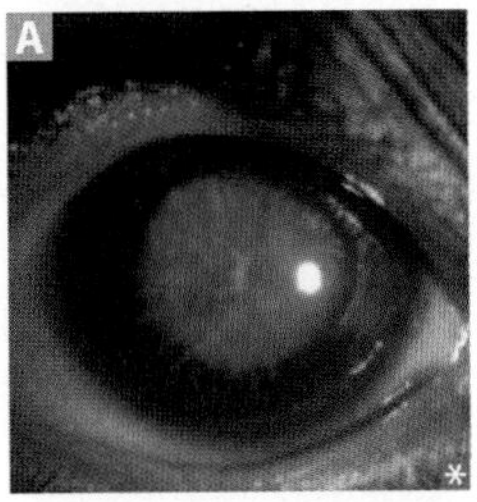

Painless, often bilateral, opacification of lens A. Can result in glare and ↓ vision, especially at night, and loss of the red reflex. Acquired risk factors: ↑ age, tobacco smoking, alcohol overuse, excessive sunlight, prolonged corticosteroid use, diabetes mellitus, trauma, infection. Congenital risk factors: classic galactosemia, galactokinase deficiency, trisomies (13, 18, 21), TORCH infections (eg, rubella), Marfan syndrome, Alport syndrome, myotonic dystrophy, neurofibromatosis 2.

Aqueous humor pathway

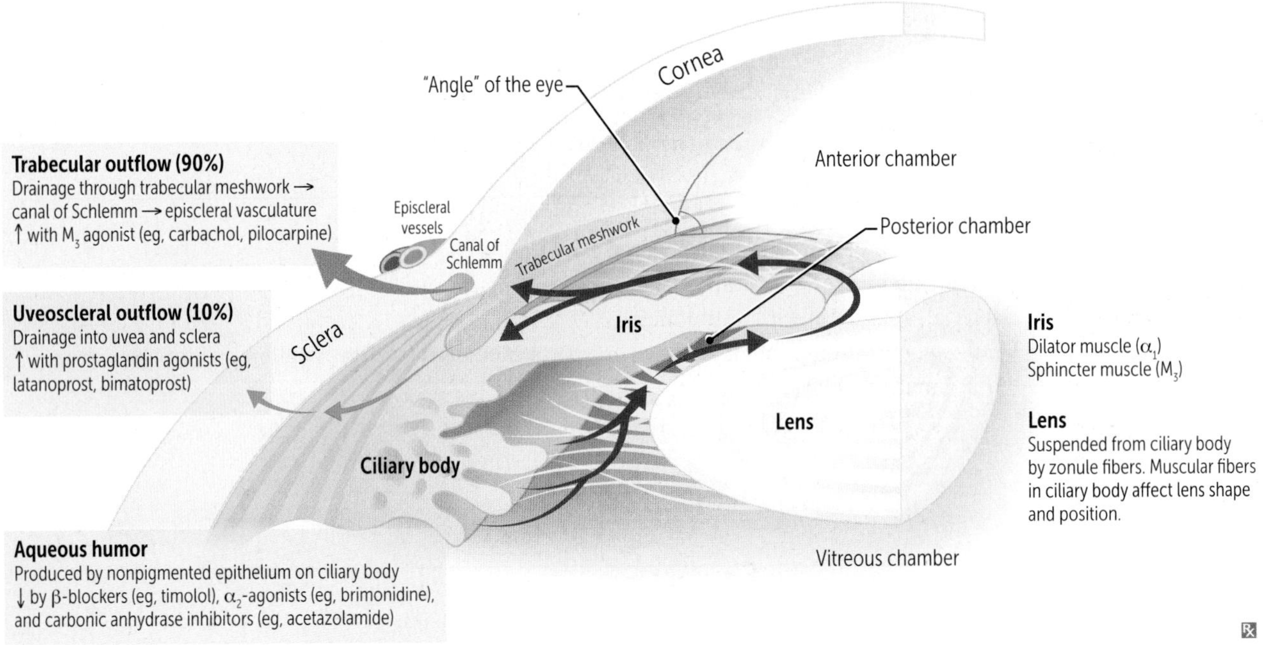
"Angle" of the eye
Cornea
Anterior chamber
Posterior chamber
Trabecular outflow (90%)
Drainage through trabecular meshwork → canal of Schlemm → episcleral vasculature
↑ with M_3 agonist (eg, carbachol, pilocarpine)
Episcleral vessels
Canal of Schlemm
Trabecular meshwork
Uveoscleral outflow (10%)
Drainage into uvea and sclera
↑ with prostaglandin agonists (eg, latanoprost, bimatoprost)
Sclera
Iris
Lens
Ciliary body
Iris
Dilator muscle (α_1)
Sphincter muscle (M_3)
Lens
Suspended from ciliary body by zonule fibers. Muscular fibers in ciliary body affect lens shape and position.
Aqueous humor
Produced by nonpigmented epithelium on ciliary body
↓ by β-blockers (eg, timolol), α_2-agonists (eg, brimonidine), and carbonic anhydrase inhibitors (eg, acetazolamide)
Vitreous chamber

Glaucoma

Optic disc atrophy with characteristic cupping (normal A versus thinning of outer rim of optic nerve head B), usually with elevated intraocular pressure (IOP) and progressive peripheral visual field loss if untreated. Treatment is through pharmacologic or surgical lowering of IOP.

Open-angle glaucoma

↑ incidence in older people, Black people, and patients with family history of condition. Painless, more common in US.

Primary—cause unclear.

Secondary—blocked trabecular meshwork from WBCs (eg, uveitis), RBCs (eg, vitreous hemorrhage), retinal elements (eg, retinal detachment).

Closed- or narrow-angle glaucoma

Primary—enlargement or anterior movement of lens against central iris (pupil margin) → obstruction of normal aqueous flow through pupil → fluid builds up behind iris, pushing peripheral iris against cornea C and impeding flow through trabecular meshwork.

Secondary—hypoxia from retinal disease (eg, diabetes mellitus, vein occlusion) induces vasoproliferation in iris that contracts angle.

Chronic closure—often asymptomatic with damage to optic nerve and peripheral vision.

Acute closure—true ophthalmic emergency. ↑ IOP pushes iris forward → angle closes abruptly. Very painful, red eye D, sudden vision loss, halos around lights, frontal headache, fixed and mid-dilated pupil, nausea and vomiting. Mydriatic agents contraindicated. **H**urts in a **h**urry with **h**alos, a **h**eadache, and a "**h**alf-dilated" pupil.

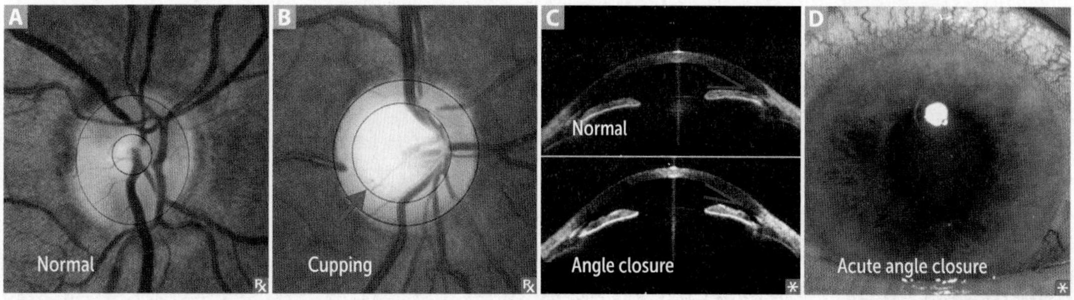

Uveitis

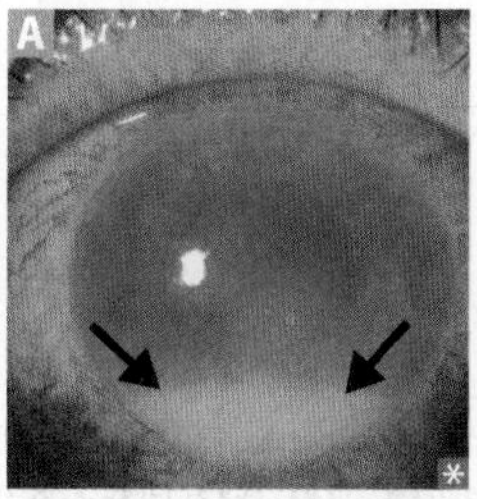

Inflammation of uvea; specific name based on location within affected eye. Anterior uveitis: iritis; posterior uveitis: choroiditis and/or retinitis. May have hypopyon (accumulation of pus in anterior chamber A) or conjunctival redness. Associated with systemic inflammatory disorders (eg, sarcoidosis, rheumatoid arthritis, juvenile idiopathic arthritis, HLA-B27–associated conditions).

Age-related macular degeneration

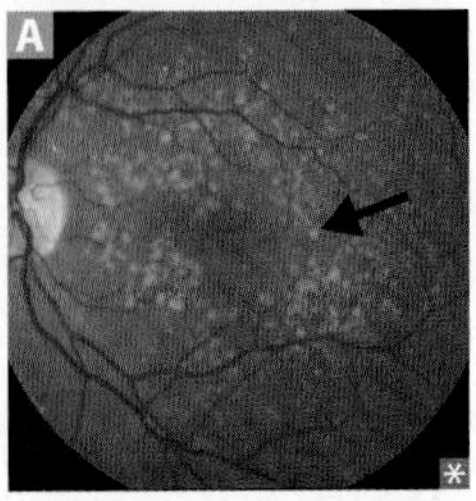

Degeneration of macula (central area of retina). Causes distortion of straight lines (metamorphopsia) and eventual loss of central vision (scotomas).

- Dry (nonexudative, > 80%)—deposition of yellowish extracellular material ("drusen") in between Bruch membrane and retinal pigment epithelium A with gradual ↓ in vision. Prevent progression with multivitamin and antioxidant supplements.
- Wet (exudative, 10–15%)—rapid loss of vision due to bleeding 2° to choroidal neovascularization. Treat with anti-VEGF (vascular endothelial growth factor) injections (eg, bevacizumab, ranibizumab).

Diabetic retinopathy

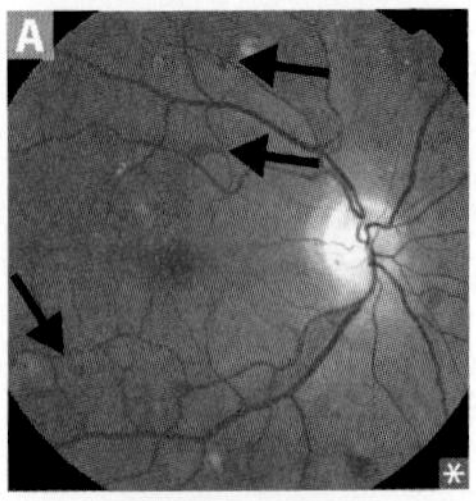

Retinal damage due to chronic hyperglycemia. Two types:

- Nonproliferative—damaged capillaries leak blood → lipids and fluid seep into retina → hemorrhages (arrows in A) and macular edema. Treatment: blood sugar control.
- Proliferative—chronic hypoxia results in new blood vessel formation with resultant traction on retina → retinal detachment. Treatment: anti-VEGF injections, peripheral retinal photocoagulation, surgery.

Hypertensive retinopathy

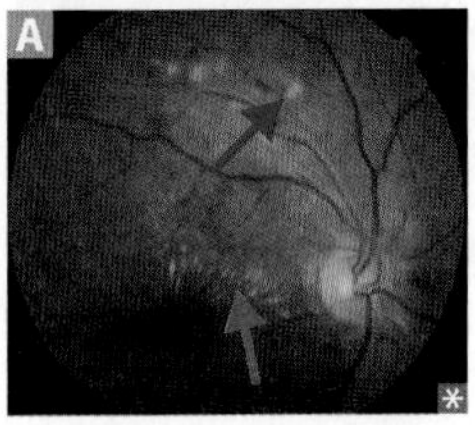

Chronic uncontrolled hypertension → endothelial disruption → fibrinoid necrosis → retinal damage.

Flame-shaped retinal hemorrhages, arteriovenous nicking, microaneurysms, macular star (exudate, red arrow in A), cotton-wool spots (blue arrow in A). Presence of papilledema requires immediate lowering of BP.

Associated with ↑ risk of stroke, CAD, kidney disease.

Retinal vein occlusion

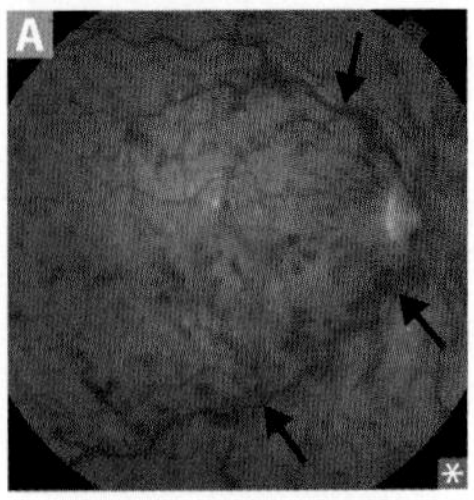

Blockage of central or branch retinal vein due to compression from nearby arterial atherosclerosis. Retinal hemorrhage and venous engorgement ("blood and thunder appearance"; arrows in A), edema in affected area.

Retinal detachment

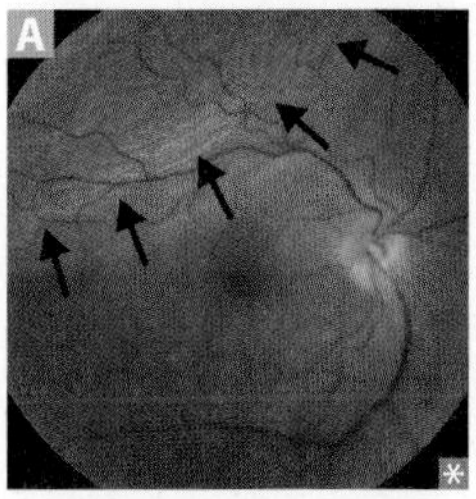

Separation of neurosensory layer of retina (photoreceptor layer with rods and cones) from outermost pigmented epithelium (normally shields excess light, supports retina) → degeneration of photoreceptors → vision loss. May be 2° to retinal breaks, diabetic traction, inflammatory effusions. Visualized on fundoscopy as crinkling of retinal tissue A and changes in vessel direction.

Breaks more common in patients with high myopia and/or history of head trauma. Often preceded by posterior vitreous detachment ("flashes" and "floaters") and eventual monocular loss of vision like a "curtain drawn down." Surgical emergency.

Central retinal artery occlusion

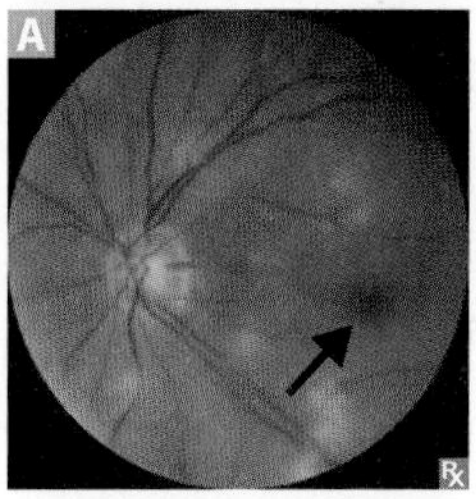

Acute, painless monocular vision loss. Retina cloudy with attenuated vessels and "cherry-red" spot at fovea (center of macula) A. Evaluate for embolic source (eg, carotid artery atherosclerosis, cardiac vegetations, patent foramen ovale).

Retinitis pigmentosa

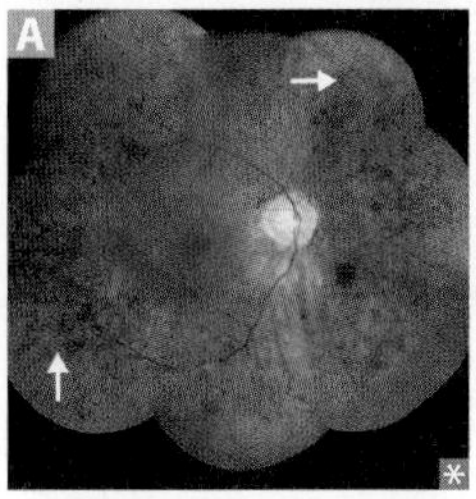

Inherited progressive dystrophy of retinal pigmented epithelium and photoreceptors. May be associated with abetalipoproteinemia. Early findings: nyctalopia (night blindness), peripheral vision loss. Fundoscopy may show triad of optic disc pallor, retinal vessel attenuation, and retinal pigmentation with bone spicule-shaped deposits A.

Papilledema

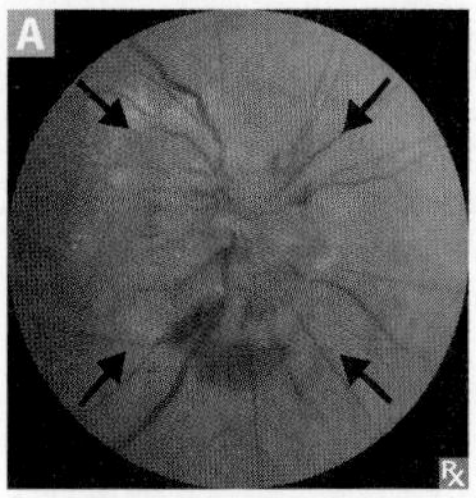

Optic disc swelling (usually bilateral) due to ↑ ICP (eg, 2° to mass effect). Enlarged blind spot and elevated optic disc with blurred margins A.

Leukocoria

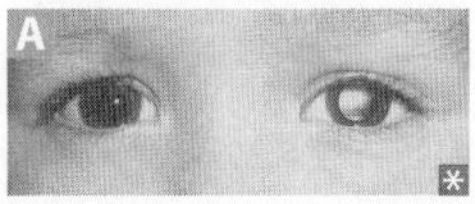

Loss (whitening) of the red reflex. Important causes in children include retinoblastoma A, congenital cataract.

Pupillary control

Miosis	Constriction, parasympathetic: ▪ 1st neuron: Edinger-Westphal nucleus to ciliary ganglion via CN III ▪ 2nd neuron: short ciliary nerves to sphincter pupillae muscles **Short** ciliary nerves **shorten** the pupil diameter.
Pupillary light reflex	Light in either retina sends a signal via CN II to pretectal nuclei (dashed lines in image) in midbrain that activates bilateral Edinger-Westphal nuclei; pupils constrict bilaterally (direct and consensual reflex). Result: illumination of 1 eye results in bilateral pupillary constriction.
Mydriasis	Dilation, sympathetic: ▪ 1st neuron: hypothalamus to ciliospinal center of Budge (C8–T2) ▪ 2nd neuron: exit at T1 to superior cervical ganglion (travels along cervical sympathetic chain near lung apex, subclavian vessels) ▪ 3rd neuron: plexus along internal carotid, through cavernous sinus; enters orbit as long ciliary nerve to pupillary dilator muscles. Sympathetic fibers also innervate smooth muscle of eyelids (minor retractors) and sweat glands of forehead and face. **Long** ciliary nerves make the pupil diameter **longer**.

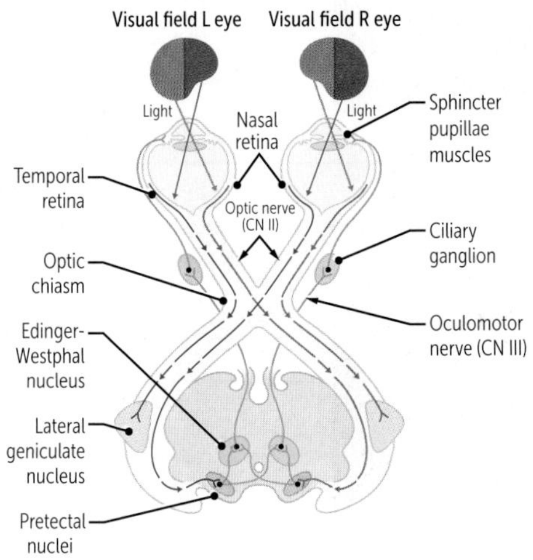

Marcus Gunn pupil

Also called relative afferent pupillary defect (RAPD). When the light shines into a normal eye, constriction of the ipsilateral (direct reflex) and contralateral eye (consensual reflex) is observed. When the light is then swung to the affected eye, both pupils dilate instead of constrict due to impaired conduction of light signal along the injured optic nerve. Associated with optic neuritis (eg, multiple sclerosis), optic neuropathies (eg, giant cell arteritis).

Horner syndrome

Sympathetic denervation of face →:
- Ptosis (slight drooping of eyelid: superior tarsal muscle)
- Anhidrosis (absence of sweating) and flushing of affected side of face
- Miosis (pupil constriction)

Associated with lesions along the sympathetic chain:
- 1st neuron: pontine hemorrhage, lateral medullary syndrome, spinal cord lesion above T1 (eg, Brown-Séquard syndrome, late-stage syringomyelia)
- 2nd neuron: stellate ganglion compression by Pancoast tumor
- 3rd neuron: carotid dissection (painful); anhidrosis is usually absent

PAM is horny (Horner).

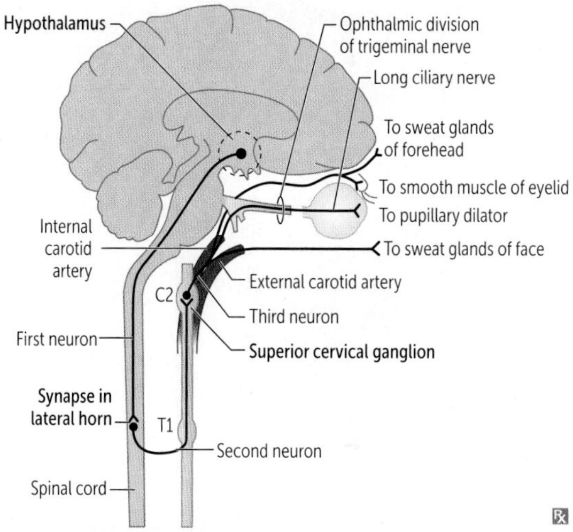

Ocular motility

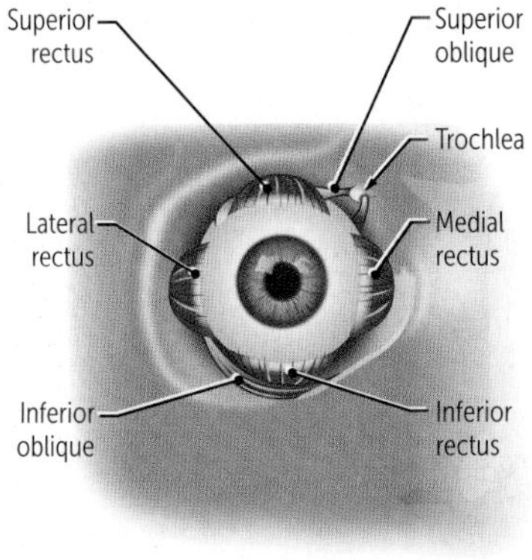

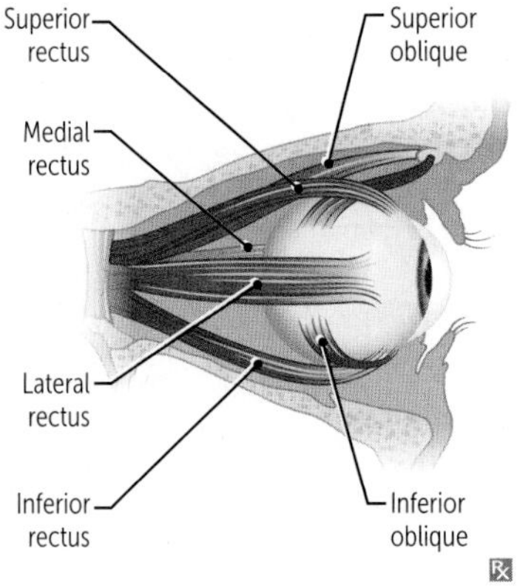

CN **VI** innervates the **L**ateral **R**ectus.
CN **IV** innervates the **S**uperior **O**blique.
CN **III** innervates the **R**est.
The "chemical formula" $\mathbf{LR_6SO_4R_3}$.

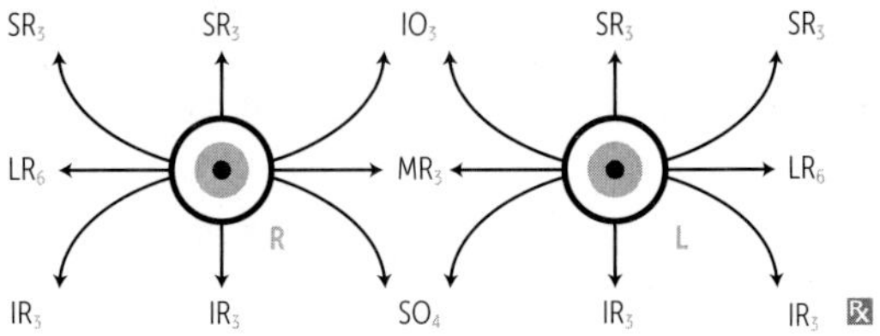

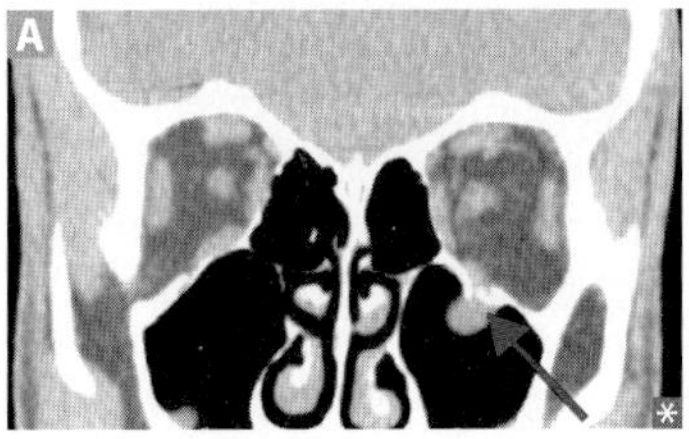

Obliques go **O**pposite (left SO and IO tested with patient looking right)
IOU: **IO** tested looking **U**p

Blowout fracture—orbital floor fracture; usually caused by direct trauma to eyeball or intraorbital rim. ↑ risk of IR muscle A and/or orbital fat entrapment. May lead to infraorbital nerve injury

CN III, IV, VI palsies

CN III damage

CN III has both motor (central) and parasympathetic (peripheral) components. Common causes include:

- Ischemia → pupil sparing (motor fibers affected more than parasympathetic fibers)
- Uncal herniation → coma
- PCom aneurysm → sudden-onset headache
- Cavernous sinus thrombosis → proptosis, involvement of CNs IV, V_1/V_2, VI
- Midbrain stroke → contralateral hemiplegia

Motor = middle (central)
Parasympathetic = peripheral

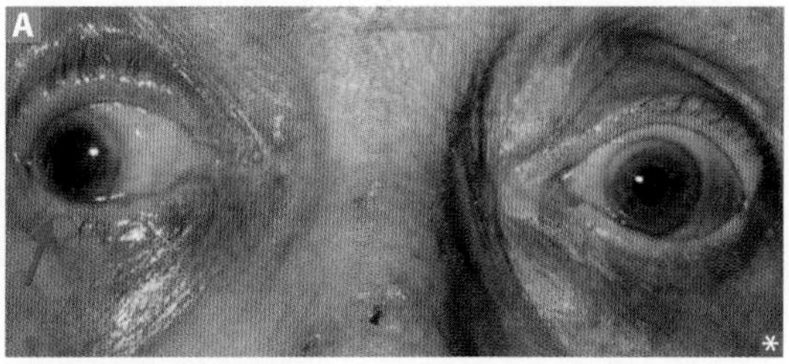

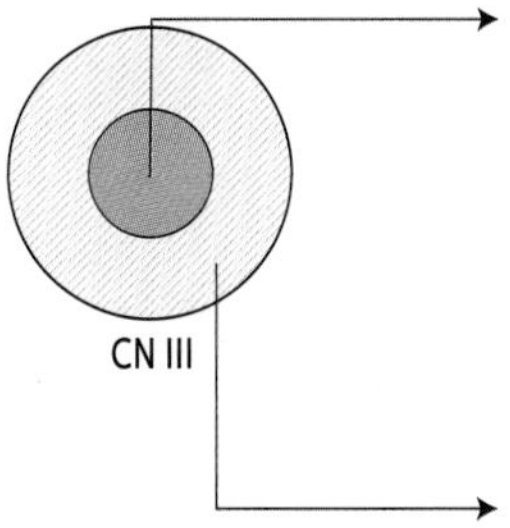

Motor output to extraocular muscles—affected primarily by vascular disease (eg, diabetes mellitus: glucose → sorbitol) due to ↓ diffusion of oxygen and nutrients to the interior fibers from compromised vasculature that resides on outside of nerve. Signs: ptosis, "down-and-out" gaze.

Parasympathetic output—fibers on the periphery are first affected by compression (eg, PCom aneurysm, uncal herniation). Signs: diminished or absent pupillary light reflex, "blown pupil" often with "down-and-out" gaze A.

CN IV damage

Pupil is higher in the affected eye B. Characteristic head tilt to contralateral/unaffected side to compensate for lack of intorsion in affected eye.

Can't see the **floor** with CN IV damage (eg, difficulty going down stairs, reading).

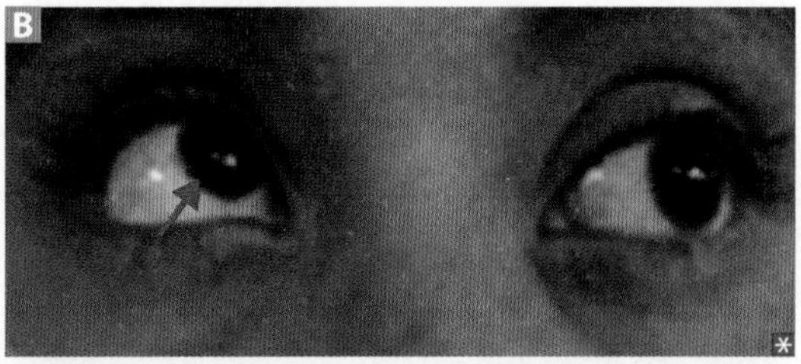

CN VI damage

Affected eye unable to abduct C and is displaced medially in primary position of gaze.

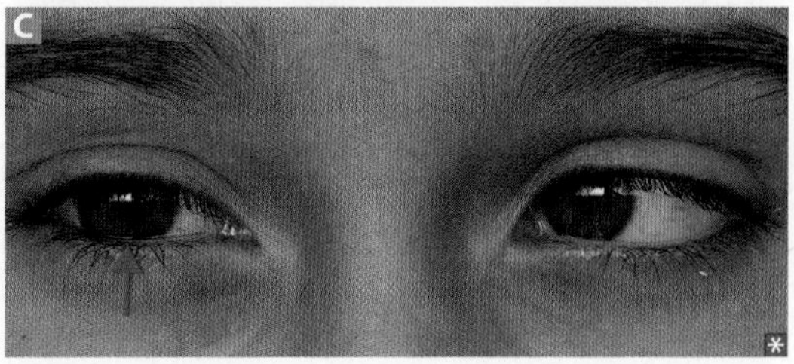

Visual field defects

1. Right anopia (monocular vision loss)
2. Bitemporal hemianopia (pituitary lesion, chiasm)
3. Left homonymous hemianopia
4. Left upper quadrantanopia (right temporal lesion, MCA)
5. Left lower quadrantanopia (right parietal lesion, MCA)
6. Left hemianopia with macular sparing (right occipital lesion, PCA)
7. Central scotoma (eg, macular degeneration)

Meyer loop—lower retina; loops around inferior horn of lateral ventricle.

Dorsal optic radiation—superior retina; takes shortest path via internal capsule.

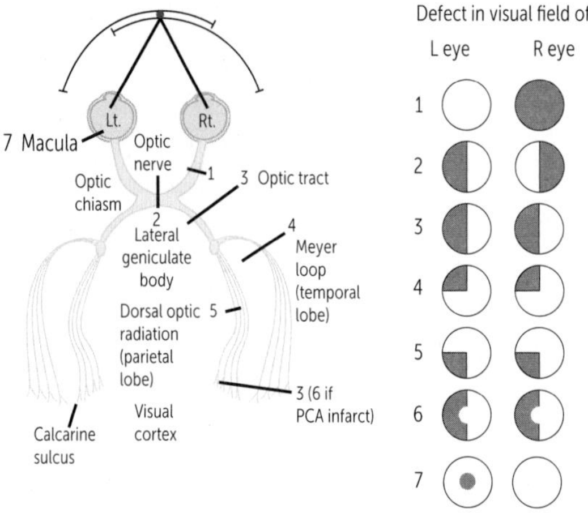

Note: When an image hits 1° visual cortex, it is upside down and left-right reversed.

Cavernous sinus

Collection of venous sinuses on either side of pituitary. Blood from eye and superficial cortex → cavernous sinus → internal jugular vein.

CNs III, IV, V_1, V_2, and VI plus postganglionic sympathetic pupillary fibers en route to orbit all pass through cavernous sinus. Cavernous portion of internal carotid artery is also here.

Cavernous sinus syndrome—presents with variable ophthalmoplegia (eg, CN III and CN VI), ↓ corneal sensation, Horner syndrome and occasional decreased maxillary sensation. 2° to pituitary tumor mass effect, carotid-cavernous fistula, or cavernous sinus thrombosis related to infection.

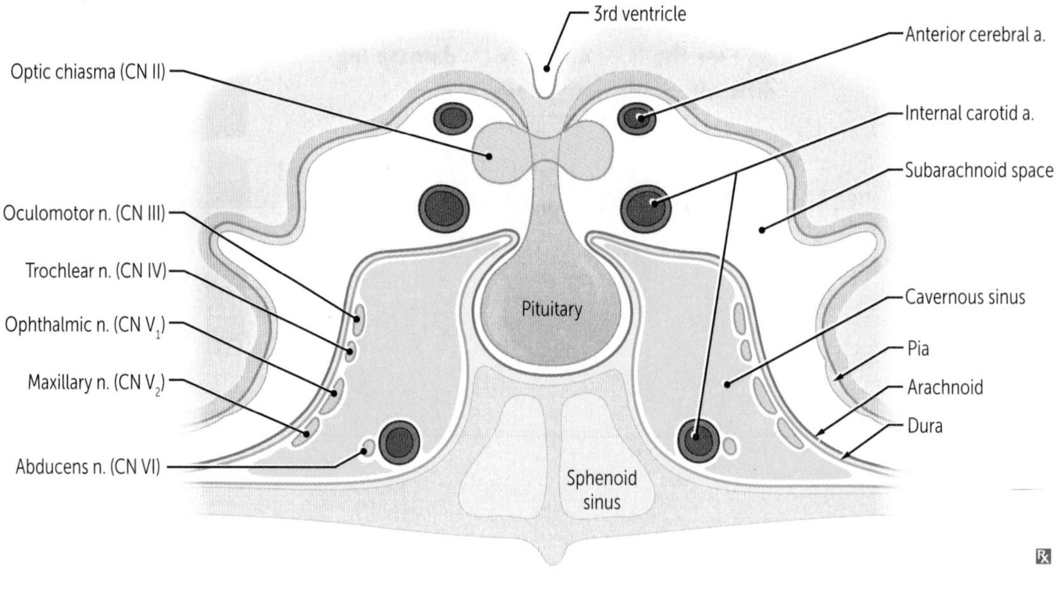

Internuclear ophthalmoplegia

Medial longitudinal fasciculus (MLF): pair of tracts that interconnect CN VI and CN III nuclei. Coordinates both eyes to move in same horizontal direction. Highly myelinated (must communicate quickly so eyes move at same time). Lesions may be unilateral or bilateral (latter classically seen in multiple sclerosis, stroke).

Lesion in MLF = internuclear ophthalmoplegia (INO), a conjugate horizontal gaze palsy. Lack of communication such that when CN VI nucleus activates ipsilateral lateral rectus, contralateral CN III nucleus does not stimulate medial rectus to contract. Abducting eye displays nystagmus (CN VI overfires to stimulate CN III). Convergence normal.

MLF in MS.

When looking left, the left nucleus of CN VI fires, which contracts the left lateral rectus and stimulates the contralateral (right) nucleus of CN III via the right MLF to contract the right medial rectus.

Directional term (eg, right INO, left INO) refers to the eye that is unable to adduct.

INO = Ipsilateral adduction failure, Nystagmus Opposite.

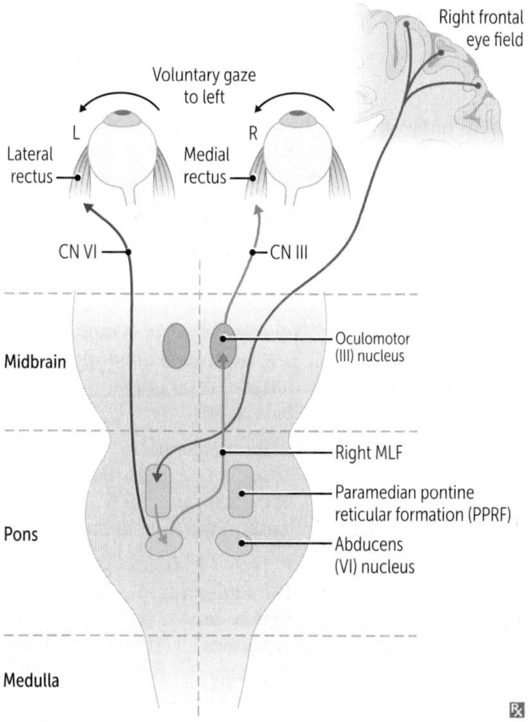
Right frontal eye field
Voluntary gaze to left
L
R
Lateral rectus
Medial rectus
CN VI
CN III
Midbrain
Oculomotor (III) nucleus
Right MLF
Paramedian pontine reticular formation (PPRF)
Pons
Abducens (VI) nucleus
Medulla

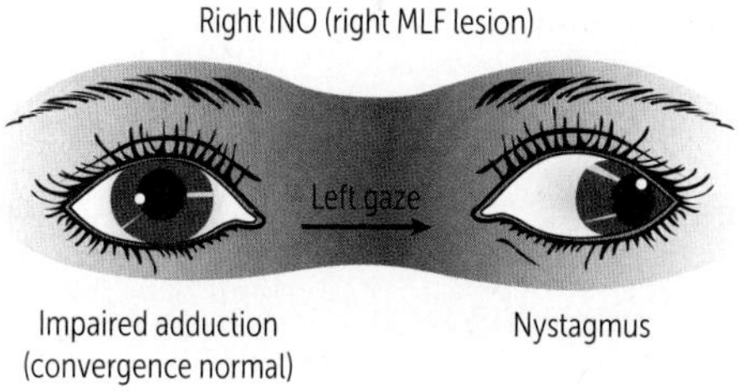
Right INO (right MLF lesion)
Left gaze
Impaired adduction (convergence normal)
Nystagmus

▶ NEUROLOGY—PHARMACOLOGY

Epilepsy therapy

	PARTIAL (FOCAL)†	1° GENERALIZED		STATUS EPILEPTICUS	MECHANISM	SIDE EFFECTS	NOTES
		TONIC-CLONIC	ABSENCE				
Benzodiazepines				** ✓	↑ $GABA_A$ action	Sedation, tolerance, dependence, respiratory depression	Also for eclampsia seizures (1st line is $MgSO_4$)
Carbamazepine	* ✓				Blocks Na^+ channels	Diplopia, ataxia, blood dyscrasias (agranulocytosis, aplastic anemia), liver toxicity, teratogenesis (cleft lip/palate, spina bifida), induction of cytochrome P-450, SIADH, SJS	1st line for trigeminal neuralgia
Ethosuximide			* ✓		Blocks thalamic T-type Ca^{2+} channels	EFGHIJ—Ethosuximide causes Fatigue, GI distress, Headache, Itching (and urticaria), SJS	Sucks to have silent (absence) seizures
Gabapentin	✓				Primarily inhibits high-voltage-activated Ca^{2+} channels; designed as GABA analog	Sedation, ataxia	Also used for peripheral neuropathy, postherpetic neuralgia
Lamotrigine	✓	✓	✓		Blocks voltage-gated Na^+ channels, inhibits the release of glutamate	SJS (must be titrated slowly), hemophagocytic lymphohistiocytosis (black box warning)	
Levetiracetam	✓	✓			SV2A receptor blocker; may modulate GABA and glutamate release, inhibit voltage-gated Ca^{2+} channels	Neuropsychiatric symptoms (eg, personality change), fatigue, drowsiness, headache	
Phenobarbital	✓	✓		✓	↑ $GABA_A$ action	Sedation, tolerance, dependence, induction of cytochrome P-450, cardiorespiratory depression	1st line in **neonates** ("phenobabytal")
Phenytoin, fosphenytoin	✓			*** ✓	Blocks Na^+ channels; zero-order kinetics	**PPHENYTOIN**: cytochrome **P**-450 induction, **P**seudolymphoma, **H**irsutism, **E**nlarged gums, **N**ystagmus, **Y**ellow-brown skin, **T**eratogenicity (fetal hydantoin syndrome), **O**steopenia, **I**nhibited folate absorption, **N**europathy. Rare: SJS, DRESS syndrome, drug-induced lupus. Toxicity leads to diplopia, ataxia, sedation.	
Topiramate	✓	✓			Blocks Na^+ channels, ↑ GABA action	Sedation, slow cognition, kidney stones, skinny (weight loss), sight threatened (glaucoma), speech (word-finding) difficulties	Also used for migraine prophylaxis
Valproic acid	✓	* ✓	✓		↑ Na^+ channel inactivation, ↑ GABA concentration by inhibiting GABA transaminase	**VALPPROaTTE**: **V**omiting, **A**lopecia, **L**iver damage (hepatotoxic), **P**ancreatitis, **P**-450 inhibition, **R**ash, **O**besity (weight gain), **T**remor, **T**eratogenesis (neural tube defects). **E**pigastric pain (GI distress).	Also used for myoclonic seizures, bipolar disorder, migraine prophylaxis
Vigabatrin	✓				↑ GABA. Irreversible GABA transaminase inhibitor	Permanent visual loss (black box warning)	Vision loss with **GABA** transaminase **inhibitor**

* = Common use, ** = 1st line for acute, *** = 1st line for recurrent seizure prophylaxis.
† Includes partial simple/complex and 2° generalized seizures.

Epilepsy therapy *(continued)*

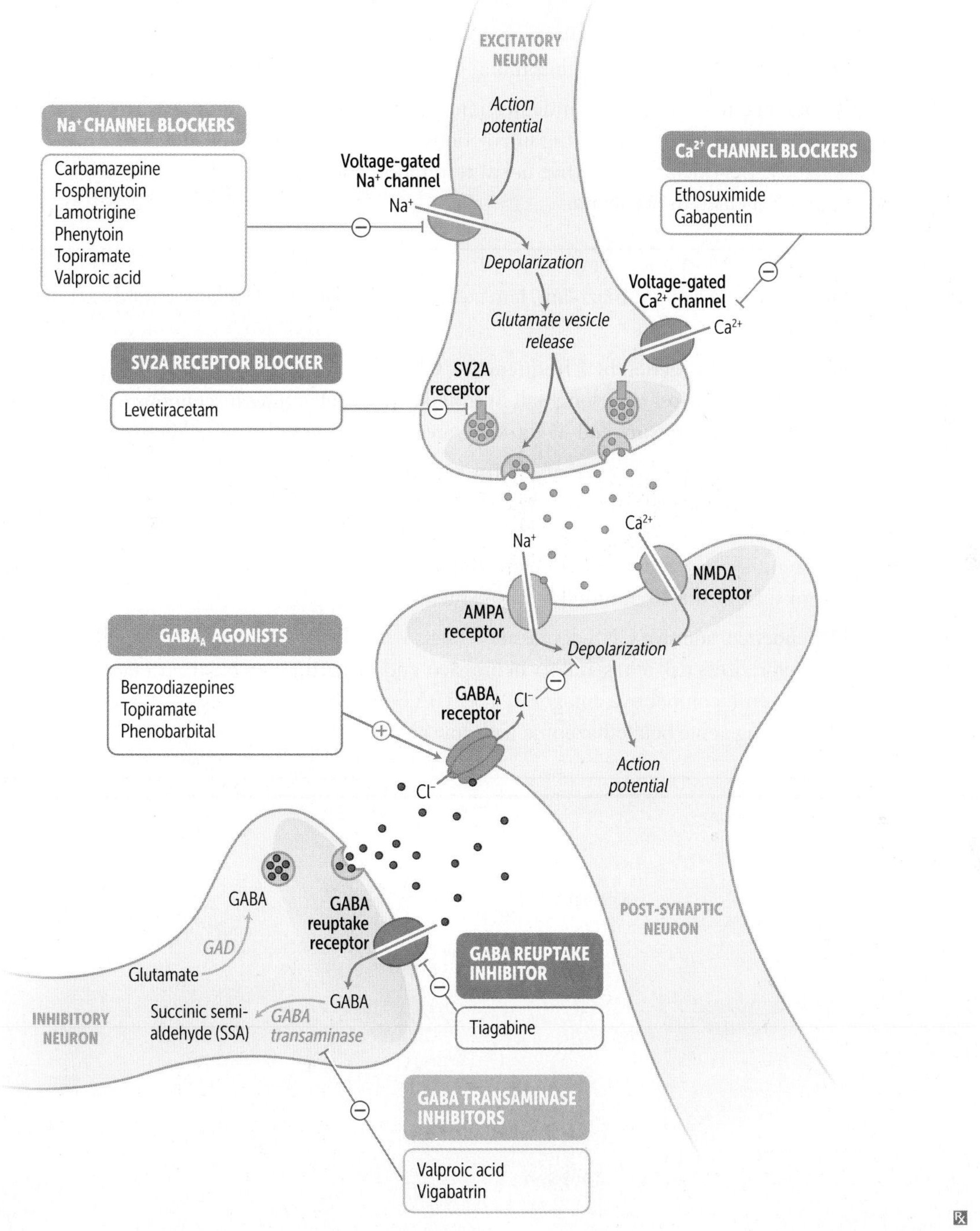

Barbiturates	Phenobarbital, pentobarbital, thiopental, secobarbital.
MECHANISM	Facilitate $GABA_A$ action by ↑ **duration** of Cl^- channel opening, thus ↓ neuron firing (barbi**durat**es ↑ **durat**ion).
CLINICAL USE	Sedative for anxiety, seizures, insomnia, induction of anesthesia (thiopental).
ADVERSE EFFECTS	Respiratory and cardiovascular depression (can be fatal); CNS depression (can be exacerbated by alcohol use); dependence; drug interactions (induces cytochrome P-450). Overdose treatment is supportive (assist respiration and maintain BP). Contraindicated in porphyria.

Benzodiazepines	Diazepam, lorazepam, triazolam, temazepam, oxazepam, midazolam, chlordiazepoxide, alprazolam.
MECHANISM	Facilitate $GABA_A$ action by ↑ **frequency** of Cl^- channel opening ("**fre**nzodiazepines" ↑ **fre**quency). ↓ REM sleep. Most have long half-lives and active metabolites (exceptions [**ATOM**]: **A**lprazolam, **T**riazolam, **O**xazepam, and **M**idazolam are short acting → higher addictive potential).
CLINICAL USE	Anxiety, panic disorder, spasticity, status epilepticus (lorazepam, diazepam, midazolam), eclampsia, detoxification (eg, alcohol withdrawal/DTs; long-acting chlordiazepoxide and diazepam are preferred), night terrors, sleepwalking, general anesthetic (amnesia, muscle relaxation), hypnotic (insomnia). **L**orazepam, **O**xazepam, and **T**emazepam can be used for those with liver disease who drink a **LOT** due to minimal first-pass metabolism.
ADVERSE EFFECTS	Dependence, additive CNS depression effects with alcohol and barbiturates (all bind the $GABA_A$ receptor). Less risk of respiratory depression and coma than with barbiturates. Treat overdose with flumazenil (competitive antagonist at GABA benzodiazepine receptor). Can precipitate seizures by causing acute benzodiazepine withdrawal.

Insomnia therapy

AGENT	MECHANISM	ADVERSE EFFECTS	NOTES
Nonbenzodiazepine hypnotics	Examples: Zolpidem, Zaleplon, esZopiclone Act via the BZ_1 subtype of GABA receptor	Ataxia, headaches, confusion Cause only modest day-after psychomotor depression and few amnestic effects (vs older sedative-hypnotics)	These **ZZZ**s put you to sleep Short duration due to rapid metabolism by liver enzymes; effects reversed by flumazenil ↓ dependency risk and ↓ sleep cycle disturbance (vs benzodiazepine hypnotics)
Suvorexant	**Orex**in (hypocretin) receptor **ant**agonist	CNS depression (somnolence), headache, abnormal sleep-related activities	Contraindications: narcolepsy, combination with strong CYP3A4 inhibitors Not recommended in patients with liver disease Limited risk of dependency
Ramelteon	**Mel**atonin receptor agonist: binds MT1 and MT2 in suprachiasmatic nucleus	Dizziness, nausea, fatigue, headache	No known risk of dependency

Triptans

	Sumatriptan	
MECHANISM	$5\text{-HT}_{1B/1D}$ agonists. Inhibit trigeminal nerve activation, prevent vasoactive peptide release, induce vasoconstriction.	A sumo wrestler **trips** and falls on their **head**.
CLINICAL USE	Acute migraine, cluster **head**ache attacks.	
ADVERSE EFFECTS	Coronary vasospasm (contraindicated in patients with CAD or vasospastic angina), mild paresthesia, serotonin syndrome (in combination with other 5-HT agonists).	

Parkinson disease therapy

The most effective treatments are non-ergot dopamine agonists which are usually started in younger patients, and Levodopa (with carbidopa) which is usually started in older patients. Deep brain stimulation of the STN or GPi may be helpful in advanced disease.

STRATEGY	AGENTS
Dopamine agonists	Non-ergot (preferred)—pramipexole, ropinirole; toxicity includes nausea, impulse control disorder (eg, gambling), postural hypotension, hallucinations, confusion. Ergot—bromocriptine rarely used due to toxicity.
↑ dopamine availability	Amantadine (↑ dopamine release and ↓ dopamine reuptake); toxicity = peripheral edema, livedo reticularis, ataxia.
↑ L-DOPA availability	Agents prevent peripheral (pre-BBB) L-DOPA degradation → ↑ L-DOPA entering CNS → ↑ central L-DOPA available for conversion to dopamine. ▪ Levodopa (L-DOPA)/carbidopa—carbidopa blocks peripheral conversion of L-DOPA to dopamine by inhibiting DOPA decarboxylase. Also reduces side effects of peripheral L-DOPA conversion into dopamine (eg, nausea, vomiting). ▪ Entacapone and tolcapone prevent peripheral L-DOPA degradation to 3-O-methyldopa (3-OMD) by inhibiting COMT. Used in conjunction with levodopa.
Prevent dopamine breakdown	Agents act centrally (post-BBB) to inhibit breakdown of dopamine. ▪ Selegiline, rasagiline—block conversion of dopamine into DOPAC by selectively inhibiting MAO-B. ▪ Tolcapone—crosses BBB and blocks conversion of dopamine to 3-methoxytyramine (3-MT) in the brain by inhibiting central COMT.
Curb excess cholinergic activity	**Benz**tropine, **tri**hexyphenidyl (Antimuscarinic; improves tremor and rigidity but has little effect on bradykinesia in **Park**inson disease). **Tri Park**ing my Mercedes-**Benz**.

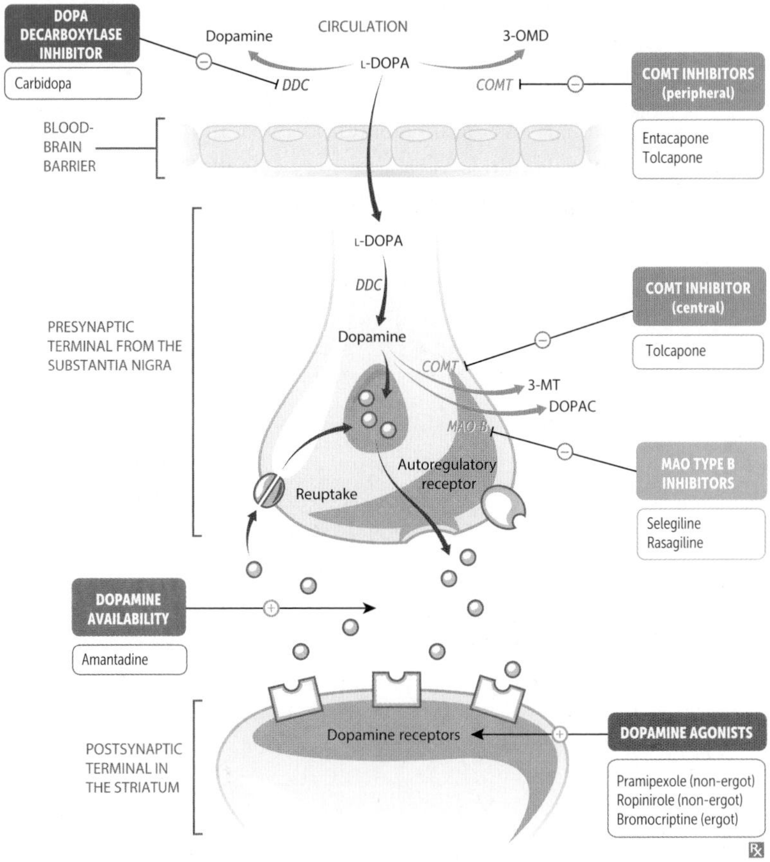

Carbidopa/levodopa

MECHANISM	↑ dopamine in brain. Unlike dopamine, L-DOPA can cross blood-brain barrier and is converted by dopa decarboxylase in the CNS to dopamine. Carbidopa, a peripheral DOPA decarboxylase inhibitor, is given with L-DOPA to ↑ bioavailability of L-DOPA in the brain and to limit peripheral side effects.
CLINICAL USE	Parkinson disease.
ADVERSE EFFECTS	Nausea, hallucinations, postural hypotension. With progressive disease, L-DOPA can lead to "on-off" phenomenon with improved mobility during "on" periods, then impaired motor function during "off" periods when patient responds poorly to L-DOPA or medication wears off.

Selegiline, rasagiline

MECHANISM	Selectively inhibit MAO-B (metabolize dopamine) → ↑ dopamine availability. **S**elegiline **s**electively inhibits MAO-**B** and is more commonly found in the **B**rain than in the periphery.
CLINICAL USE	Adjunctive agent to L-DOPA in treatment of Parkinson disease.
ADVERSE EFFECTS	May enhance adverse effects of L-DOPA.

Neurodegenerative disease therapy

DISEASE	AGENT	MECHANISM	NOTES
Alzheimer disease	Donepezil, rivastigmine, galantamine	AChE inhibitor	1st-line treatment Adverse effects: nausea, dizziness, insomnia. Contraindicated in patients with cardiac conduction abnormalities. **Dona Riva** dances at the **gala**
	Memantine	NMDA receptor antagonist; helps prevent excitotoxicity (mediated by Ca^{2+})	Used for moderate to advanced dementia Adverse effects: dizziness, confusion, hallucinations
Amyotrophic lateral sclerosis	Riluzole	↓ neuron glutamate excitotoxicity	↑ survival Treat **Lou** Gehrig disease with ri**Lou**zole
Huntington disease	Tetrabenazine	Inhibit vesicular monoamine transporter (VMAT) → ↓ dopamine vesicle packaging and release	May be used for Huntington chorea and tardive dyskinesia

Anesthetics—general principles

CNS drugs must be lipid soluble (cross the blood-brain barrier) or be actively transported.
Drugs with ↓ solubility in blood = rapid induction and recovery times.
Drugs with ↑ solubility in lipids = ↑ potency.
MAC = **M**inimum **A**lveolar **C**oncentration (of inhaled anesthetic) required to prevent 50% of subjects from moving in response to noxious stimulus (eg, skin incision). Potency = 1/MAC.
Examples: nitrous oxide (N_2O) has ↓ blood and lipid solubility, and thus fast induction and low potency. Halothane has ↑ lipid and blood solubility, and thus high potency and slow induction.

Inhaled anesthetics

Desfl**urane**, halo**thane**, enfl**urane**, isofl**urane**, sevofl**urane**, methoxyfl**urane**, N_2O.

MECHANISM	Mechanism unknown.
EFFECTS	Myocardial depression, respiratory depression, postoperative nausea/vomiting, ↑ cerebral blood flow and ICP, ↓ cerebral metabolic demand.
ADVERSE EFFECTS	**H**epatotoxicity (**h**alothane), **neph**rotoxicity (**meth**oxyflurane), proconvulsant (**en**flurane, **e**pileptogenic), expansion of trapped gas in a body cavity (N_2O). Malignant hyperthermia—rare, life-threatening condition in which inhaled anesthetics or succinylcholine induce severe muscle contractions and hyperthermia. Susceptibility is often inherited as autosomal dominant with variable penetrance. Mutations in ryanodine receptor (*RYR1*) cause ↑ Ca^{2+} release from sarcoplasmic reticulum. Treatment: dantrolene (a ryanodine receptor antagonist).

Intravenous anesthetics

AGENT	MECHANISM	ANESTHESIA USE	NOTES
Thiopental	Facilitates $GABA_A$ (barbiturate)	Anesthesia induction, short surgical procedures	↓ cerebral blood flow. High lipid solubility Effect terminated by rapid redistribution into tissue, fat
Midazolam	Facilitates $GABA_A$ (benzodiazepine)	Procedural sedation (eg, endoscopy), anesthesia induction	May cause severe postoperative respiratory depression, ↓ BP, anterograde amnesia
Propofol	Potentiates $GABA_A$	Rapid anesthesia induction, short procedures, ICU sedation	May cause respiratory depression, ↓ BP
Ketamine	NMDA receptor antagonist	Dissociative anesthesia Sympathomimetic	↑ cerebral blood flow Emergence reaction possible with disorientation, hallucination, vivid dreams

Local anesthetics

Esters—procaine, tetracaine, benzocaine, chloroprocaine.
Amides—lidocaine, mepivacaine, bupivacaine, ropivacaine, prilocaine (amides have 2 i's in name).

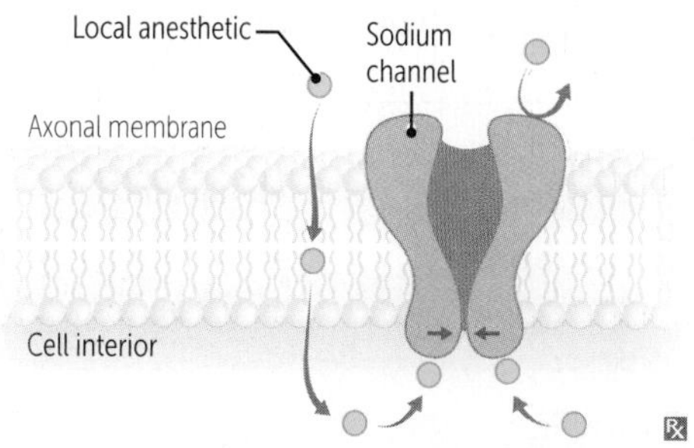

MECHANISM

Block neurotransmission via binding to voltage-gated Na^+ channels on inner portion of the channel along nerve fibers. Most effective in rapidly firing neurons. 3° amine local anesthetics penetrate membrane in uncharged form, then bind to ion channels as charged form.
Can be given with vasoconstrictors (usually epinephrine) to enhance block duration of action by ↓ systemic absorption.
In infected (acidic) tissue, alkaline anesthetics are charged and cannot penetrate membrane effectively → need more anesthetic.
Order of loss: (1) pain, (2) temperature, (3) touch, (4) pressure.

CLINICAL USE

Minor surgical procedures, spinal anesthesia. If allergic to esters, give amides.

ADVERSE EFFECTS

CNS excitation, severe cardiovascular toxicity (bupivacaine), hypertension, hypotension, arrhythmias (cocaine), methemoglobinemia (benzocaine, prilocaine).

Neuromuscular blocking drugs

Muscle paralysis in surgery or mechanical ventilation. Selective for Nm nicotinic receptors at neuromuscular junction but not autonomic Nn receptors.

Depolarizing neuromuscular blocking drugs

Succinylcholine—strong ACh receptor agonist; produces sustained depolarization and prevents muscle contraction.
Reversal of blockade:
- Phase I (prolonged depolarization)—no antidote. Block potentiated by cholinesterase inhibitors.
- Phase II (repolarized but blocked; ACh receptors are available, but desensitized)—may be reversed with cholinesterase inhibitors.

Complications include hypercalcemia, hyperkalemia, malignant hyperthermia. ↑ risk of prolonged muscle paralysis in patients with pseudocholinesterase deficiency.

Nondepolarizing neuromuscular blocking drugs

Atra**cu**rium, cisatra**cu**rium, pan**cu**ronium, ro**cu**ronium, tubo**cu**rarine, ve**cu**ronium—competitive ACh antagonist.
Reversal of blockade—sugammadex or cholinesterase inhibitors (eg, neostigmine, edrophonium). Anticholinergics (eg, atropine, glycopyrrolate) are given with cholinesterase inhibitors to prevent muscarinic effects (eg, bradycardia).

Spasmolytics, antispasmodics

DRUG	MECHANISM	CLINICAL USE	NOTES
Baclofen	$GABA_B$ receptor agonist in spinal cord	Muscle spasticity, dystonia, multiple sclerosis	Acts on the back (spinal cord)
Cyclobenzaprine	Acts within CNS, mainly at the brain stem	Muscle spasticity	Centrally acting Structurally related to TCAs May cause anticholinergic side effects, sedation
Dantrolene	Prevents release of Ca^{2+} from sarcoplasmic reticulum of skeletal muscle by inhibiting the ryanodine receptor	Malignant hyperthermia (toxicity of inhaled anesthetics and succinylcholine) and neuroleptic malignant syndrome (toxicity of antipsychotic drugs)	Acts directly on muscle
Tizanidine	α_2 agonist, acts centrally	Muscle spasticity, multiple sclerosis, ALS, cerebral palsy	

Opioid analgesics

MECHANISM	Act as agonists at opioid receptors (μ = β-endorphin, δ = enkephalin, κ = dynorphin) to modulate synaptic transmission—close presynaptic Ca^{2+} channels, open postsynaptic K^+ channels → ↓ synaptic transmission. Inhibit release of ACh, norepinephrine, 5-HT, glutamate, substance P.
EFFICACY	Full agonist: morphine, heroin, meperidine (long acting), methadone, codeine (prodrug; activated by CYP2D6), fentanyl. Partial agonist: buprenorphine. Mixed agonist/antagonist: nalbuphine, pentazocine, butorphanol. Antagonist: naloxone, naltrexone, methylnaltrexone.
CLINICAL USE	Moderate to severe or refractory pain, diarrhea (loperamide, diphenoxylate), acute pulmonary edema, maintenance programs for opiate use disorder (methadone, buprenorphine + naloxone), neonatal abstinence syndrome (methadone, morphine).
ADVERSE EFFECTS	Nausea, vomiting, pruritus (histamine release), opiate use disorder, respiratory depression, constipation, sphincter of Oddi spasm, miosis (except meperidine → mydriasis), additive CNS depression with other drugs. Tolerance does not develop to miosis and constipation. Treat toxicity with naloxone (competitive opioid receptor antagonist) and prevent relapse with naltrexone once detoxified.

Mixed agonist and antagonist opioid analgesics

DRUG	MECHANISM	CLINICAL USE	NOTES
Pentazocine	κ-opioid receptor agonist and μ-opioid receptor weak antagonist or partial agonist.	Analgesia for moderate to severe pain.	Can cause opioid withdrawal symptoms if patient is also taking full opioid agonist (due to competition for opioid receptors).
Butorphanol	κ-opioid receptor agonist and μ-opioid receptor partial agonist.	Severe pain (eg, migraine, labor).	Causes less respiratory depression than full opioid agonists. Use with full opioid agonist can precipitate withdrawal. Not easily reversed with naloxone.

Tramadol

MECHANISM	Very weak opioid agonist; also inhibits the reuptake of norepinephrine and serotonin.	Tramadol is a slight opioid agonist, and a serotonin and norepinephrine reuptake inhibitor. It is used for stubborn pain, but can lower seizure threshold, and may cause serotonin syndrome.
CLINICAL USE	Chronic pain.	
ADVERSE EFFECTS	Similar to opioids; decreases seizure threshold; serotonin syndrome.	

Glaucoma therapy

↓ IOP via ↓ amount of aqueous humor (inhibit synthesis/secretion or ↑ drainage).
BAD humor may not be politically correct.

DRUG CLASS	EXAMPLES	MECHANISM	ADVERSE EFFECTS
β-blockers	Timolol, betaxolol, carteolol	↓ aqueous humor synthesis	No pupillary or vision changes
α-agonists	Epinephrine (α_1), apraclonidine, brimonidine (α_2)	↓ aqueous humor synthesis via vasoconstriction (epinephrine) ↓ aqueous humor synthesis (apraclonidine, brimonidine)	Mydriasis (α_1); do not use in closed-angle glaucoma Blurry vision, ocular hyperemia, foreign body sensation, ocular allergic reactions, ocular pruritus
Diuretics	Acetazolamide	↓ aqueous humor synthesis via inhibition of carbonic anhydrase	No pupillary or vision changes
Prostaglandins	Bimatoprost, latanoprost ($PGF_{2\alpha}$)	↑ outflow of aqueous humor via ↓ resistance of flow through uveoscleral pathway	Darkens color of iris (browning), eyelash growth
Cholinomimetics (M_3)	Direct: pilocarpine, carbachol Indirect: physostigmine, echothiophate	↑ outflow of aqueous humor via contraction of ciliary muscle and opening of trabecular meshwork Use pilocarpine in acute angle closure glaucoma—very effective at opening meshwork into canal of Schlemm	Miosis (contraction of pupillary sphincter muscles) and cyclospasm (contraction of ciliary muscle)

▶ NOTES

HIGH-YIELD PRINCIPLES IN

Psychiatry

"Words of comfort, skillfully administered, are the oldest therapy known to man."

—Louis Nizer

"Even a happy life cannot be without a measure of darkness, and the word happy would lose its meaning if it were not balanced by sadness."

—Carl G. Jung

"The sorrow which has no vent in tears may make other organs weep."

—Henry Maudsley

"I have schizophrenia. I am not schizophrenia. I am not my mental illness. My illness is a part of me."

—Jonathan Harnisch

This chapter encompasses overlapping areas in psychiatry, psychology, sociology, and psychopharmacology. High-yield topics include schizophrenia, mood disorders, eating disorders, personality disorders, somatic symptom disorders, substance use disorders, and antipsychotic agents. Know the DSM-5 criteria for diagnosing common psychiatric disorders.

▸ PSYCHIATRY—PSYCHOLOGY

Classical conditioning

Learning in which a natural response (salivation) is elicited by a conditioned, or learned, stimulus (bell) that previously was presented in conjunction with an unconditioned stimulus (food).

Usually elicits **involuntary** responses.
Pavlov's classical experiments with dogs—ringing the bell provoked salivation.

Operant conditioning

Learning in which a particular action is elicited because it produces a punishment or reward. Usually elicits **voluntary** responses.

Reinforcement	Target behavior (response) is followed by desired reward (positive reinforcement) or removal of aversive stimulus (negative reinforcement).
Punishment	Repeated application of aversive stimulus (positive punishment) or removal of desired reward (negative punishment) to extinguish unwanted behavior.
Extinction	Discontinuation of reinforcement (positive or negative) eventually eliminates behavior. Can occur in operant or classical conditioning.

Skinner operant conditioning quadrants:

	Increase behavior	**Decrease behavior**
Add a stimulus	Positive reinforcement	Positive punishment
Remove a stimulus	Negative reinforcement	Negative punishment

Transference and countertransference

Transference	Patient projects feelings about formative or other important persons onto physician (eg, psychiatrist is seen as parent).
Countertransference	Physician projects feelings about formative or other important persons onto patient (eg, patient reminds physician of younger sibling).

Ego defenses

Thoughts and behaviors (voluntary or involuntary) used to resolve conflict and prevent undesirable feelings (eg, anxiety, depression).

IMMATURE DEFENSES	DESCRIPTION	EXAMPLE
Acting out	Subconsciously coping with stressors or emotional conflict using actions rather than reflections or feelings.	A patient skips therapy appointments after deep discomfort from dealing with his past.
Denial	Avoiding the awareness of some painful reality.	A patient with cancer plans a full-time work schedule despite being warned of significant fatigue during chemotherapy.
Displacement	Redirection of emotions or impulses to a neutral person or object (vs projection).	After being reprimanded by her principal, a frustrated teacher returns home and criticizes her wife's cooking instead of confronting the principal directly.
Dissociation	Temporary, drastic change in personality, memory, consciousness, or motor behavior to avoid emotional stress. Patient has incomplete or no memory of traumatic event.	A survivor of sexual abuse sees the abuser and suddenly becomes numb and detached.

Ego defenses *(continued)*

IMMATURE DEFENSES	DESCRIPTION	EXAMPLE
Fixation	Partially remaining at a more childish level of development (vs regression).	A surgeon throws a tantrum in the operating room because the last case ran very late.
Idealization	Expressing extremely positive thoughts of self and others while ignoring negative thoughts.	A patient boasts about his physician and his accomplishments while ignoring any flaws.
Identification	Largely unconscious assumption of the characteristics, qualities, or traits of another person or group.	A resident starts putting her stethoscope in her pocket like her favorite attending, instead of wearing it around her neck like before.
Intellectualization	Using facts and logic to emotionally distance oneself from a stressful situation.	A patient diagnosed with cancer discusses the pathophysiology of the disease.
Isolation (of affect)	Separating feelings from ideas and events.	Describing murder in graphic detail with no emotional response.
Passive aggression	Demonstrating hostile feelings in a nonconfrontational manner; showing indirect opposition.	A disgruntled employee is repeatedly late to work, but won't admit it is a way to get back at the manager.
Projection	Attributing an unacceptable internal impulse to an external source (vs displacement).	A man who wants to cheat on his wife accuses his wife of being unfaithful.
Rationalization	Asserting plausible explanations for events that actually occurred for other reasons, usually to avoid self-blame.	An employee who was recently fired claims that the job was not important anyway.
Reaction formation	Replacing a warded-off idea or feeling with an emphasis on its opposite (vs sublimation).	A stepfather treats a child he resents with excessive nurturing and overprotection.
Regression	Involuntarily turning back the maturational clock to behaviors previously demonstrated under stress (vs fixation).	A previously toilet-trained child begins bedwetting again following the birth of a sibling.
Repression	Involuntarily withholding an idea or feeling from conscious awareness (vs suppression).	A 20-year-old does not remember going to counseling during his parents' divorce 10 years earlier.
Splitting	Believing that people are either all good or all bad at different times due to intolerance of ambiguity. Common in borderline personality disorder.	A patient says that all the nurses are cold and insensitive, but the physicians are warm and friendly.
MATURE DEFENSES		
Sublimation	Replacing an unacceptable wish with a course of action that is similar to the wish but socially acceptable (vs reaction formation).	A teenager's aggression toward her parents because of their high expectations is channeled into excelling in sports.
Altruism	Alleviating negative feelings via unsolicited generosity, which provides gratification (vs reaction formation).	A mafia boss makes a large donation to charity.
Suppression	Intentionally withholding an idea or feeling from conscious awareness (vs repression); temporary.	An athlete focuses on other tasks to prevent worrying about an important upcoming match.
Humor	Lightheartedly expressing uncomfortable feelings to shift the internal focus away from the distress.	A nervous medical student jokes about the boards.
	Mature adults wear a **SASH**.	

Grief

The five stages of grief per the Kübler-Ross model are denial, anger, bargaining, depression, and acceptance (may occur in any order). Other common grief symptoms include shock, guilt, sadness, anxiety, yearning, and somatic symptoms that usually occur in waves. Auditory or visual hallucinations can occur in the context of normal bereavement (eg, hearing the deceased speaking). Duration varies widely. Persistent complex bereavement disorder is diagnosed if severe grief interferes with functioning for > 12 months.

Normal infant and child development

Milestone dates are ranges that have been approximated and vary by source. Children not meeting milestones may need assessment for potential developmental delay.

AGE	MOTOR	SOCIAL	VERBAL/COGNITIVE
Infant	**Parents**	**Start**	**Observing,**
0–12 mo	Primitive reflexes disappear—Moro (by 3 mo), rooting (by 4 mo), palmar (by 6 mo), Babinski (by 12 mo) Posture—lifts head up prone (by 1 mo), rolls and sits (by 6 mo), crawls (by 8 mo), stands (by 10 mo), walks (by 12–18 mo) Picks—passes toys hand to hand (by 6 mo), Pincer grasp (by 10 mo) Points to objects (by 12 mo)	Social smile (by 2 mo) Stranger anxiety (by 6 mo) Separation anxiety (by 9 mo)	Orients—first to voice (by 4 mo), then to name and gestures (by 9 mo) Object permanence (by 9 mo) Oratory—says "mama" and "dada" (by 10 mo)
Toddler	**Child**	**Rearing**	**Working,**
12–36 mo	Cruises, takes first steps (by 12 mo) Climbs stairs (by 18 mo) Cubes stacked (number) = age (yr) × 3 Cutlery—feeds self with fork and spoon (by 20 mo) Kicks ball (by 24 mo)	Recreation—parallel play (by 24–36 mo) Rapprochement—moves away from and returns to parent (by 24 mo) Realization—core gender identity formed (by 36 mo)	Words—uses 50-200 words (by 2 yr), uses 300+ words (by 3 yr)
Preschool	**Don't**	**Forget, they're still**	**Learning!**
3–5 yr	Drive—tricycle (3 wheels at 3 yr) Drawings—copies line or circle, stick figure (by 4 yr) Dexterity—hops on one foot by 4 yr ("4 on one foot"), uses buttons or zippers, grooms self (by 5 yr)	Freedom—comfortably spends part of day away from parent (by 3 yr) Friends—cooperative play, has imaginary friends (by 4 yr)	Language—understands 1000 (**3 zeros**) words (by 3 yr), uses complete sentences and prepositions (by 4 yr) Legends—can tell detailed stories (by 4 yr)

▸ PSYCHIATRY—PATHOLOGY

Infant deprivation effects	Long-term deprivation of affection results in: ▪ Failure to thrive ▪ Poor language/socialization skills ▪ Lack of basic trust ▪ Reactive attachment disorder (infant withdrawn/unresponsive to comfort) ▪ Disinhibited social engagement (child indiscriminately attaches to strangers)	Deprivation for > 6 months can lead to irreversible changes. Severe deprivation can result in infant death.

Child abuse

	Physical abuse	Sexual abuse	Emotional abuse
SIGNS	Nonaccidental trauma (eg, fractures, bruises, burns). Injuries often in different stages of healing or in patterns resembling possible implements of injury. Includes abusive head trauma (shaken baby syndrome), characterized by subdural hematomas or retinal hemorrhages. Caregivers may delay seeking medical attention for the child or provide explanations inconsistent with the child's developmental stage or pattern of injury.	STIs, UTIs, and genital, anal, or oral trauma. Most often, there are no physical signs; sexual abuse should not be excluded from a differential diagnosis in the absence of physical trauma. Children often exhibit sexual knowledge or behavior incongruent with their age.	Babies or young children may lack a bond with the caregiver but are overly affectionate with less familiar adults. They may be aggressive toward children and animals or unusually anxious. Older children are often emotionally labile and prone to angry outbursts. They may distance themselves from caregivers and other children. They can experience vague somatic symptoms for which a medical cause cannot be found.
EPIDEMIOLOGY	40% of deaths related to child abuse or neglect occur in children < 1 year old.	Peak incidence 9–12 years old.	~80% of young adult victims of child emotional abuse meet the criteria for ≥ 1 psychiatric illness by age 21.

Child neglect	Failure to provide a child with adequate food, shelter, supervision, education, and/or affection. Most common form of child maltreatment. Signs: poor hygiene, malnutrition, withdrawal, impaired social/emotional development, failure to thrive. As with child abuse, suspected child neglect must be reported to local child protective services.
Vulnerable child syndrome	Parents perceive the child as especially susceptible to illness or injury (vs factitious disorder imposed on another). Usually follows a serious illness or life-threatening event. Can result in missed school or overuse of medical services.

Childhood and early-onset disorders

Attention-deficit hyperactivity disorder	Onset before age 12. ≥ 6 months of limited attention span and/or poor impulse control. Characterized by hyperactivity, impulsivity, and/or inattention in ≥ 2 settings (eg, school, home, places of worship). Normal intelligence, but commonly coexists with difficulties in school. Often persists into adulthood. Commonly coexists with oppositional defiant disorder. Treatment: stimulants (eg, methylphenidate) +/– behavioral therapy; alternatives include atomoxetine and α_2-agonists (eg, clonidine, guanfacine).
Autism spectrum disorder	Onset in early childhood. Social and communication deficits, repetitive/ritualized behaviors, restricted interests. May be accompanied by intellectual disability and/or above average abilities in specific skills (eg, music). More common in males. Associated with ↑ head and/or brain size.
Conduct disorder	Repetitive, pervasive behavior violating societal norms or the basic rights of others (eg, aggression toward people and animals, destruction of property, theft). After age 18, often reclassified as antisocial personality disorder. Treatment: psychotherapy (eg, cognitive behavioral therapy [CBT]).
Disruptive mood dysregulation disorder	Onset before age 10. Severe, recurrent temper outbursts out of proportion to situation. Child is constantly angry and irritable between outbursts. Treatment: CBT, stimulants, antipsychotics.
Intellectual disability	Global cognitive deficits (vs specific learning disorder) that affect reasoning, memory, abstract thinking, judgment, language, learning. Adaptive functioning is impaired, leading to major difficulties with education, employment, communication, socialization, independence. Treatment: psychotherapy, occupational therapy, special education.
Intermittent explosive disorder	Onset after age 6. Recurrent verbal or physical outbursts representing a failure to control aggressive impulses. Outbursts are out of proportion to provocation and may lead to legal, financial, or social consequences. Episodes are not premeditated and last < 30 minutes. Treatment: psychotherapy, SSRIs.
Oppositional defiant disorder	Pattern of anger and irritability with argumentative, vindictive, and defiant behavior toward authority figures lasting ≥ 6 months. Treatment: psychotherapy (eg, CBT).
Selective mutism	Onset before age 5. Anxiety disorder lasting ≥ 1 month involving refraining from speech in certain situations despite speaking in other, usually more comfortable situations. Development (eg, speech and language) not typically impaired. Interferes with social, academic, and occupational tasks. Commonly coexists with social anxiety disorder. Treatment: behavioral, family, and play therapy; SSRIs.
Separation anxiety disorder	Overwhelming fear of separation from home or attachment figure lasting ≥ 4 weeks. Can be normal behavior up to age 3–4. May lead to factitious physical complaints to avoid school. Treatment: CBT, play therapy, family therapy.
Specific learning disorder	Onset during school-age years. Inability to acquire or use information from a specific subject (eg, math, reading, writing) near age-expected proficiency for ≥ 6 months despite focused intervention. General functioning and intelligence are normal (vs intellectual disability). Treatment: academic support, counseling, extracurricular activities.
Tourette syndrome	Onset before age 18. Sudden, recurrent, nonrhythmic, stereotyped motor and vocal tics that persist for > 1 year. Coprolalia (involuntary obscene speech) found in some patients. Associated with OCD and ADHD. Treatment: psychoeducation, behavioral therapy. For intractable and distressing tics: tetrabenazine, antipsychotics, α_2-agonists.

Orientation	Patients' ability to know the date and time, where they are, and who they are (order of loss: time → place → person). Common causes of loss of orientation: alcohol, drugs, fluid/electrolyte imbalance, head trauma, hypoglycemia, infection, nutritional deficiencies, hypoxia.

Amnesias	
Retrograde amnesia	Inability to remember things that occurred **before** a CNS insult.
Anterograde amnesia	Inability to remember things that occurred **after** a CNS insult (↓ acquisition of new memory).
Korsakoff syndrome	Amnesia (anterograde > retrograde) and disorientation caused by vitamin B_1 deficiency. Associated with disruption and destruction of the limbic system, especially mammillary bodies and anterior thalamus. Seen in chronic alcohol use as a late neuropsychiatric manifestation of Wernicke encephalopathy. Confabulations are characteristic.

Dissociative disorders	
Depersonalization/ derealization disorder	Persistent feelings of detachment or estrangement from one's own body, thoughts, perceptions, and actions (depersonalization) or one's environment (derealization). Intact reality testing (vs psychosis).
Dissociative amnesia	Inability to recall important personal information, usually following severe trauma or stress. May be accompanied by **dissociative fugue** (abrupt, unexpected travelling away from home).
Dissociative identity disorder	Formerly called multiple personality disorder. Presence of ≥ 2 distinct identities or personality states, typically with distinct memories and patterns of behavior. More common in females. Associated with history of sexual abuse, PTSD, depression, substance use, borderline personality disorder, somatic symptom disorders.

Delirium

"Waxing and waning" level of consciousness with acute onset, ↓ attention span, ↓ level of arousal. Characterized by disorganized thinking, hallucinations (often visual), misperceptions (eg, illusions), disturbance in sleep-wake cycle, cognitive dysfunction, agitation. Reversible.

Usually 2° to other identifiable illness (eg, CNS disease, infection, trauma, substance use/withdrawal, metabolic/electrolyte disturbances, hemorrhage, urinary/fecal retention), or medications (eg, anticholinergics), especially in the elderly.

Most common presentation of altered mental status in inpatient setting, especially in the ICU or during prolonged hospital stays.

Deli**rium** = changes in senso**rium**.

EEG may show diffuse background rhythm slowing.

Treatment: identification and management of underlying condition. Orientation protocols (eg, keeping a clock or calendar nearby), ↓ sleep disturbances, and ↑ cognitive stimulation to manage symptoms. Antipsychotics (eg, haloperidol) as needed. Avoid unnecessary restraints and drugs that may worsen delirium (eg, anticholinergics, benzodiazepines, opioids).

Psychosis	Distorted perception of reality characterized by delusions, hallucinations, and/or disorganized thought/speech. Can occur in patients with medical illness, psychiatric illness, or both.
Delusions	False, fixed, idiosyncratic beliefs that persist despite evidence to the contrary and are not typical of a patient's culture or religion (eg, a patient who believes that others are reading his thoughts). Types include erotomanic, grandiose, jealous, persecutory, somatic, mixed, and unspecified.
Disorganized thought	Speech may be incoherent ("word salad"), tangential, or derailed ("loose associations").
Hallucinations	Perceptions in the absence of external stimuli (eg, seeing a light that is not actually present). Contrast with misperceptions (eg, illusions) of real external stimuli. Types include: ▪ Auditory—more commonly due to psychiatric illness (eg, schizophrenia) than medical illness. ▪ Visual—more commonly due to medical illness (eg, drug intoxication, delirium) than psychiatric illness. ▪ Tactile—common in alcohol withdrawal and stimulant use (eg, "cocaine crawlies," a type of delusional parasitosis). ▪ Olfactory—often occur as an aura of temporal lobe epilepsy (eg, burning rubber) and in brain tumors. ▪ Gustatory—rare, but seen in epilepsy. ▪ Hypna**gogic**—occurs while **going** to sleep. Sometimes seen in narcolepsy. ▪ Hypno**pompic**—occurs while waking from sleep ("get **pomp**ed up in the morning"). Sometimes seen in narcolepsy. Contrast with illusions, which are misperceptions of real external stimuli (eg, mistaking a shadow for a black cat).

Mood disorder	Characterized by an abnormal range of moods or internal emotional states and loss of control over them. Severity of moods causes distress and impairment in social and occupational functioning. Includes major depressive, bipolar, dysthymic, and cyclothymic disorders. Episodic superimposed psychotic features (delusions, hallucinations, disorganized speech/behavior) may be present.

Schizophrenia spectrum disorders

Schizophrenia	Chronic illness causing profound functional impairment. Symptom categories include: ▪ Positive—excessive or distorted functioning (eg, hallucinations, delusions, unusual thought processes, disorganized speech, bizarre behavior) ▪ Negative—diminished functioning (eg, flat or blunted affect, apathy. anhedonia, alogia, social withdrawal) ▪ Cognitive—reduced ability to understand or make plans, diminished working memory, inattention Diagnosis requires ≥ 2 of the following active symptoms, including ≥ 1 from symptoms #1–3: 1. Delusions 2. Hallucinations, often auditory 3. Disorganized speech 4. Disorganized or catatonic behavior 5. Negative symptoms Symptom onset ≥ 6 months prior to diagnosis; requires ≥ 1 month of active symptoms over the past 6 months.	Associated with altered dopaminergic activity, ↑ serotonergic activity, and ↓ dendritic branching. Ventriculomegaly on brain imaging. Lifetime prevalence—1.5% (males > females). Presents earlier in males (late teens to early 20s) than in females (late 20s to early 30s). ↑ suicide risk. Heavy cannabis use in adolescence is associated with ↑ incidence and worsened course of psychotic, mood, and anxiety disorders. Treatment: atypical antipsychotics (eg, risperidone) are first line. Negative symptoms often persist after treatment, despite resolution of positive symptoms.
	Brief psychotic disorder—≥ 1 positive symptom(s) lasting < 1 month, usually stress-related. Schizophreniform disorder—≥ 2 symptoms lasting 1–6 months.	
Schizoaffective disorder	Shares symptoms with both schizophrenia and mood disorders (major depressive or bipolar disorder). To differentiate from a mood disorder with psychotic features, patient must have > 2 weeks of psychotic symptoms without a manic or depressive episode.	
Delusional disorder	≥ 1 delusion(s) lasting > 1 month, but without a mood disorder or other psychotic symptoms. Daily functioning, including socialization, may be impacted by the pathological, fixed belief but is otherwise unaffected. Can be shared by individuals in close relationships (folie à deux).	
Schizotypal personality disorder	Cluster A personality disorder that also falls on the schizophrenia spectrum. May include brief psychotic episodes (eg, delusions) that are less frequent and severe than in schizophrenia.	

Manic episode

Distinct period of abnormally and persistently elevated, expansive, or irritable mood and ↑ activity or energy lasting ≥ 1 week. Diagnosis requires hospitalization or marked functional impairment with ≥ 3 of the following (manics **DIG FAST**):

- Distractibility
- Impulsivity/Indiscretion—seeks pleasure without regard to consequences (hedonistic)
- Grandiosity—inflated self-esteem
- Flight of ideas—racing thoughts
- ↑ goal-directed Activity/psychomotor Agitation
- ↓ need for Sleep
- Talkativeness or pressured speech

Hypomanic episode	Similar to a manic episode except mood disturbance is not severe enough to cause marked impairment in social and/or occupational functioning or to necessitate hospitalization. Abnormally ↑ activity or energy usually present. No psychotic features. Lasts ≥ 4 consecutive days.
Bipolar disorder	Bipolar I—≥ 1 manic episode +/– a hypomanic or depressive episode (may be separated by any length of time). Bipolar II—a hypomanic and a depressive episode (no history of manic episodes). Patient's mood and functioning usually normalize between episodes. Use of antidepressants can destabilize mood. High suicide risk. Treatment: mood stabilizers (eg, lithium, valproic acid, carbamazepine, lamotrigine), atypical antipsychotics. **Cyclothymic disorder**—milder form of bipolar disorder fluctuating between mild depressive and hypomanic symptoms. Must last ≥ 2 years with symptoms present at least half of the time, with any remission lasting ≤ 2 months.
Major depressive disorder	Recurrent episodes lasting ≥ 2 weeks characterized by ≥ 5 of 9 diagnostic symptoms including depressed mood or anhedonia (or irritability in children). SIG E CAPS: ▪ Sleep disturbances ▪ ↓ Interest in pleasurable activities (anhedonia) ▪ Guilt or feelings of worthlessness ▪ ↓ Energy ▪ ↓ Concentration ▪ Appetite/weight changes ▪ Psychomotor retardation or agitation ▪ Suicidal ideation Screen for previous manic or hypomanic episodes to rule out bipolar disorder. Treatment: CBT and SSRIs are first line; alternatives include SNRIs, mirtazapine, bupropion, electroconvulsive therapy (ECT), ketamine. Responses to a significant loss (eg, bereavement, natural disaster, disability) may resemble a depressive episode. Diagnosis of MDD is made if criteria are met.
MDD with psychotic features	MDD + hallucinations or delusions. Psychotic features are typically mood congruent (eg, depressive themes of inadequacy, guilt, punishment, nihilism, disease, or death) and occur only in the context of major depressive episode (vs schizoaffective disorder). Treatment: antidepressant with atypical antipsychotic, ECT.
Persistent depressive disorder	Also called dysthymia. Often milder than MDD; ≥ 2 depressive symptoms lasting ≥ 2 years (≥ 1 year in children), with any remission lasting ≤ 2 months.
MDD with seasonal pattern	Formerly called seasonal affective disorder. Major depressive episodes occurring only during a particular season (usually winter) in ≥ 2 consecutive years and in most years across a lifetime. Atypical symptoms common. Treatment: standard MDD therapies + light therapy.
Depression with atypical features	Characterized by mood reactivity (transient improvement in response to a positive event), hypersomnia, hyperphagia, leaden paralysis (heavy feeling in arms and legs), long-standing interpersonal rejection sensitivity. Most common subtype of depression. Treatment: CBT and SSRIs are first line. MAO inhibitors (MAOIs) are effective but not first line because of their risk profile.

Peripartum mood disturbances	Onset during pregnancy or within 4 weeks of delivery. ↑ risk with history of mood disorders.
Postpartum blues	50–85% incidence rate. Characterized by depressed affect, tearfulness, and fatigue starting 2–3 days after delivery. Usually resolves within 2 weeks. Treatment: supportive. Follow up to assess for possible MDD with peripartum onset.
MDD with peripartum onset	10–15% incidence rate. Formerly called postpartum depression. Meets MDD criteria with onset no later than 1 year after delivery. Treatment: CBT and SSRIs are first line.
Postpartum psychosis	0.1–0.2% incidence rate. Characterized by mood-congruent delusions, hallucinations, and thoughts of harming the baby or self. Risk factors include first pregnancy, family history, bipolar disorder, psychotic disorder, recent medication change. Treatment: hospitalization and initiation of atypical antipsychotic; if insufficient, ECT may be used.

Electroconvulsive therapy

Rapid-acting method to treat refractory depression, depression with psychotic symptoms, catatonia, and acute suicidality. Induces tonic-clonic seizure under anesthesia and neuromuscular blockade. Adverse effects include disorientation, headache, partial anterograde/retrograde amnesia usually resolving in 6 months. No absolute contraindications. Safe in pregnant and elderly individuals.

Risk factors for suicide completion

Sex (male)
Age (young adult or elderly)
Depression
Previous attempt (highest risk factor)
Ethanol or drug use
Rational thinking loss (psychosis)
Sickness (medical illness)
Organized plan
No spouse or other social support
Stated future intent

SAD PERSONS are more likely to complete suicide.

Most common method in US is firearms; access to guns ↑ risk of suicide completion.

Women try more often; men complete more often.

Other risk factors include recent psychiatric hospitalization and family history of completed suicide.

Protective factors include effective care for comorbidities; medical, familial, or community connectedness; cultural/religious beliefs encouraging self-preservation; and strong problem-solving skills.

Anxiety disorders

Inappropriate experiences of fear/worry and their physical manifestations incongruent with the magnitude of the stressors. Symptoms are not attributable to another psychiatric disorder, medical condition (eg, hyperthyroidism), or substance use. Includes panic disorder, phobias, generalized anxiety disorder, and selective mutism.

Panic disorder

Recurrent panic attacks involving intense fear and discomfort +/– a known trigger. Attacks typically peak in 10 minutes with ≥ 4 of the following: palpitations, paresthesias, depersonalization or derealization, abdominal pain, nausea, intense fear of dying, intense fear of losing control, lightheadedness, chest pain, chills, choking, sweating, shaking, shortness of breath. Strong genetic component. ↑ risk of suicide.

Diagnosis requires attack followed by ≥ 1 month of ≥ 1 of the following:

- Persistent concern of additional attacks
- Worrying about consequences of attack
- Behavioral change related to attacks

Symptoms are systemic manifestations of fear.

Treatment: CBT, SSRIs, and venlafaxine are first line. Benzodiazepines occasionally used in acute setting.

Phobias

Severe, persistent (≥ 6 months) fear or anxiety due to presence or anticipation of a specific object or situation. Person often recognizes fear is excessive. Treatment: CBT with exposure therapy.

Social anxiety disorder—exaggerated fear of embarrassment in social situations (eg, public speaking, using public restrooms). Treatment: CBT, SSRIs, venlafaxine. For performance type (eg, anxiety restricted to public speaking), use β-blockers or benzodiazepines as needed.

Agoraphobia—irrational fear/anxiety while facing or anticipating ≥ 2 specific situations (eg, open/closed spaces, lines, crowds, public transport). If severe, patients may refuse to leave their homes. Associated with panic disorder. Treatment: CBT, SSRIs.

Generalized anxiety disorder

Excessive anxiety and worry about different aspects of daily life (eg, work, school, children) for most days of ≥ 6 months. Associated with ≥ 3 of the following for adults (≥ 1 for kids): restlessness, irritability, sleep disturbance, fatigue, muscle tension, difficulty concentrating. Treatment: CBT, SSRIs, SNRIs are first line. Buspirone, TCAs, benzodiazepines are second line.

Obsessive-compulsive disorders

Obsessions (recurring intrusive thoughts, feelings, or sensations) that cause severe distress, relieved in part by compulsions (performance of repetitive, often time-consuming actions). Ego-dystonic: behavior inconsistent with one's beliefs and attitudes (vs obsessive-compulsive personality disorder, ego-syntonic). Associated with Tourette syndrome. Treatment: CBT and SSRIs; clomipramine and venlafaxine are second line.

Body dysmorphic disorder—preoccupation with minor or imagined defects in appearance. Causes significant emotional distress and repetitive appearance-related behaviors (eg, mirror checking, excessive grooming). Common in eating disorders. Treatment: CBT.

Trichotillomania

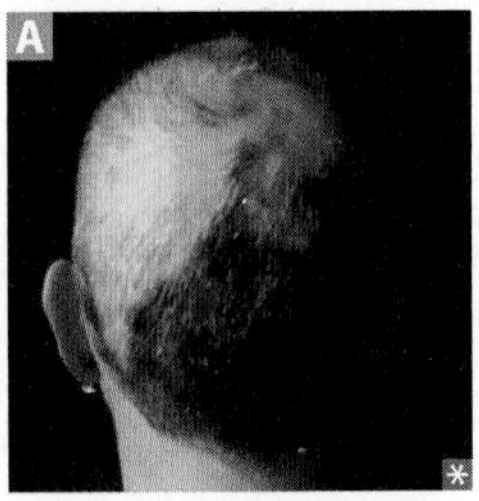

Compulsively pulling out one's hair. Causes significant distress and persists despite attempts to stop. Presents with areas of thinning hair or baldness on any area of the body, most commonly the scalp A. Remaining hair shafts are of different lengths (vs alopecia). Incidence highest in childhood but spans all ages. Treatment: psychotherapy.

Trauma and stress-related disorders

Adjustment disorder	Emotional or behavioral symptoms (eg, anxiety, outbursts) that occur within 3 months of an identifiable psychosocial stressor (eg, divorce, illness) lasting < 6 months once the stressor has ended. Symptoms do not meet criteria for another psychiatric illness. If symptoms persist > 6 months after stressor ends, reevaluate for other explanations (eg, MDD, GAD). Treatment: CBT is first line; antidepressants and anxiolytics may be considered.
Post-traumatic stress disorder	Experiencing, or discovering that a loved one has experienced, a life-threatening situation (eg, serious injury, rape, witnessing death) → persistent **H**yperarousal, **A**voidance of associated stimuli, intrusive **R**e-experiencing of the event (eg, nightmares, flashbacks), changes in cognition or mood (eg, fear, horror, **D**istress) (having PTSD is **HARD**). Disturbance lasts > 1 month with significant distress or impaired functioning. Treatment: CBT, SSRIs, and venlafaxine are first line. Prazosin can reduce nightmares. Acute stress disorder—lasts between 3 days and 1 month. Treatment: CBT; pharmacotherapy is usually not indicated.

Diagnostic criteria by symptom duration

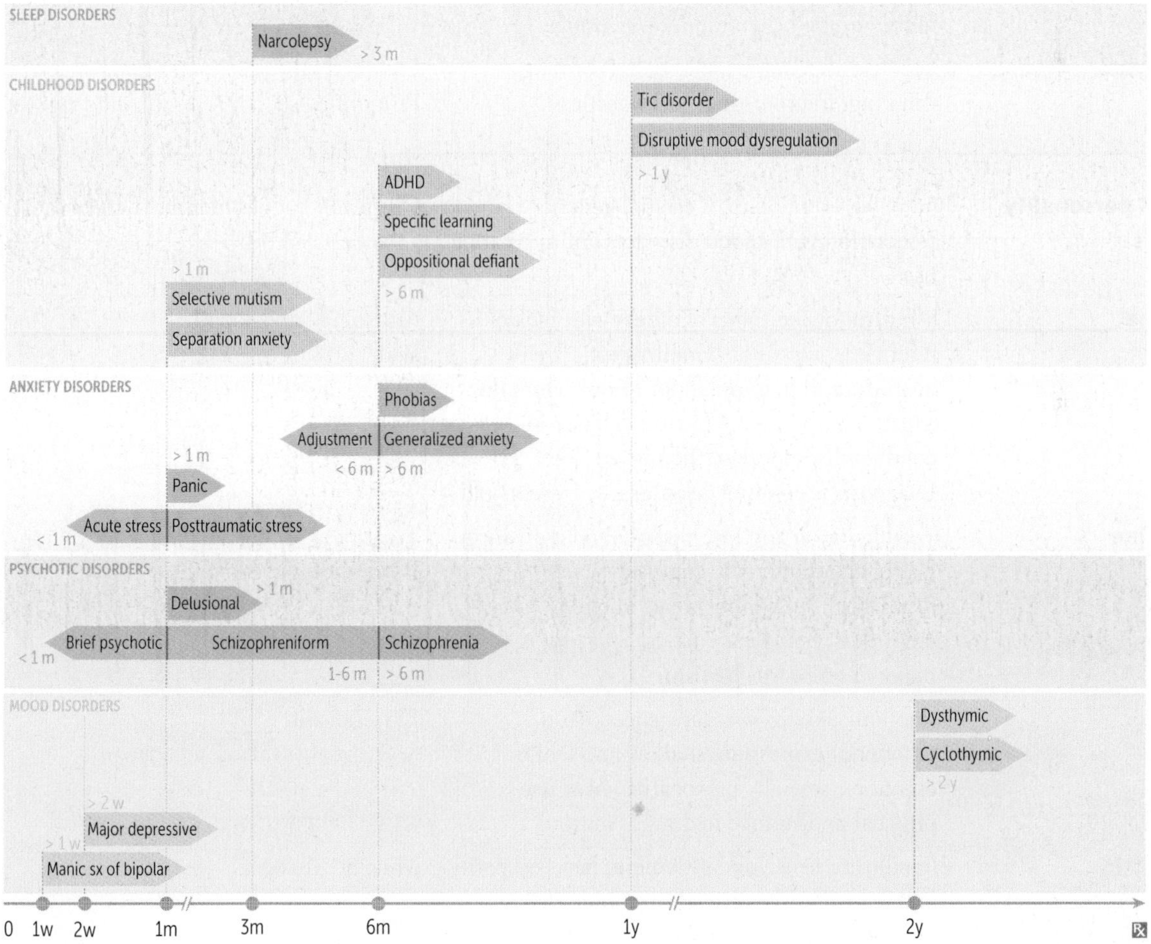

Personality

Personality trait	An enduring, repetitive pattern of perceiving, relating to, and thinking about the environment and oneself.
Personality disorder	Inflexible, maladaptive, and rigidly pervasive pattern of behavior causing subjective distress and/or impaired functioning; person is usually not aware of problem (ego-syntonic). Usually presents by early adulthood. Three clusters: **A**, **B**, **C**; remember as **weird**, **wild**, and **worried**, respectively, based on symptoms.

Cluster A personality disorders	Odd or eccentric; inability to develop meaningful social relationships. No psychosis; genetic association with schizophrenia.	Cluster **A**: accusatory, aloof, awkward. "**Weird**."
Paranoid	Pervasive distrust (**a**ccusatory), suspiciousness, hypervigilance, and a profoundly cynical view of the world.	
Schizoid	Prefers social withdrawal and solitary activities (vs avoidant), limited emotional expression, indifferent to others' opinions (**A**loof).	
Schizotypal	Eccentric appearance, odd beliefs or magical thinking, interpersonal **A**wkwardness.	Included on the schizophrenia spectrum. Pronounce schizo-**type**-al: **odd-type** thoughts.

Cluster B personality disorders	Dramatic, emotional, or erratic; genetic association with mood disorders and substance use.	Cluster **B**: **b**ad, **b**orderline, flam**b**oyant, must be the **b**est. "**Wild**."
Antisocial	Disregard for the rights of others with lack of remorse. Involves criminality, impulsivity, hostility, and manipulation. Males > females. Must be ≥ 18 years old with evidence of conduct disorder onset before age 15. Diagnosis is conduct disorder if < 18 years old.	Antisocial = **sociopath**. **B**ad.
Borderline	Unstable mood and interpersonal relationships, fear of abandonment, impulsivity, self-mutilation, suicidality, sense of emotional emptiness. Females > males. Splitting is a major defense mechanism.	Treatment: dialectical behavior therapy. **B**orderline.
Histrionic	Attention-seeking, dramatic speech and emotional expression, shallow and labile emotions, sexually provocative. May use physical appearance to draw attention.	Flam**b**oyant.
Narcissistic	Grandiosity, sense of entitlement; lacks empathy and requires excessive admiration; often demands the "best" and reacts to criticism with rage and/or defensiveness. Fragile self-esteem. Often envious of others.	Must be the **b**est.

Cluster C personality disorders	Anxious or fearful; genetic association with anxiety disorders.	Cluster C: cowardly, obsessive-compulsive, clingy. "Worried."
Avoidant	Hypersensitive to rejection and criticism, socially inhibited, timid, feelings of inadequacy, desires relationships with others (vs schizoid).	Cowardly.
Obsessive-compulsive	Preoccupation with order, perfectionism, and control; ego-syntonic: behavior consistent with one's own beliefs and attitudes (vs OCD).	
Dependent	Excessive need for support, low self-confidence. Patients often get stuck in abusive relationships.	Submissive and clingy.

Malingering	Symptoms are intentional, motivation is intentional. Patient consciously fakes, profoundly exaggerates, or claims to have a disorder in order to attain a specific 2° (external) gain (eg, avoiding work, obtaining compensation). Poor compliance with treatment or follow-up of diagnostic tests. Complaints cease after gain (vs factitious disorder).

Factitious disorders	Symptoms are intentional, motivation is unconscious. Patient consciously creates physical and/or psychological symptoms in order to assume "sick role" and to get medical attention and sympathy (1° [internal] gain).
Factitious disorder imposed on self	Formerly called Munchausen syndrome. Chronic factitious disorder with predominantly physical signs and symptoms. Characterized by a history of multiple hospital admissions and willingness to undergo invasive procedures. More common in women and healthcare workers.
Factitious disorder imposed on another	Formerly called Munchausen syndrome by proxy. Illness in a child or elderly patient is caused or fabricated by the caregiver. Motivation is to assume a sick role by proxy. Form of child/elder abuse.

Somatic symptom and related disorders	Symptoms are unconscious, motivation is unconscious. Category of disorders characterized by physical symptoms causing significant distress and impairment. Symptoms not intentionally produced or feigned.
Somatic symptom disorder	≥ 1 bodily complaints (eg, abdominal pain, fatigue) lasting months to years. Associated with excessive, persistent thoughts and anxiety about symptoms. May co-occur with medical illness. Treatment: regular office visits with the same physician in combination with psychotherapy.
Conversion disorder	Also called functional neurologic symptom disorder. Unexplained loss of sensory or motor function (eg, paralysis, blindness, mutism), often following an acute stressor; patient may be aware of but indifferent toward symptoms ("la belle indifférence"); more common in females, adolescents, and young adults.
Illness anxiety disorder	Preoccupation with acquiring or having a serious illness, often despite medical evaluation and reassurance; minimal to no somatic symptoms.

Malingering vs factitious disorder vs somatic symptom disorders

	Malingering	Factitious disorder	Somatic symptom disorders
SYMPTOMS	Intentional	Intentional	Unconscious
MOTIVATION	Intentional	Unconscious	Unconscious

Eating disorders	Most common in young women.
Anorexia nervosa	Intense fear of weight gain, overvaluation of thinness, and body image distortion leading to calorie restriction and severe weight loss resulting in inappropriately low body weight (BMI < 18.5 kg/m^2 for adults). May present with hypothyroidism, amenorrhea, osteoporosis, lanugo. Binge-eating/purging type—recurring purging behaviors (eg, laxative or diuretic abuse, self-induced vomiting) or binge eating over the last 3 months. Restricting type—primary disordered behaviors include dieting, fasting, and/or over-exercising. No recurring purging behaviors or binge eating over the last 3 months. Refeeding syndrome—often occurs in significantly malnourished patients with sudden ↑ calorie intake → ↑ insulin → ↓ PO_4^{3-}, ↓ K^+, ↓ Mg^{2+} → cardiac complications, rhabdomyolysis, seizures. Treatment: nutritional rehabilitation, psychotherapy, olanzapine.
Bulimia nervosa	Recurring episodes of binge eating with compensatory purging behaviors at least weekly over the last 3 months. BMI often normal or slightly overweight (vs anorexia). Associated with parotid gland hypertrophy (may see ↑ serum amylase), enamel erosion, Mallory-Weiss syndrome, electrolyte disturbances (eg, ↓ K^+, ↓ Cl^-), metabolic alkalosis, dorsal hand calluses from induced vomiting (Russell sign). Treatment: psychotherapy, nutritional rehabilitation, antidepressants (eg, SSRIs). Bupropion is contraindicated due to seizure risk.
Binge-eating disorder	Recurring episodes of binge eating without purging behaviors at least weekly over the last 3 months. ↑ diabetes risk. Most common eating disorder in adults. Treatment: psychotherapy (first line); SSRIs; lisdexamfetamine.
Pica	Recurring episodes of eating non-food substances (eg, ice, dirt, hair, paint chips) over ≥ 1 month that are not culturally or developmentally recognized as normal. May provide temporary emotional relief. Common in children and during pregnancy. Associated with malnutrition, iron deficiency anemia, developmental disabilities, emotional trauma. Treatment: psychotherapy and nutritional rehabilitation (first line); SSRIs (second line).

Gender dysphoria	Significant incongruence between one's experienced gender and the gender assigned at birth, lasting > 6 months and leading to persistent distress. Individuals may self-identify as another gender, pursue gender-affirming surgery, and/or live as another gender. Gender nonconformity itself is not a mental disorder. Gender identity develops at age ~3 years. **Transgender**—desiring and often making lifestyle changes to live as a different gender. Medical interventions (eg, hormone therapy, gender-affirming surgery) may be utilized during the transition to enable the individual's appearance to match their gender identity.

Sexual dysfunction	Includes sexual desire disorders (hypoactive sexual desire or sexual aversion), sexual arousal disorders (erectile dysfunction), orgasmic disorders (anorgasmia, premature ejaculation), sexual pain disorders (dyspareunia, vaginismus). Differential diagnosis includes (PENIS): ▪ Psychological (if nighttime erections still occur) ▪ Endocrine (eg, diabetes, low testosterone) ▪ Neurogenic (eg, postoperative, spinal cord injury) ▪ Insufficient blood flow (eg, atherosclerosis) ▪ Substances (eg, antihypertensives, antidepressants, ethanol)

Sleep terror disorder	Periods of inconsolable terror with screaming in the middle of the night. Most common in children. Occurs during slow-wave/deep (stage N3) non-REM sleep with no memory of the arousal episode, as opposed to nightmares that occur during **REM** sleep (**rem**embering a scary dream). Triggers include emotional stress, fever, and lack of sleep. Usually self limited.
Enuresis	Nighttime urinary incontinence ≥ 2 times/week for ≥ 3 months in person > 5 years old. First-line treatment: behavioral modification (eg, scheduled voids, nighttime fluid restriction) and positive reinforcement. For refractory cases: bedwetting alarm, oral desmopressin (ADH analog; preferred over imipramine due to fewer side effects).
Narcolepsy	Excessive daytime sleepiness (despite awakening well-rested) with recurrent episodes of rapid-onset, overwhelming sleepiness ≥ 3 times/week for the last 3 months. Due to ↓ orexin (hypocretin) production in lateral hypothalamus and dysregulated sleep-wake cycles. Associated with: ▪ Hypna**go**gic (just before **go**ing to sleep) or hypno**pomp**ic (just before awakening; get **pomp**ed up in the morning) hallucinations. ▪ Nocturnal and narcoleptic sleep episodes that start with REM sleep (sleep paralysis). ▪ Cataplexy (loss of all muscle tone following strong emotional stimulus, such as laughter). Treatment: good sleep hygiene (scheduled naps, regular sleep schedule), daytime stimulants (eg, amphetamines, modafinil) and/or nighttime sodium oxybate (GHB).
Substance use disorder	Maladaptive pattern of substance use involving ≥ 2 of the following in the past year: ▪ Tolerance ▪ Withdrawal ▪ Intense, distracting cravings ▪ Using more, or longer, than intended ▪ Persistent desire but inability to cut down ▪ Time-consuming substance acquisition, use, or recovery ▪ Impaired functioning at work, school, or home ▪ Social or interpersonal conflicts ▪ Reduced recreational activities ▪ > 1 episode of use involving danger (eg, unsafe sex, driving while impaired) ▪ Continued use despite awareness of harm
Gambling disorder	Persistent, recurrent, problematic gambling. May include preoccupation with gambling, compulsion to increase size of bet, unsuccessful attempts to decrease gambling, gambling to escape stressors, attempting to recoup losses with more gambling, lying to family or therapists to conceal extent. Treatment: psychotherapy.

Transtheoretical model of change

STAGE	FEATURES	MOTIVATIONAL STRATEGIES
Precontemplation	Denies problem and its consequences.	Encourage introspection. Use patient's personal priorities in explaining risks. Affirm your availability to the patient.
Contemplation	Acknowledges problem but is ambivalent or unwilling to change.	Discuss pros of changing and cons of maintaining current behavior. Suggest means to support behavior changes.
Preparation/ determination	Committed to and planning for behavior change.	Encourage initial changes, promote expectations for positive results, provide resources to assist in planning.
Action/willpower	Executes a plan and demonstrates a change in behavior.	Assist with strategies for self-efficacy, contingency management, and coping with situations that trigger old behaviors.
Maintenance	New behaviors become sustained, integrate into personal identity and lifestyle.	Reinforce developing habits. Evaluate and mitigate relapse risk. Praise progress.
Relapse	Regression to prior behavior (does not always occur).	Varies based on degree of regression. Encourage return to changes. Provide reassurance that change remains possible.

Psychiatric emergencies

	CAUSE	MANIFESTATION	TREATMENT
Serotonin syndrome	Any drug that ↑ 5-HT. Psychiatric drugs: MAOIs, SSRIs, SNRIs, TCAs, vilazodone, vortioxetine, buspirone Nonpsychiatric drugs: tramadol, ondansetron, triptans, linezolid, MDMA, dextromethorphan, meperidine, St. John's wort	3 A's: ↑ activity (neuromuscular; eg, clonus, hyperreflexia, hypertonia, tremor, seizure), autonomic instability (eg, hyperthermia, diaphoresis, diarrhea), altered mental status	Cyproheptadine (5-HT_2 receptor antagonist) Prevention: avoid simultaneous serotonergic drugs, and allow a washout period between them
Hypertensive crisis	Eating tyramine-rich foods (eg, aged cheeses, cured meats, wine, chocolate) while taking MAOIs	Hypertensive crisis (tyramine displaces other neurotransmitters [eg, NE] in the synaptic cleft → ↑ sympathetic stimulation)	Phentolamine
Neuroleptic malignant syndrome	Antipsychotics (typical > atypical) + genetic predisposition	Malignant **FEVER**: **M**yoglobinuria, **F**ever, **E**ncephalopathy, **V**itals unstable, ↑ **E**nzymes (eg, CK), muscle **R**igidity ("lead pipe")	Dantrolene, dopaminergics (eg, bromocriptine, amantadine), benzodiazepines; discontinue causative agent
Delirium tremens	Alcohol withdrawal; occurs 2–4 days after last drink Classically seen in hospital setting when inpatient cannot drink	Altered mental status, hallucinations, autonomic hyperactivity, anxiety, seizures, tremors, psychomotor agitation, insomnia, nausea	Longer-acting benzodiazepines
Acute dystonia	Typical antipsychotics, anticonvulsants (eg, carbamazepine), metoclopramide	Sudden onset of muscle spasms, stiffness, and/or oculogyric crisis occurring hours to days after medication use; can lead to laryngospasm requiring intubation	Benztropine or diphenhydramine
Lithium toxicity	↑ lithium dosage, ↓ renal elimination (eg, acute kidney injury), medications affecting clearance (eg, ACE inhibitors, thiazide diuretics, NSAIDs). Narrow therapeutic window.	Nausea, vomiting, slurred speech, hyperreflexia, seizures, ataxia, nephrogenic diabetes insipidus	Discontinue lithium, hydrate aggressively with isotonic sodium chloride, consider hemodialysis
Tricyclic antidepressant toxicity	TCA overdose	Respiratory depression, hyperpyrexia, prolonged QT **Tri**cy**c**lic's: convulsions, coma, cardiotoxicity (arrhythmia due to Na^+ channel inhibition)	Supportive treatment, monitor ECG, $NaHCO_3$ (prevents arrhythmia), activated charcoal

Psychoactive drug intoxication and withdrawal

DRUG	INTOXICATION	WITHDRAWAL
Depressants		
	Nonspecific: mood elevation, ↓ anxiety, sedation, behavioral disinhibition, respiratory depression.	Nonspecific: anxiety, tremor, seizures, insomnia.
Alcohol	Emotional lability, slurred speech, ataxia, coma, blackouts. Serum γ-glutamyltransferase (GGT)—sensitive indicator of alcohol use. AST value is 2× ALT value ("ToAST 2 ALcohol"). Treatment: supportive (eg, fluids, antiemetics).	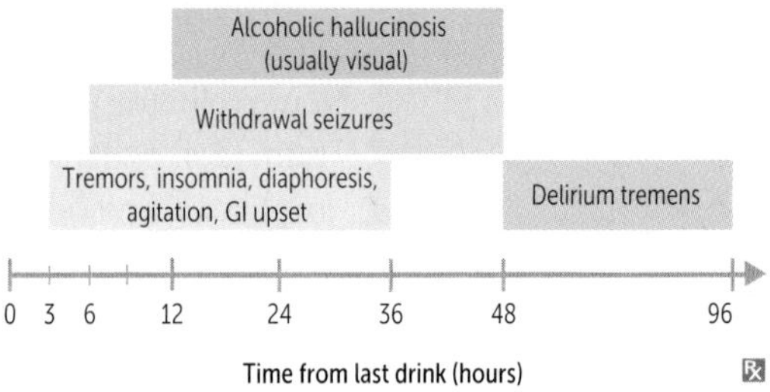 Treatment: longer-acting benzodiazepines.
Barbiturates	Low safety margin, marked respiratory depression. Treatment: symptom management (eg, assist respiration, ↑ BP).	Delirium, life-threatening cardiovascular collapse.
Benzodiazepines	Greater safety margin. Ataxia, minor respiratory depression. Treatment: flumazenil (benzodiazepine receptor antagonist, but rarely used as it can precipitate seizures).	Seizures, sleep disturbance, depression.
Opioids	Euphoria, respiratory and CNS depression, ↓ gag reflex, pupillary constriction (pinpoint pupils), seizures, ↓ GI motility. Most common cause of drug overdose death. Treatment: naloxone.	Sweating, dilated pupils, piloerection ("cold turkey"), rhinorrhea, lacrimation, yawning, nausea, stomach cramps, diarrhea ("flu-like" symptoms). Treatment: symptom management, methadone, buprenorphine.
Inhalants	Disinhibition, euphoria, slurred speech, disturbed gait, disorientation, drowsiness. Effects often have rapid onset and resolution. Perinasal/perioral rash with repeated use.	Irritability, dysphoria, sleep disturbance, headache.
Stimulants		
	Nonspecific: mood elevation, ↓ appetite, psychomotor agitation, insomnia, cardiac arrhythmias, tachycardia, anxiety.	Nonspecific: post-use "crash," including depression, lethargy, ↑ appetite, sleep disturbance, vivid nightmares.
Amphetamines	Euphoria, grandiosity, pupillary dilation, prolonged wakefulness, hyperalertness, hypertension, paranoia, fever, fractured teeth. Skin excoriations with methamphetamine use. Severe: cardiac arrest, seizures. Treatment: benzodiazepines for agitation and seizures.	
Caffeine	Palpitation, agitation, tremor, insomnia.	Headache, difficulty concentrating, flu-like symptoms.

Psychoactive drug intoxication and withdrawal *(continued)*

DRUG	INTOXICATION	WITHDRAWAL
Cocaine	Impaired judgment, pupillary dilation, diaphoresis, hallucinations (including tactile), paranoia, angina, sudden cardiac death. Chronic use may lead to perforated nasal septum due to vasoconstriction and resulting ischemic necrosis. Treatment: benzodiazepines; use of β-blockers or mixed α-/β-blockers (eg, labetalol) for hypertension and tachycardia is controversial as first-line therapy.	Restlessness, hunger, severe depression, sleep disturbance.
Nicotine	Restlessness.	Irritability, anxiety, restlessness, ↓ concentration, ↑ appetite/weight. Treatment: nicotine patch, gum, or lozenges; bupropion/varenicline.
Hallucinogens		
Lysergic acid diethylamide	Perceptual distortion (visual, auditory), depersonalization, anxiety, paranoia, psychosis, flashbacks (usually nondisturbing), mydriasis.	
Cannabis/ cannabinoids	Euphoria, anxiety, paranoid delusions, perception of slowed time, impaired judgment, social withdrawal, ↑ appetite, dry mouth, conjunctival injection, hallucinations.	Irritability, anxiety, depression, insomnia, restlessness, ↓ appetite.
MDMA	Also known as ecstasy. Euphoria, hallucinations, disinhibition, hyperactivity, ↑ thirst, bruxism, distorted sensory and time perception, mydriasis. Life-threatening effects include hypertension, tachycardia, hyperthermia, hyponatremia, serotonin syndrome.	Depression, fatigue, change in appetite, difficulty concentrating, anxiety.
Phencyclidine	Violence, nystagmus, impulsivity, psychomotor agitation, miosis, tachycardia, hypertension, analgesia, psychosis, delirium, seizures.	

Alcohol use disorder

Diagnosed using criteria for substance use disorder.

Complications: vitamin B_1 (thiamine) deficiency, alcoholic cirrhosis, hepatitis, pancreatitis, peripheral neuropathy, testicular atrophy.

Treatment: naltrexone (reduces cravings), acamprosate, disulfiram (to condition the patient to abstain from alcohol use). Support groups such as Alcoholics Anonymous are helpful in sustaining abstinence and supporting patient and family.

Wernicke-Korsakoff syndrome

Results from vitamin B_1 deficiency. Symptoms can be precipitated by administering dextrose before vitamin B_1. Triad of confusion, ophthalmoplegia, ataxia (Wernicke encephalopathy). May progress to irreversible memory loss, confabulation, personality change (Korsakoff syndrome).

Treatment: IV vitamin B_1 (before dextrose).

▸ PSYCHIATRY—PHARMACOLOGY

Psychotherapy

Behavioral therapy	Teaches patients how to identify and change maladaptive behaviors or reactions to stimuli (eg, systematic desensitization for specific phobia).
Cognitive behavioral therapy	Teaches patients to recognize distortions in their thought processes, develop constructive coping skills, and ↓ maladaptive coping behaviors → greater emotional control and tolerance of distress (eg, recognizing triggers for alcohol consumption).
Dialectical behavioral therapy	Designed for use in borderline personality disorder, but can be used in other psychiatric conditions as well (eg, depression).
Interpersonal therapy	Focused on improving interpersonal relationships and communication skills.
Motivational interviewing	Enhances intrinsic motivation to change by exploring and resolving ambivalence. Used in substance use disorder and weight loss.
Supportive therapy	Utilizes empathy to help individuals during a time of hardship to maintain optimism or hope.

Preferred medications for selected psychiatric conditions

PSYCHIATRIC CONDITION	PREFERRED DRUGS
ADHD	Stimulants (methylphenidate, amphetamines)
Alcohol withdrawal	Benzodiazepines (eg, chlordiazepoxide, lorazepam, diazepam)
Bipolar disorder	Carbamazepine, atypical antipsychotics, lithium, lamotrigine, valproate. Character a little less variable
Bulimia nervosa	SSRIs
Depression	SSRIs
Generalized anxiety disorder	SSRIs, SNRIs
Obsessive-compulsive disorder	SSRIs, venlafaxine, clomipramine
Panic disorder	SSRIs, venlafaxine, benzodiazepines
PTSD	SSRIs, venlafaxine, prazosin (for nightmares)
Schizophrenia	Atypical antipsychotics
Social anxiety disorder	SSRIs, venlafaxine Performance only: β-blockers, benzodiazepines
Tourette syndrome	Antipsychotics (eg, fluphenazine, risperidone), tetrabenazine

Central nervous system stimulants

	Methylphenidate, dextroamphetamine, methamphetamine, lisdexamfetamine.
MECHANISM	↑ catecholamines in the synaptic cleft, especially norepinephrine and dopamine.
CLINICAL USE	ADHD, narcolepsy, binge-eating disorder.
ADVERSE EFFECTS	Nervousness, agitation, anxiety, insomnia, anorexia, tachycardia, hypertension, weight loss, tics, bruxism.

Antipsychotics	Typical (1st-generation) antipsychotics—haloperidol, pimozide, trifluoperazine, fluphenazine, thioridazine, chlorpromazine. Atypical (2nd-generation) antipsychotics—aripiprazole, asenapine, clozapine, olanzapine, quetiapine, iloperidone, paliperidone, risperidone, lurasidone, ziprasidone.
MECHANISM	Block dopamine D_2 receptor (↑ cAMP). Atypical antipsychotics also block serotonin 5-HT_2 receptor. Aripiprazole is a D_2 partial agonist.
CLINICAL USE	Schizophrenia (typical antipsychotics primarily treat positive symptoms; atypical antipsychotics treat both positive and negative symptoms), disorders with concomitant psychosis (eg, bipolar disorder), Tourette syndrome, OCD, Huntington disease. Clozapine is used for treatment-resistant psychotic disorders or those with persistent suicidality.

ADVERSE EFFECTS	Antihistaminic (sedation), anti-α_1-adrenergic (orthostatic hypotension), antimuscarinic (dry mouth, constipation) (anti-**HAM**). Use with caution in dementia.
	Metabolic: weight gain, hyperglycemia, dyslipidemia. Highest risk with clozapine and olanzapine (obesity).
	Endocrine: hyperprolactinemia → galactorrhea, oligomenorrhea, gynecomastia.
	Cardiac: QT prolongation.
	Neurologic: neuroleptic malignant syndrome.
	Ophthalmologic: chlorpromazine—corneal deposits; thioridazine—retinal deposits.
	Clozapine—agranulocytosis (monitor WBCs clozely), seizures (dose related), myocarditis.
	Extrapyramidal symptoms—**ADAPT**:
	▪ Hours to days: **A**cute **D**ystonia (muscle spasm, stiffness, oculogyric crisis). Treatment: benztropine, diphenhydramine.
	▪ Days to months:
	  ▪ **A**kathisia (restlessness). Treatment: β-blockers, benztropine, benzodiazepines.
	  ▪ **P**arkinsonism (bradykinesia). Treatment: benztropine, amantadine.
	▪ Months to years: **T**ardive dyskinesia (chorea, especially orofacial). Treatment: benzodiazepines, botulinum toxin injections, valbenazine, deutetrabenazine.

NOTES	Lipid soluble → stored in body fat → slow to be removed from body. Typical antipsychotics have greater affinity for D_2 receptor than atypical antipsychotics → ↑ risk for hyperprolactinemia, extrapyramidal symptoms, neuroleptic malignant syndrome. **High**-potency typical antipsychotics: **hal**operidol, **tri**fluoperazine, **pi**mozide, **fl**uphenazine (**Hal tries pie to fly high**)—more neurologic side effects (eg, extrapyramidal symptoms). **Low**-potency typical antipsychotics: **ch**lorpromazine, **thi**oridazine (**cheating thieves are low**)—more antihistaminic, anti-α_1-adrenergic, antimuscarinic effects.

Lithium

MECHANISM	Not established; possibly related to inhibition of phosphoinositol cascade.	LiTHIUM: Low Thyroid (hypothyroidism) Heart (Ebstein anomaly) Insipidus (nephrogenic diabetes insipidus) Unwanted Movements (tremor)
CLINICAL USE	Mood stabilizer for bipolar disorder; treats acute manic episodes and prevents relapse.	
ADVERSE EFFECTS	Tremor, hypothyroidism, hyperthyroidism, polyuria (causes nephrogenic diabetes insipidus), teratogenesis (causes Ebstein anomaly). Narrow therapeutic window requires close monitoring of serum levels. Almost exclusively excreted by kidneys; most is reabsorbed at PCT via Na^+ channels. Thiazides, NSAIDs, and other drugs affecting clearance are implicated in lithium toxicity.	

Buspirone

MECHANISM	Partial 5-HT_{1A} receptor agonist.	I get **anxious** if the **bus** doesn't arrive at **one**, so I take **buspirone**.
CLINICAL USE	Generalized **anxiety** disorder. Does not cause sedation, addiction, or tolerance. Begins to take effect after 1–2 weeks. Does not interact with alcohol (vs barbiturates, benzodiazepines).	

Antidepressants

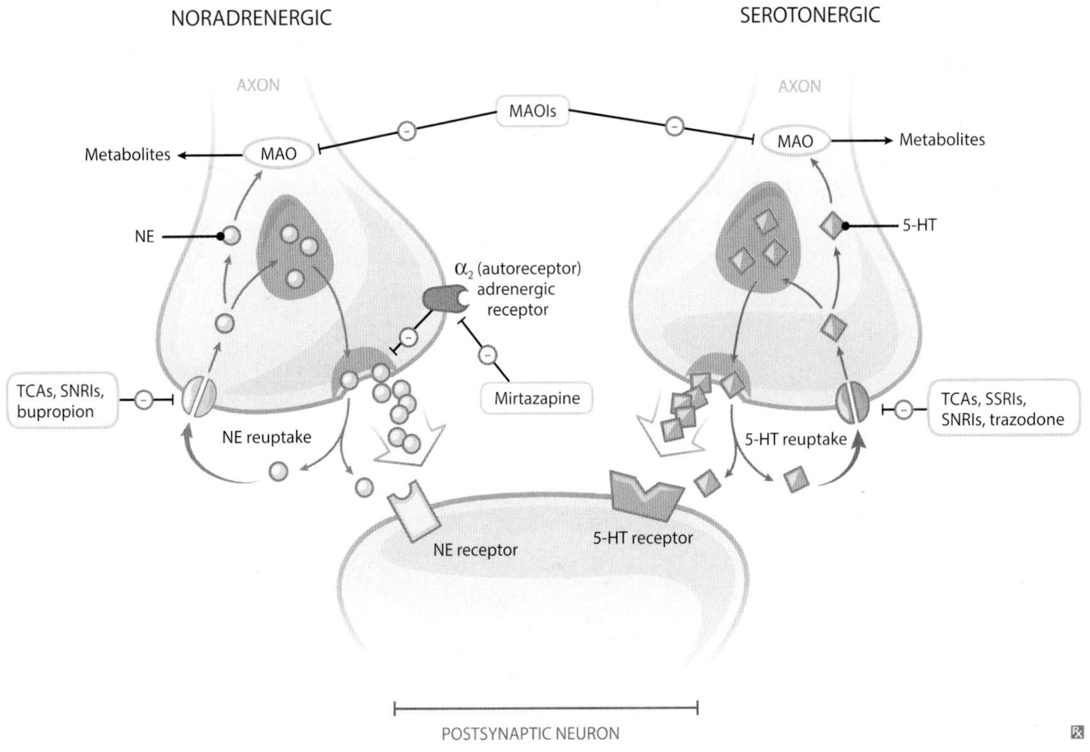

Selective serotonin reuptake inhibitors

Fluoxetine, fluvoxamine, paroxetine, sertraline, escitalopram, citalopram.

MECHANISM	Inhibit 5-HT reuptake.	It normally takes 4–8 weeks for antidepressants to show appreciable effect.
CLINICAL USE	Depression, generalized anxiety disorder, panic disorder, OCD, bulimia, binge-eating disorder, social anxiety disorder, PTSD, premature ejaculation, premenstrual dysphoric disorder.	
ADVERSE EFFECTS	Fewer than TCAs. Serotonin syndrome, GI distress, SIADH, sexual dysfunction (anorgasmia, ↓ libido), mania precipitation if underlying bipolar disorder.	

Serotonin-norepinephrine reuptake inhibitors

Venlafaxine, desvenlafaxine, duloxetine, levomilnacipran, milnacipran.

MECHANISM	Inhibit 5-HT and NE reuptake.
CLINICAL USE	Depression, generalized anxiety disorder, diabetic neuropathy. Venlafaxine is also indicated for social anxiety disorder, panic disorder, PTSD, OCD. Duloxetine and milnacipran are also indicated for fibromyalgia.
ADVERSE EFFECTS	↑ BP, stimulant effects, sedation, nausea.

Tricyclic antidepressants

Amitriptyline, nortriptyline, imipramine, desipramine, clomipramine, doxepin, amoxapine.

MECHANISM	TCAs inhibit 5-HT and NE reuptake.
CLINICAL USE	MDD, peripheral neuropathy, chronic neuropathic pain, migraine prophylaxis, OCD (clomipramine), nocturnal enuresis (imipramine).
ADVERSE EFFECTS	Sedation, α_1-blocking effects including postural hypotension, and atropine-like (anticholinergic) side effects (tachycardia, urinary retention, dry mouth). 3° TCAs (amitriptyline) have more anticholinergic effects than 2° TCAs (nortriptyline). Can prolong QT interval. Tri-CyCliC's: Convulsions, Coma, Cardiotoxicity (arrhythmia due to Na^+ channel inhibition); also respiratory depression, hyperpyrexia. Confusion and hallucinations are more common in the elderly due to anticholinergic side effects (2° amines [eg, nortriptyline] better tolerated). Treatment: $NaHCO_3$ to prevent arrhythmia.

Monoamine oxidase inhibitors

Tranylcypromine, phenelzine, isocarboxazid, selegiline (selective MAO-B inhibitor).
(MAO takes pride in Shanghai).

MECHANISM	Nonselective MAO inhibition → ↑ levels of amine neurotransmitters (norepinephrine, 5-HT, dopamine).
CLINICAL USE	Atypical depression, anxiety. Parkinson disease (selegiline).
ADVERSE EFFECTS	CNS stimulation; hypertensive crisis, most notably with ingestion of tyramine. Contraindicated with SSRIs, TCAs, St. John's wort, meperidine, dextromethorphan, pseudoephedrine, linezolid (to avoid precipitating serotonin syndrome). Wait 2 weeks after stopping MAOIs before starting serotonergic drugs or stopping dietary restrictions.

Atypical antidepressants

Bupropion	Inhibits NE and DA reuptake. Also used for smoking cessation. Toxicity: stimulant effects (tachycardia, insomnia), headache, seizures in patients with bulimia and anorexia nervosa. ↓ risk of sexual side effects and weight gain compared to other antidepressants.
Mirtazapine	α_2-antagonist (↑ release of NE and 5-HT), potent 5-HT_2 and 5-HT_3 receptor antagonist, and H_1 antagonist. Toxicity: sedation (which may be desirable in depressed patients with insomnia), ↑ appetite, weight gain (which may be desirable in underweight patients), dry mouth.
Trazodone	Primarily blocks 5-HT_2, α_1-adrenergic, and H_1 receptors; also weakly inhibits 5-HT reuptake. Used primarily for insomnia, as high doses are needed for antidepressant effects. Toxicity: sedation, nausea, priapism, postural hypotension. Think tra**ZZZobone** due to sedative and male-specific side effects.
Varenicline	Nicotinic ACh receptor partial agonist. Used for smoking cessation. Toxicity: sleep disturbance. Vare**nicline** helps **nicotine** cravings de**cline**.
Vilazodone	Inhibits 5-HT reuptake; 5-HT_{1A} receptor partial agonist. Used for MDD. Toxicity: headache, diarrhea, nausea, anticholinergic effects. May cause serotonin syndrome if taken with other serotonergic agents.
Vortioxetine	Inhibits 5-HT reuptake; 5-HT_{1A} receptor agonist and 5-HT_3 receptor antagonist. Used for MDD. Toxicity: nausea, sexual dysfunction, sleep disturbances, anticholinergic effects. May cause serotonin syndrome if taken with other serotonergic agents.

Opioid detoxification and relapse prevention	Intravenous drug users at ↑ risk for hepatitis, HIV, abscesses, bacteremia, right-heart endocarditis.
Methadone	Long-acting oral opiate used for heroin detoxification or long-term maintenance therapy.
Buprenorphine	Sublingual form (partial agonist) used to prevent relapse. Can precipitate withdrawal symptoms when combined with full agonist.
Naloxone	Short-acting opioid antagonist given IM, IV, or as a nasal spray to treat acute opioid overdose, particularly to reverse respiratory and CNS depression.
Naltrexone	Long-acting oral opioid antagonist used after detoxification to prevent relapse. May help alcohol and nicotine cessation, weight loss. Use nal**trex**one for the long **trex** back to sobriety.

Renal

"But I know all about love already. I know precious little still about kidneys."

—Aldous Huxley, *Antic Hay*

"This too shall pass. Just like a kidney stone."

—Hunter Madsen

"I drink too much. The last time I gave a urine sample it had an olive in it."

—Rodney Dangerfield

Being able to understand and apply renal physiology will be critical for the exam. Important topics include electrolyte disorders, acid-base derangements, glomerular disorders (including histopathology), acute and chronic kidney disease, urine casts, diuretics, ACE inhibitors, and AT II receptor blockers. Renal anomalies associated with various congenital defects are also high-yield associations to think about when evaluating pediatric vignettes.

▶ RENAL—EMBRYOLOGY

Kidney embryology

Pronephros—week 3 of development; then degenerates.

Mesonephros—week 4 of development; functions as interim kidney for 1st trimester; persists in the male genital system as Wolffian duct, forming ductus deferens and epididymis.

Metanephros—permanent; first appears in week 5 of development; nephrogenesis is normally completed by week 36 of gestation..

- Ureteric bud (metanephric diverticulum)—derived from caudal end of mesonephric duct; gives rise to ureter, pelvises, calyces, collecting ducts; fully canalized by week 10 of development
- Metanephric mesenchyme (ie, metanephric blastema)—ureteric bud interacts with this tissue; interaction induces differentiation and formation of glomerulus through to distal convoluted tubule (DCT)
- Aberrant interaction between these 2 tissues may result in several congenital malformations of the kidney (eg, renal agenesis, multicystic dysplastic kidney)

Ureteropelvic junction—last to canalize → congenital obstruction. Can be unilateral or bilateral. Most common pathologic cause of prenatal hydronephrosis. Detected by prenatal ultrasound.

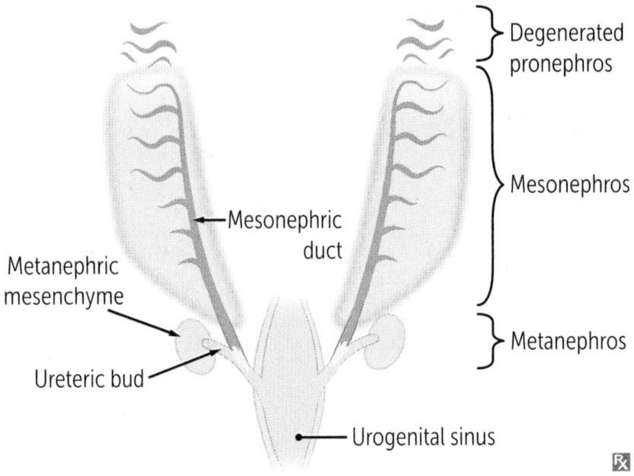

Potter sequence

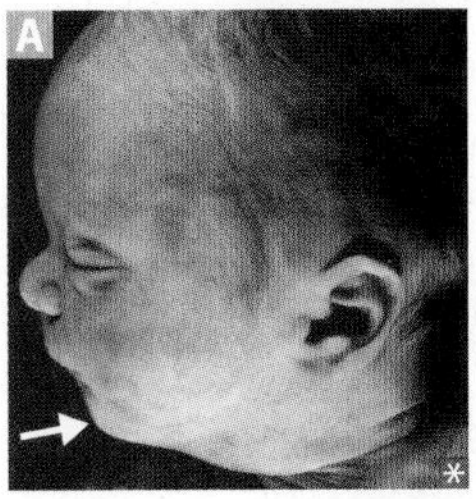

Oligohydramnios → compression of developing fetus → limb deformities, facial anomalies (eg, low-set ears and retrognathia A, flattened nose), compression of chest and lack of amniotic fluid aspiration into fetal lungs → pulmonary hypoplasia (cause of death).

Caused by chronic placental insufficiency or reduced renal output, including ARPKD, obstructive uropathy (eg, posterior urethral valves), bilateral renal agenesis.

Babies who can't "Pee" in utero develop Potter sequence.

POTTER sequence associated with:

- **P**ulmonary hypoplasia
- **O**ligohydramnios (trigger)
- **T**wisted face
- **T**wisted skin
- **E**xtremity defects
- **R**enal failure (in utero)

Horseshoe kidney

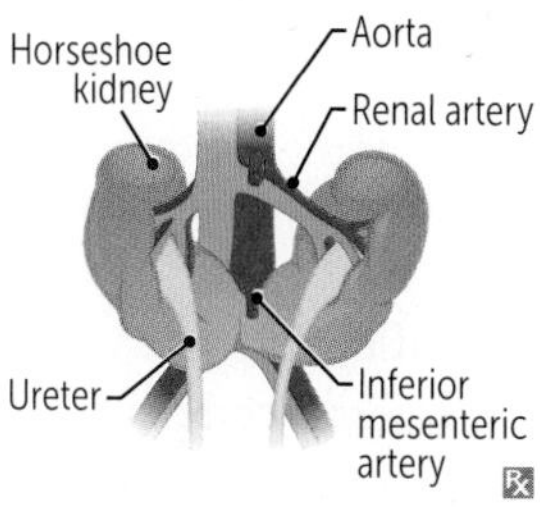
Horseshoe kidney
Aorta
Renal artery
Ureter
Inferior mesenteric artery

Inferior poles of both kidneys fuse abnormally A. As they ascend from pelvis during fetal development, horseshoe kidneys get trapped under inferior mesenteric artery and remain low in the abdomen. Kidneys can function normally, but associated with hydronephrosis (eg, ureteropelvic junction obstruction), renal stones, infection, ↑ risk of renal cancer.

Higher incidence in chromosomal aneuploidy (eg, Turner syndrome, trisomies 13, 18, 21).

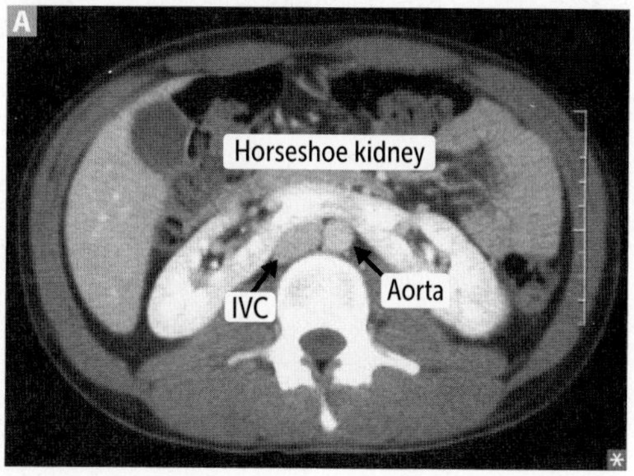
A
Horseshoe kidney
IVC
Aorta

Congenital solitary functioning kidney

Condition of being born with only one functioning kidney. Majority asymptomatic with compensatory hypertrophy of contralateral kidney, but anomalies in contralateral kidney are common. Often diagnosed prenatally via ultrasound.

Unilateral renal agenesis

Ureteric bud fails to develop and induce differentiation of metanephric mesenchyme → complete absence of kidney and ureter.

Multicystic dysplastic kidney

Ureteric bud develops, but fails to induce differentiation of metanephric mesenchyme → nonfunctional kidney consisting of cysts and connective tissue. Predominantly nonhereditary and usually unilateral; bilateral leads to Potter sequence.

Duplex collecting system

Bifurcation of ureteric bud before it enters the metanephric blastema creates a Y-shaped bifid ureter. Duplex collecting system can alternatively occur through two ureteric buds reaching and interacting with metanephric blastema. Strongly associated with vesicoureteral reflux and/or ureteral obstruction, ↑ risk for UTIs. Frequently presents with hydronephrosis.

Posterior urethral valves

Membrane remnant in the posterior (prostatic) urethra in males; its persistence can lead to urethral obstruction. Can be diagnosed prenatally by bilateral hydronephrosis and dilated or thick-walled bladder on ultrasound. Most common cause of bladder outlet obstruction in male infants. Associated with oligohydramnios in cases of severe obstruction.

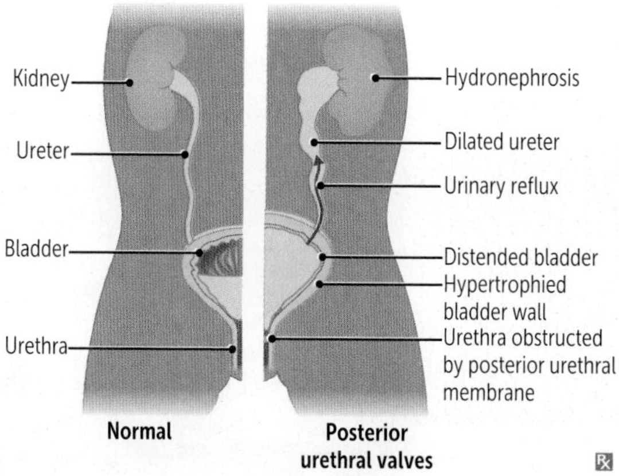
Kidney
Ureter
Bladder
Urethra
Hydronephrosis
Dilated ureter
Urinary reflux
Distended bladder
Hypertrophied bladder wall
Urethra obstructed by posterior urethral membrane
Normal
Posterior urethral valves

Vesicoureteral reflux

Retrograde flow of urine from bladder toward upper urinary tract. Can be 1° due to abnormal/insufficient insertion of the ureter within the vesicular wall (ureterovesical junction [UVJ]) or 2° due to abnormally high bladder pressure resulting in retrograde flow via the UVJ. ↑ risk of recurrent UTIs.

▶ RENAL—ANATOMY

Kidney anatomy and glomerular structure

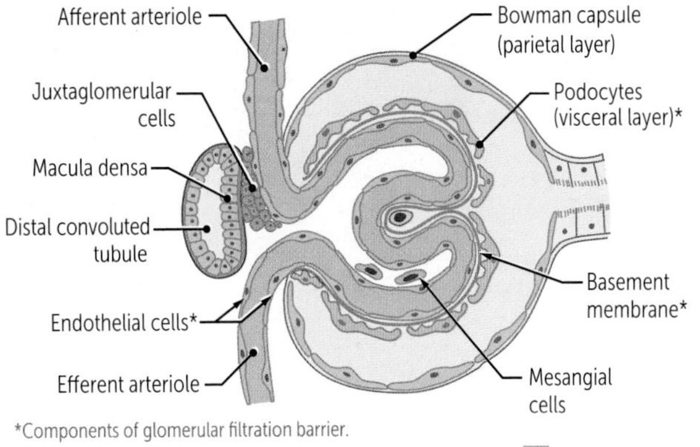

*Components of glomerular filtration barrier.

Cross-section of glomerulus A

Left renal vein receives two additional veins: left suprarenal and left gonadal veins.

Despite high overall renal blood flow, renal medulla receives significantly less blood flow than renal cortex → very sensitive to hypoxia → vulnerable to ischemic damage.

Left kidney is taken during living donor transplantation because it has a longer renal vein.

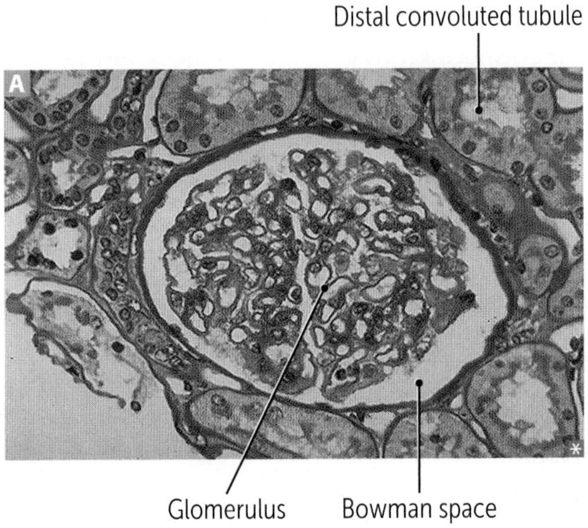

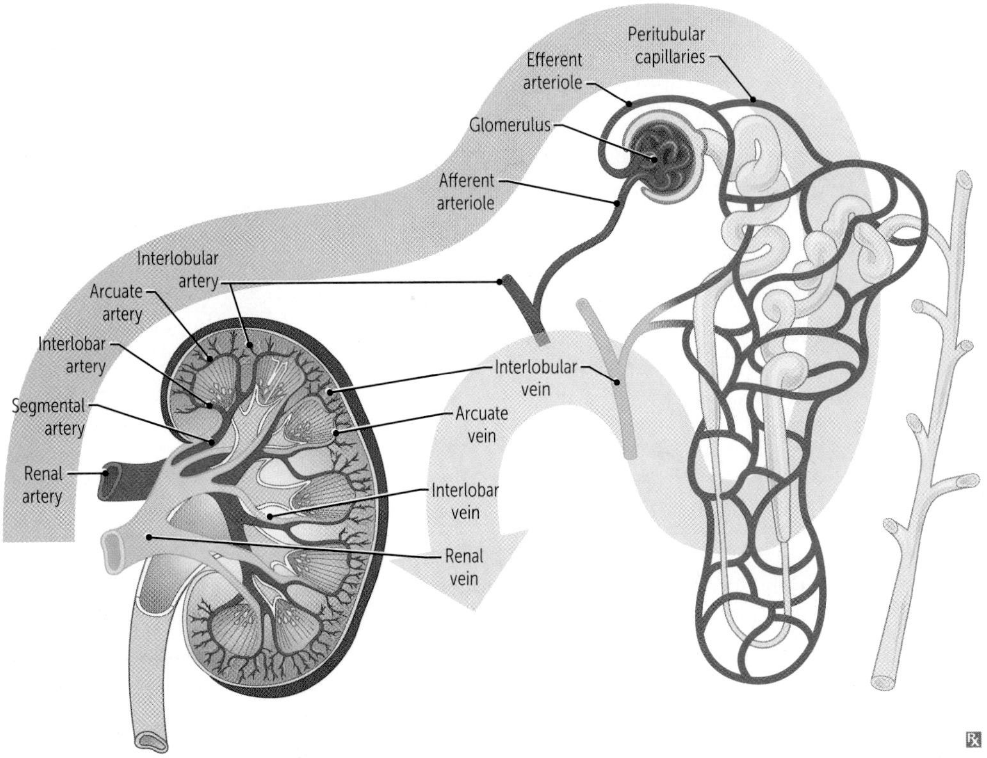

Course of ureters

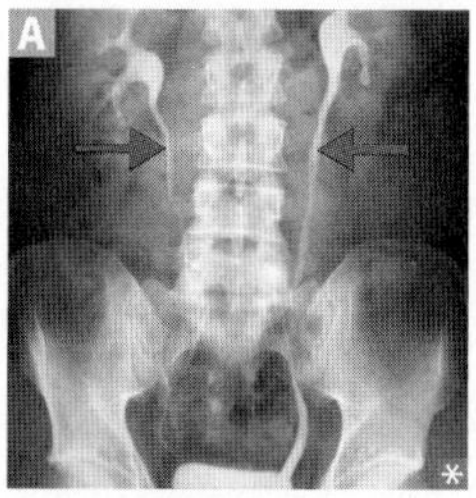

Course of ureter A: arises from renal pelvis, travels under gonadal arteries → **over** common iliac artery → **under** uterine artery/vas deferens (retroperitoneal).

Gynecologic procedures (eg, ligation of uterine or ovarian vessels) may damage ureter → ureteral obstruction or leak.

Bladder contraction compresses the intramural ureter, preventing urine reflux.

Blood supply to ureter:

- Proximal—renal arteries
- Middle—gonadal artery, aorta, common and internal iliac arteries
- Distal—internal iliac and superior vesical arteries

3 common points of ureteral obstruction: ureteropelvic junction, pelvic inlet, ureterovesical junction.

Water (ureters) flows **over** the iliacs and **under** the bridge (uterine artery or vas deferens).

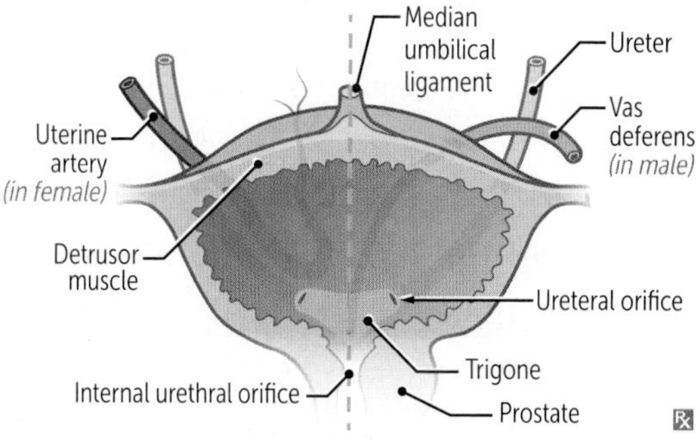

▸ RENAL—PHYSIOLOGY

Fluid compartments

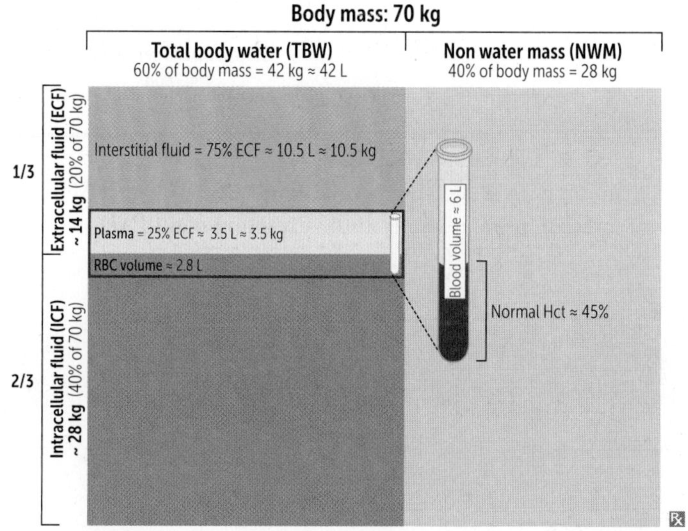

HIKIN': **HI**gh **K**$^+$ **IN**tracellularly.

60–40–20 rule (% of body weight for average person):

- 60% total body water
- 40% ICF, mainly composed of K^+, Mg^{2+}, organic phosphates (eg, ATP)
- 20% ECF, mainly composed of Na^+, Cl^-, HCO_3^-, albumin

Plasma volume can be measured by radiolabeling albumin.

Extracellular volume can be measured by inulin or mannitol.

Serum osmolality = 275–295 mOsm/kg H_2O.

Plasma volume = TBV × (1 – Hct).

Glomerular filtration barrier

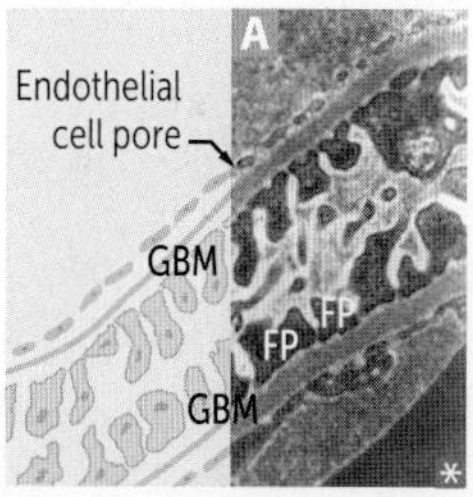

Responsible for filtration of plasma according to size and charge selectivity.

Composed of:

- Fenestrated capillary endothelium
- Basement membrane with type IV collagen chains and heparan sulfate
- Visceral epithelial layer consisting of podocyte foot processes (FPs) A

Charger barrier—glomerular filtration barrier contains ⊖ charged glycoproteins that prevent entry of ⊖ charged molecules (eg, albumin).

Size barrier—fenestrated capillary endothelium (prevents entry of > 100 nm molecules/blood cells); podocyte foot processes interpose with glomerular basement membrane (GBM); slit diaphragm (prevents entry of molecules > 4–5 nm).

Renal clearance

$C_x = (U_xV)/P_x$ = volume of plasma from which the substance is completely cleared in the urine per unit time.
If $C_x <$ GFR: net tubular reabsorption and/or not freely filtered.
If $C_x >$ GFR: net tubular secretion of X.
If $C_x =$ GFR: no net secretion or reabsorption.

C_x = clearance of X (mL/min).
U_x = urine concentration of X (eg, mg/mL).
P_x = plasma concentration of X (eg, mg/mL).
V = urine flow rate (mL/min).

Glomerular filtration rate

Inulin clearance can be used to calculate GFR because it is freely filtered and is neither reabsorbed nor secreted.

$$C_{inulin} = GFR = U_{inulin} \times V/P_{inulin} = K_f [(P_{GC} - P_{BS}) - (\pi_{GC} - \pi_{BS})]$$

(GC = glomerular capillary; BS = Bowman space; π_{BS} normally equals zero; K_f = filtration coefficient).

Normal GFR ≈ 100 mL/min.
Creatinine clearance is an approximate measure of GFR. Slightly overestimates GFR because creatinine is moderately secreted by renal tubules.

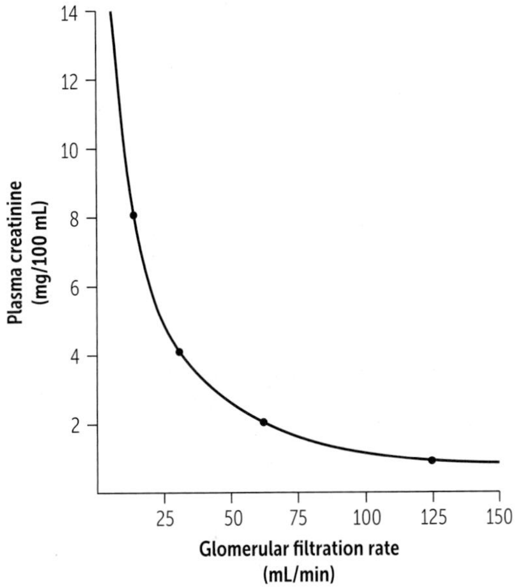

Effective renal plasma flow

Effective renal plasma flow (eRPF) can be estimated using *para*-aminohippuric acid (PAH) clearance. Between filtration and secretion, there is nearly 100% excretion of all PAH that enters the kidney.
$eRPF = U_{PAH} \times V/P_{PAH} = C_{PAH}$.
Renal blood flow (RBF) = RPF/(1 – Hct). Usually 20–25% of cardiac output, remaining constant due to autoregulation.
eRPF underestimates true renal plasma flow (RPF) slightly.

Filtration

Filtration fraction (FF) = GFR/RPF.
Normal FF = 20%.
Filtered load (mg/min) = GFR (mL/min) × plasma concentration (mg/mL).

GFR can be estimated with creatinine clearance.
RPF is best estimated with PAH clearance.
Prostaglandins **D**ilate **A**fferent arteriole (**PDA**).
Angiotensin II **C**onstricts **E**fferent arteriole (**ACE**).

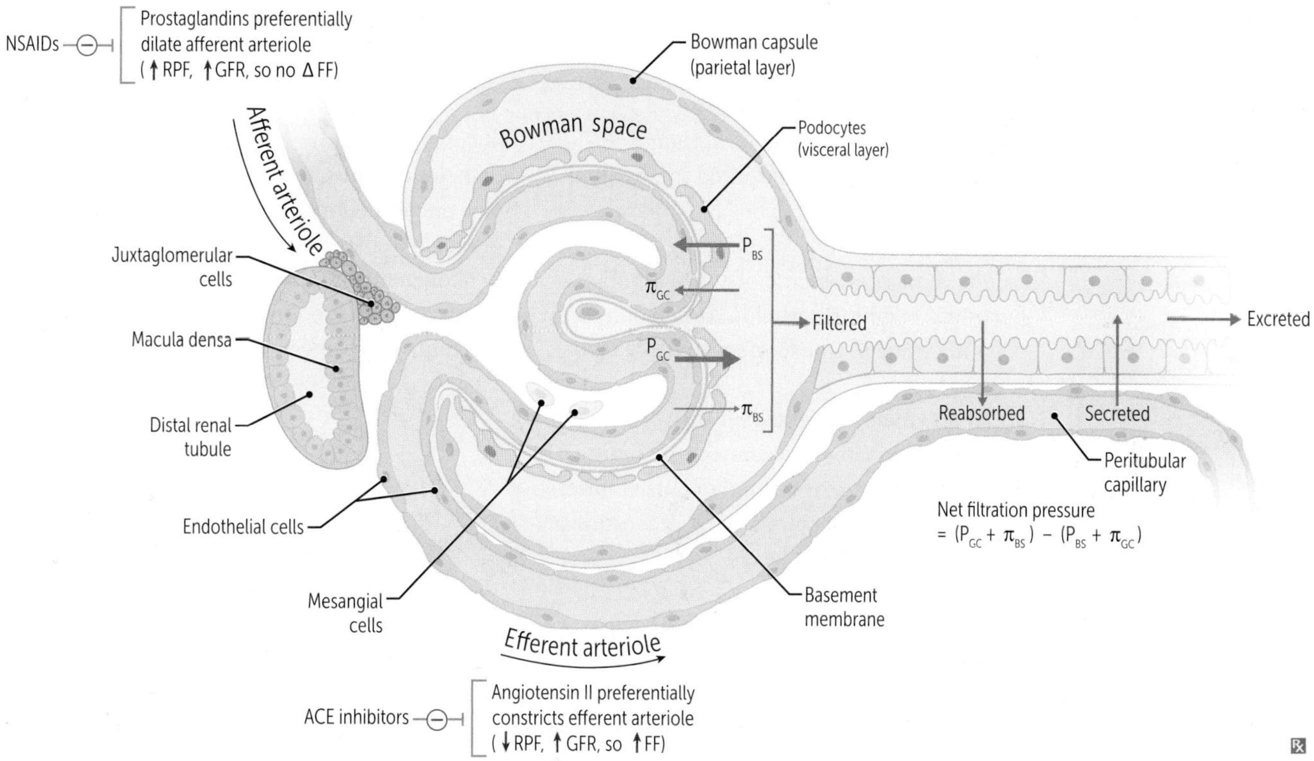

Changes in glomerular dynamics

	GFR	RPF	FF (GFR/RPF)
Afferent arteriole constriction	↓	↓	—
Efferent arteriole constriction	↑	↓	↑
↑ plasma protein concentration	↓	—	↓
↓ plasma protein concentration	↑	—	↑
Constriction of ureter	↓	—	↓
Dehydration	↓	↓↓	↑

Calculation of reabsorption and secretion rate

Filtered load = GFR × P_x.
Excretion rate = V × U_x.
Reabsorption rate = filtered – excreted.
Secretion rate = excreted – filtered.
Fe_{Na} = fractional excretion of sodium.

$$Fe_{Na} = \frac{Na^+ \text{ excreted}}{Na^+ \text{ filtered}} = \frac{V \times U_{Na}}{GFR \times P_{Na}} = \frac{P_{Cr} \times U_{Na}}{U_{Cr} \times P_{Na}} \text{ where } GFR = \frac{U_{Cr} \times V}{P_{Cr}}$$

Glucose clearance

Glucose at a normal plasma level (range 60–120 mg/dL) is completely reabsorbed in proximal convoluted tubule (PCT) by Na^+/glucose cotransport.

In adults, at plasma glucose of ~ 200 mg/dL, glucosuria begins (threshold). At rate of ~ 375 mg/min, all transporters are fully saturated (T_m).

Normal pregnancy is associated with ↑ GFR. With ↑ filtration of all substances, including glucose, the glucose threshold occurs at lower plasma glucose concentrations → glucosuria at normal plasma glucose levels.

Sodium-glucose cotransporter 2 (SGLT2) inhibitors (eg, -flozin drugs) result in glucosuria at plasma concentrations < 200 mg/dL.

Glucosuria is an important clinical clue to diabetes mellitus.

Splay phenomenon—T_m for glucose is reached gradually rather than sharply due to the heterogeneity of nephrons (ie, different T_m points); represented by the portion of the titration curve between threshold and T_m.

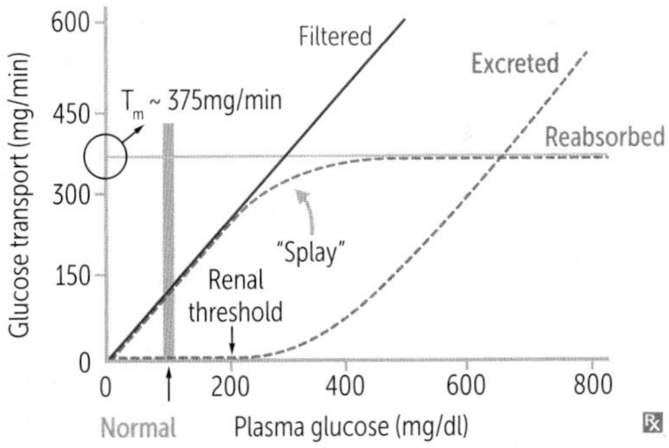

Nephron transport physiology

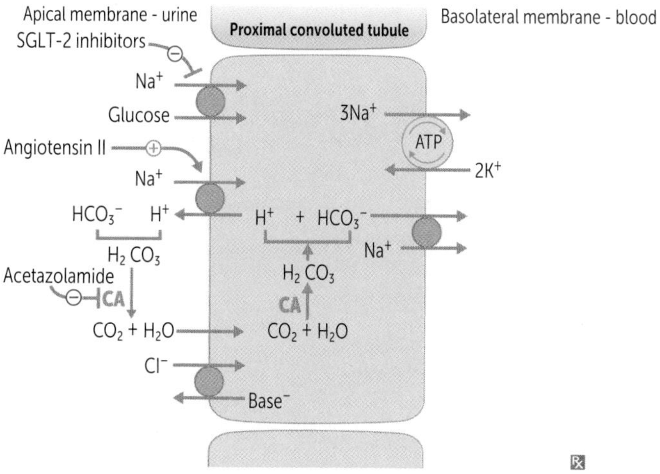

Early PCT—contains brush border. Reabsorbs all glucose and amino acids and most HCO_3^-, Na^+, Cl^-, PO_4^{3-}, K^+, H_2O, and uric acid. Isotonic absorption. Generates and secretes NH_3, which enables the kidney to secrete more H^+.

PTH—inhibits Na^+/PO_4^{3-} cotransport → ↑ PO_4^{3-} excretion.

AT II—stimulates Na^+/H^+ exchange → ↑ Na^+, H_2O, and HCO_3^- reabsorption (permitting contraction alkalosis).

65–80% Na^+ and H_2O reabsorbed.

Thin descending loop of Henle—passively reabsorbs H_2O via medullary hypertonicity (impermeable to Na^+). Concentrating segment. Makes urine hypertonic.

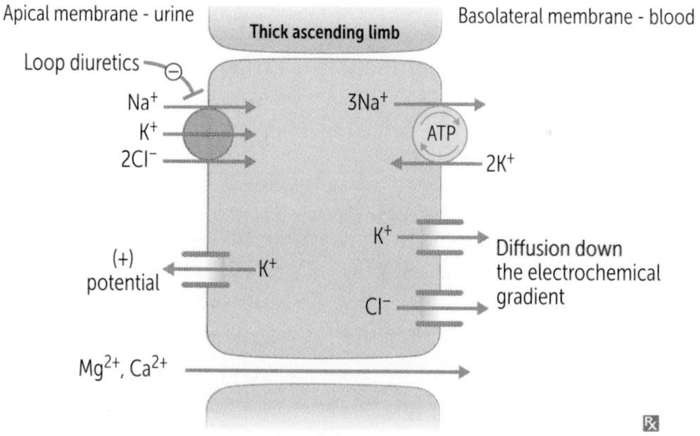

Thick ascending loop of Henle—reabsorbs Na^+, K^+, and Cl^-. Indirectly induces paracellular reabsorption of Mg^{2+} and Ca^{2+} through ⊕ lumen potential generated by K^+ backleak. Impermeable to H_2O. Makes urine less concentrated as it ascends.

10–20% Na^+ reabsorbed.

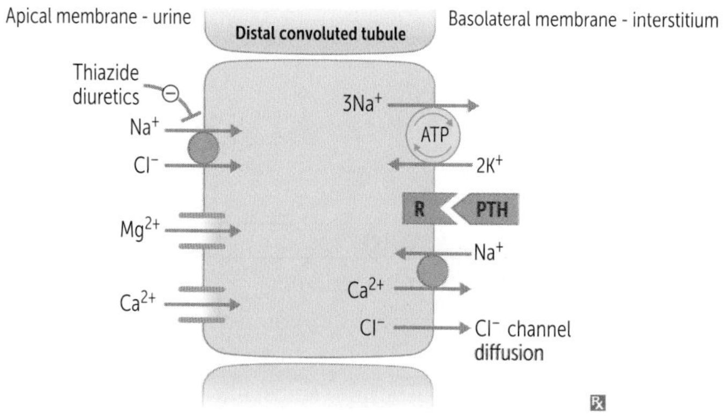

Early DCT—reabsorbs Na^+, Cl^-. Impermeable to H_2O. Makes urine fully dilute (hypotonic).

PTH—↑ Ca^{2+}/Na^+ exchange → ↑ Ca^{2+} reabsorption.

5–10% Na^+ reabsorbed.

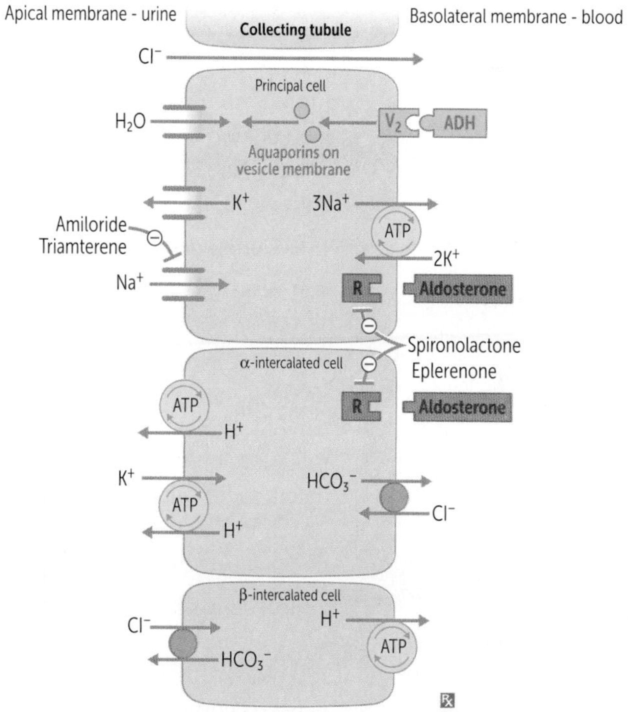

Collecting tubule—reabsorbs Na^+ in exchange for secreting K^+ and H^+ (regulated by aldosterone).

Aldosterone—acts on mineralocorticoid receptor → mRNA → protein synthesis. In principal cells: ↑ apical K^+ conductance, ↑ Na^+/K^+ pump, ↑ epithelial Na^+ channel (ENaC) activity → lumen negativity → K^+ secretion. In α-intercalated cells: lumen negativity → ↑ H^+ ATPase activity → ↑ H^+ secretion → ↑ HCO_3^-/Cl^- exchanger activity.

ADH—acts at V_2 receptor → insertion of aquaporin H_2O channels on apical side.

3–5% Na^+ reabsorbed.

Renal tubular defects Order: Fanconi's BaGeLS

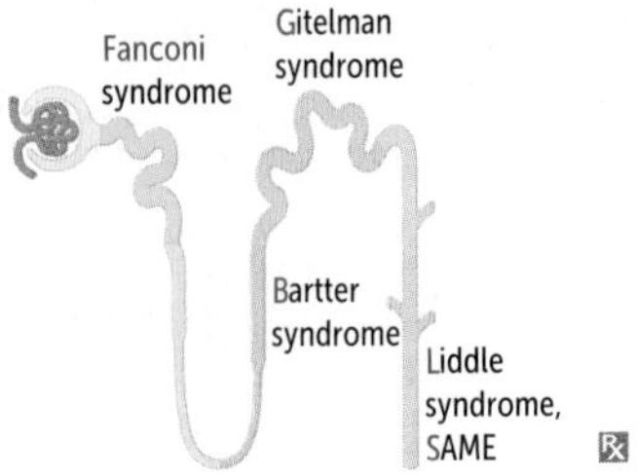

	DEFECTS	EFFECTS	CAUSES	NOTES
Fanconi syndrome	Generalized reabsorption defect in PCT → ↑ excretion of amino acids, glucose, HCO_3^-, and PO_4^{3-}, and all substances reabsorbed by the PCT	Metabolic acidosis (proximal RTA), hypophosphatemia, hypokalemia	Hereditary defects (eg, Wilson disease, tyrosinemia, glycogen storage disease), ischemia, multiple myeloma, nephrotoxins/drugs (eg, ifosfamide, cisplatin), lead poisoning	Growth retardation and rickets/osteopenia common due to hypophosphatemia Volume depletion also common
Bartter syndrome	Reabsorption defect in thick ascending loop of Henle (affects $Na^+/K^+/2Cl^-$ cotransporter)	Metabolic alkalosis, hypokalemia, hypercalciuria	Autosomal recessive	Presents similarly to chronic loop diuretic use
Gitelman syndrome	Reabsorption defect of NaCl in DCT	Metabolic alkalosis, hypomagnesemia, hypokalemia, hypocalciuria	Autosomal recessive	Presents similarly to lifelong thiazide diuretic use Less severe than Bartter syndrome
Liddle syndrome	Gain of function mutation → ↓ Na^+ channel degradation → ↑ Na^+ reabsorption in collecting tubules	Metabolic alkalosis, hypokalemia, hypertension, ↓ aldosterone	Autosomal dominant	Presents similarly to hyperaldosteronism, but aldosterone is nearly undetectable Treatment: amiloride
Syndrome of Apparent Mineralocorticoid Excess	Cortisol activates mineralocorticoid receptors; 11β-HSD converts cortisol to cortisone (inactive on these receptors) Hereditary 11β-HSD deficiency → ↑ cortisol → ↑ mineralocorticoid receptor activity	Metabolic alkalosis, hypokalemia, hypertension ↓ serum aldosterone level; cortisol tries to be the SAME as aldosterone	Autosomal recessive Can acquire disorder from glycyrrhetinic acid (present in licorice), which blocks activity of 11β-hydroxysteroid dehydrogenase	Treatment: K^+-sparing diuretics (↓ mineralocorticoid effects) or corticosteroids (exogenous corticosteroid ↓ endogenous cortisol production → ↓ mineralocorticoid receptor activation)

Relative concentrations along proximal convoluted tubules

[TF/P] > 1
when solute is reabsorbed less quickly than water or when solute is secreted

[TF/P] = 1
when solute and water are reabsorbed at the same rate

[TF/P] < 1
when solute is reabsorbed more quickly than water

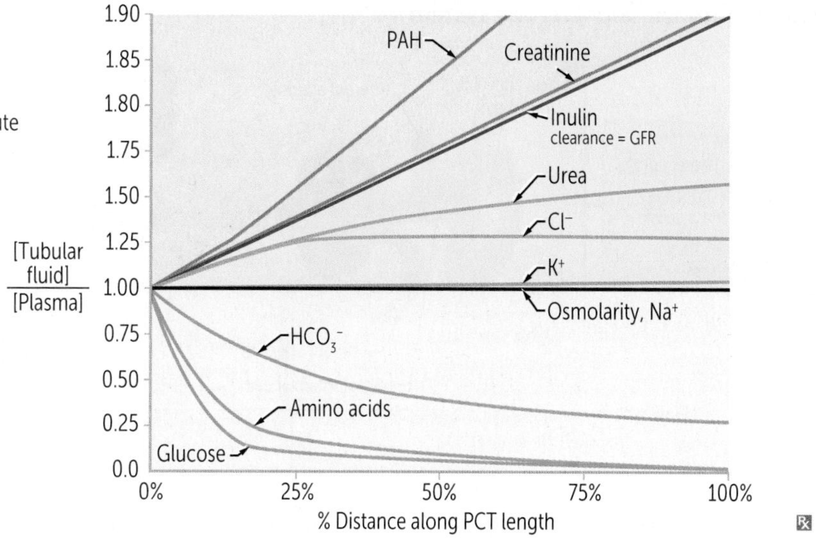

Tubular inulin ↑ in concentration (but not amount) along the PCT as a result of water reabsorption.

Cl^- reabsorption occurs at a slower rate than Na^+ in early PCT and then matches the rate of Na^+ reabsorption more distally. Thus, its relative concentration ↑ before it plateaus.

Renin-angiotensin-aldosterone system

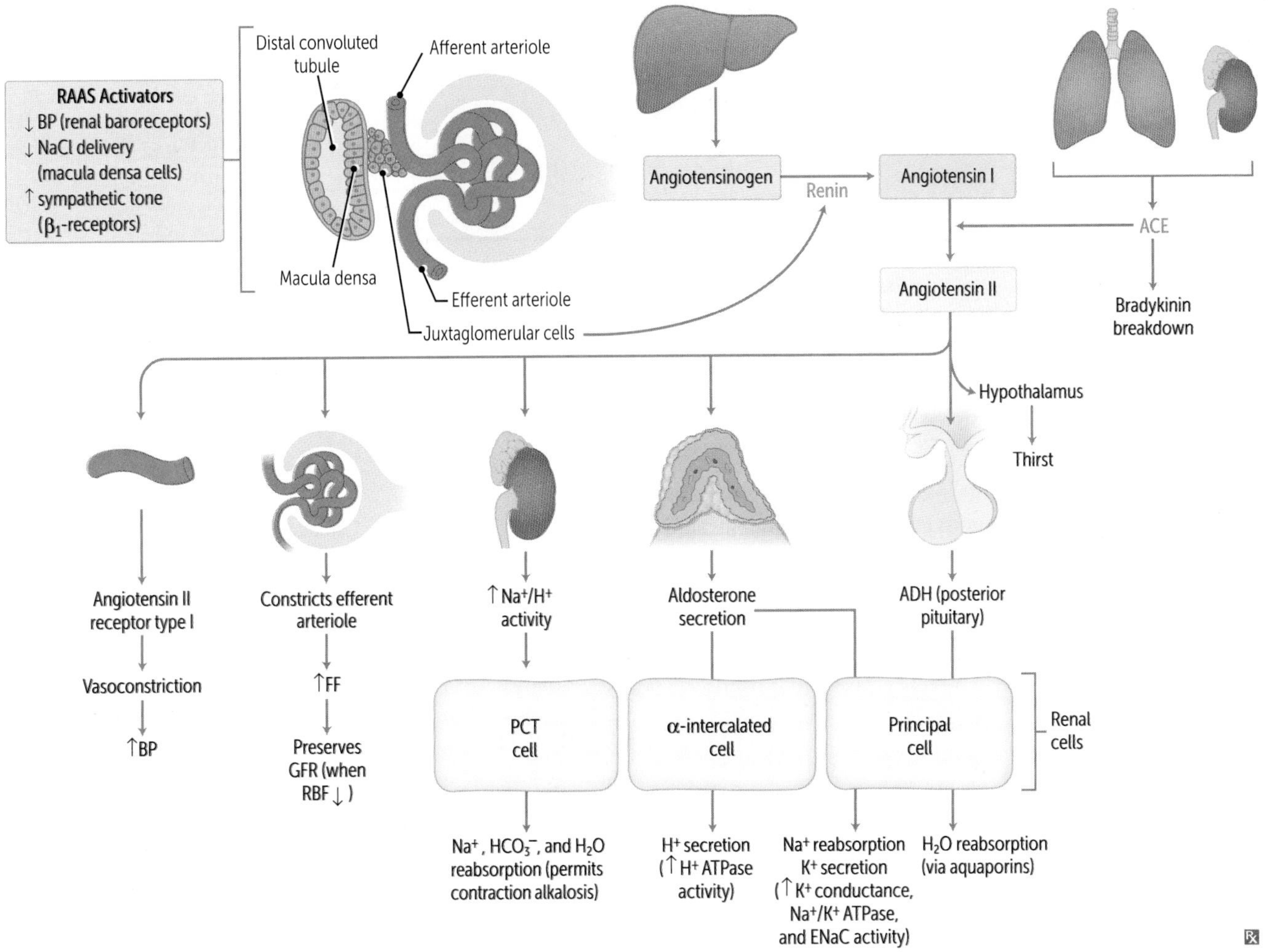

Renin	Secreted by JG cells in response to ↓ renal perfusion pressure (detected by renal baroreceptors in afferent arteriole), ↑ renal sympathetic discharge (β_1 effect), and ↓ NaCl delivery to macula densa cells.
ACE	Catalyzes conversion of angiotensin I to angiotensin II. Located in many tissues but conversion occurs most extensively in the lung. Produced by vascular endothelial cells in the lung.
AT II	Helps maintain blood volume and blood pressure. Affects baroreceptor function; limits reflex bradycardia, which would normally accompany its pressor effects.
ANP, BNP	Released from atria (ANP) and ventricles (BNP) in response to ↑ volume; inhibits renin-angiotensin-aldosterone system; relaxes vascular smooth muscle via cGMP → ↑ GFR, ↓ renin. Dilates afferent arteriole, promotes natriuresis.
ADH (vasopressin)	Primarily regulates serum osmolality; also responds to low blood volume states. Stimulates reabsorption of water in collecting ducts. Also stimulates reabsorption of urea in collecting ducts to maximize corticopapillary osmotic gradient.
Aldosterone	Primarily regulates ECF volume and Na^+ content; ↑ release in hypovolemic states. Responds to hyperkalemia by ↑ K^+ excretion.

Juxtaglomerular apparatus	Consists of mesangial cells, JG cells (modified smooth muscle of afferent arteriole), and the macula densa (NaCl sensor located at the DCT). JG cells secrete renin in response to ↓ renal blood pressure and ↑ sympathetic tone (β_1). Macula densa cells sense ↓ NaCl delivery to DCT → ↑ renin release → efferent arteriole vasoconstriction → ↑ GFR.	JGA maintains GFR via renin-angiotensin-aldosterone system. In addition to vasodilatory properties, β-blockers can decrease BP by inhibiting β_1-receptors of the JGA → ↓ renin release.

Kidney hormone functions

Erythropoietin	Released by interstitial cells in peritubular capillary bed in response to hypoxia.	Stimulates RBC proliferation in bone marrow. Administered for anemia secondary to chronic kidney disease. ↑ risk of HTN.
Calciferol (vitamin D)	PCT cells convert 25-OH vitamin D_3 to 1,25-$(OH)_2$ vitamin D_3 (calcitriol, active form). Increases calcium absorption in small bowel.	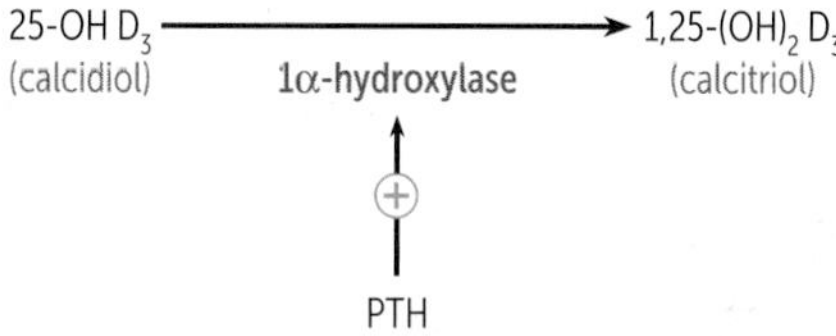
Prostaglandins	Paracrine secretion vasodilates afferent arterioles to ↑ RBF.	NSAIDs block renal-protective prostaglandin synthesis → constriction of afferent arteriole and ↓ GFR; this may result in acute kidney injury in low renal blood flow states.
Dopamine	Secreted by PCT cells, promotes natriuresis. At low doses; dilates interlobular arteries, afferent arterioles, efferent arterioles → ↑ RBF, little or no change in GFR. At higher doses; acts as vasoconstrictor.	

Hormones acting on kidney

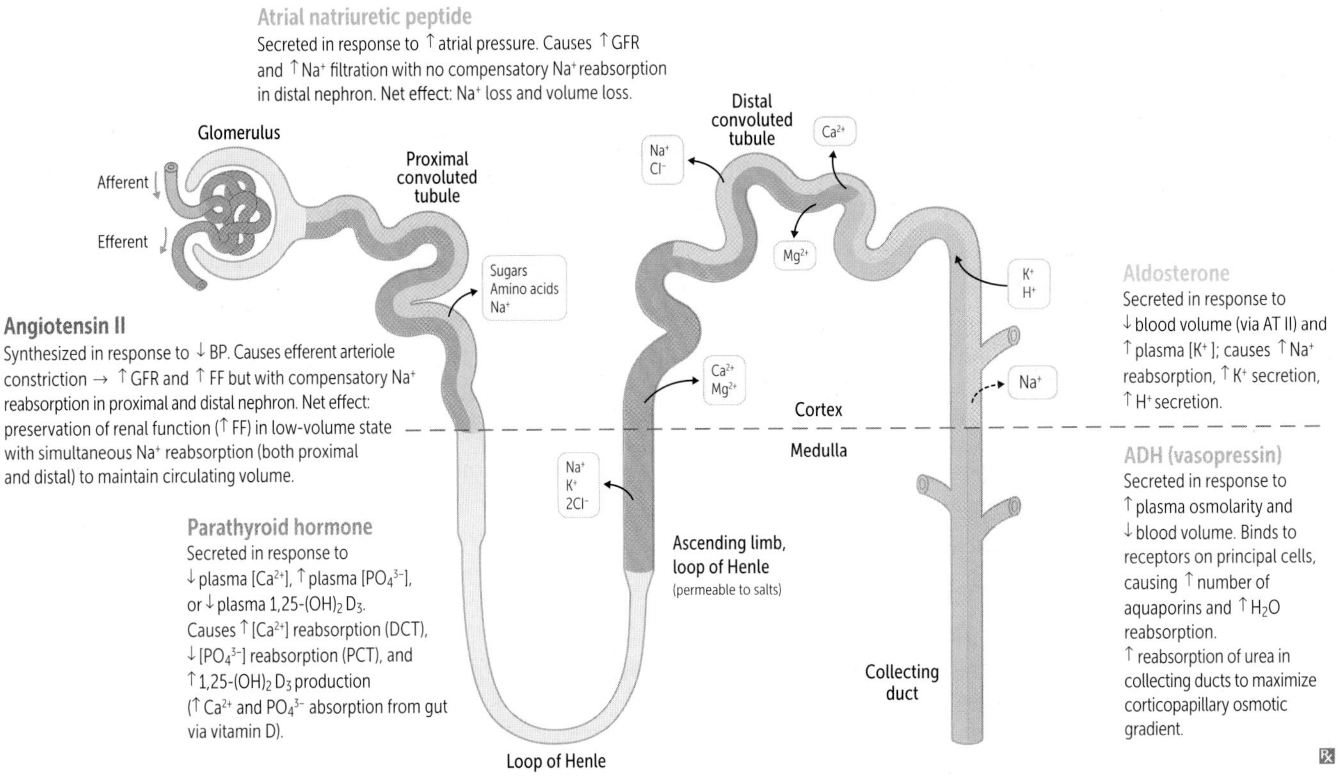
Atrial natriuretic peptide
Secreted in response to ↑ atrial pressure. Causes ↑ GFR and ↑ Na^+ filtration with no compensatory Na^+ reabsorption in distal nephron. Net effect: Na^+ loss and volume loss.
Glomerulus
Afferent
Efferent
Proximal convoluted tubule
Sugars
Amino acids
Na^+
Distal convoluted tubule
Na^+
Cl^-
Ca^{2+}
Mg^{2+}
K^+
H^+
Na^+
Angiotensin II
Synthesized in response to ↓ BP. Causes efferent arteriole constriction → ↑ GFR and ↑ FF but with compensatory Na^+ reabsorption in proximal and distal nephron. Net effect: preservation of renal function (↑ FF) in low-volume state with simultaneous Na^+ reabsorption (both proximal and distal) to maintain circulating volume.
Ca^{2+}
Mg^{2+}
Cortex
Medulla
Na^+
K^+
2Cl^-
Parathyroid hormone
Secreted in response to ↓ plasma [Ca^{2+}], ↑ plasma [PO_4^{3-}], or ↓ plasma 1,25-$(OH)_2$ D_3. Causes ↑ [Ca^{2+}] reabsorption (DCT), ↓ [PO_4^{3-}] reabsorption (PCT), and ↑ 1,25-$(OH)_2$ D_3 production (↑ Ca^{2+} and PO_4^{3-} absorption from gut via vitamin D).
Ascending limb, loop of Henle
(permeable to salts)
Collecting duct
Loop of Henle
Aldosterone
Secreted in response to ↓ blood volume (via AT II) and ↑ plasma [K^+]; causes ↑ Na^+ reabsorption, ↑ K^+ secretion, ↑ H^+ secretion.
ADH (vasopressin)
Secreted in response to ↑ plasma osmolarity and ↓ blood volume. Binds to receptors on principal cells, causing ↑ number of aquaporins and ↑ H_2O reabsorption.
↑ reabsorption of urea in collecting ducts to maximize corticopapillary osmotic gradient.

Potassium shifts

SHIFTS K^+ INTO CELL (CAUSING HYPOKALEMIA)	SHIFTS K^+ OUT OF CELL (CAUSING HYPERKALEMIA)
	Digoxin (blocks Na^+/K^+ ATPase)
Hypo-osmolarity	HyperOsmolarity
	Lysis of cells (eg, crush injury, rhabdomyolysis, tumor lysis syndrome)
Alkalosis	Acidosis
β-adrenergic agonist (↑ Na^+/K^+ ATPase)	β-blocker
Insulin (↑ Na^+/K^+ ATPase)	High blood Sugar (insulin deficiency)
Insulin shifts K^+ into cells	Succinylcholine (↑ risk in burns/muscle trauma)
	Hyperkalemia? DO LAβSS

Electrolyte disturbances

ELECTROLYTE	LOW SERUM CONCENTRATION	HIGH SERUM CONCENTRATION
Sodium	Nausea, malaise, stupor, coma, seizures	Irritability, stupor, coma
Potassium	U waves and flattened T waves on ECG, arrhythmias, muscle cramps, spasm, weakness	Wide QRS and peaked T waves on ECG, arrhythmias, muscle weakness
Calcium	Tetany, seizures, QT prolongation, twitching (eg, Chvostek sign), spasm (eg, Trousseau sign)	**Stones** (renal), **bones** (pain), **groans** (abdominal pain), **thrones** (↑ urinary frequency), **psychiatric overtones** (anxiety, altered mental status)
Magnesium	Tetany, torsades de pointes, hypokalemia, hypocalcemia (when $[Mg^{2+}] < 1.0$ mEq/L)	↓ DTRs, lethargy, bradycardia, hypotension, cardiac arrest, hypocalcemia
Phosphate	Bone loss, osteomalacia (adults), rickets (children)	Renal stones, metastatic calcifications, hypocalcemia

Features of renal disorders

CONDITION	BLOOD PRESSURE	PLASMA RENIN	ALDOSTERONE	SERUM Mg^{2+}	URINE Ca^{2+}
SIADH	—/↑	**↓**	**↓**	—	—
Primary hyperaldosteronism	**↑**	**↓**	↑	—	—
Renin-secreting tumor	**↑**	↑	**↑**	—	—
Bartter syndrome	—	**↑**	**↑**	—	**↑**
Gitelman syndrome	—	**↑**	**↑**	**↓**	**↓**
Liddle syndrome, syndrome of apparent mineralocorticoid excess	**↑**	**↓**	↓	—	—

↑ ↓ = important differentiating feature.

Acid-base physiology

	pH	P_{CO_2}	$[HCO_3^-]$	COMPENSATORY RESPONSE
Metabolic acidosis	↓	↓	↓	Hyperventilation (immediate)
Metabolic alkalosis	↑	↑	↑	Hypoventilation (immediate)
Respiratory acidosis	↓	↑	↑	↑ renal $[HCO_3^-]$ reabsorption (delayed)
Respiratory alkalosis	↑	↓	↓	↓ renal $[HCO_3^-]$ reabsorption (delayed)

Key: ↓ ↑ = compensatory response.

Henderson-Hasselbalch equation: $pH = 6.1 + \log \frac{[HCO_3^-]}{0.03\ P_{CO_2}}$

Predicted respiratory compensation for a simple metabolic acidosis can be calculated using the Winters formula. If measured P_{CO_2} > predicted P_{CO_2} → concomitant respiratory acidosis; if measured P_{CO_2} < predicted P_{CO_2} → concomitant respiratory alkalosis:

$$P_{CO_2} = 1.5\ [HCO_3^-] + 8 \pm 2$$

Acidosis and alkalosis

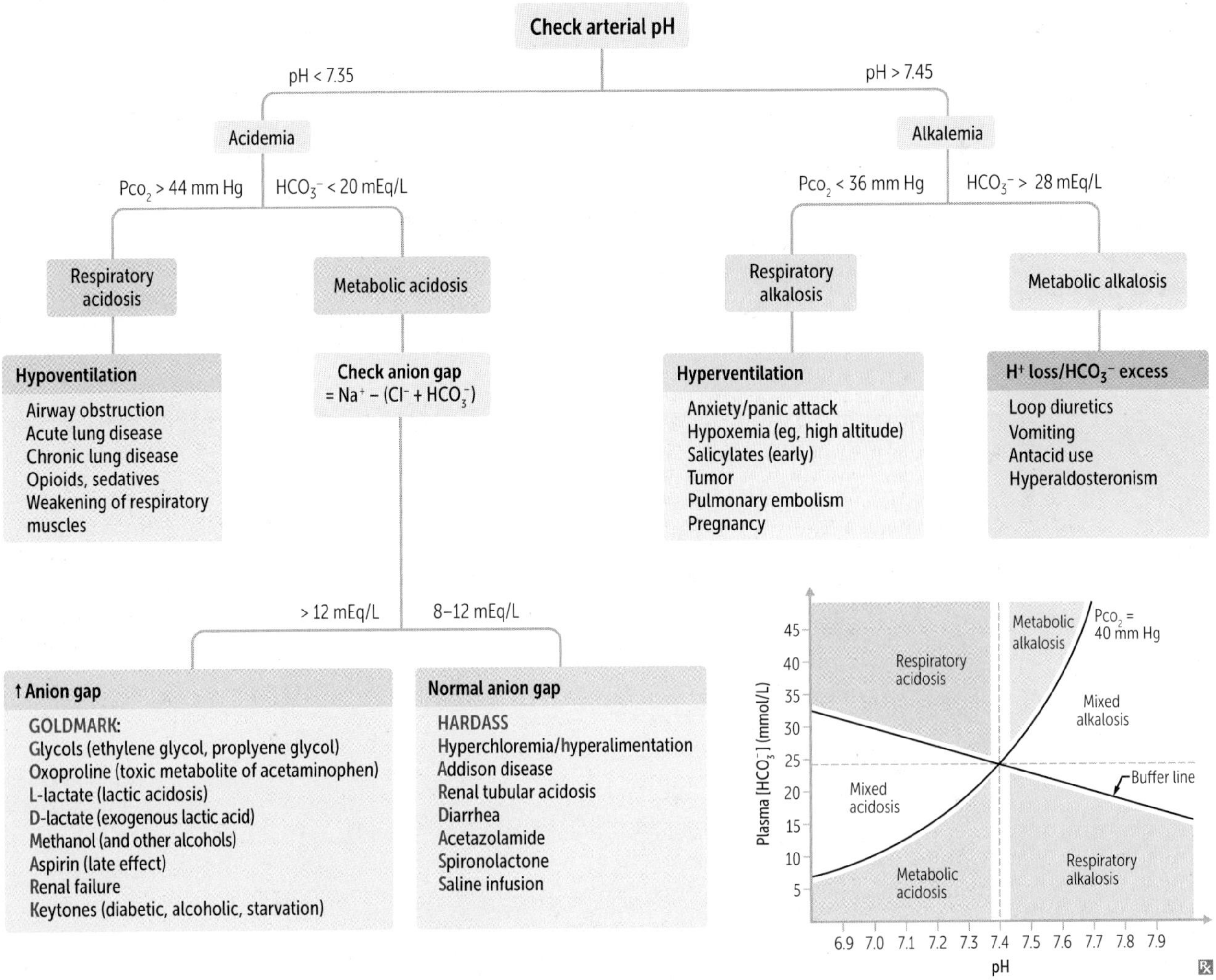

Renal tubular acidosis

	Distal renal tubular acidosis (RTA type 1)	Proximal renal tubular acidosis (RTA type 2)	Hyperkalemic tubular acidosis (RTA type 4)
	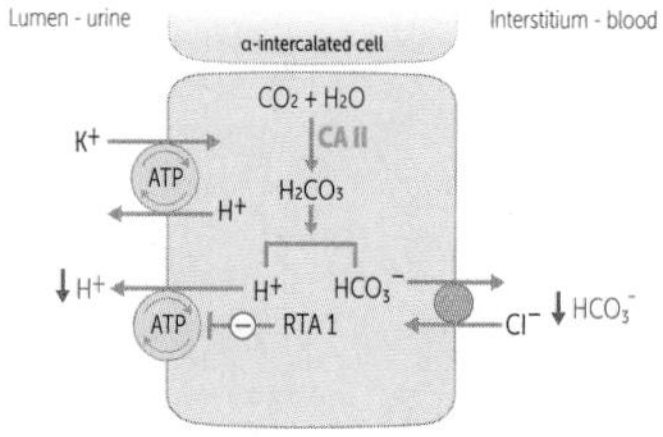	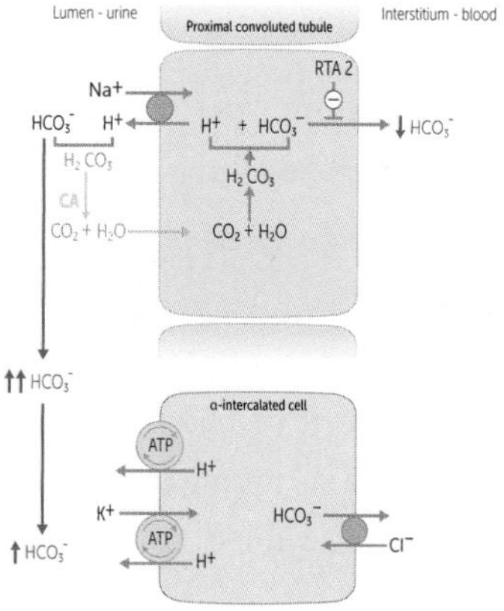	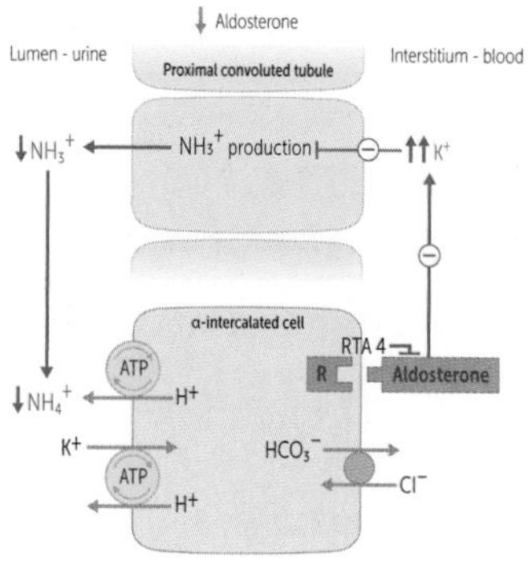
DEFECT	Inability of α-intercalated cells to secrete H^+ → no new HCO_3^- is generated → metabolic acidosis	Defect in PCT HCO_3^- reabsorption → ↑ excretion of HCO_3^- in urine → metabolic acidosis Urine can be acidified by α-intercalated cells in collecting duct, but not enough to overcome ↑ HCO_3^- excretion	Hypoaldosteronism or aldosterone resistance; hyperkalemia → ↓ NH_3 synthesis in PCT → ↓ NH_4^+ excretion
URINE pH	> 5.5	< 5.5 when plasma HCO_3^- below reduced resorption threshold > 5.5 when filtered HCO_3^- exceeds resorptive threshold	< 5.5 (or variable)
SERUM K^+	↓	↓	↑
CAUSES	Amphotericin B toxicity, analgesic nephropathy, congenital anomalies (obstruction) of urinary tract, autoimmune diseases (eg, SLE)	Fanconi syndrome, multiple myeloma, carbonic anhydrase inhibitors	↓ aldosterone production (eg, diabetic hyporeninism, ACE inhibitors, ARB, NSAIDs, heparin, cyclosporine, adrenal insufficiency) or aldosterone resistance (eg, K^+-sparing diuretics, nephropathy due to obstruction, TMP-SMX)
ASSOCIATIONS	↑ risk for calcium phosphate kidney stones (due to ↑ urine pH and ↑ bone turnover related to buffering)	↑ risk for hypophosphatemic rickets (in Fanconi syndrome)	

▶ RENAL—PATHOLOGY

Casts in urine	Presence of casts indicates that hematuria/pyuria is of glomerular or renal tubular origin. Bladder cancer, kidney stones → hematuria, no casts. Acute cystitis → pyuria, no casts.
RBC casts A	Glomerulonephritis, hypertensive emergency.
WBC casts B	Tubulointerstitial inflammation, acute pyelonephritis, transplant rejection.
Granular casts C	Acute tubular necrosis (ATN). Can be "muddy brown" in appearance.
Fatty casts ("oval fat bodies")	Nephrotic syndrome. Associated with "Maltese cross" sign D.
Waxy casts	End-stage renal disease/chronic kidney disease.
Hyaline casts E	Nonspecific, can be a normal finding with dehydration, exercise, or diuretic therapy. Form via solidification of Tamm-Horsfall mucoprotein (uromodulin), secreted by renal tubular cells to prevent UTIs.

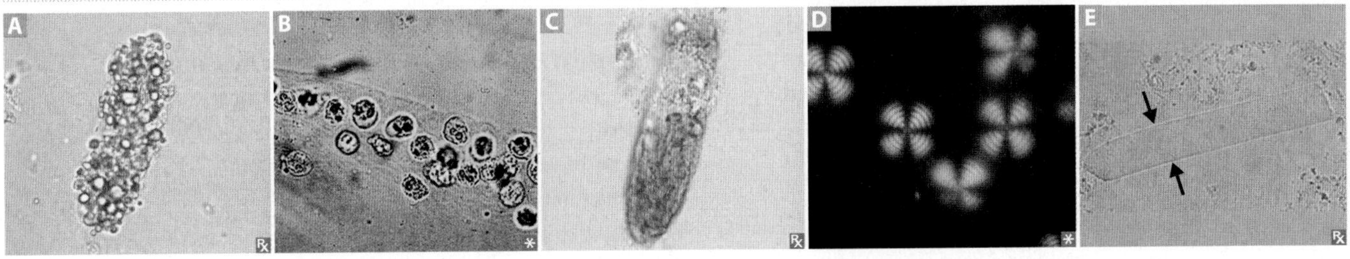

Nomenclature of glomerular disorders

TYPE	CHARACTERISTICS	EXAMPLE
Focal	< 50% of glomeruli are involved	Focal segmental glomerulosclerosis
Diffuse	> 50% of glomeruli are involved	Diffuse proliferative glomerulonephritis
Proliferative	Hypercellular glomeruli	Membranoproliferative glomerulonephritis
Membranous	Thickening of glomerular basement membrane (GBM)	Membranous nephropathy
Primary glomerular disease	1° disease of the kidney specifically impacting the glomeruli	Minimal change disease
Secondary glomerular disease	Systemic disease or disease of another organ system that also impacts the glomeruli	SLE, diabetic nephropathy

Glomerular diseases

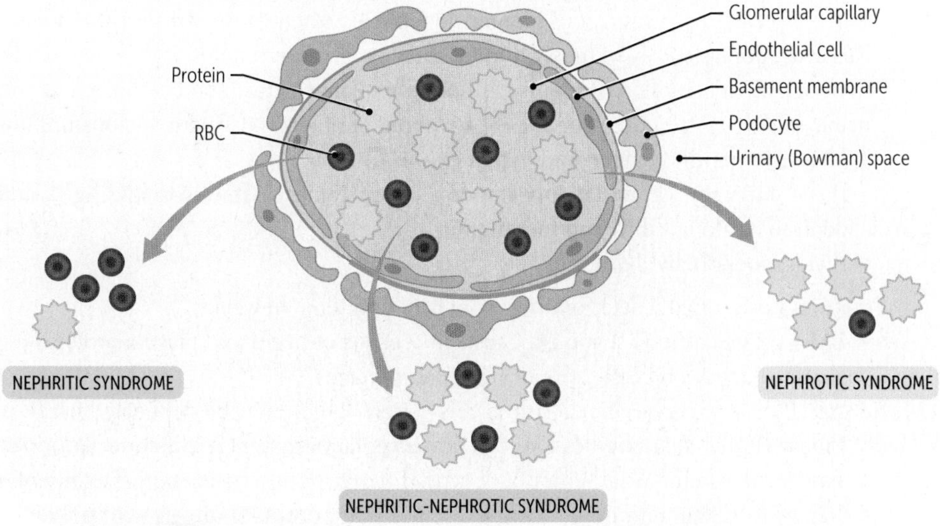

TYPE	ETIOLOGY	CLINICAL PRESENTATION	EXAMPLES
Nephritic syndrome	Glomerular inflammation → GBM damage → loss of RBCs into urine → dysmorphic RBCs, hematuria	Hematuria, RBC casts in urine ↓ GFR → oliguria, azotemia ↑ renin release, HTN Proteinuria often in the subnephrotic range (< 3.5 g/day) but in severe cases may be in nephrotic range	▪ Acute poststreptococcal glomerulonephritis ▪ Goodpasture syndrome ▪ IgA nephropathy (Berger disease) ▪ Alport syndrome ▪ Membranoproliferative glomerulonephritis
Nephrotic syndrome	Podocyte damage → impaired charge barrier → proteinuria	Massive proteinuria (> 3.5 g/day) with hypoalbuminemia, edema Frothy urine with fatty casts Associated with hypercoagulable state due to antithrombin III loss in urine and ↑ risk of infection (loss of IgGs in urine and soft tissue compromise by edema)	May be 1° (eg, direct podocyte damage) or 2° (podocyte damage from systemic process): ▪ Focal segmental glomerulosclerosis (1° or 2°) ▪ Minimal change disease (1° or 2°) ▪ Membranous nephropathy (1° or 2°) ▪ Amyloidosis (2°) ▪ Diabetic glomerulonephropathy (2°)
Nephritic-nephrotic syndrome	Severe GBM damage → loss of RBCs into urine + impaired charge barrier → hematuria + proteinuria	Nephrotic-range proteinuria (> 3.5 g/day) and concomitant features of nephritic syndrome	Can occur with any form of nephritic syndrome, but is most common with: ▪ Diffuse proliferative glomerulonephritis ▪ Membranoproliferative glomerulonephritis

Nephritic syndrome	Nephritic syndrome = inflammatory process.
Acute poststreptococcal glomerulonephritis	Most frequently seen in children. ~ 2–4 weeks after group A streptococcal infection of pharynx or skin. Also called postinfectious glomerulonephritis when caused by non-streptococcal pathogens. Resolves spontaneously in most children; may progress to renal insufficiency in adults. Type III hypersensitivity reaction. Presents with peripheral and periorbital edema, tea or cola-colored urine, HTN. ⊕ strep titers/serologies, ↓ complement levels (C3) due to consumption. ▪ LM—glomeruli enlarged and hypercellular A ▪ IF—("starry sky") granular appearance ("lumpy-bumpy") B due to IgG, IgM, and C3 deposition along GBM and mesangium ▪ EM—subepithelial IC humps
Rapidly progressive (crescentic) glomerulonephritis	Poor prognosis, rapidly deteriorating renal function (days to weeks). ▪ LM—crescent moon shape C. Crescents consist of fibrin and plasma proteins (eg, C3b) with glomerular parietal cells, monocytes, macrophages Several disease processes may result in this pattern which may be delineated via IF pattern. ▪ Linear IF due to antibodies to GBM and alveolar basement membrane: Goodpasture syndrome—hematuria/hemoptysis; type II hypersensitivity reaction. Treatment: plasmapheresis ▪ Negative IF/Pauci-immune (no Ig/C3 deposition): granulomatosis with polyangiitis (formerly Churg-Strauss syndrome)—PR3-ANCA/c-ANCA, eosinophilic granulomatosis with polyangiitis or Microscopic polyangiitis—MPO-ANCA/p-ANCA ▪ Granular IF—PSGN or DPGN
Diffuse proliferative glomerulonephritis	Often due to SLE (think "wire lupus"). DPGN and MPGN often present as nephrotic syndrome and nephritic syndrome concurrently. ▪ LM—"wire looping" of capillaries D ▪ IF—granular; EM—subendothelial, sometimes subepithelial or intramembranous IgG-based ICs often with C3 deposition
IgA nephropathy (Berger disease)	Episodic hematuria that usually occurs concurrently with respiratory or GI tract infections (IgA is secreted by mucosal linings). Renal pathology of IgA vasculitis (HSP). ▪ LM—mesangial proliferation ▪ IF—IgA-based IC deposits in mesangium; EM—mesangial IC deposition
Alport syndrome	Mutation in type IV collagen → irregular thinning and thickening and splitting of glomerular basement membrane. Most commonly X-linked dominant. Eye problems (eg, retinopathy, anterior lenticonus), glomerulonephritis, sensorineural deafness; "can't see, can't pee, can't hear a bee." ▪ EM—"basket-weave" appearance due to irregular thickening of GBM
Membrano-proliferative glomerulonephritis	MPGN is a nephritic syndrome that often co-presents with nephrotic syndrome. Type I may be 2° to hepatitis B or C infection. May also be idiopathic. ▪ Subendothelial IC deposits with granular IF Type II is associated with C3 nephritic factor (IgG autoantibody that stabilizes C3 convertase → persistent complement activation → ↓ C3 levels). ▪ Intramembranous deposits, also called dense deposit disease Both types: mesangial ingrowth → GBM splitting → "tram-track" on H&E and PAS E stains.

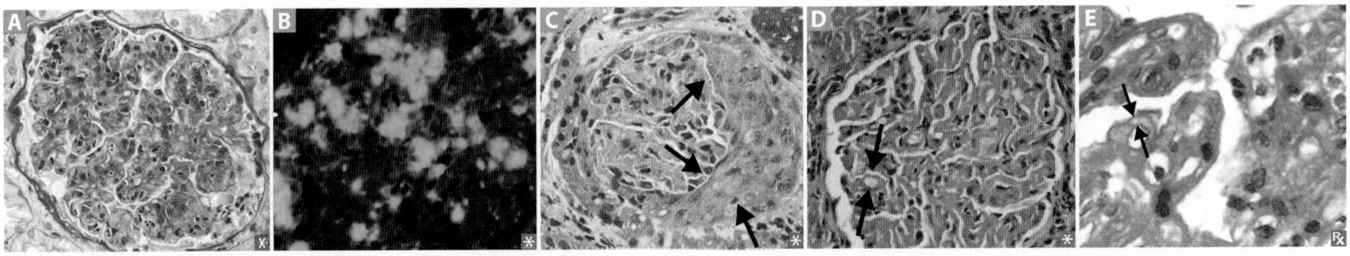

Nephrotic syndrome — Nephrotic syndrome—massive proteinuria (> 3.5 g/day)

Minimal change disease

Also known as lipoid nephrosis. Most common cause of nephrotic syndrome in children.

Often 1° (idiopathic) and may be triggered by recent infection, immunization, immune stimulus (4 I's of MCD). Rarely, may be 2° to lymphoma (eg, cytokine-mediated damage).

1° disease has excellent response to corticosteroids.

- LM—Normal glomeruli (lipid may be seen in PCT cells)
- IF—⊖
- EM—effacement of podocyte foot processes A

Focal segmental glomerulosclerosis

Higher prevalence in Black people.

Can be 1° (idiopathic) or 2° to other conditions (eg, HIV infection, sickle cell disease, heroin use, obesity, interferon treatment, or congenital malformations).

1° disease has inconsistent response to steroids. May progress to CKD.

- LM—segmental sclerosis and hyalinosis B
- IF—often ⊖ but may be ⊕ for nonspecific focal deposits of IgM, C3, C1
- EM—effacement of foot processes similar to minimal change disease

Membranous nephropathy

Also known as membranous glomerulonephritis.

Can be 1° (eg, antibodies to phospholipase A_2 receptor) or 2° to drugs (eg, NSAIDs, penicillamine, gold), infections (eg, HBV, HCV, syphilis), SLE, or solid tumors.

1° disease has poor response to steroids. May progress to CKD.

- LM—diffuse capillary and GBM thickening C
- IF—granular due to immune complex (IC) deposition
- EM—"Spike and dome" appearance of subepithelial deposits

Amyloidosis

Kidney is the most commonly involved organ (systemic amyloidosis). Associated with chronic conditions that predispose to amyloid deposition (eg, AL amyloid, AA amyloid, prolonged dialysis).

- LM—Congo red stain shows apple-green birefringence under polarized light due to amyloid deposition in the mesangium

Diabetic glomerulonephropathy

Most common cause of ESRD in the United States.

Hyperglycemia → nonenzymatic glycation of tissue proteins → mesangial expansion; GBM thickening and ↑ permeability. Hyperfiltration (glomerular HTN and ↑ GFR) → glomerular hypertrophy and glomerular scarring (glomerulosclerosis) → further progression of nephropathy.

- LM—Mesangial expansion, GBM thickening, eosinophilic nodular glomerulosclerosis (Kimmelstiel-Wilson lesions D)

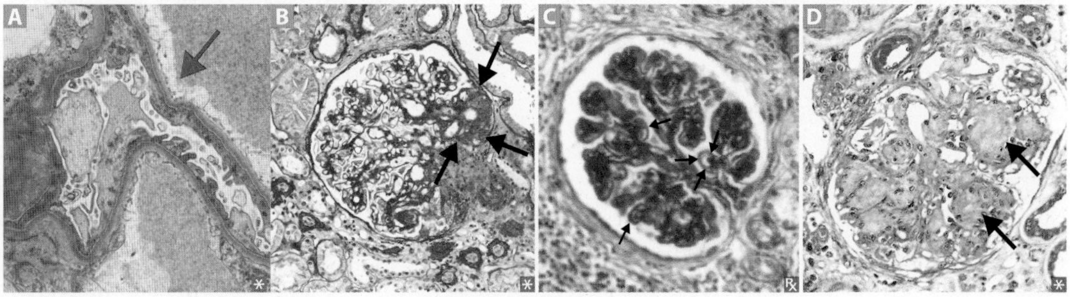

Kidney stones Can lead to severe complications such as hydronephrosis, pyelonephritis, and acute kidney injury. Obstructed stone presents with unilateral flank tenderness, colicky pain radiating to groin, hematuria. Treat and prevent by encouraging fluid intake.

CONTENT	PRECIPITATES WITH	X-RAY FINDINGS	CT FINDINGS	URINE CRYSTAL	NOTES
Calcium	Calcium oxalate: hypocitraturia	Radiopaque	Radiopaque	Shaped like envelope A or dumbbell	Calcium stones most common (80%); calcium oxalate more common than calcium phosphate stones. Can result from ethylene glycol (antifreeze) ingestion, vitamin C overuse, hypocitraturia (associated with ↓ urine pH), malabsorption (eg, Crohn disease). Treatment: thiazides, citrate, low-sodium diet.
	Calcium phosphate: ↑ pH	Radiopaque	Radiopaque	Wedge-shaped prism	Treatment: low-sodium diet, thiazides.
Ammonium magnesium phosphate (struvite)	↑ pH	Radiopaque	Radiopaque	Coffin lid B	Account for 15% of stones. Caused by infection with urease ⊕ bugs (eg, *Proteus mirabilis*, *Staphylococcus saprophyticus*, *Klebsiella*) that hydrolyze urea to ammonia → urine alkalinization. Commonly form staghorn calculi C. Treatment: eradication of underlying infection, surgical removal of stone.
Uric acid	↓ pH	Radiolucent	Visible	Rhomboid D or rosettes	About 5% of all stones. Risk factors: ↓ urine volume, arid climates, acidic pH. Strong association with hyperuricemia (eg, gout). Often seen in diseases with ↑ cell turnover (eg, leukemia). Treatment: alkalinization of urine, allopurinol.
Cystine	↓ pH	Faintly radiopaque	Moderately radiopaque	Hexagonal E	Hereditary (autosomal recessive) condition in which Cystine-reabsorbing PCT transporter loses function, causing cystinuria. Transporter defect also results in poor reabsorption of Ornithine, Lysine, Arginine (COLA). Cystine is poorly soluble, thus stones form in urine. Usually begins in childhood. Can form staghorn calculi. Sodium cyanide nitroprusside test ⊕. "Sixtine" stones have six sides. Treatment: low sodium diet, alkalinization of urine, chelating agents (eg, tiopronin, penicillamine) if refractory.

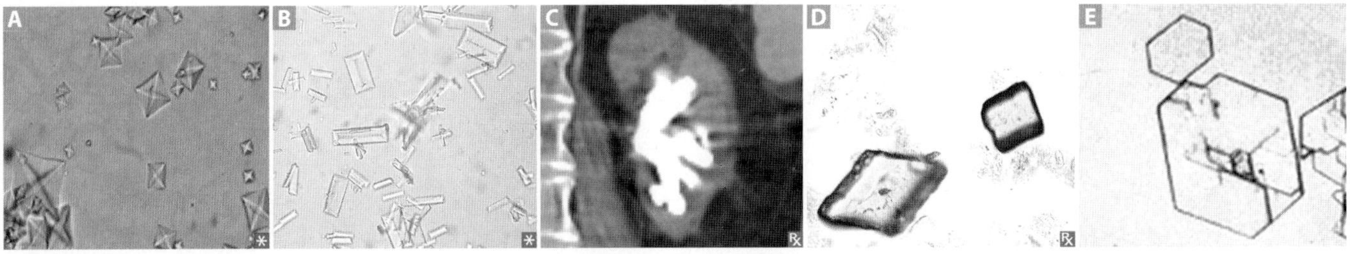

Hydronephrosis

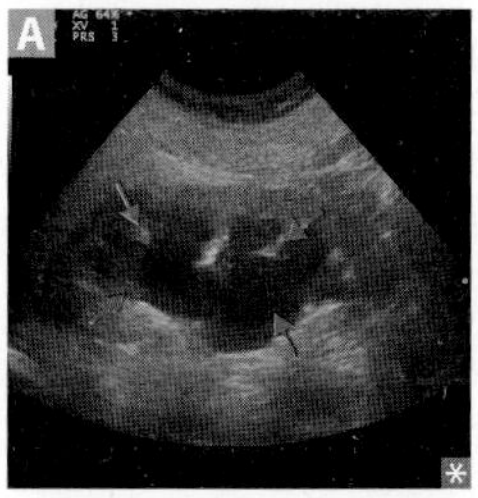

Distention/dilation of renal pelvis and/or calyces A. Usually caused by urinary tract obstruction (eg, renal stones, severe BPH, congenital obstructions, cervical cancer, injury to ureter); other causes include retroperitoneal fibrosis, vesicoureteral reflux. Dilation occurs proximal to site of pathology. Serum creatinine becomes elevated if obstruction is bilateral or if patient has an obstructed solitary kidney. Leads to compression and possible atrophy of renal cortex and medulla.

Urinary incontinence

Mixed incontinence has features of both stress and urgency incontinence.

	Stress incontinence	Urgency incontinence	Overflow incontinence
	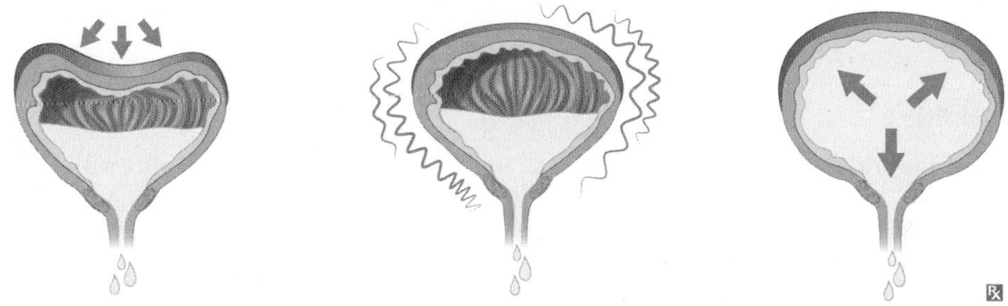		
MECHANISM	Outlet incompetence (urethral hypermobility or intrinsic sphincter deficiency) → leak with ↑ intra-abdominal pressure (eg, sneezing, lifting) ⊕ bladder stress test (directly observed leakage from urethra upon coughing or Valsalva maneuver)	Detrusor overactivity → leak with urge to void immediately	Incomplete emptying (detrusor underactivity or outlet obstruction) → leak with overfilling, ↑ postvoid residual on catheterization or ultrasound
ASSOCIATIONS	Obesity, pregnancy, vaginal delivery, prostate surgery	UTI	Polyuria (eg, diabetes), bladder outlet obstruction (eg, BPH), spinal cord injury (eg, MS)
TREATMENT	Pelvic floor muscle strengthening (Kegel) exercises, weight loss, pessaries	Kegel exercises, bladder training (timed voiding, distraction or relaxation techniques), antimuscarinics (eg, oxybutynin for overactive bladder), mirabegron	Catheterization, relieve obstruction (eg, α-blockers for BPH)

Acute cystitis

Inflammation of urinary bladder. Presents as suprapubic pain, dysuria, urinary frequency, urgency. Systemic signs (eg, high fever, chills) are usually absent.

Risk factors include female sex (short urethra), sexual intercourse, indwelling catheter, diabetes mellitus, impaired bladder emptying.

Causes:

- *E coli* (most common)
- *Staphylococcus saprophyticus*—seen in sexually active young women (*E coli* is still more common in this group)
- *Klebsiella*
- *Proteus mirabilis*—urine has ammonia scent

Labs: ⊕ leukocyte esterase. ⊕ nitrites (indicates presence of Enterobacteriaceae). Sterile pyuria (pyuria with ⊖ urine cultures) could suggest urethritis by *Neisseria gonorrhoeae* or *Chlamydia trachomatis*.

Treatment: antibiotics (eg, TMP-SMX, nitrofurantoin).

Pyelonephritis

Acute pyelonephritis

Neutrophils infiltrate renal interstitium A. Affects cortex with relative sparing of glomeruli/vessels. Presents with fevers, flank pain (costovertebral angle tenderness), nausea/vomiting, chills.

Causes include ascending UTI (*E coli* is most common), hematogenous spread to kidney. Presents with WBCs in urine +/– WBC casts. CT would show striated parenchymal enhancement B.

Risk factors include indwelling urinary catheter, urinary tract obstruction, vesicoureteral reflux, diabetes mellitus, pregnancy.

Complications include chronic pyelonephritis, renal papillary necrosis, perinephric abscess, urosepsis.

Treatment: antibiotics.

Chronic pyelonephritis

The result of recurrent or inadequately treated episodes of acute pyelonephritis. Typically requires predisposition to infection such as vesicoureteral reflux or chronically obstructing kidney stones.

Coarse, asymmetric corticomedullary scarring, blunted calyces. Tubules can contain eosinophilic casts resembling thyroid tissue C (thyroidization of kidney).

Xanthogranulomatous pyelonephritis—rare; grossly orange nodules that can mimic tumor nodules; characterized by widespread kidney damage due to granulomatous tissue containing foamy macrophages. Associated with *Proteus* infection.

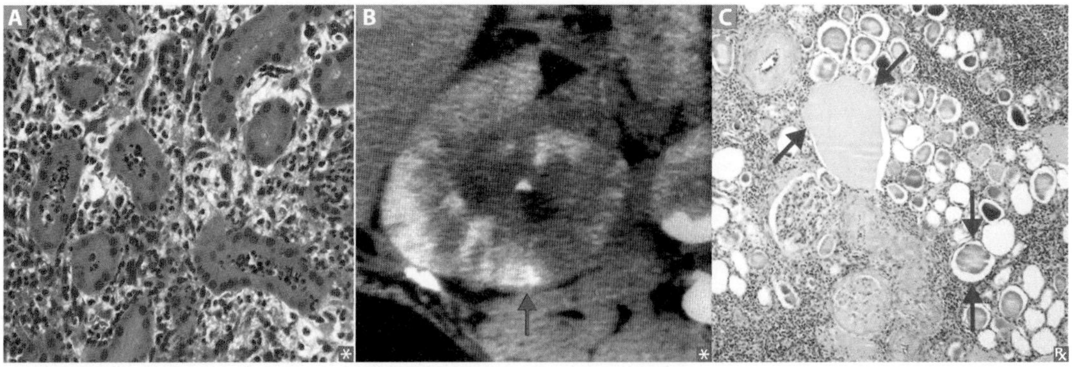

Acute kidney injury

	Prerenal azotemia	Intrinsic renal failure	Postrenal azotemia
ETIOLOGY	Hypovolemia ↓ cardiac output ↓ effective circulating volume (eg, HF, liver failure)	Tubules and interstitium: ▪ Acute tubular necrosis (ischemia, nephrotoxins) ▪ Acute interstitial nephritis Glomerulus: ▪ Acute glomerulonephritis Vascular: ▪ Vasculitis ▪ Malignant hypertension ▪ TTP-HUS	Stones BPH Neoplasm Congenital anomalies
PATHOPHYSIOLOGY	↓ RBF → ↓ GFR → ↑ reabsorption of Na^+/H_2O and urea	In ATN, patchy necrosis → debris obstructing tubules and fluid backflow → ↓ GFR	Outflow obstruction (bilateral)
URINE OSMOLALITY (mOsm/kg)	>500	<350	<350
URINE Na^+ (mEq/L)	<20	>40	Varies
FE_{Na}	<1%	>2%	Varies
SERUM BUN/Cr	>20	<15	Varies

Acute interstitial nephritis

Also called tubulointerstitial nephritis. Acute interstitial renal inflammation. Pyuria (classically eosinophils) and azotemia occurring after administration of drugs that act as haptens, inducing hypersensitivity (eg, diuretics, NSAIDs, penicillin derivatives, proton pump inhibitors, rifampin, quinolones, sulfonamides). Less commonly may be 2° to other processes such as systemic infections (eg, *Mycoplasma*) or autoimmune diseases (eg, Sjögren syndrome, SLE, sarcoidosis).

Associated with fever, rash, pyuria, hematuria, and costovertebral angle tenderness, but can be asymptomatic.

Remember these **5 P'S**:

- **P**ee (diuretics)
- **P**ain-free (NSAIDs)
- **P**enicillins and cephalosporins
- **P**roton pump inhibitors
- Rifam**P**in
- Sulfa drugs

Acute tubular necrosis

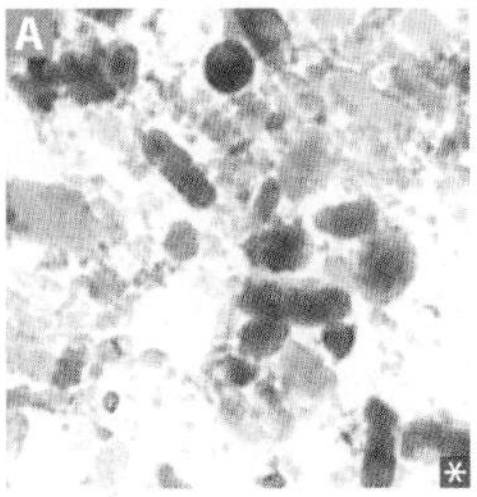

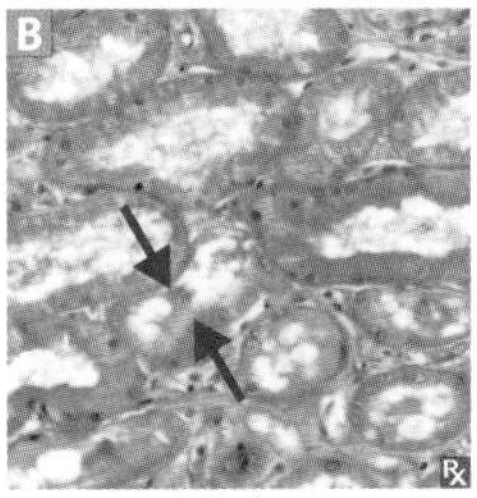

Most common cause of acute kidney injury in hospitalized patients. Spontaneously resolves in many cases. Can be fatal, especially during initial oliguric phase. ↑ FE_{Na}.

Key finding: granular casts (often muddy brown in appearance) A.

3 stages:

1. Inciting event
2. Maintenance phase—oliguric; lasts 1–3 weeks; risk of hyperkalemia, metabolic acidosis, uremia
3. Recovery phase—polyuric; BUN and serum creatinine fall; risk of hypokalemia and renal wasting of other electrolytes and minerals

Can be caused by ischemic or nephrotoxic injury:

- Ischemic—2° to ↓ renal blood flow (eg, hypotension, shock, sepsis, hemorrhage, HF). Results in death of tubular cells that may slough into tubular lumen B (PCT and thick ascending limb are highly susceptible to injury).
- Nephrotoxic—2° to injury resulting from toxic substances (eg, aminoglycosides, radiocontrast agents, lead, cisplatin, ethylene glycol), crush injury (myoglobinuria), hemoglobinuria. Proximal tubules are particularly susceptible to injury.

Diffuse cortical necrosis

Acute generalized cortical infarction of both kidneys. Likely due to a combination of vasospasm and DIC.

Associated with obstetric catastrophes (eg, abruptio placentae), septic shock.

Renal papillary necrosis

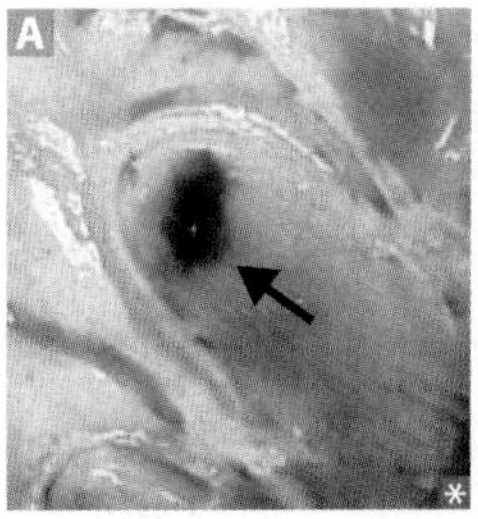

Sloughing of necrotic renal papillae A → gross hematuria. May be triggered by recent infection or immune stimulus.

Associated with:

- Sickle cell disease or trait
- Acute pyelonephritis
- Analgesics (eg, NSAIDs)
- Diabetes mellitus

SAAD papa with **papillary** necrosis.

Consequences of renal failure

Decline in renal filtration can lead to excess retained nitrogenous waste products and electrolyte disturbances.

Consequences (**MAD HUNGER**):

- **M**etabolic **A**cidosis
- **D**yslipidemia (especially ↑ triglycerides)
- **H**igh potassium
- **U**remia
- **N**a^+/H_2O retention (HF, pulmonary edema, hypertension)
- **G**rowth retardation and developmental delay
- **E**rythropoietin deficiency (anemia)
- **R**enal osteodystrophy

2 forms of renal failure: acute (eg, ATN) and chronic (eg, hypertension, diabetes mellitus, congenital anomalies).

Incremental reductions in GFR define the stages of chronic kidney disease.

Normal phosphate levels are maintained during early stages of CKD due to ↑ levels of fibroblast growth factor 23 (FGF23), which promotes renal excretion of phosphate.

Uremia—syndrome resulting from high serum urea. Can present with nausea, anorexia, encephalopathy (seen with asterixis), pericarditis, platelet dysfunction. Management: dialysis.

Renal osteodystrophy	Hypocalcemia, hyperphosphatemia, and failure of vitamin D hydroxylation associated with chronic kidney disease → 2° hyperparathyroidism → 3° hyperparathyroidism (if 2° poorly managed). High serum phosphate can bind with Ca^{2+} → tissue deposits → ↓ serum Ca^{2+}. ↓ 1,25-$(OH)_2D_3$ → ↓ intestinal Ca^{2+} absorption. Causes subperiosteal thinning of bones.

Renal cyst disorders

Autosomal dominant polycystic kidney disease	Numerous cysts in cortex and medulla A causing bilateral enlarged kidneys ultimately destroy kidney parenchyma. Presents with combinations of flank pain, hematuria, hypertension, urinary infection, progressive renal failure in ~ 50% of individuals. Mutation in *PKD1* (85% of cases, chromosome 16) or *PKD2* (15% of cases, chromosome 4). Complications include chronic kidney disease and hypertension (caused by ↑ renin production). Associated with berry aneurysms, mitral valve prolapse, benign hepatic cysts, diverticulosis. Treatment: If hypertension or proteinuria develops, treat with ACE inhibitors or ARBs.
Autosomal recessive polycystic kidney disease	Cystic dilation of collecting ducts B. Often presents in infancy. Associated with congenital hepatic fibrosis. Significant oliguric renal failure in utero can lead to Potter sequence. Concerns beyond neonatal period include systemic hypertension, progressive renal insufficiency, and portal hypertension from congenital hepatic fibrosis.
Autosomal dominant tubulointerstitial kidney disease	Also called medullary cystic kidney disease. Causes tubulointerstitial fibrosis and progressive renal insufficiency with inability to concentrate urine. Medullary cysts usually not visualized; smaller kidneys on ultrasound. Poor prognosis.
Simple vs complex renal cysts	Simple cysts are filled with ultrafiltrate (anechoic on ultrasound C). Very common and account for majority of all renal masses. Found incidentally and typically asymptomatic. Complex cysts, including those that are septated, enhanced, or have solid components on imaging require follow-up or removal due to possibility of renal cell carcinoma.

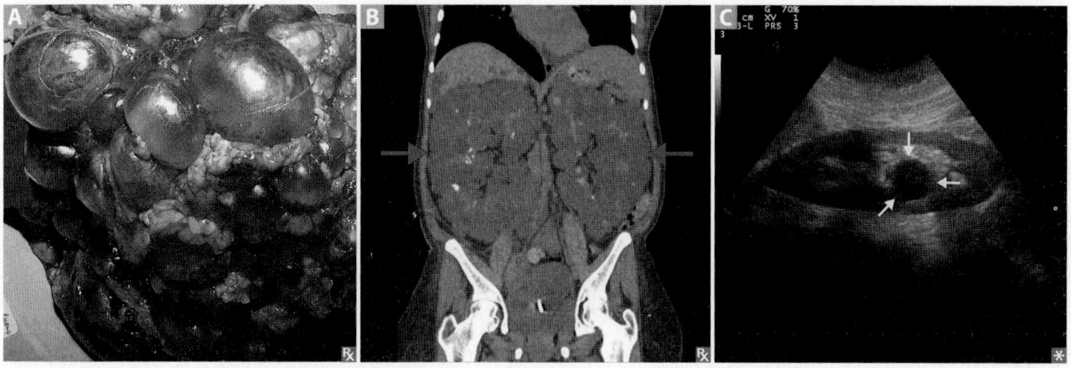

Renovascular disease

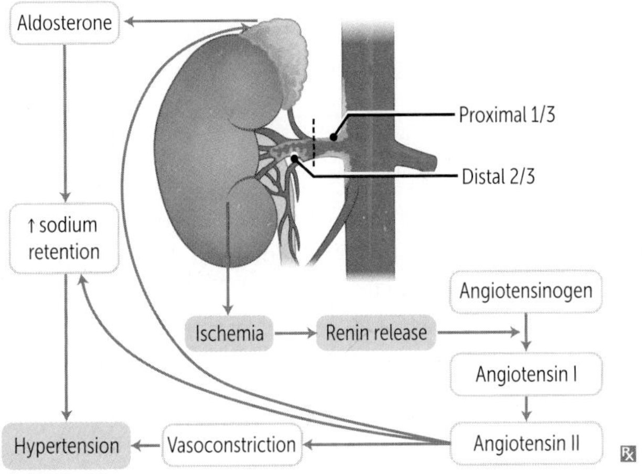

Unilateral or bilateral renal artery stenosis (RAS) → ↓ renal perfusion → ↑ renin → ↑ angiotensin → HTN. Most common cause of 2° HTN in adults.

Main causes of RAS:

- Atherosclerotic plaques: proximal 1/3 of renal artery, usually in older males, smokers.
- Fibromuscular dysplasia: distal 2/3 of renal artery or segmental branches, usually young or middle-aged females

For unilateral RAS, affected kidney can atrophy → asymmetric kidney size. Renal venous sampling will show ↑ renin in affected kidney, ↓ renin in unaffected kidney.

For bilateral RAS, patients can have a sudden rise in creatinine after starting an ACE inhibitor, ARB, or renin inhibitor, due to their interference on RAAS-mediated renal perfusion.

Can present with severe/refractory HTN, flash pulmonary edema, epigastric/flank bruit. Patients with RAS may also have stenosis in other large vessels.

Renal cell carcinoma

Polygonal clear cells A filled with accumulated lipids and carbohydrate. Often golden-yellow B due to ↑ lipid content.

Originates from PCT → invades renal vein (may develop varicocele if left sided) → IVC → hematogenous spread → metastasis to lung and bone.

Manifests with hematuria, palpable masses, 2° polycythemia, flank pain, fever, weight loss.

Treatment: surgery/ablation for localized disease. Immunotherapy (eg, ipilimumab) or targeted therapy for metastatic disease, rarely curative. Resistant to chemotherapy and radiation therapy.

Class triad: flank pain, palpable mass, hematuria.

Most common 1° renal malignancy C.

Most common in males 50–70 years old, ↑ incidence with tobacco smoking and obesity.

Associated with paraneoplastic syndromes, eg, **P**THrP, **E**ctopic EPO, **A**CTH, **R**enin ("**PEAR**"-aneoplastic).

Clear cell (most common subtype) associated with gene deletion on chromosome 3 (sporadic, or inherited as von Hippel-Lindau syndrome).

RCC = 3 letters = chromosome **3** = associated with **VHL** (also 3 letters).

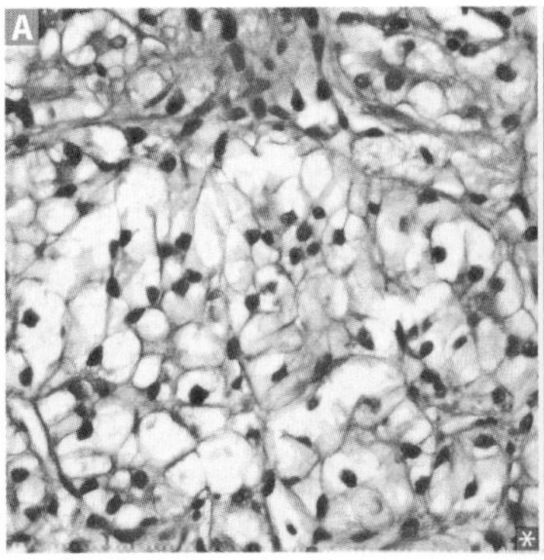

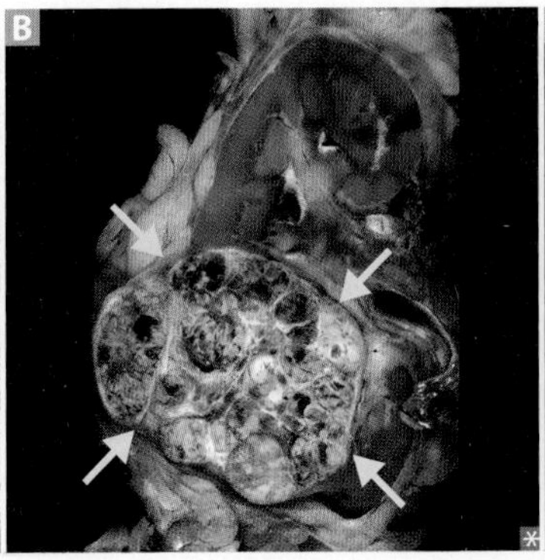

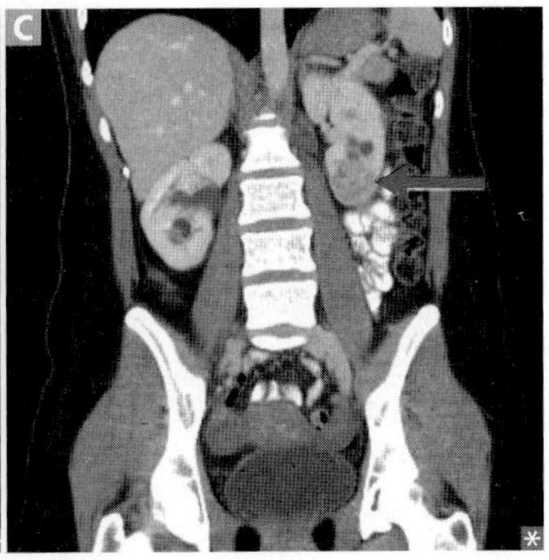

Renal oncocytoma

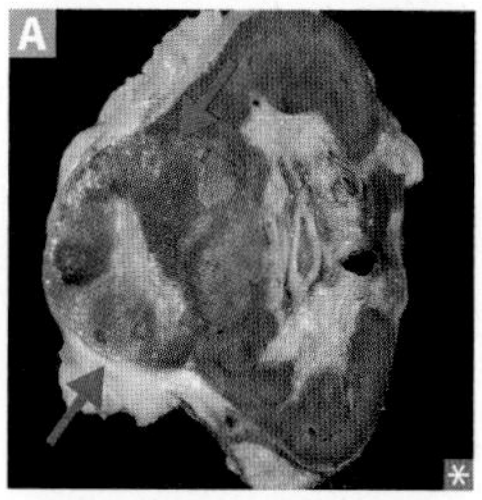

Benign epithelial cell tumor arising from collecting ducts (arrows in A point to well-circumscribed mass with central scar).
Large eosinophilic cells with abundant mitochondria without perinuclear clearing B (vs chromophobe renal cell carcinoma).
Presents with painless hematuria, flank pain, abdominal mass.
Often resected to exclude malignancy (eg, renal cell carcinoma).

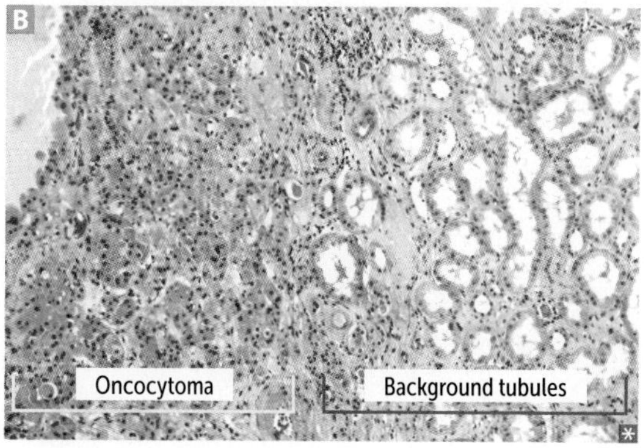
B
Oncocytoma
Background tubules

Nephroblastoma

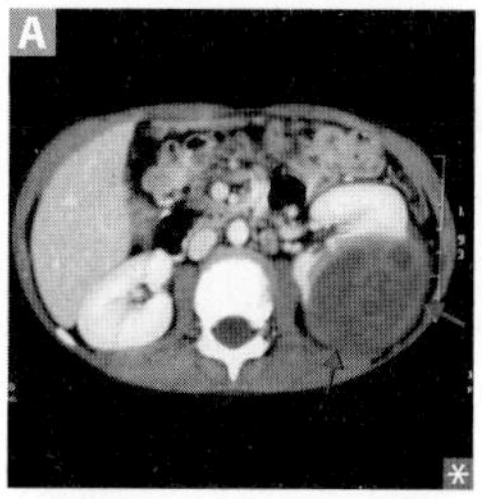

Also called Wilms tumor. Most common renal malignancy of early childhood (ages 2–4). Contains embryonic glomerular structures. Most often present with large, palpable, unilateral flank mass A and/or hematuria and possible HTN.
Can be associated with loss-of-function mutations of tumor suppressor genes *WT1* or *WT2* on chromosome 11.
May be a part of several syndromes:
- **WAGR** complex—Wilms tumor, Aniridia (absence of iris), Genitourinary malformations, Range of developmental delays (*WT1* deletion)
- **Denys-Drash** syndrome—Wilms tumor, Diffuse mesangial sclerosis (early-onset nephrotic syndrome), Dysgenesis of gonads (male pseudohermaphroditism), *WT1* mutation
- **Beckwith-Wiedemann** syndrome—Wilms tumor, macroglossia, organomegaly, hemihyperplasia (*WT2* mutation), omphalocele

Urothelial carcinoma of the bladder

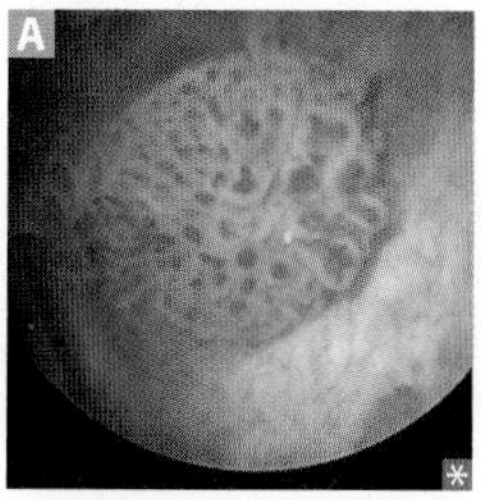

Also called transitional cell carcinoma. Most common tumor of urinary tract system (can occur in renal calyces, renal pelvis, ureters, and bladder) A B. Can be suggested by painless hematuria (no casts).
Associated with problems in your Pee SAC: Phenacetin, tobacco Smoking, Aromatic amines (found in dyes), Cyclophosphamide.

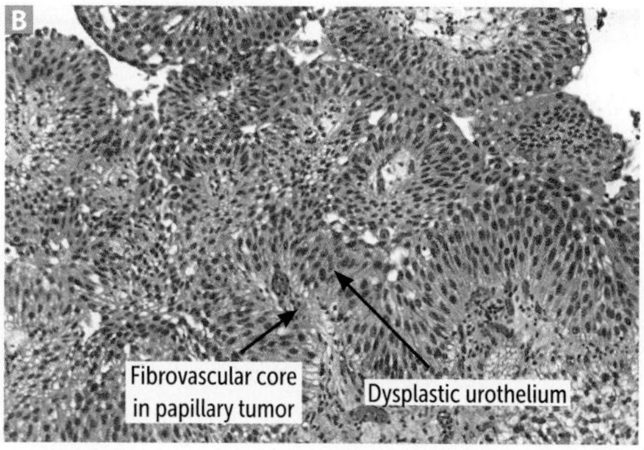
B
Fibrovascular core in papillary tumor
Dysplastic urothelium

Squamous cell carcinoma of the bladder

Chronic irritation of urinary bladder → squamous metaplasia → dysplasia and squamous cell carcinoma.
Risk factors include 4 S's: *Schistosoma haematobium* infection (Middle East), chronic cystitis ("systitis"), **smoking, chronic nephrolithiasis** (stones). Presents with painless hematuria (no casts).

▸ RENAL—PHARMACOLOGY

Diuretics site of action

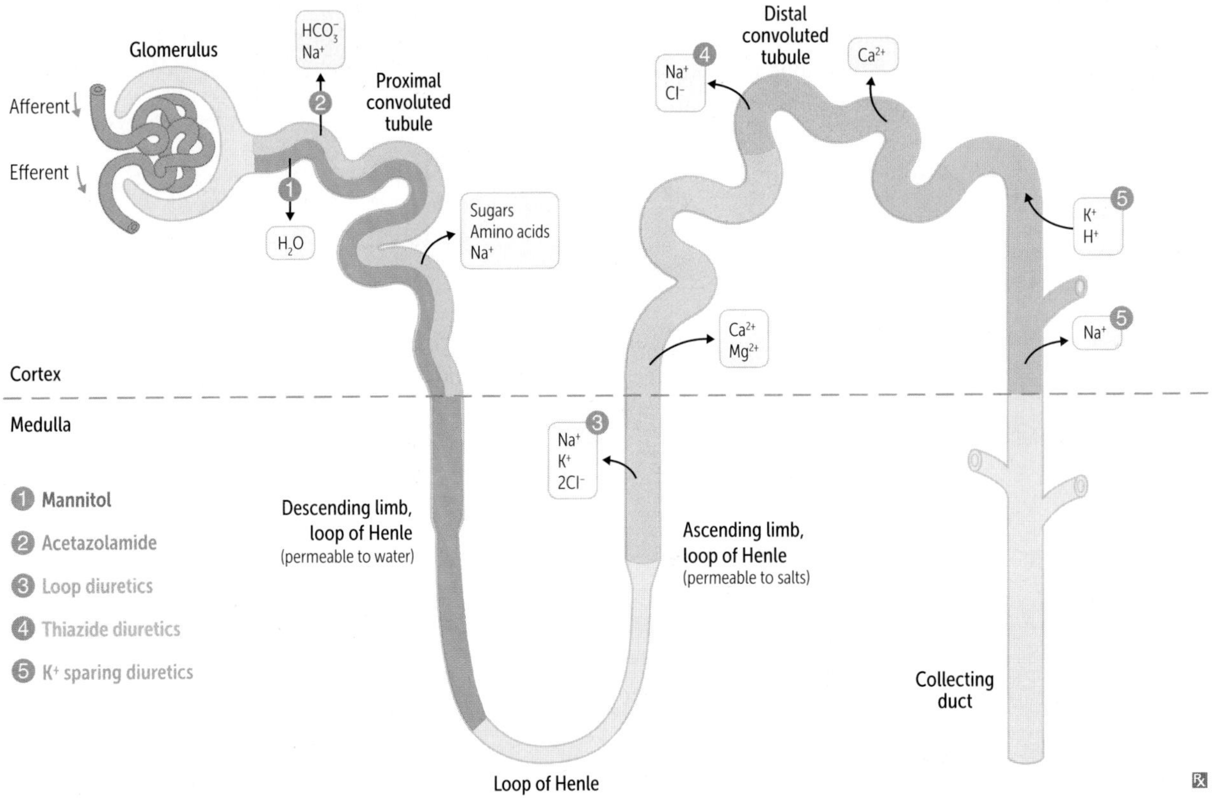

Mannitol

MECHANISM	Osmotic diuretic. ↑ tubular fluid osmolarity → ↑ urine flow, ↓ intracranial/intraocular pressure.
CLINICAL USE	Drug overdose, elevated intracranial/intraocular pressure.
ADVERSE EFFECTS	Dehydration, hypo- or hypernatremia, pulmonary edema. Contraindicated in anuria, HF.

Acetazolamide

MECHANISM	Carbonic anhydrase inhibitor. Causes self-limited $NaHCO_3$ diuresis and ↓ total body HCO_3^- stores. Alkalinizes urine.	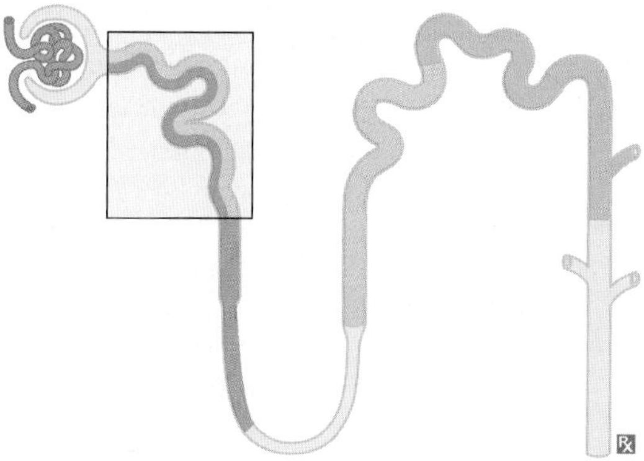
CLINICAL USE	Glaucoma, metabolic alkalosis, altitude sickness (by offsetting respiratory alkalosis), idiopathic intracranial hypertension.	
ADVERSE EFFECTS	Proximal renal tubular acidosis (type 2 RTA), paresthesias, NH_3 toxicity, sulfa allergy, hypokalemia. Promotes calcium phosphate stone formation (insoluble at high pH).	"**Acid**"azolamide causes **acid**osis.

Loop diuretics

Furosemide, bumetanide, torsemide

MECHANISM	Sulfonamide loop diuretics. Inhibit cotransport system ($Na^+/K^+/2Cl^-$) of thick ascending limb of loop of Henle. Abolish hypertonicity of medulla, preventing concentration of urine. Associated with ↑ PGE (vasodilatory effect on afferent arteriole); inhibited by NSAIDs. ↑ Ca^{2+} excretion. Loops lose Ca^{2+}.	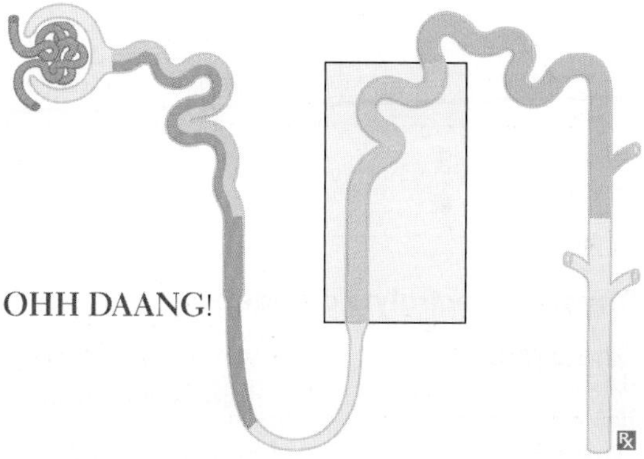
CLINICAL USE	Edematous states (HF, cirrhosis, nephrotic syndrome, pulmonary edema), hypertension, hypercalcemia.	
ADVERSE EFFECTS	**O**totoxicity, **H**ypokalemia, **H**ypomagnesemia, **D**ehydration, **A**llergy (sulfa), metabolic **A**lkalosis, **N**ephritis (interstitial), **G**out.	OHH DAANG!

Ethacrynic acid

MECHANISM	Nonsulfonamide inhibitor of cotransport system ($Na^+/K^+/2Cl^-$) of thick ascending limb of **loop** of Henle.	
CLINICAL USE	Diuresis in patients allergic to sulfa drugs.	
ADVERSE EFFECTS	Similar to furosemide, but more **ot**otoxic.	**Loop** earrings hurt your **ears**.

Thiazide diuretics	Hydrochlorothiazide, chlorthalidone, metolazone.	
MECHANISM	Inhibit NaCl reabsorption in early DCT → ↓ diluting capacity of nephron. ↓ Ca^{2+} excretion.	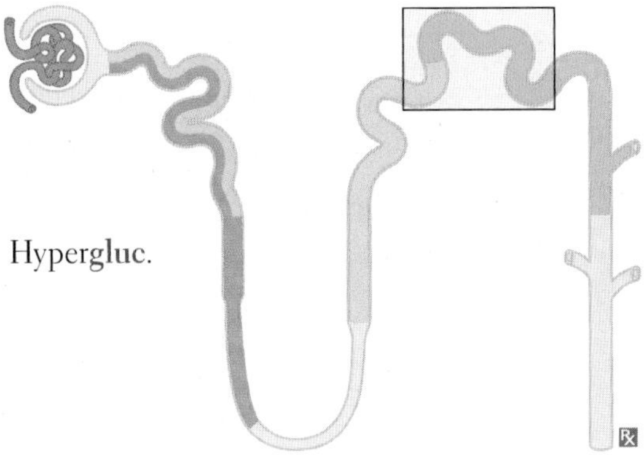
CLINICAL USE	Hypertension, HF, idiopathic hypercalciuria, nephrogenic diabetes insipidus, osteoporosis.	
ADVERSE EFFECTS	Hypokalemic metabolic alkalosis, hyponatremia, hyperglycemia, hyperlipidemia, hyperuricemia, hypercalcemia. Sulfa allergy.	Hypergluc.

Potassium-sparing diuretics	Spironolactone, Eplerenone, Amiloride, Triamterene.	Keep your SEAT.
MECHANISM	Spironolactone and eplerenone are competitive aldosterone receptor antagonists in cortical collecting tubule. Triamterene and amiloride block Na^+ channels at the same part of the tubule.	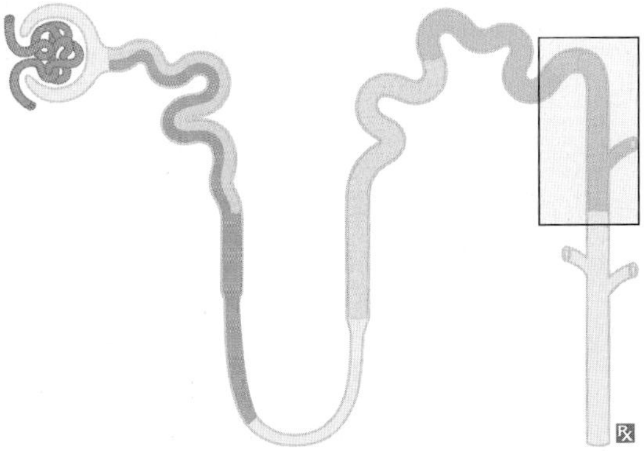
CLINICAL USE	Hyperaldosteronism, K^+ depletion, HF, hepatic ascites (spironolactone), nephrogenic DI (amiloride), antiandrogen (spironolactone).	
ADVERSE EFFECTS	Hyperkalemia (can lead to arrhythmias), endocrine effects with spironolactone (eg, gynecomastia, antiandrogen effects).	

Diuretics: electrolyte changes

Urine NaCl	↑ with all diuretics (concentration varies based on potency of diuretic effect). Serum NaCl may decrease as a result.
Urine K^+	↑ especially with loop and thiazide diuretics, excluding K^+-sparing diuretics.
Blood pH	↓ (**acidemia**): carbonic anhydrase inhibitors: ↓ HCO_3^- reabsorption. K^+ sparing: aldosterone blockade prevents K^+ secretion and H^+ secretion. Additionally, hyperkalemia leads to K^+ entering all cells (via H^+/K^+ exchanger) in exchange for H^+ exiting cells. ↑ (**alkalemia**): loop diuretics and thiazides cause alkalemia through several mechanisms: ▪ Volume contraction → ↑ AT II → ↑ Na^+/H^+ exchange in PCT → ↑ HCO_3^- reabsorption ("contraction alkalosis") ▪ K^+ loss leads to K^+ exiting all cells (via H^+/K^+ exchanger) in exchange for H^+ entering cells ▪ In low K^+ state, H^+ (rather than K^+) is exchanged for Na^+ in cortical collecting tubule → alkalosis and "paradoxical aciduria"
Urine Ca^{2+}	↑ with loop diuretics: ↓ paracellular Ca^{2+} reabsorption → hypocalcemia. ↓ with thiazides: enhanced Ca^{2+} reabsorption.

Angiotensin-converting enzyme inhibitors	Captopril, enalapril, lisinopril, ramipril.	
MECHANISM	Inhibit ACE → ↓ AT II → ↓ GFR by preventing constriction of efferent arterioles. ↑ renin due to loss of negative feedback. Inhibition of ACE also prevents inactivation of bradykinin, a potent vasodilator.	
CLINICAL USE	Hypertension, HF (↓ mortality), proteinuria, diabetic nephropathy. Prevent unfavorable heart remodeling as a result of chronic hypertension.	In chronic kidney disease (eg, diabetic nephropathy), ↓ intraglomerular pressure, slowing GBM thickening.
ADVERSE EFFECTS	**C**ough, **A**ngioedema (both due to ↑ bradykinin; contraindicated in C1 esterase inhibitor deficiency), **T**eratogen (fetal renal malformations), ↑ **C**reatinine (↓ GFR), **H**yperkalemia, and **H**ypotension. Used with caution in bilateral renal artery stenosis because ACE inhibitors will further ↓ GFR → renal failure.	Captopril's **CATCHH**.

Angiotensin II receptor blockers	Losartan, candesartan, valsartan.
MECHANISM	Selectively block binding of angiotensin II to AT_1 receptor. Effects similar to ACE inhibitors, but ARBs do not increase bradykinin.
CLINICAL USE	Hypertension, HF, proteinuria, or chronic kidney disease (eg, diabetic nephropathy) with intolerance to ACE inhibitors (eg, cough, angioedema).
ADVERSE EFFECTS	Hyperkalemia, ↓ GFR, hypotension; teratogen.

Aliskiren	
MECHANISM	Direct renin inhibitor, blocks conversion of angiotensinogen to angiotensin I. Alis**kiren kills renin**.
CLINICAL USE	Hypertension.
ADVERSE EFFECTS	Hyperkalemia, ↓ GFR, hypotension, angioedema. Relatively contraindicated in patients already taking ACE inhibitors or ARBs and contraindicated in pregnancy.

▶ NOTES

HIGH-YIELD SYSTEMS

Reproductive

"Life is always a rich and steady time when you are waiting for something to happen or to hatch."

—E.B. White, *Charlotte's Web*

"Love is only a dirty trick played on us to achieve continuation of the species."

—W. Somerset Maugham

"In pregnancy, there are two bodies, one inside the other. Two people live under one skin. When so much of life is dedicated to maintaining our integrity as distinct beings, this bodily tandem is an uncanny fact."

—Joan Raphael-Leff, *Pregnancy: The Inside Story*

"Life is a sexually transmitted disease and the mortality rate is one hundred percent."

—R.D. Laing

Organizing the reproductive system by key concepts such as embryology, endocrinology, pregnancy, and oncology can help with understanding this complex topic. Study the endocrine and reproductive chapters together, because mastery of the hypothalamic-pituitary-gonadal axis is key to answering questions on ovulation, menstruation, disorders of sexual development, contraception, and many pathologies.

Embryology is a nuanced subject that spans multiple organ systems. Approach it from a clinical perspective. For instance, make the connection between the presentation of DiGeorge syndrome and the 3rd/4th pharyngeal pouch, and between the Müllerian/Wolffian systems and disorders of sexual development.

As for oncology, don't worry about remembering screening or treatment guidelines. It is more important to recognize the clinical presentation (eg, signs and symptoms) of reproductive cancers and their associated labs, histopathology, and risk factors. In addition, some of the testicular and ovarian cancers have distinct patterns of hCG, AFP, LH, or FSH derangements that serve as helpful clues in exam questions.

▶ REPRODUCTIVE—EMBRYOLOGY

Important genes of embryogenesis

GENE	LOCATION	FUNCTION	NOTES
Sonic hedgehog (*SHH*) gene	Zone of polarizing activity at base of limb buds	Anterior-posterior axis patterning, CNS development	Mutations → holoprosencephaly
***Wnt-7* gene**	Apical ectodermal ridge at distal end of each limb	Dorsal-ventral axis patterning, limb development	"*V*nt-7"
Fibroblast growth factor (*FGF*) gene	Apical ectodermal ridge	Limb lengthening (via mitosis of mesoderm)	"Look at that Fetus, Growing Fingers"
Homeobox (*Hox*) genes	Multiple	Segmental organization in cranial-caudal direction, transcription factor coding	Mutations → appendages in wrong locations. Isotretinoin → ↑ *Hox* gene expression

Early fetal development

Timeline shown is based on developmental age (ie, time since fertilization) rather than gestational age (ie, time since first day of last menstrual period).

Early embryonic development

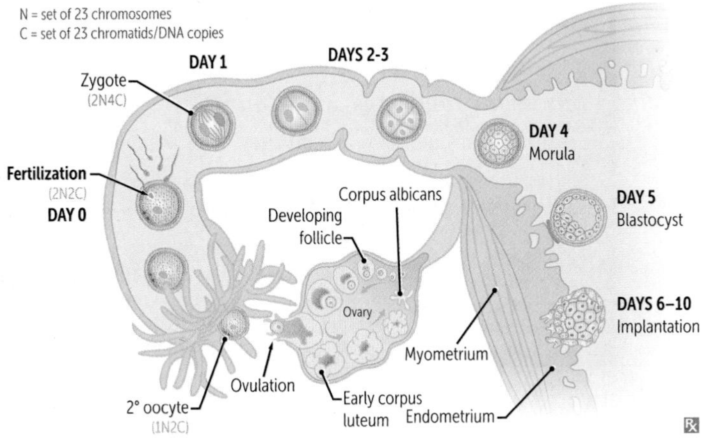

Within week 1	hCG secretion begins around the time of implantation of blastocyst.	Blastocyst "sticks" at day 6.
Within week 2	Bilaminar disc (epiblast, hypoblast).	2 weeks = 2 layers.
Within week 3	Gastrulation forms trilaminar embryonic disc. Cells from epiblast invaginate → primitive streak → endoderm, mesoderm, ectoderm. Notochord arises from midline mesoderm and induces overlying ectoderm to become neural plate.	3 weeks = 3 layers.
Weeks 3–8 (embryonic period)	Neural tube formed by neuroectoderm and closes by week 4. Organogenesis.	Extremely susceptible to teratogens.
Week 4	Heart begins to beat. Cardiac activity visible by transvaginal ultrasound. Upper and lower limb buds begin to form.	4 weeks = 4 limbs and 4 heart chambers.
Week 6	Fetal movements start.	
Week 8	Genitalia have male/female characteristics.	

Embryologic derivatives

Ectoderm		External/outer layer
Surface ectoderm	Epidermis; adenohypophysis (from Rathke pouch); lens of eye; epithelial linings of oral cavity, sensory organs of ear, and olfactory epithelium; anal canal below the pectinate line; parotid, sweat, mammary glands.	Craniopharyngioma—benign Rathke pouch tumor with cholesterol crystals, calcifications.
Neural tube	Brain (neurohypophysis, CNS neurons, oligodendrocytes, astrocytes, ependymal cells, pineal gland), retina, spinal cord.	Neuroectoderm—think CNS.
Neural crest	Enterochromaffin cells, Leptomeninges (arachnoid, pia), Melanocytes, Odontoblasts, PNS ganglia (cranial, dorsal root, autonomic), Adrenal medulla, Schwann cells, Spiral membrane (aorticopulmonary septum), Endocardial cushions (also derived partially from mesoderm), Skull bones.	ELMO PASSES Neural crest—think PNS and non-neural structures nearby.
Mesoderm	Muscle, bone, connective tissue, serous linings of body cavities (eg, peritoneum, pericardium, pleura), spleen (develops within foregut mesentery), cardiovascular structures, lymphatics, blood, wall of gut tube, upper 2/3 of vagina, kidneys, adrenal cortex, dermis, testes, ovaries, microglia, dura mater, tracheal cartilage. Notochord induces ectoderm to form neuroectoderm (neural plate); its only postnatal derivative is the nucleus pulposus of the intervertebral disc.	Middle/"meat" layer. Mesodermal defects = VACTERL association: Vertebral defects Anal atresia Cardiac defects Tracheo-Esophageal fistula Renal defects Limb defects (bone and muscle)
Endoderm	Gut tube epithelium (including anal canal above the pectinate line), most of urethra and lower 1/3 of vagina (derived from urogenital sinus), luminal epithelial derivatives (eg, lungs, liver, gallbladder, pancreas, eustachian tube, thymus, parathyroid, thyroid follicular and parafollicular [C] cells).	"Enternal" layer.

Types of errors in morphogenesis

Agenesis	Absent organ due to absent primordial tissue.
Aplasia	Absent organ despite presence of primordial tissue.
Hypoplasia	Incomplete organ development; primordial tissue present.
Disruption	2° breakdown of previously normal tissue or structure (eg, amniotic band syndrome).
Deformation	Extrinsic mechanical distortion (eg, congenital torticollis); occurs after embryonic period.
Malformation	Intrinsic developmental defect; occurs during embryonic period (weeks 3–8 of development).
Sequence	Abnormalities result from a single 1° embryologic event (eg, oligohydramnios → Potter sequence).
Field defect	Disturbance of tissues that develop in a contiguous physical space (eg, holoprosencephaly).

Teratogens Most susceptible in 3rd–8th weeks (embryonic period—organogenesis) of development. Before week 3, "all-or-none" effects. After week 8, growth and function affected.

TERATOGEN	EFFECTS ON FETUS	NOTES
Medications		
ACE inhibitors	Renal failure, oligohydramnios, hypocalvaria	
Alkylating agents	Absence of digits, multiple anomalies	
Aminoglycosides	Ototoxicity	**A mean guy** hit the baby in the **ear**
Antiepileptic drugs	Neural tube defects, cardiac defects, cleft palate, skeletal abnormalities (eg, phalanx/nail hypoplasia, facial dysmorphism)	High-dose folate supplementation recommended; most commonly valproate, carbamazepine, phenytoin, phenobarbital
Diethylstilbestrol	Vaginal clear cell adenocarcinoma, congenital Müllerian anomalies	
Fluoroquinolones	Cartilage damage	
Folate antagonists	Neural tube defects	Antiepileptics, trimethoprim, methotrexate
Isotretinoin	Craniofacial (eg, microtia, dysmorphism), CNS, cardiac, and thymic defects	Contraception mandatory. Pronounce "iso**terat**inoin."
Lithium	Ebstein anomaly	
Methimazole	Aplasia cutis congenita (congenital absence of skin, particularly on scalp)	
Tetracyclines	Discolored teeth, inhibited bone growth	"**Teeth**racyclines"
Thalidomide	Limb defects (phocomelia, micromelia—"flipper" limbs)	**Limb** defects with "tha-**limb**-domide"
Warfarin	Bone and cartilage deformities (stippled epiphyses, nasal and limb hypoplasia), optic nerve atrophy, fetal cerebral hemorrhage	Do not wage **warfare** on the baby; keep it **heppy** with **heparin** (does not cross placenta)
Substance use		
Alcohol	Fetal alcohol syndrome	
Cocaine	Low birth weight, preterm birth, IUGR, placental abruption	Cocaine → vasoconstriction
Smoking	Low birth weight (leading cause in developed countries), preterm labor, placental problems, IUGR, SIDS, ADHD	Nicotine → vasoconstriction CO → impaired O_2 delivery
Other		
Iodine lack or excess	Congenital hypothyroidism (cretinism), congenital goiter	
Diabetes in pregnancy	Caudal regression syndrome, cardiac defects (eg, VSD), neural tube defects, macrosomia, neonatal hypoglycemia (due to islet cell hyperplasia), polycythemia, neonatal respiratory distress syndrome	
Methylmercury	Neurotoxicity	Higher concentrations in top-predator fish (eg, shark, swordfish, king mackerel, tilefish)
X-rays	Microcephaly, intellectual disability	Minimized by lead shielding

Fetal alcohol syndrome

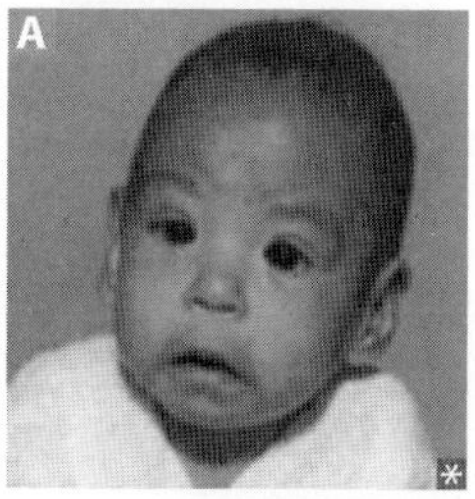

One of the leading preventable causes of intellectual disability in the US. Newborns of patients who consumed alcohol during any stage of pregnancy have ↑ incidence of congenital abnormalities, including pre- and postnatal developmental delay, microcephaly, facial abnormalities A (eg, smooth philtrum, thin vermillion border, small palpebral fissures), limb dislocation, heart defects. Heart-lung fistulas and holoprosencephaly may occur in more severe presentations. One mechanism is due to impaired migration of neuronal and glial cells.

Neonatal abstinence syndrome

Complex disorder involving CNS, ANS, and GI systems. Secondary to substance use (most commonly opioids) during pregnancy.

Universal screening for substance use is recommended in all pregnant patients.

Newborns may present with uncoordinated sucking reflexes, irritability, high-pitched crying, tremors, tachypnea, sneezing, diarrhea, and possibly seizures.

Treatment (for opiate use): methadone, morphine, buprenorphine.

Placenta	1° site of nutrient and gas exchange between pregnant patient and fetus.
Fetal component	
Cytotrophoblast	Inner layer of chorionic villi; makes cells.
Syncytiotrophoblast	Outer layer of chorionic villi; synthesizes and secretes hormones, eg, hCG (structurally similar to LH; stimulates corpus luteum to secrete progesterone during first trimester). Lacks MHC I expression → ↓ chance of attack by maternal immune system.
Parental component	
Decidua basalis	Derived from endometrium. Parental blood in lacunae.

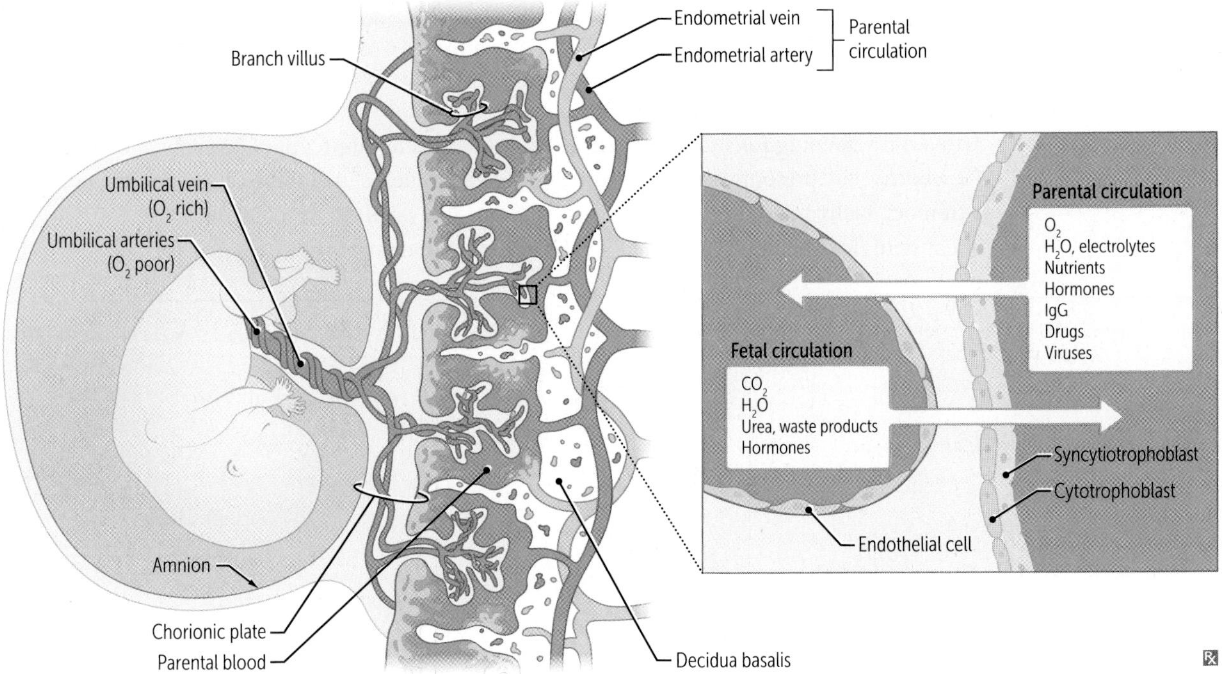

Amniotic fluid

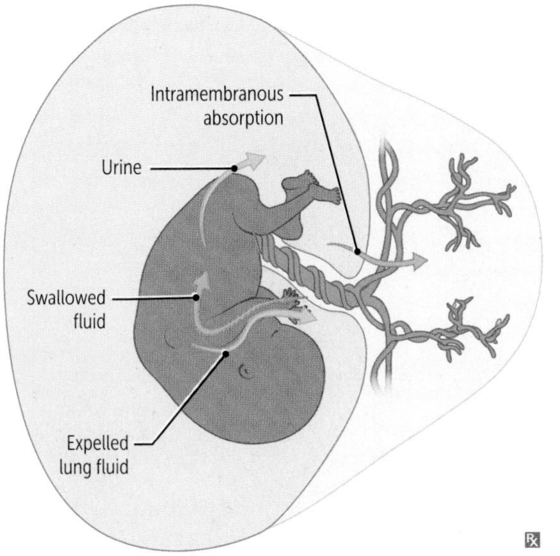

Derived from fetal urine (mainly) and fetal lung liquid.

Cleared by fetal swallowing (mainly) and intramembranous absorption.

Polyhydramnios—too much amniotic fluid. May be idiopathic or associated with fetal malformations (eg, esophageal/duodenal atresia, anencephaly; both result in inability to swallow amniotic fluid), diabetes in pregnant patient, fetal anemia, multiple gestations.

Oligohydramnios—too little amniotic fluid. Associated with placental insufficiency, bilateral renal agenesis, posterior urethral valves (in males); these result in inability to excrete urine. Profound oligohydramnios can cause Potter sequence.

Twinning

Dizygotic ("fraternal") twins arise from 2 eggs that are separately fertilized by 2 different sperm (always 2 zygotes) and will have 2 separate amniotic sacs and 2 separate placentas (chorions).

Monozygotic ("identical") twins arise from 1 fertilized egg (1 egg + 1 sperm) that splits in early pregnancy. The timing of splitting determines chorionicity (number of chorions) and amnionicity (number of amnions) (take **separate** cars or **share** a **CCAB**):

- Splitting 0–4 days: **separate** chorion and amnion (di-di)
- Splitting 4–8 days: **shared C**horion (mo-di)
- Splitting 8–12 days: **shared C**horion and **A**mnion (mo-mo)
- Splitting 13+ days: **shared B**ody (conjoined)

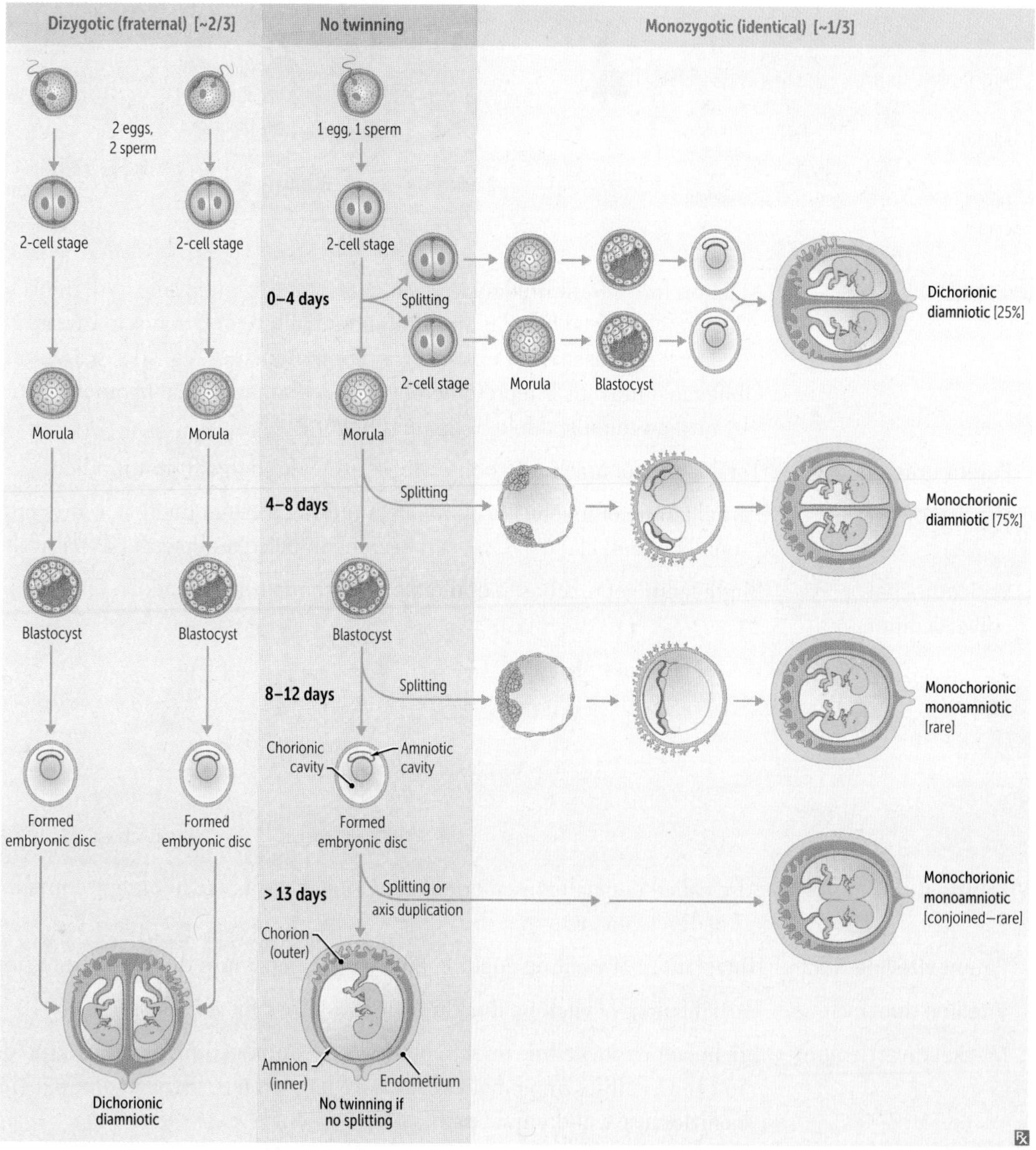

Twin-twin transfusion syndrome

Occurs in monochorionic twin gestations. Unbalanced vascular connections between twins in shared placenta → net blood flow from one twin to the other.

Donor twin → hypovolemia and oligohydramnios ("stuck twin" appearance).

Recipient twin → hypervolemia and polyhydramnios.

Umbilical cord

Two umbilical arteries return deoxygenated blood from fetal internal iliac arteries to placenta A.

One umbilical vein supplies oxygenated blood from placenta to fetus; drains into IVC via liver or via ductus venosus.

Single umbilical artery (2-vessel cord) is associated with congenital and chromosomal anomalies.

Umbilical arteries and vein are derived from allantois.

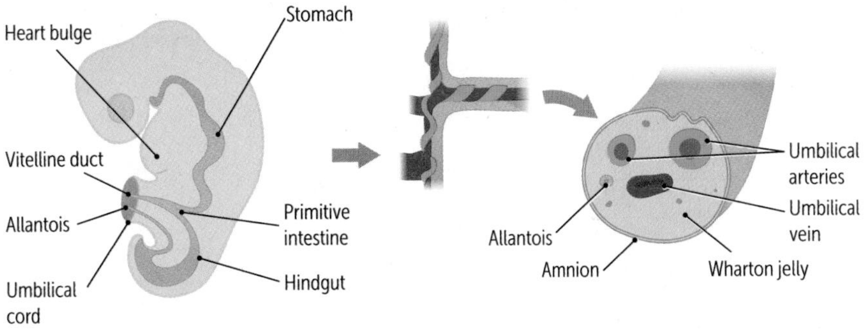

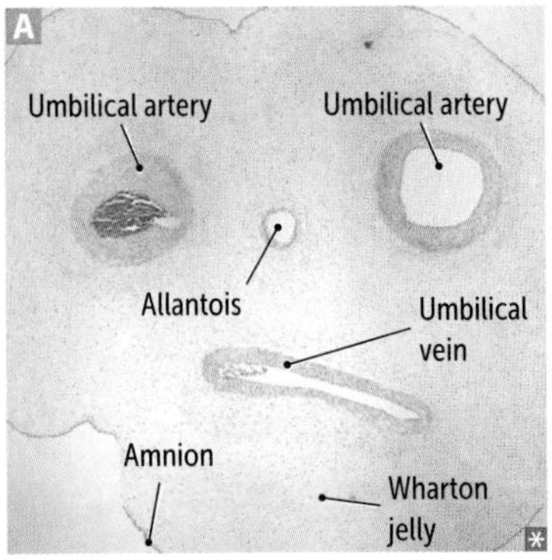

Urachus

Allantois forms from hindgut and extends into urogenital sinus. Allantois becomes the urachus, a duct between fetal bladder and umbilicus. Failure of urachus to involute can lead to anomalies that may increase risk of infection and/or malignancy (eg, adenocarcinoma) if not treated.

Obliterated urachus is represented by the median umbilical ligament after birth, which is covered by median umbilical fold of the peritoneum.

Patent urachus — Total failure of urachus to obliterate → urine discharge from umbilicus.

Urachal cyst — Partial failure of urachus to obliterate; fluid-filled cavity lined with uroepithelium, between umbilicus and bladder. Cyst can become infected and present as painful mass below umbilicus.

Vesicourachal diverticulum — Slight failure of urachus to obliterate → outpouching of bladder.

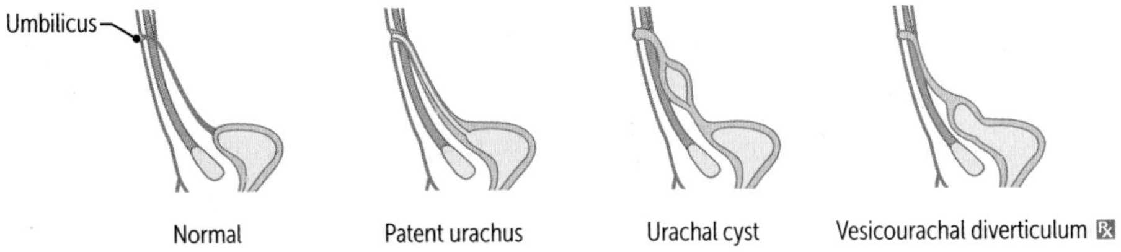

Vitelline duct

Also called omphalomesenteric duct. Connects yolk sac to midgut lumen. Obliterates during week 7 of development.

Patent vitelline duct — Total failure of vitelline duct to obliterate → meconium discharge from umbilicus.

Vitelline duct cyst — Partial failure of vitelline duct to obliterate. ↑ risk for volvulus.

Meckel diverticulum — Slight failure of vitelline duct to obliterate → outpouching of ileum (true diverticulum, arrow in B). Usually asymptomatic. May have heterotopic gastric and/or pancreatic tissue → melena, hematochezia, abdominal pain.

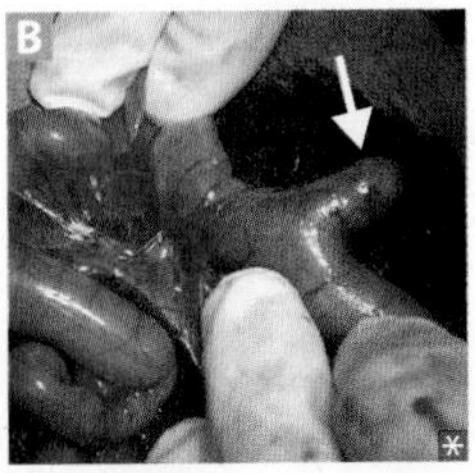

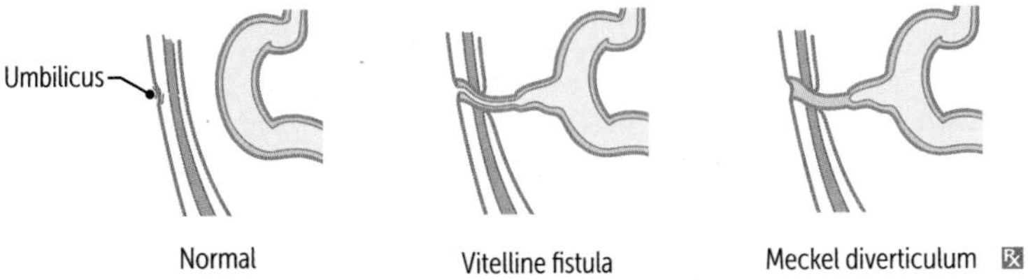

Pharyngeal apparatus

Composed of pharyngeal (branchial) clefts, arches, pouches.

Pharyngeal clefts—derived from ectoderm. Also called pharyngeal grooves.

Pharyngeal arches—derived from mesoderm (muscles, arteries) and neural crest (bones, cartilage).

Pharyngeal pouches—derived from endoderm.

CAP covers outside to inside:
Clefts = ectoderm
Arches = mesoderm + neural crest
Pouches = endoderm

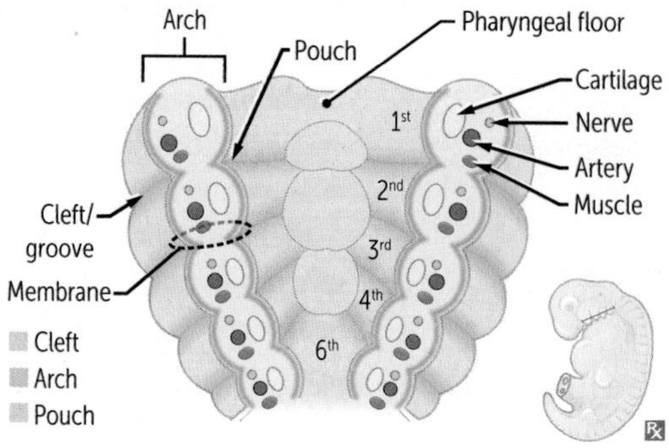

Pharyngeal cleft derivatives

1st cleft develops into external auditory meatus.

2nd through 4th clefts form temporary cervical sinuses, which are obliterated by proliferation of 2nd arch mesenchyme.

Pharyngeal cleft cyst—persistent cervical sinus; presents as lateral neck mass anterior to sternocleidomastoid muscle that does not move with swallowing (vs thyroglossal duct cyst).

Pharyngeal arch derivatives

When at the restaurant of the golden **arches**, children tend to first **chew** (1), then **smile** (2), then **swallow** stylishly (3) or **simply swallow** (4), and then **speak** (6).

ARCH	CARTILAGE	MUSCLES	NERVES[a]	NOTES
1st pharyngeal arch	Maxillary process → maxilla, zygomatic bone Mandibular process → meckel cartilage → mandible, malleus and incus, sphenomandibular ligament	Muscles of mastication (temporalis, masseter, lateral and medial pterygoids), mylohyoid, anterior belly of digastric, tensor tympani, anterior 2/3 of tongue, tensor veli palatini	CN V_3 **chew**	Pierre Robin sequence—micrognathia, glossoptosis, cleft palate, airway obstruction Treacher Collins syndrome—autosomal dominant neural crest dysfunction → craniofacial abnormalities (eg, zygomatic bone and mandibular hypoplasia), hearing loss, airway compromise
2nd pharyngeal arch	Reichert cartilage: stapes, styloid process, lesser horn of hyoid, stylohyoid ligament	Muscles of facial expression, stapedius, stylohyoid, platysma, posterior belly of digastric	CN VII (seven) **smile** (facial expression)	
3rd pharyngeal arch	Greater horn of hyoid	Stylopharyngeus	CN IX (**stylo**-pharyngeus) **swallow stylishly**	
4th and 6th pharyngeal arches	Arytenoids, Cricoid, Corniculate, Cuneiform, Thyroid (used to sing and ACCCT)	4th arch: most pharyngeal constrictors; cricothyroid, levator veli palatini 6th arch: all intrinsic muscles of larynx except cricothyroid	4th arch: CN X (superior laryngeal branch) **simply swallow** 6th arch: CN X (recurrent/inferior laryngeal branch) **speak**	Arches 3 and 4 form posterior 1/3 of tongue Arch 5 makes no major developmental contributions

[a]Sensory and motor nerves are not pharyngeal arch derivatives. They grow into the arches and are derived from neural crest (sensory) and neuroectoderm (motor).

Pharyngeal pouch derivatives

Ear, tonsils, bottom-to-top: 1 (**ear**), 2 (**tonsils**), 3 dorsal (**bottom** for inferior parathyroids), 3 ventral (**to** = thymus), 4 (**top** = **superior** parathyroids)

POUCH	DERIVATIVES	NOTES
1st pharyngeal pouch	Middle ear cavity, eustachian tube, mastoid air cells	1st pouch contributes to endoderm-lined structures of ear
2nd pharyngeal pouch	Epithelial lining of palatine tonsil	
3rd pharyngeal pouch	Dorsal wings → **inferior** parathyroids Ventral wings → thymus	**Third** pouch contributes to **th**ymus and both inferior parathyroids Structures from 3rd pouch end up **below** those from 4th pouch
4th pharyngeal pouch	Dorsal wings → **superior** parathyroids Ventral wings → ultimopharyngeal body → parafollicular (C) cells of thyroid	4th pharyngeal pouch forms para"4"llicular cells

Orofacial clefts Cleft lip and cleft palate have distinct, multifactorial etiologies, but often occur together.

Cleft lip Due to failure of fusion of the maxillary and merged medial nasal processes (formation of 1° palate).

Cleft palate Due to failure of fusion of the two lateral palatine shelves or failure of fusion of lateral palatine shelf with the nasal septum and/or 1° palate (formation of 2° palate).

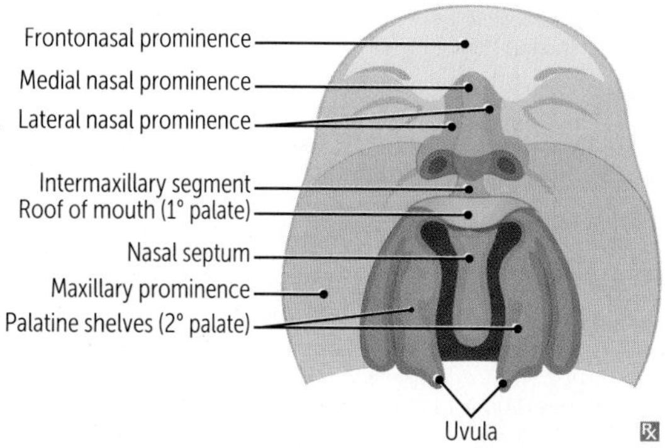

Genital embryology

Female Default development. Mesonephric duct degenerates and paramesonephric duct develops.

Male *SRY* gene on Y chromosome—produces testis-determining factor → testes development.
Sertoli cells secrete Müllerian inhibitory factor (MIF, also called antimullerian hormone) that suppresses development of paramesonephric ducts.
Leydig cells secrete androgens that stimulate development of mesonephric ducts.

Paramesonephric (Müllerian) duct Develops into female internal structures—fallopian tubes, uterus, upper portion of vagina (lower portion from urogenital sinus). Male remnant is appendix testis.
Müllerian agenesis (Mayer-Rokitansky-Küster-Hauser syndrome)—may present as 1° amenorrhea (due to a lack of uterine development) in females with fully developed 2° sexual characteristics (functional ovaries).

Mesonephric (Wolffian) duct Develops into male internal structures (except prostate)—**S**eminal vesicles, **E**pididymis, **E**jaculatory duct, **D**uctus deferens (**SEED**).
Female remnant is Gartner duct.

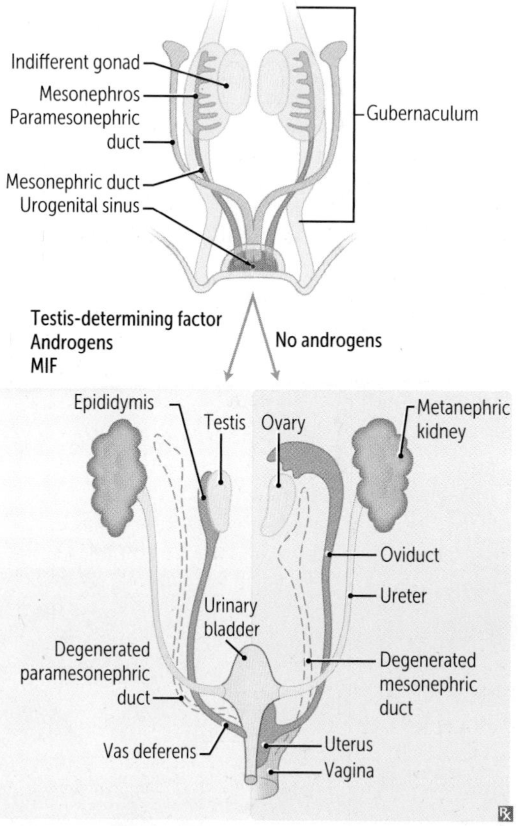

Sexual differentiation

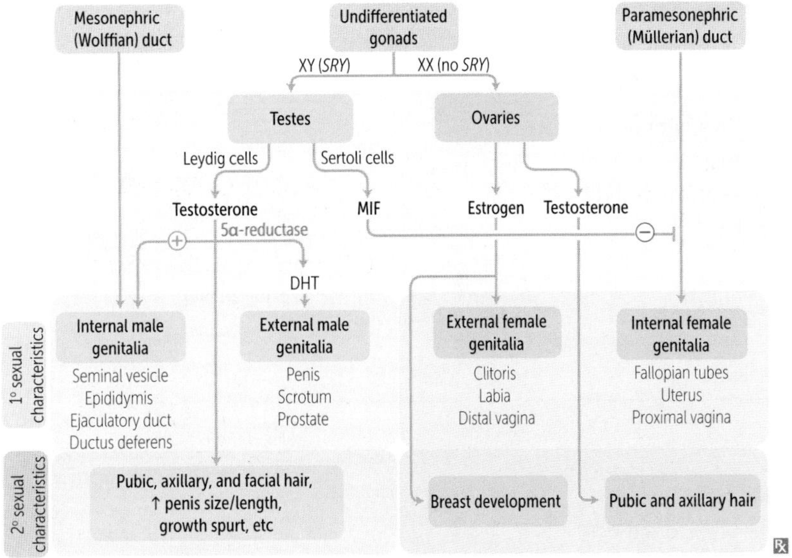

Absence of Sertoli cells or lack of Müllerian inhibitory factor → develop both male and female internal genitalia and male external genitalia (streak gonads)

5α-reductase deficiency—inability to convert testosterone into DHT → male internal genitalia, ambiguous external genitalia until puberty (when ↑ testosterone levels cause masculinization)

In the testes:

- Leydig leads to male (internal and external) sexual differentiation.
- Sertoli shuts down female (internal) sexual differentiation.

Uterine (Müllerian duct) anomalies	↓ fertility and ↑ risk of complicated pregnancy (eg, spontaneous abortion, prematurity, IUGR, malpresentation). Contrast with normal uterus A.
Septate uterus	Incomplete resorption of septum B. Common anomaly. Treat with septoplasty.
Bicornuate uterus	Incomplete fusion of Müllerian ducts C.
Uterus didelphys	Complete failure of fusion → double uterus, cervix, vagina D.

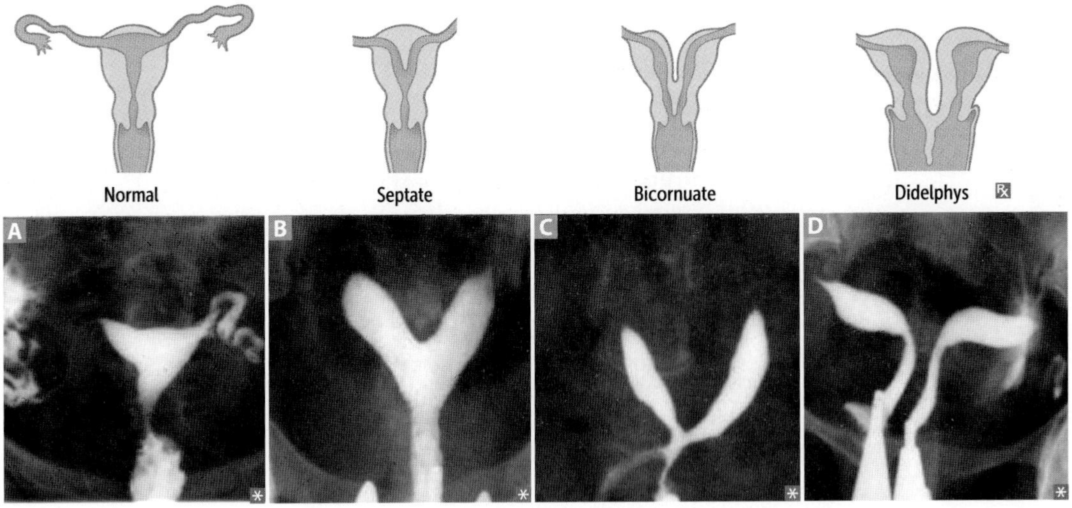

Male/female genital homologs

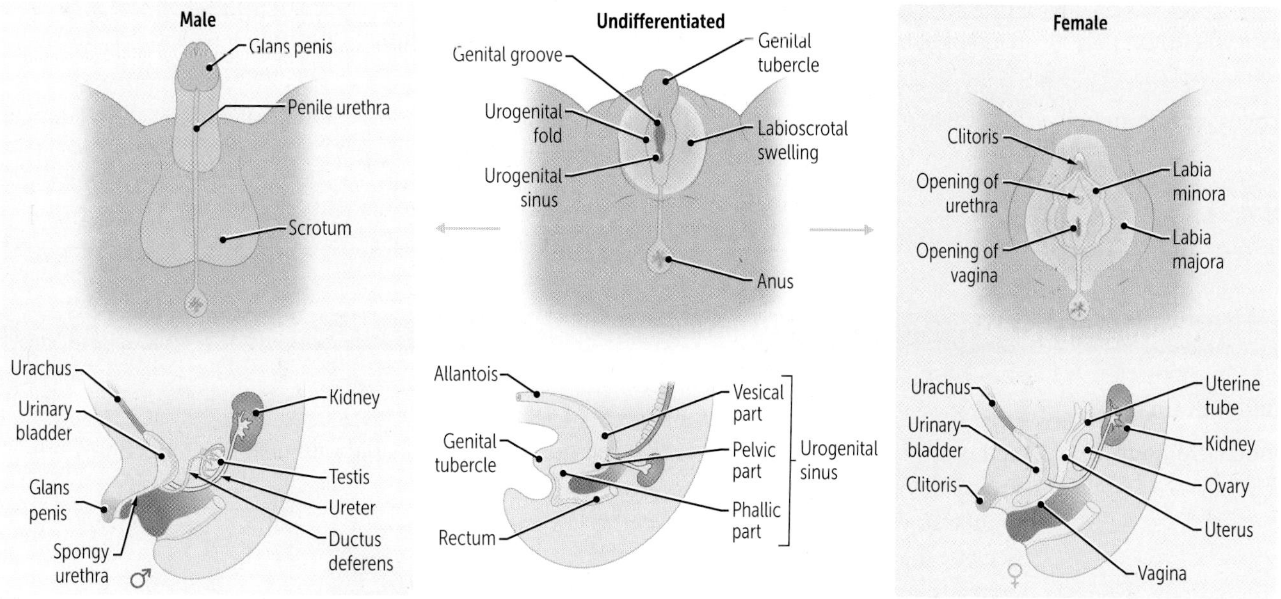

Dihydrotestosterone ←		Estrogen →
Glans penis	Genital tubercle	Glans clitoris
Corpus cavernosum and spongiosum	Genital tubercle	Vestibular bulbs
Bulbourethral glands (of Cowper)	Urogenital sinus	Greater vestibular glands (of Bartholin)
Prostate gland	Urogenital sinus	Urethral and paraurethral glands (of Skene)
Ventral shaft of penis (penile urethra)	Urogenital folds	Labia minora
Scrotum	Labioscrotal swelling	Labia majora

Congenital penile abnormalities

Hypospadias

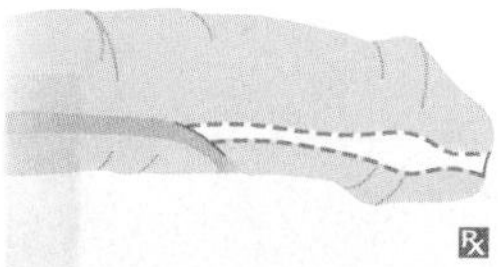

Abnormal opening of penile urethra on ventral (under) surface due to failure of urethral folds to fuse.

Hypospadias is more common than epispadias. Associated with inguinal hernia, cryptorchidism, chordee (downward or upward bending of penis).

Can be seen in 5α-reductase deficiency.

Epispadias

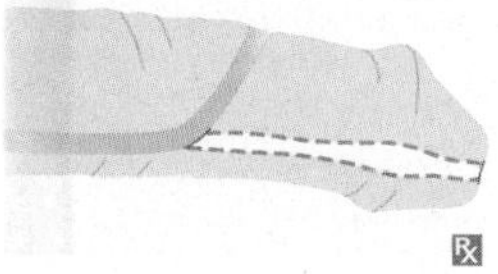

Abnormal opening of penile urethra on dorsal (top) surface due to faulty positioning of genital tubercle.

Exstrophy of the bladder is associated with epispadias.

Descent of testes and ovaries

	DESCRIPTION	MALE REMNANT	FEMALE REMNANT
Gubernaculum	Band of fibrous tissue	Anchors testes within scrotum	Ovarian ligament + round ligament of uterus
Processus vaginalis	Evagination of peritoneum	Forms tunica vaginalis Persistent patent processus vaginalis → hydrocele	Obliterated

▸ REPRODUCTIVE—ANATOMY

Gonadal drainage

Venous drainage

Left ovary/testis → left gonadal vein → left renal vein → IVC.
Right ovary/testis → right gonadal vein → IVC.
Because the left spermatic vein enters the left renal vein at a 90° angle, flow is less laminar on left than on right → left venous pressure > right venous pressure → varicocele more common on the left.

"Left gonadal vein takes the longer way."

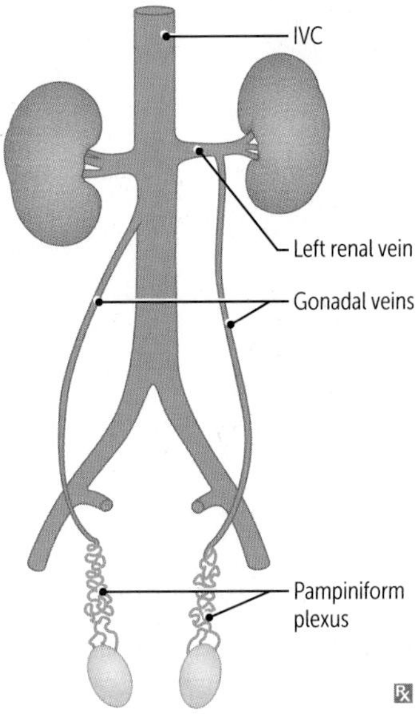

Lymphatic drainage

Ovaries/testes/fundus of uterus → para-aortic lymph nodes.
Body of uterus/cervix/superior part of bladder → external iliac nodes.
Prostate/cervix/corpus cavernosum/proximal vagina → internal iliac nodes.
Distal vagina/vulva/scrotum/distal anus → superficial inguinal nodes.
Clitoris/glans penis → deep inguinal nodes.

Female reproductive anatomy

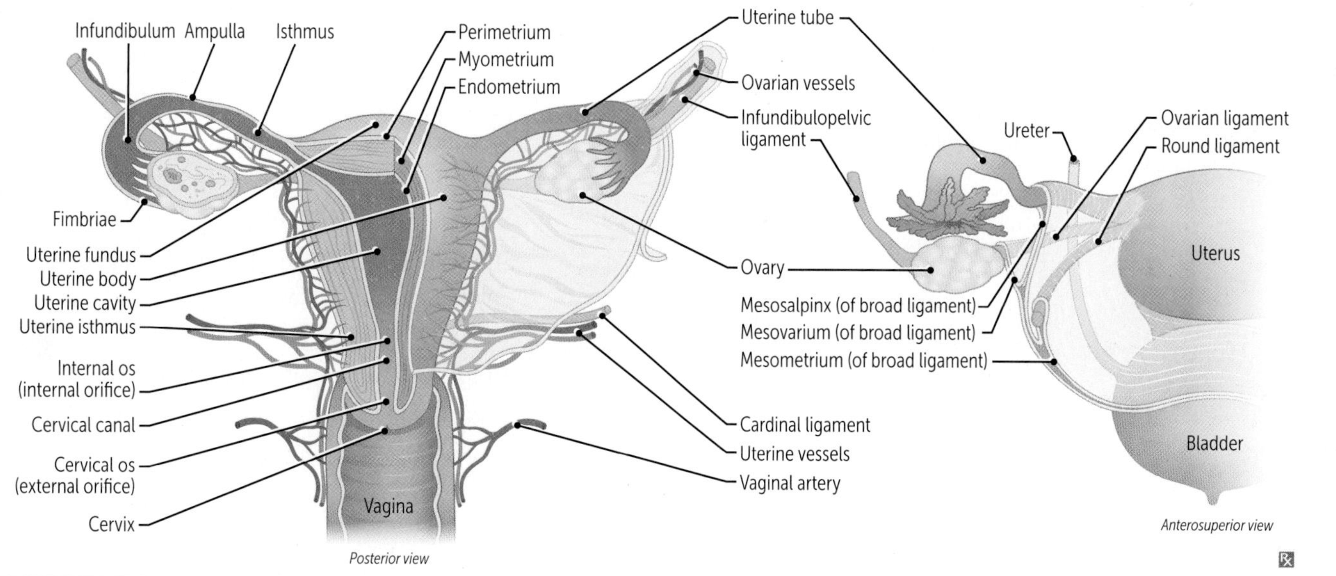

LIGAMENT	CONNECTS	STRUCTURES CONTAINED	NOTES
Infundibulopelvic (suspensory) ligament	Ovaries to lateral pelvic wall	Ovarian vessels	Ureter courses retroperitoneally, close to gonadal vessels → ligation of ovarian vessels during oophorectomy presents risk to ureter
Cardinal (transverse cervical) ligament	Cervix to side wall of pelvis	Uterine vessels	Ligation of uterine vessels during hysterectomy presents risk to ureter
Round ligament of the uterus	Uterine horn to labia majora		Derivative of gubernaculum. Travels through **round** inguinal canal; above the artery of Sampson
Broad ligament	Uterus, fallopian tubes, and ovaries to pelvic side wall	Ovaries, fallopian tubes, round ligaments of uterus	Fold of peritoneum that comprises the mesosalpinx, mesometrium, and mesovarium
Ovarian ligament	Medial pole of ovary to uterine horn		Derivative of gubernaculum Ovarian ligament latches to lateral uterus

Adnexal torsion

Twisting of ovary and fallopian tube around infundibulopelvic ligament and ovarian ligament → compression of ovarian vessels in infundibulopelvic ligament → blockage of lymphatic and venous outflow. Continued arterial perfusion → ovarian edema → complete blockage of arterial inflow → necrosis, local hemorrhage. Associated with ovarian masses. Presents with acute pelvic pain, adnexal mass, nausea/vomiting. Surgical emergency.

Pelvic organ prolapse

Herniation of pelvic organs to or beyond the vaginal walls (anterior, posterior) or apex. Associated with multiparity, ↑ age, obesity. Presents with pelvic pressure, tissue protrusion from vagina, urinary frequency, constipation, sexual dysfunction.

- Anterior compartment prolapse—bladder (cystocele). Most common.
- Posterior compartment prolapse—rectum (rectocele) or small bowel (enterocele).
- Apical compartment prolapse—uterus, cervix, or vaginal vault.

Uterine procidentia—herniation involving all 3 compartments.

Female reproductive epithelial histology

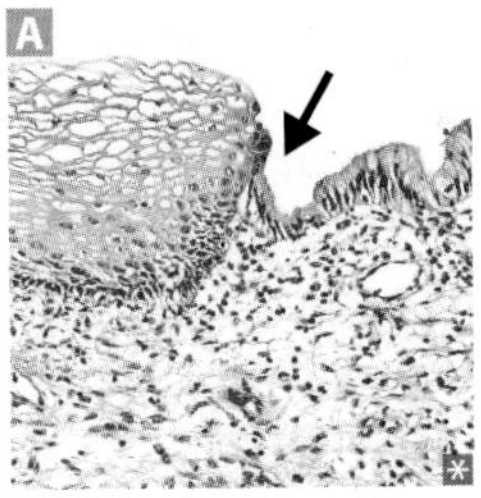

TISSUE	HISTOLOGY/NOTES
Vulva	Stratified squamous epithelium
Vagina	Stratified squamous epithelium, nonkeratinized
Ectocervix	Stratified squamous epithelium, nonkeratinized
Transformation zone	Squamocolumnar junction A (most common area for cervical cancer; sampled in Pap test)
Endocervix	Simple columnar epithelium
Uterus	Simple columnar epithelium with long tubular glands in proliferative phase; coiled glands in secretory phase
Fallopian tube	Simple columnar epithelium, ciliated
Ovary, outer surface	Simple cuboidal epithelium (germinal epithelium covering surface of ovary)

Male reproductive anatomy

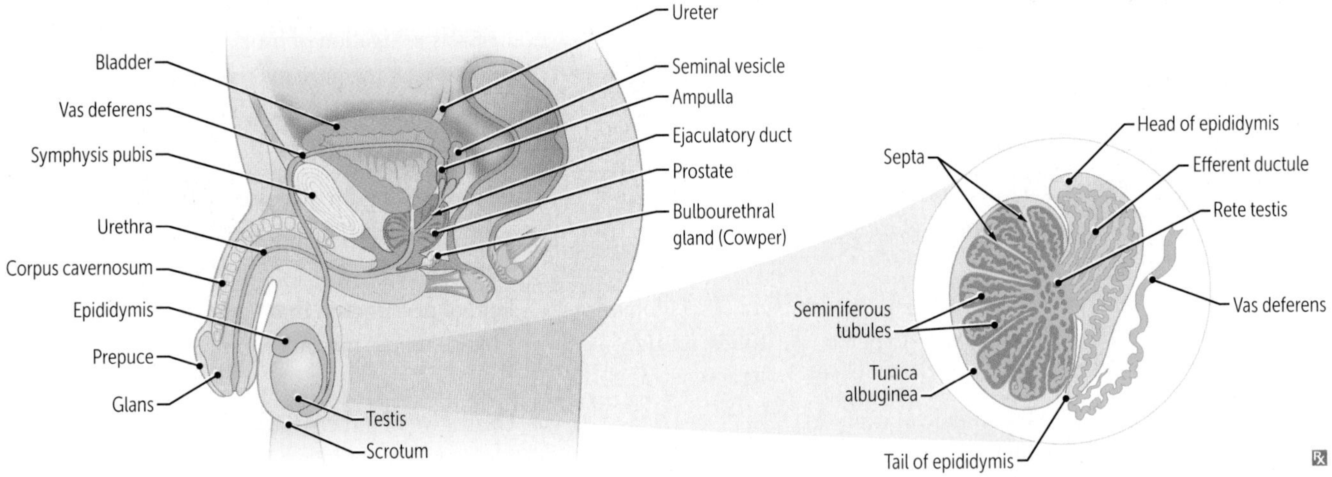

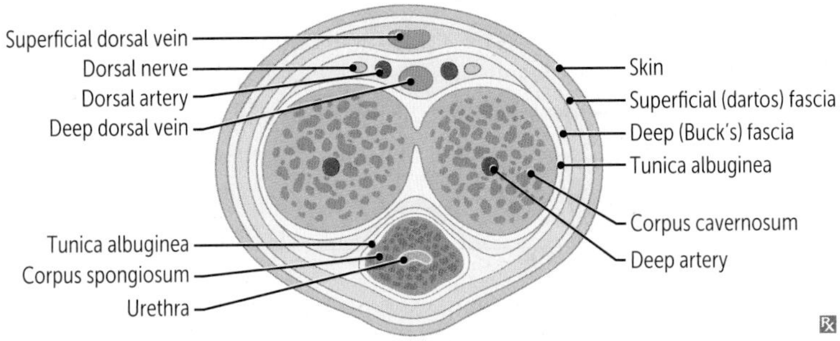

Pathway of sperm during ejaculation—
SEVEN UP:
- Seminiferous tubules
- Epididymis
- Vas deferens
- Ejaculatory ducts
- (Nothing)
- Urethra
- Penis

Genitourinary trauma	Most commonly due to blunt trauma (eg, motor vehicle collision).
Renal injury	Presents with bruises, flank pain, hematuria. Caused by direct blows or lower rib fractures.
Bladder injury	Presents with hematuria, suprapubic pain, difficulty voiding. ▪ Superior bladder wall (dome) injury—direct trauma to full bladder (eg, seatbelt) → abrupt ↑ intravesical pressure → dome rupture (weakest part) → intraperitoneal urine accumulation. Peritoneal absorption of urine → ↑ BUN, ↑ creatinine. ▪ Anterior bladder wall or neck injury—pelvic fracture → perforation by bony spicules → extraperitoneal urine accumulation (retropubic space).
Urethral injury	Occurs almost exclusively in males. Presents with blood at urethral meatus, hematuria, difficulty voiding. Urethral catheterization is relatively contraindicated. ▪ Anterior urethral injury—perineal straddle injury → disruption of bulbar (spongy) urethra → scrotal hematoma. If Buck fascia is torn, urine escapes into perineal space. ▪ Posterior urethral injury—pelvic fracture → disruption at bulbomembranous junction (weakest part) → urine leakage into retropubic space and high-riding prostate.

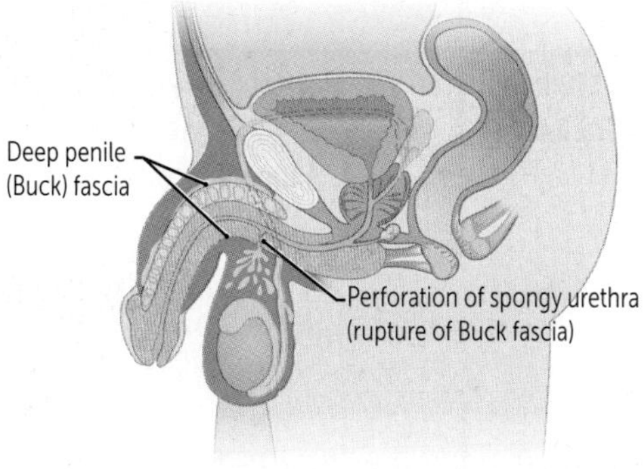
Deep penile (Buck) fascia
Perforation of spongy urethra (rupture of Buck fascia)

Anterior urethral injury

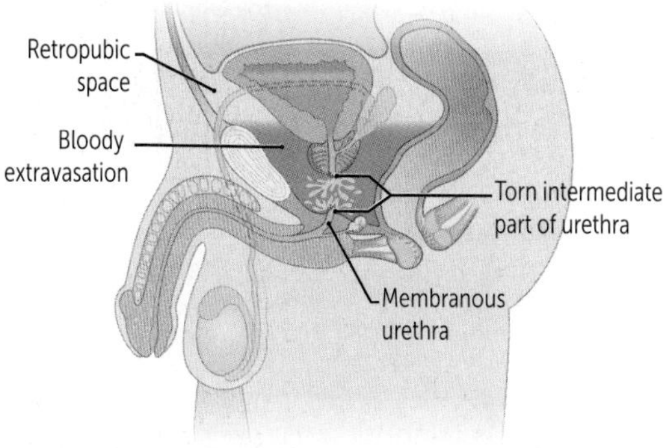
Retropubic space
Bloody extravasation
Torn intermediate part of urethra
Membranous urethra

Posterior urethral injury

Autonomic innervation of male sexual response	Erection—parasympathetic nervous system (pelvic splanchnic nerves, S2-S4): ▪ NO → ↑ cGMP → smooth muscle relaxation → vasodilation → proerectile. ▪ Norepinephrine → ↑ $[Ca^{2+}]_{in}$ → smooth muscle contraction → vasoconstriction → antierectile. Emission—sympathetic nervous system (hypogastric nerve, T11-L2). Expulsion—visceral and somatic nerves (pudendal nerve).	Point, squeeze, and shoot. S2, 3, 4 keep the penis off the floor. PDE-5 inhibitors (eg, sildenafil) → ↓ cGMP breakdown.

Seminiferous tubules

CELL	FUNCTION	LOCATION/NOTES
Spermatogonia	Maintain germ cell pool and produce 1° spermatocytes	Line seminiferous tubules A Germ cells
Sertoli cells	Secrete inhibin B → inhibit FSH Secrete androgen-binding protein → maintain local levels of testosterone Produce MIF Tight junctions between adjacent Sertoli cells form blood-testis barrier → isolate gametes from autoimmune attack Support and nourish developing spermatozoa Regulate spermatogenesis Temperature sensitive; ↓ sperm production and ↓ inhibin B with ↑ temperature	Line seminiferous tubules Non–germ cells Convert testosterone and androstenedione to estrogens via aromatase Sertoli cells are temperature sensitive, line seminiferous tubules, support sperm synthesis, and inhibit FSH Homolog of female granulosa cells ↑ temperature seen in varicocele, cryptorchidism
Leydig cells	Secrete testosterone in the presence of LH; testosterone production unaffected by temperature	Interstitium Endocrine cells Homolog of female theca interna cells

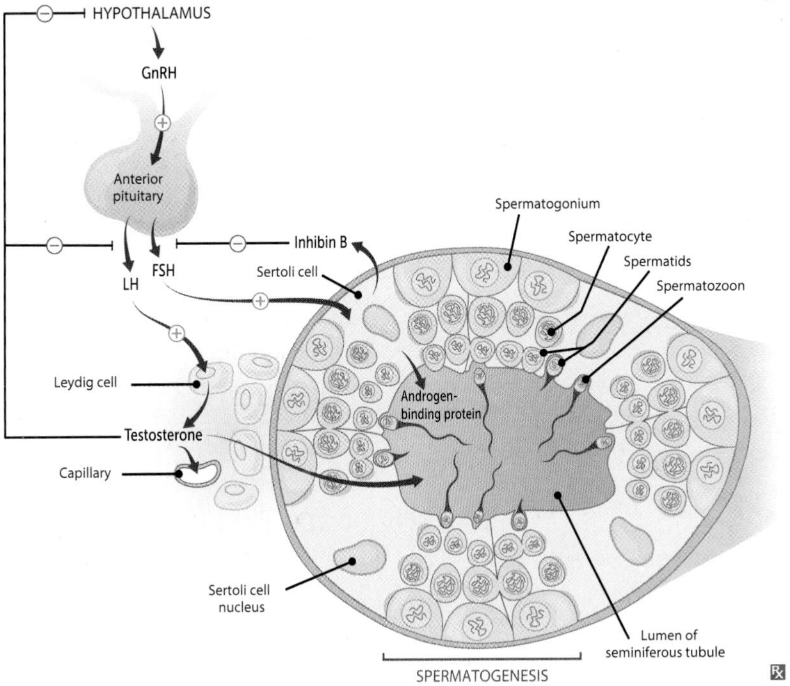

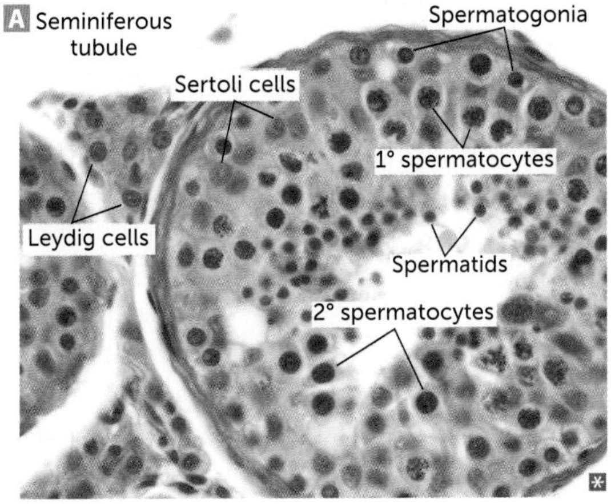

▶ REPRODUCTIVE—PHYSIOLOGY

Spermatogenesis

Begins at puberty with spermatogonia. Full development takes 2 months. Occurs in seminiferous tubules. Produces spermatids that undergo spermiogenesis (loss of cytoplasmic contents, gain of acrosomal cap) to form mature spermatozoa.

"Gonium" is going to be a sperm; "zoon" is "zooming" to egg.

Tail mobility impaired in ciliary dyskinesia/Kartagener syndrome → infertility.

Tail mobility normal in cystic fibrosis (in CF, absent vas deferens → infertility).

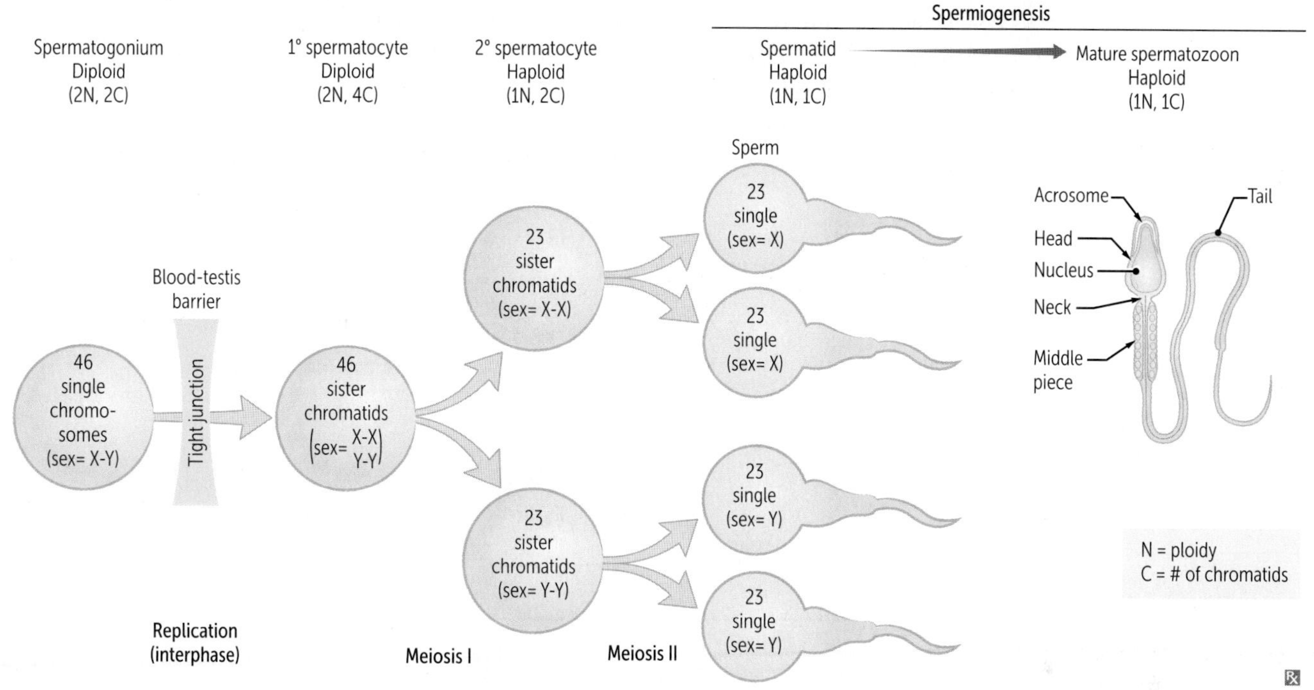

Estrogen

SOURCE	Ovary (17β-estradiol), placenta (estriol), adipose tissue (estrone via aromatization).	Potency: estradiol > estrone > estriol.
FUNCTION	Development of internal/external genitalia, breasts, female fat distribution. Growth of follicle, endometrial proliferation, ↑ myometrial excitability. Upregulation of estrogen, LH, and progesterone receptors; feedback inhibition of FSH and LH, then LH surge; stimulation of prolactin secretion, ↓ prolactin action on breasts. ↑ transport proteins, SHBG; ↑ HDL; ↓ LDL.	Pregnancy: ▪ 50-fold ↑ in estradiol and estrone ▪ 1000-fold ↑ in estriol (indicator of fetal well-being) Estrogen receptors expressed in cytoplasm; translocate to nucleus when bound by estrogen.

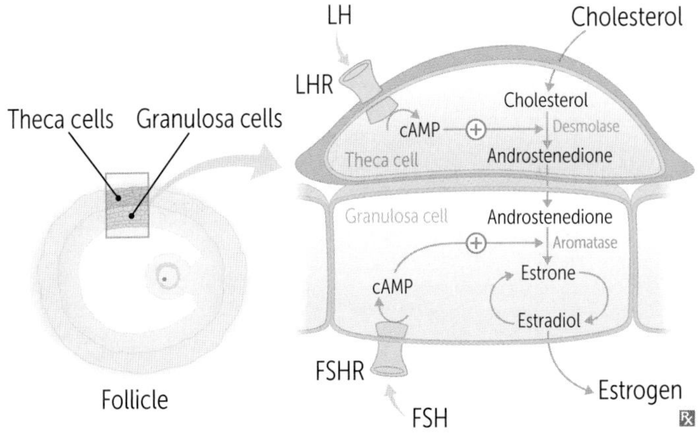

Progesterone

SOURCE	Corpus luteum, placenta, adrenal cortex, testes.	Fall in estrogen and progesterone after delivery disinhibits prolactin → lactation. ↑ progesterone is indicative of ovulation. **Progesterone** is **pro-gestation**. **Prolactin** is **pro-lactation**.
FUNCTION	During luteal phase, prepares uterus for implantation of fertilized egg: ▪ Stimulation of endometrial glandular secretions and spiral artery development ▪ Production of thick cervical mucus → inhibits sperm entry into uterus ▪ Prevention of endometrial hyperplasia ▪ ↑ body temperature ▪ ↓ estrogen receptor expression ▪ ↓ gonadotropin (LH, FSH) secretion During pregnancy: ▪ Maintenance of pregnancy ▪ ↓ myometrial excitability → ↓ contraction frequency and intensity ▪ ↓ prolactin action on breasts	

Oogenesis

1° oocytes begin meiosis I during fetal life and complete meiosis I just prior to ovulation.
Meiosis I is arrested in prophase I for years until ovulation (1° oocytes).
Meiosis II is arrested in metaphase II until fertilization (2° oocytes). "An egg met a sperm."
If fertilization does not occur within 1 day, the 2° oocyte degenerates.

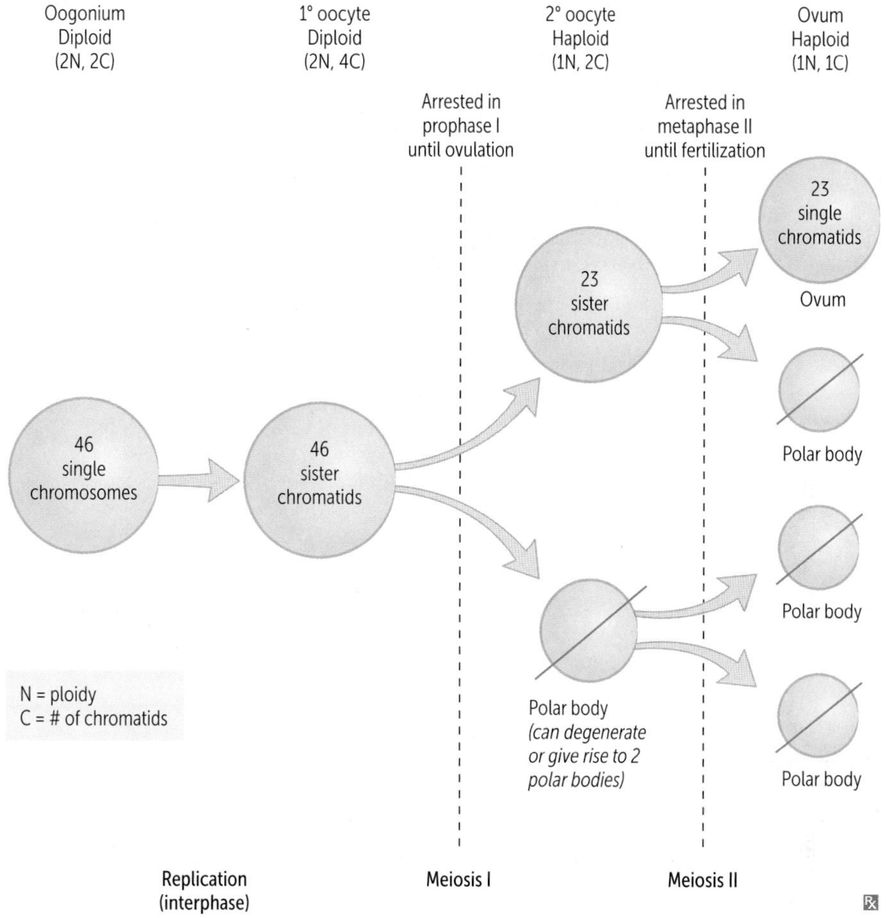

Ovulation

↑ estrogen, ↑ GnRH receptors on anterior pituitary. Estrogen rise then stimulates LH surge → ovulation (rupture of follicle).
↑ temperature (progesterone induced).

Mittelschmerz—transient mid-cycle ovulatory pain ("middle hurts"); classically associated with peritoneal irritation (eg, follicular swelling/rupture, fallopian tube contraction). Can mimic appendicitis.

Menstrual cycle

Follicular phase can fluctuate in length.
Follicular growth is fastest during 2nd week of the follicular phase.
Luteal phase is a fixed 14 days, after which menstruation occurs.
Estrogen stimulates endometrial proliferation.
Progesterone maintains endometrium to support implantation.
↓ progesterone → ↓ fertility.

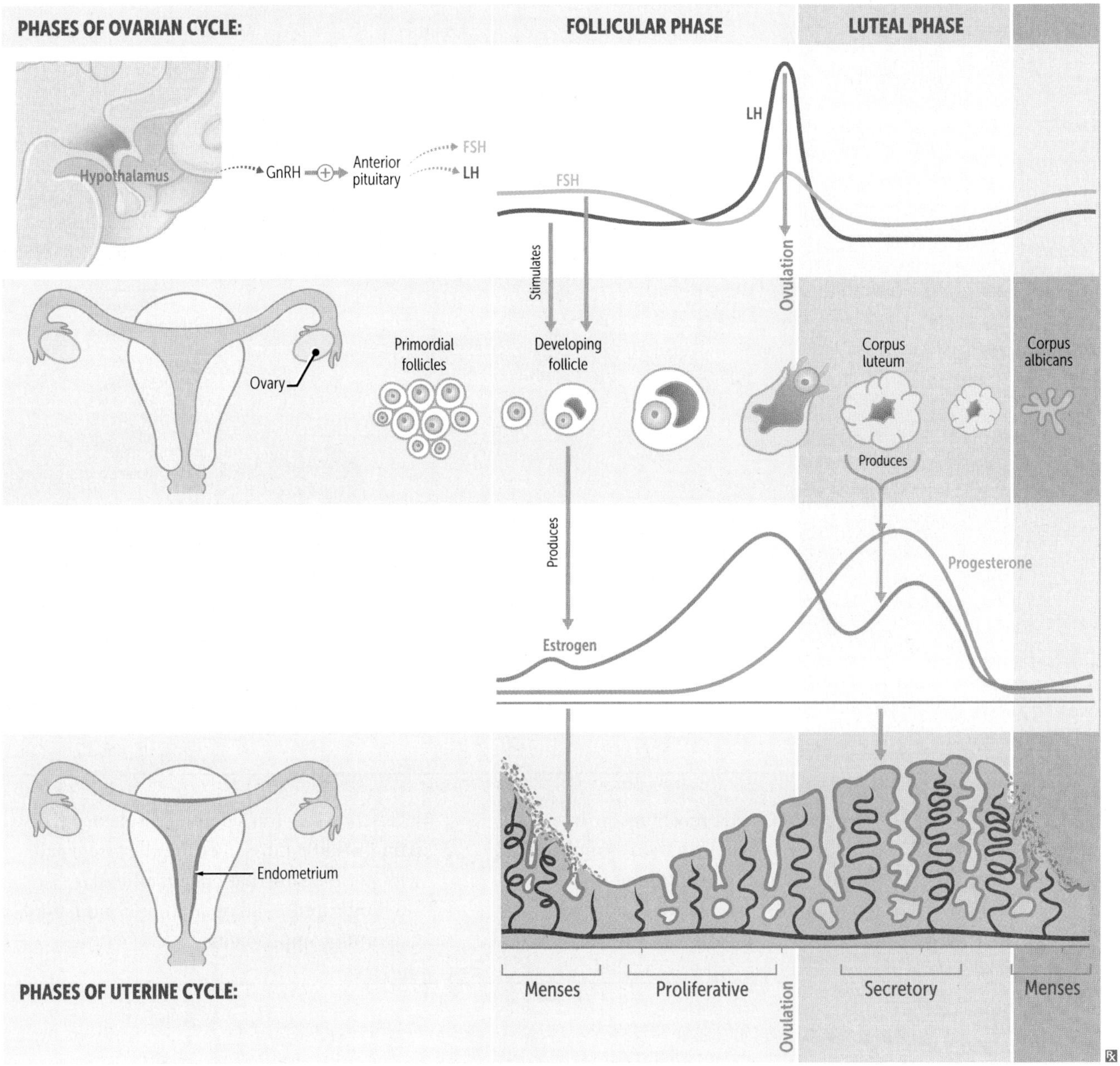

Abnormal uterine bleeding

Characterized as either heavy menstrual bleeding (AUB/HMB) or intermenstrual bleeding (AUB/IMB).

These are further subcategorized by **PALM-COEIN**:

- Structural causes (**PALM**): **P**olyp, **A**denomyosis, **L**eiomyoma, or **M**alignancy/hyperplasia
- Non-structural causes (**COEIN**): **C**oagulopathy, **O**vulatory, **E**ndometrial, **I**atrogenic, **N**ot yet classified

Terms such as dysfunctional uterine bleeding, menorrhagia, oligomenorrhea are no longer recommended.

Pregnancy

Fertilization (conception) most commonly occurs in upper end of fallopian tube (the ampulla). Occurs within 1 day of ovulation.

Implantation in the uterine wall occurs 6 days after fertilization. Syncytiotrophoblasts secrete hCG, which is detectable in blood 1 week after fertilization and on home urine tests 2 weeks after fertilization.

Embryonic/developmental age—time since fertilization. Used in embryology.

Gestational age—time since first day of last menstrual period. Used clinically.

Gravidity ("gravida")—number of pregnancies.

Parity ("para")—number of pregnancies that resulted in live births.

Placental hormone secretion generally increases over the course of pregnancy, but hCG peaks at 8–10 weeks of gestation.

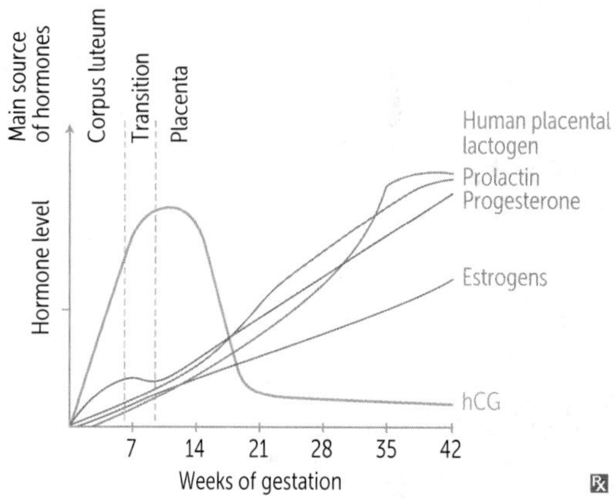

Physiologic changes in pregnancy	Changes that nurture the developing fetus and prepare the pregnant patient for labor and delivery. Mediated by ↑ hormones (eg, estrogen, progesterone) and mechanical effects of gravid uterus.
CARDIOVASCULAR	↓ SVR (↓ afterload) and ↑ blood volume (↑ preload) → ↑ SV → ↑ CO → ↑ placental perfusion. ↑ HR is the major contributor to ↑ CO in late pregnancy. Hemodilution → ↓ oncotic pressure → peripheral edema.
ENDOCRINE	Insulin resistance and hypoglycemia → ↑ lipolysis and fat utilization (to preserve glucose and amino acids for fetus). Pituitary enlargement (lactotroph hyperplasia). ↑ TBG, ↑ CBG, ↑ SHBG.
GASTROINTESTINAL	↓ GI motility, ↓ LES tone, gallbladder stasis; predispose to constipation, GERD, gallstones.
HEMATOLOGIC	Dilutional anemia (↑↑ plasma volume, ↑ RBC mass), hypercoagulable state (to ↓ blood loss at delivery). ↑ micronutrient requirements predispose to deficiency (eg, iron, folate).
MUSCULOSKELETAL	Lordosis (to realign gravity center), joint laxity (to facilitate fetal descent).
SKIN	Hyperpigmentation (eg, melasma, linea nigra, areola darkening), striae gravidarum (stretch marks), vascular changes (eg, spider angiomas, palmar erythema, varicosities).
RENAL	Vasodilation → ↑ renal plasma flow → ↑ GFR → ↓ BUN and ↓ creatinine. Mild glucosuria, proteinuria. Ureter and renal pelvis dilation (hydroureter and hydronephrosis) predisposes to pyelonephritis.
RESPIRATORY	Respiratory center stimulation → chronic hyperventilation (to ↑ fetal CO_2 elimination).

Human chorionic gonadotropin

SOURCE	Syncytiotrophoblast of placenta.
FUNCTION	Maintains corpus luteum (and thus progesterone) for first 8–10 weeks of gestation by acting like LH (otherwise no luteal cell stimulation → abortion). Luteal-placental shift is complete after 8–10 weeks; placenta synthesizes its own estriol and progesterone and corpus luteum degenerates. Used to detect pregnancy because it appears early in urine (see above). Has identical α subunit as LH, FSH, TSH (states of ↑ hCG can cause hyperthyroidism). β subunit is unique (pregnancy tests detect β subunit). hCG is ↑ in multiple gestations, hydatidiform moles, choriocarcinomas, and Down syndrome; hCG is ↓ in ectopic/failing pregnancy, Edwards syndrome, and Patau syndrome.

Human placental lactogen

Also called chorionic somatomammotropin.

SOURCE	Syncytiotrophoblast of placenta.
FUNCTION	Stimulates insulin production; overall ↑ insulin resistance. Gestational diabetes can occur if pancreatic function cannot overcome the insulin resistance.

Apgar score

	Score 2	Score 1	Score 0
Appearance	Pink	Extremities blue	Pale or blue
Pulse	$\geq$ 100 bpm	< 100 bpm	No pulse
Grimace	Cries and pulls away	Grimaces or weak cry	No response to stimulation
Activity	Active movement	Arms, legs flexed	No movement
Respiration	Strong cry	Slow, irregular	No breathing

Assessment of newborn vital signs following delivery via a 10-point scale evaluated at 1 minute and 5 minutes. **Apgar** score is based on **a**ppearance, **p**ulse, **g**rimace, **a**ctivity, and **r**espiration. Apgar scores < 7 may require further evaluation. If Apgar score remains low at later time points, there is ↑ risk the child will develop long-term neurologic damage.

Low birth weight

Defined as < 2500 g. Caused by prematurity or intrauterine growth restriction (IUGR). Associated with ↑ risk of sudden infant death syndrome (SIDS) and with ↑ overall mortality.

Lactation

After parturition and delivery of placenta, rapid ↓ in estrogen and progesterone disinhibits prolactin → initiation of lactation. Suckling is required to maintain milk production and ejection, since ↑ nerve stimulation → ↑ oxytocin and prolactin.

Prolactin—induces and maintains lactation and ↓ reproductive function.

Oxytocin—assists in milk letdown; also promotes uterine contractions.

Breast milk is the ideal nutrition for infants < 6 months old. Contains immunoglobulins (conferring passive immunity; mostly IgA), macrophages, lymphocytes. Breast milk reduces infant infections and is associated with ↓ risk for child to develop asthma, allergies, diabetes mellitus, and obesity. Guidelines recommend exclusively breastfed infants get vitamin D and possibly iron supplementation.

Breastfeeding facilitates bonding with the child. Breastfeeding or donating milk ↓ risk of breast and ovarian cancers.

Menopause

Diagnosed by amenorrhea for 12 months. ↓ estrogen production due to age-linked decline in number of ovarian follicles. Average age at onset is 51 years (earlier in people who smoke tobacco).

Usually preceded by 4–5 years of abnormal menstrual cycles. Source of estrogen (estrone) after menopause becomes peripheral conversion of androgens, ↑ androgens → hirsutism.

↑↑ FSH is specific for menopause (loss of negative feedback on FSH due to ↓ estrogen).

Hormonal changes: ↓ estrogen, ↑↑ FSH, ↑ LH (no surge), ↑ GnRH.

Causes HAVOCS: Hot flashes (most common), Atrophy of the Vagina, Osteoporosis, Coronary artery disease, Sleep disturbances.

Menopause before age 40 suggests 1° ovarian insufficiency (premature ovarian failure); may occur in females who have received chemotherapy and/or radiation therapy.

Androgens

Testosterone, dihydrotestosterone (DHT), androstenedione.

SOURCE

DHT and testosterone (testis), androstenedione (adrenal)

Potency: DHT > testosterone > androstenedione.

FUNCTION

Testosterone:
- Differentiation of epididymis, vas deferens, seminal vesicles (internal genitalia, except prostate)
- Growth spurt: penis, seminal vesicles, sperm, muscle, RBCs
- Deepening of voice
- Closing of epiphyseal plates (via estrogen converted from testosterone)
- Libido

DHT:
- Early—differentiation of penis, scrotum, prostate
- Late—prostate growth, balding, sebaceous gland activity

Testosterone is converted to DHT by 5α-reductase, which is inhibited by finasteride.

In the male, androgens are converted to estrogens by aromatase (primarily in adipose tissue and testes).

Anabolic-androgenic steroid use—↑ fat-free mass, muscle strength, performance. Suspect in males who present with changes in behavior (eg, aggression), acne, gynecomastia, ↑ Hb and Hct, small testes (exogenous testosterone → hypothalamic-pituitary-gonadal axis inhibition → ↓ intratesticular testosterone → ↓ testicular size, ↓ sperm count, azoospermia). Females may present with virilization (eg, hirsutism, acne, breast atrophy, male pattern baldness).

Tanner stages of sexual development

Tanner stage is assigned independently to genitalia, pubic hair, and breast (eg, a person can have Tanner stage 2 genitalia, Tanner stage 3 pubic hair). Earliest detectable secondary sexual characteristic is breast bud development in females, testicular enlargement in males.

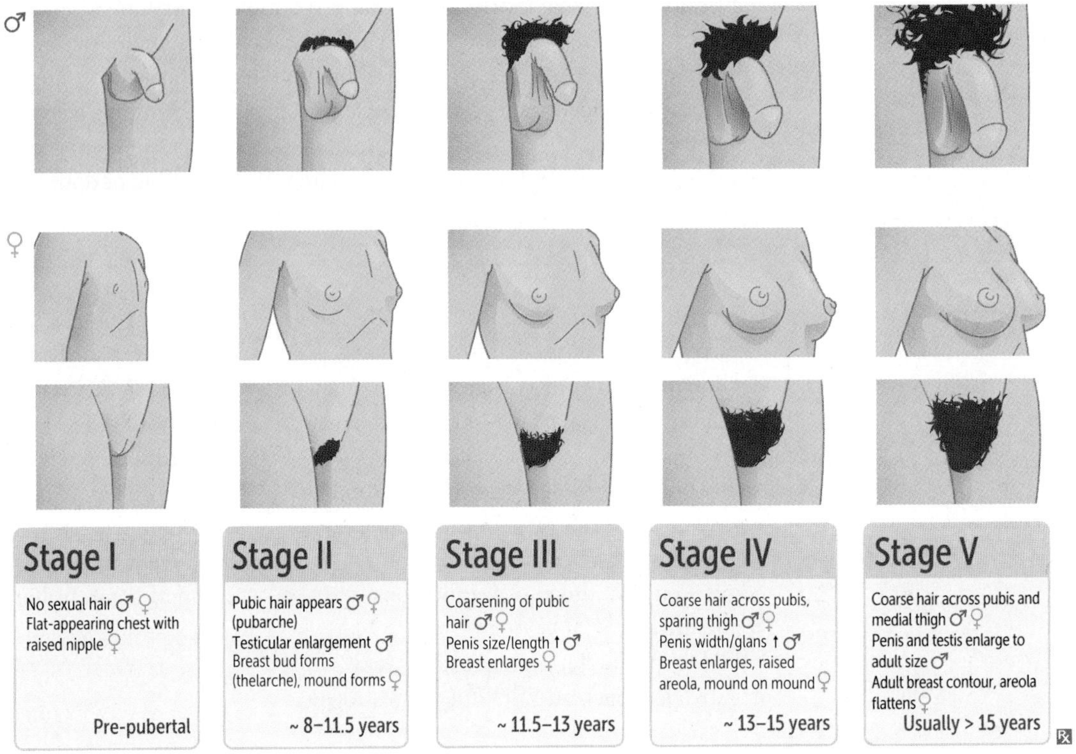
♂
♀
Stage I
No sexual hair ♂ ♀
Flat-appearing chest with raised nipple ♀
Pre-pubertal
Stage II
Pubic hair appears ♂ ♀ (pubarche)
Testicular enlargement ♂
Breast bud forms (thelarche), mound forms ♀
~ 8–11.5 years
Stage III
Coarsening of pubic hair ♂ ♀
Penis size/length ↑ ♂
Breast enlarges ♀
~ 11.5–13 years
Stage IV
Coarse hair across pubis, sparing thigh ♂ ♀
Penis width/glans ↑ ♂
Breast enlarges, raised areola, mound on mound ♀
~ 13–15 years
Stage V
Coarse hair across pubis and medial thigh ♂ ♀
Penis and testis enlarge to adult size ♂
Adult breast contour, areola flattens ♀
Usually > 15 years

Precocious puberty

Appearance of 2° sexual characteristics (eg, adrenarche, thelarche, menarche) before age 8 years in females and 9 years in males. ↑ sex hormone exposure or production → ↑ linear growth, somatic and skeletal maturation (eg, premature closure of epiphyseal plates → short stature). Types include:

- Central precocious puberty (↑ GnRH secretion): idiopathic (most common; early activation of hypothalamic-pituitary gonadal axis), CNS tumors.
- Peripheral precocious puberty (GnRH-independent; ↑ sex hormone production or exposure to exogenous sex steroids): congenital adrenal hyperplasia, estrogen-secreting ovarian tumor (eg, granulosa cell tumor), Leydig cell tumor, McCune-Albright syndrome.

▶ REPRODUCTIVE—PATHOLOGY

Sex chromosome disorders

Aneuploidy most commonly due to meiotic nondisjunction.

Klinefelter syndrome

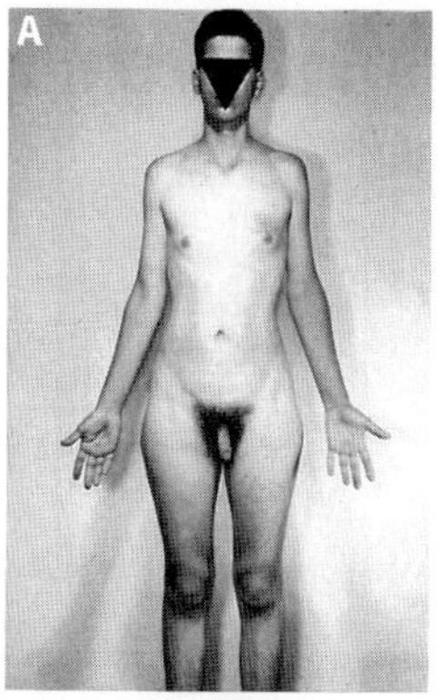

Male, 47,XXY.

Testicular atrophy (small, firm testes), tall stature with eunuchoid proportions (delayed epiphyseal closure → ↑ long bone length), gynecomastia, female hair distribution A. May present with developmental delay. Presence of inactivated X chromosome (Barr body). Common cause of hypogonadism seen in infertility workup. ↑ risk of breast cancer.

Dysgenesis of seminiferous tubules → ↓ inhibin B → ↑ FSH.

Abnormal Leydig cell function → ↓ testosterone → ↑ LH → ↑ estrogen.

Turner syndrome

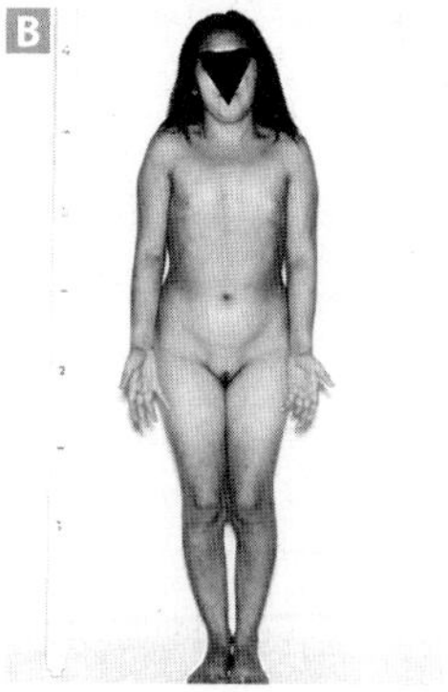

Female, 45,XO.

Short stature (associated with *SHOX* gene, preventable with growth hormone therapy), ovarian dysgenesis (streak ovary), shield chest B, bicuspid aortic valve, coarctation of the aorta (femoral < brachial pulse), lymphatic defects (result in webbed neck or cystic hygroma; lymphedema in feet, hands), horseshoe kidney, high-arched palate, shortened 4th metacarpals.

Most common cause of 1° amenorrhea. No Barr body.

Menopause before menarche.

↓ estrogen leads to ↑ LH, FSH.

Sex chromosome (X, or rarely Y) loss often due to nondisjunction during meiosis or mitosis.

Meiosis errors usually occur in paternal gametes → sperm missing the sex chromosome.

Mitosis errors occur after zygote formation → loss of sex chromosome in some but not all cells → mosaic karyotype (eg. 45,X/46XX).

(45,X/46,XY) mosaicism associated with increased risk for gonadoblastoma.

Pregnancy is possible in some cases (IVF, exogenous estradiol-17β and progesterone).

Double Y males

47, XYY.

Phenotypically normal (usually undiagnosed), very tall. Normal fertility. May be associated with severe acne, learning disability, autism spectrum disorders.

Ovotesticular disorder of sex development

46,XX > 46,XY.

Both ovarian and testicular tissue present (ovotestis); ambiguous genitalia. Previously called true hermaphroditism.

Diagnosing disorders of sex hormones

Testosterone	LH	Diagnosis
↑	↑	Defective androgen receptor
↑	↓	Testosterone-secreting tumor, exogenous steroids
↓	↑	Hypergonadotropic hypogonadism (1°)
↓	↓	Hypogonadotropic hypogonadism (2°)

Other disorders of sex development

Disagreement between the phenotypic sex (external genitalia, influenced by hormonal levels) and the gonadal sex (testes vs ovaries, corresponds with Y chromosome). Formerly called hermaphroditism and pseudohermaphroditism; now most commonly referred to as intersex.

46,XX DSD

Ovaries present, but external genitalia are virilized or ambiguous. Due to excessive and inappropriate exposure to androgenic steroids during early gestation (eg, congenital adrenal hyperplasia or exogenous administration of androgens during pregnancy).

46,XY DSD

Testes present, but external genitalia are female or ambiguous. Most common form is androgen insensitivity syndrome (testicular feminization).

Disorders by physical characteristics

UTERUS	BREASTS	DISORDERS
⊕	⊖	Hypergonadotropic hypogonadism (eg, Turner syndrome, genetic mosaicism, pure gonadal dysgenesis) Hypogonadotropic hypogonadism (eg, CNS lesions, Kallmann syndrome)
⊖	⊕	Uterovaginal agenesis in genotypic female or androgen insensitivity in genotypic male
⊖	⊖	Male genotype with insufficient production of testosterone

Placental aromatase deficiency	Inability to synthesize estrogens from androgens. Masculinization of female (46,XX DSD) infants (ambiguous genitalia), ↑ serum testosterone and androstenedione. Can present with virilization of pregnant patient (fetal androgens cross the placenta).
Androgen insensitivity syndrome	Defect in androgen receptor resulting in female-appearing genetic male (46,XY DSD); female external genitalia with scant axillary and pubic hair, rudimentary vagina; uterus and fallopian tubes absent due to persistence of anti-Müllerian hormone from testes. Patients develop normal functioning testes (often found in labia majora; surgically removed to prevent malignancy). ↑ testosterone, estrogen, LH (vs sex chromosome disorders).
5α-reductase deficiency	Autosomal recessive; sex limited to genetic males (46,XY DSD). Inability to convert testosterone to DHT. Ambiguous genitalia until puberty, when ↑ testosterone causes masculinization/↑ growth of external genitalia. Testosterone/estrogen levels are normal; LH is normal or ↑. Internal genitalia are normal.
Kallmann syndrome	Failure to complete puberty; a form of hypogonadotropic hypogonadism. Defective migration of neurons and subsequent failure of olfactory bulbs to develop → ↓ synthesis of GnRH in the hypothalamus; hyposmia/anosmia; ↓ GnRH, FSH, LH, testosterone. Infertility (low sperm count in males; amenorrhea in females).

Pregnancy complications

Abruptio placentae

Premature separation (partial or complete) of placenta from uterine wall before delivery of infant. Risk factors: trauma (eg, motor vehicle accident), smoking, hypertension, preeclampsia, cocaine use.

Presentation: **abrupt**, painful bleeding (concealed or apparent) in third trimester; possible DIC (mediated by tissue factor activation), shock, fetal distress. May be life threatening for patient and fetus.

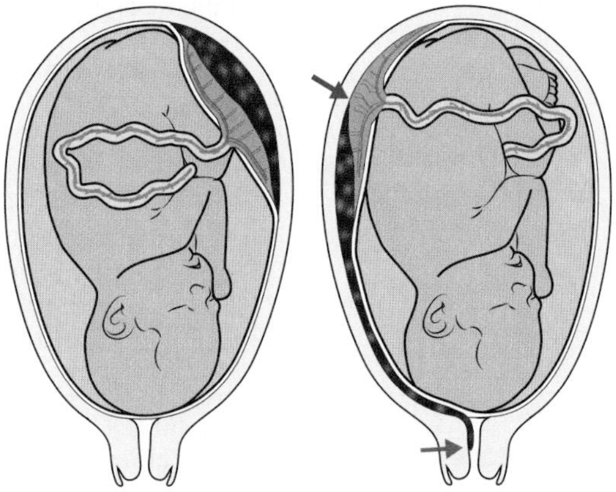

Complete abruption with concealed hemorrhage

Partial abruption (blue arrow) with apparent hemorrhage (red arrow)

Placenta accreta spectrum

Defective decidual layer → abnormal attachment and separation after delivery. Risk factors: prior C-section or uterine surgery involving myometrium, inflammation, placenta previa, advanced age during pregnancy, multiparity. Three types distinguishable by the depth of penetration:

Placenta **accreta**—placenta **attaches** to myometrium without penetrating it; most common type.

Placenta **increta**—placenta penetrates **into** myometrium.

Placenta **percreta**—placenta penetrates ("**perforates**") through myometrium and into uterine serosa (invades entire uterine wall); can result in placental attachment to rectum or bladder (can result in hematuria).

Presentation: often detected on ultrasound prior to delivery. No separation of placenta after delivery → postpartum hemorrhage (can cause Sheehan syndrome).

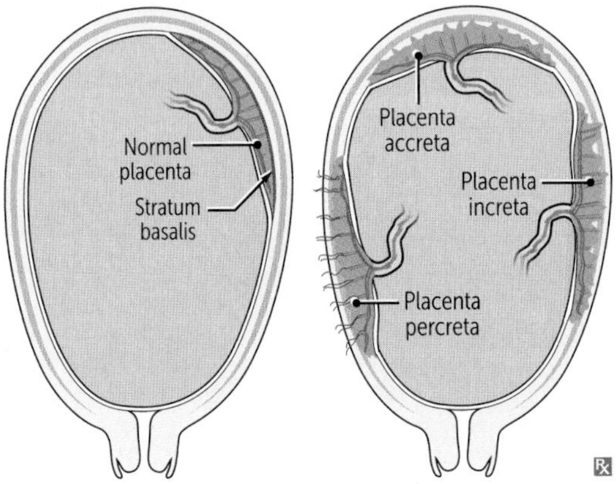

Placenta previa

Attachment of placenta over internal cervical os. Risk factors: multiparity, prior C-section. Associated with painless third-trimester bleeding. A "**preview**" of the **placenta** is visible through cervix.

Low-lying placenta is located < 2 cm from, but not covering, the internal cervical os.

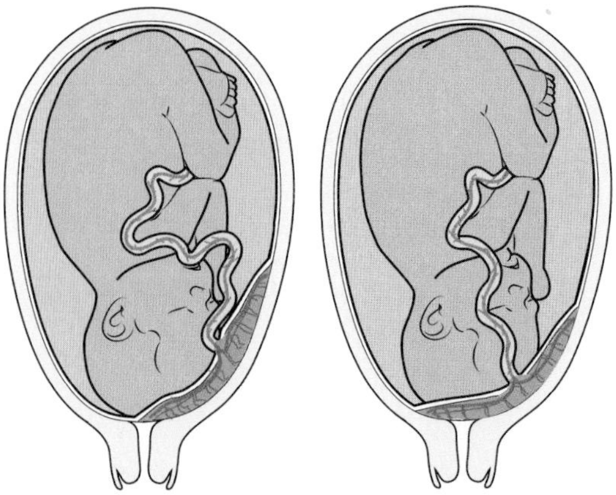

Partial placenta previa

Complete placenta previa

Pregnancy complications *(continued)*

Vasa previa	Fetal vessels run over, or in close proximity to, cervical os. May result in vessel rupture, exsanguination, fetal death. Presents with triad of membrane rupture, painless vaginal bleeding, fetal bradycardia (< 110 beats/min). Emergency C-section usually indicated. Frequently associated with velamentous umbilical cord insertion (cord inserts in chorioamniotic membrane rather than placenta → fetal vessels travel to placenta unprotected by Wharton jelly).	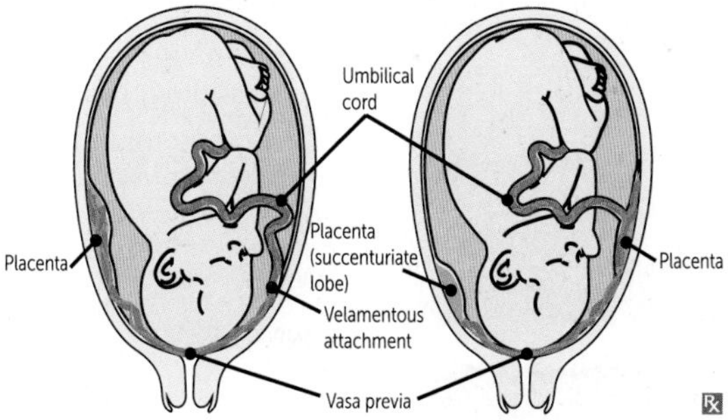
Postpartum hemorrhage	Due to 4 T's: tone (uterine atony → soft, boggy uterus; most common), trauma (lacerations, incisions, uterine rupture), thrombin (coagulopathy), tissue (retained products of conception). Treatment: uterine massage, oxytocin. If refractory, surgical ligation of uterine or internal iliac artery (will preserve fertility since ovarian arteries provide collateral circulation).	
Ectopic pregnancy 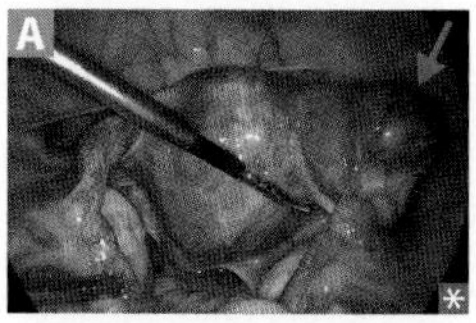	Implantation of fertilized ovum in a site other than the uterus, most often in ampulla of fallopian tube A. Risk factors: tubal pathologies (eg, scarring from salpingitis [PID] or surgery), previous ectopic pregnancy, IUD, IVF. Presents with first-trimester bleeding and/or lower abdominal pain. Often clinically mistaken for appendicitis. Suspect in patients with history of amenorrhea, lower-than-expected rise in hCG based on dates. Confirm with ultrasound, which may show extraovarian adnexal mass. Treatment: methotrexate, surgery.	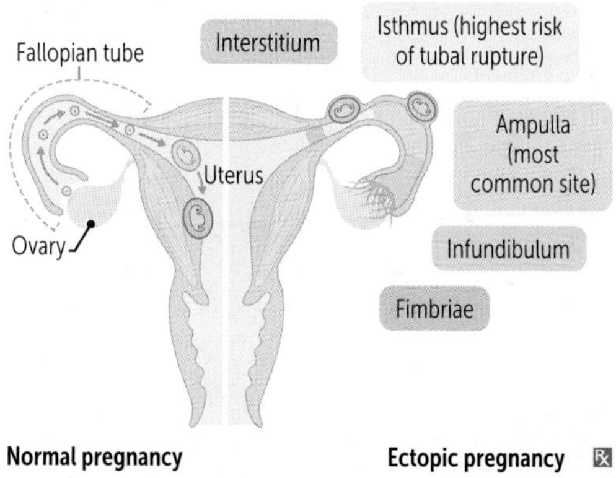

Hydatidiform mole

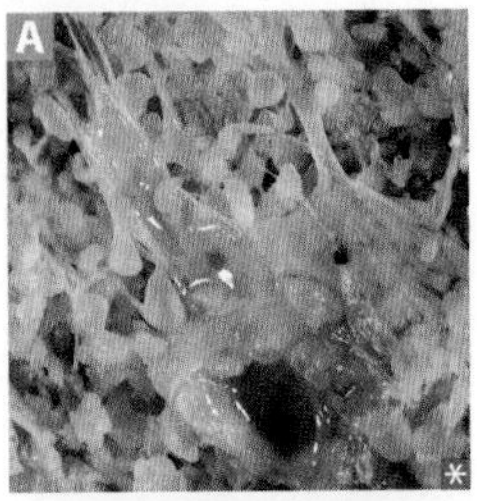

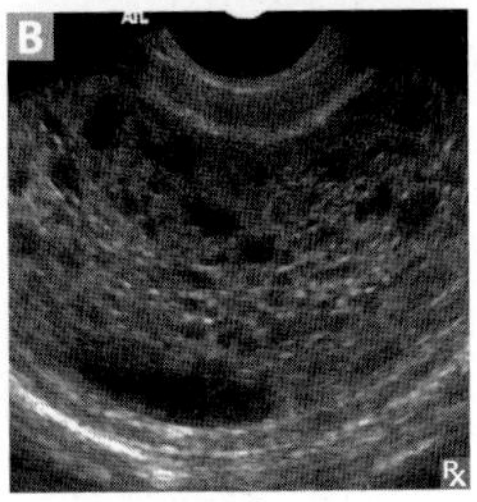

Cystic swelling of chorionic villi and proliferation of chorionic epithelium (only trophoblast).

Presents with vaginal bleeding, emesis, uterine enlargement more than expected, pelvic pressure/pain. Associated with hCG-mediated sequelae: early preeclampsia (before 20 weeks of gestation), theca-lutein cysts, hyperemesis gravidarum, hyperthyroidism.

Treatment: dilation and curettage +/– methotrexate. Monitor hCG.

	Complete mole	Partial mole
KARYOTYPE	46,XX (most common); 46,XY	69,XXX; 69,XXY; 69,XYY
COMPONENTS	Most commonly enucleated egg + single sperm (subsequently duplicates paternal DNA)	2 sperm + 1 egg
HISTOLOGY	Hydropic villi, circumferential and diffuse trophoblastic proliferation	Only some villi are hydropic, focal/minimal trophoblastic proliferation
FETAL PARTS	No	Yes (**partial** = fetal **parts**)
STAINING FOR P57 PROTEIN	⊖ (paternally imprinted)	⊕ (maternally expressed) Partial mole is P57 positive
UTERINE SIZE	↑	—
hCG	↑↑↑↑	↑
IMAGING	"Honeycombed" uterus or "clusters of grapes" A, "snowstorm" B on ultrasound	Fetal parts
RISK OF INVASIVE MOLE	15–20%	< 5%
RISK OF CHORIOCARCINOMA	2%	Rare

Choriocarcinoma

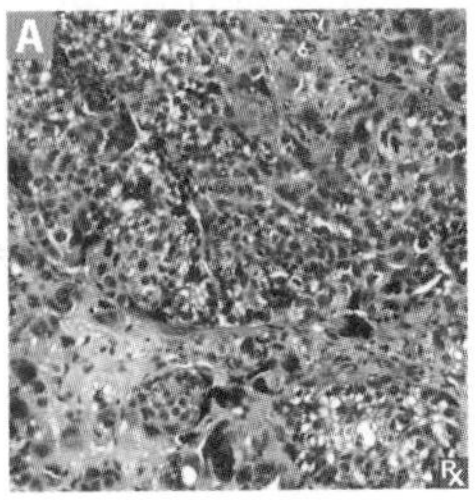

Rare; can develop during or after pregnancy in parent or baby. Malignancy of trophoblastic tissue A (cytotrophoblasts, syncytiotrophoblasts); **no** chorionic villi present. ↑ frequency of bilateral/multiple theca-lutein cysts. Presents with abnormal ↑ hCG, shortness of breath, hemoptysis. Hematogenous spread to lungs → "cannonball" metastases B.

Treatment: methotrexate.

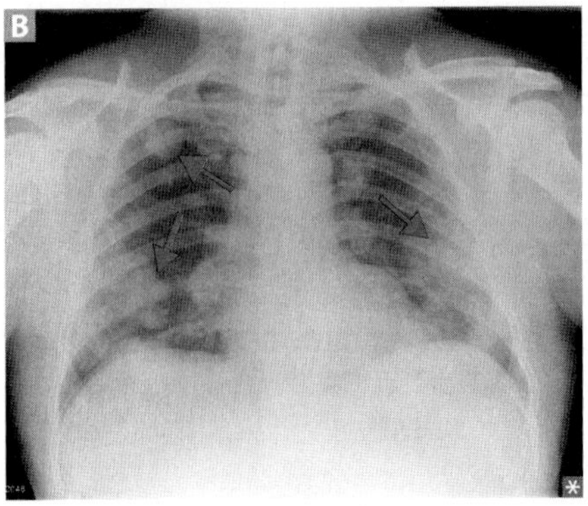

Hypertension in pregnancy	
Gestational hypertension	BP > 140/90 mm Hg after 20 weeks of gestation. No preexisting hypertension. No proteinuria or end-organ damage. Hypertension prior to 20 weeks of gestation suggests chronic hypertension. Treatment: antihypertensives (**H**ydralazine, α-**m**ethyldopa, **l**abetalol, **n**ifedipine), deliver at 37–39 weeks. **H**ypertensive **m**oms **l**ove **n**ifedipine.
Preeclampsia	New-onset hypertension with either proteinuria or end-organ dysfunction after 20 weeks' gestation (onset of preeclampsia < 20 weeks of gestation may suggest molar pregnancy). Caused by abnormal placental spiral arteries → endothelial dysfunction, vasoconstriction, ischemia. ↑ incidence in patients with history of preeclampsia, chronic hypertension, diabetes, chronic kidney disease, autoimmune disorders (eg, antiphospholipid syndrome), age > 35 years. Complications: placental abruption, coagulopathy, renal failure, pulmonary edema, uteroplacental insufficiency; may lead to eclampsia and/or HELLP syndrome. Treatment: antihypertensives, IV magnesium sulfate (to prevent seizure); definitive is delivery.
Eclampsia	Preeclampsia with seizures. Death due to stroke, intracranial hemorrhage, ARDS. Treatment: IV magnesium sulfate, antihypertensives, immediate delivery.
HELLP syndrome	Preeclampsia with thrombotic microangiopathy of the liver. **H**emolysis, **E**levated **L**iver enzymes, **L**ow **P**latelets. May occur in the absence of hypertension and proteinuria. Blood smear shows schistocytes. Can lead to hepatic subcapsular hematomas (rupture → severe hypotension) and DIC (due to release of tissue factor from injured placenta). Treatment: immediate delivery.

Supine hypotensive syndrome

Also called aortocaval compression syndrome. Seen at > 20 weeks of gestation. Supine position → compression of patient's abdominal aorta and IVC by gravid uterus → ↓ placental perfusion (can lead to pregnancy loss) and ↓ venous return (hypotension).

Gynecologic tumor epidemiology

Incidence (US)—endometrial > ovarian > cervical; cervical cancer is more common worldwide due to lack of screening or HPV vaccination.

Prognosis: Cervical (**best** prognosis, diagnosed < 45 years old) > **E**ndometrial (middle-aged, about 55 years old) > **O**varian (**worst** prognosis, > 65 years).

CEOs often go from **best** to **worst** as they get older.

Vulvar pathology

Non-neoplastic	
Bartholin cyst and abscess	Due to blockage of Bartholin gland duct causing accumulation of gland fluid. May lead to abscess 2° to obstruction and inflammation A. Usually in reproductive-age females.
Lichen sclerosus	Thinning of epidermis with fibrosis/sclerosis of dermis. Presents with porcelain-white plaques with a red or violet border. Skin fragility with erosions can be observed B. Most common in postmenopausal females. Benign, but slightly increased risk for SCC.
Lichen simplex chronicus	Hyperplasia of vulvar squamous epithelium. Presents with leathery, thick vulvar skin with enhanced skin markings due to chronic rubbing or scratching. Benign, no risk of SCC.
Neoplastic	
Vulvar carcinoma	Carcinoma from squamous epithelial lining of vulva C. Rare. Presents with leukoplakia, biopsy often required to distinguish carcinoma from other causes. HPV-related vulvar carcinoma—associated with high-risk HPV types 16, 18. Risk factors: multiple partners, early coitarche. Usually in reproductive-age females. Non-HPV vulvar carcinoma—usually from long-standing lichen sclerosus. Females > 70 years old.
Extramammary Paget disease	Intraepithelial adenocarcinoma. Carcinoma in situ, low risk of underlying carcinoma (vs Paget disease of the breast, which is always associated with underlying carcinoma). Presents with pruritus, erythema, crusting, ulcers D.

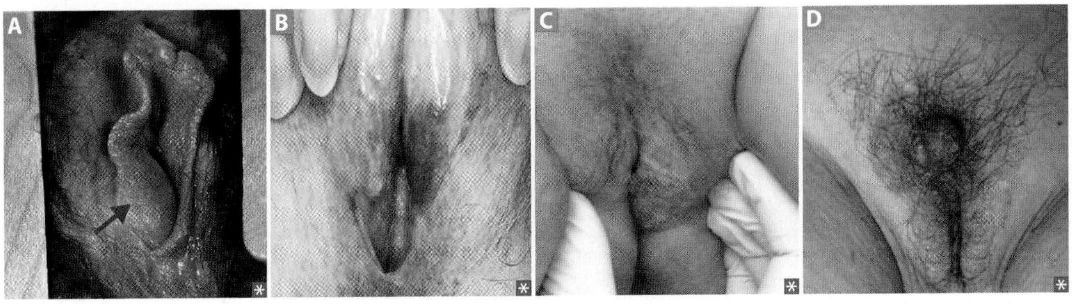

Imperforate hymen	Incomplete degeneration of the central portion of the hymen. Accumulation of vaginal mucus at birth → self-resolving bulge in introitus. If untreated, leads to 1° amenorrhea, cyclic abdominal pain, hematocolpos (accumulation of menstrual blood in vagina → bulging and bluish hymenal membrane).

Vaginal tumors

Squamous cell carcinoma	Usually 2° to cervical SCC; 1° vaginal carcinoma rare.
Clear cell adenocarcinoma	Arises from vaginal adenosis (persistence of glandular columnar epithelium in upper 2/3 of vagina), found in females who had exposure to diethylstilbestrol in utero.
Sarcoma botryoides	Embryonal rhabdomyosarcoma variant. Affects females < 4 years old; spindle-shaped cells; desmin ⊕. Presents with clear, grape-like, polypoid mass emerging from vagina.

Cervical pathology

Dysplasia and carcinoma in situ

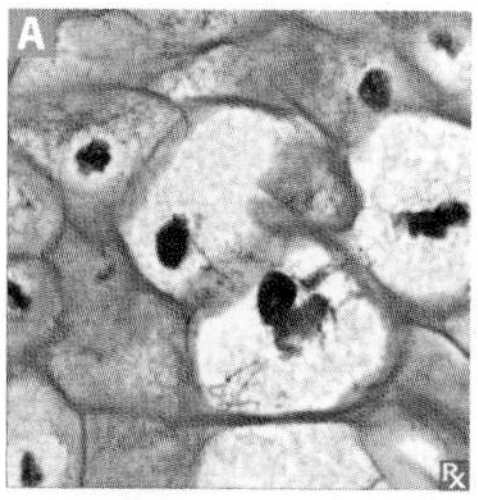

Disordered epithelial growth; begins at basal layer of squamocolumnar junction (transformation zone) and extends outward. Classified as CIN 1, CIN 2, or CIN 3 (severe, irreversible dysplasia or carcinoma in situ), depending on extent of dysplasia. Associated with HPV-16 and HPV-18, which produce both the E6 gene product (inhibits *TP53*) and E7 gene product (inhibits *pRb*) (6 before 7; P before R). Koilocytes (cells with wrinkled "raisinoid" nucleus and perinuclear halo A) are pathognomonic of HPV infection. May progress slowly to invasive carcinoma if left untreated. Typically asymptomatic (detected with Pap smear) or presents as abnormal vaginal bleeding (often postcoital).

Risk factors: multiple sexual partners, HPV, smoking, early coitarche, DES exposure, immunocompromise (eg, HIV, transplant).

Invasive carcinoma

Often squamous cell carcinoma. Pap smear can detect cervical dysplasia before it progresses to invasive carcinoma. Diagnose via colposcopy and biopsy. Lateral invasion can block ureters → hydronephrosis → renal failure.

Primary ovarian insufficiency

Also called premature ovarian failure.

Premature atresia of ovarian follicles in females of reproductive age. Most often idiopathic; associated with chromosomal abnormalities (especially in females < 30 years), autoimmunity. Need karyotype screening. Patients present with signs of menopause after puberty but before age 40. ↓ estrogen, ↑ LH, ↑ FSH.

Most common causes of anovulation

Pregnancy, polycystic ovarian syndrome, obesity, HPO axis abnormalities/immaturity, premature ovarian failure, hyperprolactinemia, thyroid disorders, eating disorders, competitive athletics, Cushing syndrome, adrenal insufficiency, chromosomal abnormalities (eg, Turner syndrome).

Functional hypothalamic amenorrhea

Also called exercise-induced amenorrhea. Severe caloric restriction, ↑ energy expenditure, and/or stress → functional disruption of pulsatile GnRH secretion → ↓ LH, FSH, estrogen. Pathogenesis includes ↓ leptin (due to ↓ fat) and ↑ cortisol (stress, excessive exercise).

Associated with eating disorders and "female athlete triad" (↓ calorie availability/excessive exercise, ↓ bone mineral density, menstrual dysfunction).

Polycystic ovarian syndrome

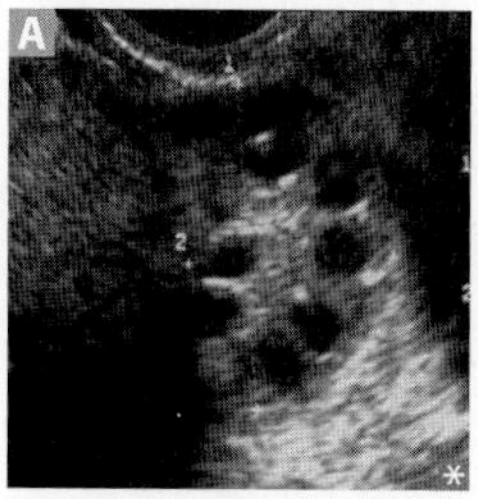

Hyperinsulinemia and/or insulin resistance hypothesized to alter hypothalamic hormonal feedback response → ↑ LH:FSH, ↑ androgens (eg, testosterone) from theca interna cells, ↓ rate of follicular maturation → unruptured follicles (cysts) + anovulation. Common cause of ↓ fertility in females.

Enlarged, bilateral cystic ovaries A; presents with amenorrhea/oligomenorrhea, hirsutism, acne, ↓ fertility. Associated with obesity, acanthosis nigricans. ↑ risk of endometrial cancer 2° to unopposed estrogen from repeated anovulatory cycles.

Treatment: cycle regulation via weight reduction (↓ peripheral estrone formation), OCPs (prevent endometrial hyperplasia due to unopposed estrogen); clomiphene (ovulation induction); spironolactone, finasteride, flutamide to treat hirsutism.

Primary dysmenorrhea Painful menses, caused by uterine contractions to ↓ blood loss → ischemic pain. Mediated by prostaglandins. Treatment: NSAIDs.

Ovarian cysts	
Follicular cyst	Distention of unruptured Graafian follicle. May be associated with hyperestrogenism, endometrial hyperplasia. Most common ovarian mass in young females.
Theca lutein cyst	Also called hyperreactio luteinalis. Often bilateral/multiple. Due to hCG overstimulation. Associated with choriocarcinoma and hydatidiform moles.

Ovarian tumors

Most common adnexal mass in females > 55 years old. Present with abdominal distention, bowel obstruction, pleural effusion.

Risk ↑ with advanced age, infertility, endometriosis, PCOS, genetic predisposition (eg, *BRCA1* or *BRCA2* mutations, Lynch syndrome, strong family history).

Risk ↓ with previous pregnancy, history of breastfeeding, OCPs, tubal ligation.

Epithelial tumors are typically serous (lined by serous epithelium natively found in fallopian tubes, and often bilateral) or mucinous (lined by mucinous epithelium natively found in cervix). Monitor response to therapy/relapse by measuring CA 125 levels (not good for screening).

Germ cell tumors can differentiate into somatic structures (eg, teratomas), or extra-embryonic structures (eg, yolk sac tumors), or can remain undifferentiated (eg, dysgerminoma).

Sex cord stromal tumors develop from embryonic sex cord (develops into theca and granulosa cells of follicle, Sertoli and Leydig cells of seminiferous tubules) and stromal (ovarian cortex) derivatives.

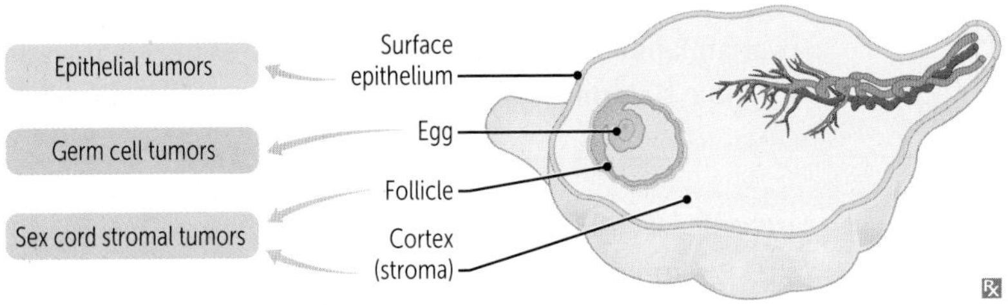

TYPE	CHARACTERISTICS
Epithelial tumors	
Serous cystadenoma	Benign. Most common ovarian neoplasm.
Mucinous cystadenoma	Benign. Multiloculated, large. Lined by mucus-secreting epithelium A. Can result in pseudomyxoma peritonei intraperitoneal accumulation of mucinous material.
Brenner tumor	Usually benign. Solid, pale yellow-tan tumor that appears encapsulated. “Coffee bean” nuclei on H&E stain.
Serous carcinoma	Most common malignant ovarian neoplasm. Psammoma bodies.
Mucinous carcinoma	Malignant. Rare. May be metastatic from appendiceal or other GI tumors.

Ovarian tumors *(continued)*

TYPE	CHARACTERISTICS
Germ cell tumors	
Mature cystic teratoma	Also called dermoid cyst. Benign. Most common ovarian tumor in young females. Cystic mass with elements from all 3 germ layers (eg, teeth, hair, sebum) B. May be painful 2° to ovarian enlargement or torsion. Monodermal form with thyroid tissue (struma ovarii C) may present with hyperthyroidism. Malignant transformation rare (usually to squamous cell carcinoma).
Immature teratoma	Malignant, aggressive. Contains fetal tissue, neuroectoderm. Commonly diagnosed before age 20. Typically represented by immature/embryonic-like neural tissue.
Dysgerminoma	Malignant. Most common in adolescents. Equivalent to male seminoma but rarer. Sheets of uniform "fried egg" cells D. Tumor markers: ↑ hCG, ↑ LDH.
Yolk sac tumor	Also called endodermal sinus tumor. Malignant, aggressive. Yellow, friable (hemorrhagic) mass. 50% have **S**chiller-Duval bodies (resemble glomeruli, arrow in E). Tumor marker: ↑ **AFP**. Occurs in children and young adult females.
Sex cord stromal tumors	
Fibroma	Benign. Bundle of spindle-shaped fibroblasts. Meigs syndrome—triad of ovarian fibroma, ascites, pleural effusion. "Pulling" sensation in groin.
Thecoma	Benign. May produce estrogen. Usually presents as abnormal uterine bleeding in a postmenopausal female.
Sertoli-Leydig cell tumor	Benign. Small, grey to yellow-brown mass. Resembles testicular histology with tubules/cords lined by pink Sertoli cells. May produce androgens → virilization (eg, hirsutism, male pattern baldness, clitoral enlargement).
Granulosa cell tumor	Most common malignant sex cord stromal tumor. Predominantly occurs in females in their 50s. Often produces estrogen and/or progesterone. Presents with postmenopausal bleeding, endometrial hyperplasia, sexual precocity (in preadolescents), breast tenderness. Histology shows **Call**-Exner bodies (granulosa cells arranged haphazardly around collections of eosinophilic fluid, resembling primordial follicles; arrow in F). Tumor marker: ↑ inhibin. "Give **Granny** a **Call**."

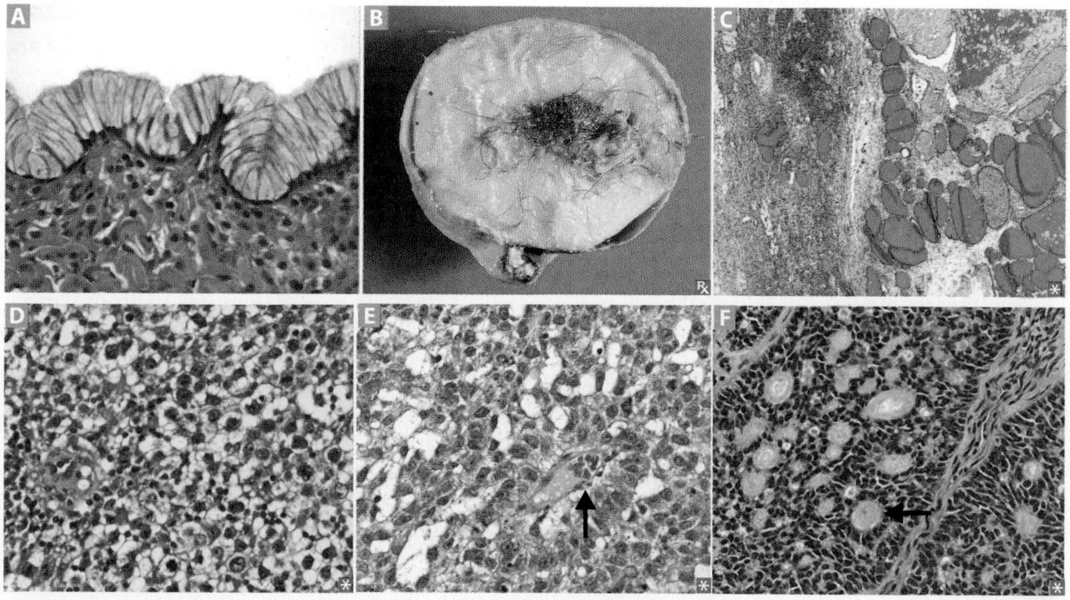

Uterine conditions

TYPE	CHARACTERISTICS
Non-neoplastic uterine conditions	
Adenomyosis	Extension of endometrial tissue (glandular) into uterine myometrium. Caused by hyperplasia of basal layer of endometrium. Presents with dysmenorrhea, AUB/HMB, and uniformly enlarged, soft, globular uterus. Treatment: GnRH agonists, hysterectomy, excision of an organized adenomyoma.
Asherman syndrome	Adhesions and/or fibrosis of the endometrium. Presents with ↓ fertility, recurrent pregnancy loss, AUB, pelvic pain. Often associated with dilation and curettage of intrauterine pregnancy.
Endometrial hyperplasia	Abnormal endometrial gland proliferation usually stimulated by excess estrogen. ↑ risk for endometrial carcinoma (especially with nuclear atypia). Presents as postmenopausal vaginal bleeding. ↑ risk with anovulatory cycles, hormone replacement therapy, PCOS, granulosa cell tumors.
Endometriosis	Endometrium-like glands/stroma outside endometrial cavity, most commonly in the ovary (frequently bilateral), pelvis, peritoneum (yellow-brown "powder burn" lesions). In ovary, appears as endometrioma (blood-filled "chocolate cysts" [oval structures above and below asterisks in A]). May be due to retrograde flow, metaplastic transformation of multipotent cells, transportation of endometrial tissue via lymphatic system. Characterized by cyclic pelvic pain, bleeding, dysmenorrhea, dyspareunia, dyschezia (pain with defecation), infertility; normal-sized uterus. Treatment: NSAIDs, OCPs, progestins, GnRH agonists, danazol, laparoscopic removal.
Endometritis	Inflammation of endometrium B associated with retained products of conception following delivery, miscarriage, abortion, or with foreign body (eg, IUD). Retained material is nidus for bacteria from vagina or GI tract. Chronic endometritis shows plasma cells on histology. Treatment: gentamicin + clindamycin +/– ampicillin.
Uterine neoplasms	
Endometrial carcinoma	Most common gynecologic malignancy. Presents with irregular vaginal bleeding. Two types: Endometrioid C—most cases caused by unopposed estrogen exposure due to obesity, but also associated with early menarche, late menopause, nulliparity. Histology shows abnormally arranged endometrial glands. Early pathogenic events include loss of PTEN or mismatch repair proteins. Serous—associated with endometrial atrophy in postmenopausal females. Aggressive. Psammoma bodies often seen on histology. Characterized by formation of papillae and tufts.
Leiomyoma (fibroid)	Most common tumor in females. Often presents with multiple discrete tumors D. ↑ incidence in Black patients. Benign smooth muscle tumor; malignant transformation to leiomyosarcoma is rare. Estrogen sensitive; tumor size ↑ with pregnancy and ↓ with menopause. Peak occurrence at 20-40 years of age. May be asymptomatic, cause AUB, or result in miscarriage. Severe bleeding may lead to iron deficiency anemia. Whorled pattern of smooth muscle bundles with well-demarcated borders on histology E.
Leiomyosarcoma	Malignant proliferation of smooth muscle arising from myometrium; arises de novo (not from leiomyomas), usually in postmenopausal females. Exam shows single lesion with areas of necrosis.

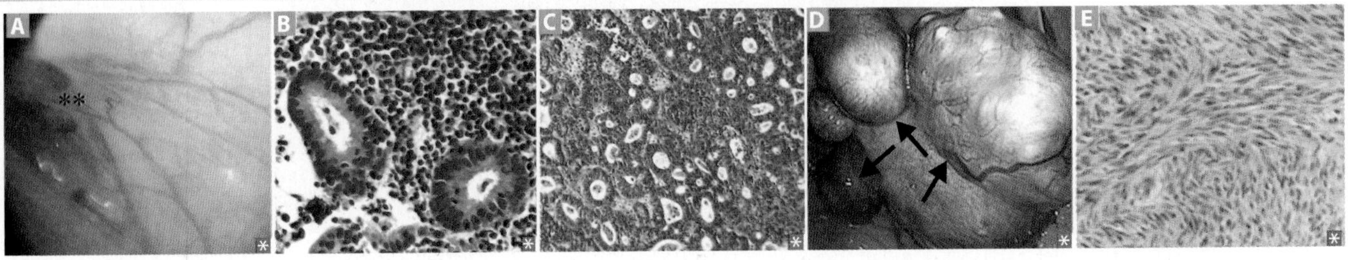

Breast pathology

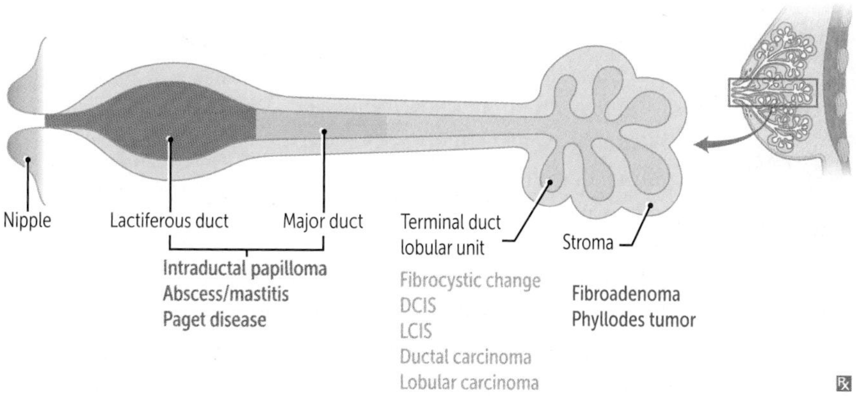

Benign breast diseases

Fibrocystic changes	Most common in premenopausal females 20-50 years old. Present with premenstrual breast pain or lumps; often bilateral and multifocal. Nonproliferative lesions include simple cysts (fluid-filled duct dilation, blue dome), papillary apocrine change/metaplasia, stromal fibrosis. Risk of cancer is usually not increased. Subtypes include: ▪ Sclerosing adenosis—acini and stromal fibrosis, associated with calcifications. Slight ↑ risk for cancer. ▪ Epithelial hyperplasia—cells in terminal ductal or lobular epithelium. ↑ risk of carcinoma with atypical cells.
Inflammatory processes	Fat necrosis—benign, usually painless, lump due to injury to breast tissue. Calcified oil cyst on mammography; necrotic fat and giant cells on biopsy. Up to 50% of patients may not report trauma. Lactational mastitis—occurs during breastfeeding, ↑ risk of bacterial infection through cracks in nipple. *S aureus* is most common pathogen. Treat with antibiotics and continue breastfeeding.
Benign tumors	Fibroadenoma—most common in females < 35 years old. Small, well-defined, mobile mass A. Tumor composed of fibrous tissue and glands. ↑ size and tenderness with ↑ estrogen (eg, pregnancy, prior to menstruation). Risk of cancer is usually not increased. Intraductal papilloma—small fibroepithelial tumor within lactiferous ducts, typically beneath areola. Most common cause of nipple discharge (serous or bloody). Slight ↑ risk for cancer. Phyllodes tumor—large mass B of connective tissue and cysts with "leaf-like" lobulations C. Most common in 5th decade. Some may become malignant.
Gynecomastia	Breast enlargement in males due to ↑ estrogen compared with androgen activity. Physiologic in newborn, pubertal, and elderly males, but may persist after puberty. Other causes include cirrhosis, hypogonadism (eg, Klinefelter syndrome), testicular tumors, and drugs (spironolactone, hormones, cimetidine, finasteride, ketoconazole).

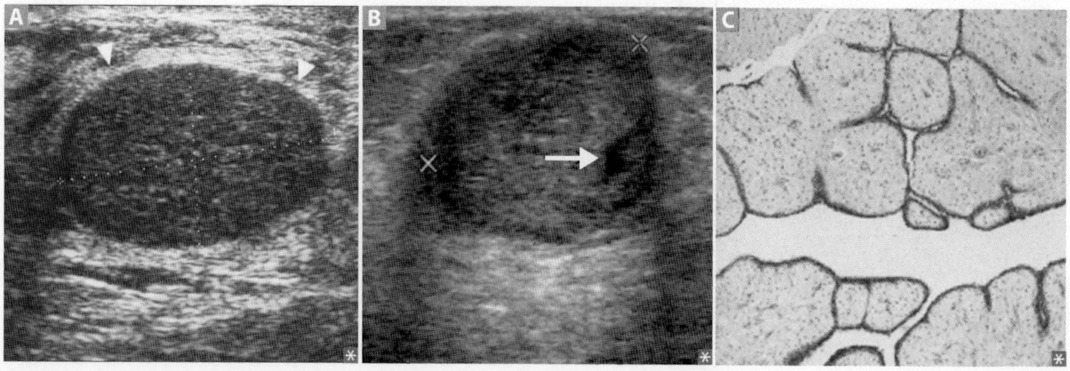

Breast cancer

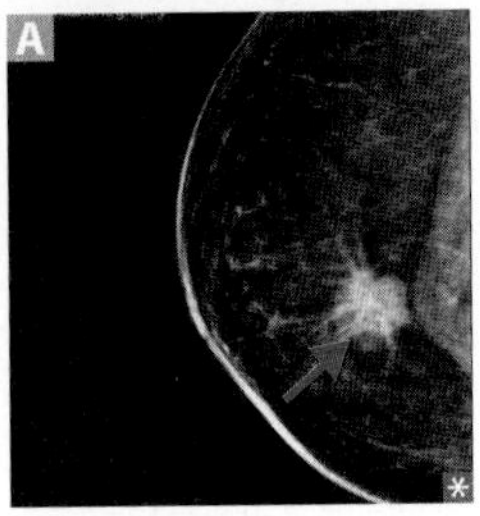

Commonly postmenopausal. Often presents as a palpable hard mass A most often in the upper outer quadrant. Invasive cancer can become fixed to pectoral muscles, deep fascia, Cooper ligaments, and overlying skin → nipple retraction/skin dimpling.

Usually arises from terminal duct lobular unit. Amplification/overexpression of estrogen/progesterone receptors or *c-erbB2* (HER2, an EGF receptor) is common; triple negative (ER ⊖, PR ⊖, and HER2/neu ⊖) form more aggressive.

Risk factors in females: ↑ age; history of atypical hyperplasia; family history of breast cancer; race (White patients at highest risk, Black patients at ↑ risk for triple ⊖ breast cancer); *BRCA1/BRCA2* mutations; ↑ estrogen exposure (eg, nulliparity); postmenopausal obesity (adipose tissue converts androstenedione to estrone); ↑ total number of menstrual cycles; absence of breastfeeding; later age of first pregnancy; alcohol intake. In males: *BRCA2* mutation, Klinefelter syndrome.

Axillary lymph node metastasis most important prognostic factor in early-stage disease.

TYPE	CHARACTERISTICS	NOTES
Noninvasive carcinomas		
Ductal carcinoma in situ	Fills ductal lumen (black arrow in B indicates neoplastic cells in duct; blue arrow shows engorged blood vessel). Arises from ductal atypia. Often seen early as microcalcifications on mammography.	Early malignancy without basement membrane penetration. Usually does not produce a mass. Comedocarcinoma—Subtype of DCIS. Cells have high-grade nuclei with extensive central necrosis C and dystrophic calcification.
Paget disease	Extension of underlying DCIS/invasive breast cancer up the lactiferous ducts and into the contiguous skin of nipple → eczematous patches over nipple and areolar skin D.	Paget cells = intraepithelial adenocarcinoma cells.
Lobular carcinoma in situ	↓ E-cadherin expression. No mass or calcifications → incidental biopsy finding.	↑ risk of cancer in either breast (vs DCIS, same breast and quadrant).
Invasive carcinomas[a]		
Invasive ductal	Firm, fibrous, "rock-hard" mass with sharp margins and small, glandular, duct-like cells in desmoplastic stroma.	Most common type of invasive breast cancer.
Invasive lobular	↓ E-cadherin expression → orderly row of cells ("single file" E) and no duct formation. Often lacks desmoplastic response.	Often bilateral with multiple lesions in the same location. Lines of cells = Lobular.
Medullary	Large, anaplastic cells growing in sheets with associated lymphocytes and plasma cells.	Well-circumscribed tumor can mimic fibroadenoma.
Inflammatory	Dermal lymphatic space invasion → breast pain with warm, swollen, erythematous skin around exaggerated hair follicles (peau d'orange) F.	Poor prognosis (50% survival at 5 years). Often mistaken for mastitis or Paget disease. Usually lacks a palpable mass.

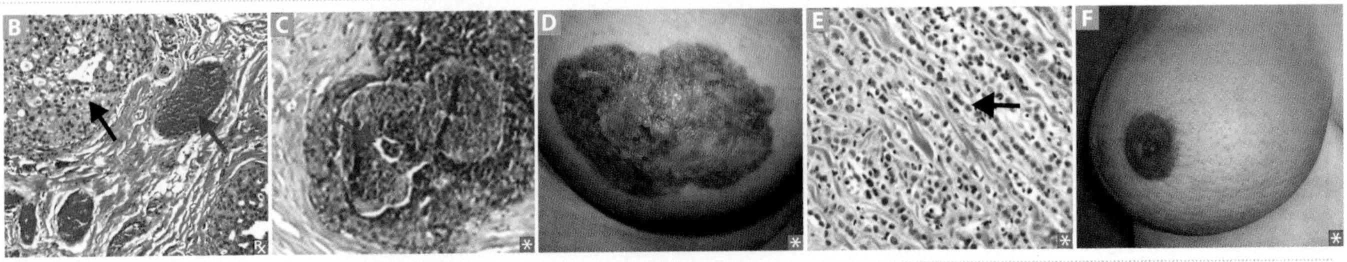

[a]All types of invasive breast carcinoma can be either of tubular subtype (well-differentiated tubules that lack myoepithelium) or mucinous subtype (abundant extracellular mucin, seen in older females).

Penile pathology

Peyronie disease

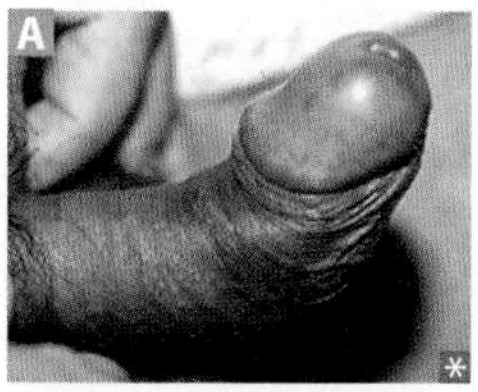

Abnormal curvature of penis A due to fibrous plaque within tunica albuginea. Associated with repeated minor trauma during intercourse. Can cause pain, anxiety, erectile dysfunction. Consider surgical repair or treatment with collagenase injections once curvature stabilizes. Distinct from penile fracture (rupture of corpora cavernosa due to forced bending).

Ischemic priapism

Painful sustained erection lasting > 4 hours. Associated with sickle cell disease (sickled RBCs block venous drainage of corpus cavernosum vascular channels), medications (eg, sildenafil, trazodone). Treat immediately with corporal aspiration, intracavernosal phenylephrine, or surgical decompression to prevent ischemia.

Squamous cell carcinoma

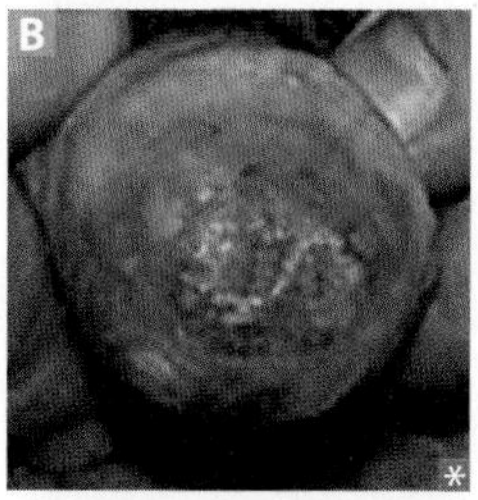

Seen in the US, but more common in Asia, Africa, South America. Precursor in situ lesions: Bowen disease (in penile shaft, presents as leukoplakia "white plaque"), erythroplasia of Queyrat (carcinoma in situ of the glans B, presents as erythroplakia "red plaque"), Bowenoid papulosis (carcinoma in situ of unclear malignant potential, presenting as reddish papules). Associated with uncircumcised males and HPV.

Cryptorchidism

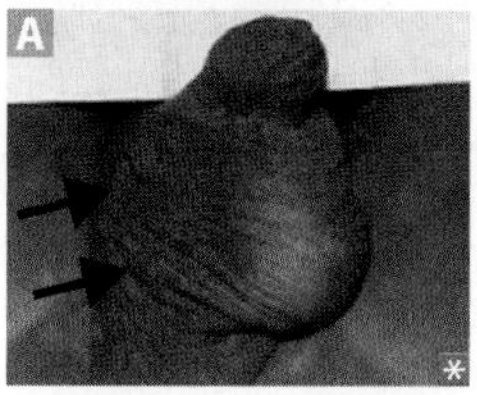

Descent failure of one A or both testes; impaired spermatogenesis (since sperm develop best at temperatures < 37°C); can have normal testosterone levels (Leydig cells are mostly unaffected by temperature); associated with ↑ risk of germ cell tumors. Prematurity ↑ risk of cryptorchidism. ↓ inhibin B, ↑ FSH, ↑ LH; testosterone ↓ in bilateral cryptorchidism, normal in unilateral. Most cases resolve spontaneously; otherwise, orchiopexy performed before 2 years of age.

Testicular torsion

Rotation of testicle around spermatic cord and vascular pedicle. Commonly presents in males 12–18 years old. Associated with congenital horizontal positioning of testes ("bell clapper" deformity). May occur after an inciting event (eg, trauma) or spontaneously. Characterized by acute, severe pain, high-riding testis, and absent cremasteric reflex. ⊖ Prehn sign.

Treatment: surgical correction (orchiopexy) within 6 hours, manual detorsion if surgical option unavailable in timeframe. If testis is not viable, orchiectomy. Orchiopexy, when performed, should be bilateral because the contralateral testis is at risk for subsequent torsion.

Varicocele

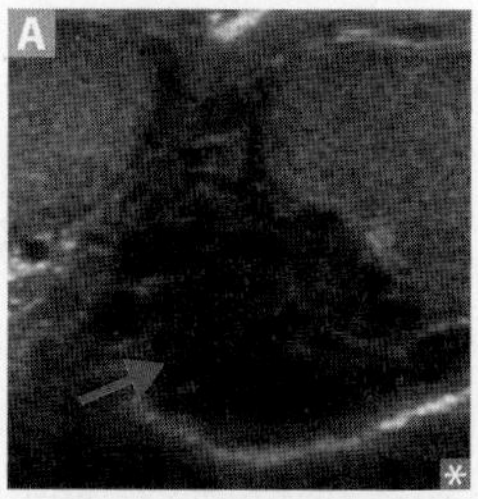

Dilated veins in pampiniform plexus due to ↑ venous pressure; most common cause of scrotal enlargement in adult males; most often on left side because of ↑ resistance to flow from left gonadal vein drainage into left renal vein; can cause infertility because of ↑ temperature; diagnosed by standing clinical exam/Valsalva maneuver (distension on inspection and "bag of worms" on palpation; augmented by Valsalva) or ultrasound A; does not transilluminate.

Treatment: consider surgical ligation or embolization if associated with pain or infertility.

Extragonadal germ cell tumors Arise in midline locations. In adults, most commonly in retroperitoneum, mediastinum, pineal, and suprasellar regions. In infants and young children, sacrococcygeal teratomas are most common.

Benign scrotal lesions Testicular masses that can be transilluminated (vs solid testicular tumors).

Congenital hydrocele 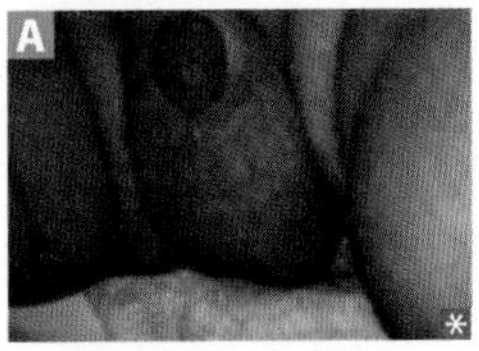	Common cause of scrotal swelling A in infants, due to incomplete obliteration of processus vaginalis. Most spontaneously resolve within 1 year.	Communicating hydrocele.
Acquired hydrocele	Scrotal fluid collection usually 2° to infection, trauma, tumor. If bloody → hematocele.	Noncommunicating hydrocele.
Spermatocele	Cyst due to dilated epididymal duct or rete testis.	Paratesticular fluctuant nodule.

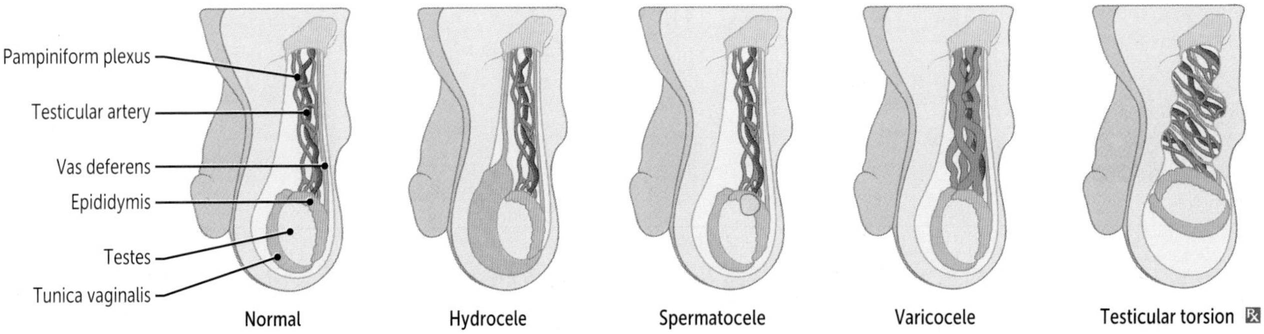
Pampiniform plexus
Testicular artery
Vas deferens
Epididymis
Testes
Tunica vaginalis
Normal
Hydrocele
Spermatocele
Varicocele
Testicular torsion

Testicular tumors Germ cell tumors account for ~ 95% of all testicular tumors. Arise from germ cells that produce sperm. Most often occur in young males. Risk factors: cryptorchidism, Klinefelter syndrome. Can present as a mixed germ cell tumor. Do not transilluminate. Usually not biopsied (risk of seeding scrotum), removed via radical orchiectomy.

Sex cord stromal tumors develop from embryonic sex cord (develops into Sertoli and Leydig cells of seminiferous tubules, theca and granulosa cells of follicle) derivatives. 5% of all testicular tumors. Mostly benign.

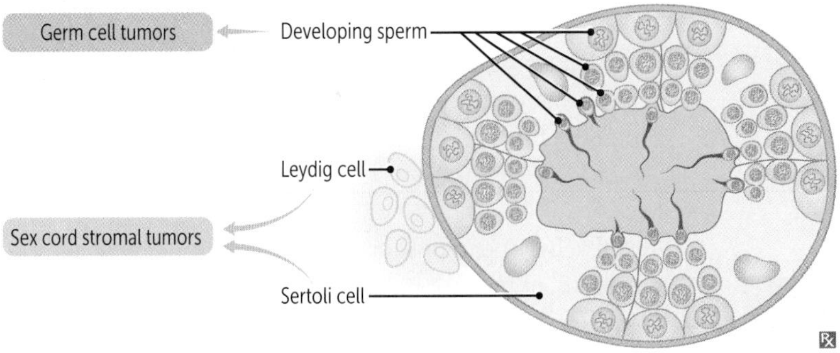
Germ cell tumors
Developing sperm
Leydig cell
Sex cord stromal tumors
Sertoli cell

Testicular tumors *(continued)*

TYPE	CHARACTERISTICS
Germ cell tumors	
Seminoma	Malignant. Painless, homogenous testicular enlargement. Most common testicular tumor. Analogous to ovarian dysgerminoma. Does not occur in infancy. Large cells in lobules with watery cytoplasm and "fried egg" appearance on histology, ↑ placental ALP (PALP). Highly radiosensitive. Late metastasis, excellent prognosis.
Embryonal carcinoma	Malignant. Painful, hemorrhagic mass with necrosis. Often glandular/papillary morphology. "Pure" embryonal carcinoma is rare; most commonly mixed with other tumor types. May present with metastases. May be associated with ↑ hCG and normal AFP levels when pure (↑ AFP when mixed). Worse prognosis than seminoma.
Teratoma	**M**ature teratoma may be **m**alignant in adult **m**ales. Benign in children and females.
Yolk sac tumor	Also called endodermal sinus tumor. Malignant, aggressive. Yellow, mucinous. Analogous to ovarian yolk sac tumor. **S**chiller-Duval bodies resemble primitive glomeruli. ↑ **A**FP is highly characteristic. Most common testicular tumor in **c**hildren < 3 years old.
Choriocarcinoma	Malignant. Disordered syncytiotrophoblastic and cytotrophoblastic elements. Hematogenous metastases to lungs and brain. ↑ hCG. May produce gynecomastia, symptoms of hyperthyroidism (α-subunit of hCG is identical to α-subunit of LH, FSH, TSH).
Non–germ cell tumors	
Leydig cell tumor	Mostly benign. Golden brown color; contains Reinke crystals (eosinophilic cytoplasmic inclusions). Produces androgens or estrogens → precocious puberty, gynecomastia.
Sertoli cell tumor	Also called androblas**toma** (arises from sex cord **stroma**). Mostly benign.
Primary testicular lymphoma	Malignant, aggressive. Typically diffuse large B-cell lymphoma. Most common testicular cancer in older males.

Hormone levels in germ cell tumors

	SEMINOMA	YOLK SAC TUMOR	CHORIOCARCINOMA	TERATOMA	EMBRYONAL CARCINOMA
PALP	↑	–	–	–	–
AFP	–	↑↑	–	–/↑	–/↑ (when mixed)
β-hCG	–/↑	–/↑	↑↑	–	↑

Epididymitis and orchitis

Most common causes:
- *C trachomatis* and *N gonorrhoeae* (young males)
- *E coli* and *Pseudomonas* (older males, associated with UTI and BPH)
- Autoimmune (eg, granulomas involving seminiferous tubules)

Epididymitis

Inflammation of epididymis. Presents with localized pain and tenderness over posterior testis. ⊕ Prehn sign (pain relief with scrotal elevation). May progress to involve testis.

Orchitis

Inflammation of testis. Presents with testicular pain and swelling. Mumps orchitis ↑ infertility risk. Rare in males < 10 years old.

Benign prostatic hyperplasia

Common in males > 50 years old.
Characterized by smooth, elastic, firm nodular enlargement (hyperplasia not hypertrophy) of periurethral (lateral and middle) lobes, which compress the urethra into a vertical slit. Not premalignant.
Often presents with ↑ frequency of urination, nocturia, difficulty starting and stopping urine stream, dysuria. May lead to distention and hypertrophy of bladder, hydronephrosis, UTIs.
↑ total PSA, with ↑ fraction of free PSA. PSA is made by prostatic epithelium stimulated by androgens.
Treatment: α_1-antagonists (terazosin, tamsulosin), which cause relaxation of smooth muscle; 5α-reductase inhibitors (eg, finasteride); PDE-5 inhibitors (eg, tadalafil); surgical resection (eg, TURP, ablation).

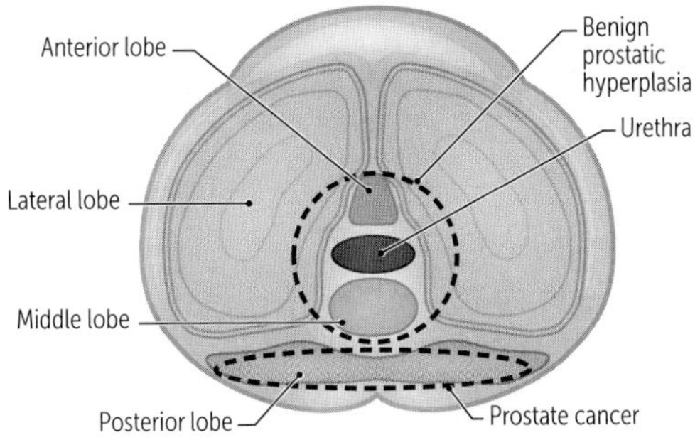

Prostatitis

Characterized by dysuria, frequency, urgency, low back pain. Warm, tender, enlarged prostate.
Acute bacterial prostatitis—in older males most common bacterium is *E coli*; in young males consider *C trachomatis*, *N gonorrhoeae*.
Chronic prostatitis—either bacterial or nonbacterial (eg, 2° to previous infection, nerve problems, chemical irritation).

Prostatic adenocarcinoma

Common in males > 50 years old. Arises most often from posterior lobe (peripheral zone) of prostate gland and is most frequently diagnosed by ↑ PSA and subsequent needle core biopsies (transrectal, ultrasound-guided). Histologically graded using **Gl**eason grade, which is based on **gl**andular architecture and correlates closely with metastatic potential. Prostatic acid phosphatase (PAP) and PSA are useful tumor markers (↑ total PSA, with ↓ fraction of free PSA). Osteoblastic metastases in bone may develop in late stages, as indicated by lower back pain and ↑ serum ALP and PSA. Metastasis to the spine often occurs via Batson (vertebral) venous plexus.

▸ REPRODUCTIVE—PHARMACOLOGY

Control of reproductive hormones

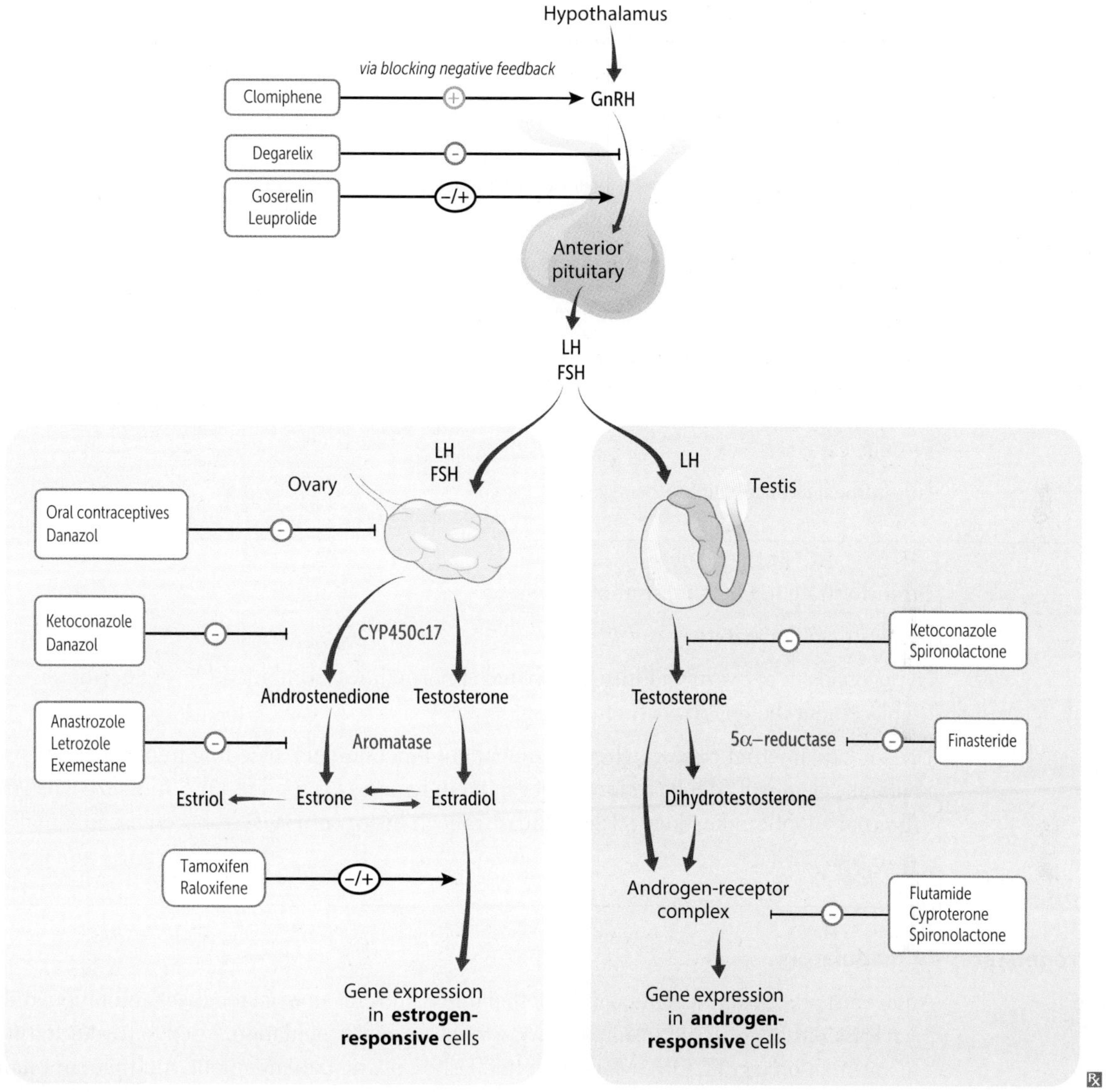

Gonadotropin-releasing hormone analogs	Leuprolide, goserelin, nafarelin, histrelin.
MECHANISM	Act as GnRH agonists when used in pulsatile fashion. When used in continuous fashion, first transiently act as GnRH agonists (tumor flare), but subsequently act as GnRH antagonists (downregulate GnRH receptor in pituitary → ↓ FSH and ↓ LH). Can be used in **lieu** of GnRH.
CLINICAL USE	Uterine fibroids, endometriosis, precocious puberty, prostate cancer, infertility. Pulsatile for pregnancy, continuous for cancer.
ADVERSE EFFECTS	Hypogonadism, ↓ libido, erectile dysfunction, nausea, vomiting.

Degarelix	
MECHANISM	GnRH antagonist. No start-up flare.
CLINICAL USE	Prostate cancer.
ADVERSE EFFECTS	Hot flashes, liver toxicity.

Estrogens	Ethinyl estradiol, DES, mestranol.
MECHANISM	Bind estrogen receptors.
CLINICAL USE	Hypogonadism or ovarian failure, menstrual abnormalities (combined OCPs), hormone replacement therapy in postmenopausal females.
ADVERSE EFFECTS	↑ risk of endometrial cancer (when given without progesterone), bleeding in postmenopausal patients, clear cell adenocarcinoma of vagina in females exposed to DES in utero, ↑ risk of thrombi. Contraindications—ER ⊕ breast cancer, history of DVTs, tobacco use in females > 35 years old.

Selective estrogen receptor modulators	
Clomiphene	Antagonist at estrogen receptors in hypothalamus. Prevents normal feedback inhibition and ↑ release of LH and FSH from pituitary, which stimulates ovulation. Used to treat infertility due to anovulation (eg, PCOS). May cause hot flashes, ovarian enlargement, multiple simultaneous pregnancies, visual disturbances.
Tamoxifen	Antagonist at breast, partial agonist at uterus, bone. Hot flashes, ↑ risk of thromboembolic events (especially with tobacco smoking), and endometrial cancer. Used to treat and prevent recurrence of ER/PR ⊕ breast cancer and to prevent gynecomastia in patients undergoing prostate cancer therapy.
Raloxifene	Antagonist at breast, uterus; agonist at bone; hot flashes, ↑ risk of thromboembolic events (especially with tobacco smoking), but no increased risk of endometrial cancer (vs tamoxifen, so you can "**relax**"); used primarily to treat osteoporosis.

Aromatase inhibitors	Anastrozole, letrozole, exemestane.
MECHANISM	Inhibit peripheral conversion of androgens to estrogen.
CLINICAL USE	ER ⊕ breast cancer in postmenopausal females.

Hormone replacement therapy	Used for relief or prevention of menopausal symptoms (eg, hot flashes, vaginal atrophy), osteoporosis (↑ estrogen, ↓ osteoclast activity). Unopposed estrogen replacement therapy ↑ risk of endometrial cancer, progesterone/progestin is added. Possible increased cardiovascular risk.

Progestins	Levonorgestrel, medroxyprogesterone, etonogestrel, norethindrone, megestrol.
MECHANISM	Bind progesterone receptors, ↓ growth and ↑ vascularization of endometrium, thicken cervical mucus.
CLINICAL USE	Contraception (forms include pill, intrauterine device, implant, depot injection), endometrial cancer, abnormal uterine bleeding. Progestin challenge: presence of bleeding upon withdrawal of progestins excludes anatomic defects (eg, Asherman syndrome) and chronic anovulation without estrogen.

Antiprogestins	Mifepristone, ulipristal.
MECHANISM	Competitive inhibitors of progestins at progesterone receptors.
CLINICAL USE	Termination of pregnancy (mifepristone with misoprostol); emergency contraception (ulipristal).

Combined contraception	Progestins and ethinyl estradiol; forms include pill, patch, vaginal ring. Estrogen and progestins inhibit LH/FSH and thus prevent estrogen surge. No estrogen surge → no LH surge → no ovulation. Progestins cause thickening of cervical mucus, thereby limiting access of sperm to uterus. Progestins also inhibit endometrial proliferation → endometrium is less suitable to the implantation of an embryo. Adverse effects: breakthrough menstrual bleeding, breast tenderness, VTE, hepatic adenomas. Contraindications: people > 35 years old who smoke tobacco (↑ risk of cardiovascular events), patients with ↑ risk of cardiovascular disease (including history of venous thromboembolism, coronary artery disease, stroke), migraine (especially with aura), breast cancer, liver disease.

Copper intrauterine device	
MECHANISM	Produces local inflammatory reaction toxic to sperm and ova, preventing fertilization and implantation; hormone free.
CLINICAL USE	Long-acting reversible contraception. Most effective emergency contraception.
ADVERSE EFFECTS	Heavier or longer menses, dysmenorrhea. Insertion contraindicated in active PID (IUD may impede PID resolution).

Tocolytics	Medications that relax the uterus; include terbutaline (β_2-agonist action), nifedipine (Ca^{2+} channel blocker), indomethacin (NSAID). Used to ↓ contraction frequency in preterm labor and allow time for administration of steroids (to promote fetal lung maturity) or transfer to appropriate medical center with obstetrical care.

Danazol

MECHANISM	Synthetic androgen that acts as partial agonist at androgen receptors.
CLINICAL USE	Endometriosis, hereditary angioedema.
ADVERSE EFFECTS	Weight gain, edema, acne, hirsutism, masculinization, ↓ HDL levels, hepatotoxicity, idiopathic intracranial hypertension.

Testosterone, methyltestosterone

MECHANISM	Agonists at androgen receptors.
CLINICAL USE	Treat hypogonadism and promote development of 2° sex characteristics; stimulate anabolism to promote recovery after burn or injury.
ADVERSE EFFECTS	Masculinization in females; ↓ intratesticular testosterone in males by inhibiting release of LH (via negative feedback) → gonadal atrophy. Premature closure of epiphyseal plates. ↑ LDL, ↓ HDL.

Antiandrogens

DRUG	MECHANISM	CLINICAL USE	ADVERSE EFFECTS
Abiraterone	17α-hydroxylase/17,20-lyase inhibitor (↓ steroid synthesis)	Prostate cancer	Hypertension, hypokalemia (↑ mineralocorticoids)
Finasteride	5α-reductase inhibitor (↓ conversion of testosterone to DHT)	BPH, male-pattern baldness	Gynecomastia, sexual dysfunction
Flutamide, bicalutamide	Nonsteroidal competitive inhibitors at androgen receptor (↓ steroid binding)	Prostate cancer	Gynecomastia, sexual dysfunction
Ketoconazole	17α-hydroxylase/17,20-lyase inhibitor	Prostate cancer	Gynecomastia
Spironolactone	Androgen receptor and 17α-hydroxylase/17,20-lyase inhibitor	PCOS	Amenorrhea

Tamsulosin

α_1-antagonist used to treat BPH by inhibiting smooth muscle contraction. Selective for $\alpha_{1A/D}$ receptors (found on prostate) vs vascular α_{1B} receptors.

Minoxidil

MECHANISM	Direct arteriolar vasodilator.
CLINICAL USE	Androgenetic alopecia (pattern baldness), severe refractory hypertension.

Respiratory

"There's so much pollution in the air now that if it weren't for our lungs, there'd be no place to put it all."

—Robert Orben

"Freedom is the oxygen of the soul."

—Moshe Dayan

"Whenever I feel blue, I start breathing again."

—L. Frank Baum

"Life is not the amount of breaths you take; it's the moments that take your breath away."

—Will Smith, *Hitch*

Group key respiratory, cardiovascular, and renal concepts together for study whenever possible. Respiratory physiology is challenging but high yield, especially as it relates to the pathophysiology of respiratory diseases. Develop a thorough understanding of normal respiratory function. Know obstructive vs restrictive lung disorders, $\dot{V}/\dot{Q}$ mismatch, lung volumes, mechanics of respiration, and hemoglobin physiology. Lung cancers and other causes of lung masses are also high yield. Be comfortable reading basic chest x-rays, CT scans, and PFTs.

▶ RESPIRATORY—EMBRYOLOGY

Lung development Occurs in five stages. Begins with the formation of lung bud from distal end of respiratory diverticulum during week 4 of development. Every pulmonologist can see alveoli.

STAGE	STRUCTURAL DEVELOPMENT	NOTES
Embryonic (weeks 4–7)	Lung bud → trachea → bronchial buds → mainstem bronchi → secondary (lobar) bronchi → tertiary (segmental) bronchi.	Errors at this stage can lead to tracheoesophageal fistula.
Pseudoglandular (weeks 5–17)	Endodermal tubules → terminal bronchioles. Surrounded by modest capillary network.	Respiration impossible, incompatible with life.
Canalicular (weeks 16–25)	Terminal bronchioles → respiratory bronchioles → alveolar ducts. Surrounded by prominent capillary network.	Airways increase in diameter. Pneumocytes develop starting at week 20 of development. Respiration capable at ~ week 25.
Saccular (week 24–birth)	Alveolar ducts → terminal sacs. Terminal sacs separated by 1° septae.	
Alveolar (week 36–8 years)	Terminal sacs → adult alveoli (due to 2° septation). In utero, "breathing" occurs via aspiration and expulsion of amniotic fluid → ↑ pulmonary vascular resistance through gestation. At birth, air replaces fluid → ↓ pulmonary vascular resistance.	

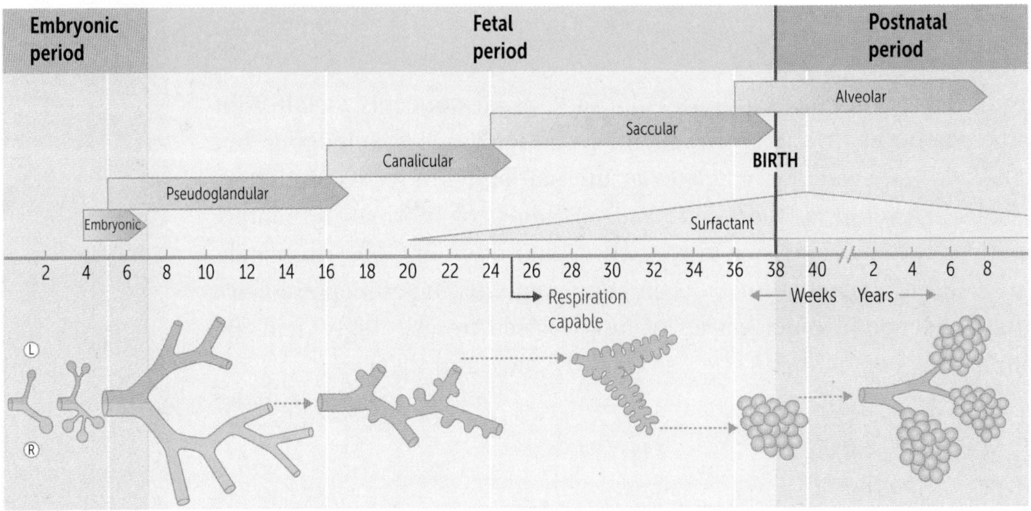

Congenital lung malformations

Pulmonary hypoplasia	Poorly developed bronchial tree with abnormal histology. Associated with congenital diaphragmatic hernia (usually left-sided), bilateral renal agenesis (Potter sequence).
Bronchogenic cysts	Caused by abnormal budding of the foregut and dilation of terminal or large bronchi. Discrete, round, sharply defined, fluid-filled densities on CXR (air-filled if infected). Generally asymptomatic but can drain poorly → airway compression, recurrent respiratory infections.

Club cells

Nonciliated; low columnar/cuboidal with secretory granules. Located in bronchioles. Degrade toxins via cytochrome P-450; secrete component of surfactant; progenitor cells for club and ciliated cells.

Alveolar cell types

Type I pneumocytes

Squamous. 97% of alveolar surfaces. Thinly line the alveoli (two black arrows in A) for optimal gas exchange.

Type II pneumocytes

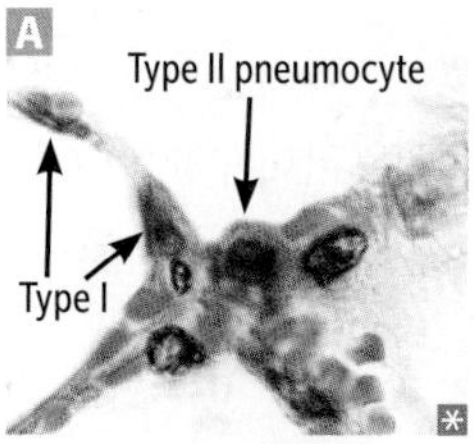

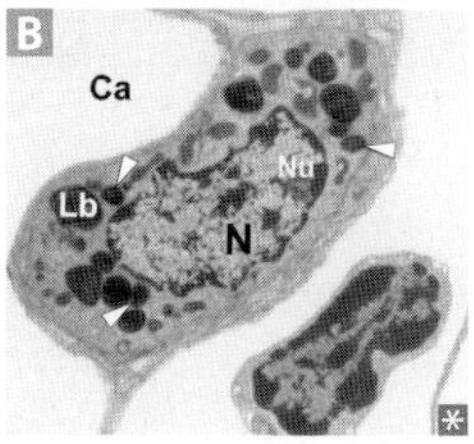

Cuboidal and clustered A.
2 functions:
1. Serve as stem cell precursors for 2 cell types (type I and type II cells); proliferate during lung damage.
2. Secrete surfactant from lamellar bodies (arrowheads in B).

Surfactant— ↓ alveolar surface tension, ↓ alveolar collapse, ↓ lung recoil, and ↑ compliance.

Composed of multiple lecithins, mainly dipalmitoylphosphatidylcholine (DPPC).
Synthesis begins ~20 weeks' gestation and achieves mature levels ~35 weeks of gestation.
Corticosteroids important for fetal surfactant synthesis and lung development.

$$\text{Collapsing pressure } (P) = \frac{2\text{ (surface tension)}}{\text{radius}}$$

Law of Laplace—Alveoli have ↑ tendency to collapse on expiration as radius ↓.

Alveolar macrophages

Phagocytose foreign materials; release cytokines and alveolar proteases. Hemosiderin-laden macrophages (heart failure cells) may be found in the setting of pulmonary edema or alveolar hemorrhage.

Neonatal respiratory distress syndrome

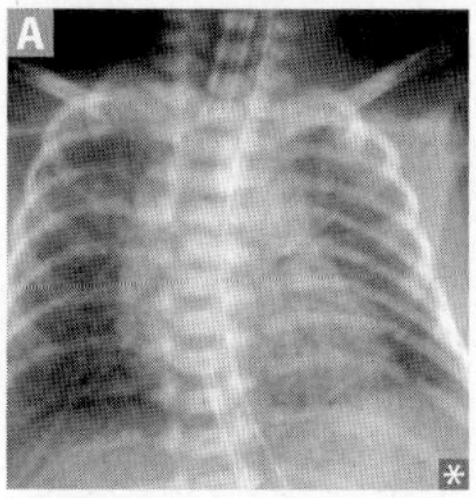

Surfactant deficiency → ↑ surface tension → alveolar collapse ("ground-glass" appearance of lung fields) A.

Risk factors: prematurity, diabetes during pregnancy (due to ↑ fetal insulin), C-section delivery (↓ release of fetal glucocorticoids; less stressful than vaginal delivery).

Treatment: maternal steroids before birth; exogenous surfactant for infant.

Therapeutic supplemental O_2 can result in **R**etinopathy of prematurity, **I**ntraventricular hemorrhage, **B**ronchopulmonary dysplasia (**RIB**).

Screening tests for fetal lung maturity: lecithin-sphingomyelin (L/S) ratio in amniotic fluid (≥ 2 is healthy; < 1.5 predictive of NRDS), foam stability index, surfactant-albumin ratio.

Persistently low O_2 tension → risk of PDA.

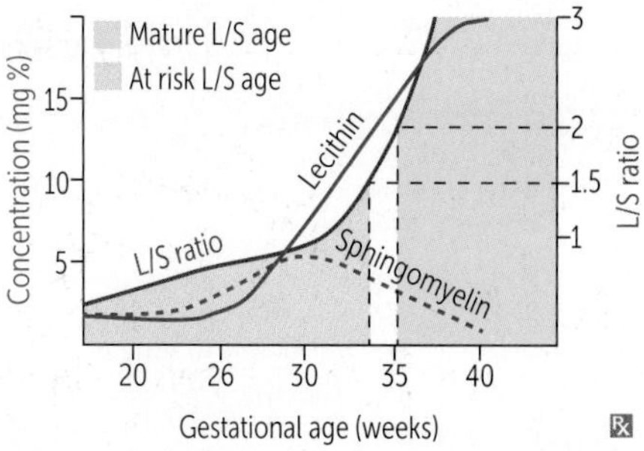

▶ RESPIRATORY—ANATOMY

Respiratory tree

Conducting zone	Large airways consist of nose, pharynx, larynx, trachea, and bronchi. Airway resistance highest in the large- to medium-sized bronchi. Small airways consist of bronchioles that further divide into terminal bronchioles (large numbers in parallel → least airway resistance). Warms, humidifies, and filters air but does not participate in gas exchange → "anatomic dead space." Cartilage and goblet cells extend to the end of bronchi. Pseudostratified ciliated columnar cells primarily make up epithelium of bronchus and extend to beginning of terminal bronchioles, then transition to cuboidal cells. Clear mucus and debris from lungs (mucociliary escalator). Airway smooth muscle cells extend to end of terminal bronchioles (sparse beyond this point).
Respiratory zone	Lung parenchyma; consists of respiratory bronchioles, alveolar ducts, and alveoli. Participates in gas exchange. Mostly cuboidal cells in respiratory bronchioles, then simple squamous cells up to alveoli. Cilia terminate in respiratory bronchioles. Alveolar macrophages clear debris and participate in immune response.

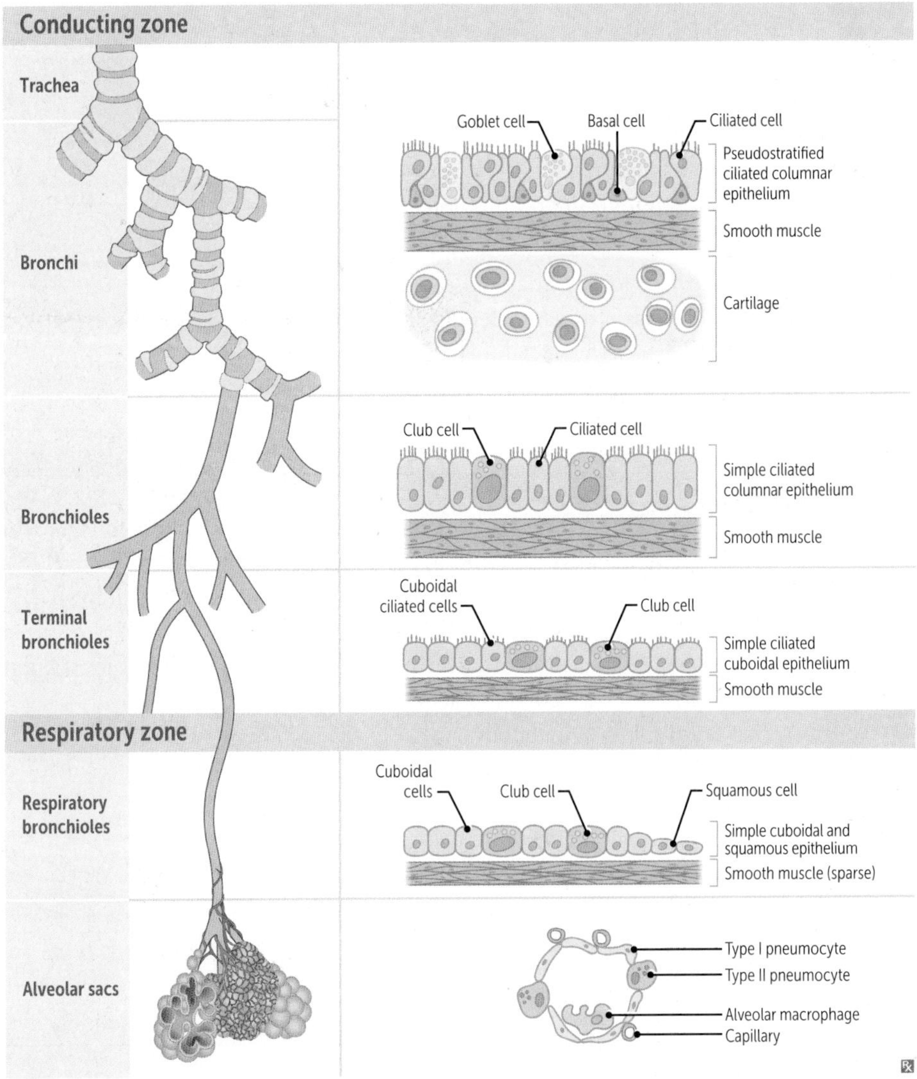

Lung anatomy

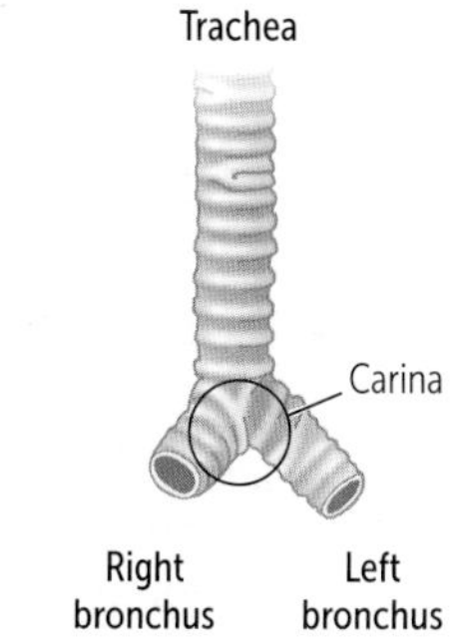
Trachea
Carina
Right bronchus
Left bronchus

Right lung has 3 lobes; Left has less lobes (2) and lingula (homolog of right middle lobe). Instead of a middle lobe, left lung has a space occupied by the heart A.

Relation of the pulmonary artery to the bronchus at each lung hilum is described by **RALS**—**R**ight **A**nterior; **L**eft **S**uperior. Carina is posterior to ascending aorta and anteromedial to descending aorta B.

Right lung is a more common site for inhaled foreign bodies because right main stem bronchus is wider, more vertical, and shorter than the left. If you aspirate a peanut:

- While supine—usually enters superior segment of right lower lobe.
- While lying on right side—usually enters right upper lobe.
- While upright—usually enters right lower lobe.

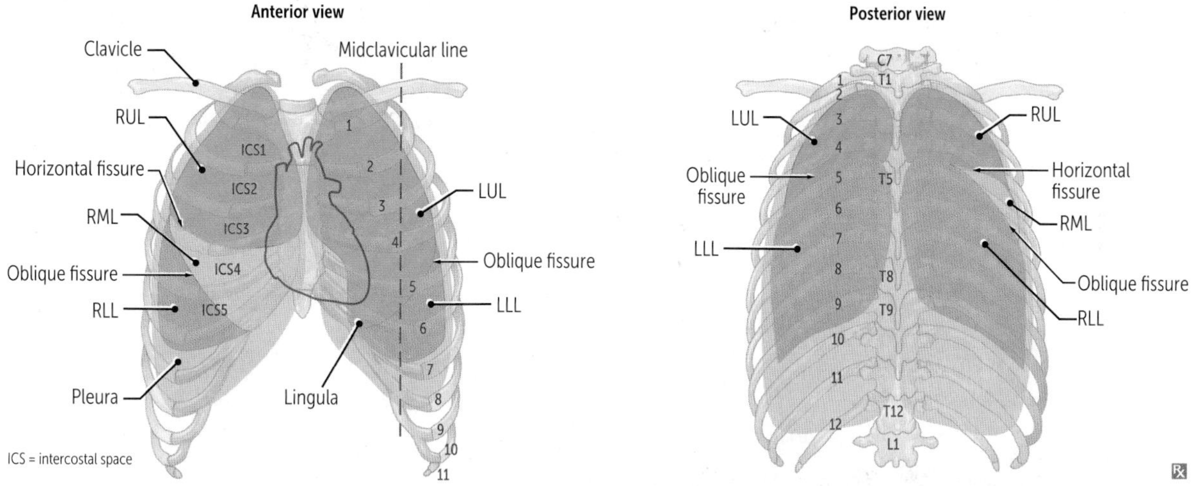
Anterior view
Clavicle
Midclavicular line
RUL
Horizontal fissure
RML
Oblique fissure
RLL
Pleura
ICS1
ICS2
ICS3
ICS4
ICS5
LUL
Oblique fissure
LLL
Lingula
ICS = intercostal space
Posterior view
C7
T1
T5
T8
T9
T12
L1
LUL
Oblique fissure
LLL
RUL
Horizontal fissure
RML
Oblique fissure
RLL

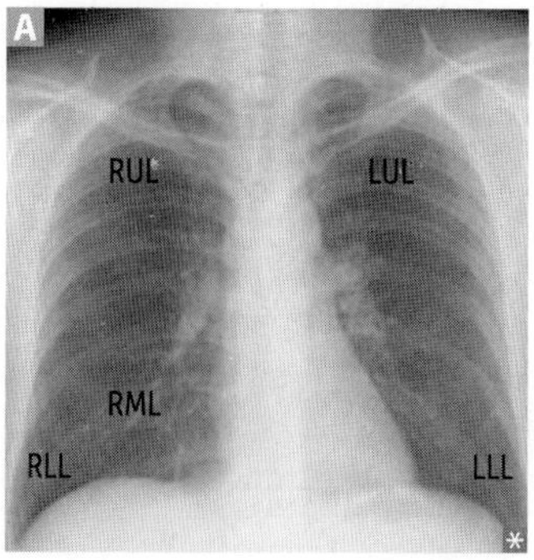
A
RUL
LUL
RML
RLL
LLL

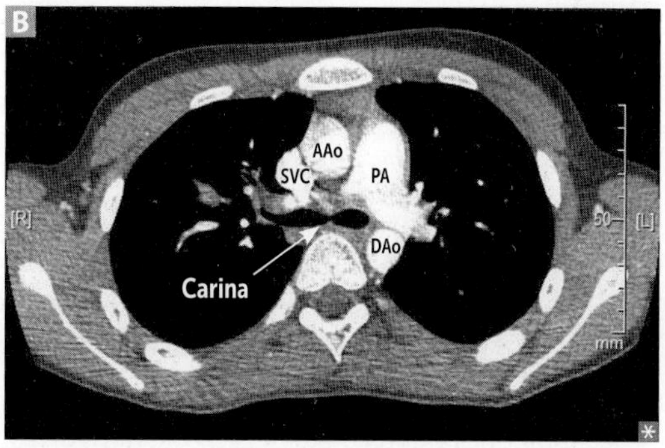
B
AAo
SVC
PA
DAo
Carina

Diaphragm structures

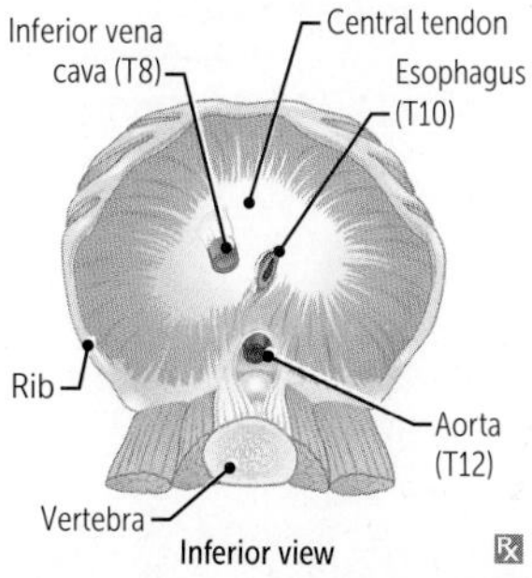
Inferior vena cava (T8)
Central tendon
Esophagus (T10)
Rib
Aorta (T12)
Vertebra
Inferior view

Structures perforating diaphragm:

- At T8: IVC, right phrenic nerve
- At T10: esophagus, vagus (CN 10; 2 trunks)
- At T12: aorta (red), thoracic duct (white), azygos vein (blue) ("At **T-1-2** it's the **red, white, and blue**")

Diaphragm is innervated by C3, 4, and 5 (phrenic nerve). Pain from diaphragm irritation (eg, air, blood, or pus in peritoneal cavity) can be referred to shoulder (C5) and trapezius ridge (C3, 4).

Number of letters = T level:

T8: vena cava (IVC)
T10: (O)esophagus
T12: aortic hiatus

I ate (8) **ten eggs at twelve.**

C3, 4, 5 keeps the diaphragm **alive.**

Other bifurcations:

- The **C**ommon **C**arotid **bifour**cates at **C4**.
- The **T**rachea **bifour**cates at **T4**.
- The abdominal aorta **bifour**cates at **L4**.

▸ RESPIRATORY—PHYSIOLOGY

Lung volumes and capacities — Note: a capacity is a sum of ≥ 2 physiologic volumes.

Tidal volume	Air that moves into lung with each quiet inspiration, typically 500 mL
Inspiratory reserve volume	Air that can still be breathed in after normal inspiration
Expiratory reserve volume	Air that can still be breathed out after normal expiration
Residual volume	Air in lung after maximal expiration; RV and any lung capacity that includes RV cannot be measured by spirometry
Inspiratory capacity	IRV + TV Air that can be breathed in after normal exhalation
Functional residual capacity	RV + ERV Volume of gas in lungs after normal expiration; outward pulling force of chest wall is balanced with inward collapsing force of lungs
Vital capacity	IRV + TV + ERV Maximum volume of gas that can be expired after a maximal inspiration
Total lung capacity	IRV + TV + ERV + RV = VC + RV Volume of gas present in lungs after a maximal inspiration

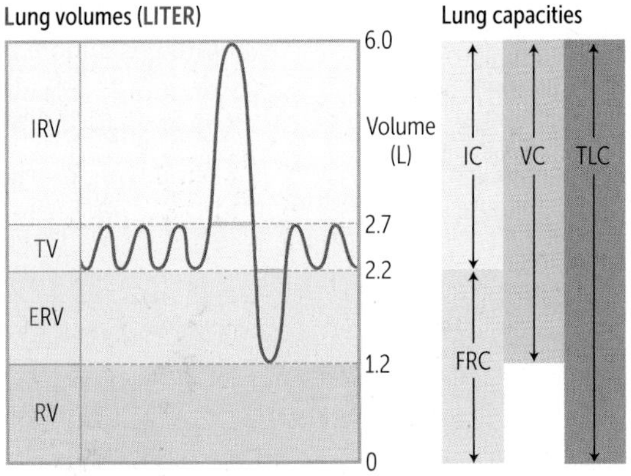

IRV = inspiratory reserve volume
TV = tidal volume
ERV = expiratory reserve volume
RV = residual volume
IC = inspiratory capacity
FRC = functional residual capacity
VC = vital capacity
TLC = total lung capacity

Determination of physiologic dead space

$$V_D = V_T \times \frac{Pa_{CO_2} - Pe_{CO_2}}{Pa_{CO_2}}$$

V_D = physiologic dead space = anatomic dead space of conducting airways plus alveolar dead space; apex of healthy lung is largest contributor of alveolar dead space. Volume of inspired air that does not take part in gas exchange.

V_T = tidal volume.

Pa_{CO_2} = arterial P_{CO_2}.

Pe_{CO_2} = expired air P_{CO_2}.

Physiologic dead space—approximately equivalent to anatomic dead space in normal lungs. May be greater than anatomic dead space in lung diseases with $\dot{V}/\dot{Q}$ mismatch.

Ventilation

Minute ventilation	Abbreviated as V_E. Total volume of gas entering lungs per minute $V_E = V_T \times RR$	Normal values: ▪ Respiratory rate (RR) = 12–20 breaths/min ▪ V_T = 500 mL/breath ▪ V_D = 150 mL/breath
Alveolar ventilation	Abbreviated as V_A. Volume of gas that reaches alveoli each minute $V_A = (V_T - V_D) \times RR$	

Lung and chest wall

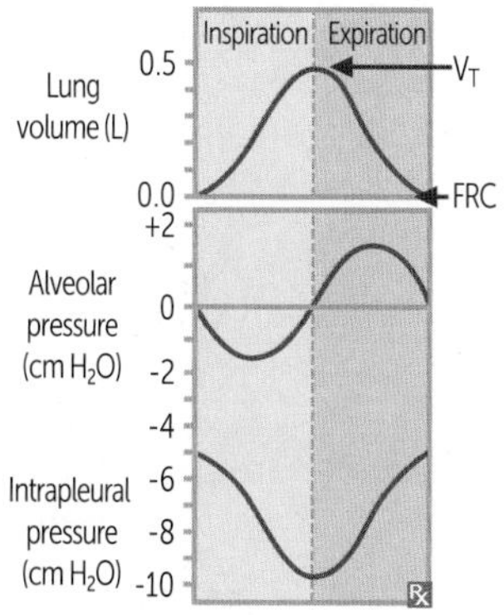

Elastic recoil	Tendency for lungs to collapse inward and chest wall to spring outward. At FRC, airway and alveolar pressures equal atmospheric pressure (called zero), and intrapleural pressure is negative (preventing atelectasis). The inward pull of the lung is balanced by the outward pull of the chest wall. System pressure is atmospheric. Pulmonary vascular resistance (PVR) is at a minimum.
Compliance	Change in lung volume for a change in pressure ($\Delta V/\Delta P$). Inversely proportional to wall stiffness and increased by surfactant. ▪ ↑ compliance = lung easier to fill (eg, emphysema, aging) ▪ ↓ compliance = lung harder to fill (eg, pulmonary fibrosis, pneumonia, ARDS, pulmonary edema)
Hysteresis	Lung inflation follows a different pressure-volume curve than lung deflation due to need to overcome surface tension forces in inflation.

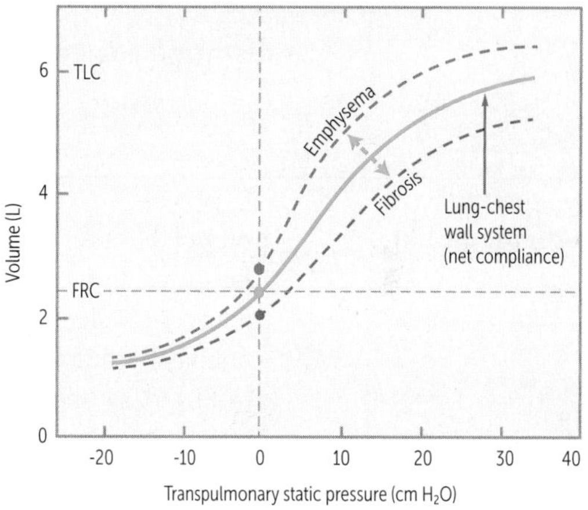

Respiratory system changes in the elderly

Aging is associated with progressive ↓ in lung function. TLC remains the same.

INCREASED	DECREASED
Lung compliance (loss of elastic recoil)	Chest wall compliance (↑ chest wall stiffness)
RV	FVC and FEV_1
$\dot{V}/\dot{Q}$ mismatch	Respiratory muscle strength (can impair cough)
A-a gradient	Ventilatory response to hypoxia/hypercapnia

Hemoglobin

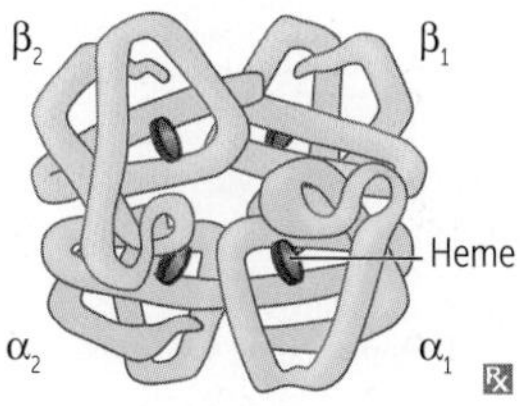

Normal adult hemoglobin (Hb) is composed of 4 polypeptide subunits (2 α and 2 β) that each bind one O_2 molecule. Hb is an allosteric protein that exhibits positive cooperativity when binding to O_2, such that:

- Oxygenated Hb has high affinity for O_2 (300×).
- Deoxygenated Hb has low affinity for O_2 → promotes release/unloading of O_2.

The protein component of hemoglobin acts as buffer for H^+ ions.

Myoglobin is composed of a single polypeptide chain associated with one heme moiety. Higher affinity for oxygen than Hb.

Oxygen content of blood

O_2 content = (1.34 × Hb × Sao_2) + (0.003 × Pao_2).
Hb = hemoglobin concentration; Sao_2 = arterial O_2 saturation.
Pao_2 = partial pressure of O_2 in arterial blood.

Normally 1 g Hb can bind 1.34 mL O_2; normal Hb amount in blood is 15 g/dL.
O_2 binding capacity ≈ 20 mL O_2/dL of blood.
With ↓ Hb there is ↓ O_2 content of arterial blood, but no change in O_2 saturation and Pao_2.
O_2 delivery to tissues = cardiac output × O_2 content of blood.

	Hb CONCENTRATION	% O_2 SAT OF Hb	DISSOLVED O_2 (Pao_2)	TOTAL O_2 CONTENT
CO poisoning	Normal	↓ (CO competes with O_2)	Normal	↓
Anemia	↓	Normal	Normal	↓
Polycythemia	↑	Normal	Normal	↑
Methemoglobinemia	Normal	↓ (Fe^{3+} poor at binding O_2)	Normal	↓
Cyanide toxicity	Normal	Normal	Normal	Normal

Methemoglobin

Iron in Hb is normally in a reduced state (ferrous Fe^{2+}; "just the 2 of **us**"). Oxidized form of Hb (ferric, Fe^{3+}) does not bind O_2 as readily as Fe^{2+}, but has ↑ affinity for cyanide → tissue hypoxia from ↓ O_2 saturation and ↓ O_2 content.
Methemoglobinemia may present with cyanosis (does not improve with supplemental O_2) or with chocolate-colored blood.

Dapsone, local anesthetics (eg, benzocaine), and nitrites (eg, from dietary intake or polluted/high-altitude water sources) cause poisoning by oxidizing Fe^{2+} to Fe^{3+}.
Methemoglobinemia can be treated with **meth**ylene blue and vitamin C.

Oxygen-hemoglobin dissociation curve

ODC has sigmoidal shape due to positive cooperativity (ie, tetrameric Hb molecule can bind 4 O_2 molecules and has higher affinity for each subsequent O_2 molecule bound). Myoglobin is monomeric and thus does not show positive cooperativity; curve lacks sigmoidal appearance.
Shifting ODC to the right → ↓ Hb affinity for O_2 (facilitates unloading of O_2 to tissue) → ↑ P_{50} (higher Po_2 required to maintain 50% saturation). In peripheral tissue, ↑ H^+ from tissue metabolism shifts curve to right, unloading O_2 (Bohr effect).
Shifting ODC to the left → ↓ O_2 unloading → renal hypoxia → ↑ EPO synthesis → compensatory erythrocytosis.
Fetal Hb (2 α and 2 γ subunits) has higher affinity for O_2 than adult Hb (due to ↓ affinity for 2,3-BPG) → dissociation curve is shifted left, driving diffusion of O_2 across the placenta from pregnant patient to fetus.

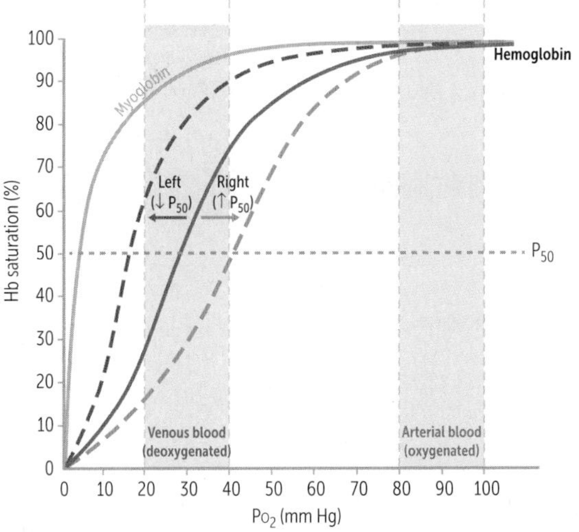

Left shift (↓ O_2 unloading to tissue) Left = lower	Right shift (↑ O_2 unloading to tissues) ACE BATs right handed
↓ H^+ (↑ pH, base) ↓ Pco_2 ↓ 2,3-BPG ↓ Temperature ↑ CO ↑ MetHb ↑ HbF	↑ H^+ (↓ pH, **A**cid) ↑ Pco_2 **E**xercise ↑ 2,3-**BP**G High **A**ltitude ↑ **T**emperature

Cyanide vs carbon monoxide poisoning	Both inhibit aerobic metabolism via inhibition of complex IV of ETC (cytochrome c oxidase) → hypoxia that does not fully correct with supplemental O_2 and ↑ anaerobic metabolism.	
	Cyanide	**Carbon monoxide**
EXPOSURE	Synthetic product combustion, amygdalin ingestion (found in apricot seeds), cyanide ingestion (eg, in suicide attempts), fire victims.	Motor exhaust, gas heaters, fire victims.
PRESENTATION	Headache, dyspnea, drowsiness, seizure, coma. May have cherry red skin. Breath may have bitter almond odor.	Headache, vomiting, confusion, visual disturbances, coma. May have cherry-red skin with bullous skin lesions. Multiple victims may be involved (eg, family due to faulty furnace).
LABS 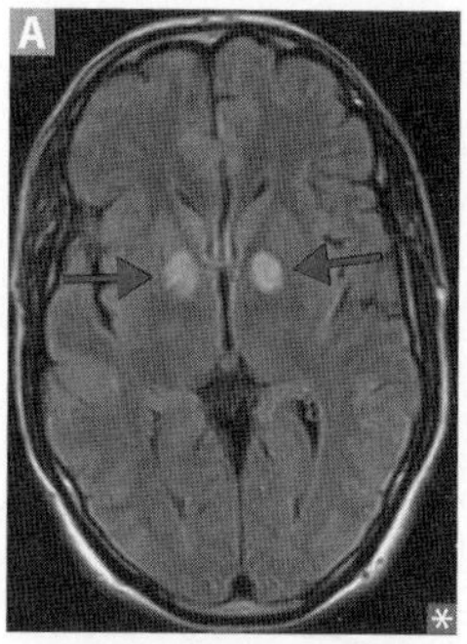	Normal PaO_2. Elevated lactate → metabolic acidosis.	Normal PaO_2. Elevated carboxyhemoglobin on co-oximetry. Classically associated with bilateral globus pallidus lesions on MRI A, although can rarely be seen with cyanide toxicity.
EFFECT ON OXYGEN-HEMOGLOBIN CURVE	Curve normal. Oxygen saturation may appear normal initially. Despite ample O_2 supply, it cannot be used due to ineffective oxidative phosphorylation.	Left shift in curve → ↑ affinity for O_2 → ↓ O_2 unloading in tissues. Binds competitively to Hb with > 200× greater affinity than O_2 to form carboxyhemoglobin → ↓ %O_2 saturation of Hb.
TREATMENT	Decontamination (eg, remove clothing). Hydroxocobalamin (binds cyanide → cyanocobalamin → renal excretion). Nitrites (oxidize Hb → methemoglobin → binds cyanide → cyanomethemoglobin → ↓ toxicity). Sodium thiosulfate (↑ cyanide conversion to thiocyanate → renal excretion).	100% O_2. Hyperbaric oxygen if severe.

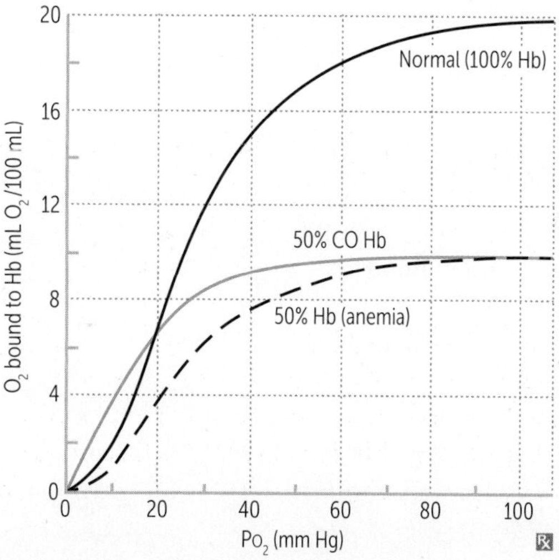
Normal (100% Hb)
50% CO Hb
50% Hb (anemia)
O2 bound to Hb (mL O2/100 mL)
Po2 (mm Hg)
0
4
8
12
16
20
0
20
40
60
80
100

Pulmonary circulation

Normally a low-resistance, high-compliance system. A ↓ in PAO_2 causes a hypoxic vasoconstriction that shifts blood away from poorly ventilated regions of lung to well-ventilated regions of lung.

Perfusion limited—O_2 (normal health), CO_2, N_2O. Gas equilibrates early along the length of the capillary. Exchange can be ↑ only if blood flow ↑.

Diffusion limited—O_2 (emphysema, fibrosis, exercise), CO. Gas does not equilibrate by the time blood reaches the end of the capillary.

O_2 diffuses slowly, while CO_2 diffuses very rapidly across the alveolar membrane. Disease states that lead to diffusion limitation (eg, pulmonary fibrosis) are more likely to cause early hypoxia than hypercapnia.

Chronic hypoxic vasoconstriction may lead to pulmonary hypertension +/– cor pulmonale.

Diffusion: $\dot{V}_{gas} = A \times D_k \times \frac{P_1 - P_2}{\Delta_x}$ where

A = area, Δ_x = alveolar wall thickness, D_k = diffusion coefficient of gas, $P_1 - P_2$ = difference in partial pressures.

- A ↓ in emphysema.
- Δ_x ↑ in pulmonary fibrosis.

DLCO is the extent to which CO passes from air sacs of lungs into blood.

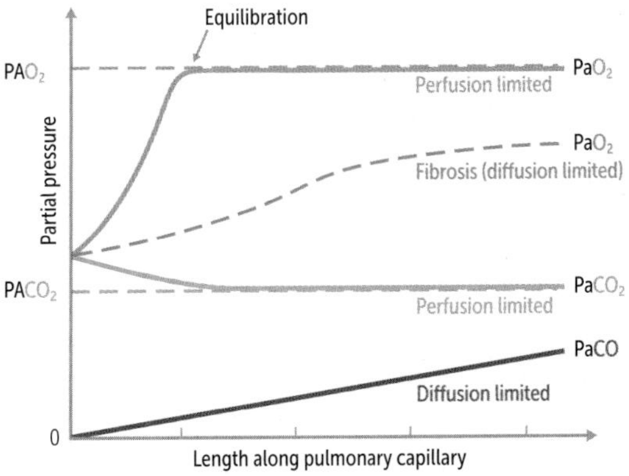

Pa = partial pressure of gas in pulmonary capillary blood
PA = partial pressure of gas in alveolar air

Pulmonary vascular resistance

$$PVR = \frac{P_{pulm\ artery} - P_{L\ atrium}}{Q}$$

Remember: $\Delta P = Q \times R$, so $R = \Delta P / Q$

$$R = \frac{8\eta l}{\pi r^4}$$

$P_{pulm\ artery}$ = pressure in pulmonary artery

$P_{L\ atrium}$ ≈ pulmonary artery occlusion pressure (also called pulmonary capillary wedge pressure)

Q = cardiac output (flow)

R = resistance

η = viscosity of blood

l = vessel length

r = vessel radius

Alveolar gas equation

$$PAO_2 = PIO_2 - \frac{PaCO_2}{R}$$

$$\approx 150 \text{ mm Hg}^{a} - \frac{PaCO_2}{0.8}$$

[a]At sea level breathing room air

PAO_2 = alveolar PO_2 (mm Hg)

PIO_2 = PO_2 in inspired air (mm Hg)

$PaCO_2$ = arterial PCO_2 (mm Hg)

R = respiratory quotient = CO_2 produced/O_2 consumed

A-a gradient = $PAO_2 - PaO_2$. Normal A-a gradient estimated as (age/4) + 4 (eg, for a person <40 years old, gradient should be <14).

Oxygen deprivation

Hypoxia (↓ O_2 delivery to tissue)	Hypoxemia (↓ Pao_2)	Ischemia (loss of blood flow)
↓ cardiac output Hypoxemia Ischemia Anemia CO/cyanide poisoning	Normal A-a gradient ▪ High altitude (↓ barometric pressure) ▪ Hypoventilation (eg, opioid use, obesity hypoventilation syndrome) ↑ A-a gradient ▪ $\dot{V}/\dot{Q}$ mismatch ▪ Diffusion limitation (eg, fibrosis) ▪ Right-to-left shunt	Impeded arterial flow ↓ venous drainage

Ventilation/perfusion mismatch

Ideally, ventilation is matched to perfusion (ie, $\dot{V}/\dot{Q} = 1$) for adequate gas exchange.

Lung zones:
- $\dot{V}/\dot{Q}$ at apex of lung = 3 (wasted ventilation)
- $\dot{V}/\dot{Q}$ at base of lung = 0.6 (wasted perfusion)

Both ventilation and perfusion are greater at the base of the lung than at the apex of the lung.

With exercise (↑ cardiac output), there is vasodilation of apical capillaries → $\dot{V}/\dot{Q}$ ratio approaches 1.

Certain organisms that thrive in high O_2 (eg, TB) flourish in the apex.

$\dot{V}/\dot{Q} = 0$ = "oirway" obstruction (shunt). In shunt, 100% O_2 does not improve Pao_2 (eg, foreign body aspiration).

$\dot{V}/\dot{Q} = \infty$ = blood flow obstruction (physiologic dead space). Assuming < 100% dead space, 100% O_2 improves Pao_2 (eg, pulmonary embolus).

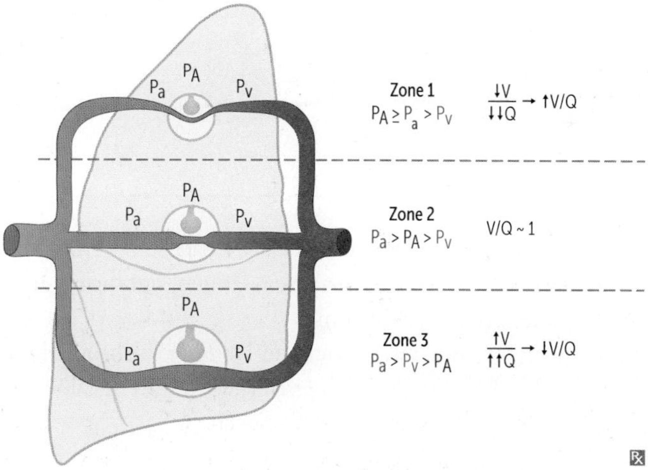

Carbon dioxide transport

CO_2 is transported from tissues to lungs in 3 forms:

❶ HCO_3^- (70%). HCO_3^-/Cl^- transporter on RBC membrane allows HCO_3^- to diffuse out to plasma and Cl^- to diffuse into RBC (chloride shift).

❷ Carbaminohemoglobin or $HbCO_2$ (21–25%). CO_2 bound to Hb at N-terminus of globin (not heme). CO_2 favors deoxygenated form (O_2 unloaded).

❸ Dissolved CO_2 (5–9%).

In lungs, oxygenation of Hb promotes dissociation of H^+ from Hb. This shifts equilibrium toward CO_2 formation; therefore, CO_2 is released from RBCs (Haldane effect).

Majority of blood CO_2 is carried as HCO_3^- in the plasma.

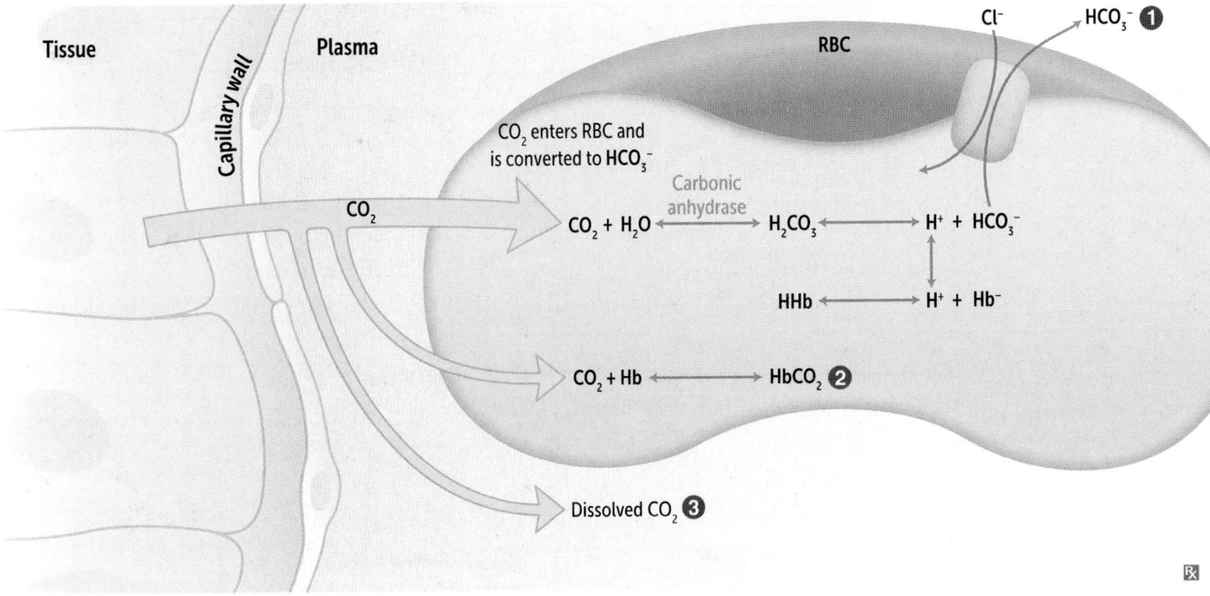

Response to high altitude

↓ atmospheric oxygen (PiO_2) → ↓ Pao_2 → ↑ ventilation → ↓ $Paco_2$ → respiratory alkalosis → altitude sickness (headaches, nausea, fatigue, lightheadedness, sleep disturbance).

Chronic ↑ in ventilation.

↑ erythropoietin → ↑ Hct and Hb (due to chronic hypoxia).

↑ 2,3-BPG (binds to Hb → rightward shift of ODC dissociation curve → ↑ O_2 release).

Cellular changes (↑ mitochondria).

↑ renal excretion of HCO_3^- to compensate for respiratory alkalosis (can augment with acetazolamide).

Chronic hypoxic pulmonary vasoconstriction → ↑ pulmonary vascular resistance → pulmonary hypertension, RVH.

Response to exercise

↑ CO_2 production.

↑ O_2 consumption.

Right shift of ODC.

↑ ventilation to meet O_2 demand and remove excess CO_2.

$\dot{V}/\dot{Q}$ ratio from apex to base becomes more uniform.

↑ pulmonary blood flow due to ↑ cardiac output.

↓ pH during strenuous exercise (2° to lactic acidosis).

No change in Pao_2 and $Paco_2$, but ↑ in venous CO_2 content and ↓ in venous O_2 content.

▶ RESPIRATORY—PATHOLOGY

Rhinosinusitis

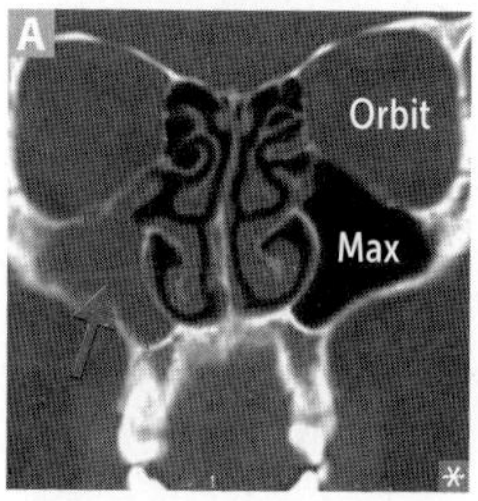

Obstruction of sinus drainage into nasal cavity → inflammation and pain over affected area. Typically affects maxillary sinuses, which drain against gravity due to ostia located superomedially (red arrow points to fluid-filled right maxillary sinus in A).

Superior meatus—drains sphenoid, posterior ethmoid; middle meatus—drains frontal, maxillary, and anterior ethmoid; inferior meatus—drains nasolacrimal duct.

Acute rhinosinusitis is most commonly caused by viruses (eg, rhinovirus); may lead to superimposed bacterial infection, most commonly *H influenzae*, *S pneumoniae*, *M catarrhalis.*

Paranasal sinus infections may extend to the orbits, cavernous sinus, and brain, causing complications (eg, orbital cellulitis, cavernous sinus syndrome, meningitis).

Epistaxis

Nose bleed. Most commonly occurs in anterior segment of nostril (**Kiesselbach plexus**). Life-threatening hemorrhages occur in posterior segment (sphenopalatine artery, a branch of maxillary artery). Common causes include foreign body, trauma, allergic rhinitis, and nasal angiofibromas (common in adolescent males).

Kiesselbach drives his **Lexus** with his **LEGS**: superior **L**abial artery, anterior and posterior **E**thmoidal arteries, **G**reater palatine artery, **S**phenopalatine artery.

Head and neck cancer

Mostly squamous cell carcinoma. Risk factors include tobacco, alcohol, HPV-16 (oropharyngeal), EBV (nasopharyngeal). Field cancerization: carcinogen damages wide mucosal area → multiple tumors that develop independently after exposure.

Nasopharyngeal carcinoma may present with unilateral nasal obstruction, discharge, epistaxis. Eustachian tube obstruction may lead to otitis media +/– effusion, hearing loss.

Deep venous thrombosis

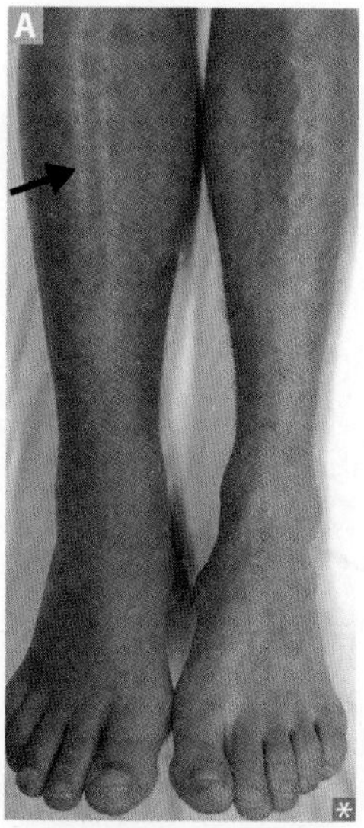

Blood clot within a deep vein → swelling, redness A, warmth, pain. Predisposed by Virchow triad (**SHE**):
- **S**tasis (eg, post-op, long drive/flight)
- **H**ypercoagulability (eg, defect in coagulation cascade proteins, such as factor V Leiden; oral contraceptive use; pregnancy)
- **E**ndothelial damage (exposed collagen triggers clotting cascade)

Most pulmonary emboli arise from proximal deep veins of lower extremity (iliac, femoral, popliteal veins).

D-dimer test may be used clinically to rule out DVT if disease probability is low or moderate (high sensitivity, low specificity).

Imaging test of choice is compression ultrasound with Doppler.

Use unfractionated heparin or low-molecular weight heparins (eg, enoxaparin) for prophylaxis and acute management.

Use direct anticoagulants (eg, rivaroxaban, apixaban) for treatment and long-term prevention.

Pulmonary emboli

Obstruction of the pulmonary artery or its branches by foreign material (usually thrombus) that originated elsewhere. Affected alveoli are ventilated but not perfused ($\dot{V}/\dot{Q}$ mismatch). May present with sudden-onset dyspnea, pleuritic chest pain, tachypnea, tachycardia, hypoxemia, respiratory alkalosis. Large emboli or saddle embolus A may cause sudden death due to electromechanical dissociation (pulseless electrical activity). CT pulmonary angiography is imaging test of choice for PE (look for filling defects) B. ECG may show sinus tachycardia or, less commonly, S1Q3T3 abnormality.

Lines of Zahn C are interdigitating areas of pink (platelets, fibrin) and red (RBCs) found only in thrombi formed before death; help distinguish pre- and postmortem thrombi.

Treatment: anticoagulation (eg, heparin, direct thrombin/factor Xa inhibitors), IVC filter (if anticoagulation is contraindicated).

Types: **F**at, **A**ir, **T**hrombus, **B**acteria, **A**mniotic fluid, **T**umor. An embolus moves like a **FAT BAT**.

Fat emboli—associated with long bone fractures and liposuction; classic triad of hypoxemia, neurologic abnormalities, petechial rash.

Air emboli—nitrogen bubbles precipitate in ascending divers (caisson disease/decompression sickness); treat with hyperbaric O_2; or, can be iatrogenic 2° to invasive procedures (eg, central line placement).

Amniotic fluid emboli—typically occurs during labor or postpartum, but can be due to uterine trauma. Can lead to DIC. Rare, but high mortality.

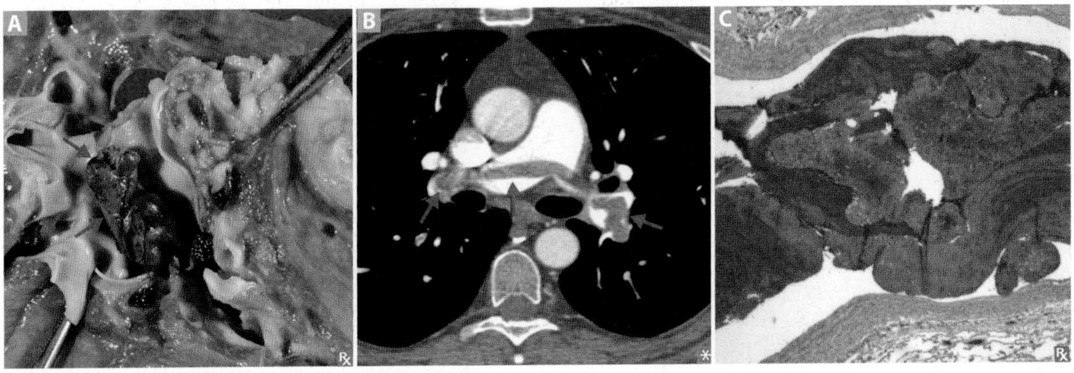

Mediastinal pathology

Normal mediastinum contains heart, thymus, lymph nodes, esophagus, and aorta.

Mediastinal masses

Some pathologies (eg, lymphoma, lung cancer, abscess) can occur in any compartment, but there are common associations:

- Anterior—4 T's: thyroid (substernal goiter), thymic neoplasm, teratoma, "terrible" lymphoma.
- Middle—esophageal carcinoma, metastases, hiatal hernia, bronchogenic cysts.
- Posterior—neurogenic tumor (eg, neurofibroma), multiple myeloma.

Mediastinitis

Inflammation of mediastinal tissues. Commonly due to postoperative complications of cardiothoracic procedures (≤ 14 days), esophageal perforation, or contiguous spread of odontogenic/retropharyngeal infection.

Chronic mediastinitis—also known as fibrosing mediastinitis; due to ↑ proliferation of connective tissue in mediastinum. *Histoplasma capsulatum* is common cause.

Clinical features: fever, tachycardia, leukocytosis, chest pain, and sternal wound drainage.

Pneumomediastinum

Presence of gas (usually air) in the mediastinum. Can either be spontaneous (due to rupture of pulmonary bleb) or 2° (eg, trauma, iatrogenic, Boerhaave syndrome).

Ruptured alveoli allow tracking of air into the mediastinum via peribronchial and perivascular sheaths.

Clinical features: chest pain, dyspnea, voice change, subcutaneous emphysema, ⊕ Hamman sign (crepitus on cardiac auscultation).

Flow-volume loops

FLOW-VOLUME PARAMETER	Obstructive lung disease	Restrictive lung disease
RV	↑	↓
FRC	↑	↓
TLC	↑	↓
FEV_1	↓↓	↓
FVC	↓	↓
FEV_1/FVC	↓ FEV_1 decreased more than FVC	Normal or ↑ FEV_1 decreased proportionately to FVC

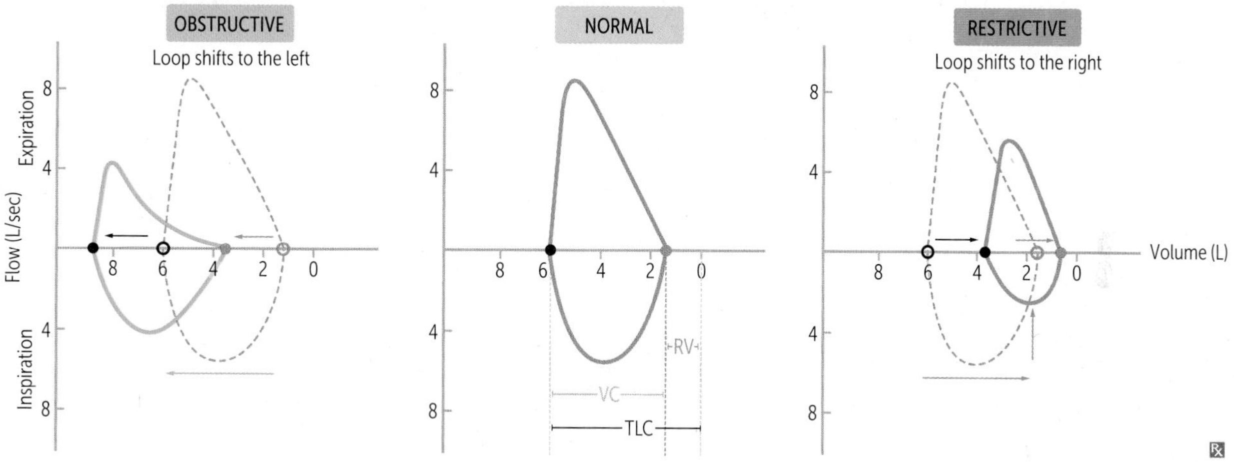

Obstructive lung diseases Obstruction of air flow (↑ FRC, ↑ RV, ↑ TLC) → air trapping in lungs with premature airway closure at high lung volumes (↓↓ FEV_1, ↓ FVC ↓ FEV_1/FVC ratio). Leads to $\dot{V}/\dot{Q}$ mismatch.

TYPE	PRESENTATION	PATHOLOGY	OTHER
Chronic bronchitis	Wheezing, crackles, cyanosis (hypoxemia due to shunting), dyspnea, CO_2 retention, 2° polycythemia.	Hypertrophy and hyperplasia of mucus-secreting glands in bronchi → Reid index (thickness of mucosal gland layer to thickness of wall between epithelium and cartilage) > 50%. DLCO may be normal.	Diagnostic criteria: productive cough for ≥ 3 months in a year for > 2 consecutive years.
Emphysema 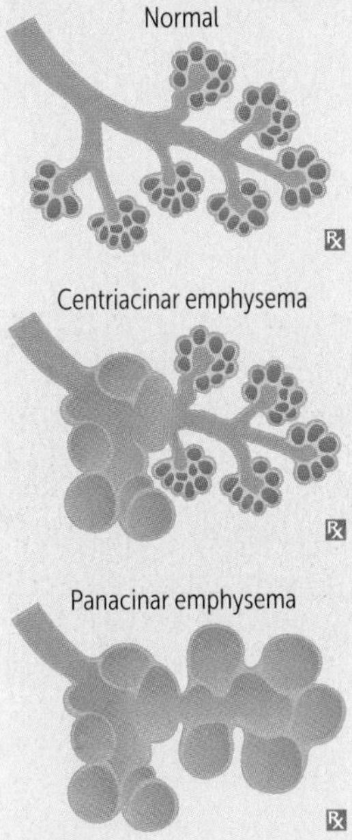 Normal Centriacinar emphysema Panacinar emphysema	Barrel-shaped chest A, expiration is prolonged and/or through pursed lips (increases airway pressure and prevents airway collapse).	Centriacinar—affects respiratory bronchioles while sparing distal alveoli, associated with tobacco **smoking** B C. Frequently in **upper** lobes (**smoke** rises **up**). Panacinar—affects respiratory bronchioles and alveoli, associated with α_1-antitrypsin deficiency. Frequently in lower lobes. Enlargement of air spaces ↓ recoil, ↑ compliance, ↓ DLCO from destruction of alveolar walls (arrow in D) and ↓ blood volume in pulmonary capillaries. Imbalance of proteases and antiproteases → ↑ elastase activity → ↑ loss of elastic fibers → ↑ lung compliance.	CXR: ↑ AP diameter, flattened diaphragm, ↑ lung field lucency. Chronic inflammation is mediated by $CD8^+$ T cells, neutrophils, and macrophages.
Asthma	Asymptomatic baseline with intermittent episodes of coughing, wheezing, tachypnea, dyspnea, hypoxemia, ↓ inspiratory/expiratory ratio, mucus plugging E. Severe attacks may lead to pulsus paradoxus. Triggers: viral URIs, allergens, stress.	Hyperresponsive bronchi → reversible bronchoconstriction. Smooth muscle hypertrophy and hyperplasia, Curschmann spirals F (shed epithelium forms whorled mucous plugs), and Charcot-Leyden crystals G (eosinophilic, hexagonal, double-pointed crystals formed from breakdown of eosinophils in sputum). DLCO normal or ↑.	Type I hypersensitivity reaction. Diagnosis supported by spirometry +/– methacholine challenge. NSAID-exacerbated respiratory disease is a combination of COX inhibition (leukotriene overproduction → airway constriction), chronic sinusitis with nasal polyps, and asthma symptoms.

Obstructive lung diseases *(continued)*

TYPE	PRESENTATION	PATHOLOGY	OTHER
Bronchiectasis	Daily purulent sputum, recurrent infections (most often *P aeruginosa*), hemoptysis, digital clubbing.	Chronic necrotizing infection of bronchi or obstruction → permanently dilated airways.	Associated with bronchial obstruction, poor ciliary motility (eg, tobacco smoking, Kartagener syndrome), cystic fibrosis (arrows in H show dilated airway with mucus plug), allergic bronchopulmonary aspergillosis.

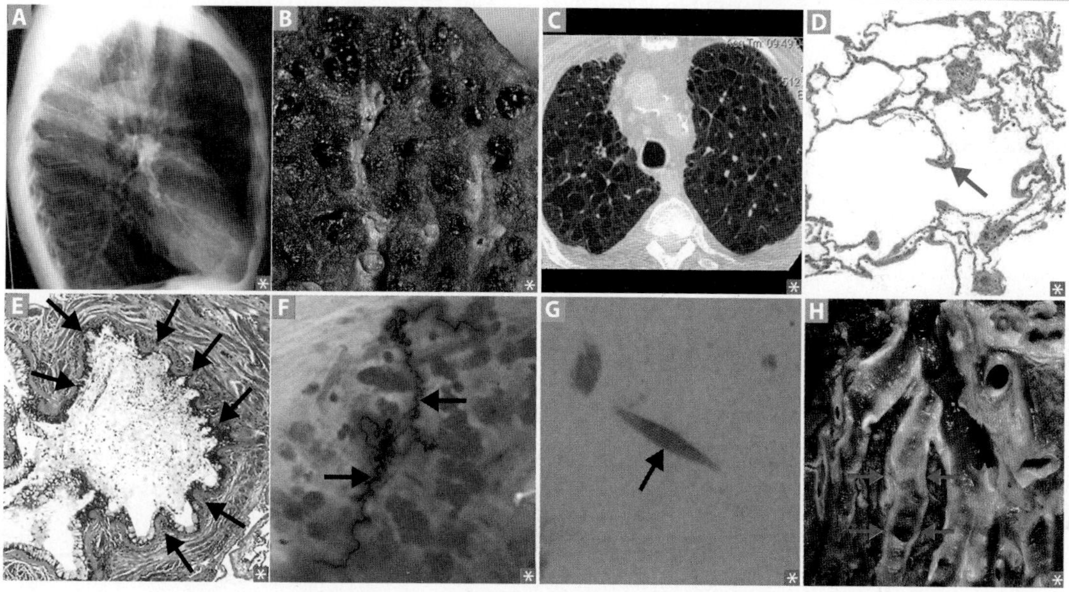

Restrictive lung diseases

May lead to ↓ lung volumes (↓ FVC and TLC). PFTs: normal or ↑ FEV_1/FVC ratio. Patient presents with short, shallow breaths.

Types:
- Altered respiratory mechanics (extrapulmonary, normal D_{LCO}, normal A-a gradient):
  - Respiratory muscle weakness—polio, myasthenia gravis, Guillain-Barré syndrome, ALS
  - Chest wall abnormalities—scoliosis, severe obesity
- Diffuse parenchymal lung diseases, also known as interstitial lung diseases (pulmonary, ↓ D_{LCO}, ↑ A-a gradient):
  - Pneumoconioses (eg, coal workers' pneumoconiosis, silicosis, asbestosis)
  - Sarcoidosis: bilateral hilar lymphadenopathy, noncaseating granulomas; ↑ ACE and Ca^{2+}
  - Idiopathic pulmonary fibrosis
  - Granulomatosis with polyangiitis
  - Pulmonary Langerhans cell histiocytosis (eosinophilic granuloma)
  - Hypersensitivity pneumonitis
  - Drug toxicity (eg, bleomycin, busulfan, amiodarone, methotrexate)
  - Acute respiratory distress syndrome
  - **Radiation-induced lung injury**—Associated with proinflammatory cytokine release (eg, TNF-α, IL-1, IL-6). May be asymptomatic but most common symptoms are dry cough and dyspnea ± low-grade fever. Acute radiation pneumonitis develops within 3–12 weeks (exudative phase); radiation fibrosis may develop after 6–12 months.

Idiopathic pulmonary fibrosis

Progressive fibrotic lung disease of unknown etiology. May involve multiple cycles of lung injury, inflammation, and fibrosis. Associated with cigarette smoking, environmental pollutants, genetic defects.

Findings: progressive dyspnea, fatigue, nonproductive cough, crackles, clubbing. Imaging shows peripheral reticular opacities with traction bronchiectasis +/– "honeycomb" appearance of lung (advanced disease). Histologic pattern: usual interstitial pneumonia.

Complications: pulmonary hypertension, respiratory failure, lung cancer, arrhythmias.

Hypersensitivity pneumonitis

Mixed type III/IV hypersensitivity reaction to environmental antigens. Often seen in farmers and bird-fanciers. Acutely, causes dyspnea, cough, chest tightness, fever, headache. Often self-limiting if stimulus is removed. Chronically, leads to irreversible fibrosis with noncaseating granuloma, alveolar septal thickening, traction bronchiectasis.

Sarcoidosis

Characterized by immune-mediated, widespread noncaseating granulomas A, elevated serum ACE levels, and elevated CD4/CD8 ratio in bronchoalveolar lavage fluid. More common in Black females. Often asymptomatic except for enlarged lymph nodes. CXR shows bilateral adenopathy and coarse reticular opacities B; CT of the chest better demonstrates the extensive hilar and mediastinal adenopathy C.

Associated with Bell palsy, uveitis, granulomas (noncaseating epithelioid, containing microscopic Schaumann and asteroid bodies), lupus pernio (skin lesions on face resembling lupus), interstitial fibrosis (restrictive lung disease), erythema nodosum, rheumatoid arthritis-like arthropathy, hypercalcemia (due to ↑ 1α-hydroxylase–mediated vitamin D activation in macrophages).

Treatment: steroids (if symptomatic).

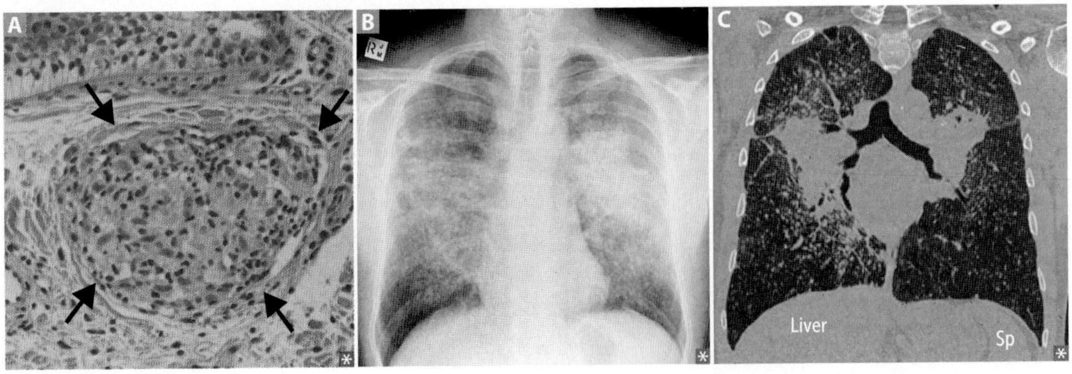

Inhalation injury and sequelae

Complication of inhalation of noxious stimuli (eg, smoke). Caused by heat, particulates (< 1 μm diameter), or irritants (eg, NH_3) → chemical tracheobronchitis, edema, pneumonia, ARDS. Many patients present 2° to burns, CO inhalation, cyanide poisoning, or arsenic poisoning. Singed nasal hairs or soot in oropharynx common on exam.

Bronchoscopy shows severe edema, congestion of bronchus, and soot deposition (A, 18 hours after inhalation injury; B, resolution at 11 days after injury).

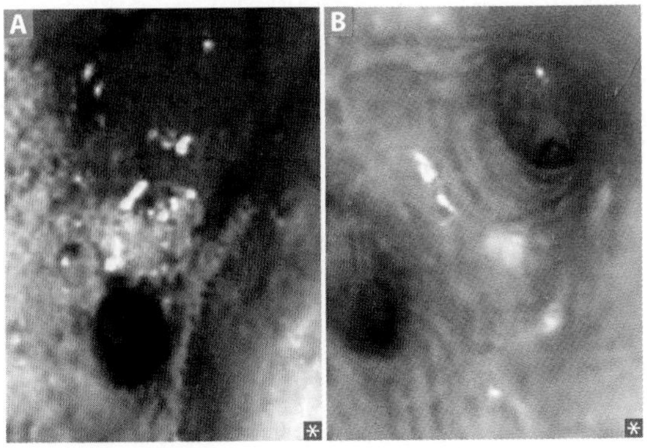

Pneumoconioses	**Asbestos** is from the **roof** (was common in insulation), but affects the **base** (lower lobes). **Silica**, **coal**, and **berries** are from the **base** (earth), but affect the **roof** (upper lobes).	
Asbestos-related disease	Asbestos causes asbestosis (pulmonary fibrosis), pleural disease, malignancies. Associated with shipbuilding, roofing, plumbing. "Ivory white," calcified, supradiaphragmatic A and pleural B plaques are pathognomonic. Risk of bronchogenic carcinoma > risk of mesothelioma. ↑ risk of Caplan syndrome (rheumatoid arthritis and pneumoconioses with intrapulmonary nodules).	Affects lower lobes. Asbestos (ferruginous) bodies are golden-brown fusiform rods resembling dumbbells C, found in alveolar sputum sample, visualized using Prussian blue stain, often obtained by bronchoalveolar lavage. ↑ risk of pleural effusions.
Berylliosis	Associated with exposure to beryllium in aerospace and manufacturing industries. Granulomatous (noncaseating) D on histology and therefore occasionally responsive to steroids. ↑ risk of cancer and cor pulmonale.	Affects upper lobes.
Coal workers' pneumoconiosis	Prolonged coal dust exposure → macrophages laden with carbon → inflammation and fibrosis. Also known as black lung disease. ↑ risk of Caplan syndrome.	Affects upper lobes. Small, rounded nodular opacities seen on imaging. Anthracosis—asymptomatic condition found in many urban dwellers exposed to sooty air.
Silicosis	Associated with **sand**blasting, **found**ries, **mines**. Macrophages respond to silica and release fibrogenic factors, leading to fibrosis. It is thought that silica may disrupt phagolysosomes and impair macrophages, increasing susceptibility to TB. ↑ risk of cancer, cor pulmonale, and Caplan syndrome.	Affects upper lobes. "Eggshell" calcification of hilar lymph nodes on CXR. The **silly egg sandwich** I **found** is **mine**!

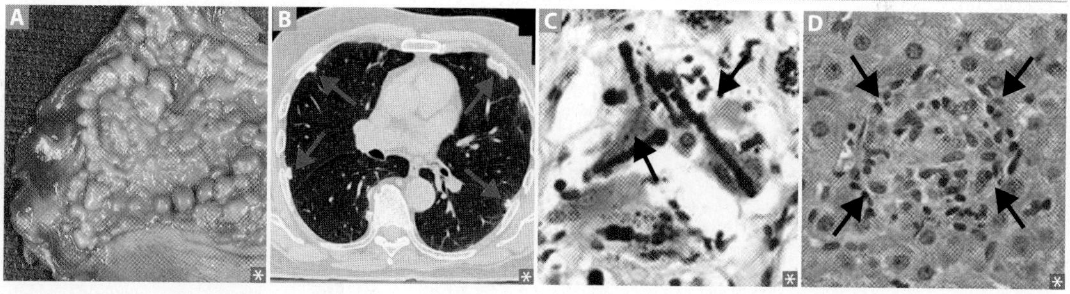

Mesothelioma

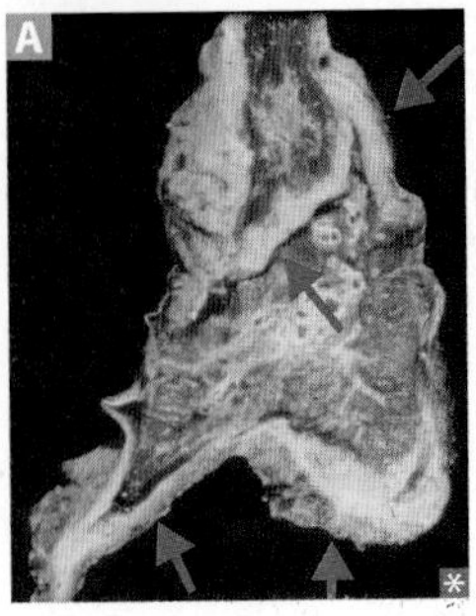

Malignancy of the pleura associated with asbestosis. May result in hemorrhagic pleural effusion (exudative), pleural thickening A.

Histology may show psammoma bodies. EM may show polygonal tumor cells with microvili, desmosomes, tonofilaments.

Calretinin and cytokeratin 5/6 ⊕ in almost all mesotheliomas, ⊖ in most carcinomas.

Tobacco smoking is not a risk factor.

Acute respiratory distress syndrome

PATHOPHYSIOLOGY	Alveolar insult → release of pro-inflammatory cytokines → neutrophil recruitment, activation, and release of toxic mediators (eg, reactive oxygen species, proteases, etc) → capillary endothelial damage and ↑ vessel permeability → leakage of protein-rich fluid into alveoli → formation of intra-alveolar hyaline membranes (arrows in A) and noncardiogenic pulmonary edema (normal PCWP). Loss of surfactant also contributes to alveolar collapse.
CAUSES	Sepsis (most common), aspiration, pneumonia, trauma, pancreatitis.
DIAGNOSIS	Diagnosis of exclusion with the following criteria (**ARDS**): ▪ **A**bnormal chest X-ray (bilateral lung opacities) B ▪ **R**espiratory failure within 1 week of alveolar insult ▪ **D**ecreased Pa_{O_2}/Fi_{O_2} (ratio < 300, hypoxemia due to ↑ intrapulmonary shunting and diffusion abnormalities) ▪ **S**ymptoms of respiratory failure are not due to HF/fluid overload
CONSEQUENCES	Impaired gas exchange, ↓ lung compliance; pulmonary hypertension.
MANAGEMENT	Treat the underlying cause. Mechanical ventilation: ↓ tidal volume, ↑ PEEP (keeps alveoli open during expiration).

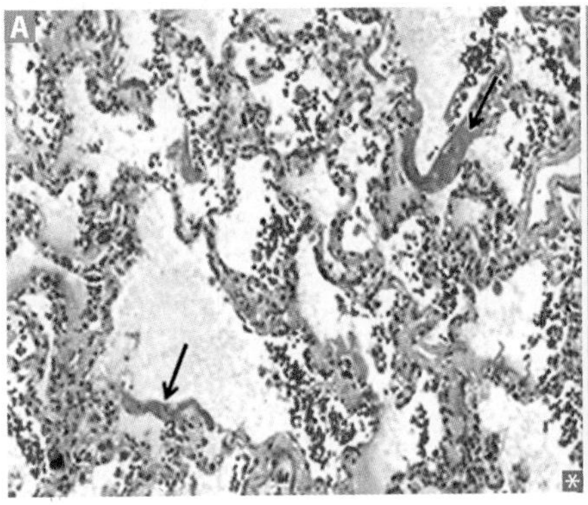

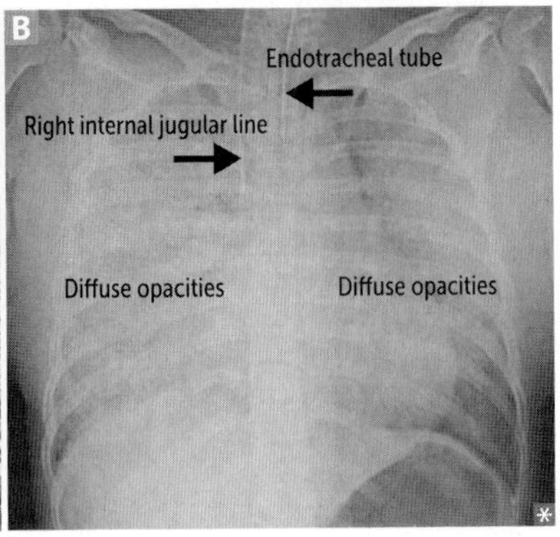

Sleep apnea	Repeated cessation of breathing > 10 seconds during sleep → disrupted sleep → daytime somnolence. Diagnosis confirmed by sleep study. Nocturnal hypoxia → systemic and pulmonary hypertension, arrhythmias (atrial fibrillation/flutter), sudden death. Hypoxia → ↑ EPO release → ↑ erythropoiesis.
Obstructive sleep apnea	Respiratory effort against airway obstruction. $Pa{O_2}$ is usually normal during the day. Associated with obesity, loud snoring, daytime sleepiness. Usually caused by excess parapharyngeal/oropharyngeal tissue in adults, adenotonsillar hypertrophy in children. Treatment: weight loss, CPAP, dental devices, hypoglossal nerve stimulation, upper airway surgery.
Central sleep apnea	Impaired respiratory effort due to CNS injury/toxicity, Congestive HF, opioids. May be associated with Cheyne-Stokes respirations (oscillations between apnea and hyperpnea). Treatment: positive airway pressure.
Obesity hypoventilation syndrome	Also called Pickwickian syndrome. Obesity (BMI ≥ 30 kg/m^2) → hypoventilation → ↑ $Pa{CO_2}$ during waking hours (retention); ↓ $Pa{O_2}$ and ↑ $Pa{CO_2}$ during sleep. Treatment: weight loss, positive airway pressure.

Pulmonary hypertension	Elevated mean pulmonary artery pressure (> 20 mm Hg) at rest. Results in arteriosclerosis, medial hypertrophy, intimal fibrosis of pulmonary arteries, plexiform lesions. ↑ pulmonary vascular resistance → ↑ RV pressure → RVH, RV failure.
ETIOLOGIES	
Pulmonary arterial hypertension	Often idiopathic. Females > males. Heritable PAH can be due to an inactivating mutation in *BMPR2* gene (normally inhibits vascular smooth muscle proliferation); poor prognosis. Pulmonary vasculature endothelial dysfunction results in ↑ vasoconstrictors (eg, endothelin) and ↓ vasodilators (eg, NO and prostacyclins). Other causes include drugs (eg, amphetamines, cocaine), connective tissue disease, HIV infection, portal hypertension, congenital heart disease, schistosomiasis.
Left heart disease	Causes include systolic/diastolic dysfunction and valvular disease.
Lung diseases or hypoxia	Destruction of lung parenchyma (eg, COPD), lung inflammation/fibrosis (eg, interstitial lung diseases), hypoxemic vasoconstriction (eg, obstructive sleep apnea, living in high altitude).
Chronic thromboembolic	Recurrent microthrombi → ↓ cross-sectional area of pulmonary vascular bed.
Multifactorial	Causes include hematologic, systemic, and metabolic disorders, along with compression of the pulmonary vasculature by a tumor.

Physical findings in select lung diseases

ABNORMALITY	BREATH SOUNDS	PERCUSSION	FREMITUS	TRACHEAL DEVIATION
Pleural effusion	↓	Dull	↓	None if small Away from side of lesion if large
Atelectasis	↓	Dull	↓	Toward side of lesion
Simple pneumothorax	↓	Hyperresonant	↓	None
Tension pneumothorax	↓	Hyperresonant	↓	Away from side of lesion
Consolidation (lobar pneumonia, pulmonary edema)	Bronchial breath sounds; late inspiratory crackles, egophony, whispered pectoriloquy	Dull	↑	None

Digital clubbing

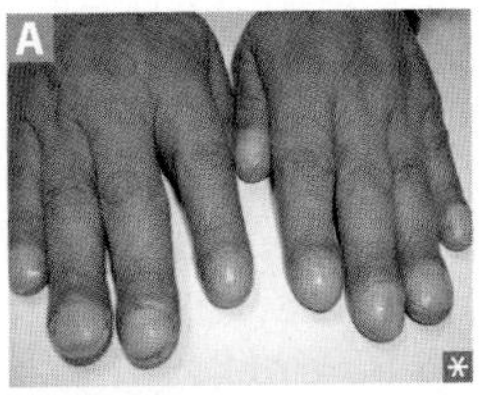

Increased angle between nail bed and nail plate (> 180°) A. Pathophysiology not well understood; in patients with intrapulmonary shunt, platelets and megakaryocytes become lodged in digital vasculature → local release of PDGF and VEGF. Can be hereditary or acquired. Causes include respiratory diseases (eg, idiopathic pulmonary fibrosis, cystic fibrosis, bronchiectasis, lung cancer), cardiovascular diseases (eg, cyanotic congenital heart disease), infections (eg, lung abscess, TB), and others (eg, IBD). Not typically associated with COPD or asthma.

Atelectasis

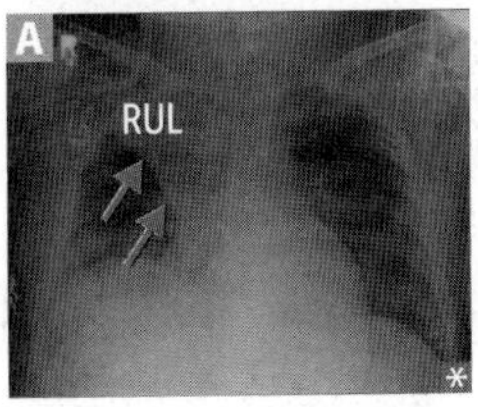

Alveolar collapse (right upper lobe collapse against mediastinum in A). Multiple causes:
- Obstructive—airway obstruction prevents new air from reaching distal airways, old air is resorbed (eg, foreign body, mucous plug, tumor)
- Compressive—external compression on lung decreases lung volumes (eg, space-occupying lesion, pleural effusion)
- Contraction (cicatrization)—scarring of lung parenchyma that distorts alveoli (eg, sarcoidosis)
- Adhesive—due to lack of surfactant (eg, NRDS in premature babies)

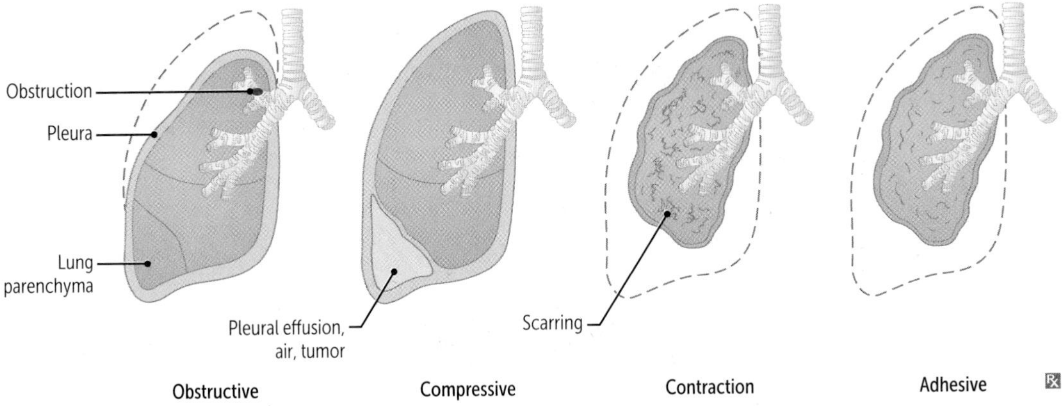

Pleural effusions	Excess accumulation of fluid A between pleural layers → restricted lung expansion during inspiration. Can be treated with thoracentesis to remove/reduce fluid B. Based on the Light criteria, fluid is exudate if pleural fluid protein/serum protein > 0.5, pleural fluid LDH/serum LDH > 0.6, or pleural fluid LDH > 2/3 upper limit of normal serum LDH.
Exudate	Cloudy fluid (cellular). Due to malignancy, inflammation/infection (eg, pneumonia, collagen vascular disease), trauma (occurs in states of ↑ vascular permeability). Often needs to be drained due to risk of infection.
Transudate	Clear fluid (hypocellular). Due to ↑ hydrostatic pressure (eg, HF, Na^+ retention) and/or ↓ oncotic pressure (eg, nephrotic syndrome, cirrhosis).
Lymphatic	Also known as chylothorax. Due to thoracic duct injury from trauma or malignancy. Milky-appearing fluid; ↑ triglycerides.

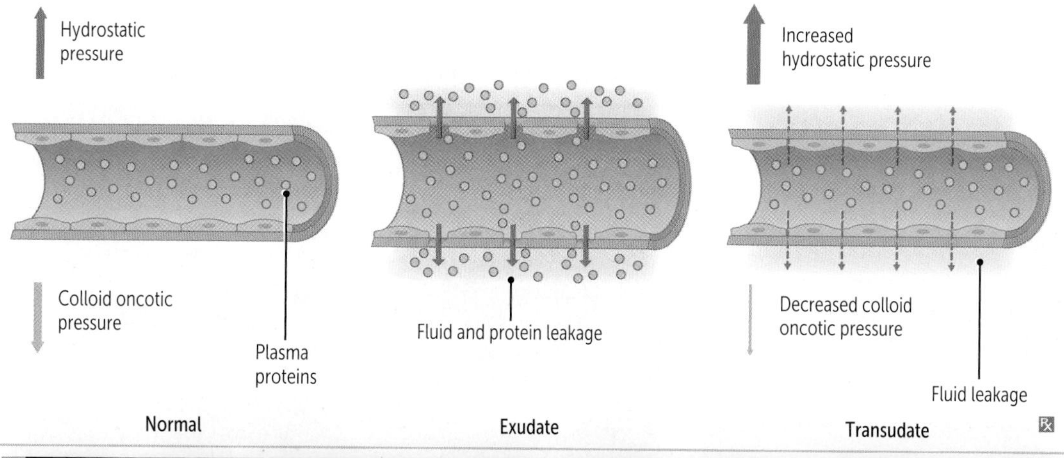

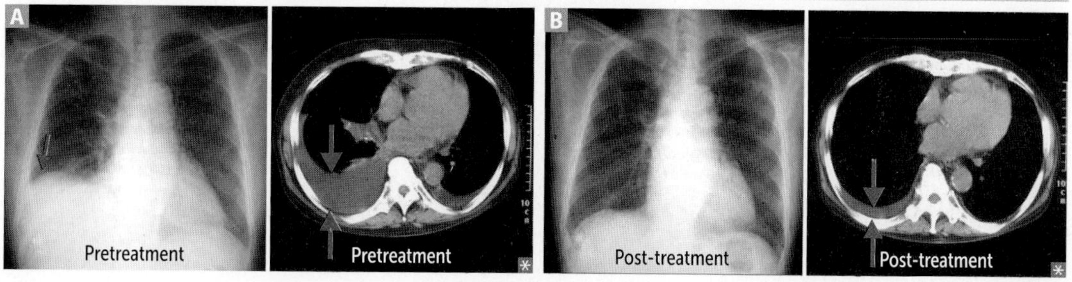

Pneumothorax	Accumulation of air in pleural space A. Dyspnea, uneven chest expansion. Chest pain, ↓ tactile fremitus, hyperresonance, and diminished breath sounds, all on the affected side.
Primary spontaneous pneumothorax	Due to rupture of apical subpleural bleb or cysts. Occurs most frequently in tall, thin, young males. Associated with tobacco smoking.
Secondary spontaneous pneumothorax	Due to diseased lung (eg, bullae in emphysema, Marfan syndrome, infections), mechanical ventilation with use of high pressures → barotrauma.
Traumatic pneumothorax	Caused by blunt (eg, rib fracture), penetrating (eg, gunshot), or iatrogenic (eg, central line placement, lung biopsy, barotrauma due to mechanical ventilation) trauma.
Tension pneumothorax	Can be from any of the above. Air enters pleural space but cannot exit. Increasing trapped air → tension pneumothorax. Trachea deviates away from affected lung B. May lead to increased intrathoracic pressure → mediastinal displacement → kinking of IVC → ↓ venous return → ↓ cardiac output, obstructive shock (hypotension, tachycardia), jugular venous distention. Needs immediate needle decompression and chest tube placement.

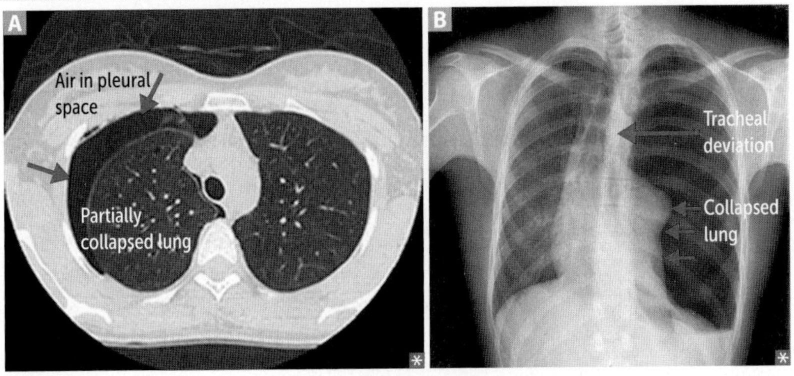

Pneumonia

TYPE	TYPICAL ORGANISMS	CHARACTERISTICS
Lobar pneumonia	*S pneumoniae* (most common), *Legionella*, *Klebsiella*	Intra-alveolar exudate → consolidation A; may involve entire lobe B or the whole lung.
Bronchopneumonia	*S pneumoniae*, *S aureus*, *H influenzae*, *Klebsiella*	Acute inflammatory infiltrates C from bronchioles into adjacent alveoli; patchy distribution involving ≥ 1 lobe D.
Interstitial (atypical) pneumonia	*Mycoplasma*, *Chlamydophila pneumoniae*, *Chlamydophila psittaci*, *Legionella*, *Coxiella burnetii*, viruses (RSV, CMV, influenza, adenovirus)	Diffuse patchy inflammation localized to interstitial areas at alveolar walls; CXR shows bilateral multifocal opacities E. Generally follows a more indolent course ("walking" pneumonia).
Cryptogenic organizing pneumonia	Etiology unknown. ⊖ sputum and blood cultures, often responds to steroids but not to antibiotics.	Formerly known as bronchiolitis obliterans organizing pneumonia (BOOP). Noninfectious pneumonia characterized by inflammation of bronchioles and surrounding structure.

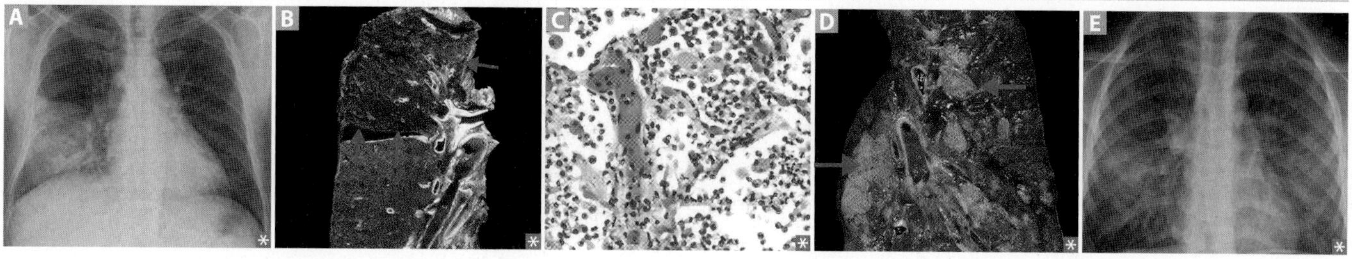
A
B
C
D
E

Natural history of lobar pneumonia

	Congestion	Red hepatization	Gray hepatization	Resolution
DAYS	1–2	3–4	5–7	8+
FINDINGS	Red-purple, partial consolidation of parenchyma Exudate with mostly bacteria	Red-brown consolidation Exudate with fibrin, bacteria, RBCs, WBCs Reversible	Uniformly gray Exudate full of WBCs, lysed RBCs, and fibrin	Enzymatic digestion of exudate by macrophages

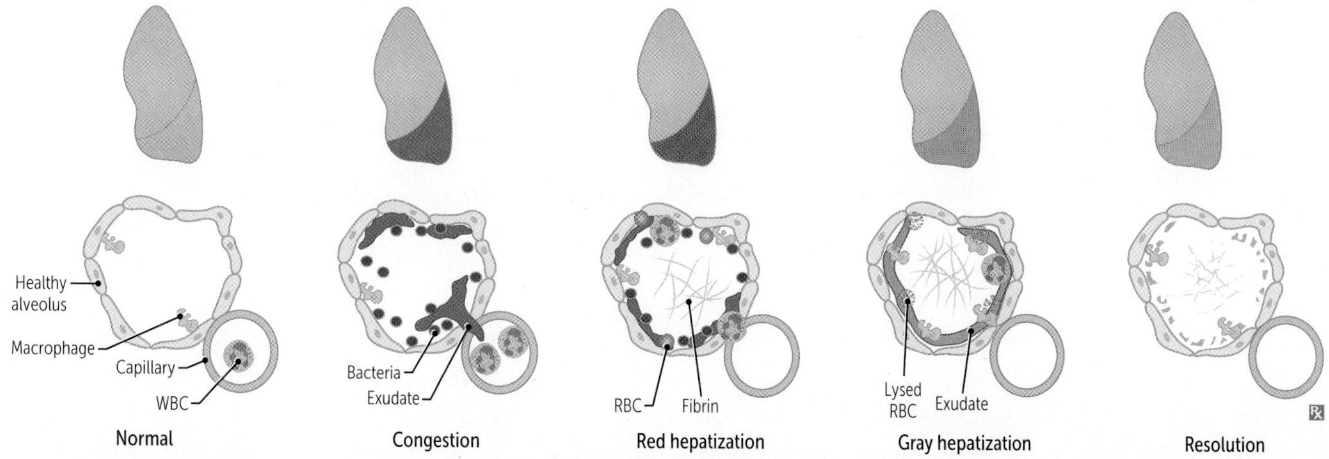
Healthy alveolus
Macrophage
Capillary
WBC
Normal
Bacteria
Exudate
Congestion
RBC
Fibrin
Red hepatization
Lysed RBC
Exudate
Gray hepatization
Resolution

Lung abscess

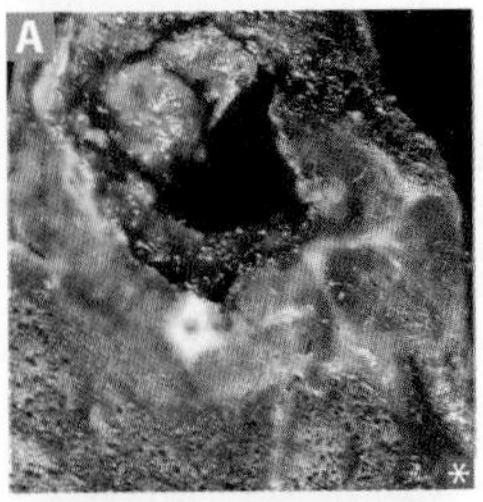

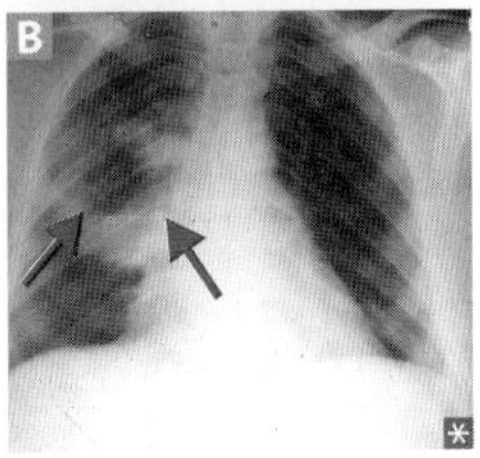

Localized collection of pus within parenchyma A. Caused by aspiration of oropharyngeal contents (especially in patients predisposed to loss of consciousness [eg, alcohol overuse, epilepsy]) or bronchial obstruction (eg, cancer).

Air-fluid levels B often seen on CXR; presence suggests cavitation. Due to anaerobes (eg, *Bacteroides*, *Fusobacterium*, *Peptostreptococcus*) or *S aureus*.

Treatment: antibiotics, drainage, or surgery.

Lung abscess 2° to aspiration is most often found in right lung. Location depends on patient's position during aspiration: RLL if upright, RUL or RML if recumbent.

Lung cancer

Leading cause of cancer death.
Presentation: cough, hemoptysis, bronchial obstruction, wheezing, pneumonic "coin" lesion on CXR or noncalcified nodule on CT.
Sites of metastases from lung cancer: **l**iver (jaundice, hepatomegaly), adrenals, **bone** (pathologic fracture), **brain**; "Lung 'mets' Love affective **bone**heads and **brain**iacs."
In the lung, metastases (usually multiple lesions) are more common than 1° neoplasms. Most often from breast, colon, prostate, and bladder cancer.

SPHERE of complications: **S**uperior vena cava/thoracic outlet syndromes, **P**ancoast tumor, **H**orner syndrome, **E**ndocrine (paraneoplastic), **R**ecurrent laryngeal nerve compression (hoarseness), **E**ffusions (pleural or pericardial).
Risk factors include tobacco smoking, secondhand smoke, radiation, environmental exposures (eg, radon, asbestos), pulmonary fibrosis, family history.
Squamous and **s**mall cell carcinomas are **s**entral (central) and often caused by **s**moking.

TYPE	LOCATION	CHARACTERISTICS	HISTOLOGY
Small cell			
Small cell (oat cell) carcinoma	Central	Undifferentiated → very aggressive. May produce ACTH (Cushing syndrome), ADH (SIADH), or **A**ntibodies against presynaptic Ca^{2+} channels (Lambert-Eaton myasthenic syndrome) or neurons (paraneoplastic myelitis, encephalitis, subacute cerebellar degeneration). **A**mplification of *myc* oncogenes common. Managed with chemotherapy +/– radiation.	Neoplasm of neuroendocrine Kulchitsky cells → small dark blue cells **A**. Chromogranin A ⊕, neuron-specific enolase ⊕, synaptophysin ⊕.
Non-small cell			
Adenocarcinoma	Peripheral	Most common 1° lung cancer. Most common subtype in people who do not smoke. More common in females than males. Activating mutations include *KRAS*, *EGFR*, and *ALK*. Associated with hypertrophic osteoarthropathy (clubbing). Bronchioloalveolar subtype (adenocarcinoma in situ): CXR often shows hazy infiltrates similar to pneumonia; better prognosis.	Glandular pattern, often stains mucin ⊕ **B**. Bronchioloalveolar subtype: grows along alveolar septa → apparent "thickening" of alveolar walls. Tall, columnar cells containing mucus.
Squamous cell carcinoma	Central	Hilar mass **C** arising from bronchus; cavitation; cigarettes; hypercalcemia (produces PTHrP).	Keratin pearls **D** and intercellular bridges (desmosomes).
Large cell carcinoma	Peripheral	Highly anaplastic undifferentiated tumor. Strong association with tobacco smoking. May produce hCG → gynecomastia. Less responsive to chemotherapy; removed surgically. Poor prognosis.	Pleomorphic **giant** cells **E**.
Bronchial carcinoid tumor	Central or peripheral	Excellent prognosis; metastasis rare. Symptoms due to mass effect or carcinoid syndrome (flushing, diarrhea, wheezing).	Nests of neuroendocrine cells; chromogranin A ⊕.

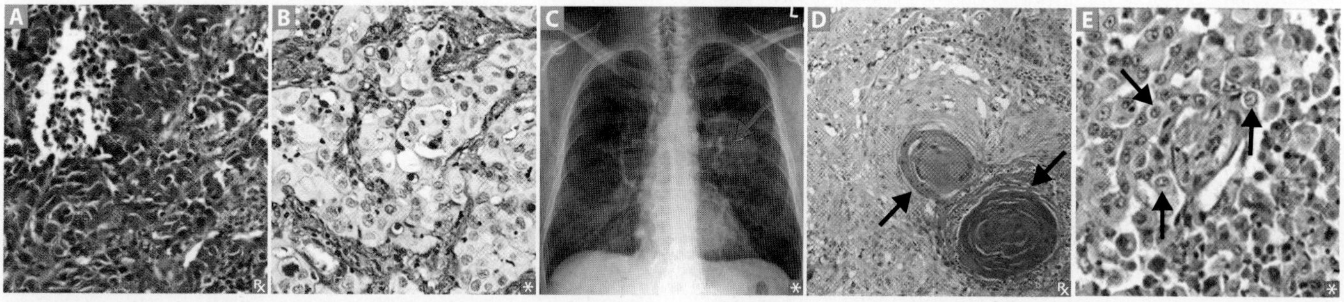

Pancoast tumor

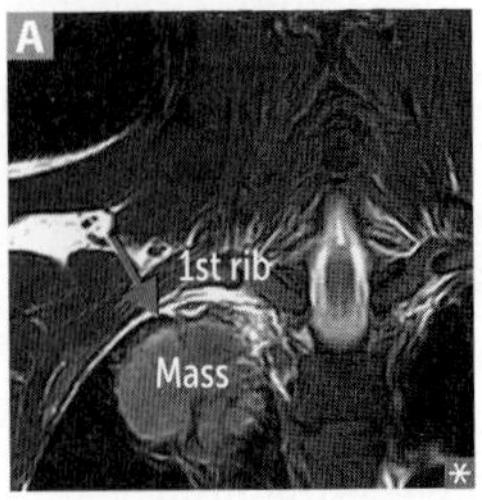

Also known as superior sulcus tumor. Carcinoma that occurs in the apex of lung A may cause Pancoast syndrome by invading/compressing local structures.

Compression of locoregional structures may cause array of findings:

- Recurrent laryngeal nerve → hoarseness
- Stellate ganglion → Horner syndrome (ipsilateral ptosis, miosis, anhidrosis)
- Superior vena cava → SVC syndrome
- Brachiocephalic vein → brachiocephalic syndrome (unilateral symptoms)
- Brachial plexus → shoulder pain, sensorimotor deficits (eg, atrophy of intrinsic muscles of the hand)
- Phrenic nerve → hemidiaphragm paralysis (hemidiaphragm elevation on CXR)

Superior vena cava syndrome

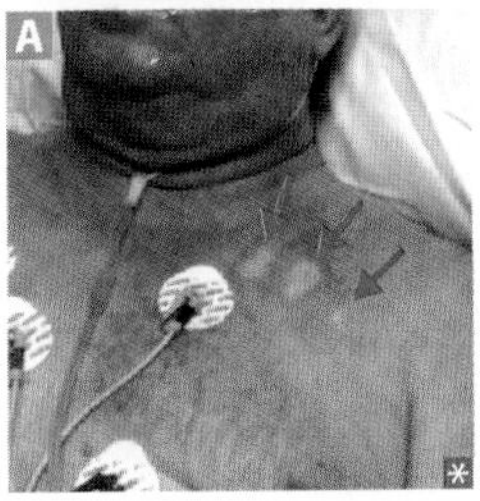

An obstruction of the SVC that impairs blood drainage from the head ("facial plethora"; note blanching after fingertip pressure in A), neck (jugular venous distention), and upper extremities (edema). Commonly caused by malignancy (eg, mediastinal mass, Pancoast tumor) and thrombosis from indwelling catheters B. Medical emergency. Can raise intracranial pressure (if obstruction is severe) → headaches, dizziness, ↑ risk of aneurysm/rupture of intracranial arteries.

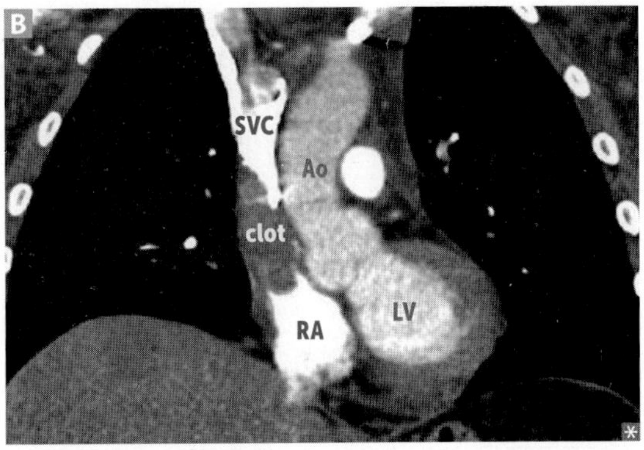

▸ RESPIRATORY—PHARMACOLOGY

H_1-blockers	Also called antihistamines. Reversible inhibitors of H_1 histamine receptors. May function as neutral antagonists or inverse agonists.	
First generation	Diphen**hydramine**, dimen**hydrinate**, chlorphenir**amine**, doxyl**amine**.	Names usually contain "-en/-ine" or "-en/-ate."
CLINICAL USE	Allergy, motion sickness, vomiting in pregnancy, sleep aid.	
ADVERSE EFFECTS	Sedation, antimuscarinic, anti-α-adrenergic.	
Second generation	Lorat**adine**, fexofen**adine**, desloratadine, cetirizine.	Names usually end in "-adine." Setirizine (cetirizine) is second-generation agent.
CLINICAL USE	Allergy.	
ADVERSE EFFECTS	Far less sedating than 1st generation because of ↓ entry into CNS.	

Dextromethorphan Antitussive (antagonizes NMDA glutamate receptors). Synthetic codeine analog. Has mild opioid effect when used in excess. Naloxone can be given for overdose. Mild abuse potential. May cause serotonin syndrome if combined with other serotonergic agents.

Pseudoephedrine, phenylephrine

MECHANISM	Activation of α-adrenergic receptors in nasal mucosa → local vasoconstriction.
CLINICAL USE	Reduce hyperemia, edema (used as nasal decongestants); open obstructed eustachian tubes.
ADVERSE EFFECTS	Hypertension. Rebound congestion (rhinitis medicamentosa) if used more than 4–6 days. Associated with tachyphylaxis. Can also cause CNS stimulation/anxiety (pseudoephedrine).

Pulmonary hypertension drugs

DRUG	MECHANISM	CLINICAL NOTES
Endothelin receptor antagonists	Competitively antagonizes endothelin-1 receptors → ↓ pulmonary vascular resistance.	Hepatotoxic (monitor LFTs). Example: bosentan.
PDE-5 inhibitors	Inhibits PDE-5 → ↑ cGMP → prolonged vasodilatory effect of NO.	Also used to treat erectile dysfunction. Contraindicated when taking nitroglycerin or other nitrates (due to risk of severe hypotension). Example: sildenafil.
Prostacyclin analogs	PGI_2 (prostacyclin) with direct vasodilatory effects on pulmonary and systemic arterial vascular beds. Inhibits platelet aggregation.	Side effects: flushing, jaw pain. Examples: epoprostenol, iloprost.

Asthma drugs	Bronchoconstriction is mediated by (1) inflammatory processes and (2) parasympathetic tone; therapy is directed at these 2 pathways.
Inhaled β_2-agonists	**Albuterol**—relaxes bronchial smooth muscle (short acting β_2-agonist). For acute exacerbations. Can cause tremor, arrhythmia. **Salmeterol, formoterol**—long-acting agents for prophylaxis. Can cause tremor, arrhythmia.
Inhaled corticosteroids	**Fluticasone, budesonide**—inhibit the synthesis of virtually all cytokines. Inactivate NF-κB, the transcription factor that induces production of TNF-α and other inflammatory agents. 1st-line therapy for chronic asthma. Use a spacer or rinse mouth after use to prevent oral thrush.
Muscarinic antagonists	**Tiotropium, ipratropium**—competitively block muscarinic receptors, preventing bronchoconstriction. Also used for COPD. Tiotropium is long acting.
Antileukotrienes	**Montelukast, zafirlukast**—block leukotriene receptors (CysLT1). Especially good for aspirin-induced and exercise-induced asthma. **Zileuton**—5-lipoxygenase pathway inhibitor. Blocks conversion of arachidonic acid to leukotrienes. Hepatotoxic.
Anti-IgE monoclonal therapy	**Omalizumab**—binds mostly unbound serum IgE and blocks binding to FcεRI. Used in allergic asthma with ↑ IgE levels resistant to inhaled steroids and long-acting β_2-agonists.
Methylxanthines	**Theophylline**—likely causes bronchodilation by inhibiting phosphodiesterase → ↑ cAMP levels due to ↓ cAMP hydrolysis. Limited use due to narrow therapeutic index (cardiotoxicity, neurotoxicity); metabolized by cytochrome P-450. Blocks actions of adenosine.
Chromones	**Cromolyn**—prevents mast cell degranulation. Prevents acute asthma symptoms. Rarely used.
Anti-IL-5 monoclonal therapy	Prevents eosinophil differentiation, maturation, activation, and survival mediated by IL-5 stimulation. For maintenance therapy in severe eosinophilic asthma. **Mepolizumab, reslizumab**—against IL-5. **Benralizumab**—against IL-5 receptor α.

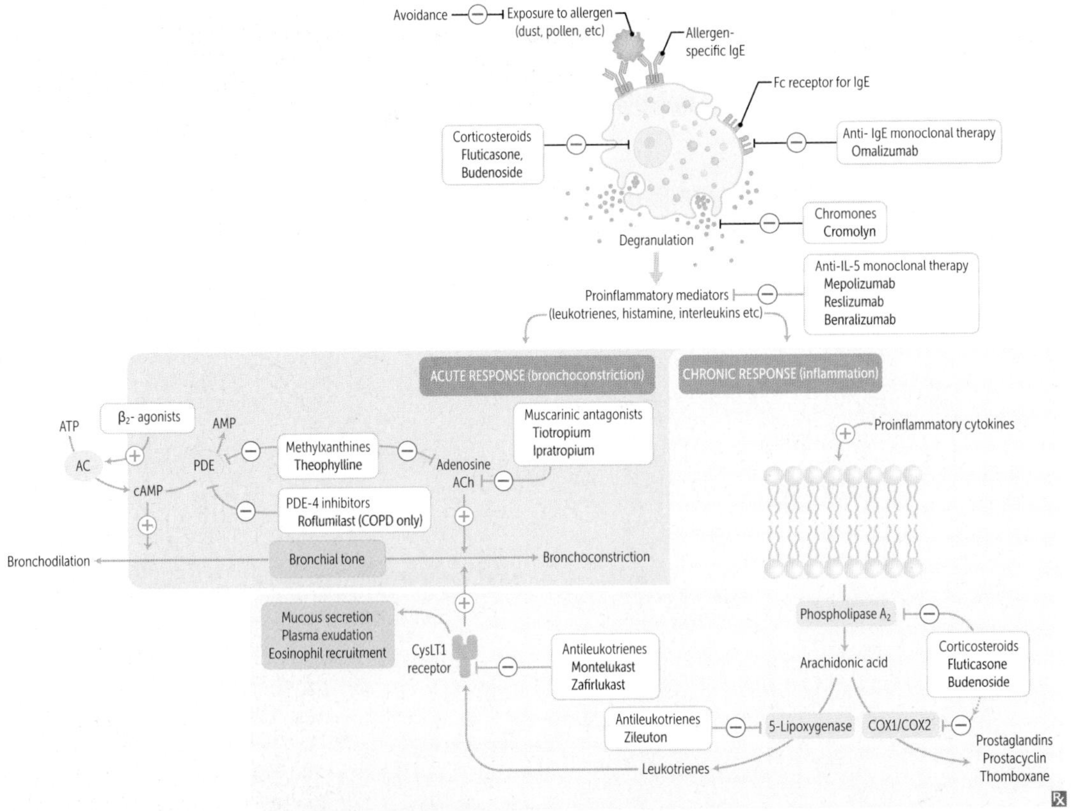

HIGH-YIELD SYSTEMS

Rapid Review

"Study without thought is vain: thought without study is dangerous."
—Confucius

"It is better, of course, to know useless things than to know nothing."
—Lucius Annaeus Seneca

"For every complex problem there is an answer that is clear, simple, and wrong."
—H. L. Mencken

The following tables represent a collection of high-yield associations between diseases and their clinical findings, treatments, and key associations. They can be quickly reviewed in the days before the exam.

▶ CLASSIC PRESENTATIONS

CLINICAL PRESENTATION	DIAGNOSIS/DISEASE	PAGE
Gout, intellectual disability, self-mutilating behavior in a boy	Lesch-Nyhan syndrome (HGPRT deficiency, X-linked recessive)	37
Situs inversus, chronic ear infections, sinusitis, bronchiectasis, infertility	Kartagener syndrome (dynein arm defect affecting cilia)	49
Blue sclera	Osteogenesis imperfecta (type I collagen defect)	51
Elastic skin, hypermobility of joints, ↑ bleeding tendency	Ehlers-Danlos syndrome (type V collagen defect, type III collagen defect seen in vascular subtype of ED)	51
Arachnodactyly, lens dislocation (upward and temporal), aortic dissection, hyperflexible joints	Marfan syndrome (fibrillin defect)	52
Arachnodactyly, pectus deformity, lens dislocation (downward)	Homocystinuria (autosomal recessive)	52
Café-au-lait spots (unilateral), polyostotic fibrous dysplasia, precocious puberty, multiple endocrine abnormalities	McCune-Albright syndrome (G_s-protein activating mutation)	57
Meconium ileus in neonate, recurrent pulmonary infections, nasal polyps, pancreatic insufficiency, infertility/subfertility	Cystic fibrosis (*CFTR* gene defect, chr 7, Phe508 deletion)	60
Calf pseudohypertrophy	Muscular dystrophy (most commonly Duchenne, due to X-linked recessive frameshift mutation of dystrophin gene)	61
Child uses arms to stand up from squat	Duchenne muscular dystrophy (Gowers sign)	61
Slow, progressive muscle weakness in boys	Becker muscular dystrophy (X-linked non-frameshift deletions in dystrophin; less severe than Duchenne)	61
Infant with cleft lip/palate, microcephaly or holoprosencephaly, polydactyly, cutis aplasia	Patau syndrome (trisomy 13)	63
Infant with microcephaly, rocker-bottom feet, clenched hands, and structural heart defect	Edwards syndrome (trisomy 18)	63
Single palmar crease	Down syndrome	63
Confusion, ophthalmoplegia/nystagmus, ataxia	Wernicke encephalopathy	66
Dilated cardiomyopathy/high-output heart failure, edema, alcoholism or malnutrition	Wet beriberi (thiamine [vitamin B_1] deficiency)	66
Burning feet syndrome	Vitamin B_5 deficiency	67
Dermatitis, dementia, diarrhea	Pellagra (niacin [vitamin B_3] deficiency)	67
Swollen gums, mucosal bleeding, poor wound healing, petechiae	Scurvy (vitamin C deficiency: can't hydroxylate proline/lysine for collagen synthesis); tea and toast diet	69
Bowlegs in children, bone pain, and muscle weakness	Rickets (children), osteomalacia (adults); vitamin D deficiency	70
Hemorrhagic disease of newborn with ↑ PT, ↑ PTT	Vitamin K deficiency	71
Bluish-black connective tissue, ear cartilage, sclerae; urine turns black on prolonged exposure to air	Alkaptonuria (homogentisate oxidase deficiency; ochronosis)	84
Chronic exercise intolerance with myalgia, fatigue, painful cramps, myoglobinuria	McArdle disease (skeletal muscle glycogen phosphorylase deficiency)	87

CLINICAL PRESENTATION	DIAGNOSIS/DISEASE	PAGE
Infant with hypoglycemia, hepatomegaly	Cori disease (debranching enzyme deficiency) or Von Gierke disease (glucose-6-phosphatase deficiency, more severe)	87
Myopathy (infantile hypertrophic cardiomyopathy), exercise intolerance	Pompe disease (lysosomal α-1,4-glucosidase deficiency)	87
"Cherry-red spots" on macula	Tay-Sachs (ganglioside accumulation) or Niemann-Pick (sphingomyelin accumulation), central retinal artery occlusion	88, 557
Hepatosplenomegaly, pancytopenia, osteoporosis, avascular necrosis of femoral head, bone crises	Gaucher disease (glucocerebrosidase [β-glucosidase] deficiency)	88
Achilles tendon xanthoma	Familial hypercholesterolemia (↓ LDL receptor signaling)	94
Recurrent *Neisseria* infection	Terminal complement deficiencies (C5-C9)	107
Anaphylaxis following blood transfusion	IgA deficiency	116
Male child, recurrent infections, no mature B cells	Bruton disease (X-linked agammaglobulinemia)	116
Recurrent cold (noninflamed) abscesses, eczema, high serum IgE, ↑ eosinophils	Hyper-IgE syndrome (Job syndrome: neutrophil chemotaxis abnormality)	116
Late separation (>30 days) of umbilical cord, no pus, recurrent skin and mucosal bacterial infections	Leukocyte adhesion deficiency (type 1; defective LFA-1 integrin)	117
Recurrent infections and granulomas with catalase ⊕ organisms	Chronic granulomatous disease (defect of NAPDH oxidase)	117
Fever, vomiting, diarrhea, desquamating rash following use of nasal pack or tampon	Staphylococcal toxic shock syndrome	135
"Strawberry tongue"	Scarlet fever Kawasaki disease	136, 314
Colon cancer diagnosed a few years after endocarditis	*Streptococcus bovis*	137
Abdominal pain, diarrhea, leukocytosis, recent antibiotic use	*Clostridium difficile* infection	138
Flaccid paralysis in newborn after ingestion of honey	*Clostridium botulinum* infection (floppy baby syndrome)	138
Tonsillar pseudomembrane with "bull's neck" appearance	*Corynebacterium diphtheria* infection	139
Back pain, fever, night sweats	Pott disease (vertebral TB)	140
Adrenal insufficiency, fever, DIC	Waterhouse-Friderichsen syndrome (meningococcemia)	142, 357
Red "currant jelly" sputum in patients with alcohol overuse or diabetes	*Klebsiella pneumoniae* pneumonia	145
Large rash with bull's-eye appearance	Erythema migrans from *Ixodes* tick bite (Lyme disease: *Borrelia*)	146
Ulcerated genital lesion	Nonpainful, indurated: chancre (1° syphilis, *Treponema pallidum*) Painful, with exudate: chancroid (*Haemophilus ducreyi*)	147, 184
Pupil accommodates but doesn't react to light	Neurosyphilis (Argyll Robertson pupil)	147
Smooth, moist, painless, wart-like white lesions on genitals	Condylomata lata (2° syphilis)	147
Fever, chills, headache, myalgia following antibiotic treatment for syphilis	Jarisch-Herxheimer reaction (due to host response to sudden release of bacterial antigens)	148

CLINICAL PRESENTATION	DIAGNOSIS/DISEASE	PAGE
Dog or cat bite resulting in infection (cellulitis, osteomyelitis)	*Pasteurella multocida* (cellulitis at inoculation site)	149
Atypical "walking pneumonia" with x-ray looking worse than the patient	*Mycoplasma pneumoniae* infection	150
Rash on palms and soles	Coxsackie A, 2° syphilis, Rocky Mountain spotted fever	150
Black eschar on face of patient with diabetic ketoacidosis and/or neutropenia	*Mucor* or *Rhizopus* fungal infection	153
Chorioretinitis, hydrocephalus, intracranial calcifications	Congenital toxoplasmosis	156
Pruritus, serpiginous rash after walking barefoot	Hookworm (*Ancylostoma* spp, *Necator americanus*)	159
Child with fever later develops red rash on face that spreads to body	Erythema infectiosum/fifth disease ("slapped cheeks" appearance, caused by parvovirus B19)	164
Fever, cough, conjunctivitis, coryza, diffuse rash	Measles	170
Small, irregular red spots on buccal/lingual mucosa with blue-white centers	Koplik spots (measles [rubeola] virus)	170
Bounding pulses, wide pulse pressure, diastolic heart murmur, head bobbing	Aortic regurgitation	300
Systolic ejection murmur (crescendo-decrescendo), narrow pulse pressure, pulsus parvus et tardus	Aortic stenosis	300
Continuous "machine-like" heart murmur	PDA (close with indomethacin; keep open with PGE analogs)	300
Chest pain on exertion	Angina (stable: with moderate exertion; unstable: with minimal exertion or at rest)	312
Chest pain with ST depressions on ECG	Angina (⊖ troponins) or NSTEMI (⊕ troponins)	312
Chest pain, pericardial effusion/friction rub, persistent fever following MI	Dressler syndrome (autoimmune-mediated post-MI fibrinous pericarditis, 2 weeks to several months after acute episode)	317
Distant heart sounds, distended neck veins, hypotension	Beck triad of cardiac tamponade	320
Painful, raised red lesions on pads of fingers/toes	Osler nodes (infective endocarditis, immune complex deposition)	321
Painless erythematous lesions on palms and soles	Janeway lesions (infective endocarditis, septic emboli/microabscesses)	321
Splinter hemorrhages in fingernails	Bacterial endocarditis	321
Retinal hemorrhages with pale centers	Roth spots (bacterial endocarditis)	321
Telangiectasias, recurrent epistaxis, skin discoloration, arteriovenous malformations, GI bleeding, hematuria	Hereditary hemorrhagic telangiectasia (Osler-Weber-Rendu syndrome)	324
Polyuria (water diuresis), polydipsia	Primary polydipsia, diabetes insipidus (central, nephrogenic)	346
No lactation postpartum, absent menstruation, cold intolerance	Sheehan syndrome (postpartum hemorrhage leading to pituitary infarction)	347
Heat intolerance, weight loss, palpitations	Hyperthyroidism	348
Cold intolerance, weight gain, brittle hair	Hypothyroidism	348
Cutaneous/dermal edema due to deposition of mucopolysaccharides in connective tissue	Myxedema (caused by hypothyroidism, Graves disease [pretibial])	348

CLINICAL PRESENTATION	DIAGNOSIS/DISEASE	PAGE
Facial muscle spasm upon tapping	Chvostek sign (hypocalcemia)	352
Carpal spasm upon inflation of BP cuff	Trousseau sign (hypocalcemia)	352
Deep, labored breathing/hyperventilation	Diabetic ketoacidosis (Kussmaul respirations)	355
Skin hyperpigmentation, orthostatic hypotension, fatigue, weakness, muscle aches, weight loss, GI disturbances	Chronic 1° adrenal insufficiency (Addison disease) → ↑ ACTH, ↑ α-MSH	357
Shock, altered mental status, vomiting, abdominal pain, weakness, fatigue	Acute adrenal insufficiency (adrenal crisis)	357
Pancreatic, pituitary, parathyroid tumors	MEN 1 (autosomal dominant *MEN1* mutation)	360
Thyroid tumors, pheochromocytoma, ganglioneuromatosis, Marfanoid habitus	MEN 2B (autosomal dominant *RET* mutation)	360
Thyroid and parathyroid tumors, pheochromocytoma	MEN 2A (autosomal dominant *RET* mutation)	360
Cutaneous flushing, diarrhea, bronchospasm, heart murmur	Carcinoid syndrome (↑ 5-HIAA)	361
Jaundice, palpable distended non-tender gallbladder	Courvoisier sign (distal malignant obstruction of biliary tree)	378
Vomiting blood following gastroesophageal lacerations	Mallory-Weiss syndrome (alcohol use disorder, bulimia nervosa)	387
Dysphagia (esophageal webs), glossitis, iron deficiency anemia	Plummer-Vinson syndrome (may progress to esophageal squamous cell carcinoma)	387
Enlarged, hard left supraclavicular node	Virchow node (abdominal metastasis)	389
Hematemesis, melena	Upper GI bleeding (eg, peptic ulcer disease)	390
Hematochezia	Lower GI bleeding (eg, colonic diverticulosis)	390
Arthralgias, adenopathy, cardiac and neurological symptoms, diarrhea	Whipple disease (*Tropheryma whipplei*)	391
Severe RLQ pain with palpation of LLQ	Rovsing sign (acute appendicitis)	393
Severe RLQ pain with deep tenderness	McBurney sign (acute appendicitis)	393
Hamartomatous GI polyps, hyperpigmented macules on mouth, feet, hands, genitalia	Peutz-Jeghers syndrome (inherited, benign polyposis can cause bowel obstruction; ↑ cancer risk, mainly GI)	397
Multiple colon polyps, osteomas/soft tissue tumors, impacted/supernumerary teeth	Gardner syndrome (subtype of FAP)	397
Severe jaundice in neonate	Crigler-Najjar syndrome (congenital unconjugated hyperbilirubinemia)	404
Golden brown rings around peripheral cornea	Wilson disease (Kayser-Fleischer rings due to copper accumulation)	405
Female, fat, fertile, forty	Cholelithiasis (gallstones)	406
Painless jaundice with enlarged gallbladder	Cancer of the pancreatic head obstructing bile duct	408
Bluish line on gingiva	Burton line (lead poisoning)	429
Short stature, café-au-lait spots, thumb/radial defects, ↑ incidence of tumors/leukemia, aplastic anemia	Fanconi anemia (genetic loss of DNA crosslink repair; often progresses to AML)	431
Red/pink urine, fragile RBCs	Paroxysmal nocturnal hemoglobinuria	432
Painful blue fingers/toes, hemolytic anemia	Cold agglutinin disease (autoimmune hemolytic anemia caused by *Mycoplasma pneumoniae*, infectious mononucleosis, CLL)	433

CLINICAL PRESENTATION	DIAGNOSIS/DISEASE	PAGE
Petechiae, mucosal bleeding, prolonged bleeding time	Platelet disorders (eg, Glanzmann thrombasthenia, Bernard Soulier, HUS, TTP, ITP)	437
Fever, night sweats, weight loss	B symptoms of malignancy	438
Skin patches/plaques, Pautrier microabscesses, atypical T cells	Mycosis fungoides (cutaneous T-cell lymphoma) or Sézary syndrome (mycosis fungoides + malignant T cells in blood)	439
Neonate with arm paralysis following difficult birth, arm in "waiter's tip" position	Erb-Duchenne palsy (superior trunk [C5–C6] brachial plexus injury)	458
Anterior drawer sign ⊕	Anterior cruciate ligament injury	464
Bone pain, bone enlargement, arthritis	Osteitis deformans (Paget disease of bone, ↑ osteoblastic and osteoclastic activity)	475
Swollen, hard, painful finger joints in an elderly individual, pain worse with activity	Osteoarthritis (osteophytes on PIP [Bouchard nodes], DIP [Heberden nodes])	478
Sudden swollen/painful big toe joint, tophi	Gout/podagra (hyperuricemia)	479
Dry eyes, dry mouth, arthritis	Sjögren syndrome (autoimmune destruction of exocrine glands)	480
Urethritis, conjunctivitis, arthritis in a male	Reactive arthritis associated with HLA-B27	481
"Butterfly" facial rash, arthritis, cytopenia, and fever in a young female	Systemic lupus erythematosus	482
Cervical lymphadenopathy, desquamating rash, coronary aneurysms, red conjunctivae and tongue, hand-foot changes	Kawasaki disease (mucocutaneous lymph node syndrome, treat with IVIG and aspirin)	484
Palpable purpura on buttocks/legs, joint pain, abdominal pain (child), hematuria	Immunoglobulin A vasculitis (Henoch-Schönlein purpura, affects skin and kidneys)	485
Painful fingers/toes changing color from white to blue to red with cold or stress	Raynaud phenomenon (vasospasm in extremities)	486
Dark purple skin/mouth nodules in a patient with AIDS	Kaposi sarcoma, associated with HHV-8	492
Pruritic, purple, polygonal planar papules and plaques (6 P's)	Lichen planus	496
Ataxia, nystagmus, vertigo, dysarthria	Cerebellar lesion (lateral affects voluntary movement of extremities; medial affects axial and proximal movement)	515
Dorsiflexion of large toe with fanning of other toes upon plantar scrape	Babinski sign (UMN lesion)	527
Hyperphagia, hypersexuality, hyperorality	Klüver-Bucy syndrome (bilateral amygdala lesion)	528
Resting tremor, athetosis, chorea	Basal ganglia lesion	528
Lucid interval after traumatic brain injury	Epidural hematoma (middle meningeal artery rupture; branch of maxillary artery)	531
"Worst headache of my life"	Subarachnoid hemorrhage	531
Dysphagia, hoarseness, ↓ gag reflex, nystagmus, ipsilateral Horner syndrome	Lateral medullary syndrome (posterior inferior cerebellar artery lesion)	533
Resting tremor, rigidity, akinesia, postural instability, shuffling gait, micrographia	Parkinson disease (loss of dopaminergic neurons in substantia nigra pars compacta)	538
Chorea, dementia, caudate degeneration	Huntington disease (autosomal dominant CAG repeat expansion)	538

CLINICAL PRESENTATION	DIAGNOSIS/DISEASE	PAGE
Urinary incontinence, gait apraxia, cognitive dysfunction	Normal pressure hydrocephalus	540
Nystagmus, intention tremor, scanning speech, bilateral internuclear ophthalmoplegia	Multiple sclerosis	541
Rapidly progressive limb weakness that ascends following GI/upper respiratory infection	Guillain-Barré syndrome (acute inflammatory demyelinating polyneuropathy)	542
Café-au-lait spots, Lisch nodules (iris hamartoma), cutaneous neurofibromas, pheochromocytomas, optic gliomas	Neurofibromatosis type I	543
Vascular birthmark (port-wine stain) of the face	Nevus flammeus (benign, but associated with Sturge-Weber syndrome)	543
Renal cell carcinoma (bilateral), hemangioblastomas, angiomatosis, pheochromocytoma	von Hippel-Lindau disease (deletion of *VHL* gene on chromosome 3p)	543
Bilateral vestibular schwannomas	Neurofibromatosis type 2	543
Hyperreflexia, hypertonia, Babinski sign present	UMN damage	547
Hyporeflexia, hypotonia, atrophy, fasciculations	LMN damage	547
Flaccid limb weakness, fasciculations, atrophy, bulbar palsy	UMN and LMN deficits	548
Staggering gait, frequent falls, nystagmus, hammer toes, diabetes mellitus, hypertrophic cardiomyopathy	Friedreich ataxia	549
Unilateral facial drooping involving forehead	LMN facial nerve (CN VII) palsy; UMN lesions spare the forehead	550
Episodic vertigo, tinnitus, sensorineural hearing loss	Ménière disease	552
Ptosis, miosis, anhidrosis	Horner syndrome (sympathetic chain lesion)	559
Conjugate horizontal gaze palsy, horizontal diplopia	Internuclear ophthalmoplegia (damage to MLF; may be unilateral or bilateral)	563
"Waxing and waning" level of consciousness (acute onset), ↓ attention span, ↓ level of arousal	Delirium (usually 2° to other cause)	581
Polyuria, renal tubular acidosis type II, growth retardation, electrolyte imbalances, hypophosphatemic rickets	Fanconi syndrome (multiple combined dysfunction of the proximal convoluted tubule)	610
Periorbital and/or peripheral edema, proteinuria (> 3.5g/day), hypoalbuminemia, hypercholesterolemia	Nephrotic syndrome	619
Hereditary nephritis, sensorineural hearing loss, retinopathy, lens dislocation	Alport syndrome (mutation in type IV collagen)	620
Wilms tumor, macroglossia, organomegaly, hemihyperplasia, omphalocele	Beckwith-Wiedemann syndrome (*WT2* mutation)	629
Streak ovaries, congenital heart disease, horseshoe kidney, cystic hygroma, short stature, webbed neck, lymphedema	Turner syndrome (45,XO)	661
Red, itchy, swollen rash of nipple/areola	Paget disease of the breast (sign of underlying neoplasm)	674
Ovarian fibroma, ascites, pleural effusion	Meigs syndrome	671
Fibrous plaques in tunica albuginea of penis with abnormal curvature	Peyronie disease (connective tissue disorder)	675
Hypoxemia, polycythemia, hypercapnia	Chronic bronchitis (hypertrophy and hyperplasia of mucous cells, "blue bloater")	698

CLINICAL PRESENTATION	DIAGNOSIS/DISEASE	PAGE
Pink complexion, dyspnea, hyperventilation	Emphysema ("pink puffer," centriacinar [smoking] or panacinar [α_1-antitrypsin deficiency])	698
Bilateral hilar adenopathy, uveitis	Sarcoidosis (noncaseating granulomas)	700

▶ CLASSIC LABS/FINDINGS

LAB/DIAGNOSTIC FINDING	DIAGNOSIS/DISEASE	PAGE
Colonies of mucoid *Pseudomonas* in lungs	Cystic fibrosis (autosomal recessive mutation in *CFTR* gene → fat-soluble vitamin deficiency and mucous plugs)	60
↓ AFP in amniotic fluid/maternal serum	Down syndrome, Edwards syndrome	63
↑ β-hCG, ↓ PAPP-A on first trimester screening	Down syndrome	63
↑ serum homocysteine, ↑ mehtylmalonic acid, ↓ folate	Vitamin B_{12} deficiency	69
Anti-histone antibodies	Drug-induced SLE (eg, hydralazine, isoniazid, phenytoin, TNF-α inhibitors)	115, 501
↓ T cells, ↓ PTH, ↓ Ca^{2+}, absent thymic shadow on CXR	Thymic aplasia (DiGeorge syndrome, velocardiofacial syndrome)	116
Large granules in phagocytes, immunodeficiency	Chédiak-Higashi disease (congenital failure of phagolysosome formation)	117
Recurrent infections, eczema, thrombocytopenia	Wiskott-Aldrich syndrome	117
Optochin sensitivity	Sensitive: *S pneumoniae*; resistant: viridans streptococci (*S mutans*, *S sanguis*)	134
Novobiocin response	Sensitive: *S epidermidis*; resistant: *S saprophyticus*	134
Bacitracin response	Sensitive: *S pyogenes* (group A); resistant: *S agalactiae* (group B)	134
Branching gram ⊕ rods with sulfur granules	*Actinomyces israelii*	139
Hilar lymphadenopathy, peripheral granulomatous lesion in middle or lower lung lobes (can calcify)	Ghon complex (1° TB: *Mycobacterium* bacilli)	140
"Thumb sign" on lateral neck x-ray	Epiglottitis (*Haemophilus influenzae*)	142
Bacteria-covered vaginal epithelial cells	"Clue cells" (*Gardnerella vaginalis*)	148
Dilated cardiomyopathy with apical atrophy	Chagas disease (*Trypanosoma cruzi*)	158
Atypical lymphocytes, heterophile antibodies	Infectious mononucleosis (EBV infection)	165
Eosinophilic intranuclear inclusions with perinuclear halo	Cells infected by herpesviruses (eg, HSV, VZV, CMV)	165, 166
"Steeple" sign on frontal CXR	Croup (parainfluenza virus)	170
Eosinophilic inclusion bodies in cytoplasm of hippocampal and cerebellar neurons	Negri bodies of rabies	171
Ring-enhancing brain lesion on CT/MRI in AIDS	*Toxoplasma gondii*, CNS lymphoma	177
Psammoma bodies	Meningiomas, papillary thyroid carcinoma, mesothelioma, papillary serous carcinoma of the endometrium and ovary	228

LAB/DIAGNOSTIC FINDING	DIAGNOSIS/DISEASE	PAGE
"Delta wave" on ECG, short PR interval, supraventricular tachycardia	Wolff-Parkinson-White syndrome (bundle of Kent bypasses AV node)	315
"Boot-shaped" heart on x-ray	Tetralogy of Fallot (due to RVH)	306
Rib notching (inferior surface, on x-ray)	Coarctation of the aorta	307
Granuloma with giant cells after pharyngeal infection	Aschoff bodies (rheumatic fever)	322
Electrical alternans (alternating amplitude on ECG)	Cardiac tamponade	320
Enlarged thyroid cells with ground-glass nuclei with central clearing	"Orphan Annie" eyes nuclei (papillary carcinoma of the thyroid)	351
"Brown" tumor of bone	Hyperparathyroidism or osteitis fibrosa cystica (deposited hemosiderin from hemorrhage gives brown color)	353, 476
Hypertension, hypokalemia, metabolic alkalosis	1° hyperaldosteronism (eg, Conn syndrome)	358
Mucin-filled cell with peripheral nucleus	"Signet ring" (gastric carcinoma)	389
Anti-transglutaminase/anti-gliadin/anti-endomysial antibodies	Celiac disease (diarrhea, weight loss)	391
Narrowing of bowel lumen on barium x-ray	"String sign" (Crohn disease)	392
"Lead pipe" appearance of colon on abdominal imaging	Ulcerative colitis (loss of haustra)	392
Thousands of polyps on colonoscopy	Familial adenomatous polyposis (autosomal dominant, mutation of APC gene)	397
"Apple core" lesion on barium enema x-ray	Colorectal cancer (usually left-sided)	398
Eosinophilic cytoplasmic inclusion in liver cell	Mallory body (alcoholic liver disease)	401
Triglyceride accumulation in liver cell vacuoles	Fatty liver disease (alcoholic or metabolic syndrome)	401
Anti-smooth muscle antibodies (ASMAs), anti-liver/kidney microsomal-1 (anti-LKM1) antibodies	Autoimmune hepatitis	401
"Nutmeg" appearance of liver	Chronic passive congestion of liver due to right heart failure or Budd-Chiari syndrome	402
Antimitochondrial antibodies (AMAs)	1° biliary cholangitis (female, cholestasis, portal hypertension)	405
Low serum ceruloplasmin	Wilson disease (hepatolenticular degeneration; Kayser-Fleischer rings due to copper accumulation)	405
Migratory thrombophlebitis (leading to migrating DVTs and vasculitis)	Trousseau syndrome (adenocarcinoma of pancreas or lung)	408
Hypersegmented neutrophils	Megaloblastic anemia (B_{12} deficiency: neurologic symptoms; folate deficiency: no neurologic symptoms)	416
Basophilic nuclear remnants in RBCs	Howell-Jolly bodies (due to splenectomy or nonfunctional spleen)	426
Basophilic stippling of RBCs	Lead poisoning or sideroblastic anemia	426
Hypochromic, microcytic anemia	Iron deficiency anemia, lead poisoning, thalassemia (fetal hemoglobin sometimes present)	427, 428
"Hair on end" ("crew cut") appearance on x-ray	β-thalassemia, sickle cell disease (marrow expansion)	428, 432
Anti-GpIIb/IIIa antibodies	Immune thrombocytopenia	436
High level of D-dimers	DVT, DIC	437, 695

LAB/DIAGNOSTIC FINDING	DIAGNOSIS/DISEASE	PAGE
Giant B cells with bilobed nuclei with prominent inclusions ("owl's eye")	Reed-Sternberg cells (Hodgkin lymphoma)	438
Sheets of medium-sized lymphoid cells with scattered pale, tingible body–laden macrophages ("starry sky" histology)	Burkitt lymphoma (t[8:14] c-*myc* activation, associated with EBV; "starry sky" made up of malignant cells)	439
Lytic ("punched-out") bone lesions on x-ray	Multiple myeloma	440
Monoclonal spike on serum protein electrophoresis	▪ Multiple myeloma (usually IgG or IgA) ▪ Waldenström macroglobulinemia (IgM) ▪ Monoclonal gammopathy of undetermined significance	440
Stacks of RBCs	Rouleaux formation (high ESR, multiple myeloma)	440
Azurophilic peroxidase ⊕ granular inclusions in granulocytes and myeloblasts	Auer rods (APL)	442
WBCs that look "smudged"	CLL	442
"Tennis racket"-shaped cytoplasmic organelles (EM) in Langerhans cells	Birbeck granules (Langerhans cell histiocytosis)	444
"Soap bubble" in femur or tibia on x-ray	Giant cell tumor of bone (generally benign)	476
Raised periosteum (creating a "Codman triangle")	Aggressive bone lesion (eg, osteosarcoma, Ewing sarcoma)	477
"Onion skin" periosteal reaction	Ewing sarcoma (malignant small blue cell tumor)	477
Anti-IgG antibodies	Rheumatoid arthritis (systemic inflammation, joint pannus, boutonniere and swan neck deformities)	478
Rhomboid crystals, ⊕ birefringent	Pseudogout (calcium pyrophosphate dihydrate crystals)	479
Needle-shaped, ⊖ birefringent crystals	Gout (monosodium urate crystals)	479
↑ uric acid levels	Gout, Lesch-Nyhan syndrome, tumor lysis syndrome, loop and thiazide diuretics	479
"Bamboo spine" on x-ray	Ankylosing spondylitis (chronic inflammatory arthritis: HLA-B27)	481
Antinuclear antibodies (ANAs: anti-Smith and anti-dsDNA)	SLE (type III hypersensitivity)	482
Antineutrophil cytoplasmic antibodies (ANCAs)	Microscopic polyangiitis and eosinophilic granulomatosis with polyangiitis (MPO-ANCA/p-ANCA); granulomatosis with polyangiitis (PR3-ANCA/c-ANCA); primary sclerosing cholangitis (MPO-ANCA/p-ANCA)	485
Anticentromere antibodies	Scleroderma (CREST syndrome)	487
Anti-topoisomerase antibodies	Diffuse scleroderma	487
Anti-desmoglein (anti-desmosome) antibodies	Pemphigus vulgaris (blistering)	494
Keratin pearls on a skin biopsy	Squamous cell carcinoma	498
↑ AFP in amniotic fluid/maternal serum	Dating error, anencephaly, spina bifida (open neural tube defects)	505
Bloody or yellow tap on lumbar puncture	Xanthochromia (due to subarachnoid hemorrhage)	531
Eosinophilic cytoplasmic inclusion in neuron	Lewy body (Parkinson disease and Lewy body dementia)	538, 539
Extracellular amyloid deposition in gray matter of brain	Senile plaques (Alzheimer disease)	538

LAB/DIAGNOSTIC FINDING	DIAGNOSIS/DISEASE	PAGE
Depigmentation of neurons in substantia nigra	Parkinson disease (basal ganglia disorder: rigidity, resting tremor, bradykinesia)	538
Protein aggregates in neurons from hyperphosphorylation of tau protein	Neurofibrillary tangles (Alzheimer disease) and Pick bodies (Pick disease)	538
Silver-staining spherical aggregation of tau proteins in neurons	Pick bodies (frontotemporal dementia: progressive dementia, changes in personality)	538
Pseudopalisading pleomorphic tumor cells on brain biopsy	Glioblastoma multiforme	544
Circular grouping of dark tumor cells surrounding pale neurofibrils	Homer-Wright rosettes (neuroblastoma, medulloblastoma)	546
"Waxy" casts with very low urine flow	Chronic end-stage renal disease	618
WBC casts in urine	Acute pyelonephritis, transplant rejection, tubulointerstitial inflammation	618
RBC casts in urine	Glomerulonephritis	618
"Tram-track" appearance of capillary loops of glomerular basement membranes on light microscopy	Membranoproliferative glomerulonephritis	620
Anti–glomerular basement membrane antibodies	Goodpasture syndrome (glomerulonephritis and hemoptysis)	620
Cellular crescents in Bowman capsule	Rapidly progressive (crescentic) glomerulonephritis	620
"Wire loop" glomerular capillary appearance on light microscopy	Diffuse proliferative glomerulonephritis (usually seen with lupus)	620
Linear appearance of IgG deposition on glomerular and alveolar basement membranes	Goodpasture syndrome	620
"Lumpy bumpy" appearance of glomeruli on immunofluorescence	Poststreptococcal glomerulonephritis (due to deposition of IgG, IgM, and C3)	620
Necrotizing vasculitis (lungs) and necrotizing glomerulonephritis	Granulomatosis with polyangiitis (PR3-ANCA/c-ANCA) and Goodpasture syndrome (anti–basement membrane antibodies)	620
Nodular hyaline deposits in glomeruli	Kimmelstiel-Wilson nodules (diabetic nephropathy)	621
Podocyte fusion or "effacement" on electron microscopy	Minimal change disease (child with nephrotic syndrome)	621
"Spikes" on basement membrane, "dome-like" subepithelial deposits	Membranous nephropathy (nephrotic syndrome)	621
Thyroid-like appearance of kidney	Chronic pyelonephritis (usually due to recurrent infections)	624
Granular casts in urine	Acute tubular necrosis (eg, ischemia or toxic injury)	626
hCG elevated	Multiple gestations, hydatidiform moles, choriocarcinomas, Down syndrome	658
Dysplastic squamous cervical cells with "raisinoid" nuclei and hyperchromasia	Koilocytes (HPV: predisposes to cervical cancer)	669
Sheets of uniform "fried egg" cells, ↑ hCG, ↑ LDH	Dysgerminoma	671
Disarrayed granulosa cells arranged around collections of eosinophilic fluid	Call-Exner bodies (granulosa cell tumor of the ovary)	671
"Chocolate cyst" of ovary	Endometriosis (frequently involves both ovaries)	672
Mammary gland ("blue domed") cyst	Fibrocystic change of the breast	673

LAB/DIAGNOSTIC FINDING	DIAGNOSIS/DISEASE	PAGE
Glomerulus-like structure surrounding vessel in germ cells	Schiller-Duval bodies (yolk sac tumor)	671
Rectangular, crystal-like, cytoplasmic inclusions in Leydig cells	Reinke crystals (Leydig cell tumor)	677
Thrombi made of white/red layers	Lines of Zahn (arterial thrombus, layers of platelets/ RBCs)	696
Hexagonal, double-pointed, needle-like crystals in bronchial secretions	Bronchial asthma (Charcot-Leyden crystals: eosinophilic granules)	698
Desquamated epithelium casts in sputum	Curschmann spirals (bronchial asthma; can result in whorled mucous plugs)	698
"Honeycomb lung" on x-ray or CT	Idiopathic pulmonary fibrosis	700
Iron-containing nodules in alveolar septum	Ferruginous bodies (asbestosis: ↑ chance of lung cancer)	701
Bronchogenic apical lung tumor on imaging	Pancoast tumor (can compress cervical sympathetic chain and cause Horner syndrome)	709

▶ CLASSIC/RELEVANT TREATMENTS

CONDITION	COMMON TREATMENT(S)	PAGE
Ethylene glycol/methanol intoxication	Fomepizole (alcohol dehydrogenase inhibitor)	72
Chronic hepatitis B or C	IFN-α (HBV and HCV); ribavirin, simeprevir, sofosbuvir (HCV)	121, 204
Streptococcus bovis	Penicillin prophylaxis; evaluation for colon cancer if linked to endocarditis	137
Clostridium botulinum	Human botulinum immunoglobulin	138
Clostridium tetani	Antitoxin and wound debridement	138
Clostridium difficile	Oral metronidazole; if refractory, oral vancomycin. Refractory cases: repeat regimen or fecal microbiota transplant	138
Haemophilus influenzae (B)	Amoxicillin ± clavulanate (mucosal infections), ceftriaxone (meningitis), rifampin (prophylaxis)	142
Neisseria gonorrhoeae	Ceftriaxone (add azithromycin or doxycycline to cover likely concurrent *C trachomatis*)	142
Neisseria meningitidis	Penicillin/ceftriaxone, rifampin/ciprofloxacin/ceftriaxone (prophylaxis)	142
Legionella pneumophila	Macrolides (eg, azithromycin or fluoroquinolones)	143
Pseudomonas aeruginosa	Piperacillin-tazobactam, cephalosporins, monobactams, fluoroquinolones, carbapenems	143
Treponema pallidum	Penicillin G	147
Chlamydia trachomatis	Azithromycin or doxycycline (+ ceftriaxone for gonorrhea coinfection), oral erythromycin to treat chlamydial conjunctivitis in infants	148

CONDITION	COMMON TREATMENT(S)	PAGE
Candida albicans	Topical azoles (vaginitis); nystatin, fluconazole, caspofungin (oral); fluconazole, caspofungin, amphotericin B (esophageal or systemic)	153
Cryptococcus neoformans	Induction with amphotericin B and flucytosine, maintenance with fluconazole (in AIDS patients)	153
Sporothrix schenckii	Itraconazole, oral potassium iodide	154
Pneumocystis jirovecii	TMP-SMX (prophylaxis and treatment in immunosuppressed patients, CD4 < $200/mm^3$)	154
Toxoplasma gondii	Sulfadiazine + pyrimethamine	156
Malaria	Chloroquine, mefloquine, atovaquone/proguanil (for blood schizont), primaquine (for liver hypnozoite)	157
Trichomonas vaginalis	Metronidazole (patient and partner[s])	158
Streptococcus pyogenes	Penicillin prophylaxis	187
Streptococcus pneumoniae	Penicillin/cephalosporin (systemic infection, pneumonia), vancomycin (meningitis)	187, 190
Staphylococcus aureus	MSSA: nafcillin, oxacillin, dicloxacillin (antistaphylococcal penicillins); MRSA: vancomycin, daptomycin, linezolid, ceftaroline	188, 190, 198
Enterococci	Vancomycin, aminopenicillins/cephalosporins. VRE: daptomycin, linezolid, tigecycline, streptogramins	189, 198
Rickettsia rickettsii	Doxycycline, chloramphenicol	192
Mycobacterium tuberculosis	RIPE (rifampin, isoniazid, pyrazinamide, ethambutol)	196
UTI prophylaxis	TMP-SMX	198
Influenza	Oseltamivir, zanamivir	201
CMV	Ganciclovir, foscarnet, cidofovir	202
Patent ductus arteriosus	Close with indomethacin; keep open with PGE analogs	291
Stable angina	Sublingual nitroglycerin	312
Hypercholesterolemia	Statin (first-line)	328
Hypertriglyceridemia	Fibrate	328
Arrhythmia in damaged cardiac tissue	Class IB antiarrhythmic (lidocaine, mexiletine)	330
Prolactinoma	Cabergoline/bromocriptine (dopamine agonists)	338
Diabetes insipidus	Desmopressin (central); hydrochlorothiazide, indomethacin, amiloride (nephrogenic)	346
SIADH	Fluid restriction, IV hypertonic saline, conivaptan/tolvaptan, demeclocycline	346
Diabetic ketoacidosis/hyperosmolar hyperglycemic state	Fluids, insulin, K^+	355
Pheochromocytoma	α-antagonists (eg, phenoxybenzamine)	359
Carcinoid syndrome	Octreotide, telotristat	361
Diabetes mellitus type 1	Dietary intervention (low carbohydrate) + insulin replacement	362
Diabetes mellitus type 2	Dietary intervention, oral hypoglycemics, and insulin (if refractory)	362

CONDITION	COMMON TREATMENT(S)	PAGE
Crohn disease	Corticosteroids, infliximab, azathioprine	392
Ulcerative colitis	5-ASA preparations (eg, mesalamine), 6-mercaptopurine, infliximab, colectomy	392
Sickle cell disease	Hydroxyurea (↑ fetal hemoglobin)	432
Chronic myelogenous leukemia	BCR-ABL tyrosine kinase inhibitors (eg, imatinib)	442
Acute promyelocytic leukemia (M3)	All-*trans* retinoic acid, arsenic trioxide	442
Drug of choice for anticoagulation in pregnancy	Low-molecular-weight heparin	445
Immediate anticoagulation	Heparin	445
Long-term anticoagulation	Warfarin, dabigatran, direct factor Xa inhibitors	446
Heparin reversal	Protamine sulfate	447
Warfarin reversal	Vitamin K (slow) +/– fresh frozen plasma or prothrombin complex concentrate (rapid)	447
Dabigatran reversal	Idarucizumab	447
Direct factor Xa inhibitor reversal	Andexanet alfa	447
HER2 ⊕ breast cancer	Trastuzumab	452
Hemorrhagic cystitis from cyclophosphamide/ifosfamide	Mesna	453
Nephrotoxicity from platinum compounds	Amifostine	453
Cardiotoxicity from anthracyclines	Dexrazoxane	453
Myelosuppression from methotrexate	Leucovorin	453
Osteoporosis	Calcium/vitamin D supplementation (prophylaxis); bisphosphonates, PTH analogs, SERMs, calcitonin, denosumab (treatment)	474
Osteomalacia/rickets	Vitamin D supplementation	475
Chronic gout	Xanthine oxidase inhibitors (eg, allopurinol, febuxostat); pegloticase; probenecid	479
Acute gout attack	NSAIDs, colchicine, glucocorticoids	479
Buerger disease	Smoking cessation	484
Kawasaki disease	IVIG, aspirin	484
Temporal arteritis	High-dose glucocorticoids	484
Granulomatosis with polyangiitis	Cyclophosphamide, glucocorticoids	485
Neural tube defect prevention	Prenatal folic acid	505
Migraine	Abortive therapies (eg, sumatriptan, NSAIDs); prophylaxis (eg, propranolol, topiramate, anti-CGRP antibodies, amitriptyline)	536
Multiple sclerosis	Disease-modifying therapies (eg, β-interferon, glatiramer, natalizumab); for acute flares, use IV steroids	541
Tonic-clonic seizures	Levetiracetam, phenytoin, valproate, carbamazepine	564
Absence seizures	Ethosuximide	564
Trigeminal neuralgia (tic douloureux)	Carbamazepine	536

CONDITION	COMMON TREATMENT(S)	PAGE
Malignant hyperthermia	Dantrolene	572
Anorexia	Nutrition, psychotherapy, SSRIs	590
Bulimia nervosa	Nutrition rehabilitation, psychotherapy, SSRIs	590
Alcohol use disorder	Disulfiram, acamprosate, naltrexone, supportive care	595
ADHD	Methylphenidate, amphetamines, behavioral therapy, atomoxetine, guanfacine, clonidine	580, 596
Alcohol withdrawal	Long-acting benzodiazepines	596
Bipolar disorder	Mood stabilizers (eg, lithium, valproic acid, carbamazepine), atypical antipsychotics	596
Depression	SSRIs (first-line)	596
Generalized anxiety disorder	SSRIs, SNRIs (first line); buspirone (second line)	596
Schizophrenia	Atypical antipsychotics	583, 596
Hyperaldosteronism	Spironolactone	632
Benign prostatic hyperplasia	α_1-antagonists, 5α-reductase inhibitors, PDE-5 inhibitors, TURP	678
Infertility	Leuprolide, GnRH (pulsatile), clomiphene	680
Breast cancer in postmenopausal woman	Aromatase inhibitor (anastrozole)	680
ER/PR ⊕ breast cancer	Tamoxifen	680
Uterine fibroids	Leuprolide, GnRH (continuous)	680
Medical abortion	Mifepristone	681
Prostate adenocarcinoma	Flutamide, GnRH (continuous), degarelix, ketoconazole	680, 682
Erectile dysfunction	Sildenafil	711
Pulmonary arterial hypertension (idiopathic)	Sildenafil, bosentan, epoprostenol, iloprost	711

▸ KEY ASSOCIATIONS

DISEASE/FINDING	MOST COMMON/IMPORTANT ASSOCIATIONS	PAGE
Mitochondrial inheritance	Disease occurs in both males and females, inherited through females only	59
Intellectual disability	Down syndrome, fragile X syndrome	62, 63
Vitamin deficiency (USA)	Folate (pregnant women are at high risk; body stores only 3- to 4-month supply; prevents neural tube defects)	68
Lysosomal storage disease	Gaucher disease	88
Bacterial meningitis (> 6 months old)	*S pneumoniae*	180
Bacterial meningitis (newborns and kids)	Group B streptococcus/*E coli*/*Listeria monocytogenes* (newborns)	180

DISEASE/FINDING	MOST COMMON/IMPORTANT ASSOCIATIONS	PAGE
HLA-DR3	Diabetes mellitus type 1, SLE, Graves disease, Hashimoto thyroiditis (also associated with HLA-DR5), Addison disease	100
HLA-DR4	Diabetes mellitus type 1, rheumatoid arthritis, Addison disease	100
Bacteria associated with gastritis, peptic ulcer disease, and gastric malignancies (eg, adenocarcinoma, MALToma)	*H pylori*	146
Opportunistic respiratory infection in AIDS	*Pneumocystis jirovecii* pneumonia	154
Helminth infection (US)	*Enterobius vermicularis*	159
Viral encephalitis affecting temporal lobe	HSV-1	164
Infection 2° to blood transfusion	Hepatitis C	173
Food poisoning (exotoxin mediated)	*S aureus*, *B cereus*	178
Osteomyelitis	*S aureus* (most common overall)	180
Osteomyelitis in sickle cell disease	*Salmonella*	180
Osteomyelitis with IV drug use	*S aureus*, *Pseudomonas*, *Candida*	180
UTI	*E coli*, *Staphylococcus saprophyticus* (young women)	181
Sexually transmitted disease	*C trachomatis* (usually coinfected with *N gonorrhoeae*)	184
Nosocomial pneumonia	*S aureus*, *Pseudomonas*, *Klebsiella*, *Acinetobacter*	185
Pelvic inflammatory disease	*C trachomatis*, *N gonorrhoeae*	185
Metastases to bone	Prostate, breast > kidney, thyroid, lung	224
Metastases to brain	Lung > breast > melanoma, colon, kidney	224
Metastases to liver	Colon >> stomach > pancreas	224
S3 heart sound	↑ ventricular filling pressure (eg, mitral regurgitation, HF), common in dilated ventricles	296
S4 heart sound	Stiff/hypertrophic ventricle (aortic stenosis, restrictive cardiomyopathy)	296
Constrictive pericarditis	TB (developing world); idiopathic, viral illness (developed world)	296, 320
Holosystolic murmur	VSD, tricuspid regurgitation, mitral regurgitation	299
Ejection click	Aortic stenosis	300
Mitral valve stenosis	Rheumatic heart disease	300
Opening snap	Mitral stenosis	300
Heart murmur, congenital	Mitral valve prolapse	300
Chronic arrhythmia	Atrial fibrillation (associated with high risk of emboli)	316
Cyanosis (early; less common)	Tetralogy of Fallot, transposition of great vessels, truncus arteriosus, total anomalous pulmonary venous return, tricuspid atresia	306
Late cyanotic shunt (uncorrected left to right becomes right to left)	Eisenmenger syndrome (caused by ASD, VSD, PDA; results in pulmonary hypertension/polycythemia)	307
Congenital cardiac anomaly	VSD	307

DISEASE/FINDING	MOST COMMON/IMPORTANT ASSOCIATIONS	PAGE
Hypertension, 2°	Renal artery stenosis, chronic kidney disease (eg, polycystic kidney disease, diabetic nephropathy), hyperaldosteronism	308
Aortic aneurysm, thoracic	Marfan syndrome (idiopathic cystic medial degeneration)	310
Aortic aneurysm, abdominal	Atherosclerosis, smoking is major risk factor	310
Aortic aneurysm, ascending or arch	3° syphilis (syphilitic aortitis), vasa vasorum destruction	310
Sites of atherosclerosis	Abdominal aorta > coronary artery > popliteal artery > carotid artery	310
Aortic dissection	Hypertension	311
Right heart failure due to a pulmonary cause	Cor pulmonale	319
Heart valve in bacterial endocarditis	Mitral > aortic (rheumatic fever), tricuspid (IV drug abuse)	321
Endocarditis presentation associated with bacterium	*S aureus* (acute, IVDA, tricuspid valve), viridans streptococci (subacute, dental procedure), *S bovis* (colon cancer), culture negative (*Coxiella*, *Bartonella*, HACEK)	321
Temporal arteritis	Risk of ipsilateral blindness due to occlusion of ophthalmic artery; polymyalgia rheumatica	484
Recurrent inflammation/thrombosis of small/medium vessels in extremities	Buerger disease (strongly associated with tobacco)	484
Cardiac 1° tumor (kids)	Rhabdomyoma, often seen in tuberous sclerosis	324
Cardiac tumor (adults)	Metastasis, myxoma (90% in left atrium; "ball valve")	324
Congenital adrenal hyperplasia, hypotension	21-hydroxylase deficiency	343
Hypopituitarism	Pituitary adenoma (usually benign tumor)	347
Congenital hypothyroidism (cretinism)	Thyroid dysgenesis/dyshormonogenesis, iodine deficiency	349
Thyroid cancer	Papillary carcinoma (childhood irradiation)	351
Hypoparathyroidism	Accidental excision during thyroidectomy	352
1° hyperparathyroidism	Adenomas, hyperplasia, carcinoma	353
2° hyperparathyroidism	Hypocalcemia of chronic kidney disease	353
Cushing syndrome	▪ Iatrogenic (from corticosteroid therapy) ▪ Adrenocortical adenoma (secretes excess cortisol) ▪ ACTH-secreting pituitary adenoma (Cushing disease) ▪ Paraneoplastic (due to ACTH secretion by tumors)	356
1° hyperaldosteronism	Adrenal hyperplasia or adenoma	358
Tumor of the adrenal medulla (kids)	Neuroblastoma (malignant)	358
Tumor of the adrenal medulla (adults)	Pheochromocytoma (usually benign)	359
Refractory peptic ulcers and high gastrin levels	Zollinger-Ellison syndrome (gastrinoma of duodenum or pancreas), associated with MEN1	360, 361
Esophageal cancer	Squamous cell carcinoma (worldwide); adenocarcinoma (US)	388
Acute gastric ulcer associated with CNS injury	Cushing ulcer (↑ intracranial pressure stimulates vagal gastric H^+ secretion)	389
Acute gastric ulcer associated with severe burns	Curling ulcer (greatly reduced plasma volume results in sloughing of gastric mucosa)	389

DISEASE/FINDING	MOST COMMON/IMPORTANT ASSOCIATIONS	PAGE
Bilateral ovarian metastases from gastric carcinoma	Krukenberg tumor (mucin-secreting signet ring cells)	389
Chronic atrophic gastritis (autoimmune)	Predisposition to gastric carcinoma (can also cause pernicious anemia)	389
Alternating areas of transmural inflammation and normal colon	Skip lesions (Crohn disease)	392
Site of diverticula	Sigmoid colon	393
Diverticulum in pharynx	Zenker diverticulum (diagnosed by barium swallow)	394
Hepatocellular carcinoma	HBV (+/– cirrhosis) or other causes of cirrhosis (eg, alcoholic liver disease, hemochromatosis), aflatoxins	402
Congenital conjugated hyperbilirubinemia (black liver)	Dubin-Johnson syndrome (inability of hepatocytes to secrete conjugated bilirubin into bile)	404
Hereditary harmless jaundice	Gilbert syndrome (benign congenital unconjugated hyperbilirubinemia)	404
Wilson disease	Hereditary *ATP7B* mutation (copper buildup in liver, brain, cornea, kidneys)	405
Hemochromatosis	Multiple blood transfusions or hereditary *HFE* mutation (can result in heart failure, "bronze diabetes," and ↑ risk of hepatocellular carcinoma)	405
Pancreatitis (acute)	Gallstones, alcohol	407
Pancreatitis (chronic)	Alcohol (adults), cystic fibrosis (kids)	407
Microcytic anemia	Iron deficiency	428
Autosplenectomy (fibrosis and shrinkage)	Sickle cell disease (hemoglobin S)	432
Bleeding disorder with GpIb deficiency	Bernard-Soulier syndrome (defect in platelet adhesion to von Willebrand factor)	436
Bleeding disorder with GpIIb/IIIa deficiency	Glanzmann thrombasthenia (defect in platelet-to-platelet aggregation)	436
Hereditary bleeding disorder	von Willebrand disease	437
Hereditary thrombophilia	Factor V Leiden	437
DIC	Severe sepsis, obstetric complications, cancer, burns, trauma, major surgery, acute pancreatitis, APL	437
Malignancy associated with noninfectious fever	Hodgkin lymphoma	438
Type of Hodgkin lymphoma	Nodular sclerosis	438
t(14;18)	Follicular lymphoma (*BCL-2* activation, anti-apoptotic oncogene)	439, 444
t(8;14)	Burkitt lymphoma (c-*myc* fusion, transcription factor oncogene)	439, 444
Type of non-Hodgkin lymphoma	Diffuse large B-cell lymphoma	439
1° bone tumor (adults)	Multiple myeloma	440
Age ranges for patient with ALL/CLL/AML/CML	ALL: child, CLL: adult > 60, AML: adult ~ 65, CML: adult 45–85	442
Malignancy (kids)	Leukemia, brain tumors	442, 546

DISEASE/FINDING	MOST COMMON/IMPORTANT ASSOCIATIONS	PAGE
Death in CML	Blast crisis	442
t(9;22)	Philadelphia chromosome, CML (*BCR-ABL* oncogene, tyrosine kinase activation), more rarely associated with ALL	442, 444
Vertebral compression fracture	Osteoporosis	474
HLA-B27	Psoriatic arthritis, ankylosing spondylitis, IBD-associated arthritis, reactive arthritis	481
Death in SLE	Lupus nephropathy	482
Tumor of infancy	Strawberry hemangioma (grows rapidly and regresses spontaneously by childhood)	492
Actinic (solar) keratosis	Precursor to squamous cell carcinoma	496
Herald patch	Pityriasis rosea	496
Cerebellar tonsillar herniation	Chiari I malformation	506
Atrophy of the mammillary bodies	Wernicke encephalopathy (thiamine deficiency causing ataxia, ophthalmoplegia, and confusion)	528
Epidural hematoma	Rupture of middle meningeal artery (trauma; lentiform shaped)	531
Subdural hematoma	Rupture of bridging veins (crescent shaped)	531
Dementia	Alzheimer disease, multiple infarcts (vascular dementia)	538, 539
Demyelinating disease in young women	Multiple sclerosis	541
Brain tumor (adults)	Supratentorial: metastasis, astrocytoma (including glioblastoma multiforme), meningioma, schwannoma	544
Pituitary tumor	Prolactinoma, somatotropic adenoma	545
Brain tumor (children)	Infratentorial: medulloblastoma (cerebellum) or supratentorial: craniopharyngioma	546
Mixed (UMN and LMN) motor neuron disease	Amyotrophic lateral sclerosis	548
Degeneration of dorsal column fibers	Tabes dorsalis (3° syphilis), subacute combined degeneration (dorsal columns, lateral corticospinal, spinocerebellar tracts affected)	548
Glomerulonephritis (adults)	Berger disease (IgA nephropathy)	620
Nephrotic syndrome (adults)	Membranous nephropathy	621
Nephrotic syndrome (children)	Minimal change disease	621
Kidney stones	▪ Calcium = radiopaque ▪ Struvite (ammonium) = radiopaque (formed by urease ⊕ organisms such as *Proteus mirabilis, S saprophyticus, Klebsiella*) ▪ Uric acid = radiolucent ▪ Cystine = faintly radiopaque	622
Renal tumor	Renal cell carcinoma: associated with von Hippel-Lindau and cigarette smoking; paraneoplastic syndromes (EPO, renin, PTHrP, ACTH)	628
1° amenorrhea	Turner syndrome (45,XO or 45,XO/46,XX mosaic)	661

DISEASE/FINDING	MOST COMMON/IMPORTANT ASSOCIATIONS	PAGE
Neuron migration failure	Kallmann syndrome (hypogonadotropic hypogonadism and anosmia)	662
Clear cell adenocarcinoma of the vagina	DES exposure in utero	668
Ovarian tumor (benign, bilateral)	Serous cystadenoma	670
Ovarian tumor (malignant)	Serous carcinoma	670
Tumor in women	Leiomyoma (estrogen dependent, not precancerous)	672
Gynecologic malignancy	Endometrial carcinoma (most common in US); cervical carcinoma (most common worldwide)	672
Breast mass	Fibrocystic change, carcinoma (in postmenopausal women)	673
Breast tumor (benign, young woman)	Fibroadenoma	673
Breast cancer	Invasive ductal carcinoma	674
Testicular tumor	Seminoma (malignant, radiosensitive), ↑ placental ALP	677
Obstruction of male urinary tract	BPH	678
Hypercoagulability, endothelial damage, blood stasis	Virchow triad (↑ risk of thrombosis)	695
Pulmonary hypertension	Idiopathic, heritable, left heart disease (eg, HF), lung disease (eg, COPD), hypoxemic vasoconstriction (eg, OSA), thromboembolic (eg, PE)	703
SIADH	Small cell carcinoma of the lung	709

▶ EQUATION REVIEW

TOPIC	EQUATION	PAGE
Volume of distribution	$V_d = \dfrac{\text{amount of drug in the body}}{\text{plasma drug concentration}}$	233
Half-life	$t_{1/2} = \dfrac{0.7 \times V_d}{CL}$	233
Drug clearance	$CL = \dfrac{\text{rate of elimination of drug}}{\text{plasma drug concentration}} = V_d \times K_e$ (elimination constant)	233
Loading dose	$LD = \dfrac{C_p \times V_d}{F}$	233
Maintenance dose	$D = \dfrac{C_p \times CL \times \tau}{F}$	233
Therapeutic index	TI = median toxic dose/median effective dose = TD_{50}/ED_{50}	237
Odds ratio (for case-control studies)	$OR = \dfrac{a/c}{b/d} = \dfrac{ad}{bc}$	262
Relative risk	$RR = \dfrac{a/(a+b)}{c/(c+d)}$	262

TOPIC	EQUATION	PAGE
Attributable risk	$AR = \frac{a}{a+b} - \frac{c}{c+d}$	262
Relative risk reduction	RRR = 1 – RR	262
Absolute risk reduction	$ARR = \frac{c}{c+d} - \frac{a}{a+b}$	262
Number needed to treat	NNT = 1/ARR	262
Number needed to harm	NNH = 1/AR	262
Likelihood ratio +	LR+ = sensitivity/(1 – specificity) = TP rate/FP rate	263
Likelihood ratio –	LR– = (1 – sensitivity)/specificity = FN rate/TN rate	263
Sensitivity	Sensitivity = TP / (TP + FN)	264
Specificity	Specificity = TN / (TN + FP)	264
Positive predictive value	PPV = TP / (TP + FP)	264
Negative predictive value	NPV = TN / (FN + TN)	264
Cardiac output	$CO = \frac{\text{rate of } O_2 \text{ consumption}}{(\text{arterial } O_2 \text{ content} - \text{venous } O_2 \text{ content})}$ CO = stroke volume × heart rate	294 294
Mean arterial pressure	MAP = cardiac output × total peripheral resistance MAP = ⅔ diastolic + ⅓ systolic	294 294
Stroke volume	SV = EDV – ESV	294
Ejection fraction	$EF = \frac{SV}{EDV} = \frac{EDV - ESV}{EDV}$	294
Resistance	$\text{Resistance} = \frac{\text{driving pressure } (\Delta P)}{\text{flow } (Q)} = \frac{8\eta \text{ (viscosity)} \times \text{length}}{\pi r^4}$	295
Capillary fluid exchange	J_v = net fluid flow = $K_f[(P_c - P_i) - \sigma(\pi_c - \pi_i)]$	305
Reticulocyte production index	$RPI = \frac{\text{reticulocyte \%} \times \text{actual Hct}}{\text{normal Hct } (\approx 45\%)}$	427
Renal clearance	$C_x = (U_x V)/P_x$	606
Glomerular filtration rate	$C_{inulin} = GFR = U_{inulin} \times V/P_{inulin}$ $= K_f [(P_{GC} - P_{BS}) - (\pi_{GC} - \pi_{BS})]$	606
Effective renal plasma flow	$eRPF = U_{PAH} \times \frac{V}{P_{PAH}} = C_{PAH}$	606
Renal blood flow	$RBF = \frac{RPF}{1 - Hct}$	606
Filtration fraction	$FF = \frac{GFR}{RPF}$	607
Henderson-Hasselbalch equation (for extracellular pH)	$pH = 6.1 + \log \frac{[HCO_3^-]}{0.03\ Pco_2}$	616
Winters formula	$Pco_2 = 1.5\ [HCO_3^-] + 8 \pm 2$	616

TOPIC	EQUATION	PAGE
Anion gap	$Na^+ - (Cl^- + HCO_3^-)$	616
Physiologic dead space	$V_D = V_T \times \frac{PaCO_2 - PECO_2}{PaCO_2}$	688
Pulmonary vascular resistance	$PVR = \frac{P_{pulm\ artery} - P_{L\ atrium}}{cardiac\ output}$	692
Alveolar gas equation	$PAO_2 = PIO_2 - \frac{PaCO_2}{R}$	692

▶ EASILY CONFUSED MEDICATIONS

DRUG	CLINICAL USE/MECHANISM OF ACTION
Amiloride	K^+-sparing diuretic
Amiodarone	Class III antiarrhythmic
Amlodipine	Dihydropyridine Ca^{2+} channel blocker
Benztropine	Cholinergic antagonist
Bromocriptine	Dopamine agonist
Buspirone	Generalized anxiety disorder (5-HT_{1A}-receptor agonist)
Bupropion	Depression, smoking cessation (NE-DA reuptake inhibitor)
Cimetidine	H_2-receptor antagonist
Cetirizine	2nd-generation antihistamine
Chloramphenicol	Antibiotic (blocks 50S subunit)
Chlordiazepoxide	Long-acting benzodiazepine
Chlorpromazine	Typical antipsychotic
Chlorpropamide	1st-generation sulfonylurea
Chlorpheniramine	1st-generation antihistamine
Chlorthalidone	Thiazide diuretic
Clozapine	Atypical antipsychotic
Clomipramine	Tricyclic antidepressant
Clomiphene	Selective estrogen receptor modulator
Clonidine	α_2-agonist
Doxepin	Tricyclic antidepressant
Doxazosin	α_1-antagonist
Eplerenone	K^+-sparing diuretic
Propafenone	Class IC antiarrhythmic
Fluoxetine	Selective serotonin reuptake inhibitor
Fluphenazine	Typical antipsychotic
Duloxetine	Serotonin-norepinephrine reuptake inhibitor
Mifepristone	Progesterone receptor antagonist

DRUG	CLINICAL USE/MECHANISM OF ACTION
Misoprostol	PGE_1 synthetic analog
Naloxone	Opioid receptor antagonist (treats toxicity)
Naltrexone	Opioid receptor antagonist (prevents relapse)
Nitroprusside	Hypertensive emergency (↑ cGMP/NO)
Nitroglycerin	Antianginal (↑ cGMP/NO)
Omeprazole	Proton pump inhibitor
Ketoconazole	Antifungal (inhibits fungal sterol synthesis)
Aripiprazole	Atypical antipsychotic
Anastrozole	Aromatase inhibitor
Rifaximin	Hepatic encephalopathy (↓ ammoniagenic bacteria)
Rifampin	Antimicrobial (inhibits DNA-dependent RNA polymerase)
Sertraline	Selective serotonin reuptake inhibitor
Selegiline	MAO-B inhibitor
Trazodone	Insomnia (blocks $5\text{-}HT_2$, α_1-adrenergic, and H_1 receptors)
Tramadol	Chronic pain (weak opioid agonist)
Varenicline	Smoking cessation (nicotinic ACh receptor partial agonist)
Venlafaxine	Serotonin-norepinephrine reuptake inhibitor

▶ NOTES

SECTION IV

Top-Rated Review Resources

"Some books are to be tasted, others to be swallowed, and some few to be chewed and digested."

—Sir Francis Bacon

"Always read something that will make you look good if you die in the middle of it."

—P.J. O'Rourke

"So many books, so little time."

—Frank Zappa

"If one cannot enjoy reading a book over and over again, there is no use in reading it at all."

—Oscar Wilde

"Start where you are. Use what you have. Do what you can."

—Arthur Ashe

▶ HOW TO USE THE DATABASE

This section is a database of top-rated basic science review books, sample examination books, websites, apps, and commercial review courses that have been marketed to medical students studying for the USMLE Step 1. For each recommended resource, we list (where applicable) the **Title**, the **First Author** (or editor), the **Series Name** (where applicable), the **Current Publisher**, the **Copyright Year**, the **Number of Pages**, the **ISBN**, the **Approximate List Price**, the **Format** of the resource, and the **Number of Test Questions**. We also include **Summary Comments** that describe their style and overall utility for studying. Finally, each recommended resource receives a **Rating**. Within each section, resources are arranged first by Rating and then alphabetically by the first author within each Rating group.

A letter rating scale with six different grades reflects the detailed student evaluations for **Rated Resources**. Each rated resource receives a rating as follows:

A+	Excellent for boards review.
A A–	Very good for boards review; choose among the group.
B+ B	Good, but use only after exhausting better resources.
B–	Fair, but there are many better resources in the discipline; or low-yield subject material.

The Rating is meant to reflect the overall usefulness of the resource in helping medical students prepare for the USMLE Step 1. This is based on a number of factors, including:

- The importance of the discipline for the USMLE Step 1
- The appropriateness and accuracy of the material
- The readability of the text
- The quality and number of sample questions
- The quality of written answers to sample questions
- The cost
- The quality of the user interface and learning experience, for web and mobile apps
- The quality and appropriateness of the images and illustrations
- The length of the text (longer is not necessarily better)
- The quality and number of other resources available in the same discipline

Please note that ratings do not reflect the quality of the resources for purposes other than reviewing for the USMLE Step 1. Many books with lower ratings are well written and informative but are not ideal for boards preparation. We have not listed or commented on general textbooks available for the basic sciences.

Evaluations are based on the cumulative results of formal and informal surveys of thousands of medical students at many medical schools across the country. The summary comments and overall ratings represent a consensus opinion, but there may have been a broad range of opinion or limited student feedback on any particular resource.

Please note that the data listed are subject to change in that:

- Publisher and app store prices change frequently.
- Retail and online bookstores may set their own prices.
- New editions and app versions come out frequently, and the quality of updating varies.
- The same book may be reissued through another publisher.

We actively encourage medical students and faculty to submit their opinions and ratings of these basic science review materials so that we may update our database. In addition, we ask that publishers and authors submit for evaluation review copies of basic science review books, including new editions and books not included in our database. We also solicit reviews of new books, mobile apps, websites, flash cards, and commercial review courses.

Disclaimer/Conflict of Interest Statement

None of the ratings reflects the opinion or influence of the publisher. All errors and omissions will gladly be corrected if brought to the attention of the authors through our blog at firstaidteam.com. Please note that USMLE-Rx, ScholarRx, and the entire *First Aid for the USMLE* series are publications by certain authors of *First Aid for the USMLE Step 1*; the following ratings are based solely on recommendations from the student authors of *First Aid for the USMLE Step 1* as well as data from the student survey and feedback forms.

TOP-RATED REVIEW RESOURCES

Question Banks

		AUTHOR	PUBLISHER	TYPE	PRICE
A+	*UWorld Qbank*	UWorld	uworld.com	Test/3000+ q	$269–$799
A	*NBME Practice Exams*	National Board of Medical Examiners	nbme.org/students/sas/Comprehensive.html	Test/200 q	$60
A−	*AMBOSS*	Amboss	amboss.com	Test/3500 q	$59–$286
A−	*USMLE-Rx Qmax*	USMLE-Rx	usmle-rx.com	Test/2300+ q	$79–$349
B+	*Kaplan Qbank*	Kaplan	kaptest.com	Test/3300 q	$99–$599
B+	*TrueLearn Review*		truelearn.com	Test/2200 q	$160–$400
B	*BoardVitals*		boardvitals.com	Test/3150 q	Free–$189
B	*Pastest*		pastest.com	Test/2100 q	$79–$249

Web and Mobile Apps

		AUTHOR	PUBLISHER	TYPE	PRICE
A	*Anki*		ankisrs.net	Flash cards	Free
A	*Boards and Beyond*		boardsbeyond.com	Review/Test/2300 q	$19–$299
A	*SketchyMedical*		sketchymedical.com	Review	$100–$550
A	*Rx Bricks*		usmle-rx.scholarrx.com/rx-bricks	Study plan	$15–$199
A−	*Physeo*		physeo.com	Review	$30–$150
A−	*USMLE-Rx Step 1 Express*		usmle-rx.com	Review/Test	$49–$199
A−	*USMLE-Rx Step 1 Flash Facts*		usmle-rx.com	Flash cards	$29–$149
A−	*Dirty Medicine*		youtube.com/c/DirtyMedicine		Free
B+	*USMLE Step 1 Mastery*		builtbyhlt.com/medical/usmle-step-1-mastery	Test/1400 q	$10–$30
B+	*Cram Fighter*		cramfighter.com	Study plan	$29–$159
B+	*Medical School Pathology*		medicalschoolpathology.com	Review	Free
B+	*OnlineMedEd*		onlinemeded.org	Review	Free
B+	*Osmosis*		osmosis.org	Test	$299–$399
B+	*Medbullets*		step1.medbullets.com	Review/Test/1000 q	Free–$250
B+	*Ninja Nerd Medicine*		youtube.com/c/NinjaNerdMedicine		Free
B+	*WebPath: The Internet Pathology Laboratory*		webpath.med.utah.edu	Review/Test/1300 q	Free
B	*Digital Anatomist Project: Interactive Atlases*		da.si.washington.edu/da.html	Review	Free

B	***Dr. Najeeb Lectures***	drnajeeblectures.com	Review	$199
B	***Firecracker***	firecracker.lww.com	Review/ Test/2800 q	$99–$499
B	***KISSPrep***	kissprep.com	Review	$30–$150
B	***Memorang***	memorangapp.com	Flash cards	$19–$239
B	***Picmonic***	picmonic.com	Review	$25–$480
B	***Radiopaedia.org***	radiopaedia.org	Cases/Test	Free
B⁻	***Innerbody Research***	innerbody.com/htm/body.html	Review	Free
B⁻	***Lecturio***	lecturio.com/usmle-step-1	Review/ Test/2150 q	$105–$720

Comprehensive

		AUTHOR	PUBLISHER	TYPE	PRICE
A	***First Aid for the Basic Sciences: General Principles***	Le	McGraw-Hill, 2017, 528 pages, ISBN 9781259587016	Review	$75
A	***First Aid Cases for the USMLE Step 1***	Le	McGraw-Hill, 2018, 496 pages, ISBN 9781260143133	Cases	$50
A⁻	***First Aid for the Basic Sciences: Organ Systems***	Le	McGraw-Hill, 2017, 912 pages, ISBN 9781259587030	Review	$72
A⁻	***Cracking the USMLE Step 1***	Princeton Review	Princeton Review, 2013, 832 pages, ISBN 9780307945068	Review	$45
B⁺	***USMLE Step 1 Secrets in Color***	Brown	Elsevier, 2016, 800 pages, ISBN 9780323396790	Review	$43
B⁺	***USMLE Step 1 Lecture Notes 2020***	Kaplan	Kaplan Medical, 2019, 2624 pages, ISBN 9781506254944	Review	$330
B⁺	***Crush Step 1: The Ultimate USMLE Step 1 Review***	O'Connell	Elsevier, 2017, 704 pages, 9780323481632	Review	$45
B	***Kaplan USMLE Step 1 Qbook***	Kaplan	Kaplan Medical, 2017, 468 pages, ISBN 9781506223544	Test/850 q	$50
B	***medEssentials for the USMLE Step 1***	Kaplan	Kaplan Medical, 2019, 528 pages, ISBN 9781506223599	Review	$55
B	***Step-Up to USMLE Step 1 2015***	McInnis	Lippincott Williams & Wilkins, 2015, 528 pages, ISBN 9781469894690	Review	$60
B⁻	***USMLE Step 1 Made Ridiculously Simple***	Carl	MedMaster, 2017, 416 pages, ISBN 9781935660224	Review/Test 1000 q	$30

Anatomy, Embryology, and Neuroscience

		AUTHOR	PUBLISHER	TYPE	PRICE
A⁻	***High-Yield Gross Anatomy***	Dudek	Lippincott Williams & Wilkins, 2015, 320 pages, ISBN 9781451190236	Review	$45
A⁻	***Clinical Anatomy Made Ridiculously Simple***	Goldberg	MedMaster, 2016, 175 pages, ISBN 9780940780972	Review	$30

Anatomy, Embryology, and Neuroscience *(continued)*

		AUTHOR	PUBLISHER	TYPE	PRICE
B+	*BRS Embryology*	Dudek	Lippincott Williams & Wilkins, 2014, 336 pages, ISBN 9781451190380	Review/Test/220 q	$56
B+	*High-Yield Embryology*	Dudek	Lippincott Williams & Wilkins, 2013, 176 pages, ISBN 9781451176100	Review	$43
B+	*Clinical Neuroanatomy Made Ridiculously Simple*	Goldberg	MedMaster, 2014, 99 pages, ISBN 9781935660194	Review/Test/Few q	$26
B+	*High-Yield Neuroanatomy*	Gould	Lippincott Williams & Wilkins, 2015, 208 pages, ISBN 9781451193435	Review/Test/50 q	$42
B+	*Crash Course: Anatomy and Physiology*	Stephens	Elsevier, 2019, 350 pages, ISBN 9780702073755	Review	$40
B	*Anatomy—An Essential Textbook*	Gilroy	Thieme, 2017, 528 pages, ISBN 9781626234390	Text/Test/400 q	$50
B	*Netter's Anatomy Flash Cards*	Hansen	Elsevier, 2018, 688 flash cards, ISBN 9780323530507	Flash cards	$40
B	*Case Files: Anatomy*	Toy	McGraw-Hill, 2014, 416 pages, ISBN 9780071794862	Cases	$35
B-	*Case Files: Neuroscience*	Toy	McGraw-Hill, 2014, 432 pages, ISBN 9780071790253	Cases	$35

Behavioral Science

		AUTHOR	PUBLISHER	TYPE	PRICE
A-	*BRS Behavioral Science*	Fadem	Lippincott Williams & Wilkins, 2020, 384 pages, ISBN 9781975118365	Review/Test/600 q	$55
B	*Biostatistics and Epidemiology: A Primer for Health and Biomedical Professionals*	Wassertheil-Smoller	Springer, 2015, 4th edition, 280 pages, 9781493921331	Review	$75

Biochemistry

		AUTHOR	PUBLISHER	TYPE	PRICE
A-	*Pixorize*		pixorize.com	Review	$130–$200
B+	*Lippincott Illustrated Reviews: Biochemistry*	Ferrier	Lippincott Williams & Wilkins, 2017, 560 pages, ISBN 9781496344496	Review/Test/200 q	$78
B+	*BRS Biochemistry, Molecular Biology, and Genetics*	Lieberman	Lippincott Williams & Wilkins, 2019, 448 pages, ISBN 9781496399236	Review/Test/500 q	$55
B+	*PreTest Biochemistry and Genetics*	Wilson	McGraw-Hill, 2013, 592 pages, ISBN 9780071791441	Test/500 q	$38
B	*Lange Flash Cards Biochemistry and Genetics*	Baron	McGraw-Hill, 2017, 184 flash cards, ISBN 9781259837210	Flash cards	$40
B	*Case Files: Biochemistry*	Toy	McGraw-Hill, 2014, 480 pages, ISBN 9780071794886	Cases	$35

Cell Biology and Histology

		AUTHOR	PUBLISHER	TYPE	PRICE
B+	*Blue Histology*		www.lab.anhb.uwa.edu.au/mb140	Test	Free
B+	*Crash Course: Cell Biology and Genetics*	Stubbs	Mosby, 2015, 216 pages, ISBN 9780723438762	Review/Print + online	$47
B	*BRS Cell Biology and Histology*	Gartner	Lippincott Williams & Wilkins, 2018, 448 pages, ISBN 9781496396358	Review/ Test/320 q	$54

Microbiology and Immunology

		AUTHOR	PUBLISHER	TYPE	PRICE
A−	*Medical Microbiology and Immunology Flash Cards*	Rosenthal	Elsevier, 2016, 192 flash cards, ISBN 9780323462242	Flash cards	$40
B+	*Basic Immunology*	Abbas	Elsevier, 2019, 336 pages, ISBN 9780323549431	Review	$70
B+	*Clinical Microbiology Made Ridiculously Simple*	Gladwin	MedMaster, 2019, 418 pages, ISBN 9781935660330	Review	$38
B+	*Microcards: Microbiology Flash Cards*	Harpavat	Lippincott Williams & Wilkins, 2015, 312 flash cards, ISBN 9781451192353	Flash cards	$53
B+	*Review of Medical Microbiology and Immunology*	Levinson	McGraw-Hill, 2020, 864 pages, ISBN 9781260116717	Review/ Test/650 q	$77
B+	*Lange Microbiology and Infectious Diseases Flash Cards, 3e*	Somers	McGraw-Hill, 2017, ISBN 9781259859823	Flash cards	$55
B	*Case Studies in Immunology: Clinical Companion*	Geha	W. W. Norton & Company, 2016, 384 pages, ISBN 9780815345121	Cases	$62
B	*How the Immune System Works*	Sompayrac	Wiley-Blackwell, 2019, 168 pages, ISBN 9781119542124	Review	$50
B	*Case Files: Microbiology*	Toy	McGraw-Hill, 2014, 416 pages, ISBN 9780071820233	Cases	$36
B−	*Lippincott Illustrated Reviews: Microbiology*	Cornelissen	Lippincott Williams & Wilkins, 2019, 448 pages, ISBN 9781496395856	Review/Test/ Few q	$74

Pathology

		AUTHOR	PUBLISHER	TYPE	PRICE
A+	*Pathoma: Fundamentals of Pathology*	Sattar	Pathoma, 2021, 226 pages, ISBN 9780983224648	Review/ Lecture	$85–$120
A−	*Crash Course: Pathology*	McKinney	Elsevier, 2019, 438 pages, ISBN 9780702073540	Review	$40
B+	*Rapid Review: Pathology*	Goljan	Elsevier, 2018, 864 pages, ISBN 9780323476683	Review/ Test/500 q	$65
B+	*Robbins and Cotran Review of Pathology*	Klatt	Elsevier, 2014, 504 pages, ISBN 9781455751556	Test/1100 q	$55
B	*BRS Pathology*	Gupta	Lippincott Williams & Wilkins, 2020, 496 pages, ISBN 9781975136628	Review/ Test/450 q	$55
B	*Pathophysiology of Disease: Introduction to Clinical Medicine*	Hammer	McGraw-Hill, 2018, 832 pages, ISBN 9781260026504	Text	$90

Pathology (continued)

B	*Haematology at a Glance*	Mehta	Wiley-Blackwell, 2014, 136 pages, ISBN 9781119969228	Review	$51
B	*Pocket Companion to Robbins and Cotran Pathologic Basis of Disease*	Mitchell	Elsevier, 2016, 896 pages, ISBN 9781455754168	Review	$39

Pharmacology

		AUTHOR	PUBLISHER	TYPE	PRICE
B^+	*Master the Boards USMLE Step 1 Pharmacology Flashcards*	Fischer	Kaplan, 2015, 200 flash cards, ISBN 9781618657947	Flash cards	$55
B^+	*Crash Course: Pharmacology*	Page	Elsevier, 2019, 336 pages, ISBN 9780702073441	Review	$40
B^+	*Katzung & Trevor's Pharmacology: Examination and Board Review*	Trevor	McGraw-Hill, 2018, 592 pages, ISBN 9781259641022	Review/ Test/800 q	$54
B	*Lange Pharmacology Flash Cards*	Baron	McGraw-Hill, 2017, 266 flash cards, ISBN 9781259837241	Flash cards	$39
B	*Pharmacology Flash Cards*	Brenner	Elsevier, 2017, 230 flash cards, ISBN 9780323355643	Flash cards	$45
B	*BRS Pharmacology*	Lerchenfeldt	Lippincott Williams & Wilkins, 2019, 384 pages, ISBN 9781975105495	Review/ Test/200 q	$55
B^-	*Lippincott Illustrated Reviews: Pharmacology*	Whalen	Lippincott Williams & Wilkins, 2018, 576 pages, ISBN 9781496384133	Review/ Test/380 q	$76

Physiology

		AUTHOR	PUBLISHER	TYPE	PRICE
A^-	*Physiology*	Costanzo	Elsevier, 2017, 528 pages, ISBN 9780323478816	Text	$60
A^-	*Color Atlas of Physiology*	Silbernagl	Thieme, 2015, 472 pages, ISBN 9783135450070	Review	$50
A^-	*Pulmonary Pathophysiology: The Essentials*	West	Lippincott Williams & Wilkins, 2017, 264 pages, ISBN 9781496339447	Review/ Test/75 q	$57
B^+	*BRS Physiology*	Costanzo	Lippincott Williams & Wilkins, 2018, 304 pages, ISBN 9781496367617	Review/ Test/350 q	$55
B^+	*Vander's Renal Physiology*	Eaton	McGraw-Hill, 2018, 224 pages, ISBN 9781260019377	Text	$49
B^+	*Pathophysiology of Heart Disease*	Lilly	Lippincott Williams & Williams, 2020, 480 pages, ISBN 9781975120597	Review	$57
B^+	*Acid-Base, Fluids, and Electrolytes Made Ridiculously Simple*	Preston	MedMaster, 2017, 166 pages, ISBN 9781935660293	Review	$24
B	*Endocrine Physiology*	Molina	McGraw-Hill, 2018, 320 pages, ISBN 9781260019353	Review	$59
B	*Netter's Physiology Flash Cards*	Mulroney	Saunders, 2015, 450 flash cards, ISBN 9780323359542	Flash cards	$40

SECTION IV

Abbreviations and Symbols

ABBREVIATION	MEANING
1st MC*	1st metacarpal
A-a	alveolar-arterial [gradient]
AA	Alcoholics Anonymous, amyloid A
AAMC	Association of American Medical Colleges
AAo*	ascending aorta
Ab	antibody
ABPA	allergic bronchopulmonary aspergillosis
AC	adenylyl cyclase
ACA	anterior cerebral artery
Acetyl-CoA	acetyl coenzyme A
ACD	anemia of chronic disease
ACE	angiotensin-converting enzyme
ACh	acetylcholine
AChE	acetylcholinesterase
ACL	anterior cruciate ligament
ACom	anterior communicating [artery]
ACTH	adrenocorticotropic hormone
AD	Alzheimer disease, autosomal dominant
ADA	adenosine deaminase, Americans with Disabilities Act
ADH	antidiuretic hormone
ADHD	attention-deficit hyperactivity disorder
ADP	adenosine diphosphate
ADPKD	autosomal-dominant polycystic kidney disease
AFP	α-fetoprotein
Ag	antigen, silver
AICA	anterior inferior cerebellar artery
AIDS	acquired immunodeficiency syndrome
AIHA	autoimmune hemolytic anemia
AKI	acute kidney injury
AKT	protein kinase B
AL	amyloid light [chain]
ALA	aminolevulinate
ALI	acute lung injury
ALL	acute lymphoblastic (lymphocytic) leukemia
ALP	alkaline phosphatase
ALS	amyotrophic lateral sclerosis
ALT	alanine transaminase
AMA	American Medical Association, antimitochondrial antibody
AML	acute myelogenous (myeloid) leukemia
AMP	adenosine monophosphate
ANA	antinuclear antibody
ANCA	antineutrophil cytoplasmic antibody
ANOVA	analysis of variance

ABBREVIATION	MEANING
ANP	atrial natriuretic peptide
ANS	autonomic nervous system
Ant*	anterior
anti-CCP	anti-cyclic citrullinated peptide
Ao*	aorta
AOA	American Osteopathic Association
AP	action potential, A & P [ribosomal binding sites]
APC	antigen-presenting cell, activated protein C
APL	Acute promyelocytic leukemia
Apo	apolipoprotein
APP	amyloid precursor protein
APRT	adenine phosphoribosyltransferase
aPTT	activated partial thromboplastin time
APUD	amine precursor uptake decarboxylase
AR	attributable risk, autosomal recessive, aortic regurgitation
ARB	angiotensin receptor blocker
ARDS	acute respiratory distress syndrome
Arg	arginine
ARPKD	autosomal-recessive polycystic kidney disease
ART	antiretroviral therapy
AS	aortic stenosis
ASA	anterior spinal artery
Asc*	ascending
Asc Ao*	ascending aorta
ASD	atrial septal defect
ASO	anti–streptolysin O
AST	aspartate transaminase
AT	angiotensin, antithrombin
ATN	acute tubular necrosis
ATP	adenosine triphosphate
ATPase	adenosine triphosphatase
ATTR	transthyretin-mediated amyloidosis
AUB	abnormal uterine bleeding
AV	atrioventricular
AZT	azidothymidine
BAL	British anti-Lewisite [dimercaprol]
BBB	blood-brain barrier
BCG	bacille Calmette-Guérin
BD*	bile duct
BH_4	tetrahydrobiopterin
BM	basement membrane
BOOP	bronchiolitis obliterans organizing pneumonia
BP	bisphosphate, blood pressure
BPG	bisphosphoglycerate

*Image abbreviation only

ABBREVIATION	MEANING
BPH	benign prostatic hyperplasia
BT	bleeding time
BUN	blood urea nitrogen
C*	caudate
Ca*	capillary
Ca^{2+}	calcium ion
CAD	coronary artery disease
CAF	common application form
cAMP	cyclic adenosine monophosphate
CBG	corticosteroid-binding globulin
Cbm*	cerebellum
CBSE	Comprehensive Basic Science Examination
CBSSA	Comprehensive Basic Science Self-Assessment
CBT	computer-based test, cognitive behavioral therapy
CC*	corpus callosum
CCA*	common carotid artery
CCK	cholecystokinin
CCS	computer-based case simulation
CD	cluster of differentiation
CDK	cyclin-dependent kinase
cDNA	complementary deoxyribonucleic acid
CEA	carcinoembryonic antigen
CETP	cholesteryl-ester transfer protein
CF	cystic fibrosis
CFTR	cystic fibrosis transmembrane conductance regulator
CGD	chronic granulomatous disease
cGMP	cyclic guanosine monophosphate
CGRP	calcitonin gene–related peptide
C_H1–C_H3	constant regions, heavy chain [antibody]
ChAT	choline acetyltransferase
CHD*	common hepatic duct
χ^2	chi-squared
CI	confidence interval
CIN	candidate identification number, carcinoma in situ, cervical intraepithelial neoplasia
CIS	Communication and Interpersonal Skills
CK	clinical knowledge, creatine kinase
CKD	chronic kidney disease
CK-MB	creatine kinase, MB fraction
C_L	constant region, light chain [antibody]
CL	clearance
Cl^-	chloride ion
CLL	chronic lymphocytic leukemia
CMC	carpometacarpal (joint)
CML	chronic myelogenous (myeloid) leukemia
CMV	cytomegalovirus
CN	cranial nerve
CN^-	cyanide ion
CNS	central nervous system
CNV	copy number variation
CO	carbon monoxide, cardiac output
CO_2	carbon dioxide
CoA	coenzyme A
Coarct*	coarctation

*Image abbreviation only

ABBREVIATION	MEANING
COL1A1	collagen, type I, alpha 1
COL1A2	collagen, type I, alpha 2
COMT	catechol-O-methyltransferase
COP	coat protein
COPD	chronic obstructive pulmonary disease
CoQ	coenzyme Q
COVID-19	Coronavirus disease 2019
COX	cyclooxygenase
C_p	plasma concentration
CPAP	continuous positive airway pressure
CPR	cardiopulmonary resuscitation
Cr	creatinine
CRC	colorectal cancer
CREST	calcinosis, Raynaud phenomenon, esophageal dysfunction, sclerosis, and telangiectasias [syndrome]
CRH	corticotropin-releasing hormone
CRP	C-reactive protein
CS	clinical skills
C-section	cesarean section
CSF	cerebrospinal fluid
CT	computed tomography
CTP	cytidine triphosphate
CXR	chest x-ray
DA	dopamine
DAF	decay-accelerating factor
DAG	diacylglycerol
DAo*	descending aorta
dATP	deoxyadenosine triphosphate
DCIS	ductal carcinoma in situ
DCT	distal convoluted tubule
ddI	didanosine
DES	diethylstilbestrol
Desc Ao*	descending aorta
DHAP	dihydroxyacetone phosphate
DHEA	dehydroepiandrosterone
DHF	dihydrofolic acid
DHT	dihydrotestosterone
DI	diabetes insipidus
DIC	disseminated intravascular coagulation
DIP	distal interphalangeal [joint]
DKA	diabetic ketoacidosis
DLCO	diffusing capacity for carbon monoxide
DM	diabetes mellitus
DNA	deoxyribonucleic acid
DNR	do not resuscitate
dNTP	deoxynucleotide triphosphate
DO	doctor of osteopathy
DPGN	diffuse proliferative glomerulonephritis
DPM	doctor of podiatric medicine
DPP-4	dipeptidyl peptidase-4
DPPC	dipalmitoylphosphatidylcholine
DS	double stranded
dsDNA	double-stranded deoxyribonucleic acid
dsRNA	double-stranded ribonucleic acid
DRG	dorsal root ganglion

ABBREVIATION	MEANING
d4T	didehydrodeoxythymidine [stavudine]
dTMP	deoxythymidine monophosphate
DTR	deep tendon reflex
DTs	delirium tremens
dUDP	deoxyuridine diphosphate
dUMP	deoxyuridine monophosphate
DVT	deep venous thrombosis
E*	euthromatin, esophagus
EBV	Epstein-Barr virus
ECA*	external carotid artery
ECF	extracellular fluid
ECFMG	Educational Commission for Foreign Medical Graduates
ECG	electrocardiogram
ECL	enterochromaffin-like [cell]
ECM	extracellular matrix
ECT	electroconvulsive therapy
ED_{50}	median effective dose
EDRF	endothelium-derived relaxing factor
EDTA	ethylenediamine tetra-acetic acid
EDV	end-diastolic volume
EEG	electroencephalogram
EF	ejection fraction
EGF	epidermal growth factor
EHEC	enterohemorrhagic *E coli*
EIEC	enteroinvasive *E coli*
ELISA	enzyme-linked immunosorbent assay
EM	electron micrograph/microscopy
EMB	eosin–methylene blue
EPEC	eneteropathogenic *E coli*
Epi	epinephrine
EPO	erythropoietin
EPS	extrapyramidal system
ER	endoplasmic reticulum, estrogen receptor
ERAS	Electronic Residency Application Service
ERCP	endoscopic retrograde cholangiopancreatography
ERP	effective refractory period
eRPF	effective renal plasma flow
ERT	estrogen replacement therapy
ERV	expiratory reserve volume
ESR	erythrocyte sedimentation rate
ESRD	end-stage renal disease
ESV	end-systolic volume
ETEC	enterotoxigenic *E coli*
EtOH	ethyl alcohol
EV	esophageal vein
F	bioavailability
FA	fatty acid
Fab	fragment, antigen-binding
FAD	flavin adenine dinucleotide
$FADH_2$	reduced flavin adenine dinucleotide
FAP	familial adenomatous polyposis
F1,6BP	fructose-1,6-bisphosphate
F2,6BP	fructose-2,6-bisphosphate
FBPase	fructose bisphosphatase

ABBREVIATION	MEANING
FBPase-2	fructose bisphosphatase-2
Fc	fragment, crystallizable
FcR	Fc receptor
5f-dUMP	5-fluorodeoxyuridine monophosphate
Fe^{2+}	ferrous ion
Fe^{3+}	ferric ion
Fem*	femur
FENa	excreted fraction of filtered sodium
FEV_1	forced expiratory volume in 1 second
FF	filtration fraction
FFA	free fatty acid
FGF	fibroblast growth factor
FGFR	fibroblast growth factor receptor
FISH	fluorescence in situ hybridization
FIT	fecal immunochemical testing
FKBP	FK506 binding protein
fMet	formylmethionine
FMG	foreign medical graduate
FMN	flavin mononucleotide
FN	false negative
FP, FP*	false positive, foot process
FRC	functional residual capacity
FSH	follicle-stimulating hormone
FSMB	Federation of State Medical Boards
FTA-ABS	fluorescent treponemal antibody—absorbed
FTD*	frontotemporal dementia
5-FU	5-fluorouracil
FVC	forced vital capacity
GABA	γ-aminobutyric acid
GAG	glycosaminoglycan
Gal	galactose
GBM	glomerular basement membrane
GC	glomerular capillary
G-CSF	granulocyte colony-stimulating factor
GERD	gastroesophageal reflux disease
GFAP	glial fibrillary acid protein
GFR	glomerular filtration rate
GGT	γ-glutamyl transpeptidase
GH	growth hormone
GHB	γ-hydroxybutyrate
GHRH	growth hormone–releasing hormone
G_I	G protein, I polypeptide
GI	gastrointestinal
GIP	gastric inhibitory peptide
GIST	gastrointestinal stromal tumor
GLUT	glucose transporter
GM	granulocyte macrophage
GM-CSF	granulocyte-macrophage colony stimulating factor
GMP	guanosine monophosphate
GnRH	gonadotropin-releasing hormone
Gp	glycoprotein
G6P	glucose-6-phosphate
G6PD	glucose-6-phosphate dehydrogenase
GPe	globus pallidus externa

*Image abbreviation only

ABBREVIATION	MEANING
GPi	globus pallidus interna
GPI	glycosyl phosphatidylinositol
GRP	gastrin-releasing peptide
G_S	G protein, S polypeptide
GSH	reduced glutathione
GSSG	oxidized glutathione
GTP	guanosine triphosphate
GTPase	guanosine triphosphatase
GU	genitourinary
H*	heterochromatin
H^+	hydrogen ion
H_1, H_2	histamine receptors
H_2S	hydrogen sulfide
HA*	hepatic artery
HAV	hepatitis A virus
HAVAb	hepatitis A antibody
Hb	hemoglobin
HBcAb/HBcAg	hepatitis B core antibody/antigen
HBeAb/HBeAg	hepatitis B early antibody/antigen
HBsAb/HBsAg	hepatitis B surface antibody/antigen
$HbCO_2$	carbaminohemoglobin
HBV	hepatitis B virus
HCC	hepatocellular carcinoma
hCG	human chorionic gonadotropin
HCO_3^-	bicarbonate
Hct	hematocrit
HCTZ	hydrochlorothiazide
HCV	hepatitis C virus
HDL	high-density lipoprotein
HDN	hemolytic disease of the newborn
HDV	hepatitis D virus
H&E	hematoxylin and eosin
HEV	hepatitis E virus
HF	heart failure
Hfr	high-frequency recombination [cell]
HFpEF	heart failure with preserved ejection fraction
HFrEF	heart failure with reduced ejection fraction
HGPRT	hypoxanthine-guanine phosphoribosyltransferase
HHb	deoxygenated hemoglobin
HHS	hyperosmolar hyperglycemic state
HHV	human herpesvirus
5-HIAA	5-hydroxyindoleacetic acid
HIT	heparin-induced thrombocytopenia
HIV	human immunodeficiency virus
HL	hepatic lipase
HLA	human leukocyte antigen
HMG-CoA	hydroxymethylglutaryl-coenzyme A
HMP	hexose monophosphate
HMWK	high-molecular-weight kininogen
HNPCC	hereditary nonpolyposis colorectal cancer
hnRNA	heterogeneous nuclear ribonucleic acid
H_2O_2	hydrogen peroxide
HOCM	hypertrophic obstructive cardiomyopathy
HPA	hypothalamic-pituitary-adrenal [axis]

*Image abbreviation only

ABBREVIATION	MEANING
HPO	hypothalamic-pituitary-ovarian [axis]
HPV	human papillomavirus
HR	heart rate
HSP	Henoch-Schönlein purpura
HSV	herpes simplex virus
5-HT	5-hydroxytryptamine (serotonin)
HTLV	human T-cell leukemia virus
HTN	hypertension
HUS	hemolytic-uremic syndrome
HVA	homovanillic acid
IBD	inflammatory bowel disease
IBS	irritable bowel syndrome
IC	inspiratory capacity, immune complex
I_{Ca}	calcium current [heart]
I_f	funny current [heart]
ICA	internal carotid artery
ICAM	intercellular adhesion molecule
ICD	implantable cardioverter defibrillator
ICE	Integrated Clinical Encounter
ICF	intracellular fluid
ICP	intracranial pressure
ID	identification
ID_{50}	median infective dose
IDL	intermediate-density lipoprotein
IF	immunofluorescence, initiation factor
IFN	interferon
Ig	immunoglobulin
IGF	insulin-like growth factor
I_K	potassium current [heart]
IL	interleukin
IM	intramuscular
IMA	inferior mesenteric artery
IMG	international medical graduate
IMP	inosine monophosphate
IMV	inferior mesenteric vein
I_{Na}	sodium current [heart]
INH	isoniazid
INO	internuclear ophthalmoplegia
INR	International Normalized Ratio
IO	inferior oblique [muscle]
IOP	intraocular pressure
IP_3	inositol triphosphate
IPV	inactivated polio vaccine
IR	current × resistance [Ohm's law], inferior rectus [muscle]
IRV	inspiratory reserve volume
ITP	idiopathic thrombocytopenic purpura
IUD	intrauterine device
IUGR	intrauterine growth restriction
IV	intravenous
IVC	inferior vena cava
IVDU	intravenous drug use
IVIG	intravenous immunoglobulin
JAK/STAT	Janus kinase/signal transducer and activator of transcription [pathway]

ABBREVIATION	MEANING
JGA	juxtaglomerular apparatus
JVD	jugular venous distention
JVP	jugular venous pulse
K^+	potassium ion
KatG	catalase-peroxidase produced by *M tuberculosis*
K_e	elimination constant
K_f	filtration constant
KG	ketoglutarate
Kid*	kidney
K_m	Michaelis-Menten constant
KOH	potassium hydroxide
L	left, lentiform, liver
LA	left atrial, left atrium
LAD	left anterior descending coronary artery
LAP	leukocyte alkaline phosphatase
Lat cond*	lateral condyle
Lb*	lamellar body
LCA	left coronary artery
LCAT	lecithin-cholesterol acyltransferase
LCC*	left common carotid artery
LCFA	long-chain fatty acid
LCL	lateral collateral ligament
LCME	Liaison Committee on Medical Education
LCMV	lymphocytic choriomeningitis virus
LCX	left circumflex coronary artery
LD	loading dose
LD_{50}	median lethal dose
LDH	lactate dehydrogenase
LDL	low-density lipoprotein
LES	lower esophageal sphincter
LFA	leukocyte function–associated antigen
LFT	liver function test
LH	luteinizing hormone
Liv*	liver
LLL*	left lower lobe (of lung)
LLQ	left lower quadrant
LM	lateral meniscus, left main coronary artery, light microscopy
LMN	lower motor neuron
LOS	lipooligosaccharide
LPA*	left pulmonary artery
LPL	lipoprotein lipase
LPS	lipopolysaccharide
LR	lateral rectus [muscle]
LT	labile toxin, leukotriene
LUL*	left upper lobe (of lung)
LV	left ventricle, left ventricular
M_1-M_5	muscarinic (parasympathetic) ACh receptors
MAC	membrane attack complex, minimum alveolar concentration
MALT	mucosa-associated lymphoid tissue
MAO	monoamine oxidase
MAOI	monoamine oxidase inhibitor
MAP	mean arterial pressure, mitogen-activated protein
Max*	maxillary sinus

ABBREVIATION	MEANING
MC	midsystolic click, metacarpal
MCA	middle cerebral artery
MCAT	Medical College Admissions Test
MCHC	mean corpuscular hemoglobin concentration
MCL	medial collateral ligament
MCP	metacarpophalangeal [joint]
MCV	mean corpuscular volume
MD	maintenance dose
MDD	major depressive disorder
Med cond*	medial condyle
MELAS syndrome	mitochondrial encephalopathy, lactic acidosis, and stroke-like episodes
MEN	multiple endocrine neoplasia
MERS	Middle East respiratory syndrome
Mg^{2+}	magnesium ion
$MgSO_4$	magnesium sulfate
MHC	major histocompatibility complex
MI	myocardial infarction
MIF	müllerian inhibiting factor
MIRL	membrane inhibitor of reactive lysis
MLCK	myosin light-chain kinase
MLF	medial longitudinal fasciculus
MMC	migrating motor complex
MMR	measles, mumps, rubella [vaccine]
MODY	maturity onset diabetes of the young
6-MP	6-mercaptopurine
MPGN	membranoproliferative glomerulonephritis
MPO	myeloperoxidase
MPO-ANCA/p-ANCA	myeloperoxidase/perinuclear antineutrophil cytoplasmic antibody
MR	medial rectus [muscle], mitral regurgitation
MRI	magnetic resonance imaging
miRNA	microribonucleic acid
mRNA	messenger ribonucleic acid
MRSA	methicillin-resistant *S aureus*
MS	mitral stenosis, multiple sclerosis
MSH	melanocyte-stimulating hormone
mtDNA	mitochondrial DNA
mTOR	mammalian target of rapamycin
MTP	metatarsophalangeal [joint]
MTX	methotrexate
MVO_2	myocardial oxygen consumption
MVP	mitral valve prolapse
N*	nucleus
Na^+	sodium ion
NAT	nucleic acid testing
NAD	nicotinamide adenine dinucleotide
NAD^+	oxidized nicotinamide adenine dinucleotide
NADH	reduced nicotinamide adenine dinucleotide
$NADP^+$	oxidized nicotinamide adenine dinucleotide phosphate
NADPH	reduced nicotinamide adenine dinucleotide phosphate
NBME	National Board of Medical Examiners
NBOME	National Board of Osteopathic Medical Examiners
NBPME	National Board of Podiatric Medical Examiners

*Image abbreviation only

ABBREVIATION	MEANING
NE	norepinephrine
NF	neurofibromatosis
NFAT	nuclear factor of activated T-cell
NH_3	ammonia
NH_4^+	ammonium
NK	natural killer [cells]
N_M	muscarinic ACh receptor in neuromuscular junction
NMDA	N-methyl-d-aspartate
NMJ	neuromuscular junction
NMS	neuroleptic malignant syndrome
N_N	nicotinic ACh receptor in autonomic ganglia
NRMP	National Residency Matching Program
NNRTI	non-nucleoside reverse transcriptase inhibitor
NO	nitric oxide
N_2O	nitrous oxide
NPH	neutral protamine Hagedorn, normal pressure hydrocephalus
NPV	negative predictive value
NRTI	nucleoside reverse transcriptase inhibitor
NSAID	nonsteroidal anti-inflammatory drug
NSE	neuron-specific enolase
NSTEMI	non–ST-segment elevation myocardial infarction
Nu*	nucleolus
OAA	oxaloacetic acid
OCD	obsessive-compulsive disorder
OCP	oral contraceptive pill
ODC	oxygen-hemoglobin dissociation curve
OH	hydroxy
1,25-OH D_3	calcitriol (active form of vitamin D)
25-OH D_3	storage form of vitamin D
OPV	oral polio vaccine
OR	odds ratio
OS	opening snap
OSA	obstructive sleep apnea
OVLT	organum vasculosum of the lamina terminalis
P-body	processing body (cytoplasmic)
P-450	cytochrome P-450 family of enzymes
PA	posteroanterior, pulmonary artery
PABA	*para*-aminobenzoic acid
$Paco_2$	arterial Pco_2
P_{ACO_2}	alveolar Pco_2
PAH	*para*-aminohippuric acid
PAN	polyarteritis nodosa
Pao_2	partial pressure of oxygen in arterial blood
P_{AO_2}	partial pressure of oxygen in alveolar blood
PAP	Papanicolaou [smear], prostatic acid phosphatase, posteromedial papillary muscle
PAPPA	pregnancy-associated plasma protein A
PAS	periodic acid–Schiff
Pat*	patella
PBP	penicillin-binding protein
PC	platelet count, pyruvate carboxylase
PCA	posterior cerebral artery
PCC	prothrombin complex concentrate
PCL	posterior cruciate ligament
Pco_2	partial pressure of carbon dioxide
PCom	posterior communicating [artery]
PCOS	polycystic ovarian syndrome
PCP	phencyclidine hydrochloride, *Pneumocystis jirovecii* pneumonia
PCR	polymerase chain reaction
PCT	proximal convoluted tubule
PCV13	pneumococcal conjugate vaccine
PCWP	pulmonary capillary wedge pressure
PDA	patent ductus arteriosus, posterior descending artery
PDE	phosphodiesterase
PDGF	platelet-derived growth factor
PDH	pyruvate dehydrogenase
PE	pulmonary embolism
PECAM	platelet–endothelial cell adhesion molecule
P_{ECO_2}	expired air Pco_2
PEP	phosphoenolpyruvate
PF	platelet factor
PFK	phosphofructokinase
PFK-2	phosphofructokinase-2
PFT	pulmonary function test
PG	phosphoglycerate
P_i	plasma interstitial osmotic pressure, inorganic phosphate
PICA	posterior inferior cerebellar artery
PID	pelvic inflammatory disease
P_{IO_2}	Po_2 in inspired air
PIP	proximal interphalangeal [joint]
PIP_2	phosphatidylinositol 4,5-bisphosphate
PIP_3	phosphatidylinositol 3,4,5-bisphosphate
PKD	polycystic kidney disease
PKR	interferon-α–induced protein kinase
PKU	phenylketonuria
PLP	pyridoxal phosphate
PML	progressive multifocal leukoencephalopathy
PMN	polymorphonuclear [leukocyte]
P_{net}	net filtration pressure
PNET	primitive neuroectodermal tumor
PNS	peripheral nervous system
Po_2	partial pressure of oxygen
PO_4^{3-}	phosphate
Pop*	popliteal artery
Pop a*	popliteal artery
Post*	posterior
PPAR	peroxisome proliferator-activated receptor
PPD	purified protein derivative
PPI	proton pump inhibitor
PPM	parts per million
PPSV23	pneumococcal polysaccharide vaccine
PPV	positive predictive value
PR3-ANCA/c-ANCA	cytoplasmic antineutrophil cytoplasmic antibody
PrP	prion protein
PRPP	phosphoribosylpyrophosphate

*Image abbreviation only

ABBREVIATION	MEANING
PSA	prostate-specific antigen
PSS	progressive systemic sclerosis
PT	prothrombin time
PTEN	phosphatase and tensin homolog
PTH	parathyroid hormone
PTHrP	parathyroid hormone–related protein
PTSD	post-traumatic stress disorder
PTT	partial thromboplastin time
PV	plasma volume, venous pressure, portal vein
Pv*	pulmonary vein
PVC	polyvinyl chloride
PVR	pulmonary vascular resistance
R	correlation coefficient, right, R variable [group]
R_3	Registration, Ranking, & Results [system]
RA	right atrium
RAAS	renin-angiotensin-aldosterone system
RANK-L	receptor activator of nuclear factor-κ B ligand
RAS	reticular activating system
RBF	renal blood flow
RCA	right coronary artery
REM	rapid eye movement
RER	rough endoplasmic reticulum
Rh	*rhesus* antigen
RLL*	right lower lobe (of lungs)
RLQ	right lower quadrant
RML*	right middle lobe (of lung)
RNA	ribonucleic acid
RNP	ribonucleoprotein
ROS	reactive oxygen species
RPF	renal plasma flow
RPGN	rapidly progressive glomerulonephritis
RPR	rapid plasma reagin
RR	relative risk, respiratory rate
rRNA	ribosomal ribonucleic acid
RS	Reed-Sternberg [cells]
RSC*	right subclavian artery
RSV	respiratory syncytial virus
RTA	renal tubular acidosis
RUL*	right upper lobe (of lung)
RUQ	right upper quadrant
RV	residual volume, right ventricle, right ventricular
RVH	right ventricular hypertrophy
[S]	substrate concentration
SA	sinoatrial
SAA	serum amyloid–associated [protein]
SAM	S-adenosylmethionine
SARS	severe acute respiratory syndrome
SARS-CoV-2	severe acute respiratory syndrome coronavirus 2 (virus)
SCC	squamous cell carcinoma
SCD	sudden cardiac death
SCID	severe combined immunodeficiency disease
SCJ	squamocolumnar junction
SCM	sternocleidomastoid muscle
SCN	suprachiasmatic nucleus

ABBREVIATION	MEANING
SD	standard deviation
SE	standard error [of the mean]
SEP	Spoken English Proficiency
SER	smooth endoplasmic reticulum
SERM	selective estrogen receptor modulator
SGLT	sodium-glucose transporter
SHBG	sex hormone–binding globulin
SIADH	syndrome of inappropriate [secretion of] antidiuretic hormone
SIDS	sudden infant death syndrome
SJS	Stevens-Johnson syndrome
SLE	systemic lupus erythematosus
SLL	small lymphocytic lymphoma
SLT	Shiga-like toxin
SMA	superior mesenteric artery
SMX	sulfamethoxazole
SNARE	soluble NSF attachment protein receptor
SNc	substantia nigra pars compacta
SNP	single nucleotide polymorphism
SNr	substantia nigra pars reticulata
SNRI	serotonin and norepinephrine receptor inhibitor
snRNA	small nuclear RNA
snRNP	small nuclear ribonucleoprotein
SO	superior oblique [muscle]
SOAP	Supplemental Offer and Acceptance Program
Sp*	spleen
spp	species
SR	superior rectus [muscle]
SS	single stranded
ssDNA	single-stranded deoxyribonucleic acid
SSPE	subacute sclerosing panencephalitis
SSRI	selective serotonin reuptake inhibitor
ssRNA	single-stranded ribonucleic acid
St*	stomach
ST	Shiga toxin
StAR	steroidogenic acute regulatory protein
STEMI	ST-segment elevation myocardial infarction
STI	sexually transmitted infection
STN	subthalamic nucleus
SV	splenic vein, stroke volume
SVC	superior vena cava
SVR	systemic vascular resistance
SVT	supraventricular tachycardia
T*	thalamus, trachea
$t_{1/2}$	half-life
T_3	triiodothyronine
T_4	thyroxine
TAPVR	total anomalous pulmonary venous return
TB	tuberculosis
TBG	thyroxine-binding globulin
TBV	total blood volume
3TC	dideoxythiacytidine [lamivudine]
TCA	tricarboxylic acid [cycle], tricyclic antidepressant
Tc cell	cytotoxic T cell
TCR	T-cell receptor

*Image abbreviation only

ABBREVIATION	MEANING
TDF	tenofovir disoproxil fumarate
TdT	terminal deoxynucleotidyl transferase
TE	tracheoesophageal
TFT	thyroid function test
TG	triglyceride
TGF	transforming growth factor
Th cell	helper T cell
THF	tetrahydrofolic acid
TI	therapeutic index
TIA	transient ischemic attack
Tib*	tibia
TIBC	total iron-binding capacity
TIPS	transjugular intrahepatic portosystemic shunt
TLC	total lung capacity
T_m	maximum rate of transport
TMP	trimethoprim
TN	true negative
TNF	tumor necrosis factor
TNM	tumor, node, metastases [staging]
TOP	topoisomerase
ToRCHeS	*Toxoplasma gondii*, rubella, CMV, HIV, HSV-2, syphilis
TP	true positive
tPA	tissue plasminogen activator
TPO	thyroid peroxidase, thrombopoietin
TPP	thiamine pyrophosphate
TPPA	*Treponema pallidum* particle agglutination assay
TPR	total peripheral resistance
TR	tricuspid regurgitation
TRAP	tartrate-resistant acid phosphatase
TRECs	T-cell receptor excision circles
TRH	thyrotropin-releasing hormone
tRNA	transfer ribonucleic acid
TSH	thyroid-stimulating hormone
TSI	triple sugar iron
TSS	toxic shock syndrome
TSST	toxic shock syndrome toxin
TTP	thrombotic thrombocytopenic purpura
TTR	transthyretin
TV	tidal volume
TXA_2	thromboxane A_2
UDP	uridine diphosphate

*Image abbreviation only

ABBREVIATION	MEANING
UMN	upper motor neuron
UMP	uridine monophosphate
UPD	uniparental disomy
URI	upper respiratory infection
USMLE	United States Medical Licensing Examination
UTI	urinary tract infection
UTP	uridine triphosphate
UV	ultraviolet
V_1, V_2	vasopressin receptors
VC	vital capacity
V_d	volume of distribution
VD	physiologic dead space
V(D)J	variable, (diversity), joining gene segments rearranged to form Ig genes
VDRL	Venereal Disease Research Laboratory
VEGF	vascular endothelial growth factor
V_H	variable region, heavy chain [antibody]
VHL	von Hippel-Lindau [disease]
VIP	vasoactive intestinal peptide
VIPoma	vasoactive intestinal polypeptide-secreting tumor
VJ	light-chain hypervariable region [antibody]
V_L	variable region, light chain [antibody]
VLCFA	very-long-chain fatty acids
VLDL	very low density lipoprotein
VMA	vanillylmandelic acid
VMAT	vesicular monoamine transporter
V_{max}	maximum velocity
VPL	ventral posterior nucleus, lateral
VPM	ventral posterior nucleus, medial
VPN	vancomycin, polymyxin, nystatin [media]
$\dot{V}/\dot{Q}$	ventilation/perfusion [ratio]
VRE	vancomycin-resistant enterococcus
VSD	ventricular septal defect
V_T	tidal volume
VTE	venous thromboembolism
vWF	von Willebrand factor
VZV	varicella-zoster virus
VMAT	vesicular monoamine transporter
XR	X-linked recessive
XX/XY	normal complement of sex chromosomes for female/male
ZDV	zidovudine [formerly AZT]

SECTION IV

Image Acknowledgments

In this edition, in collaboration with MedIQ Learning, LLC, and a variety of other partners, we are pleased to include the following clinical images and diagrams for the benefit of integrative student learning.

Portions of this book identified with the symbol are copyright © USMLE-Rx.com (MedIQ Learning, LLC).

Portions of this book identified with the symbol are copyright © Dr. Richard Usatine and are provided under license through MedIQ Learning, LLC.

Portions of this book identified with the symbol are listed below by page number.

This symbol refers to material that is available in the public domain.

This symbol refers to the Creative Commons Attribution license, full text at http://creativecommons.org/licenses/by/4.0/legalcode.

This symbol refers to the Creative Commons Attribution-Share Alike license, full text at: http://creativecommons.org/licenses/by-sa/4.0/legalcode.

Biochemistry

34 **Chromatin structure.** Electron micrograph showing heterochromatin, euchromatin, and nucleolus. This image is a derivative work, adapted from the following source, available under : Roller RA, Rickett JD, Stickle WB. The hypobranchial gland of the estuarine snail *Stramonita haemastoma canaliculata* (Gray) (Prosobranchia: Muricidae): a light and electron microscopical study. *Am Malac Bull.* 1995;11(2):177-190. Available at https://archive.org/details/americanml01119931994amer.

49 **Cilia structure: Image A.** Nine doublet + 2 singlet arrangement of microtubule. Courtesy of Louisa Howard and Michael Binder. The image may have been modified by cropping, labeling, and/or captions. All rights to this adaptation by MedIQ Learning, LLC are reserved.

49 **Cilia structure: Image B.** Cilia structure of basal body. This image is a derivative work, adapted from the following source, available under : Riparbelli MG, Cabrera OA, Callaini G, et al. Unique properties of *Drosophila* spermatocyte primary cilia. *Biol Open.* 2013 Nov 15; 2(11): 1137–1147. DOI: 10.1242/bio.20135355.

49 **Cilia structure: Image C.** Dextrocardia. This image is a derivative work, adapted from the following source, available under : Oluwadare O, Ayoka AO, Akomolafe RO, et al. The role of electrocardiogram in the diagnosis of dextrocardia with mirror image atrial arrangement and ventricular position in a young adult Nigerian in Ile-Ife: a case report. *J Med Case Rep.* 2015;9:222. DOI: 10.1186/s13256-015-0695-4.

51 **Osteogenesis imperfecta: Image A.** Skeletal deformities in upper extremity of child. This image is a derivative work, adapted from the following source, available under : Vanakker OM, Hemelsoet D, De Paepe. Hereditary connective tissue diseases in young adult stroke: a comprehensive synthesis. *Stroke Res Treat.* 2011;712903. DOI: 10.4061/2011/712903. The image may have been modified by cropping, labeling, and/or captions. All rights to this adaptation by MedIQ Learning, LLC are reserved.

51 **Osteogenesis imperfecta: Image B.** Blue sclera. This image is a derivative work, adapted from the following source, available under : Wheatley K, Heng EL, Sheppard M, et al. A case of spontaneous intestinal perforation in osteogenesis imperfects. *J Clin Med Res.* 2010;2(4):198–200. DOI: 10.4021/jocmr369w.

51 **Ehlers-Danlos syndrome: Images A and B.** Hyperextensibility of skin (A) and DIP joint (B). These images are a derivative work, adapted from the following source, available under : Whitaker JK, Alexander, P, Chau DYS, et al. Severe conjunctivochalasis in association with classic type Ehlers-Danlos syndrome. *BMC Ophthalmol.* 2012;2:47. DOI: 10.1186/1471-2415-12-47.

52 **Elastin.** Pes escavatum. This image is a derivative work, adapted from the following source, available under : De Maio F, Fichera A, De Luna V, et al. Orthopaedic aspects of Marfan syndrome: the experience of a referral center for diagnosis of rare diseases. *Adv Orthop.* 2016; 2016: 8275391. DOI 10.1155/2016/8275391.

55 **Karyotyping.** Paar C, Herber G, Voskova, et al. This image is a derivative work, adapted from the following source, available under : A case of acute myeloid leukemia (AML) with an unreported combination of chromosomal abnormalities: gain of isochromosome 5p, tetrasomy 8 and unbalanced translocation der(19)t(17;19)(q23;p13). *Mol Cytogenet.* 2013;6:40. DOI: 10.1186/1755-8166-6-40.

55 **Fluorescence in situ hybridization.** This image is a derivative work, adapted from the following source, available under : Paar C, Herber G, Voskova, et al. A case of acute myeloid leukemia (AML) with an unreported combination of chromosomal abnormalities: gain of isochromosome 5p, tetrasomy 8 and unbalanced translocation der(19)t(17;19)(q23;p13). *Mol Cytogenet.* 2013;6:40. DOI: 10.1186/1755-8166-6-40.

57 **Genetic terms.** Café-au-lait spots. This image is a derivative work, adapted from the following source, available under : Dumitrescu CE and Collins MT. *Orphanet J Rare Dis.* 2008;3:12. DOI: 10.1186/1750-1172-3-12.

61 **Muscular dystrophies.** Fibrofatty replacement of muscle. Courtesy of the Department of Health and Human Services and Dr. Edwin P. Ewing, Jr. The image may have been modified by cropping, labeling, and/or captions. All rights to this adaptation by MedIQ Learning, LLC are reserved.

66 **Vitamin A.** Bitot sponts on conjunctiva. This image is a derivative work, adapted from the following source, available under : Baiyeroju A, Bowman R, Gilbert C, et al. Managing eye health in young children. *Comm Eye Health.* 2010;23(72):4-11. Available at https://www.ncbi.nlm.nih.gov/pmc/articles/PMC2873666.

67 **Vitamin B_3.** Pellagra. This image is a derivative work, adapted from the following source, available under : van Dijk HA, Fred H. Images of memorable cases: case 2. Connexions Web site. Dec 4, 2008. Available at: http://cnx.org/contents/3d3dcb2e-8e98-496f-91c2-fe94e93428a1@3@3/.

70 **Vitamin D.** X-ray of lower extremity in child with rickets. This image is a derivative work, adapted from the following source, available

under: Dr. Michael L. Richardson. The image may have been modified by cropping, labeling, and/or captions. MedIQ Learning, LLC makes this available under.

71 **Protein-energy malnutrition: Image A.** Child with kwashiorkor. Courtesy of the Department of Health and Human Services and Dr. Lyle Conrad.

71 **Protein-energy malnutrition: Image B.** Child with marasmus. Courtesy of the Department of Health and Human Services.

84 **Alkaptonuria.** Pigment granules on dorsum of hand. This image is a derivative work, adapted from the following source, available under: Vasudevan B, Sawhney MPS, Radhakrishnan S. Alkaptonuria associated with degenerative collagenous palmar plaques. *Indian J Dermatol.* 2009;54:299-301. DOI: 10.4103/0019-5154.55650.

85 **Cystinuria.** Hexagonal cystine stones in urine. This image is a derivative work, adapted from the following source, available under: Courtesy of Cayla Devine.

88 **Lysosomal storage diseases: Image A.** "Cherry-red" spot on macula in Tay-Sachs disease. This image is a derivative work, adapted from the following source, available under: Courtesy of Dr. Jonathan Trobe.

88 **Lysosomal storage diseases: Image B.** Angiokeratomas. This image is a derivative work, adapted from the following source, available under: Burlina AP, Sims KB, Politei JM, et al. Early diagnosis of peripheral nervous system involvement in Fabry disease and treatment of neuropathic pain: the report of an expert panel. *BMC Neurol.* 2011;11:61. DOI: 10.1186/1471-2377-11-61. The image may have been modified by cropping, labeling, and/or captions. All rights to this adaptation by MedIQ Learning, LLC are reserved.

88 **Lysosomal storage diseases: Image C.** Gaucher cells in Gaucher disease. This image is a derivative work, adapted from the following source, available under: Sokołowska B, Skomra D, Czartoryska B. et al. Gaucher disease diagnosed after bone marrow trephine biopsy—a report of two cases. *Folia Histochem Cytobiol.* 2011;49:352-356. DOI: 10.5603/FHC.2011.0048. The image may have been modified by cropping, labeling, and/or captions. All rights to this adaptation by MedIQ Learning, LLC are reserved.

88 **Lysosomal storage diseases: Image D.** Foam cells in Niemann-Pick disease. This image is a derivative work, adapted from the following source, available under: Prieto-Potin I, Roman-Blas JA, Martinez-Calatrava MJ, et al. Hypercholesterolemia boosts joint destruction in chronic arthritis. An experimental model aggravated by foam macrophage infiltration. *Arthritis Res Ther.* 2013;15:R81. DOI: 10.1186/ar4261.

94 **Abetalipoproteinemia.** Small bowel mucosa shows clear enterocytes. Courtesy of Dr. Michael Bonert.

Immunology

96 **Lymph node: Images A and B.** Lymph node histology. These images are a derivative work, adapted from the following source, available under: Navid Golpur.

98 **Thymus.** "Sail sign" on x-ray of normal thymus in neonate. This image is a derivative work, adapted from the following source, available under: Di Serafino M, Esposito F, Severino R, et al. Think thymus, think well: the chest x-ray thymic signs. *J Pediatr Moth Care.* 2016;1(2):108-109. DOI: 10.19104/japm.2016.108.

107 **Complement disorders.** Urine discoloration in paroxysmal nocturnal hemoglobinuria. This image is a derivative work, adapted from the following source, available under: Nakamura N, Sugawara T, Shirato K, et al. *J Med Case Reports.* 2011;5:550. doi: 10.1186/1752-1947-5-550

117 **Immunodeficiencies: Image A.** Spider angioma (telangiectasia). This image is a derivative work, adapted from the following source, available under: Liapakis IE, Englander M, Sinani R, et al. Management of facial telangiectasias with hand cautery. *World J Plast Surg.* 2015 Jul;4(2):127-133.

117 **Immunodeficiencies: Image B.** Giant granules in granulocytes in Chédiak-Higashi syndrome. This image is a derivative work, adapted from the following source, available under: Bharti S, Bhatia P, Bansal D, et al. The accelerated phase of Chediak-Higashi syndrome: the importance of hematological evaluation. *Turk J Haematol.* 2013;30:85-87. DOI: 10.4274/tjh.2012.0027. The image may have been modified by cropping, labeling, and/or captions. All rights to this adaptation by MedIQ Learning, LLC are reserved.

Microbiology

125 **Stains: Image A.** *Trypanosoma lewisi* on Giemsa stain. Courtesy of the Department of Health and Human Services and Dr. Mae Melvin.

125 **Stains: Image B.** Periodic acid–Schiff stain reveals *Tropheryma whipplei* infection. This image is a derivative work, adapted from the following source, available under: Courtesy of Dr. Ed Uthman.

125 **Stains: Image C.** *Mycobacterium tuberculosis* on Ziehl-Neelsen stain. Courtesy of the Department of Health and Human Services and Dr. George P. Kubica.

125 **Stains: Image D.** *Cryptococcus neoformans* on India ink stain. Courtesy of the Department of Health and Human Services.

125 **Stains: Image E.** *Coccidioides immitis* on silver stain. Courtesy of the Department of Health and Human Services and Dr. Edwin P. Ewing, Jr.

127 **Encapsulated bacteria.** Capsular swelling of *Streptococcus pneumoniae* using the Neufeld-Quellung test. Courtesy of the Department of Health and Human Services.

128 **Catalase-positive organisms.** Oxygen bubbles released during catalase reaction. This image is a derivative work, adapted from the following source, available under: Stefano Nase. The image may have been modified by cropping, labeling, and/or captions. MedIQ Learning, LLC makes this available under.

129 **Spore-forming bacteria.** This image is a derivative work, adapted from the following source, available under: Jones SW, Paredes CJ, Tracy B. The transcriptional program underlying the physiology of clostridial sporulation. *Genome Biol.* 2008;9:R114. DOI: 10.1186/gb-2008-9-7-r114.

135 **α-hemolytic bacteria.** α-hemolysis. This image is a derivative work, adapted from the following source, available under: Y. Tambe. The image may have been modified by cropping, labeling, and/or captions. MedIQ Learning, LLC makes this available under.

135 **β-hemolytic bacteria.** β-hemolysis. This image is a derivative work, adapted from the following source, available under: Wikimedia Commons.

135 ***Staphylococcus aureus.*** Courtesy of the Department of Health and Human Services and Dr. Richard Facklam.

136 ***Streptococcus pneumoniae.*** Courtesy of the Department of Health and Human Services and Dr. Mike Miller.

136 ***Streptococcus pyogenes:* (group A streptococci).** This image is a derivative work, adapted from the following source, available under: Y. Tambe. The image may have been modified by cropping, labeling, and/or captions. MedIQ Learning, LLC makes this available under.

137 ***Bacillus anthracis.*** Ulcer with black eschar. Courtesy of the Department of Health and Human Services and James H. Steele.

138 **Clostridia: Image A.** Gas gangrene due to *Clostridium perfringens.* This image is a derivative work, adapted from the following source, available under: Schröpfer E, Rauthe S, Meyer T. Diagnosis and misdiagnosis of necrotizing soft tissue infections: three case reports. *Cases J.* 2008;1:252. DOI: 10.1186/1757-1626-1-252.

138 **Clostridia: Image B.** Pseudomembranous enterocolitis on colonoscopy. This image is a derivative work, adapted from the following source, available under [cc-by-sa]: Klinikum Dritter Orden für die Überlassung des Bildes zur Veröffentlichu. The image may have been modified by cropping, labeling, and/or captions. MedIQ Learning, LLC makes this available under [cc-by-sa].

139 ***Corynebacterium diphtheriae.*** Pseudomembranous pharyngitis. This image is a derivative work, adapted from the following source, available under [cc-by-sa]: Wikimedia Commons. The image may have been modified by cropping, labeling, and/or captions. MedIQ Learning, LLC makes this available under [cc-by-sa].

139 ***Listeria monocytogenes.*** Actin rockets. This image is a derivative work, adapted from the following source, available under [cc-by]: Schuppler M, Loessner MJ. The opportunistic pathogen *Listeria monocytogenes*: pathogenicity and interaction with the mucosal immune system. *Int J Inflamm.* 2010;2010:704321. DOI: 10.4061/2010/704321. The image may have been modified by cropping, labeling, and/or captions. All rights to this adaptation by MedIQ Learning, LLC are reserved.

139 ***Nocardia* vs *Actinomyces*: Image A.** *Nocardia* on acid-fast stain. This image is a derivative work, adapted from the following source, available under [cc-by]: Venkataramana K. Human *Nocardia* infections: a review of pulmonary nocardiosis. *Cereus.* 2015;7(8):e304. DOI: 10.7759/cureus.304.

139 ***Nocardia* vs *Actinomyces*: Image B.** *Actinomyces israelii* on Gram stain. [public domain] Courtesy of the Department of Health and Human Services.

140 **Mycobacteria.** Acid-fast stain. [public domain] Courtesy of the Department of Health and Human Services and Dr. George P. Kubica

140 **Tuberculosis.** Langhans giant cell in caseating granuloma. [public domain] Courtesy of J. Hayman.

141 **Leprosy: Image A.** "Glove and stocking" distribution. This image is a derivative work, adapted from the following source, available under [cc-by]: Courtesy of Bruno Jehle.

142 ***Neisseria*: Image A.** Intracellular *N gonorrhoeae*. [public domain] Courtesy of the Department of Health and Human Services and Bill Schwartz.

142 ***Haemophilus influenzae*: Image A.** Epiglottitis. This image is a derivative work, adapted from the following source, available under [cc-by]: Wikimedia Commons. The image may have been modified by cropping, labeling, and/or captions. All rights to this adaptation by MedIQ Learning, LLC are reserved.

143 ***Legionella pneumophila.*** Lung findings of unilateral and lobar infiltrate. This image is a derivative work, adapted from the following source, available under [cc-by]: Robbins NM, Kumar A, Blair BM. *Legionella pneumophila* infection presenting as headache, confusion and dysarthria in a human immunodeficiency virus-1 (HIV-1) positive patient: case report. *BMC Infect Dis.* 2012;12:225. DOI: 10.1186/1471-2334-12-225.

143 ***Pseudomonas aeruginosa*: Image A.** Blue-green pigment on centrimide agar. This image is a derivative work, adapted from the following source, available under [cc-by-sa]: Hansen. The image may have been modified by cropping, labeling, and/or captions. MedIQ Learning, LLC makes this available under [cc-by-sa].

143 ***Pseudomonas aeruginosa*: Image B.** Ecthyma gangrenosum. This image is a derivative work, adapted from the following source, available under [cc-by]: Uludokumaci S, Balkan II, Mete B, et al. Ecthyma gangrenosum-like lesions in a febrile neutropenic patient with simultaneous *Pseudomonas* sepsis and disseminated fusariosis. *Turk J Haematol.* 2013 Sep;30(3):321-4. DOI: 10.4274/Tjh.2012.0030.

145 ***Klebsiella.*** [public domain] Courtesy of the Department of Health and Human Services.

145 ***Campylobacter jejuni.*** [public domain] Courtesy of the Department of Health and Human Services.

146 ***Vibrio cholerae.*** This image is a derivative work, adapted from the following source, available under [cc-by]: Phetsouvanh R, Nakatsu M, Arakawa E, et al. Fatal bacteremia due to immotile *Vibrio cholerae* serogroup O21 in Vientiane, Laos—a case report. *Ann Clin Microbiol Antimicrob.* 2008;7:10. DOI: 10.1186/1476-0711-7-10.

146 ***Helicobacter pylori.*** [public domain] Courtesy of the Department of Health and Human Services, Dr. Patricia Fields, and Dr. Collette Fitzgerald.

146 **Spirochetes.** Appearance on darkfield microscopy. [public domain] Courtesy of the Department of Health and Human Services.

146 **Lyme disease: Image A.** *Ixodes* tick. [public domain] Courtesy of the Department of Health and Human Services and Dr. Michael L. Levin.

146 **Lyme disease: Image B.** Erythema migrans. [public domain] Courtesy of the Department of Health and Human Services and James Gathany.

147 **Syphilis: Image A.** Painless chancre in primary syphilis. [public domain] Courtesy of the Department of Health and Human Services and M. Rein.

147 **Syphilis: Image B.** Treponeme on darkfield microscopy. [public domain] Courtesy of the Department of Health and Human Services and Renelle Woodall.

147 **Syphilis: Image D.** Rash on palms. This image is a derivative work, adapted from the following source, available under [cc-by]: Drahansky M, Dolezel M, Urbanek J, et al. Influence of skin diseases on fingerprint recognition. *J Biomed Biotechnol.* 2012;626148. DOI: 10.1155/2012/626148.

147 **Syphilis: Image E.** Condyloma lata. [public domain] Courtesy of the Department of Health and Human Services and Susan Lindsley.

147 **Syphilis: Image F.** Gumma. This image is a derivative work, adapted from the following source, available under [cc-by]: Chakir K, Benchikhi H. Granulome centro-facial révélant une syphilis tertiaire. *Pan Afr Med J.* 2013;15:82. DOI: 10.11604/pamj.2013.15.82.3011.

147 **Syphilis: Image G.** Congenital syphilis. [public domain] Courtesy of the Department of Health and Human Services and Dr. Norman Cole.

147 **Syphilis: Image H.** Hutchinson teeth. [public domain] Courtesy of the Department of Health and Human Services and Susan Lindsley.

148 ***Gardnerella vaginalis.*** [public domain] Courtesy of the Department of Health and Human Services and M. Rein.

150 **Rickettsial diseases and vector-borne illnesses: Image A.** Rash of Rocky Mountain spotted fever. [public domain] Courtesy of the Department of Health and Human Services.

150 **Rickettsial diseases and vector-borne illnesses: Image B.** *Ehrlichia* morulae. This image is a derivative work, adapted from the following source, available under [cc-by]: Dantas-Torres F. Canine vector-borne diseases in Brazil. *Parasit Vectors.* 2008;1:25. DOI: 10.1186/1756-3305-1-25. The image may have been modified by cropping, labeling, and/or captions. All rights to this adaptation by MedIQ Learning, LLC are reserved.

150 **Rickettsial diseases and vector-borne illnesses: Image C.** *Anaplasma phagocytophilium* in neutrophil. [public domain] Courtesy of the Department of Health and Human Services and Dumler JS, Choi K, Garcia-Garcia JC, et al. Human granulocytic anaplasmosis. *Emerg Infect Dis.* 2005. DOI 10.3201/eid1112.050898.

150 ***Mycoplasma pneumoniae.*** This image is a derivative work, adapted from the following source, available under [cc-by]: Rottem S, Kosower ND, Kornspan JD. Contamination of tissue cultures by *Mycoplasma*. In: Ceccherini-Nelli L, ed: *Biomedical tissue culture.* 2016. DOI: 10.5772/51518.

151 **Systemic mycoses: Image A.** *Histoplasma.* [public domain] Courtesy of the Department of Health and Human Services and Dr. D.T. McClenan.

151 **Systemic mycoses: Image B.** *Blastomyces dermatitidis* undergoing broad-base budding. [public domain] Courtesy of the Department of Health and Human Services and Dr. Libero Ajello.

151 **Systemic mycoses: Image C.** Coccidiomycosis with endospheres. Courtesy of the Department of Health and Human Services.

151 **Systemic mycoses: Image D.** "Captain's wheel" shape of *Paracoccidioides.*. Courtesy of the Department of Health and Human Services and Dr. Lucille K. Georg.

152 **Cutaneous mycoses: Image G.** Tinea versicolor. This image is a derivative work, adapted from the following source, available under : Sarah (Rosenau) Korf. The image may have been modified by cropping, labeling, and/or captions. MedIQ Learning, LLC makes this available under .

153 **Opportunistic fungal infections: Image A.** Budding yeast of *Candida albicans*. This image is a derivative work, adapted from the following source, available under : Y. Tambe. The image may have been modified by cropping, labeling, and/or captions. MedIQ Learning, LLC makes this available under .

153 **Opportunistic fungal infections: Image B.** Germ tubes of *Candida albicans.*. This image is a derivative work, adapted from the following source, available under : Y. Tambe. The image may have been modified by cropping, labeling, and/or captions. MedIQ Learning, LLC makes this available under .

153 **Opportunistic fungal infections: Image C.** Oral thrush. Courtesy of the Department of Health and Human Services and Dr. Sol Silverman, Jr.

153 **Opportunistic fungal infections: Image E.** Conidiophores of *Aspergillus fumigatus*. Courtesy of the Department of Health and Human Services.

153 **Opportunistic fungal infections: Image F.** Aspergilloma in left lung. This image is a derivative work, adapted from the following source, available under : Souilamas R, Souilamas JI, Alkhamees K, et al. Extra corporal membrane oxygenation in general thoracic surgery: a new single veno-venous cannulation. *J Cardiothorac Surg.* 2011;6:52. DOI: 10.1186/1749-8090-6-52.

153 **Opportunistic fungal infections: Image G.** *Cryptococcus neoformans*. Courtesy of the Department of Health and Human Services and Dr. Leanor Haley.

153 **Opportunistic fungal infections: Image H.** *Cryptococcus neoformans* on mucicarmine stain. Courtesy of the Department of Health and Human Services and Dr. Leanor Haley.

153 **Opportunistic fungal infections: Image I.** Mucor. Courtesy of the Department of Health and Human Services and Dr. Lucille K. Georg.

153 **Opportunistic fungal infections: Image J.** Mucormycosis. This image is a derivative work, adapted from the following source, available under : Jiang N, Zhao G, Yang S, et al. A retrospective analysis of eleven cases of invasive rhino-orbito-cerebral mucormycosis presented with orbital apex syndrome initially. *BMC Ophthalmol.* 2016; 16: 10. DOI: 10.1186/s12886-016-0189-1.

154 ***Pneumocystis jirovecii*: Image A.** Interstitial opacities in lung. This image is a derivative work, adapted from the following source, available under : Chuang C, Zhanhong X, Yinyin G, et al. Unsuspected *Pneumocystis* pneumonia in an HIV-seronegative patient with untreated lung cancer: circa case report. *J Med Case Rep.* 2007;1:15. DOI: 10.1186/1752-1947-1-115.

154 ***Pneumocystis jirovecii*: Image B.** CT of lung. This image is a derivative work, adapted from the following source, available under : Allen CM, Al-Jahdali HH, Irion KL, et al. Imaging lung manifestations of HIV/AIDS. *Ann Thorac Med.* 2010 Oct-Dec; 5(4): 201–216. DOI: 10.4103/1817-1737.69106.

154 ***Pneumocystis jiroveci*: Image C.** Disc-shaped yeast. This image is a derivative work, adapted from the following source, available under : Kirby S, Satoskar A, Brodsky S, et al. Histological spectrum of pulmonary manifestations in kidney transplant recipients on sirolimus inclusive immunosuppressive regimens. *Diagn Pathol.* 2012;7:25. DOI: 10.1186/1746-1596-7-25.

154 ***Sporothrix schenckii*.** Subcutaneous mycosis. This image is a derivative work, adapted from the following source, available under : Govender NP, Maphanga TG, Zulu TG, et al. An outbreak of lymphocutaneous sporotrichosis among mine-workers in South Africa. *PLoS Negl Trop Dis.* 2015 Sep; 9(9): e0004096. DOI: 10.1371/journal.pntd.0004096.

155 **Protozoa—gastrointestinal infections: Image A.** *Giardia lamblia* trophozoite. This image is a derivative work, adapted from the following source, available under : Lipoldová M. Giardia and Vilém Dušan Lambl. *PLoS Negl Trop Dis.* 2014;8:e2686. DOI: 10.1371/journal.pntd.0002686.

155 **Protozoa—gastrointestinal infections: Image B.** *Giardia lamblia* cyst. Courtesy of the Department of Health and Human Services.

155 **Protozoa—gastrointestinal infections: Image C.** *Entamoeba histolytica* trophozoites. Courtesy of the Department of Health and Human Services.

155 **Protozoa—gastrointestinal infections: Image D.** *Entamoeba histolytica* cyst. Courtesy of the Department of Health and Human Services.

155 **Protozoa—gastrointestinal infections: Image E.** *Cryptosporidium* oocysts. Courtesy of the Department of Health and Human Services.

156 **Protozoa—CNS infections: Image A.** Ring-enhancing lesions in brain due to *Toxoplasma gondii*. This image is a derivative work, adapted from the following source, available under : Agrawal A, Bhake A, Sangole VM, et al. Multiple-ring enhancing lesions in an immunocompetent adult. *J Glob Infect Dis.* 2010 Sep-Dec;2(3):313-4. DOI: 10.4103/0974-777X.68545.

156 **Protozoa—CNS infections: Image B.** *Toxoplasma gondii* tachyzoite. Courtesy of the Department of Health and Human Services and Dr. L.L. Moore, Jr.

156 **Protozoa—CNS infections: Image C.** *Naegleria fowleri* amoebas. Courtesy of the Department of Health and Human Services.

156 **Protozoa—CNS infections: Image D.** *Trypanosoma brucei gambiense*. Courtesy of the Department of Health and Human Services and Dr. Mae Melvin.

157 **Protozoa—hematologic infections: Image A.** *Plasmodium* trophozoite ring form. Courtesy of the Department of Health and Human Services.

157 **Protozoa—hematologic infections: Image B.** *Plasmodium* schizont containing merozoites. Courtesy of the Department of Health and Human Services and Steven Glenn.

157 **Protozoa—hematologic infections: Image C.** *Babesia* with ring form and with "Maltese cross" form. Courtesy of the Department of Health and Human Services.

158 **Protozoa—others: Image A.** *Trypanosoma cruzi*. Courtesy of the Department of Health and Human Services and Dr. Mae Melvin.

158 **Protozoa—others: Image B.** Cutaneous leishmaniasis. This image is a derivative work, adapted from the following source, available under : Sharara SL, Kanj SS. War and infectious diseases: challenges of the Syrian civil war. *PLoS Pathog.* 2014 Nov;10(11):e1004438. DOI: 10.1371/journal.ppat.1004438.

158 **Protozoa—others: Image C.** *Leishmania* spp. Courtesy of the Department of Health and Human Services and Dr. Francis W. Chandler. The image may have been modified by cropping, labeling, and/or captions. All rights to this adaptation by MedIQ Learning, LLC are reserved.

158 **Protozoa—others: Image D.** *Trichomonas vaginalis*. Courtesy of the Department of Health and Human Services.

159 **Nematodes (roundworms): Image A.** *Enterobius vermicularis* eggs. Courtesy of the Department of Health and Human Services, BG Partin, and Dr. Moore.

159 Nematodes (roundworms): Image B. *Ascaris lumbricoides* egg. Courtesy of the Department of Health and Human Services.

159 Nematodes (roundworms): Image C. *Ancylostoma* spp rash. This image is a derivative work, adapted from the following source, available under: Archer M. Late presentation of cutaneous larva migrans: a case report. *Cases J.* 2009; 2: 7553. doi:10.4076/1757-1626-2-7553.

159 Nematodes (roundworms): Image D. *Trichinella spiralis* cysts in muscle. This image is a derivative work, adapted from the following source, available under: Franssen FFJ, Fonville M, Takumi K, et al. *Vet Res.* 2011; 42(1): 113. DOI: 10.1186/1297-9716-42-113.

159 Nematodes (roundworms): Image E. Elephantiasis. Courtesy of the Department of Health and Human Services.

160 Cestodes (tapeworms): Image A. *Taenia solium.* Courtesy of the Department of Health and Human Services Robert J. Galindo. The image may have been modified by cropping, labeling, and/or captions. MedIQ Learning, LLC makes this available under.

160 Cestodes (tapeworms): Image B. Neurocysticercosis. This image is a derivative work, adapted from the following source, available under: Coyle CM, Tanowitz HB. Diagnosis and treatment of neurocysticercosis. *Interdiscip Perspect Infect Dis.* 2009;2009:180742. DOI: 10.1155/2009/180742. The image may have been modified by cropping, labeling, and/or captions. All rights to this adaptation by MedIQ Learning, LLC are reserved.

160 Cestodes (tapeworms): Image C. *Echinococcus granulosus.* Courtesy of the Department of Health and Human Services.

160 Cestodes (tapeworms): Image D. Hyatid cyst of *Echinococcus granulosus.* Courtesy of the Department of Health and Human Services and Dr. I. Kagan.

160 Cestodes (tapeworms): Image E. *Echinococcus granulosus* cyst in liver. This image is a derivative work, adapted from the following source, available under: Ma Z, Yang W, Yao Y, et al. The adventitia resection in treatment of liver hydatid cyst: a case report of a 15-year-old boy. *Case Rep Surg.* 2014;2014:123149. DOI: 10.1155/2014/123149.

160 Trematodes (flukes): Image A. *Schistosoma mansoni* egg with lateral spine. Courtesy of the Department of Health and Human Services.

160 Trematodes (flukes): Image B. *Schistosoma haematobium* egg with terminal spine. Courtesy of the Department of Health and Human Services.

161 Ectoparasites: Image A. Scabies. This image is a derivative work, adapted from the following source, available under: Siegfried EC, Hebert AA. Diagnosis of atopic dermatitis: mimics, overlaps, and complications. *Clin Med.* 2015 May; 4(5): 884–917. DOI: 10.3390/jcm4050884.

161 Ectoparasites: Image B. Nit of a louse. Courtesy of the Department of Health and Human Services and Joe Miller.

164 DNA viruses. Febrile pharyngitis. This image is a derivative work, adapted from the following source, available under: Balfour HH Jr, Dunmire SK, Hogquist KA. *Clin Transl Immunology.*2015 Feb 27. DOI: 10.1038/cti.2015.1.

165 Herpesviruses: Image A. Keratoconjunctivitis in HSV-1 infection. This image is a derivative work, adapted from the following source, available under: Yang HK, Han YK, Wee WR, et al. Bilateral herpetic keratitis presenting with unilateral neurotrophic keratitis in pemphigus foliaceus: a case report. *J Med Case Rep.* 2011;5:328. DOI: 10.1186/1752-1947-5-328.

165 Herpesviruses: Image B. Herpes labialis. Courtesy of the Department of Health and Human Services and Dr. Herrmann.

165 Herpesviruses: Image E. Shingles (varicella-zoster virus infection). This image is a derivative work, adapted from the following source, available under: Fisle. The image may have been modified by cropping, labeling, and/or captions. MedIQ Learning, LLC makes this available under.

165 Herpesviruses: Image F. Hepatosplenomegaly due to EBV infection. This image is a derivative work, adapted from the following source, available under: Gow NJ, Davidson RN, Ticehurst R, et al. Case report: no response to liposomal daunorubicin in a patient with drug-resistant HIV-associated visceral leishmaniasis. *PLoS Negl Trop Dis.* 2015 Aug; 9(8):e0003983. DOI: 10.1371/journal.pntd.0003983.

165 Herpesviruses: Image G. Atypical lymphocytes in Epstein-Barr virus infection. This image is a derivative work, adapted from the following source, available under: Coutesy of Dr. Ed Uthman. The image may have been modified by cropping, labeling, and/or captions. All rights to this adaptation by MedIQ Learning, LLC are reserved.

165 Herpesviruses: Image I. Roseola. Courtesy of Emiliano Burzagli.

165 Herpesviruses: Image J. Kaposi sarcoma. Courtesy of the Department of Health and Human Services.

166 HSV identification. Positive Tzanck smear in HSV-2 infection. This image is a derivative work, adapted from the following source, available under: Dr. Yale Rosen. The image may have been modified by cropping, labeling, and/or captions. MedIQ Learning, LLC makes this available under.

168 Rotavirus. Courtesy of the Department of Health and Human Services and Erskine Palmer.

169 Rubella virus. Rubella rash. Courtesy of the Department of Health and Human Services.

170 Acute laryngotracheobronchitis. Steeple sign. Reproduced, with permission, from Dr. Frank Gaillard and www.radiopaedia.org.

170 Measles (rubeola) virus: Image A. Koplik spots. Courtesy of the Department of Health and Human Services. The image may have been modified by cropping, labeling, and/or captions. All rights to this adaptation by MedIQ Learning, LLC are reserved.

170 Measles (rubeola) virus: Image B. Rash of measles. Courtesy of the Department of Health and Human Services.

170 Mumps virus. Swollen neck and parotid glands. Courtesy of the Department of Health and Human Services.

171 Rabies virus: Image A. Transmission electron micrograph. Courtesy of the Department of Health and Human Services Dr. Fred Murphy, and Sylvia Whitfield.

171 Rabies virus: Image B. Negri bodies. Courtesy of the Department of Health and Human Services and Dr. Daniel P. Perl.

171 Ebola virus. Courtesy of the Department of Health and Human Services and Cynthia Goldsmith.

172 Zika virus. This image is a derivative work, adapted from the following source, available under: Rocha YRR, Costa JRC, Costa PA, et al. Radiological characterization of cerebral phenotype in newborn microcephaly cases from 2015 outbreak in Brazil. *PLoS Currents* 2016 Jun 8;8. DOI: 10.1371/currents.outbreaks.e854dbf51b8075431a05b39042c00244.

180 Osteomyelitis. X-ray (left) and MRI (right) views. This image is a derivative work, adapted from the following source, available under: Huang P-Y, Wu P-K, Chen C-F, et al. Osteomyelitis of the femur mimicking bone tumors: a review of 10 cases. *World J Surg Oncol.* 2013;11:283. DOI: 10.1186/1477-7819-11-283.

181 Common vaginal infections: Image B. Motile trichomonads. Courtesy of Joe Miller.

181 Common vaginal infections: Image C. *Candida* vulvovaginitis. Courtesy of Mikael Häggström.

182 TORCH infections: Image A. "Blueberry muffin" rash. This image is a derivative work, adapted from the following source, available under

: Benmiloud S, Elhaddou G, Belghiti ZA, et al. Blueberry muffin syndrome. *Pan Afr Med J*. 2012;13:23.

182 **TORCH infections: Image B.** Cataract in infant with contenital rubella. Courtesy of the Department of Health and Human Services .

182 **TORCH infections: Image C.** Periventricular calcifications in congenital cytomegalovirus infection. This image is a derivative work, adapted from the following source, available under : Bonthius D, Perlman S. Congenital viral infections of the brain: lessons learned from lymphocytic choriomeningitis virus in the neonatal rat. *PLoS Pathog*. 2007;3:e149. DOI: 10.1371/journal.ppat.0030149. The image may have been modified by cropping, labeling, and/or captions. All rights to this adaptation by MedIQ Learning, LLC are reserved.

183 **Red rashes of childhood: Image C.** Child with scarlet fever. This image is a derivative work, adapted from the following source, available under : www.badobadop.co.uk.

183 **Red rashes of childhood: Image D.** Chicken pox. Courtesy of the Department of Health and Human Services and Dr. JD Millar.

184 **Sexually transmitted infections: Image A.** Chancroid. Courtesy of the Department of Health and Human Services and Dr. Greg Hammond.

184 **Sexually transmitted infections: Image B.** Donovanosis. Courtesy of the Department of Health and Human Services and Dr. Pinozzi.

185 **Pelvic inflammatory disease: Image A.** Purulent cervical discharge. This image is a derivative work, adapted from the following source, available under : SOS-AIDS Amsterdam The image may have been modified by cropping, labeling, and/or captions. MedIQ Learning, LLC makes this available under .

185 **Pelvic inflammatory disease: Image B.** Adhesions in Fitz-Hugh–Curtis syndrome. Courtesy of Hic et nunc.

190 **Vancomycin.** Red man syndrome. This image is a derivative work, adapted from the following source, available under : O'Meara P, Borici-Mazi R, Morton R, et al. DRESS with delayed onset acute interstitial nephritis and profound refractory eosinophilia secondary to vancomycin. *Allergy Asthma Clin Immunol*. 2011;7:16. DOI: 10.1186/1710-1492-7-16.

Pathology

209 **Necrosis: Image A.** Coagulative necrosis. Courtesy of the Department of Health and Human Services and Dr. Steven Rosenberg.

209 **Necrosis: Image B.** Liquefactive necrosis. Courtesy of Daftblogger.

209 **Necrosis: Image C.** Caseous necrosis. This image is a derivative work, adapted from the following source, available under : Dr. Yale Rosen. The image may have been modified by cropping, labeling, and/or captions. MedIQ Learning, LLC makes this available under .

209 **Necrosis: Image D.** Fat necrosis. This image is a derivative work, adapted from the following source, available under : Patho. The image may have been modified by cropping, labeling, and/or captions. MedIQ Learning, LLC makes this available under .

209 **Necrosis: Image E.** Fibrinoid necrosis. This image is a derivative work, adapted from the following source, available under : Dr. Yale Rosen. The image may have been modified by cropping, labeling, and/or captions. MedIQ Learning, LLC makes this available under .

209 **Necrosis: Image F.** Acral gangrene. Courtesy of the Department of Health and Human Services and William Archibald.

210 **Ischemia.** This image is a derivative work, adapted from the following source, available under : Van Assche LM, Kim HW, Jensen CJ, et al. A new CMR protocol for non-destructive, high resolution, ex-vivo assessment of the area at risk simultaneous with infarction: validation with histopathology. *J Cardiovasc Magn Reson*. 2012; 14(Suppl 1): O7. DOI: 10.1186/1532-429X-14-S1-O7.

210 **Types of infarcts: Image B.** Pale infarct. Courtesy of the Department of Health and Human Services and the Armed Forces Institute of Pathology.

212 **Types of calcification.** Dystrophic calcification. This image is a derivative work, adapted from the following source, available under : Chun J-S, Hong R, Kim J-A. Osseous metaplasia with mature bone formation of the thyroid gland: three case reports. *Oncol Lett*. 2013;6:977-979. DOI: 10.3892/ol.2013.1475. The image may have been modified by cropping, labeling, and/or captions. All rights to this adaptation by MedIQ Learning, LLC are reserved.

212 **Lipofuscin.** This image is a derivative work, adapted from the following source, available under : Dr. Michael Bonert. The image may have been modified by cropping, labeling, and/or captions. MedIQ Learning, LLC makes this available under .

213 **Amyloidosis: Image A.** Amyloid deposits on Congo red stain. This image is a derivative work, adapted from the following source, available under : Dr. Ed Uthman.

213 **Amyloidosis: Image B.** Apple green birefringence under polarized light. This image is a derivative work, adapted from the following source, available under : Dr. Ed Uthman.

215 **Acute inflammation.** Pericardium with severe inflammation, neutrophilic infiltration and fibrin with entrapped clusters of bacteria. This image is a derivative work, adapted from the following source, available under : Faida Ajili, et al. Coexistence of pyoderma gangrenosum and sweet's syndrome in a patient with ulcerative colitis. *Pan Afr Med J*. 2015 Jun 24. DOI: 10.11604/pamj.2015.21.151.6364.

218 **Granulomatous diseases.** Granuloma. Courtesy of Sanjay Mukhopadhyay.

219 **Scar formation: Image A.** Hypertrophic scar. This image is a derivative work, adapted from the following source, available under : Baker R, Urso-Baiarda F, Linge C, et al. Cutaneous scarring: a clinical review. *Dermatol Res Pract*. 2009;2009:625376. DOI: 10.1155/2009/625376.

219 **Scar formation: Image B.** Keloid scar. This image is a derivative work, adapted from the following source, available under : Dr. Andreas Settje. The image may have been modified by cropping, labeling, and/or captions. MedIQ Learning, LLC makes this available under .

220 **Neoplasia and neoplastic progression.** Cervical tissue. This image is a derivative work, adapted from the following source, available under : Courtesy of Dr. Ed Uthman. The image may have been modified by cropping, labeling, and/or captions. All rights to this adaptation by MedIQ Learning, LLC are reserved.

224 **Common metastases: Image A.** Brain metastases from breast cancer. This image is a derivative work, adapted from the following source, available under : Jmarchn. The image may have been modified by cropping, labeling, and/or captions. MedIQ Learning, LLC makes this available under .

224 **Common metastases: Image B.** Brain metastasis. Courtesy of the Department of Health and Human Services and the Armed Forces Institute of Pathology.

224 **Common metastases: Image C.** Liver metastasis. This image is a derivative work, adapted from the following source, available under : Dr. James Heilman The image may have been modified by cropping, labeling, and/or captions. MedIQ Learning, LLC makes this available under .

224 **Common metastases: Image D.** Liver metastasis. Courtesy of J. Hayman.

224 **Common metastases: Image E.** Bone metastasis. This image is a derivative work, adapted from the following source, available under : Dr. Paul Hellerhoff.

224 **Common metastases: Image F.** Bone metastasis. This image is a derivative work, adapted from the following source, available under : Courtesy of M Emmanuel.

228 **Psammoma bodies.** Courtesy of the Department of Health and Human Services and the Armed Forces Institute of Pathology.

Cardiovascular

292 **Anatomy of the heart: Image A.** MRI showing normal cardiac anatomy. This image is a derivative work, adapted from the following source, available under : Zhang J, Chen L, Wang X, et al. Compounding local invariant features and global deformable geometry for medical image registration. *PLoS One.* 2014;9(8):e105815. DOI: 10.1371/journal.pone.0105815.

292 **Anatomy of the heart: Image B.** X-ray showing normal cardiac anatomy. This image is a derivative work, adapted from the following source, available under : Karippacheril JG, Joseph TT. Negative pressure pulmonary oedema and haemorrhage, after a single breath-hold: Diaphragm the culprit? *Indian J Anaesth.* 2010 Jul-Aug;54(4):361–363. DOI: 10.4103/0019-5049.68391.

306 **Congenital heart diseases: Image A.** "Egg on string" appearance on x-ray of the chest in D-transposition of the great vessels. This image is a derivative work, adapted from the following source, available under : Aloriany IA, Barlas NB, Al-Boukai AA. Pictorial essay: Infants of diabetic mothers. *Indian J Radiol Imaging.* 2010 Aug;20(3):174–181. DOI: 10.4103/0971-3026.69349.

306 **Congenital heart diseases: Image B.** Tetralogy of Fallot. This image is a derivative work, adapted from the following source, available under : Rashid AKM: Heart diseases in Down syndrome. In: Dey S, ed: Down syndrome. DOI: 10.5772/46009. The image may have been modified by cropping, labeling, and/or captions. All rights to this adaptation by MedIQ Learning, LLC are reserved.

307 **Congenital heart diseases: Image C.** Ventricular septal defect. This image is a derivative work, adapted from the following source, available under : Bardo DME, Brown P. Cardiac multidetector computed tomography: basic physics of image acquisition and clinical applications. *Curr Cardiol Rev.* 2008 Aug;4(3):231–243. DOI: 10.2174/157340308785160615.

307 **Congenital heart diseases: Image D.** Atrial septal defect. This image is a derivative work, adapted from the following source, available under : Teo KSL, Dundon BK, Molaee P, et al. Percutaneous closure of atrial septal defects leads to normalisation of atrial and ventricular volumes. *J Cardiovasc Magn Reson.* 2008;10(1):55. DOI: 10.1186/1532-429X-10-55.

307 **Congenital heart diseases: Image E.** Patent ductus arteriosus. This image is a derivative work, adapted from the following source, available under : Henjes CR, Nolte I, Wesfaedt P. Multidetector-row computed tomography of thoracic aortic anomalies in dogs and cats: patent ductus arteriosus and vascular rings. *BMC Vet Res.* 2011;7:57. DOI: 10.1186/1746-6148-7-57.

307 **Congenital heart diseases: Image F.** MRI showing coarctation of the aorta. This image is a derivative work, adapted from the following source, available under : Vergales JE, Gangemi JJ, Rhueban KS, Lim DS. Coarctation of the aorta — the current state of surgical and transcatheter therapies. *Curr Cardiol Rev.* 2013 Aug; 9(3): 211–219. DOI: 10.2174/1573403X113099990032

308 **Hypertension.** "String of beads" appearance in fibromuscular dysplasia. This image is a derivative work, adapted from the following source, available under : Plouin PF, Perdu J, LaBatide-Alanore A, et al. Fibromuscular dysplasia. *Orphanet J Rare Dis.* 2007;7:28. DOI: 10.1186/1750-1172-2-28. The image may have been modified by cropping, labeling, and/or captions. All rights to this adaptation by MedIQ Learning, LLC are reserved.

309 **Hyperlipidemia signs: Image C.** Tendinous xanthoma. This image is a derivative work, adapted from the following source, available under : Raffa W, Hassam B. Xanthomes tendineux et tubéreux révélant une hypercholestérolémie familiale. *Pan Afr Med J.* 2013; 15: 49. DOI: 10.11604/pamj.2013.15.49.2636.

309 **Arteriosclerosis: Image A.** Hyaline type. This image is a derivative work, adapted from the following source, available under : Dr. Michael Bonert. The image may have been modified by cropping, labeling, and/or captions. MedIQ Learning, LLC makes this available under .

309 **Arteriosclerosis: Image B.** Hyperplastic type. This image is a derivative work, adapted from the following source, available under : Paco Larosa. The image may have been modified by cropping, labeling, and/or captions. MedIQ Learning, LLC makes this available under .

309 **Arteriosclerosis: Image C.** Monckeberg sclerosis (medial calcific sclerosis). This image is a derivative work, adapted from the following source, available under : Couri CE, da Silva GA, Martinez JA, et al. The image may have been modified by cropping, labeling, and/or captions. All rights to this adaptation by MedIQ Learning, LLC are reserved.

311 **Aortic dissection.** This image is a derivative work, adapted from the following source, available under : Qi Y, Ma X, Li G, et al. Three-dimensional visualization and imaging of the entry tear and intimal flap of aortic dissection using CT virtual intravascular endoscopy. *PLoS One.* 2016; 11(10): e0164750. DOI: 10.1371/journal.pone.0164750.

313 **Evolution of myocardial infarction: Images A and B.** Heart tissue at 0-24 hours (image A) and 1-3 days (image B) after myocardial infarction. These images are a derivative work, adapted from the following source, available under : Chang J, Nair V, Luk A, et al. Pathology of myocardial infarction. *Diagn Histopath.* 2013;19:7-12. DOI: https://doi.org/10.1016/j.mpdhp.2012.11.001.

313 **Evolution of myocardial infarction: Image C.** Heart tissue 3-14 days after myocardial infarction. This image is a derivative work, adapted from the following source, available under : Diarmid AK, Pellicori P, Cleland JG, et al. Taxonomy of segmental myocardial systolic dysfunction. *Eur Heart J.* 2017 Apr 1;38(13):942–954. DOI: 10.1093/eurheartj/ehw140.

313 **Evolution of myocardial infarction: Image D.** Heart tissue after myocardial infarction showing dense fibrous scar replacing myocyte loss. This image is a derivative work, adapted from the following source, available under : Michaud K, Basso C, d'Amati G, et al on behalf of the Association for European Cardiovascular Pathology. Diagnosis of myocardial infarction at autopsy: AECVP reappraisal in the light of the current clinical classification. *Virchows Arch.* 2020;476:179–194.

317 **Myocardial infarction complications: Image A.** Papillary muscle rupture. This image is a derivative work, adapted from the following source, available under : Routy B, Huynh T, Fraser R, et al. Vascular endothelial cell function in catastrophic antiphospholipid syndrome: a case report and review of the literature. *Case Rep Hematol.* 2013;2013:710365. DOI: 10.1155/2013/710365.

317 **Myocardial infarction complications: Image B.** Drawing of pseudoaneurysm. This image is a derivative work, adapted from the following source, available under : Patrick J. Lynch and Dr. C. Carl Jaffe.

317 **Myocardial infarction complications: Image C.** Free wall rupture of left ventricle. This image is a derivative work, adapted from the following source, available under : Zacarias ML, da Trindade H, Tsutsu J, et al. Left ventricular free wall impeding rupture in post-myocardial infarction period diagnosed by myocardial contrast echocardiography: case report. *Cardiovasc Ultrasound.* 2006;4:7. DOI: 10.1186/1476-7120-4-7.

318 **Cardiomyopathies: Image A.** Dilated cardiomyopathy. This image is a derivative work, adapted from the following source, available under : Gho JMIH, van Es R, Stathonikos N, et al. High resolution systematic digital histological quantification of cardiac fibrosis and

adipose tissue in phospholamban p.Arg14del mutation associated cardiomyopathy. *PLoS One.* 2014;9:e94820. DOI: 10.1371/journal.pone.0094820.

318 **Cardiomyopathies: Image B.** Hypertrophic obstructive cardiomyopathy. This image is a derivative work, adapted from the following source, available under : Benetti MA, Belo Nunes RA, Benvenuti LA. Case 2/2016 - 76-year-old male with hypertensive heart disease, renal tumor and shock. *Arq Bras Cardiol.* 2016 May; 106(5): 439–446. DOI: 10.5935/abc.20160067.

319 **Heart failure.** Pedal edema. This image is a derivative work, adapted from the following source, available under : Dr. James Heilman. The image may have been modified by cropping, labeling, and/or captions. MedIQ Learning, LLC makes this available under .

320 **Cardiac tamponade: Image A.** CT showing cardiac tamponade. This image is a derivative work, adapted from the following source, available under : Yousuf T, Kramer J, Kopiec A, et al. A rare case of cardiac tamponade induced by chronic rheumatoid arthritis. *J Clin Med Res.* 2015 Sep;7(9):720–723. DOI: 10.14740/jocmr2226w.

320 **Cardiac tamponade: Image B.** ECG showing cardiac tamponade. This image is a derivative work, adapted from the following source, available under : Maharaj SS, Chang SM. Cardiac tamponade as the initial presentation of systemic lupus erythematosus: a case report and review of the literature. *Pediatr Rheumatol Online J.* 2015; 13: 9. DOI: 10.1186/s12969-015-0005-0.

321 **Bacterial endocarditis: Image A.** Vegetations on heart valves. Courtesy of the Department of Health and Human Services and Dr. Edwin P. Ewing, Jr.

321 **Bacterial endocarditis: Image C.** Osler nodes. This image is a derivative work, adapted from the following source, available under : Yang ML, Chen YH, Lin WR, et al. Case report: infective endocarditis caused by Brevundimonas vesicularis. *BMC Infect Dis.* 2006;6:179. DOI: 10.1186/1471-2334-6-179.

321 **Bacterial endocarditis: Image D.** Janeway lesions on sole. This image is a derivative work, adapted from the following source, available under : Courtesy of DeNanneke.

322 **Rheumatic fever.** Aschoff body and Anitschkow cells. This image is a derivative work, adapted from the following source, available under : Dr. Ed Uthman. The image may have been modified by cropping, labeling, and/or captions. All rights to this adaptation by MedIQ Learning, LLC are reserved.

323 **Acute pericarditis.** This image is a derivative work, adapted from the following source, available under : Bogaert J, Francone M. Cardiovascular magnetic resonance in pericardial diseases. *J Cardiovasc Magn Reson.* 2009;11:14. DOI: 10.1186/1532-429X-11-14. The image may have been modified by cropping, labeling, and/or captions. All rights to this adaptation by MedIQ Learning, LLC are reserved.

Endocrine

334 **Thyroid development.** Thyroglossal duct cyst. This image is a derivative work, adapted from the following source, available under : Adelchi C, Mara P, Melissa L, et al. Ectopic thyroid tissue in the head and neck: a case series. *BMC Res Notes.* 2014;7:790. DOI: 10.1186/1756-0500-7-790.

348 **Hypothyroidism vs hyperthyroidism: Image A.** Pretibial myxedema. This image is a derivative work, adapted from the following source, available under : Fred H, van Dijk HA. Images of memorable cases: case 144. Connexions Web site. Dec 8, 2008. Available at: https://cnx.org/contents/SCJeD6JM@3/Images-of-Memorable-Cases-Case-144.

348 **Hypothyroidism vs hyperthyroidism: Image B.** Onycholysis. This image is a derivative work, adapted from the following source, available under : Alborz Fallah. This image may have been modified by cropping, labeling, and/or captions. MedIQ Learning, LLC makes this available under .

348 **Hypothyroidism vs hyperthyroidism: Image C.** Periorbital myxedema. This image is a derivative work, adapted from the following source, available under : Dandekar F, Camacho M, Valerio J, et al. *Case Rep Ophthalmol Med.* 2015;2015:126501. DOI: 10.1155/2015/126501.

349 **Hypothyroidism: Image B.** Hashimoto thyroiditis histology. This image is a derivative work, adapted from the following source, available under : Librepath. This image may have been modified by cropping, labeling, and/or captions. MedIQ Learning, LLC makes this available under .

349 **Hypothyroidism: Image C.** Subacute granulomatous thyroiditis histology. This image is a derivative work, adapted from the following source, available under : Dr. Michael Bonert. This image may have been modified by cropping, labeling, and/or captions. MedIQ Learning, LLC makes this available under .

349 **Hypothyroidism: Image E.** Before and after treatment of congenital hypothyroidism. Courtesy of the Department of Health and Human Services.

349 **Hypothyroidism: Image F.** Congenital hypothyroidism. This image is a derivative work, adapted from the following source, available under : Sadasiv Swain. The image may have been modified by cropping, labeling, and/or captions. All rights to this adaptation by MedIQ Learning, LLC are reserved.

350 **Thyroid adenoma.** This image is a derivative work, adapted from the following source, available under : Terada T. Brain metastasis from thyroid adenomatous nodules or an encapsulated thyroid follicular tumor without capsular and vascular invasion: a case report. *Cases J.* 2009; 2: 7180. DOI: 10.4076/1757-1626-2-7180.

352 **Hypoparathyroidism.** Shortened 4th and 5th digits. This image is a derivative work, adapted from the following source, available under : Ferrario C, Gastaldi G, Portmann L, et al. Bariatric surgery in an obese patient with Albright hereditary osteodystrophy: a case report. *J Med Case Rep.* 2013; 7: 111. DOI: 10.1186/1752-1947-7-111.

353 **Hyperparathyroidism.** Multiple lytic lesions. This image is a derivative work, adapted from the following source, available under : Khaoula BA, Kaouther BA, Ines C, et al. An unusual presentation of primary hyperparathyroidism: pathological fracture. *Case Rep Orthop.* 2011;2011:521578. DOI: 10.1155/2011/521578. The image may have been modified by cropping, labeling, and/or captions. All rights to this adaptation by MedIQ Learning, LLC are reserved.

357 **Adrenal insufficiency.** Mucosal hyperpigmentation in primary adrenal insufficiency. Courtesy of FlatOut. The image may have been modified by cropping, labeling, and/or captions. All rights to this adaptation by MedIQ Learning, LLC are reserved.

359 **Pheochromocytoma.** This image is a derivative work, adapted from the following source, available under : Dr. Michael Feldman.

360 **Multiple endocrine neoplasias.** Mucosal neuroma. This image is a derivative work, adapted from the following source, available under : Martucciello G, Lerone M, Bricco L, et al. Multiple endocrine neoplasias type 2B and RET proto-oncogene. *Ital J Pediatr.* 2012;38:9. DOI: 10.1186/1824-7288-38-9.

361 **Carcinoid syndrome.** Courtesy of the Department of Health and Human Services and the Armed Forces Institute of Pathology.

Gastrointestinal

368 **Ventral wall defects: Image A.** Gastroschisis. This image is a derivative work, adapted from the following source, available under : Zvizdic Z. Gastroschisis with concomitant jejuno-ileal atresia complicated by jejunal perforation. *J Neonatal Surg.* 2016 Apr-Jun; 5(2): 25.

368 **Ventral wall defects: Image B.** Omphalocele. This image is a derivative work, adapted from the following source, available under : Khan YA, Qureshi MA, Akhtar J. Omphalomesenteric duct cyst

in an omphalocele: a rare association. *Pak J Med Sci.* 2013 May-Jun; 29(3): 866–868.

368 **Ventral wall defects.** Drawings of gastroschisis (left) and omphalocele (right). Courtesy of the Department of Health and Human Services.

368 **Ventral wall defects: Image C.** Congenital diaphragmatic hernia. This image is a derivative work, adapted from the following source, available under : Rastogi MV, LaFranchi SH. Congenital hypothyroidism. *Orphanet J Rare Dis.* 2010;5:17. DOI: 10.1186/1750-1172-5-17.

369 **Intestinal atresia.** This image is a derivative work, adapted from the following source, available under : Saha M. Alimentary tract atresias associated with anorectal malformations: 10 years' experience. *J Neonatal Surg.* 2016 Oct-Dec; 5(4): 43. DOI: 10.21699/jns.v5i4.449.

369 **Hypertrophic pyloric stenosis.** This image is a derivative work, adapted from the following source, available under : Hassan RAA, Choo YU, Noraida R, et al. Infantile hypertrophic pyloric stenosis in postoperative esophageal atresia with tracheoesophageal fistula. *J Neonatal Surg.* 2015 Jul-Sep;4(3):32.

370 **Pancreas and spleen embryology.** Annular pancreas. This image is a derivative work, adapted from the following source, available under : Mahdi B, Selim S, Hassen T, et al. A rare cause of proximal intestinal obstruction in adults—annular pancreas: a case report. *Pan Afr Med J.* 2011;10:56. The image may have been modified by cropping, labeling, and/or captions. All rights to this adaptation by MedIQ Learning, LLC are reserved.

370 **Retroperitoneal structures.** This image is a derivative work, adapted from the following source, available under : Sammut J, Ahiaku E, Williams DT. Complete regression of renal tumour following ligation of an accessory renal artery during repair of an abdominal aortic aneurysm. *Ann R Coll Surg Engl.* 2012 Sep; 94(6): e198–e200. DOI: 10.1308/003588412X13373405384972.

372 **Digestive tract anatomy.** Histology of stomach wall. This image is a derivative work, adapted from the following source, available under : Alexander Klepnev.

372 **Digestive tract histology: Image A.** Gastric glands Courtesy of Dr. Michale Bonert.

372 **Digestive tract histology: Image B.** Parietal cells and chief cells. This image is a derivative work, adapted from the following source, available under : Ziołkowska N, Lewczuk B, Petrynski P, et al. Light and electron microscopy of the European Beaver (*Castor fiber*) stomach reveal unique morphological features with possible general biological significance. *PLoS One.* 2014;9(4):e94590. DOI: 10.1371/journal.pone.0094590. This image may have been modified by cropping, labeling, and/or captions. MedIQ Learning, LLC makes this available under .

372 **Digestive tract histology: Image C.** Jejunum histology. This image is a derivative work, adapted from the following source, available under : Dr. Ed Uthman. This image may have been modified by cropping, labeling, and/or captions. MedIQ Learning, LLC makes this available under .

372 **Digestive tract histology: Image D.** Ileum histology and Peyer patches. This image is a derivative work, adapted from the following source, available under : CoRus13. This image may have been modified by cropping, labeling, and/or captions. MedIQ Learning, LLC makes this available under .

372 **Digestive tract histology: Image E.** Colon histology. This image is a derivative work, adapted from the following source, available under : Athikhun.suw. This image may have been modified by cropping, labeling, and/or captions. MedIQ Learning, LLC makes this available under .

377 **Liver tissue architecture: Image A.** Portal triad. This image is a derivative work, adapted from the following source, available under : Liver development. In: Zorn AM. Stem book. Cambridge: Harvard Stem Cell Institute, 2008.

377 **Liver tissue architecture: Image B.** Kupffer cells. This image is a derivative work, adapted from the following source, available under : Dr. Michael Bonert. The image may have been modified by cropping, labeling, and/or captions. MedIQ Learning, LLC makes this available under .

378 **Biliary structures.** Gallstones. This image is a derivative work, adapted from the following source, available under : J. Guntau. The image may have been modified by cropping, labeling, and/or captions. MedIQ Learning, LLC makes this available under .

380 **Hernias: Image A.** Congenital diaphragmatic hernia. This image is a derivative work, adapted from the following source, available under : Tovar J. Congenital diaphragmatic hernia. *Orphanet J Rare Dis.* 2012;7:1. DOI: 10.1186/1750-1172-7-1.

382 **Gastrointestinal secretory products.** Histology of gastric pit. This image is a derivative work, adapted from the following source, available under : Dr. Michael Bonert. The image may have been modified by cropping, labeling, and/or captions. MedIQ Learning, LLC makes this available under .

384 **Peyer patches.** This image is a derivative work, adapted from the following source, available under : Plainpaper. The image may have been modified by cropping, labeling, and/or captions. MedIQ Learning, LLC makes this available under .

386 **Sialolithiasis.** This image is a derivative work, adapted from the following source, available under : Pastor-Ramos V, Cuervo-Diaz A, Aracil-Kessler L. Sialolithiasis. Proposal for a new minimally invasive procedure: piezoelectric surgery. *J Clin Exp Dent.* 2014 Jul;6(3):e295–e298. DOI: 10.4317/jced.51253.

386 **Salivary gland tumors.** Pleomorphic adenoma histology. This image is a derivative work, adapted from the following source, available under : Wikimedia Commons. The image may have been modified by cropping, labeling, and/or captions. MedIQ Learning, LLC makes this available under .

386 **Achalasia.** This image is a derivative work, adapted from the following source, available under : Farnoosh Farrokhi and Michael F. Vaezi. The image may have been modified by cropping, labeling, and/or captions. All rights to this adaptation by MedIQ Learning, LLC are reserved.

387 **Esophageal pathologies: Image A.** White pseudomembrane of *Candida* infection in esophagitis. This image is a derivative work, adapted from the following source, available under : Takahashi Y, Nagata N, Shimbo T. Long-term trends in esophageal candidiasis prevalence and associated risk factors with or without HIV infection: lessons from an endoscopic study of 80,219 patients. *PLoS One.* 2015; 10(7): e0133589. DOI: 10.1371/journal.pone.0133589.

387 **Esophageal pathologies: Image B.** Esophageal varices on endoscopy. This image is a derivative work, adapted from the following source, available under : Costaguta A, Alvarez F. Etiology and management of hemorrhagic complications of portal hypertension in children. *Int J Hepatol.* 2012;2012:879163. DOI: 10.1155/2012/879163.

387 **Esophageal pathologies: Image C.** Esophageal varices on CT. This image is a derivative work, adapted from the following source, available under : Dr. Paul Hellerhoff. The image may have been modified by cropping, labeling, and/or captions. MedIQ Learning, LLC makes this available under .

387 **Esophageal pathologies: Image D.** Pneumomediastinum. This image is a derivative work, adapted from the following source, available under : Wikimedia Commons. The image may have been modified by cropping, labeling, and/or captions. MedIQ Learning, LLC makes this available under .

388 **Barrett esophagus: Image A.** Endoscopy image. This image is a derivative work, adapted from the following source, available under

: Japan Esophageal Society. Japanese classification of esophageal cancer, 11th edition: part I. *Esophagus.* 2017;14(1):1–36. DOI: 10.1007/s10388-016-0551-7.

388 **Barrett esophagus: Image B.** Goblet cells. This image is a derivative work, adapted from the following source, available under : Dr. Michael Bonert. The image may have been modified by cropping, labeling, and/or captions. MedIQ Learning, LLC makes this available under .

389 **Ménétrier disease.** This image is a derivative work, adapted from the following source, available under : Dr. Paul Hellerhoff. The image may have been modified by cropping, labeling, and/or captions. MedIQ Learning, LLC makes this available under .

389 **Gastric cancer.** This image is a derivative work, adapted from the following source, available under : Tan Y, Fu J, Li X. A minor (<50%) signet-ring cell component associated with poor prognosis in colorectal cancer patients: a 26-year retrospective study in China. *PLoS One.* 2015; 10(3): e0121944. DOI: 10.1371/journal.pone.0121944.

390 **Ulcer complications.** Free air under diaphragm in perforated ulcer. Reproduced, with permission, from Dr. Frank Gaillard and www.radiopaedia.org.

391 **Malabsorption syndromes: Image A.** Celiac disease. This image is a derivative work, adapted from the following source, available under : Celiac disease. Sedda S, Caruso R, Marafini I, et al. Pyoderma gangrenosum in refractory celiac disease: a case report. *BMC Gastroenterol.* 2013; 13: 162. DOI: 10.1186/1471-230X-13-162.

391 **Malabsorption syndromes: Image B.** *Tropheryma whippeli* on PAS stain. This image is a derivative work, adapted from the following source, available under : Tran HA. Reversible hypothyroidism and Whipple's disease. *BMC Endocr Disord.* 2006;6:3. DOI: 10.1186/1472-6823-6-3.

392 **Inflammatory bowel diseases: Image A.** "String sign" on barium swallow in Crohn disease. This image is a derivative work, adapted from the following source, available under : Al-Mofarreh MA, Al Mofleh IA, Al-Teimi IN, et al. Crohn's disease in a Saudi outpatient population: is it still rare? *Saudi J Gastroenterol.* 2009;15:111-116. DOI: 10.4103/1319-3767.45357. The image may have been modified by cropping, labeling, and/or captions. All rights to this adaptation by MedIQ Learning, LLC are reserved.

392 **Inflammatory bowel diseases: Images B and C.** Normal mucosa (B) and punched-out ulcers (C) in ulcerative colitis. These images are a derivative work, adapted from the following source, available under : Ishikawa D, Ando T, Watanabe O, et al. Images of colonic real-time tissue sonoelastography correlate with those of colonoscopy and may predict response to therapy in patients with ulcerative colitis. *BMC Gastroenterol.* 2011;11:29. DOI: 10.1186/1471-230X-11-29.

393 **Appendicitis.** Fecalith on CT. This image is a derivative work, adapted from the following source, available under : Dr. James Heilman. The image may have been modified by cropping, labeling, and/or captions. MedIQ Learning, LLC makes this available under .

393 **Diverticula of the gastrointestinal tract: Image B.** Diverticulosis. This image is a derivative work, adapted from the following source, available under : Sartelli M, Moore FA, Ansaloni L, et al. A proposal for a CT driven classification of left colon acute diverticulitis. *World J Emerg Surg.* 2015;10:3. DOI: 10.1186/1749-7922-10-3.

393 **Diverticula of the gastrointestinal tract: Image C.** Diverticulitis. This image is a derivative work, adapted from the following source, available under : Hupfeld L, Burcharth J, Pommergaard HC, Rosenberg J. The best choice of treatment for acute colonic diverticulitis with purulent peritonitis is uncertain. *Biomed Res Int.* 2014; 2014: 380607. DOI: 10.1155/2014/380607.

394 **Zenker diverticulum.** This image is a derivative work, adapted from the following source, available under : Courtesy of Bernd Brägelmann.

395 **Maltotation.** This image is a derivative work, adapted from the following source, available under : Mathews R, Thenabadu S, Jaiganesh T. Abdominal pain with a twist. *Int J Emerg Med.* 2011;4:21. DOI: 10.1186/1865-1380-4-21.

395 **Intussusception: Image A.** Interoperative image of intussusception. This image is a derivative work, adapted from the following source, available under : Vasiliadis K, Kogopoulos E, Katsamakas M, et al. Ileoileal intussusception induced by a gastrointestinal stromal tumor. *World J Surg Oncol.* 2008;6:133. DOI: 10.1186/1477-7819-6-133.

395 **Intussusception: Image B.** Ultrasound showing target sign. This image is a derivative work, adapted from the following source, available under : Abbo O, Pinnagoda K, Micol LA. Osteosarcoma metastasis causing ileo-ileal intussusception. *World J Surg Oncol.* 2013 Aug 12;11(1):188. DOI: 10.1186/1477-7819-11-188.

396 **Volvulus.** Coffee bean sign. This image is a derivative work, adapted from the following source, available under : Yigit M, Turkdogan KA. Coffee bean sign, whirl sign and bird's beak sign in the diagnosis of sigmoid volvulus. *Pan Afr Med J.* 1014;19:56. DOI: 10.11604/pamj.2014.19.56.5142.

396 **Other intestinal disorders: Image A.** Necrosis due to occlusion of SMA. This image is a derivative work, adapted from the following source, available under : Van De Winkel N, Cheragwandi A, Nieboer K, et al. Superior mesenteric arterial branch occlusion causing partial jejunal ischemia: a case report. *J Med Case Rep.* 2012;6:48. DOI: 10.1186/1752-1947-6-48.

396 **Other intestinal disorders: Image B.** Loops of dilated bowel suggestive of small bowel obstruction. This image is a derivative work, adapted from the following source, available under : Welte FJ, Crosso M. Left-sided appendicitis in a patient with congenital gastrointestinal malrotation: a case report. *J Med Case Rep.* 2007;1:92. DOI: 10.1186/1752-1947-1-92.

396 **Other intestinal disorders: Image C.** Endoscopy showing dilated vessels in colonic ischemia. This image is a derivative work, adapted from the following source, available under : Gunjan D, Sharma V, Rana SS, et al. Small bowel bleeding: a comprehensive review. *Gastroenterol Rep.* 2014 Nov;2(4):262-75. DOI: 10.1093/gastro/gou025.

396 **Other intestinal disorders: Image D.** Pneumatosis intestinalis. This image is a derivative work, adapted from the following source, available under : Pelizzo G, Nakib G, Goruppi I, et al. Isolated colon ischemia with norovirus infection in preterm babies: a case series. *J Med Case Rep.* 2013;7:108. DOI: 10.1186/1752-1947-7-108.

397 **Colonic polyps: Image A.** This image is a derivative work, adapted from the following source, available under : M. Emannuel.

397 **Colonic polyps: Image B.** Adenomatous polyps in tubular adenoma. This image is a derivative work, adapted from the following source, available under : Shussman N, Wexner SD. Colorectal polyps and polyposis syndromes. *Gastroenterol Rep (Oxf).* 2014 Feb;2(1):1-15. DOI: 10.1093/gastro/got041.

397 **Colonic polyps: Image C.** Adenomatous polyps in villous adenoma. This image is a derivative work, adapted from the following source, available under : Rehani B, Chasen RM, Dowdy Y, et al. Advanced adenoma diagnosis with FDG PET in a visibly normal mucosa: a case report. *J Med Case Reports.* 2007; 1: 99. DOI: 10.1186/1752-1947-1-99.

398 **Colorectal cancer: Image A.** Polyp. This image is a derivative work, adapted from the following source, available under : Takiyama A, Nozawa H, Ishihara S, et al. Secondary metastasis in the lymph node of the bowel invaded by colon cancer: a report of three cases. *World J Surg Oncol.* 2016; 14: 273. DOI: 10.1186/s12957-016-1026-y.

399 **Cirrhosis and portal hypertension.** Hepatocellular carcinoma. This image is a derivative work, adapted from the following source, available under : Blackburn PR, Hickey RD, Nace RA, et al. Silent tyrosinemia type I without elevated tyrosine or succinylacetone associated with liver cirrhosis and hepatocellular carcinoma. *Hum Mutat.* 2016 Oct; 37(10): 1097–1105.DOI: 10.1002/humu.23047.

401 Alcoholic liver disease: Image B. Mallory bodies. This image is a derivative work, adapted from the following source, available under: Dr. Michael Bonert. The image may have been modified by cropping, labeling, and/or captions. MedIQ Learning, LLC makes this available under.

401 Alcoholic liver disease: Image C. Sclerosis in alcoholic cirrhosis. This image is a derivative work, adapted from the following source, available under: Dr. Michael Bonert. The image may have been modified by cropping, labeling, and/or captions. MedIQ Learning, LLC makes this available under.

401 Nonalcoholic fatty liver disease. This image is a derivative work, adapted from the following source, available under: El-Karaksy HM, El-Koofy NM, Anwar GM, et al. Predictors of non-alcoholic fatty liver disease in obese and overweight Egyptian children: single center study. *Saudi J Gastroenterol.* 2011;17:40-46. DOI: 10.4103/1319-3767.74476.

402 Liver tumors: Image A. Cavernous liver hemangioma. This image is a derivative work, adapted from the following source, available under: Dr. Michael Bonert. This image may have been modified by cropping, labeling, and/or captions. MedIQ Learning, LLC makes this available under.

402 Liver tumors: Image B. Hepatocellular carcinoma/hepatoma. Reproduced, with permission, from Jean-Christophe Fournet and Humpath.

403 α_1-antitrypsin deficiency. Liver histology. This image is a derivative work, adapted from the following source, available under: Dr. Jerad M. Gardner. The image may have been modified by cropping, labeling, and/or captions. MedIQ Learning, LLC makes this available under.

403 Jaundice. Yellow sclera. Courtesy of the Department of Health and Human Services and Dr. Thomas F. Sellers.

405 Wilson disease. Kayser-Fleischer rings. This image is a derivative work, adapted from the following source, available under: Kodama H, Fujisawa C, Bhadhprasit W. Inherited copper transport disorders: biochemical mechanisms, diagnosis, and treatment. *Curr Drug Metab.* 2012 Mar; 13(3): 237–250. DOI: 10.2174/138920012799320455.

405 Hemochromatosis. Hemosiderin deposits. This image is a derivative work, adapted from the following source, available under: Mathew J, Leong MY, Morley N, et al. A liver fibrosis cocktail? Psoriasis, methotrexate and genetic hemochromatosis. *BMC Dermatol.* 2005;5:12. DOI: 10.1186/1471-5945-5-12.

406 Cholelithiasis and related pathologies: Image A. Gross specimen of gallstones. This image is a derivative work, adapted from the following source, available under: Courtesy of M. Emmanuel.

406 Cholelithiasis and related pathologies: Image B. Large gallstone. This image is a derivative work, adapted from the following source, available under: Spangler R, Van Pham T, Khoujah D, et al. Abdominal emergencies in the geriatric patient. *Int J Emerg Med.* 2014; 7: 43. DOI: 10.1186/s12245-014-0043-2.

407 Cholelithiasis and related pathologies: Image C. Porcelain gallbladder. This image is a derivative work, adapted from the following source, available under: Fred H, van Dijk H. Images of memorable cases: case 19. Connexions Web site. December 4, 2008. Available at: http://cnx.org/content/m14939/1.3/. The image may have been modified by cropping, labeling, and/or captions. All rights to this adaptation by MedIQ Learning, LLC are reserved.

407 Acute pancreatitis: Image A. Acute exudative pancreatitis. This image is a derivative work, adapted from the following source, available under: Dr. Paul Hellerhoff. The image may have been modified by cropping, labeling, and/or captions. MedIQ Learning, LLC makes this available under.

407 Acute pancreatitis: Image B. Pancreatic pseudocyst. This image is a derivative work, adapted from the following source, available under: Thomas Zimmerman. The image may have been modified by cropping, labeling, and/or captions. MedIQ Learning, LLC makes this available under.

407 Chronic pancreatitis. This image is a derivative work, adapted from the following source, available under: Dr. Paul Hellerhoff. The image may have been modified by cropping, labeling, and/or captions. MedIQ Learning, LLC makes this available under.

408 Pancreatic adenocarcinoma: Image A. Histology. This image is a derivative work, adapted from the following source, available under: KGH. The image may have been modified by cropping, labeling, and/or captions. MedIQ Learning, LLC makes this available under.

408 Pancreatic adenocarcinoma: Image B. CT scan. Courtesy of MBq. The image may have been modified by cropping, labeling, and/or captions. All rights to this adaptation by MedIQ Learning, LLC are reserved.

Hematology and Oncology

416 Neutrophils: Image A. Courtesy of B. Lennert.

416 Neutrophils: Image B. Dohle bodies. This image is a derivative work, adapted from the following source, available under: isis325.

417 Erythrocytes. Courtesy of the Department of Health and Human Services and Drs. Noguchi, Rodgers, and Schechter.

417 Thrombocytes (platelets). This image is a derivative work, adapted from the following source, available under: Dr. Ed Uthman. The image may have been modified by cropping, labeling, and/or captions. MedIQ Learning, LLC makes this available under.

417 Monocytes. This image is a derivative work, adapted from the following source, available under: Dr. Graham Beards. The image may have been modified by cropping, labeling, and/or captions. MedIQ Learning, LLC makes this available under.

417 Macrophages. This image is a derivative work, adapted from the following source, available under: De Tommasi AS, Otranto D, Furlanello T, et al. Evaluation of blood and bone marrow in selected canine vector-borne diseases. *Parasit Vectors.* 2014;7:534. DOI: 10.1186/s13071-014-0534-2.

418 Eosinophils. This image is a derivative work, adapted from the following source, available under: Dr. Ed Uthman.

418 Basophils. This image is a derivative work, adapted from the following source, available under: Dr. Erhabor Osaro. The image may have been modified by cropping, labeling, and/or captions. MedIQ Learning, LLC makes this available under.

418 Mast cells. Courtesy of Wikimedia Commons.

418 Dendritic cells. This image is a derivative work, adapted from the following source, available under: Cheng J-H, Lee S-Y, Lien Y-Y, et al. Immunomodulating activity of *Nymphaea rubra* roxb. extracts: activation of rat dendritic cells and improvement of the TH1 immune response. *Int J Mol Sci.* 2012;13:10722-10735. DOI: 10.3390/ijms130910722.

419 Lymphocytes. This image is a derivative work, adapted from the following source, available under: Fickleandfreckled.

419 Plasma cells. Courtesy of the Department of Health and Human Services and Dr. Francis W. Chandler. The image may have been modified by cropping, labeling, and/or captions. All rights to this adaptation by MedIQ Learning, LLC are reserved.

425 RBC morphology. Sickle cell. Courtesy of the Department of Health and Human Services and the Sickle Cell Foundation of Georgia, Jackie George, and Beverly Sinclair.

426 RBC inclusions. Ringed sideroblast. This image is a derivative work, adapted from the following source, available under: Paulo

Henrique Orlandi Mourao. The image may have been modified by cropping, labeling, and/or captions. MedIQ Learning, LLC makes this available under .

426 **RBC inclusions.** Howell-Jolly bodies. This image is a derivative work, adapted from the following source, available under : Serio B, Pezzullo L, Giudice V, et al. OPSI threat in hematological patients. *Transl Med UniSa.* 2013 May-Aug;6:2-10.

426 **RBC inclusions.** Basophilic stippling. This image is a derivative work, adapted from the following source, available under : Prof. Erhabor Osaro. This image may have been modified by cropping, labeling, and/or captions. MedIQ Learning, LLC makes this available under .

426 **RBC inclusions.** Pappenheimer bodies. This image is a derivative work, adapted from the following source, available under : Paulo Henrique Orlandi Mourao. The image may have been modified by cropping, labeling, and/or captions. MedIQ Learning, LLC makes this available under .

429 **Microcytic, hypochromic anemias: Image A.** This image is a derivative work, adapted from the following source, available under : Bock F, Borucki K, Vorwerk P, et al. A two-and-a-half-year-old breastfed toddler presenting with anemia: a case report. *BMC Res Notes.* 2014; 7: 917. DOI: 10.1186/1756-0500-7-917.

429 **Microcytic, hypochromic anemia: Image D.** Lead lines in lead poisoning. Reproduced, with permission, from Dr. Frank Gaillard and www.radiopaedia.org.

429 **Microcytic, hypochromic anemia: Image E.** Sideroblastic anemia. This image is a derivative work, adapted from the following source, available under : Paulo Henrique Orlandi Moura. The image may have been modified by cropping, labeling, and/or captions. MedIQ Learning, LLC makes this available under .

430 **Macrocytic anemias.** Megaloblastic anemia. This image is a derivative work, adapted from the following source, available under : Courtesy of Dr. Ed Uthman.

432 **Intrinsic hemolytic anemias.** This image is a derivative work, adapted from the following source, available under : El Ariss AB, Younes M, Matar J. Prevalence of sickle cell trait in the southern suburb of Beirut, Lebanon. *Mediterr J Hematol Infect Dis.* 2016; 8(1): e2016015. DOI: 10.4084/MJHID.2016.015.

434 **Heme synthesis, porphyrias, and lead poisoning: Image A.** Basophilic stippling in lead poisoning. This image is a derivative work, adapted from the following source, available under : van Dijk HA, Fred HL. Images of memorable cases: case 81. Connexions Web site. December 3, 2008. Available at http://cnx.org/contents/3196bf3e-1e1e-4c4d-a1ac-d4fc9ab65443@4@4.

434 **Heme synthesis, porphyrias, and lead poisoning: Image B.** Porphyria cutanea tarda. This image is a derivative work, adapted from the following source, available under : Bovenschen HJ, Vissers WHPM. Primary hemochromatosis presented by porphyria cutanea tarda: a case report. *Cases J.* 2009;2:7246. DOI: 10.4076/1757-1626-2-7246.

435 **Coagulation disorders.** Hemarthrosis. This image is a derivative work, adapted from the following source, available under : Lakjiri S, Mernissi FZ. Tabetic arthropathy revealing neurosyphilis: a new observation. *Pan Afr Med J.* 2014; 18: 198. DOI: 10.11604/pamj.2014.18.198.4893.

438 **Hodgkin lymphoma.** Reed-Sternberg cells. This image is a derivative work, adapted from the following source, available under : Knecht H, Righolt C, Mai S. Genomic instability: the driving force behind refractory/relapsing Hodgkin's lymphoma. *Cancers (Basel).* 2013 Jun; 5(2): 714–725. DOI: 10.3390/cancers5020714.

439 **Non-Hodgkin lymphoma: Image B.** Jaw lesion in Burkitt lymphoma. This image is a derivative work, adapted from the following source, available under : Bi CF, Tang Y, Zhang WY, et al. Sporadic Burkitt lymphomas of children and adolescents in Chinese: a clinicopathological study of 43 cases. *Diagn Pathol.* 2012;7:72. DOI:10.1186/1746-1596-7-72.

439 **Non-Hodgkin lymphoma: Image C.** Primary CNS lymphoma. This image is a derivative work, adapted from the following source, available under : Mansour A, Qandeel M, Abdel-Razeq H, et al. MR imaging features of intracranial primary CNS lymphoma in immune competent patients. *Cancer Imaging.* 2014;14(1):22. DOI: 10.1186/1470-7330-14-22.

439 **Non-Hodgkin lymphoma: Image D.** Mycosis fungoides/Sézary syndrome. This image is a derivative work, adapted from the following source, available under : Chaudhary S, Bansal C, Ranga U, et al. Erythrodermic mycosis fungoides with hypereosinophilic syndrome: a rare presentation. *Ecancermedicalscience.* 2013;7:337. DOI:10.3332/ecancer.2013.337

440 **Plasma cell dyscrasias: Image C.** This image is a derivative work, adapted from the following source, available under : Mehrotra R, Singh M, Singh PA, et al. Should fine needle aspiration biopsy be the first pathological investigation in the diagnosis of a bone lesion? An algorithmic approach with review of literature. *Cytojournal.* 2007; 4: 9. DOI: 10.1186/1742-6413-4-9.

441 **Myelodysplastic syndromes.** Neutrophil with bilobed nuclei. This image is a derivative work, adapted from the following source, available under : Lukaszewska J, Allison RW, Stepkowska J. Congenital Pelger-Huët anomaly in a Danish/Swedish farmdog: case report. *Acta Vet Scand.* 2011; 53(1): 14. DOI: 10.1186/1751-0147-53-14.

442 **Leukemias: Image A.** This image is a derivative work, adapted from the following source, available under : Chiaretti S, Zini G, Bassan R. Diagnosis and subclassification of acute lymphoblastic leukemia. *Mediterr J Hematol Infect Dis.* 2014; 6(1): e2014073. DOI: 10.4084/MJHID.2014.073.

442 **Leukemias: Image C.** Hairy cell leukemia. This image is a derivative work, adapted from the following source, available under : Chan SM, George T, Cherry AM, et al. Complete remission of primary plasma cell leukemia with bortezomib, doxorubicin, and dexamethasone: a case report. *Cases J.* 2009;2:121. DOI: 10.1186/1757-1626-2-121.

443 **Myeloproliferative neoplasms: Image A.** Erythromelalgia in polycythemia vera. This image is a derivative work, adapted from the following source, available under : Fred H, van Dijk H. Images of memorable cases: case 151. Connexions Web site. December 4, 2008. Available at http://cnx.org/content/m14932/1.3/.

443 **Myeloproliferative neoplasms: Image C.** Myelofibrosis. This image is a derivative work, adapted from the following source, available under : Courtesy of Dr. Ed Uthman.

444 **Langerhans cell histiocytosis: Image A.** Lytic bone lesion. This image is a derivative work, adapted from the following source, available under : Dehkordi NR, Rajabi P, Naimi A, et al. Langerhans cell histiocytosis following Hodgkin lymphoma: a case report from Iran. *J Res Med Sci.* 2010;15:58-61. PMCID PMC3082786.

444 **Langerhans cell histiocytosis: Image B.** Birbeck granules. This image is a derivative work, adapted from the following source, available under : Dr. Yale Rosen. The image may have been modified by cropping, labeling, and/or captions. MedIQ Learning, LLC makes this available under .

445 **Hemophagocytic lymphohistiocytosis.** This image is a derivative work, adapted from the following source, available under : Kashif M, Tariq H, Ijaz M. Disseminated histoplasmosis and secondary hemophagocytic syndrome in a non-HIV patient. *Case Rep Crit Care.* 2015; 2015: 295735. DOI: 10.1155/2015/295735.

446 **Warfarin.** This image is a derivative work, adapted from the following source, available under : Bakoyiannis C, Karaolanis G, Patelis N. Dabigatran in the treatment of warfarin-induced skin necrosis: A new hope. *Case Rep Dermatol Med.* 2016; 2016: 3121469. DOI: 10.1155/2016/3121469.

Musculoskeletal, Skin, and Connective Tissue

456 **Rotator cuff muscles.** Glenohumeral instability. This image is a derivative work, adapted from the following source, available under : Koike Y, Sano H, Imamura I, et al. Changes with time in skin temperature of the shoulders in healthy controls and a patient with shoulder-hand syndrome. *Ups J Med Sci* 2010;115:260-265. DOI: 10.3109/03009734.2010.503354. The image may have been modified by cropping, labeling, and/or captions. All rights to this adaptation by MedIQ Learning, LLC are reserved.

458 **Brachial plexus lesions: Image A.** Cervical rib. This image is a derivative work, adapted from the following source, available under : Dahlin LB, Backman C, Duppe H, et al. Compression of the lower trunk of the brachial plexus by a cervical rib in two adolescent girls: case reports and surgical treatment. *J Brachial Plex Peripher Nerve Inj*. 2009;4:14. DOI: 10.1186/1749-7221-4-14.

458 **Brachial plexus lesions: Image B.** Winged scapula. This image is a derivative work, adapted from the following source, available under : Boukhris J, Boussouga M, Jaafar A, et al. Stabilisation dynamique d'un winging scapula (à propos d'un cas avec revue de la littérature). *Pan Afr Med J*. 2014; 19: 331. DOI: 10.11604/pamj.2014.19.331.3429.

459 **Wrist region: Image B.** Anatomic snuff box. This image is a derivative work, adapted from the following source, available under : Rhemrev SJ, Ootes D, Beeres FJP, et al. Current methods ofdiagnosis and treatment of scaphoid fractures. *Int J Emerg Med*. 2011;4:4. DOI: 10.1186/1865-1380-4-4.

466 **Motoneuron action potential to muscle contraction.** Two muscle sarcomeres in parallel. This image is a derivative work, adapted from the following source, available under : Ottenheijm CAC, Heunks LMA, Dekhuijzen RPN. Diaphragm adaptations in patients with COPD. *Respir Res*. 2008; 9(1): 12. DOI: 10.1186/1465-9921-9-12.

470 **Clavicle fractures.** X-ray of clavicle fracture. This image is a derivative work, adapted from the following source, available under : Paladini P, Pellegrini A, Merolla G, et al. Treatment of clavicle fractures. *Transl Med UniSa*. 2012 Jan-Apr;2:47–58.

470 **Wrist and hand injuries: Image A.** Thenar eminence atrophy in carpal tunnel syndrome. Courtesy of Dr. Harry Gouvas.

470 **Wrist and hand injuries: Image B.** Metacarpal neck fracture. This image is a derivative work, adapted from the following source, available under : Bohr S, Pallua N. Early functional treatment and modern cast making for indications in hand surgery. *Adv Orthop*. 2016; 2016: 5726979. DOI: 10.1155/2016/5726979.

471 **Common knee conditions: Image A.** ACL tear. This image is a derivative work, adapted from the following source, available under : Chang MJ, Chang CB, Choi J-Y, et al. Can magnetic resonance imaging findings predict the degree of knee joint laxity in patients undergoing anterior cruciate ligament reconstruction? *BMC Musculoskelet Disord*. 2014;15:214. DOI: 10.1186/1471-2474-15-214. The image may have been modified by cropping, labeling, and/or captions. All rights to this adaptation by MedIQ Learning, LLC are reserved.

471 **Common knee conditions: Images B and C.** Prepatellar bursitis (B) and Baker cyst (C). These images are a derivative work, adapted from the following source, available under : Hirji Z, Hunhun JS, Choudur HN. Imaging of the bursae. *J Clin Imaging Sci*. 2011;1:22. DOI: 10.4103/2156-7514.80374. The images may have been modified by cropping, labeling, and/or captions. All rights to this adaptation by MedIQ Learning, LLC are reserved.

474 **Common pediatric fractures: Image A.** Greenstick fracture. This image is a derivative work, adapted from the following source, available under : Randsborg PH, Sivertsen EA. Classification of distal radius fractures in children: good inter- and intraobserver reliability, which improves with clinical experience. *BMC Musculoskelet Disord*. 2013;13:6. DOI: 10.1186/1471-2474-13-6.

474 **Common pediatric fractures: Image B.** Torus (buckle) fracture. This image is a derivative work, adapted from the following source, available under : Aksel Seyahi, et al. Tibial torus and toddler's fractures misdiagnosed as transient synovitis: a case series. *J Med Case Reports*. 2011; 5: 305. DOI: 10.1186/1752-1947-5-305.

474 **Osteoporosis.** Vertebral compression fractures of spine. This image is a derivative work, adapted from the following source, available under : Imani F, Gharaei H, Rahimzadeh P, et al. Management of painful vertebral compression fracture with kyphoplasty in a sever cardio-respiratory compromised patient. *Anesth Pain Med*. 2012 summer;2(1):42–45. DOI: 10.5812/aapm.5030.

475 **Osteopetrosis.** This image is a derivative work, adapted from the following source, available under : Kant P, Sharda N, Bhowate RR. Clinical and radiological findings of autosomal dominant osteopetrosis type II: a case report. *Case Rep Dent*. 2013;2013:707343. DOI: 10.1155/2013/707343.

475 **Osteomalacia/rickets: Image A.** Clinical photo and x-ray of leg deformity in rickets. This image is a derivative work, adapted from the following source, available under : Linglart A, Biosse-Duplan M, Briot K, et al. Therapeutic management of hypophosphatemic rickets from infancy to adulthood. *Endocr Connect*. 2014;3:R13-R30. DOI: 10.1530/EC-13-0103.

475 **Osteomalacia/rickets: Image B.** Rachitic rosary on chest x-ray. This image is a derivative work, adapted from the following source, available under : Ayadi ID, Hamida EB, Rebeh RB, et al. Perinatal lethal type II osteogenesis imperfecta: a case report. *Pan Afr Med J*. 2015;21:11. DOI: 10.11604/pamj.2015.21.11.6834.

475 **Osteitis deformans.** Thickened calvarium. This image is a derivative work, adapted from the following source, available under : Dawes L. Paget's disease. [Radiology Picture of the Day Website]. Published June 21, 2007. Available at http://www.radpod.org/2007/06/21/pagets-disease/.

475 **Avascular necrosis of bone.** Bilateral necrosis of femoral head. This image is a derivative work, adapted from the following source, available under : Ding H, Chen S-B, Lin S, et al. The effect of postoperative corticosteroid administration on free vascularized fibular grafting for treating osteonecrosis of the femoral head. *Sci World J*. 2013;708014. DOI: 10.1155/2013/708014. The image may have been modified by cropping, labeling, and/or captions. All rights to this adaptation by MedIQ Learning, LLC are reserved.

477 **Primary bone tumors: Image A.** Osteochondroma. This image is a derivative work, adapted from the following source, available under : Lucien Monfils. The image may have been modified by cropping, labeling, and/or captions. MedIQ Learning, LLC makes this available under .

477 **Primary bone tumors: Image B.** Osteoid osteoma. This image is a derivative work, adapted from the following source, available under : Jankharia B, Burute N. Percutaneous radiofrequency ablation for osteoid osteoma: how we do it. *Indian J Radiol Imaging*. 2009 Feb; 19(1): 36–42. DOI: 10.4103/0971-3026.44523.

477 **Primary bone tumors: Image C.** Giant cell tumor. Reproduced, with permission, from Dr. Frank Gaillard and www.radiopaedia.org.

477 **Primary bone tumors: Image D.** Codman triangle in osteosarcoma. This image is a derivative work, adapted from the following source, available under : Xu SF, Yu XC, Zu M, et al. Limb function and quality of life after various reconstruction methods according to tumor location following resection of osteosarcoma in distal femur. *BMC Musculoskelet Disord*. 2014; 15: 453. DOI: 10.1186/1471-2474-15-453.

477 **Primary bone tumors: Image E.** Starburst pattern in osteosarcoma. This image is a derivative work, adapted from the following source, available under : Ding H, Yu G, Tu Q, et al. Computer-aided resection and endoprosthesis design for the management of malignant bone tumors around the knee: outcomes of 12 cases. *BMC Musculoskelet Disord*. 2013; 14: 331. DOI: 10.1186/1471-2474-14-331.

478 **Osteoarthritis vs rheumatoid arthritis: Image A.** Osteoarthritis. This image is a derivative work, adapted from the following source, available under : Visser J, Busch VJJF, de Kievit-van der Heijden IM, et al. Non-Hodgkin's lymphoma of the synovium discovered in total knee arthroplasty: a case report. *BMC Res Notes.* 2012;5:449. DOI: 10.1186/1756-0500-5-449.

478 **Osteoarthritis vs rheumatoid arthritis: Image B.** Rheumatoid arthritis. This image is a derivative work, adapted from the following source, available under : Clement ND, Breusch SJ, Biant LC. Lower limb joint replacement in rheumatoid arthritis. *J Orthop Surg Res.* 2012; 7: 27. DOI: 10.1186/1749-799X-7-27.

478 **Osteoarthritis vs rheumatoid arthritis: Image C.** Histology of rheumatoid nodule. This image is a derivative work, adapted from the following source, available under : Gomez-Rivera F, El-Naggar AK, Guha-Thakurta N, et al. Rheumatoid arthritis mimicking metastatic squamous cell carcinoma. *Head Neck Oncol.* 2011;3:26. DOI: 10.1186/1758-3284-3-26.

479 **Gout: Image B.** Uric acid crystals under polarized light. This image is a derivative work, adapted from the following source, available under : Robert J. Galindo. The image may have been modified by cropping, labeling, and/or captions. MedIQ Learning, LLC makes this available under .

479 **Gout: Image C.** Podagra. This image is a derivative work, adapted from the following source, available under : Roddy E. Revisiting the pathogenesis of podagra: why does gout target the foot? *J Foot Ankle Res.* 2011;4:13. DOI: 10.1186/1757-1146-4-13.

479 **Calcium pyrophosphate deposition disease.** Calcium phosphate crystals. This image is a derivative work, adapted from the following source, available under : Dieppe P, Swan A. Identification of crystals in synovial fluid. *Ann Rheum Dis.* 1999 May;58(5):261–263.

480 **Sjögren syndrome: Image A.** Lymphocytic infiltration. Courtesy of the Department of Health and Human Services.

480 **Sjögren syndrome: Image B.** Dry tongue. This image is a derivative work, adapted from the following source, available under : Negrato CA, Tarzia O. Buccal alterations in diabetes mellitus. *Diabetol Metab Syndr.* 2010;2:3. DOI: 10.1186/1758-5996-2-3.

480 **Septic arthritis.** Joint effusion. This image is a derivative work, adapted from the following source, available under : Dr. James Heilman. The image may have been modified by cropping, labeling, and/or captions. MedIQ Learning, LLC makes this available under .

481 **Seronegative spondyloarthropathies: Image C, left.** Bamboo spine. This image is a derivative work, adapted from the following source, available under : Stevenfruitsmaak. The image may have been modified by cropping, labeling, and/or captions. MedIQ Learning, LLC makes this available under .

481 **Seronegative spondyloarthropathies: Image C, right.** Bamboo spine. Courtesy of Heather Hawker.

483 **Polymyositis/dermatomyositis: Image A.** Groton papules of dermatomyositis. This image is a derivative work, adapted from the following source, available under : *Pan Afr Med J.*2015; 21: 89. DOI: 10.11604/pamj.2015.21.89.6971.

485 **Vasculitides: Image A.** Temporal arteritis histology. This image is a derivative work, adapted from the following source, available under : Marvin. The image may have been modified by cropping, labeling, and/or captions. MedIQ Learning, LLC makes this available under .

485 **Vasculitides: Image B.** Angiogram in patient with Takayasu arteritis. Courtesy of the Department of Health and Human Services and Justin Ly.

485 **Vasculitides: Image C.** Gangrene as a consequence of Buerger disease. This image is a derivative work, adapted from the following source, available under : Afsjarfard A, Mozaffar M, Malekpour F, et al. The wound healing effects of iloprost in patients with Buerger's disease: claudication and prevention of major amputations. *Iran Red Crescent Med J.* 2011;13:420-423.

485 **Vasculitides: Image D.** Strawberry tongue in patient with Kawasaki disease. This image is a derivative work, adapted from the following source, available under : Courtesy of Natr.

485 **Vasculitides: Image E.** Coronary artery aneurysm in Kawasaki disease. This image is a derivative work, adapted from the following source, available under : Wikimedia Commons. The image may have been modified by cropping, labeling, and/or captions. All rights to this adaptation by MedIQ Learning, LLC are reserved.

485 **Vasculitides: Image F.** Polyarteritis nodosa. Reproduced, with permission, from Dr. Frank Gaillard and www.radiopaedia.org.

485 **Vasculitides: Image G.** Churg-Strauss syndrome histology. This image is a derivative work, adapted from the following source, available under : Dr. Michael Bonert. The image may have been modified by cropping, labeling, and/or captions. MedIQ Learning, LLC makes this available under .

485 **Vasculitides: Image H.** Granulomatosis with polyangiitis (formerly Wegener) and PR3-ANCA/c-ANCA. Courtesy of M.A. Little.

485 **Vasculitides: Image I.** Henoch-Schönlein purpura. Courtesy of Okwikikim.

485 **Vasculitides: Image J.** MPO-ANCA/p-ANCA in microscopic polyangiitis. Courtesy of and M.A. Little.

486 **Raynaud phenomenon.** This image is a derivative work, adapted from the following source, available under : Jamclaassen. The image may have been modified by cropping, labeling, and/or captions. MedIQ Learning, LLC makes this available under .

488 **Epithelial cell junctions: Image A.** Intracellular membrane. This image is a derivative work, adapted from the following source, available under : Tang VW. Proteomic and bioinformatic analysis of epithelial tight junction reveals an unexpected cluster of synaptic molecules. *Biol Direct.* 2006; 1: 37. DOI: 10.1186/1745-6150-1-37.

488 **Epithelial cell junctions: Image B.** Large, electron-dense actin structures within adherens junction. This image is a derivative work, adapted from the following source, available under : Taylor RR, Jagger DJ, Saeed SR, et al. Characterizing human vestibular sensory epithelia for experimental studies: new hair bundles on old tissue and implications for therapeutic interventions in ageing. *Neurobiol Aging.* 2015 Jun;36(6):2068–2084. DOI: 10.1016/j.neurobiolaging.2015.02.013.

488 **Epithelial cell junctions: Image C.** Desmosome. This image is a derivative work, adapted from the following source, available under : Massa F, Devader C, Lacas-Gervais S, et al. Impairement of HT29 cancer cells cohesion by the soluble form of neurotensin receptor-3. *Genes Cancer.* 2014 Jul; 5(7-8):240–249. DOI: 10.18632/genesandcancer.22.

488 **Epithelial cell junctions: Image D.** Gap junction. This image is a derivative work, adapted from the following source, available under : Shu X, Lev-Ram V, Deerinck TJ. A Genetically encoded tag for correlated light and electron microscopy of intact cells, tissues, and organisms. *PLoS Biol.* 2011 Apr; 9(4): e1001041. DOI: 10.1371/journal.pbio.1001041.

488 **Epithelial cell junctions: Image E.** Hemidesmosome. This image is a derivative work, adapted from the following source, available under : Nguyen NM, Pulkkinen L, Schlueter JA, et al. Lung development in laminin gamma2 deficiency: abnormal tracheal hemidesmosomes with normal branching morphogenesis and epithelial differentiation. *Respir Res.* 2006 Feb 16;7:28. DOI: 10.1186/1465-9921-7-28.

490 **Seborrheic dermatitis.** This image is a derivative work, adapted from the following source, available under : Roymishali.

491 **Common skin disorders: Image O.** Urticaria. This image is a derivative work, adapted from the following source, available

under : Dr. James Heilman. The image may have been modified by cropping, labeling, and/or captions. MedIQ Learning, LLC makes this available under .

492 Vascular tumors of skin: Image C. Glomus tumor under fingernail. This image is a derivative work, adapted from the following source, available under : Hazani R, Houle JM, Kasdan ML, et al. Glomus tumors of the hand. *Eplasty*. 2008;8:e48. The image may have been modified by cropping, labeling, and/or captions. All rights to this adaptation by MedIQ Learning, LLC are reserved.

493 Skin infections: Image C. Erysipelas. This image is a derivative work, adapted from the following source, available under : Courtesy of Klaus D. Peter.

494 Autoimmune blistering skin disorders: Image D. Bullous pemphigoid on immunofluorescence. This image is a derivative work, adapted from the following source, available under : Courtesy of M. Emmanuel.

495 Lower extremity ulcers: Image A. Venous ulcer. This image is a derivative work, adapted from the following source, available under : Motolese A, Vignati F, Brambilla R, et al. Interaction between a regenerative matrix and wound bed in nonhealing ulcers: results with 16 cases. *Biomed Res Int*. 2013;849321. DOI: 10.1155/2013/849321.

495 Lower extremity ulcers: Image B. Arterial ulcer. This image is a derivative work, adapted from the following source, available under : Metcalf DG, Bowler PG. Biofilm delays wound healing: a review of the evidence. *Burns Trauma*. 2013;1(1):5–12. DOI: 10.4103/2321-3868.113329.

495 Lower extremity ulcers: Image C. Neuropathic ulcer. This image is a derivative work, adapted from the following source, available under : Moretti B, Notarnicola A. Maggio G, et al. The management of neuropathic ulcers of the foot in diabetes by shock wave therapy. *BMC Musculoskelet Disord*. 2009;10:54. DOI: 10.1186/1471-2474-10-54.

498 Skin cancer: Image D. Basal cell palisading nuclei. This image is a derivative work, adapted from the following source, available under : Yuri T. Jadotte, MD, et al. Superficial spreading basal cell carcinoma of the face: a surgical challenge. *Eplasty*. 2010; 10: e46. Published online 2010 Jun 21.

Neurology and Special Senses

505 Holoprosencephaly. This image is a derivative work, adapted from the following source, available under : Alorainy IA, Barlas NB, Al-Boukai AA. Pictorial essay: infants of diabetic mothers. *Indian J Radiol Imaging*. 2010 Aug;20(3):174-81. DOI: 10.4103/0971-3026.69349.

505 Lissencephaly. This image is a derivative work, adapted from the following source, available under : Tian G, Cristancho AG, Dubbs HA, et al. A patient with lissencephaly, developmental delay, and infantile spasms, due to de novo heterozygous mutation of *KIF2A*. *Mol Genet Genomic Med*. 2016 Nov;4(6):599–603. DOI: 10.1002/mgg3.236.

506 Posterior fossa malformations: Image A. Chiari I malformation. This image is a derivative work, adapted from the following source, available under : Toldo I, De Carlo D, Mardari R, et al. Short lasting activity-related headaches with sudden onset in children: a case-based reasoning on classification and diagnosis. *J Headache Pain*. 2013;14(1):3. DOI: 10.1186/1129-2377-14-3.

506 Posterior fossa malformations: Image B. Dandy-Walker malformation. This image is a derivative work, adapted from the following source, available under : Krupa K, Bekiesinska-Figatowska M. Congenital and acquired abnormalities of the corpus callosum: a pictorial essay. *Biomed Res Int*. 2013;2013:265619. DOI: 10.1155/2013/265619.

506 Syringomyelia. Reproduced, with permission, from Dr. Frank Gaillard and www.radiopaedia.org.

508 Myelin. Myelinated neuron. Courtesy of the Electron Microscopy Facility at Trinity College.

510 Chromatolysis. This image is a derivative work, adapted from the following source, available under : Dr. Michael Bonert. The image may have been modified by cropping, labeling, and/or captions. MedIQ Learning, LLC makes this available under .

514 Limbic system. This image is a derivative work, adapted from the following source, available under : Schopf V, Fischmeister FP, Windischberger C, et al. Effects of individual glucose levels on the neuronal correlates of emotions. *Front Hum Neurosci*. 2013 May 21;7:212. DOI: 10.3389/fnhum.2013.00212.

515 Cerebellum. This image is a derivative work, adapted from the following source, available under : Jarius S, Wandinger KP, Horn S, et al. A new Purkinje cell antibody (anti-Ca) associated with subacute cerebellar ataxia: immunological characterization. *J Neuroinflammation*. 2010;7: 21. DOI: 10.1186/1742-2094-7-21.

516 Basal ganglia. This image is a derivative work, adapted from the following source, available under : Rudger P, Jaunmuktane Z, Adlard P, et al. Iatrogenic CJD due to pituitary-derived growth hormone with genetically determined incubation times of up to 40 years. *Brain*. 2015 Nov; 138(11): 3386–3399. DOI: 10.1093/brain/awv235.

518 Cerebral arteries—cortical distribution. Cortical watershed areas. This image is a derivative work, adapted from the following source, available under : Isabel C, Lecler A, Turc G, et al. Relationship between watershed infarcts and recent intra plaque haemorrhage in carotid atherosclerotic plaque. *PLoS One*. 2014;9(10):e108712. DOI: 10.1371/journal.pone.0108712.

519 Dural venous sinuses. This image is a derivative work, adapted from the following source, available under : Cikla U, Aagaard-Kienitz B, Turski PA, et al. Familial perimesencephalic subarachnoid hemorrhage: two case reports. *J Med Case Rep*. 2014;8. DOI: 10.1186/1752-1947-8-380. The image may have been modified by cropping, labeling, and/or captions. All rights to this adaptation by MedIQ Learning, LLC are reserved.

525 Spinal cord and associated tracts. Spinal cord cross-section. This image is a derivative work, adapted from the following source, available under : Regents of University of Michigan Medical School.

530 Neonatal intraventricular hemorrhage. This image is a derivative work, adapted from the following source, available under : Shooman D, Portess H, Sparrow O. A review of the current treatment methods for posthaemorrhagic hydrocephalus of infants. *Cerebrospinal Fluid Res*. 2009;6:1. DOI: 10.1186/1743-8454-6-1.

531 Intracranial hemorrhage: Images A and B. Axial CT of brain showing epidural blood. These images are a derivative work, adapted from the following source, available under : Dr. Paul Hellerhoff. The image may have been modified by cropping, labeling, and/or captions. MedIQ Learning, LLC makes this available under .

531 Intracranial hemorrhage: Image C. Subdural hematoma. This image is a derivative work, adapted from the following source, available under : Dr. James Heilman. The image may have been modified by cropping, labeling, and/or captions. MedIQ Learning, LLC makes this available under .

531 Intracranial hemorrhage: Image E. Subarachnoid hemorrhage. This image is a derivative work, adapted from the following source, available under : Hakan T, Turk CC, Celik H. Intra-operative real time intracranial subarachnoid haemorrhage during glial tumour resection: a case report. *Cases J*. 2008;1:306. DOI: 10.1186/1757-1626-1-306. The image may have been modified by cropping, labeling, and/or captions. All rights to this adaptation by MedIQ Learning, LLC are reserved.

533 Effects of strokes: Image A. Large abnormality of the left middle cerebral artery territory. This image is a derivative work, adapted from the following source, available under : Hakimelahi R, Yoo AJ, He

J, et al. Rapid identification of a major diffusion/perfusion mismatch in distal internal carotid artery or middle cerebral artery ischemic stroke. *BMC Neurol.* 2012 Nov 5;12:132. DOI: 10.1186/1471-2377-12-132. The image may have been modified by cropping, labeling, and/or captions. All rights to this adaptation by MedIQ Learning, LLC are reserved.

533 **Effects of strokes: Image B.** Lacunar infarct of lenticulostriate artery. This image is a derivative work, adapted from the following source, available under: Zhou L, Ni J, Yao M, et al. High-resolution MRI findings in patients with capsular warning syndrome. *BMC Neurol.* 2014;14:16. DOI: 10.1186/1471-2377-14-16.

533 **Effects of strokes: Image C.** Infarction of posterior cerebellar artery. This image is a derivative work, adapted from the following source, available under: Nouh A, Remke J, Ruland S. Ischemic posterior circulation stroke: a review of anatomy, clinical presentations, diagnosis, and current management. *Front Neurol.* 2014 Apr 7;5:30. DOI: 10.3389/fneur.2014.00030.

533 **Effects of strokes: Image D.** Infarction of posterior inferior cerebellar artery. This image is a derivative work, adapted from the following source, available under: Mittal P, Kalia V, Dua S. Pictorial essay: Susceptibility-weighted imaging in cerebral ischemia. *Indian J Radiol Imaging.* 2010 Nov; 20(4): 250–253. DOI: 10.4103/0971-3026.73530.

533 **Diffuse axonal injury.** This image is a derivative work, adapted from the following source, available under: Moenninghoff C, Kraff O, Maderwald S, et al. Diffuse axonal injury at ultra-high field MRI. *PLoS One.* 2015;10(3):e0122329. DOI: 10.1371/journal.pone.0122329.

534 **Aneurysms.** Saccular aneurysm. This image is a derivative work, adapted from the following source, available under: Kayhan A, Koc O, Keskin S. The role of bone subtraction computed tomographic angiography in determining intracranial aneurysms in non-traumatic subarachnoid hemorrhage. *Iran J Radiol.* 2014 May; 11(2): e12670. DOI: 10.5812/iranjradiol.12670.

539 **Neurodegenerative disorders: Image A.** Lewy body in substantia nigra. This image is a derivative work, adapted from the following source, available under: Werner CJ, Heyny-von Haussen R, Mall G, et al. Parkinson's disease. *Proteome Sci.* 2008;6:8. DOI: 10.1186/1477-5956-6-8. The image may have been modified by cropping, labeling, and/or captions. All rights to this adaptation by MedIQ Learning, LLC are reserved.

539 **Neurodegenerative disorders: Image B.** Gross specimen of normal brain. This image is a derivative work, adapted from the following source, available under: Niedowicz DM, Nelson PT, Murphy MP. Alzheimer's disease: pathological mechanisms and recent insights. *Curr Neuropharmacol.* 2011 Dec;9(4):674-84. DOI: 10.2174/157015911798376181.

539 **Neurodegenerative disorders: Images C and F.** Brain atrophy in Alzheimer disease (C) and frontotemporal dementia (F). These images are a derivative work, adapted from the following source, available under: Niedowicz DM, Nelson PT, Murphy MP. Alzheimer's disease: pathological mechanisms and recent insights. *Curr Neuropharmacol.* 2011 Dec;9(4):674-84. DOI: 10.2174/157015911798376181.

539 **Neurodegenerative disorders: Image G.** Frontotemporal dementia: Pick bodies in frontotemporal demendia (Pick disease). This image is a derivative work, adapted from the following source, available under: Neumann M. Molecular neuropathology of TDP-43 proteinopathies. *Int J Mol Sci.* 2009 Jan; 10(1): 232–246. DOI: 10.3390/ijms10010232.

539 **Neurodegenerative disorders: Image H.** Spongiform changes in brain in Creutzfeld-Jacob disease. This image is a derivative work, adapted from the following source, available under: DRdoubleB. The image may have been modified by cropping, labeling, and/or captions. MedIQ Learning, LLC makes this available under.

540 **Hydrocephalus: Image B.** Communicating hydrocephalus. This image is a derivative work, adapted from the following source, available under: Torres-Martin M, Pena-Granero C, Carceller F, et al. Homozygous deletion of *TNFRSF4*, *TP73*, *PPAP2B* and *DPYD* at 1p and *PDCD5* at 19q identified by multiplex ligation-dependent probe amplification (MLPA) analysis in pediatric anaplastic glioma with questionable oligodendroglial component. *Mol Cytogenet.* 2014;7:1. DOI: 10.1186/1755-8166-7-1.

540 **Hydrocephalus: Image C.** Ex vacuo ventriculomegaly. This image is a derivative work, adapted from the following source, available under: Ghetti B, Oblak AL, Boeve BF, et al. Frontotemporal dementia caused by microtubule-associated protein tau gene (*MAPT*) mutations: a chameleon for neuropathology and neuroimaging. Neurophathol Appl Neurobiol. 2015 Feb;41(1):24-46. DOI: 10.1111/nan.12213.

541 **Multiple sclerosis.** Periventricular plaques. This image is a derivative work, adapted from the following source, available under: Dooley MC, Foroozan R. Optic neuritis. *J Ophthalmic Vis Res.* 2010 Jul;5(3):182–187.

542 **Other demyelinated and dysmyelinating disorders: Image A.** Central pontine myelinolysis. This image is a derivative work, adapted from the following source, available under: Wikimedia Commons. The image may have been modified by cropping, labeling, and/or captions. MedIQ Learning, LLC makes this available under.

542 **Other demyelinating and dysmyelinating disorders: Image B.** Progressive multifocal leukoencephalopathy. This image is a derivative work, adapted from the following source, available under: Garrote H, de la Fuente A, Ona R, et al. Long-term survival in a patient with progressive multifocal leukoencephalopathy after therapy with rituximab, fludarabine and cyclophosphamide for chronic lymphocytic leukemia. *Exp Hematol Oncol.* 2015;4:8. DOI: 10.1186/s40164-015-0003-4.

543 **Neurocutaneous disorders: Image A.** Sturge-Weber syndrome and port wine stain. This image is a derivative work, adapted from the following source, available under: Babaji P, Bansal A, Krishna G, et al. Sturge-Weber syndrome with osteohypertrophy of maxilla. *Case Rep Pediatr.* 2013. DOI: 10.1155/2013/964596.

543 **Neurocutaneous disorders: Image B.** Leptomeningeal angioma in Sturge-Weber syndrome. Reproduced, with permission, from Dr. Frank Gaillard and www.radiopaedia.org.

543 **Neurocutaneous disorders: Image C.** Tuberous sclerosis. This image is a derivative work, adapted from the following source, available under: Fred H, van Dijk H. Images of memorable cases: case 143. Connexions Web site. December 4, 2008. Available at: http://cnx.org/content/m14923/1.3/.

543 **Neurocutaneous disorders: Image D.** Ash leaf spots in tuberous sclerosis. This image is a derivative work, adapted from the following source, available under: Tonekaboni SH, Tousi P, Ebrahimi A, et al. Clinical and para clinical manifestations of tuberous sclerosis: a cross sectional study on 81 pediatric patients. *Iran J Child Neurol.* 2012;6:25-31. PMCID PMC3943027.

543 **Neurocutaneous disorders: Image E.** Angiomyolipoma in tuberous sclerosis. This image is a derivative work, adapted from the following source, available under: KGH. The image may have been modified by cropping, labeling, and/or captions. MedIQ Learning, LLC makes this available under.

543 **Neurocutaneous disorders: Image F.** Café-au-lait spots in neurofibromatosis. This image is a derivative work, adapted from the following source, available under: Wikimedia Commons. The image may have been modified by cropping, labeling, and/or captions. MedIQ Learning, LLC makes this available under.

543 **Neurocutaneous disorders: Image H.** Cutaneous neurofibromas. This image is a derivative work, adapted from the following source, available under: Kim BK, Choi YS, Gwoo S, et al. Neurofibromatosis type 1 associated with papillary thyroid carcinoma

incidentally detected by thyroid ultrasonography: a case report. *J Med Case Rep*. 2012;6:179. DOI: 10.1186/1752-1947-6-179.

543 **Neurocutaneous disorders: Image I.** Cerebellar hemangioblastoma histology. This image is a derivative work, adapted from the following source, available under : Dr. Michael Bonert. The image may have been modified by cropping, labeling, and/or captions. MedIQ Learning, LLC makes this available under .

543 **Neurocutaneous disorders: Image J.** Brainstem and spinal cord hemangioblastomas in von Hippel-Lindau disease. This image is a derivative work, adapted from the following source, available under : Park DM, Zhuang Z, Chen L, et al. von Hippel-Lindau disease-associated hemangioblastomas are derived from embryologic multipotent cells. *PLoS Med.* 2007 Feb;4(2):e60. DOI: 10.1371/journal.pmed.0040060.

544 **Adult primary brain tumors: Image A.** Butterfly glioma. This image is a derivative work, adapted from the following source, available under : Rossmeisl JH, Clapp K, Pancotto TE. Canine butterfly glioblastomas: A neuroradiological review. *Front Vet Sci.* 2016; 3: 40. DOI: 10.3389/fvets.2016.00040.

544 **Adult primary brain tumors: Image B.** Glioblastoma multiforme histology. This image is a derivative work, adapted from the following source, available under : Wikimedia Commons. The image may have been modified by cropping, labeling, and/or captions. MedIQ Learning, LLC makes this available under .

544 **Adult primary brain tumors: Image C.** Oligodendroglioma in frontal lobes. This image is a derivative work, adapted from the following source, available under : Celzo FG, Venstermans C, De Belder F, et al. Brain stones revisited—between a rock and a hard place. *Insights Imaging.* 2013 Oct;4(5):625-35. DOI: 10.1007/s13244-013-0279-z.

544 **Adult primary brain tumors: Image D.** Oligodendroglioma, "fried egg" cells. This image is a derivative work, adapted from the following source, available under : Dr. Michael Bonert. The image may have been modified by cropping, labeling, and/or captions. MedIQ Learning, LLC makes this available under .

544 **Adult primary brain tumors: Image E.** Meningioma with dural tail. This image is a derivative work, adapted from the following source, available under : Smits A, Zetterling M, Lundin M, et al. Neurological impairment linked with cortico-subcortical infiltration of diffuse low-grade gliomas at initial diagnosis supports early brain plasticity. *Front Neurol.* 2015;6:137. DOI: 10.3389/fneur.2015.00137.

544 **Adult primary brain tumors: Image F.** Meningioma, psammoma bodies. This image is a derivative work, adapted from the following source, available under : Dr. Michael Bonert. The image may have been modified by cropping, labeling, and/or captions. MedIQ Learning, LLC makes this available under .

544 **Adult primary brain tumors: Image G.** Cerebellar hemangioblastoma. This image is a derivative work, adapted from the following source, available under : Park DM, Zhengping Z, Chen L, et al. von Hippel-Lindau disease-associated hemangioblastomas are derived from embryologic multipotent cells. *PLoS Med.* 2007 Feb;4(2):e60. DOI: 10.1371/journal.pmed.0040060.

544 **Adult primary brain tumors: Image H.** Minimal parenchyma in hemangioblastoma. This image is a derivative work, adapted from the following source, available under : Marvin 101. The image may have been modified by cropping, labeling, and/or captions. MedIQ Learning, LLC makes this available under .

545 **Adult primary brain tumors: Image I.** Field of vision in bitemporal hemianopia. This image is a derivative work, adapted from the following source, available under : Wikimedia Commons. The image may have been modified by cropping, labeling, and/or captions. MedIQ Learning, LLC makes this available under .

545 **Adult primary brain tumors: Image J.** Prolactinoma. This image is a derivative work, adapted from the following source, available under : Wang CS, Yeh TC, Wu TC, et al. Pituitary macroadenoma co-existent with supraclinoid internal carotid artery cerebral aneurysm: a case report and review of the literature. *Cases J.* 2009;2:6459. DOI: 10.4076/1757-1626-2-6459.

545 **Adult primary brain tumors: Image K.** Schwannoma at cerebellopontine angle. Courtesy of MRT-Bild.

545 **Adult primary brain tumors: Image L.** Schwannoma. This image is a derivative work, adapted from the following source, available under : Shah AA, Latoo S, Ahmad I, et al. Schwannoma causing resorption of zygomatic arch. *J Oral Maxillofac Pathol.* 2011;15(1):80–84. DOI: 10.4103/0973-029X.80020.

546 **Childhood primary brain tumors: Image A.** MRI of pilocytic astrocytoma. This image is a derivative work, adapted from the following source, available under : Hafez RFA. Stereotaxic gamma knife surgery in treatment of critically located pilocytic astrocytoma: preliminary result. *World J Surg Oncol.* 2007;5:39. doi 10.1186/1477-7819-5-39.

546 **Childhood primary brain tumors: Image C.** CT of medulloblastoma. Courtesy of the Department of Health and Human Services and the Armed Forces Institute of Pathology.

546 **Childhood primary brain tumors: Image D.** Medulloblastoma histology. This image is a derivative work, adapted from the following source, available under : KGH. The image may have been modified by cropping, labeling, and/or captions. MedIQ Learning, LLC makes this available under .

546 **Childhood primary brain tumors: Image E.** MRI of ependymoma. This image is a derivative work, adapted from the following source, available under : Dr. Paul Hellerhoff. The image may have been modified by cropping, labeling, and/or captions. MedIQ Learning, LLC makes this available under .

546 **Childhood primary brain tumors: Image F.** Ependymoma histology. This image is a derivative work, adapted from the following source, available under : Dr. Michael Bonert. The image may have been modified by cropping, labeling, and/or captions. MedIQ Learning, LLC makes this available under .

546 **Childhood primary brain tumors: Image G.** CT of craniopharyngioma. This image is a derivative work, adapted from the following source, available under : Garnet MR, Puget S, Grill J, et al. Craniopharyngioma. *Orphanet J Rare Dis.* 2007;2:18. DOI: 10.1186/1750-1172-2-18.

546 **Childhood primary brain tumors: Image H.** Craniopharyngioma histology. This image is a derivative work, adapted from the following source, available under : Dr. Michael Bonert. The image may have been modified by cropping, labeling, and/or captions. MedIQ Learning, LLC makes this available under .

549 **Friedreich ataxia.** Clinical kyphoscoliosis. This image is a derivative work, adapted from the following source, available under : Axelrod FB, Gold-von Simson. Hereditary sensory and autonomic neuropathies: types II, III, and IV. *Orphanet J Rare Dis.* 2007;2:39. DOI: 10.1186/1750-1172-2-39.

550 **Facial nerve lesions.** Facial nerve palsy. This image is a derivative work, adapted from the following source, available under : Socolovsky M, Paez MD, Di Masi G, et al. Bell's palsy and partial hypoglossal to facial nerve transfer: Case presentation and literature review. *Surg Neurol Int.* 2012;3:46. DOI: 10.4103/2152-7806.95391.

552 **Cholesteatoma.** This image is a derivative work, adapted from the following source, available under : Welleschik. The image may have been modified by cropping, labeling, and/or captions. MedIQ Learning, LLC makes this available under .

553 **Normal eye anatomy.** This image is a derivative work, adapted from the following source, available under : Jan Kaláb. The image may have been modified by cropping, labeling, and/or captions. MedIQ Learning, LLC makes this available under .

553 **Conjunctivitis.** This image is a derivative work, adapted from the following source, available under : Baiyeroju A, Bowman R,

Gilbert C, et al. Managing eye health in young children. *Community Eye Health*. 2010;23:4-11.

554 **Cataract.** Juvenile cataract. This image is a derivative work, adapted from the following source, available under : Roshan M, Vijaya PH, Lavanya GR, et al. A novel human CRYGD mutation in a juvenile autosomal dominant cataract. *Mol Vis*. 2010;16:887-896. PMCID PMC2875257.

555 **Glaucoma: Image C.** Closed/narrow angle glaucoma. This image is a derivative work, adapted from the following source, available under : Low S, Davidson AE, Holder GE, et al. Autosomal dominant Best disease with an unusual electrooculographic light rise and risk of angle-closure glaucoma: a clinical and molecular genetic study. *Mol Vis*. 2011;17:2272-2282. PMCID PMC3171497. The image may have been modified by cropping, labeling, and/or captions. All rights to this adaptation by MedIQ Learning, LLC are reserved.

555 **Glaucoma: Image D.** Acute angle closure glaucoma. This image is a derivative work, adapted from the following source, available under :. Courtesy of Dr. Jonathan Trobe.

555 **Uveitis.** This image is a derivative work, adapted from the following source, available under : Weber AC, Levison AL, Srivastava, et al. A case of *Listeria monocytogenes* endophthalmitis with recurrent inflammation and novel management. *J Ophthalmic Inflamm Infect*. 2015;5(1):28. DOI: 10.1186/s12348-015-0058-8.

556 **Age-related macular degeneration.** Courtesy of the Department of Health and Human Services.

556 **Diabetic retinopathy.** This image is a derivative work, adapted from the following source, available under : Sundling V, Gulbrandsen P, Straand J. Sensitivity and specificity of Norwegian optometrists' evaluation of diabetic retinopathy in single-field retinal images – a cross-sectional experimental study. *BMC Health Services Res*. 2013;13:17. DOI: 10.1186/1472-6963-13-17.

556 **Hypertensive retinopathy.** This image is a derivative work, adapted from the following source, available under : Diallo JW, Méda N, Tougouma SJB, et al. Intérêts de l'examen du fond d'œil en pratique de ville: bilan de 438 cas. *Pan Afr Med J*. 2015;20:363. DOI: 10.11604/pamj.2015.20.363.6629.

556 **Retinal vein occlusion.** This image is a derivative work, adapted from the following source, available under : Alasil T, Rauser ME. Intravitreal bevacizumab in the treatment of neovascular glaucoma secondary to central retinal vein occlusion: a case report. *Cases J*. 2009;2:176. DOI: 10.1186/1757-1626-2-176. The image may have been modified by cropping, labeling, and/or captions. All rights to this adaptation by MedIQ Learning, LLC are reserved.

557 **Retinal detachment.** Courtesy of EyeRounds.

557 **Retinitis pigmentosa.** Courtesy of EyeRounds.

557 **Leukocoria.** This image is a derivative work, adapted from the following source, available under : Aerts I, Lumbroso-Le Rouic L, Gauthier-Villars M, et al. Retinoblastoma. *Orphanet J Rare Dis*. 2006 Aug 25;1:31. DOI: 10.1186/1750-1172-1-31.

560 **Ocular motility.** Blowout fracture of orbit with entrapment of superior rectus muscle. This image is a derivative work, adapted from the following source, available under : Gonzalez MO, Durairaj VD. Indirect orbital floor fractures: a meta-analysis. *Middle East Afr J Ophthalmol*. 2010;17(2):138–141. DOI: 10.4103/0974-9233.63076.

561 **CN III, IV, VI palsies: Image A.** Cranial nerve III damage. This image is a derivative work, adapted from the following source, available under : Hakim W, Sherman R, Rezk T, et al. An acute case of herpes zoster ophthalmicus with ophthalmoplegia. *Case Rep Ophthalmol Med*. 1012; 2012:953910. DOI: 10.1155/2012/953910.

561 **CN III, IV, VI palsies: Image B.** Cranial nerve IV damage. This image is a derivative work, adapted from the following source, available under : Mendez JA, Arias CR, Sanchez D, et al. Painful ophthalmoplegia of the left eye in a 19-year-old female, with an emphasis in Tolosa-Hunt syndrome: a case report. *Cases J*. 2009; 2: 8271. DOI: 10.4076/1757-1626-2-8271.

561 **CN III, IV, VI palsies: Image C.** Cranial nerve VI damage. This image is a derivative work, adapted from the following source, available under : Jordi March i Nogué. The image may have been modified by cropping, labeling, and/or captions. MedIQ Learning, LLC makes this available under .

Psychiatry

586 **Trichotillomania.** Courtesy of Robodoc.

Renal

602 **Potter sequence.** Courtesy of the Department of Health and Human Services and the Armed Forces Institute of Pathology.

603 **Horseshoe kidney.** This image is a derivative work, adapted from the following source, available under : Rispoli P, Destefanis P, Garneri P, et al. Inferior vena cava prosthetic replacement in a patient with horseshoe kidney and metastatic testicular tumor: technical considerations and review of the literature. *BMC Urol*. 2014;14:40. DOI: 10.1186/1471-2490-14-40.

604 **Kidney anatomy and glomerular structure.** This image is a derivative work, adapted from the following source, available under : Ramidi GA, Kurukumbi MK, Sealy PL. Collapsing glomerulopathy in sickle cell disease: a case report. *J Med Case Reports*. 2011; 5: 71. DOI: 10.1186/1752-1947-5-71.

605 **Course of ureters.** This image is a derivative work, adapted from the following source, available under : Wikimedia Commons. The image may have been modified by cropping, labeling, and/or captions. MedIQ Learning, LLC makes this available under .

605 **Glomerular filtration barrier.** This image is a derivative work, adapted from the following source, available under : Feng J, Wei H, Sun Y, et al. Regulation of podocalyxin expression in the kidney of streptozotocin-induced diabetic rats with Chinese herbs (Yishen capsule). *BMC Complement Altern Med*. 2013;13:76. DOI: 10.1186/1472-6882-13-76.

618 **Casts in urine: Image B.** WBC casts. This image is a derivative work, adapted from the following source, available under : Perazella MA. Diagnosing drug-induced AIN in the hospitalized patient: a challenge for the clinician. *Clin Nephrol*. 2014 Jun; 81(6): 381-8. DOI: 10.5414/CN108301.

618 **Casts in urine: Image D.** Fatty casts. This image is a derivative work, adapted from the following source, available under : Li S, Wang ZJ, Chang TT. Temperature oscillation modulated self-assembly of periodic concentric layered magnesium carbonate microparticles. *PLoS One*. 2014;9(2):e88648. DOI:10.1371/journal.pone.0088648

620 **Nephritic syndrome: Image A.** Histology of acute poststreptococcal glomerulonephritis. This image is a derivative work, adapted from the following source, available under : Dr. Michael Bonert. The image may have been modified by cropping, labeling, and/or captions. MedIQ Learning, LLC makes this available under .

620 **Nephritic syndrome: Image B.** Immunofluorescence of acute poststreptococcal glomerulonephritis. This image is a derivative work, adapted from the following source, available under : Immunofluorescence of acute poststreptococcal glomerulonephritis. Oda T, Yoshizawa N, Yamakami K, et al. The role of nephritis-associated plasmin receptor (naplr) in glomerulonephritis associated with streptococcal infection. *Biomed Biotechnol*. 2012;2012:417675. DOI 10.1155/2012/417675.

620 **Nephritic syndrome: Image C.** Histology of rapidly progressive glomerulonephritis. Courtesy of the Department of Health and Human Services and Uniformed Services University of the Health Sciences.

620 **Nephritic syndrome: Image D.** "Tram tracks" in membranoproliverative glomerulonephritis. This image is a derivative work, adapted from the following source, available under : Kiremitci S, Ensari A. Classifying lupus nephritis: an ongoing story. *Scientific World Journal.* 2014; 2014: 580620. DOI: 10.1155/2014/580620.

621 **Nephrotic syndrome: Image A.** Effacement of podocyte foot processes in minimal change disease. This image is a derivative work, adapted from the following source, available under : Teoh DCY, El-Modir A. Managing a locally advanced malignant thymoma complicated by nephrotic syndrome: a case report. *J Med Case Reports.* 2008; 2: 89. DOI: 10.1186/1752-1947-2-89.

621 **Nephrotic syndrome: Image B.** Histology of focal segmental glomerulosclerosis. This image is a derivative work, adapted from the following source, available under : Dr. Michael Bonert. The image may have been modified by cropping, labeling, and/or captions. MedIQ Learning, LLC makes this available under .

621 **Nephrotic syndrome: Image D.** Diabetic glomerulosclerosis with Kimmelstiel-Wilson lesions. This image is a derivative work, adapted from the following source, available under : Doc Mari. The image may have been modified by cropping, labeling, and/or captions. MedIQ Learning, LLC makes this available under .

622 **Kidney stones: Image A.** Nair S, George J, Kumar S, et al. Acute oxalate nephropathy following ingestion of *Averrhoa bilimbi* juice. *Case Rep Nephrol.* 2014; 2014: DOI: 10.1155/2014/240936.

622 **Kidney stones: Image B.** This image is a derivative work, adapted from the following source, available under : Joel Mills. The image may have been modified by cropping, labeling, and/or captions. MedIQ Learning, LLC makes this available under .

623 **Hydronephrosis.** Ultrasound. This image is a derivative work, adapted from the following source, available under : Wikimedia Commons. The image may have been modified by cropping, labeling, and/or captions. MedIQ Learning, LLC makes this available under .

624 **Pyelonephritis: Image A.** This image is a derivative work, adapted from the following source, available under : Dr. Michael Bonert. The image may have been modified by cropping, labeling, and/or captions. MedIQ Learning, LLC makes this available under .

624 **Pyelonephritis: Image B.** CT scan. Courtesy of the Department of Health and Human Services and the Armed Forces Institute of Pathology.

626 **Acute tubular necrosis: Image A.** Muddy brown casts. This image is a derivative work, adapted from the following source, available under : Dr. Serban Nicolescu.

626 **Renal papillary necrosis.** Courtesy of the Department of Health and Human Services and William D. Craig, Dr. Brent J. Wagner, and Mark D. Travis.

627 **Renal cyst disorders: Image C.** Ultrasound of simple cyst. This image is a derivative work, adapted from the following source, available under : Nevit Dilmen. The image may have been modified by cropping, labeling, and/or captions. MedIQ Learning, LLC makes this available under .

628 **Renal cell carcinoma: Image A.** Histology. This image is a derivative work, adapted from the following source, available under : Dr. Yale Rosen. The image may have been modified by cropping, labeling, and/or captions. MedIQ Learning, LLC makes this available under .

628 **Renal cell carcinoma: Image B.** Gross specimen. This image is a derivative work, adapted from the following source, available under : Dr. Ed Uthman. This image may have been modified by cropping, labeling, and/or captions. MedIQ Learning, LLC makes this available under .

628 **Renal cell carcinoma: Image C.** CT scan. This image is a derivative work, adapted from the following source, available under : Behnes CL, Schlegel C, Shoukier M, et al. Hereditary papillary renal cell carcinoma primarily diagnosed in a cervical lymph node: a case report of a 30-year-old woman with multiple metastases. *BMC Urol.* 2013;13:3. DOI: 10.1186/1471-2490-13-3.

629 **Renal oncocytoma: Image A.** Gross specimen. This image is a derivative work, adapted from the following source, available under : Courtesy of M. Emmanuel.

629 **Renal oncocytoma: Image B.** Histology. This image is a derivative work, adapted from the following source, available under : Dr. Michael Bonert. The image may have been modified by cropping, labeling, and/or captions. MedIQ Learning, LLC makes this available under .

629 **Nephroblastoma.** This image is a derivative work, adapted from the following source, available under : Refaie H, Sarhan M, Hafez A. Role of CT in assessment of unresectable Wilms tumor response after preoperative chemotherapy in pediatrics. *Sci World J.* 2008;8:661-669. doi 10.1100/tsw.2008.96.

629 **Urothelial carcinoma of the bladder: Image A.** This image is a derivative work, adapted from the following source, available under : Geavlete B, Stanescu F, Moldoveanu C, et al. NBI cystoscopy and bipolar electrosurgery in NMIBC management—an overview of daily practice. *J Med Life.* 2013;6:140-145. PMCID PMC3725437.

Reproductive

639 **Fetal alcohol syndrome.** This image is a derivative work, adapted from the following source, available under : Courtesy of Teresa Kellerman. The image may have been modified by cropping, labeling, and/or captions. MedIQ Learning, LLC makes this available under .

642 **Umbilical cord: Image A.** Cross-section of umbilical cord. This image is a derivative work, adapted from the following source, available under : Dr. Ed Uthman. The image may have been modified by cropping, labeling, and/or captions. MedIQ Learning, LLC makes this available under .

642 **Umbilical cord: Image B.** Meckel diverticulum. This image is a derivative work, adapted from the following source, available under : Mathur P, Gupta R, Simlot A, et al. Congenital pouch colon with double Meckel's diverticulae. *J Neonatal Surg.* 2013 Oct-Dec; 2(4): 48.

646 **Uterine (Müllerian) duct anomalies: Images A-D.** Normal uterus (A), septate uterus (B), bicornuate uterus (C), and uterus didelphys (D). This image is a derivative work, adapted from the following source, available under : Ahmadi F, Zafarani F, Haghighi H, et al. Application of 3D ultrasonography in detection of uterine abnormalities. *Int J Fertil Steril.* 2011; 4:144-147. PMCID PMC4023499.

650 **Female reproductive epithelial histology.** Transformation zone. This image is a derivative work, adapted from the following source, available under : Courtesy of Dr. Ed Uthman. The image may have been modified by cropping, labeling, and/or captions. All rights to this adaptation by MedIQ Learning, LLC are reserved.

652 **Seminiferous tubules.** This image is a derivative work, adapted from the following source, available under : Dr. Anlt Rao. The image may have been modified by cropping, labeling, and/or captions. MedIQ Learning, LLC makes this available under .

665 **Pregnancy complications.** Ectopic pregnancy. This image is a derivative work, adapted from the following source, available under : Li W, Wang G, Lin T, et al. Misdiagnosis of bilateral tubal pregnancy: a case report. *J Med Case Rep.* 2014;8:342. DOI: 10.1186/1752-1947-8-342.

666 **Hydatidiform mole: Image A.** Cluster of cluster of grapes appearance in complete hydatidiform mole. This image is a derivative work, adapted from the following source, available under : Dr. Ed Uthman

666 **Choriocarcinoma: Image B.** "Cannonball" metastases. This image is a derivative work, adapted from the following source, available under : Lekanidi K, Vlachou PA, Morgan B, et al. Spontaneous regression of metastatic renal cell carcinoma: case report. *J Med Case Rep*. 2007;1:89. DOI: 10.1186/1752-1947-1-89.

668 **Vulvar pathology: Image A.** Bartholin cyst. Courtesy of the Department of Health and Human Services and Susan Lindsley.

668 **Vulvar pathology: Image B.** Lichen sclerosis. This image is a derivative work, adapted from the following source, available under : Lambert J. Pruritus in female patients. *Biomed Res Int*. 2014;2014:541867. DOI: 10.1155/2014/541867.

668 **Vulvar pathology: Image C.** Vulvar carcinoma. This image is a derivative work, adapted from the following source, available under : Ramli I, Hassam B. Carcinome épidermoïde vulvaire: pourquoi surveiller un lichen scléro-atrophique. *Pan Afr Med J*. 2015;21:48. DOI: 10.11604/pamj.2015.21.48.6018.

668 **Vulvar pathology: Image D.** Extramallary Paget disease. This image is a derivative work, adapted from the following source, available under : Wang X, Yang W, Yang J. Extramammary Paget's disease with the appearance of a nodule: a case report. *BMC Cancer*. 2010;10:405. DOI: 10.1186/1471-2407-10-405.

669 **Polycystic ovarian syndrome.** This image is a derivative work, adapted from the following source, available under : Kopera D, Wehr E, Obermayer-Pietsch B. Endocrinology of hirsutism. Int J Trichology. 2010;2(1):30–35. doi:10.4103/0974-7753.66910

671 **Ovarian tumors: Image C.** Dysgerminoma. This image is a derivative work, adapted from the following source, available under : Montesinos L, Acien P, Martinez-Beltran M, et al. Ovarian dysgerminoma and synchronic contralateral tubal pregnancy followed by normal intra-uterine gestation: a case report. *J Med Rep*. 2012;6:399. DOI: 10.1186/1752-1947-6-399.

671 **Ovarian tumors: Image D.** Mature cystic teratoma. This image is a derivative work, adapted from the following source, available under : Dr. Michael Bonert. The image may have been modified by cropping, labeling, and/or captions. MedIQ Learning, LLC makes this available under .

671 **Ovarian tumors: Image E.** Yolk sac tumor. This image is a derivative work, adapted from the following source, available under : Jensflorian. The image may have been modified by cropping, labeling, and/or captions. MedIQ Learning, LLC makes this available under .

671 **Ovarian tumors: Image F.** Call-Exner bodies. This image is a derivative work, adapted from the following source, available under : Katoh T, Yasuda M, Hasegawa K, et al. Estrogen-producing endometrioid adenocarcinoma resembling sex cord-stromal tumor of the ovary: a review of four postmenopausal cases. *Diagn Pathol*. 2012;7:164. DOI: 10.1186/1746-1596-7-164.

672 **Uterine conditions: Image A.** Endometrial tissue found outside the uterus. This image is a derivative work, adapted from the following source, available under : Hastings JM, Fazleabas AT. A baboon model for endometriosis: implications for fertility. *Reprod Biol Endocrinol*. 2006;4(suppl 1):S7. DOI: 10.1186/1477-7827-4-S1-S7.

672 **Uterine conditions: Image B.** Endometritis with inflammation of the endometrium. This image is a derivative work, adapted from the following source, available under : Montesinos L, Acien P, Martinez-Beltran M, et al. Ovarian dysgerminoma and synchronic contralateral tubal pregnancy followed by normal intra-uterine gestation: a case report. *J Med Rep*. 2012;6:399. DOI: 10.1186/1752-1947-6-399.

672 **Uterine conditions: Image C.** Endometrial carcinoma. This image is a derivative work, adapted from the following source, available under : Izadi-Mood N, Yarmohammadi M, Ahmadi SA, et al. Reproducibility determination of WHO classification of endometrial hyperplasia/well differentiated adenocarcinoma and comparison with computerized morphometric data in curettage specimens in Iran. *Diagn Pathol*. 2009;4:10. DOI:10.1186/1746-1596-4-10.

672 **Uterine conditions: Image D.** Leiomyoma (fibroid), gross specimen. This image is a derivative work, adapted from the following source, available under : Courtesy of Hic et nunc.

672 **Uterine conditions: Image E.** Leiomyoma (fibroid) histology. This image is a derivative work, adapted from the following source, available under : Londero AP, Perego P, Mangioni C, et al. Locally relapsed and metastatic uterine leiomyoma: a case report. *J Med Case Rep*. 2008;2:308. DOI: 10.1186/1752-1947-2-308. The image may have been modified by cropping, labeling, and/or captions. All rights to this adaptation by MedIQ Learning, LLC are reserved.

673 **Benign breast disease: Image A.** Fibroadenomas. This image is a derivative work, adapted from the following source, available under : Gokhale S. Ultrasound characterization of breast masses. *Indian J Radiol Imaging*. 2009 Aug;19(3):242-7. DOI: 10.4103/0971-3026.54878.

673 **Benign breast disease: Images B and C.** Phyllodes tumor (B) and phyllodes cyst (C) on ultrasound. These images are a derivative work, adapted from the following source, available under : Muttarak MD, Lerttumnongtum P, Somwangjaroen A, et al. Phyllodes tumour of the breast. *Biomed Imaging Interv J*. 2006 Apr-Jun;2(2):e33. DOI: 10.2349/biij.2.2.e33.

674 **Breast cancer: Image A.** Mammography of breast cancer. This image is a derivative work, adapted from the following source, available under : Molino C, Mocerino C, Braucci A, et al. Pancreatic solitary and synchronous metastasis from breast cancer: a case report and systematic review of controversies in diagnosis and treatment. World J Surg Oncol. 2014;12:2. DOI:10.1186/1477-7819-12-2

674 **Breast cancer: Image C.** Comedocarcinoma. This image is a derivative work, adapted from the following source, available under : Costarelli L, Campagna D, Mauri M, et al. Intraductal proliferative lesions of the breast—terminology and biology matter: premalignant lesions or preinvasive cancer? *Int J Surg Oncol*. 2012;501904. DOI: 10.1155/2012/501904. The image may have been modified by cropping, labeling, and/or captions. All rights to this adaptation by MedIQ Learning, LLC are reserved.

674 **Breast cancer: Image D.** Paget disease of breast. This image is a derivative work, adapted from the following source, available under : Muttarak M, Siriya B, Kongmebhol P, et al. Paget's disease of the breast: clinical, imaging and pathologic findings: a review of 16 patients. *Biomed Imaging Interv J*. 2011;7:e16. DOI: 10.2349/biij.7.2.e16.

674 **Breast cancer: Image E.** Invasive lobular carcinoma. This image is a derivative work, adapted from the following source, available under : Franceschini G, Manno A, Mule A, et al. Gastro-intestinal symptoms as clinical manifestation of peritoneal and retroperitoneal spread of an invasive lobular breast cancer: report of a case and review of the literature. *BMC Cancer*. 2006;6:193. DOI: 10.1186/1471-2407-6-193.

674 **Breast cancer: Image F.** Peau d'orange of inflammatory breast cancer. This image is a derivative work, adapted from the following source, available under : Levine PH, Zolfaghari L, Young H, et al. What Is inflammatory breast cancer? Revisiting the case definition. *Cancers (Basel)*. 2010 Mar;2(1):143–152. DOI: 10.3390/cancers2010143.

675 **Penile pathology: Image A.** Peyronie disease. This image is a derivative work, adapted from the following source, available under : Tran VQ, Kim DH, Lesser TF, et al. Review of the surgical approaches for Peyronie's disease: corporeal plication and plaque incision with grafting. *Adv Urol*. 2008; 2008: 263450. DOI: 10.1155/2008/263450.

675 **Penile pathology: Image B.** Squamous cell carcinoma. This image is a derivative work, adapted from the following source, available under : Antônio JR, Antônio CR, Trídico LA. Erythroplasia of queyrat

treated with topical 5-fluorouracil. *An Bras Dermatol.* 2016 Sep-Oct; 91(5 Suppl 1): 42–44. DOI: 10.1590/abd1806-4841.20164595.

675 Cryptorchidism. This image is a derivative work, adapted from the following source, available under : Pandey A, Gangopadhyay AN, Kumar V. High anorectal malformation in a five-month-old boy: a case report. *J Med Case Reports.* 2010; 4: 296. DOI: 10.1186/1752-1947-4-296.

675 Varicocele. This image is a derivative work, adapted from the following source, available under : Mak CW, Tzeng WS. Sonography of the scrotum. DOI: 10.5772/27586.

676 Benign scrotal lesions. Congenital hydrocele. This image is a derivative work, adapted from the following source, available under : Leonardi S, Barone P, Gravina G, et al. Severe Kawasaki disease in a 3-month-old patient: a case report. *BMC Res Notes.* 2013;6:500. DOI: 10.1186/1756-0500-6-500.

Respiratory

685 Alveolar cell types: Image A. Electron micrograph of type II pneumocyte. This image is a derivative work, adapted from the following source, available under : Fehrenbach H, Tews S, Fehrenbach A, et al. Improved lung preservation relates to an increase in tubular myelin-associated surfactant protein A. *Respir Res.* 2005 Jun 21;6:60. The image may have been modified by cropping, labeling, and/or captions. All rights to this adaptation by MedIQ Learning, LLC are reserved.

685 Alveolar cell types: Image B. Micrograph of type II pneumocyte. This image is a derivative work, adapted from the following source, available under : Courtesy of Dr. Thomas Caceci.

685 Neonatal respiratory distress syndrome. This image is a derivative work, adapted from the following source, available under : Alorainy IA, Balas NB, Al-Boukai AA. Pictorial essay: infants of diabetic mothers. *Indian J Radiol Imaging.* 2010;20:174-181. DOI: 10.4103/0971-3026.69349.

687 Lung anatomy: Image A. X-ray of normal lung. This image is a derivative work, adapted from the following source, available under : Namkoong H, Fujiwara H, Ishii M, et al. Immune reconstitution inflammatory syndrome due to *Mycobacterium avium* complex successfully followed up using 18 F-fluorodeoxyglucose positron emission tomography-computed tomography in a patient with human immunodeficiency virus infection: A case report. *BMC Med Imaging.* 2015;15:24. DOI 10.1186/s12880-015-0063-2.

687 Lung anatomy: Image B. CT scan of the chest. This image is a derivative work, adapted from the following source, available under : Wang JF, Wang B, Jansen JA, et al. Primary squamous cell carcinoma of lung in a 13-year-old boy: a case report. *Cases J.* 2008 Aug 22;1(1):123. DOI: 10.1186/1757-1626-1-123. The image may have been modified by cropping, labeling, and/or captions. All rights to this adaptation by MedIQ Learning, LLC are reserved.

691 Cyanide vs carbon monoxide poisoning. FLAIR axial image showing bilateral symmetrical basal ganglia lesions in patients with carbon monoxide poisoning. This image is a derivative work, adapted from the following source, available under : Subhaschandra S, Jatishwor W, Suraj Th. Isolated symmetrical bilateral basal ganglia T2 hyperintensity in carbon monoxide poisoning. *Ann Indian Acad Neurol.* 2008 Oct-Dec; 11(4): 251–253. DOI: 10.4103/0972-2327.44563.

695 Rhinosinusitis. This image is a derivative work, adapted from the following source, available under : Strek P, Zagolski O, Sktadzien J. Fatty tissue within the maxillary sinus: a rare finding. *Head Face Med.* 2006;2:28. DOI: 10.1186/1746-160X-2-28.

695 Deep venous thrombosis. This image is a derivative work, adapted from the following source, available under : Dr. James Heilman. The image may have been modified by cropping, labeling, and/or captions. MedIQ Learning, LLC makes this available under .

696 Pulmonary emboli: Image B. CT scan. This image is a derivative work, adapted from the following source, available under : Dr. Carl Chartrand-Lefebvre. The image may have been modified by cropping, labeling, and/or captions. MedIQ Learning, LLC makes this available under .

699 Obstructive lung diseases: Image A. Barrel-shaped chest in emphysema. This image is a derivative work, adapted from the following source, available under : Dr. James Heilman. The image may have been modified by cropping, labeling, and/or captions. MedIQ Learning, LLC makes this available under .

699 Obstructive lung diseases: Image B. Lung tissue with enlarged alveoli in emphysema. This image is a derivative work, adapted from the following source, available under : Dr. Michael Bonert.

699 Obstructive lung diseases: Image C. CT of centriacinar emphysema. Courtesy of the Department of Health and Human Services and Dr. Edwin P. Ewing, Jr.

699 Obstructive lung diseases: Image D. Emphysema histology. This image is a derivative work, adapted from the following source, available under : Dr. Michael Bonert. The image may have been modified by cropping, labeling, and/or captions. MedIQ Learning, LLC makes this available under .

699 Obstructive lung diseases: Image E. Mucus plugs in asthma. This image is a derivative work, adapted from the following source, available under : Courtesy of Dr. Yale Rosen. The image may have been modified by cropping, labeling, and/or captions. MedIQ Learning, LLC makes this available under .

699 Obstructive lung disease: Image F. Curschmann spirals. The image may have been modified by cropping, labeling, and/or captions. MedIQ Learning, LLC makes this available under . Dr. James Heilman.

699 Obstructive lung diseases: Image G. Charcot-Leyden crystals on bronchalverolar lavage. This image is a derivative work, adapted from the following source, available under : Gholamnejad M, Rezaie N. Unusual presentation of chronic eosinophilic pneumonia with "reversed halo sign": a case report. *Iran J Radiol.* 2014 May;11(2):e7891. DOI: 10.5812/iranjradiol.7891.

699 Obstructive lung disease: Image H. Bronchiectasis in cystic fibrosis. This image is a derivative work, adapted from the following source, available under : Dr. Yale Rosen. The image may have been modified by cropping, labeling, and/or captions. MedIQ Learning, LLC makes this available under .

700 Sarcoidosis: Image A. Kajal B, Harvey J, Alowami S. Melkerrson-Rosenthal Syndrome, a rare case report of chronic eyelid swelling. *Diagn Pathol.* 2013; 8: 188. DOI: 10.1186/1746-1596-8-188.

700 Sarcoidosis: Images B and C. X-ray (B) and CT (C) of the chest. These images are a derivative work, adapted from the following source, available under : Lønborg J, Ward M, Gill A, et al. Utility of cardiac magnetic resonance in assessing right-sided heart failure in sarcoidosis. *BMC Med Imaging.* 2013;13:2. DOI: 10.1186/1471-2342-13-2.

700 Inhalational injury and sequelae: Images A and B. 18 hours (A) 11 days (B) after inhalational injury. These images are a derivative work, adapted from the following source, available under : Bai C, Huang H, Yao X, et al. Application of flexible bronchoscopy in inhalation lung injury. *Diagn Pathol.* 2013;8:174. DOI: 10.1186/1746-1596-8-174.

701 Pneumoconioses: Image A. Pleural plaques in asbestosis. This image is a derivative work, adapted from the following source, available under : Dr. Yale Rosen. The image may have been modified by cropping, labeling, and/or captions. MedIQ Learning, LLC makes this available under .

701 Pneumoconioses: Image B. CT scan of asbestosis. This image is a derivative work, adapted from the following source, available under : Miles SE, Sandrini A, Johnson AR, et al. Clinical consequences of asbestos-related diffuse pleural thickening: a review. *J Occup Med Toxicol*. 2008;3:20. DOI: 10.1186/1745-6673-3-20.

701 **Pneumoconioses: Image C.** Ferruginous bodies in asbestosis. This image is a derivative work, adapted from the following source, available under : Dr, Michael Bonert. The image may have been modified by cropping, labeling, and/or captions. MedIQ Learning, LLC makes this available under .

701 **Pneumoconioses: Image D.** Berylliosis: non-caseous granuloma. *Ann Saudi Med.*2009 Nov-Dec; 29(6): 485–486. DOI: 10.4103/0256-4947.57175.

702 **Mesothelioma.** This image is a derivative work, adapted from the following source, available under : Weiner SJ, Neragi-Miandoab S. Pathogenesis of malignant pleural mesothelioma and the role of environmental and genetic factors. *J Carcinog*. 2008;7:3. DOI: 10.1186/1477-3163-7-3.

702 **Acute respiratory distress syndrome: Image A.** Alveolar fluid. This image is a derivative work, adapted from the following source, available under : Pires-Neto RC, Del Carlo Bernardi F, de Araujo PA. The expression of water and ion channels in diffuse alveolar damage is not dependent on DAD etiology. *PLoS One*. 2016; 11(11): e0166184. DOI: 10.1371/journal.pone.0166184.

702 **Acute respiratory distress syndrome: Image B.** Bilateral lung opacities. This image is a derivative work, adapted from the following source, available under : Imanaka H, Takahara B, Yamaguchi H, et al. Chest computed tomography of a patient revealing severe hypoxia due to amniotic fluid embolism: a case report. *J Med Case Reports*. 2010;4:55. DOI: 10.1186/1752-1947-4-55.

704 **Digital clubbing.** This image is a derivative work, adapted from the following source, available under : Desherinka. This image may have been modified by cropping, labeling, and/or captions. MedIQ Learning, LLC makes this available under .

704 **Atelectasis.** This image is a derivative work, adapted from the following source, available under : Khan AN, Al-Jahdali H, Al-Ghanem S, et al. Reading chest radiographs in the critically ill (Part II): Radiography of lung pathologies common in the ICU patient. Ann Thorac Med. 2009;4(3):149–157. DOI:10.4103/1817-1737.53349

705 **Pleural effusions: Images A and B.** Before (A) and after (B) treatment. These images are a derivative work, adapted from the following source, available under : Toshikazu A, Takeoka H, Nishioka K, et al. Successful management of refractory pleural effusion due to systemic immunoglobulin light chain amyloidosis by vincristine adriamycin dexamethasone chemotherapy: a case report. *Med Case Rep*. 2010;4:322. DOI: 10.1186/1752-1947-4-322.

706 **Pneumothorax: Image A.** This image is a derivative work, adapted from the following source, available under : Miura K, Kondo R, Kurai M, et al. Birt-Hogg-Dubé syndrome detected incidentally by asymptomatic bilateral pneumothorax in health screening: a case of a young Japanese woman. *Surg Case Rep*. 2015 Dec; 1: 17. DOI: 10.1186/s40792-015-0014-8.

706 **Pneumothorax: Image B.** Tension pneumothorax. This image is a derivative work, adapted from the following source, available under : Rosat A, Díaz C. Reexpansion pulmonary edema after drainage of tension pneumothorax. *Pan Afr Med J*. 2015; 22: 143.DOI: 10.11604/pamj.2015.22.143.8097.

707 **Pneumonia: Image A.** Lobar pneumonia on chest x-ray. This image is a derivative work, adapted from the following source, available under : Yoon BW, Song YG, Lee SH. Severe community-acquired adenovirus pneumonia treated with oral ribavirin: a case report. *BMC Res Notes*. 2017; 10: 47. DOI: 10.1186/s13104-016-2370-2.

707 **Pneumonia: Image B.** Lobar pneumonia, gross specimen. This image is a derivative work, adapted from the following source, available under : Dr. Yale Rosen. The image may have been modified by cropping, labeling, and/or captions. MedIQ Learning, LLC makes this available under .

707 **Pneumonia: Image C.** Acute inflammatory infiltrates in bronchopneumonia. This image is a derivative work, adapted from the following source, available under : Dr. Yale Rosen. The image may have been modified by cropping, labeling, and/or captions. MedIQ Learning, LLC makes this available under .

707 **Pneumonia: Image D.** Bronchopneumonia, gross specimen. This image is a derivative work, adapted from the following source, available under : Dr. Yale Rosen. The image may have been modified by cropping, labeling, and/or captions. MedIQ Learning, LLC makes this available under .

707 **Pneumonia: Image E.** Interstitial pneumonia. This image is a derivative work, adapted from the following source, available under : Allen CM, AL-Jahdali HH, Irion KL, et al. Imaging lung manifestations of HIV/AIDS. *Ann Thorac Med*. 2010 Oct-Dec; 5(4): 201–216. DOI: 10.4103/1817-1737.69106.

708 **Lung abscess: Image A.** Gross specimen. This image is a derivative work, adapted from the following source, available under : Dr. Yale Rosen. The image may have been modified by cropping, labeling, and/or captions. MedIQ Learning, LLC makes this available under .

708 **Lung abscess: Image B.** X-ray. This image is a derivative work, adapted from the following source, available under : Courtesy of Dr. Yale Rosen.

709 **Lung cancer: Image B.** Adenocarcinoma histology. Courtesy of the Department of Health and Human Services and the Armed Forces Institute of Pathology.

709 **Lung cancer: Image C.** Squamous cell carcinoma. This image is a derivative work, adapted from the following source, available under : Dr. James Heilman. The image may have been modified by cropping, labeling, and/or captions. MedIQ Learning, LLC makes this available under .

709 **Lung cancer: Image E.** Large cell lung cancer. This image is a derivative work, adapted from the following source, available under : Jala VR, Radde BN, Haribabu B, et al. Enhanced expression of G-protein coupled estrogen receptor (GPER/GPR30) in lung cancer. *BMC Cancer*. 2012;12:624. doi 10.1186/1471-2407-12-624.

710 **Pancoast tumor.** This image is a derivative work, adapted from the following source, available under : Manenti G, Raguso M, D'Onofrio S, et al. Pancoast tumor: the role of magnetic resonance imaging. *Case Rep Radiol*. 2013; 2013:479120. DOI: 10.1155/2013/479120.

710 **Superior vena cava syndrome: Images A and B.** Blanching of skin with pressure (A) and CT of chest (B). These images are a derivative work, adapted from the following source, available under : Shaikh I, Berg K, Kman N. Thrombogenic catheter-associated superior vena cava syndrome. *Case Rep Emerg Med*. 2013; 2013: 793054. DOI 10.1155/2013/793054.

Index

for fibromyalgia, 483
long QT interval with, 315
monoamine oxidase inhibitors, **599**
selective serotonin reuptake inhibitors, **599**
serotonin-norepinephrine reuptake inhibitors, **599**
torsades de pointes, 251
tricyclic antidepressants, **599**
Anti-desmoglein (anti-desmosome) autoantibody, 115
Anti-digoxin Fab fragments
for cardiac glycoside toxicity, 329
specific toxicity treatments, 251
Antidiuretic hormone (ADH)
antagonists, 364
function of, 335, 336
hypothalamus synthesis, 513
naming conventions for antagonist, 257
renin-angiotensis-aldosterone system, 612
signaling pathways of, 345
source, function, and regulation, **337**
Anti-DNA topoisomerase I autoantibody, 115
Anti-dsDNA antibody, 115
Antiemetic drugs
aprepitant, 410
long QT interval with, 315
metoclopramide, 410
ondansetron, 410
torsades de pointes, 251
Antiepileptic drugs
rash from, 253
teratogenicity, 638
antierectile, 651
Antifungal drugs
griseofulvin, 48
seborrheic dermatitis, 490
tinea versicolor, 152
Antifungals
Long QT with, 315
Antifungal therapy, **198**
Antigenic shift/drift, 169
Antigen-presenting cells (APCs)
B cells as, 418
CD28, 110
Antigens
active immunity, 110
chronic mucocutaneous candidiasis, 116
HLA I and II, 100
type and memory, **105**
Anti-glomerular basement membrane autoantibody, 115
Anti-glutamic acid decarboxylase autoantibody, 115
Antigout drugs
colchicine, 48
Anti-growth signal, 222
Anti-HBe, 174
Anti-helicase autoantibody, 115
Antihelminthic therapy, **200**
mebendazole, 48
naming conventions for, 256
Anti-hemidesmosome autoantibody, 115
Antihistamines
for scombroid poisoning, 250
Antihistone autoantibody, 115
Anti-histone antibody, 115
Antihypertensive drugs
hypertension in pregnancy, 667
Antihypertensives, 667
Anti-IgE monoclonal therapy, 712
Anti-IL-5 monoclonal therapy, 712
Anti-inflammatory drugs, 499
Anti-intrinsic factor autoantibody, 115
Anti-La/SSB autoantibody, 115, 480
Antileukotrienes for asthma, 712
Antimetabolites, **450**
Antimicrobial drugs
naming conventions for, 256
pregnancy contraindications, 204
prophylaxis, 198
Antimicrobials
embryotoxic, 204
Antimicrosomal autoantibody, 115
Anti-mite/louse therapy, **200**
Antimitochondrial autoantibody, 115
Antimuscarinic drugs
Parkinson disease, 568
reactions to, 254
Antimycin A
electron transport chain, 78
Antimycobacterial therapy
prophylaxis and treatment, **196**
Antineoplastics
naming conventions for, 256
Anti-NMDA receptor paraneoplastic syndrome encephalitis, 229
Antinuclear (ANA) antibody, 115
Sjögren syndrome, 478
Antioxidants
free radical elimination by, 210
Antiparasitic drugs
naming convention for, 256
Antiparietal cell autoantibody, 115
Anti-phospholipase A2 receptor autoantibody, 115
Antiphospholipid syndrome, **482**
autoantibody, 115
autoantibody in, 115
Antiplatelet drugs
for acute coronary syndromes, 317
mechanism and clinical use, 447
Anti-postsynaptic ACh receptor, autoantibody, 115
Anti-presynaptic voltage-gated calcium channel, autoantibody, 115
Antiprogestins, **681**
Antiprotozoal therapy
drugs for, **200**
Antiprotozoan drugs, 200
Antipseudomonal drugs
fluoroquinolones, 195
penicillins, **188**
Antipsychotic drugs
antimuscarinic reaction, 254
disruptive mood dysregulation disorder, 580
dopaminergic pathways, 514
dystonia with, 593
long QT interval with, 315
mechanism, use and adverse effects, **597**
Parkinson-like syndrome, 254
tardive dyskinesia, 254
torsades de pointes, 251
Tourette syndrome, 596
Antiretroviral therapy (ART)
HIV therapy, 203
Antiribonucleoprotein antibodies
Sjögren syndrome, 480
Anti-Ro/SSA autoantibody, 480
anti-Saccharomyces cerevisiae antibodies (ASCA), 392
Anti-Scl-70 autoantibody, 115
Anti-Smith autoantibody, 115
Anti-smooth muscle antibody, 115
Anti-smooth muscle autoantibody, 115
Antisocial personality disorder, 588
early-onset disorder, 580
Antispasmodics, **572**
Anti-SRP autoantibody, 115
Anti-streptolysin O (ASO) titers, 322
Antithrombin
coagulation cascade and, 423
deficiency of, 437
Antitoxins
as passive immunity, 110
Anti-TSH receptor autoantibody, 115
Antitumor antibiotics, **449**
Anti-U1 RNP antibodies, 115, 482
Anti-U1 RNP (ribonucleoprotein) autoantibody, 115
Antiviral therapy
hepatitis C, 204
mechanism and use, 201
Anti-β2 glycoprotein autoantibody, 115
Anti-β_2 glycoprotein
antiphospholipid syndrome, 482
Anxiety
drug therapy, 566
neurotransmitter changes with, 510
Anxiety disorders, **585**
Aorta
branches, 373
coarctation of, 307
diaphragm, 687
syphilitic heart disease, 322
traumatic rupture, 311
traumatic rupture of, 311
"tree bark" appearance, 322
Aortic aneurysm, **310**
hypertension, 308
Marfan syndrome, 308
syphilitic heart disease, 322
Aortic arch
derivatives, **289**
receptors, 303
Aortic dissection, 308, **311**
hypertension, 308
Marfan syndrome, 310
Aortic insufficiency
syphilis, 322
Aorticopulmonary septum, 289
embryologic derivatives, 637
Aortic regurgitation, 297
aortic dissection, 311
heart murmurs with, 300
Marfan syndrome, 308
Aortic root dilation
heart murmur with, 300
Aortic stenosis, 297, 300
heart murmurs, 300
macroangiopathic anemia, 433
Williams syndrome, 308
Aortic valve
cardiac cycle, 296
embryological development of, 289
Aortitis
syphilis, 147, 184
Aortocaval compression syndrome, 667
APC gene
adenomatous colonic polyps and, 397
colorectal cancer and, 399
Familial adenomatous polyposis, 397
tumor suppression, **225**
"Ape hand", 457
Apgar score, **658**
α (type I) error, 268
Aphasia
MCA stroke, 532
types of, **534**
Apixaban, 446
factor Xa inhibitors, 446
Aplasia, 637
Aplasia cutis
methimazole, 364
Aplastic anemia, 431
chloramphenicol, 192
drug reaction and, 253
HBV, 174
neutropenia with, 431
thionamides, 364
Aplastic crisis
hereditary spherocytosis, 432
sickle cell anemia, 432
Apolipoproteins
functions, 93
functions of, 93
Apoptosis
BCL-2 gene, 225
corticosteroids, 433
evasion of, 222
malignant tumors, 221
of keratocytes, 496
pathways for, **208**
vs necrosis, 209
Appendicitis
causes, signs and treatment, **393**
mittelschmerz vs, 655
Appetite regulation
endocannabinoids, 344
ghrelin, 344, 381
leptin, 344
"Apple core" lesion (X-ray), 398
Apraclonidine, 573
Aprepitant
mechanism and clinical use, **410**
with chemotherapy, 453
Aquagenic pruritus, 443
Aqueous humor pathway, 554
Arabinosyltransferase, 197
Arachidonic acid pathways, **499**
Arachnodactyly, 52
Arachnoid granulations, 519, 540
Arachnoid mater
derivation, 511
meningioma, 543
Area postrema, 513
Area under the curve, 233
Arenaviruses
characteristics and medical importance, 167
Argatroban, 446
Arginine
classification, 81
cystinuria, 85
kidney stones and, 622
Argyll Robertson pupil
syphilis, 147
Argyll Robertson pupils
in syphilis, 184
tabes dorsalis, 548
Aripiprazole, 597
Arm abduction
muscles and nerves, **456**
Arm adduction, 457
Armadillos (disease vectors), 149

Croup, 169
acute laryngotracheobronchitis, **170**
paramyxoviruses, 167, 169
pulsus paradoxus in, 320
Crust (skin)
basal cell carcinoma, 498
characteristics, 489
impetigo, 493
varicella zoster virus, 493
Cryoprecipitate
transfusion of, 438
Cryptococcal meningitis, 199
Cryptococcosis, 153
Cryptococcus spp
in immunodeficiency, 118
meningitis, 180
treatment, 199
urease-positive, 127
Cryptococcus neoformans, 153
HIV-positive adults, 177
stains for, 125
Cryptogenic organizing pneumonia, 707
cryptorchidism, 675
Cryptorchidism, **675**
Cryptosporidium spp, 155
in HIV positive adults, 177
stains for, 125
watery diarrhea, 179
Crypts of Lieberkühn, 372
C-section deliveries
neonatal flora, 178
risk factors after, 664
Culture requirements, **126**
"Currant jelly" stools, 396
acute mesenteric ischemia, 395
intussusception, 395
Curschmann spirals, 698
Cushing disease, 356
Cushing-like symptoms, 201
Cushing reflex, 303, 517
Cushing syndrome, 229
anovulation with, 669
corticosteroids, 120
eosinopenia, 433
etiology and diagnosis, 356
small cell lung cancer, 709
Cushing ulcers
gastritis, 389
Cutaneous anthrax, 137
Cutaneous flushing
drug reaction and, 251
drugs causing, 251
Cutaneous larva migrans, 158
Cutaneous leishmaniasis, 158
Cutaneous mycoses, 152
Cutaneous paraneoplastic syndromes, 229
Cutaneous small-vessel vasculitis, 484
Cutis aplasia
Patau syndrome, 63
CXCR4/CCR5 protein
presence on cells, 110
viral receptor, 166
Cyanide toxicity
blood oxygen in, 690
nitroprusside, 326
oxygen deprivation, 693
treatment for, 251
vs carbon monoxide poisoning, **691**
Cyanosis
"blue kids", 306
Eisenmenger syndrome, 307
esophageal atresia, 369
methemoglobinemia, 690
patent ductus arteriosus, 307
tetralogy of Fallot, 306
Cyclin-CDK complexes, **46**
Cyclin-dependent kinases, 46
Cyclobenzaprine, 572
Cyclooxygenase
aspirin effect on, 421
Cyclooxygenase inhibition
irreversible, 500
reversible, 499
selective, 500
Cyclophosphamide
hemorrhagic cystitis with, 254
mechanism, use and adverse effects, 451
SIADH with, 252
transitional cell carcinoma and, 629
Cyclopia, 505
Cycloplegia
atropine, 244
muscarinic antagonists for, 244
Cyclosporine
gingival hyperplasia, 253
gout, 253
immunosuppression, 120
Cyclothymic disorder, 584
Cystathionine
vitamin B_6 and, 67
Cystathionine synthase deficiency, 85
Cyst disorders (renal), 627
Cystic duct, 378
Cysticercosis, 160
Cystic fibrosis, **60**
Aspergillus fumigatus, 153
meconium ileus and, 396
organisms causing pneumonia in, 179
pancreatic insufficiency, 391
vitamin deficiencies and, 65
Cystine
kidney stones, 622
Cystinuria, **85**
Cystitis
acute bacterial, 624
Cytarabine
mechanism and clinical use, 450
Cytochrome C, 208
Cytochrome P-450
azoles, 199
drug interactions with, **255**
griseofulvin, 200
macrolides, 193
phenobarbital effect on, 564
rifamycins, 196
ritonavir, 203
Cytokeratin, 228, 702
Cytokines, **108**
acute, 108
corticosteroids and, 120
Graves disease and, 350
rejection reactions, 119, 120
Type IV hypersensitivity, 113
Cytokinesis, 46
Cytomegalovirus (CMV)
AIDS retinitis, 165
cholecystitis and, 406
clinical significance, 165
esophagitis, 387
HIV-positive adults, 177
immunodeficient patients, 117, 118
in HIV positive adults, 177
pneumonia, 707
TORCH infection, 182
transmission and clinical significance, 165
treatment, 202
Cytoplasm
cell cycle phase, 46
cytoskeletal elements, 48
glycolysis, 76
metabolism in, 74
Cytoplasmic ANCA (c-ANCA) autoantibody, 115
Cytoplasmic membrane (bacteria), 124
Cytoplasmic processing bodies (P-bodies), 41
Cytoskeletal elements, **48**
Cytotoxic T cells, **102**
cell surface proteins, 110
MHC I and II, 100
Cytotrophoblast, 640

D

Dabigatran, 446
reversal of, 447
Dabrafenib, 453
Dacrocytes
associated pathology, 424
Dactinomycin
RNA polymerase inhibition, 42
Dactinomycin (actinomycin D)
mechanism and clinical use, 449
Dactylitis
seronegative spondyloarthritis, 481
sickle cell anemia, 432
Dalfopristin
VRE, 198
Danazol, **682**
pseudotumor cerebri, 540
"Dancing eyes dancing feet", 229
Dandy-Walker malformation, 506
Dantrolene, 570
malignant hyperthermia treatment, 570
mechanism and use, 572
Dapagliflozin, 363
Dapsone
hemolysis in G6PD deficiency, 253
Mycobacterium leprae, 196
Pneumocystis jirovecii, 154
Leprosy treatment, 141
mechanism and use, **194**
Daptomycin
mechanism and clinical use, **195**
MRSA, 198
Darkfield microscopy
for Treponema, 146
Darunavir
HIV therapy, 203
Dasatinib, 453
Datura, 244
Daunorubicin
dilated cardiomyopathy, 251
DCC gene, 225
D cells
somatostatin production, 381
Deacetylation
histones, 34
Deafness
Alport syndrome, 620
congenital long QT syndromes, 315
congenital syphilis, 147
rubella, 182
syphilis, 182
Deamination
base excision repair, 39
Death
children explaining to, 277
common causes by age, **279**
diabetes mellitus, 354
sudden cardiac death, 312
thyroid storm, 350
Debranching enzyme
glycogen metabolism, 87
Decay-accelerating factor (DAF), 106
Deceleration injury, 311
Decerebrate (extensor) posturing, 528
Decidua basalis, 640
Decision-making capacity, **271**
surrogate for, 272
Decorticate (flexor) posturing, 528
Decussation
in spinal tracts, 526
Deep brachial artery, 465
Deeper injury burn, 497
Deep inguinal lymph nodes, 648
Deep partial-thickness burn, 497
Deep venous thrombosis, **695**
direct factor Xa inhibitors for, 446
glucagonomas and, 361
tamoxifen/raloxifene and, 452
Defense mechanisms
immature, 576
mature, 577
Defensins, 99
Deferasirox, 251
Deferiprone, 251
Deferoxamine, 251
Deformation (morphogenesis), 637
Degarelix, **680**
Degenerate/redundant genetic code, 37
Degmacytes
associated pathology, 424
Dehydration
gout exacerbation, 479
loop diuretics and, 631
osmotic laxatives, 411
salivary stones with, 386
shock, 320
Dehydrogenase, 73
Delavirdine
HIV therapy, 203
Delayed hemolytic transfusion reaction, 114
Delirium, **581**
barbiturate withdrawal, 594
PCP, 595
thyroid storm, 350
Delirium tremens (DTs)
alcohol withdrawal, 593
Delivering bad news, **274**
δ cells
pancreatic tumors, 361
Delta virus
characteristics and medical significance, 167
Deltoid muscle
Erb palsy, 458
Delusional disorder, 583
Delusions
mesolimbic pathway, 514
types of, 582
Demeclocycline, 364
diabetes insipidus and, 252, 346
Dementia
HIV-positive adults, 177
metachromatic leukodystrophy, 88
neurodegenerative disorders, 538
prion disease, 178
vitamin B_3 deficiency, 67
Demyelinating/dysmyelinating disorders, **542**
acute disseminated (postinfectious) encephalomyelitis, 542
Charcot-Marie-Tooth disease, 542

S

Z

NOTES

▶ NOTES

▶ NOTES

NOTES

NOTES

NOTES

▶ NOTES

▶ NOTES

NOTES

NOTES

NOTES

NOTES

▶ NOTES

About the Editors

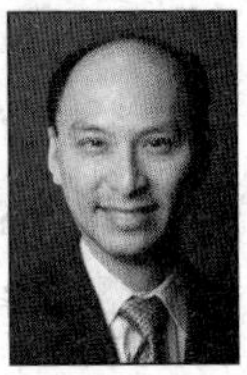

Tao Le, MD, MHS

Tao developed a passion for medical education as a medical student. He currently edits more than 15 titles in the *First Aid* series. In addition, he is Founder and Chief Education Officer of USMLE-Rx for exam preparation and ScholarRx for undergraduate medical education. As a medical student, he was editor-in-chief of the University of California, San Francisco (UCSF) *Synapse*, a university newspaper with a weekly circulation of 9000. Tao earned his medical degree from UCSF in 1996 and completed his residency training in internal medicine at Yale University and fellowship training at Johns Hopkins University. Tao subsequently went on to cofound Medsn, a medical education technology venture, and served as its chief medical officer. He is currently chief of adult allergy and immunology at the University of Louisville.

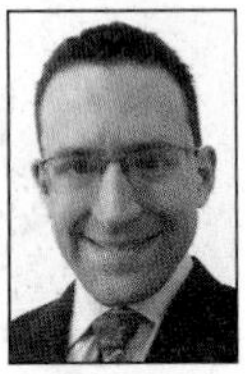

Matthew Sochat, MD

Matthew practices general hematology/oncology in North Carolina. He completed his fellowship training in 2020 at St. Louis University in St. Louis, after an internal medicine residency at Temple University Hospital in Philadelphia. Matt earned his medical degree from the Warren Alpert Medical School of Brown University, and earned undergraduate degrees in biochemistry and the classics from the University of Massachusetts. Matt's pastimes include skiing, cooking and baking, traveling, the company of friends and loved ones (especially his wonderful wife), the Spanish language, and video gaming. Be warned: Matt also loves to come up with corny jokes at (in)opportune moments.

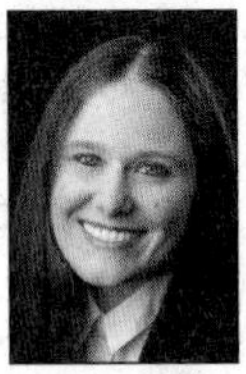

Kristina Damisch, MD

Kristina earned a degree in mathematics from Lake Forest College in 2011 and had a brief career as a software development consultant in Chicago. She graduated from the University of Iowa Carver College of Medicine in 2020 and is applying to the 2021 Match for residency. She has a lifelong passion for emergency medicine with other strong interests including medical education and mental health. Outside of medicine, Kristina's family includes husband Kevin and cats Lemma and Kylo. She enjoys a wide variety of games, trivia, puzzles, escape rooms, trying new recipes, stargazing, and percussion.

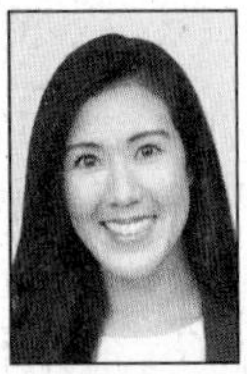

Connie Qiu, MD/PhD Candidate

Connie is in her final year of the MD/PhD program at the Lewis Katz School of Medicine at Temple University. She earned her bachelors degree at Johns Hopkins University, double majoring in molecular biology and philosophy. Connie's hard work is motivated by ensuring her dog a luxurious life. In her spare time, she enjoys mid-distance running, mountain hiking, modern art, movies, and memes. Her greatest achievement is winning a blue ribbon in the novice succulent category at the 2018 Philadelphia Flower Show. After medical school, she hopes to pursue a residency and academic career in dermatology.

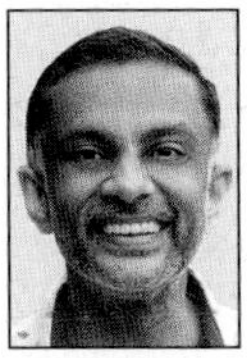

Vikas Bhushan, MD

Vikas is a writer, editor, entrepreneur, and teleradiologist on extended sabbatical. In 1990 he conceived and authored the original *First Aid for the USMLE Step 1*. His entrepreneurial endeavors included a student-focused medical publisher (S2S), an e-learning company (medschool.com), and an ER teleradiology practice (24/7 Radiology). Trained on the Left Coast, Vikas completed a bachelor's degree at the University of California Berkeley; an MD with thesis at UCSF; and a diagnostic radiology residency at UCLA. His eclectic interests include cryptoeconomics, information design, and avoiding a day job. Always finding the long shortcut, Vikas is an adventurer, knowledge seeker, and occasional innovator. He enjoys intermediate status as a kiteboarder and father, and strives to raise his three children as global citizens.

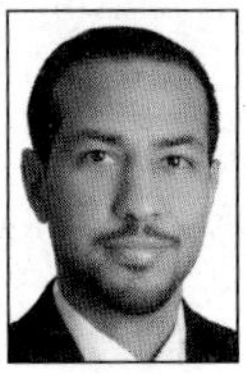

Humood Boqambar, MB BCh BAO

Humood is an orthopedic assistant registrar in Kuwait. He earned his medical degree from the Royal College of Surgeons in Ireland and is pursuing a residency in orthopedic surgery in North America. Academically, Humood serves as a senior editor at ScholarRx and is passionate about medical education and peer-led teaching. In his spare time, Humood enjoys playing sports and is a CrossFit enthusiast. He is also an avid traveler and loves learning about countries' history, tradition, and culture.

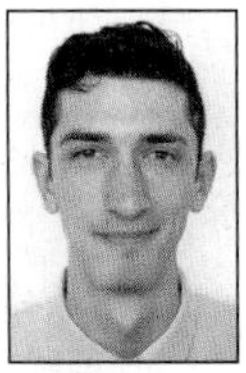

Jordan Abrams, MD

Jordan is a first-year anesthesiology resident at Mount Sinai West and Mount Sinai Morningside Hospitals in New York City. He graduated summa cum laude from St. George's University School of Medicine. Jordan is the founder and creator of theHYMedicine.com, an educational website that offers free medical study guides and resources for students worldwide. Aside from medicine, Jordan enjoys traveling, reading, soccer, and playing with his dog, Yara.

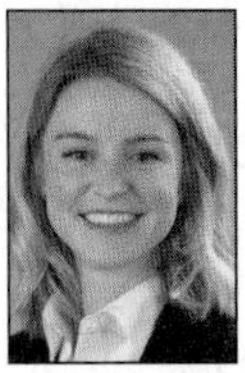

Caroline Coleman, MD

Caroline is a first-year internal medicine resident at Emory University School of Medicine. She was a Foundation Fellow at the University of Georgia and earned a degree in economics before earning her medical degree at Emory, where she was a member of Alpha Omega Alpha honor society. She is interested in a career in critical care medicine, medical education, and investing in underserved populations. Caroline spends her free time hiking in the north Georgia mountains with her dog, Beau.

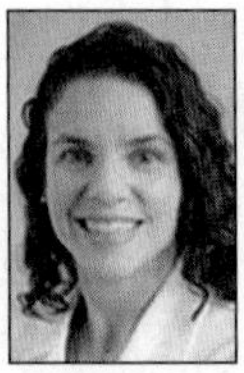

Kimberly Kallianos, MD

Originally from Atlanta, Kimberly graduated from the University of North Carolina at Chapel Hill in 2006 and from Harvard Medical School in 2011. She completed her radiology residency and fellowship at UCSF and is currently an Assistant Professor of Clinical Radiology at UCSF in the Cardiac and Pulmonary Imaging section.